Movement Disorders in Neurology and Neuropsychiatry

SECOND EDITION

Movement Disorders in Neurology and Neuropsychiatry

SECOND EDITION

Edited by

ANTHONY B. JOSEPH, MD
Medical Director
The Center for Neurobehavioral Rehabilitation
Olympus Specialty Hospital
Waltham, Massachusetts
Consultant Neuropsychiatrist
McLean Hospital
Belmont, Massachusetts
Associate Clinical Professor of Psychiatry
Harvard Medical School
Boston, Massachusetts

ROBERT R. YOUNG, MD
Professor and Vice Chairman
Department of Neurology
Medical Director, Movement Disorders Program
University of California at Irvine
Irvine, California

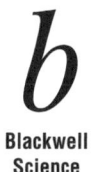
Blackwell
Science

© 1999 by Blackwell Science, Inc.

Editorial Offices:
350 Main Street, Malden, MA 02148-5018, USA
Osney Mead, Oxford OX2 0EL, England
25 John Street, London WC1N 2BL, England
23 Ainslie Place, Edinburgh EH3 6AJ, Scotland
54 University Street, Carlton, Victoria 3053, Australia

Other Editorial Offices:
Blackwell Wissenschafts-Verlag GmbH
Kurfürstendamm 57
10707 Berlin, Germany

Blackwell Science KK
MG Kodenmacho Building
7–10 Kodenmacho Nihombashi
Chuo-ku, Tokyo 104, Japan

Distributors:

USA

Blackwell Science, Inc.
Commerce Place
350 Main Street
Malden, Massachusetts 02148
    (Telephone orders: 800-215-1000 or 781-388-8250;
    fax orders: 781-388-8270)

CANADA

Copp Clark, Ltd.
200 Adelaide St. West, 3rd Floor
Toronto, Ontario
Canada, M5H 1W7
    (Telephone orders: 416-597-1616 or 800-815-9417;
    fax orders: 416-597-1617)

AUSTRALIA

Blackwell Science Pty, Ltd.
54 University Street
Carlton, Victoria 3053
    (Telephone orders: 03-9347-0300;
    fax orders: 03-9349-3016)

OUTSIDE NORTH AMERICA AND AUSTRALIA

Blackwell Science, Ltd.
c/o Marston Book Services, Ltd.
P.O. Box 269
Abingdon
Oxon OX14 4YN
England
    (Telephone orders: 44-01235-465500;
    fax orders: 44-01235-465555)

The Blackwell Science logo is a trade mark of Blackwell Science Ltd, registered at the United Kingdom Trade Marks Registry

Acquisitions: Chris Davis
Production: Kevin Sullivan
Manufacturing: Lisa Flanagan
Typeset by Best-set Typesetter Ltd., Hong Kong
Printed and bound by Maple-Vail Book Manufacturing Group
Printed in the United States of America
99 00 01 02 5 4 3 2 1

All rights reserved. No part of this book may be reproduced in any form or by any electronic or mechanical means, including information storage and retrieval systems, without permission in writing from the publisher, except by a reviewer who may quote brief passages in a review.

Library of Congress Cataloging-In-Publication Data

Movement disorders in neurology and neuropsychiatry /
    edited by Anthony B. Joseph and Robert R. Young.
    —2nd ed.
        p.   cm.
    Includes bibliographical references and index.
    ISBN 0-86542-523-X (alk. paper)
    1. Movement disorders.   2. Movement disorders in children.   3. Psychomotor disorders.   I. Joseph, Anthony B.   II. Young, Robert R., 1934–
RC376.5   M685   1998
616.8′3—ddc21
                                                    98-8767
                                                    CIP

CONTENTS

PART III

Mood and Movement

PART IV

Other Psychiatric Disorders

PART X
Special Topics

Raymond D. Adams, MD
Bullard Professor of Neuropathology, Emeritus
Harvard Medical School
Senior Neurologist
Massachusetts General Hospital
Boston, Massachusetts

Michael P. Alexander, MD
Uville Hospital
Cambridge, Massachusetts
Department of Behavioral Neurology
Beth Israel Deaconess Medical Center
Boston, Massachusetts

Norberto Alvarez, MD
Assistant Professor of Neurology
Harvard Medical School
Boston, Massachusetts
Medical Director
Wrentham Developmental Center
Wrentham, Massachusetts

Eva Andermann, MD
Montreal Neurological Hospital and Institute
Montreal, Quebec, Canada

Frederick Andermann, MD, FRCP(C)
Montreal Neurological Hospital and Institute
Montreal, Quebec, Canada

Lawrence Annable, MD
Associate Professor of Psychiatry
McGill University
Clinical Pharmacology Unit
Allan Memorial Institute
Montreal, Quebec, Canada

George W. Arana, MD
Veterans Affairs Medical Center
Charleston, South Carolina

Tarif Bakdash, MD
Assistant Professor
Department of Pediatric Neurology
Rainbow Babies and Children's Hospital
Case Western Reserve University School of Medicine
Cleveland, Ohio

Margaret L. Bauman, MD
Assistant Professor of Neurology
Harvard Medical School
Assistant Pediatrician and Assistant Neurologist
Massachusetts General Hospital
Boston, Massachusetts

Sheldon Benjamin, MD
Associate Professor of Psychiatry and Neurology
University of Massachusetts Medical School
Director, Neuropsychiatry
Director, Psychiatric Education and Training
University of Massachusetts Medical Center
Worcester, Massachusetts

D. Frank Benson, MD★
Professor Emeritus of Neurology
University of California, Los Angeles, School of Medicine
Los Angeles, California

Samuel F. Berkovic, MD
Department of Neurology
Austin and Repatriation Medical Center
Melbourne, Victoria, Australia

★ Deceased.

Stephen A. Berman, MD
Department of Neurology
Louisiana State University School of Medicine
  in Shreveport
Shreveport, Louisiana

Andrea Bernasconi
Montreal Neurological Hospital and Institute
Montreal, Quebec, Canada

James L. Bernat, MD
Neurology Section
Dartmouth-Hitchcock Medical Center
Lebanon, New Hampshire

Jerrold G. Bernstein, MD
Assistant Clinical Professor of Psychiatry
Harvard Medical School
Assistant Psychiatrist
Massachusetts General Hospital
Boston, Massachusetts

Peter M. Black, MD, PhD
Franc D. Ingraham Professor of Neurosurgery
Harvard Medical School
Neurosurgeon-in-Chief
Brigham and Women's Hospital and
Children's Hospital
Boston, Massachusetts

Joseph Bossom, MD
Retired; Formerly:
Neurology Services
West Roxbury Veterans Administration Medical
  Center
West Roxbury, Massachusetts

Robert H. Brown, Jr., MD, DPhil
Cecil B. Day Laboratory for Neuromuscular
  Research
Massachusetts General Hospital East
Charlestown, Massachusetts

Aron S. Buchman, MD
Associate Professor of Neurology
Rush Medical College of Rush University
Department of Neurological Sciences
Rush-Presbyterian-St. Luke's Medical Center
Chicago, Illinois

Donald B. Calne, DM, FRCP(C)
Professor of Medicine
Division of Neurology
University of British Columbia
Director, Neurodegenerative Disorders Centre
Vancouver Hospital and Health Sciences Centre
Vancouver, British Columbia, Canada

Daniel E. Casey, MD
Professor of Psychiatry and Neurology
Oregon Health Sciences University
Chief, Psychiatry Research/Psychopharmacology
Department of Veterans Affairs Medical Center
Portland, Oregon

**Guy Chouinard, MD, MSc (Pharm), FRCP(C),
  FAPA**
Professeur Titulaire
Université de Montreal
Professor of Psychiatry
McGill University
Hôpital Louis H. Lafontaine
Royal Victoria Hospital
Montreal, Quebec, Canada

Jonathan O. Cole, MD
Professor of Psychiatry
Harvard Medical School
Boston, Massachusetts
Senior Consultant
McLean Hospital
Belmont, Massachusetts

Cynthia L. Comella, MD
Associate Professor
Department of Neurological Sciences
Rush Medical College of Rush University
Rush-Presbyterian-St. Luke's Medical Center
Chicago, Illinois

Merit E. Cudkowicz, MD
Instructor in Neurology
Harvard Medical School
Assistant in Neurology
Massachusetts General Hospital
Boston, Massachusetts

Jeffrey L. Cummings, MD
Augustus S. Rose Professor of Neurology
Professor of Psychiatry and Behavioral Sciences
University of California, Los Angeles, School of
  Medicine
Reed Neurological Research Center
Los Angles, California

Michael Daras, MD
Professor of Clinical Neurology
New York Medical College
Valhalla New York
Chief, Neurology Department
Metropolitan Hospital
New York, New York

David M. Dawson, MD
Professor of Neurology
Harvard Medical School
Brigham and Women's Hospital
Boston, Massachusetts

Peter P. De Deyn, MD, PhD, MMPR
Professor of Neurology
University of Antwerp, UIA
Wilrijk, Belgium
Chairperson, Neurology
Algemeen Ziekenhuis Middelheim
Antwerpen, Belgium

Orrin Devinsky, MD
Professor of Neurology
New York University School of Medicine
Chief, Department of Neurology
Hospital for Joint Diseases Orthopaedic Institute
Director, NYU-HJD Comprehensive Epilepsy Center
New York, New York

Leon S. Dure IV, MD
Assistant Professor of Pediatrics and Neurology
University of Alabama School of Medicine
Attending Pediatric Neurologist
The Children's Hospital of Alabama
Birmingham, Alabama

Herbert F. Durwen, MD
Neurologische Universitatsklinik
Knappschafts-Krankenhaus
Ruhr-Universitat Bochum
Bochum, Germany

Roger C. Duvoisin, MD
Professor and Chairman, Emeritus
Department of Neurology
University of Medicine and Dentistry of New Jersey—
    Robert Wood Johnson Medical School
New Brunswick, New Jersey

Bruce L. Ehrenberg, MD
Assistant Professor of Neurology
Tufts University School of Medicine
Senior Neurologist
New England Medical Center
Boston, Massachusetts

Stanley Fahn, MD
H. Houston Merritt Professor of Neurology
Columbia University College of Physicians and Surgeons
New York, New York

Robert G. Feldman, MD
Professor and Chairman
Department of Neurology
Boston University School of Medicine
Chief of Neurology Service
Veterans Administration Medical Center
Neurologist-in-Chief
Boston University Medical Center Hospital
Boston, Massachusetts

J. Stephen Fink, MD
Medical Director
Neurology Program
GENZYME Corporation
Cambridge, Massachusetts

Seth P. Finklestein, MD
Associate Professor of Neurology
Harvard Medical School
CNS Growth Factor Research Laboratory
Massachusetts General Hospital
Boston, Massachusetts

**Pierre Flor-Henry, MD, ChB, MD (Edin), Acad
    DPM (Lond), FRCPsych, CSPQ (Psych)**
Clinical Professor of Psychiatry
University of Alberta
Clinical Director, General Psychiatry
Director, Clinical Diagnostics and Research Centre
Alberta Hospital Edmonton
Edmonton, Alberta, Canada

Albert M. Galaburda, MD
Emily Fisher Landau Professor of
    Neurology/Neuroscience
Harvard Medical School
Beth Israel Deaconess Medical Center
Boston, Massachusetts

George Gardos, MD
Associate Clinical Professor of Psychiatry
Harvard Medical School
Boston, Massachusetts

Bruce D. Geller, MD
St. Luke's Hospital
Kansas City, Missouri

Anita L. Gerhard, MD
Department of Psychiatry
University of Hawaii Medical School
Honolulu, Hawaii

Gilbert H. Glaser, MD
Professor Emeritus of Neurology
Yale University School of Medicine
Honorary Neurologist
Yale-New Haven Hospital
New Haven, Connecticut

Christopher G. Goetz, MD
Professor and Associate Chairman
Department of Neurological Sciences
Rush Medical College of Rush University
Senior Attending
Rush-Presbyterian-St. Luke's Medical Center
Chicago, Illinois

Robert C. Green, MD
Director, Neurobehavioral Program
Assistant Professor of Neurology
Emory University School of Medicine
Atlanta, Georgia

Ronald L. Green, MD
Director of Training and Education
Associate Professor of Psychiatry
Dartmouth-Hitchcock Medical Center
Dartmouth Medical School
Lebanon, New Hampshire

Penny Greenstein, MBBCh
Instructor in Neurology
Division of Neurogenetics
Beth Israel Deaconess Medical Center
Boston, Massachusetts

Thomas G. Gutheil, MD
Professor of Psychiatry
Harvard Medical School
Co-Director, Program in Psychiatry and the Law
Massachusetts Mental Health Center
Boston, Massachusetts

Michel H. Habib, MD
Director, Revue de Neuropsychologie
Cognitive Neurology Laboratory and Neurologic
 Clinic
University Hospital Timone
Marseille, France

**Graeme D. Hammond-Tooke, MBBCh, MSc,
 FCP(SA)**
Senior Lecturer in Medicine
University of Otago Medical School
Neurologist
Dunedin Hospital
Dunedin, New Zealand

Kenneth M. Heilman, MD
Professor of Neurology and Clinical Psychology
University of Florida College of Medicine
Chief, Neurology Service
Veterans Affairs Medical Center
Gainesville, Florida

Andrew G. Herzog, MD
Associate Professor of Neurology
Harvard Medical School
Neurological Unit
Beth Israel Deaconess Medical Center
Boston, Massachusetts

Jonathan M. Himmelhoch, MD
Tenured Professor of Psychiatry
University of Pittsburgh Medical School
Director, Research Affective Disorders Clinic
Western Psychiatric Institute
Pittsburgh, Pennsylvania

Reiji Iizuka MD
Emeritus Professor of Neuropsychiatry
Juntendo University School of Medicine
Tokyo, Japan

Joseph Jankovic, MD
Professor of Neurology
Director, Parkinson's Disease Center and Movement
 Disorders Clinic
Baylor College of Medicine
Houston, Texas

Anthony B. Joseph, MD
Medical Director
The Center for Neurobehavioral Rehabilitation
Olympus Specialty Hospital
Waltham, Massachusetts
Consultant Neuropsychiatrist
McLean Hospital
Belmont, Massachusetts
Associate Clinical Professor of Psychiatry
Harvard Medical School
Boston, Massachusetts

John M. Kane, MD
Chairman, Department of Psychiatry
Long Island Jewish Medical Center
Chief of Staff
Hillside Hospital
Glen Oaks, New York

Craig N. Karson, MD
Professor of Psychiatry and Pathology
Associate Dean for Veterans Health Services
University of Arkansas College of Medicine
Chief of Staff
Department of Veterans Affairs Medical Center
Little Rock, Arkansas

Ronald C. Kim, MD
Department of Pathology (Neuropathology)
University of California at Irvine
Irvine, California

Marcel Kinsbourne, MD
Center for Cognitive Studies
Tufts University
Medford, Massachusetts

Asha Kishore, MD, DM
Clinical Research Fellow
Division of Neurology
Department of Medicine
University of British Columbia
Neurodegenerative Disorders Centre
Vancouver Hospital and Health Sciences Centre
Vancouver, British Columbia, Canada

Barbara S. Koppel, MD
Professor of Clinical Neurology
New York Medical College
Valhalla, New York
Assistant Chief of Neurology
Metropolitan Hospital
New York, New York

Amos D. Korczyn, MD, MSc
Sieratzki Professor of Neurology
Sackler Faculty of Medicine
Tel Aviv University
Ramat Aviv, Israel
Tel Aviv Medical Center
Tel Aviv, Israel

Walter J. Koroshetz, MD
Associate Professor of Neurology
Harvard Medical School
Medical Director, Neurointensive Care Unit
Massachusetts General Hospital
Boston, Massachusetts

Neil W. Kowall, MD
Departments of Neurology and Pathology
Boston University School of Medicine
Boston, Massachusetts
Geriatrics Research Education and Clinical Center
Veterans Affairs Medical Center
Bedford, Massachusetts

Roger Kurlan, MD
Professor of Neurology
University of Rochester School of Medicine
and Dentistry
Strong Memorial Hospital
Rochester, New York

Janet M. Lawrence, MD
Assistant Attending Psychiatrist
Affective Disorders Unit
McLean Hospital
Belmont, Massachusetts

Carmen Z. Lemus, MD

James L. Levenson, MD
Associate Professor of Psychiatry and Medicine
Chairman, Division of Consultation-Liaison Psychiatry
Virginia Commonwealth University—Medical College
of Virginia
Richmond, Virginia

David N. Levine, MD
Professor of Neurology
New York University School of Medicine
New York University Medical Center
New York, New York

Morgan L. Levy, MD
Assistant Professor
Department of Psychiatry
Wake Forest School of Medicine
Winston-Salem, North Carolina

Jeffrey A. Lieberman, MD

J. Gila Lindsley, PhD, ACP
Sleepwell
Lexington, Massachusetts

Armand Lowenthal, MD, PhD
Professor Emeritus of Neurology and Neurochemistry
Algemeen Ziekenhuis Middelheim
Antwerpen, Belgium

Joseph B. Martin, MD, PhD
Dean
Harvard Medical School
Boston, Massachusetts

Prakash S. Masand, MD
Professor of Psychiatry
State University of New York Health Science Center
at Syracuse
Syracuse, New York

John H. Menkes, MD
Director of Pediatric Neurology
Cedars-Sinai Medical Center
Los Angeles, California

Lucinda G. Miller, PharmD
Professor and Vice Chairman, Primary Care
Interim Associate Dean for Clinical Research
School of Pharmacy
Texas Technical University Health Sciences Center
Amarillo, Texas

Gary S. Moak, MD
Assistant Professor of Psychiatry
University of Massachusetts Medical School
Boston Road Clinic
Worcester, Massachusetts

Hirotaro Narabayashi, MD, PhD
Professor Emeritus
Neurological Clinic
Meguro-ku
Tokyo, Japan

P. Nisipeanu, MD
Department of Neurology
Tel Aviv Medical Center
Tel Aviv, Israel

Torbjoern G. Nygaard, MD

David N. Osser, MD
Instructor in Psychiatry
Harvard Medical School and Massachusetts Mental
    Health Center
Boston, Massachusetts
Director of Psychopharmacology Consultation Service
Taunton State Hospital
Taunton, Massachusetts

Ananda K. Pandurangi, MD
Associate Professor of Psychiatry
Assistant Professor of Radiology
Virginia Commonwealth University—Medical College
    of Virginia
Richmond, Virginia

Anthony L. Pelonero, MD
Associate Professor of Psychiatry
Virginia Commonwealth University—Medical College
    of Virginia
Richmond, Virginia

Alan K. Percy, MD
Professor and Director
Pediatric Neurology
University of Alabama School of Medicine
Attending Pediatric Neurologist
The Children's Hospital of Alabama
Birmingham, Alabama

Roderick W. Pettis, JD, MD
Private practice in general and forensic psychiatry
San Francisco, California

Martin Pollock, MD, FRACP
Assistant Professor
University of Otago Medical School
Neurology Unit
Dunedin Hospital
Dunedin, New Zealand

Frank W. Putnam, MD
Chief, Unit of Developmental Traumatology
National Institute of Mental Health
Bethesda, Maryland

Michael Ronthal, MBBCh, FRCPE, MRCP
Department of Neurology
Beth Israel Deaconess Medical Center
Boston, Massachusetts

Leslie J. Gonzalez Rothi, PhD
Associate Professor of Neurology
University of Florida College of Medicine
Staff Speech Pathologist
Veterans Administration Medical Center
Gainesville, Florida

Robert N. Rubey, MD
Department of Veterans Affairs
Ralph H. Johnson Medical Center
Charleston, South Carolina

Thomas D. Sabin, MD
Lecturer on Neurology
Harvard Medical School
Clinical Professor and Vice Chairman of Neurology
Tufts University School of Medicine
Department of Neurology
New England Medical Center
Boston, Massachusetts

Marie-Helene Saint-Hilaire, MD, FRCP(C)
Assistant Professor of Neurology
Boston University School of Medicine
Clinical Director, Parkinson Day Program and
Staff Neurologist
Boston University Medical Center Hospital
Neurology Service
Veterans Administration Medical Center
Boston, Massachusetts

Maria Salam-Adams, MD★
Department of Neurology
Harvard Medical School
Massachusetts General Hospital
Boston, Massachusetts

★ Deceased.

Bruce L. Saltz, MD

Karen Santa Cruz, MD
University of Kansas Medical Center
Kansas City, Kansas

Jeremy D. Schmahmann, MD
Department of Neurology
Massachusetts General Hospital
Boston, Massachusetts

Michael A. Schwarzschild, MD, PhD
Instructor in Neurology
Harvard Medical School
Clinical and Research Fellow
Department of Neurology
Massachusetts General Hospital
Boston, Massachusetts

Jeremy M. Shefner, MD
Associate Professor
Department of Neurology
Director, EMG Laboratory and MDA-ALS Clinic
State University of New York Health Science Center
   at Syracuse
Syracuse, New York

Barry J. Snow, MD
Neurologist
Neuroservices Unit
Auckland Hospital
Auckland, New Zealand

Philip A. Starr, MD
Veterans Administration Medical Center
Surgical Service/Neurosurgery
San Francisco, California

Lewis Sudarsky, MD
Assistant Professor of Neurology
Harvard Medical School
Boston, Massachusetts
Neurology Services
West Roxbury Veterans Administration Medical
   Center
West Roxbury, Massachusetts

Caroline M. Tanner, MD
Associate Professor
Clinical Center of Parkinson's Disease and Movement
   Disorders
San Jose, California
Department of Neurological Services
Rush Medical College of Rush University
Chicago Illinois

Edward Tarlov, MD
Department of Neurosurgery
Lahey Clinic
Burlington, Massachusetts

Daniel Tarsy, MD
Associate Professor of Neurology
Harvard Medical School
Chief, Division of Neurology
Beth Israel Deaconess Medical Center
Boston, Massachusetts

Martin H. Teicher, MD
Associate Professor of Psychiatry
Harvard Medical School
Boston, Massachusetts
Director, Hall Mercer Snider Developmental Biopsychiatry
   Research Program
Director, Clinical Chronobiology Laboratory
McLean Hospital
Belmont, Massachusetts

Craig G. van Horne, MD, PhD
Clinical Fellow in Surgery
Harvard Medical School
Neurosurgical Resident
Brigham and Women's Hospital
Boston, Massachusetts

Nagagopal Venna, MD
Department of Neurology
Massachusetts General Hospital
Boston, Massachusetts

Jean Paul G. Vonsattel, MD
Associate Professor
Harvard Medical School
Director, Neuroscience Center
Massachusetts General Hospital—East
Charlestown, Massachusetts

Robert T. Watson, MD
Professor of Neurology
University of Florida College of Medicine
Staff Neurologist
Veterans Administration Medical Center
Gainesville, Florida

Jeffrey B. Weilburg, MD
Associate Professor
Harvard Medical School
Boston, Massachusetts

William C. Wirshing, MD
Professor of Clinical Psychiatry and Biobehavioral
    Sciences
University of California, Los Angeles, School of
    Medicine
Chief, Schizophrenia Treatment Unit
West Los Angeles Veterans Administration Medical Center
Los Angeles, California

Jonathan H. Woodcock, MD
Assistant Clinical Professor of Neurology
University of Colorado School of Medicine
Denver, Colorado
Medical Director
Mediplex Rehab—Denver
Thornton, Colorado

Bryan T. Woods, MD
Professor of Medicine
Texas A&M University College of Medicine
College Station, Texas
Chief, Neurology Section
Olin E. Teague Veterans' Center
Temple, Texas

Mark T. Wright, MD
Charter Behavioral Health System
Mobile, Alabama

Robert R. Young, MD
Professor and Vice Chairman
Department of Neurology
Medical Director, Movement Disorders Program
University of California at Irvine
Irvine, California

Richard M. Zweig, MD
Department of Neurology
Louisiana State University School of Medicine
    in Shreveport
Shreveport, Louisiana

Disorders of movement are frequent among neurologic and psychiatric patients. They, in turn, often have a behavioral, or psychiatric, component. For example, depressed patients may have apathetic facies and a paucity of spontaneous movements; it is often difficult to be certain early in the course of an illness that later turns out to be Parkinson's disease (PD) whether the patient has PD or is depressed. Neuroleptic medications, which created a revolution in the treatment of psychiatric patients, sometimes produce a PD-like syndrome or the hyperkinetic movements of tardive dyskinesia. Neurochemical changes have been described underlying such prototypical psychiatric disorders as manic–depressive illness and schizophrenia; they also underlie typical neurologic diseases such as PD, Huntington's disease, and Wilson's disease. Each of these disorders has a different neurochemical substratum and the consensus now is that neurochemical changes in the brain can also manifest themselves as psychiatric disease. This apparently trivial statement, which we now take for granted, would have been categorically denied a generation or two ago by our forebears. In summary, there is little argument that "the brain's the same" whether one is interested in its psychiatric or its neurologic disorders.

Mental influences such as stressful circumstances, fear, anxiety, or hypnosis clearly produce brain-mediated physical changes in the body, even affecting seemingly autonomous entities such as the immune system. A new discipline called psychoneuroimmunology has been formalized to investigate recently described aspects of what were earlier termed psychosomatic or mind–body problems, and another new field, psychocardiology, seeks to explore the relationship between behavior, the brain, and heart disease.

Mental influences such as stage fright or anxiety produce or exacerbate movement disorders. Enhanced physiologic tremor appears under these circumstances and because tremors are additive, may greatly worsen, albeit temporarily, an underlying essential–familial or parkinsonian tremor. Patients with Huntington's disease or those with PD who are overmedicated with L-dopa appear restless and are therefore often thought to be anxious or upset. The boundary zone between the study of movement disorders and psychiatry is ill-defined, porous, and ever changing.

The most difficult movement disorders to diagnose or to treat are those due to or associated with malingering, hysteria, or Munchausen's syndrome. Debates as to whether or not some unusual abnormal movement is factitious or "psychogenic" (an unfortunate term) often become the most heated in movement disorder clinics. Unfortunately, very little light is generated in these discussions. Ahlskog (1989), in a book review in which he was discussing movement disorders, said, "A few decades ago, many of these conditions were thought to be psychogenic. We now recognize that this spectrum of diseases is primarily organic. Nevertheless, in some patients the disorder has a functional basis, and it is these patients, especially, that present some of the greatest challenges."

An illustrative example is the young woman described by Batshaw et al (1985). At age 29, she presented with dystonic posturing of one foot and torticollis of 2 months' duration. Wilson's disease was ruled out and because of a history of "other illnesses of questionable authenticity," including chemotherapy for lymphoma 7 years before and intrathecal steroid therapy for multiple sclerosis at 28, she was admitted to a psychiatric unit for 2 months with a provisional diagnosis of a conversion disorder. Following discharge, she received regular psychotherapy for the next 3 years but her dystonia worsened and affected both arms and legs. She developed painful spasms, lost the ability to walk, and moved to a home for the handicapped. She was admitted to the National Institutes of Health where fixed contractures were found and a diagnosis of idiopathic torsion dystonia was made. This diagnosis was corroborated by three other medical centers with experience in caring for patients with torsion dystonia. She received appropriate drugs (L-dopa–carbidopa, carbamazepine, trihexyphenidyl, bromocriptine, diazepam) without improvement. She then underwent a left followed by a right ventrolateral thalamotomy. Her right arm improved but not the left. Two months later she became dysarthric and was aphonic for 18 months. She developed trismus and had to be fed by nasogastric and then gastrostomy tubes. She lost 13.6 kg and had a small-bowel biopsy. Psychotherapy continued. Periodic breathing developed and opisthotonic posturing lasted up to 6 hours associated with tonic–clonic movements and decreased levels of consciousness. She had a respiratory arrest during intravenous diazepam therapy for a "seizure" and required a tracheostomy. She was in constant pain from the dystonic spasms, required narcotics, and lost upward gaze.

Just before she was to be transferred to a nursing home, she awoke and began to speak normally. One day later she sat up, within a week she used both arms and walked for the first time in 2 years. Medications were stopped, she ate normally, her tracheostomy was closed, and all symptoms of dystonia disappeared except for shortening of the right Achilles tendon. She admitted she had feigned this illness to avoid work and to obtain sympathy and attention from family and friends. A diagnosis of chronic factitious disorder with physical symptoms (Munchausen's syndrome) was made; it was differentiated from malingering and conversion disorders. Not all patients with movement disorders are this difficult to treat, but in many cases it is unclear where the neurology ends and the psychiatry begins. One lesson to be learned from patients like this is that we should all beware of those, even those recognized as experts, who are absolutely certain about the diagnosis in a complex case. Equally august experts will often be equally certain about the correctness of a completely different diagnosis in the same patient. The wise and honest physician is not afraid to say "I don't know," and that is more often correct than one might imagine. As the field of movement disorders matures, one hopes the leaders will become increasingly critical and less dogmatic.

Although movement disorders have sometimes been thought to be the same as extrapyramidal disorders, we prefer the former terminology because it does not imply involvement of a certain (albeit vague) neural system and because it permits us to discuss disorders of incoordination and even corticospinal tract dysfunction including spasticity. Historically, the study of all these syndromes has been somewhat fragmented and, although consensus is beginning to emerge in the psychiatric and neurologic communities on some issues, many basic questions remain unresolved. There is also much confusion and overlap among terms used to describe or define many movement disorders. Similarly, etiology and treatment are often not well-understood and there are no objective diagnostic aids.

For those interested in these disorders, three levels of literature exist: basic texts that tend to be very general; journal articles that present new data and understanding, but are narrowly focused; and advanced texts that are either comprehensive, but only treat a limited number of topics, or overwhelmingly research-oriented and thus unsuitable for rapid clinical reference and use.

The purpose of *Movement Disorders in Neurology and Neuropsychiatry* is to address some of the needs of the practicing clinician when confronted with movement disorders. Two further examples are illustrative. Faced with a patient with an unusual disorder of movement, a physician can either refer the patient to an expert or attempt a diagnosis. In order to formulate a diagnosis and initiate management, it is necessary to be able to provisionally classify the type of abnormal movement, and then find appropriate clinical reference material. With the majority of movement disorders, this is a cumbersome job requiring a library search, often made even more difficult without a provisional diagnosis with which to begin.

A specialist seeing the same patient may well have a clearer idea of classification, but full access to comprehensive references on clinical diagnosis, management, and the thoughtful consideration of other diagnostically similar entities would still require a computerized search. This is not the case in other fields of medicine, where advanced general textbooks that offer a useful state-of-the-art overview for specialists, and an invaluable practical clinical guide for generalists, are usually available. *Movement Disorders in Neurology and Neuropsychiatry*, we hope, will meet this need in the area of movement disorders. In order to do so, the following goals have been set:

1. To broadly cover the field of movement disorders, not just to discuss familiar topics. In attempting to do this, one finds that not all students of movement disorders will agree that each topic in this book is a movement disorder, but some do, for all of them. Thus, this volume will make available a wide range of expert views on what constitutes a movement disorder and why.
2. To be both scientifically and clinically useful by concentrating on authoritatively written chapters that convey a high level of both theoretical understanding and practical guidance.
3. To avoid being so overly comprehensive that an unwieldy multivolume set would be required.

To attain these goals a large number of distinguished colleagues were asked to contribute individual chapters on various topics, and most were kind enough to do so. These chapters have been written so as to provide an expert's understanding of each topic, without an overwhelming array of detail. At the same time, individual points of view have been stressed and controversies within the field have been highlighted.

The authors have also usually provided an overview of therapeutic approaches, and attempted to place each movement disorder in an appropriate scientific context.

The basic thrust of this book has been to "split" rather than "lump." Inevitably, a certain amount of overlap has occurred, but this is general in nature, and each chapter has been designed either to stand alone, or to be read with its neighbors to provide a more comprehensive view of the subject.

A final point is that some authorities will no doubt disagree with aspects of the nomenclature and chapter groupings found in this book. For these choices we must take full responsibility. At this time the nomenclature of movement disorders is not well-defined, and we also note that the chapters could have been grouped in several ways. To us, the choices you see here are the most clinically and scientifically appealing. We hope this book will raise these topics for lively debate.

ABJ
RRY

REFERENCES

Ahlskog JE. Movement Disorders: A Comprehensive Survey (Weiner WJ, Lang AE). Futura Publishing, 1989 (Book review). Mayo Clin Proc 1989;64:1459–1460.

Batshaw ML, Wachtel RC, Deckel AW, et al. Munchausen's syndrome simulating torsion dystonia. New Engl J Med 1985;312:1437–1439.

This new edition of *Movement Disorders in Neurology and Neuorpsychiatry* arrives at a time when our field is growing as never before. Important new understandings are being generated from a myriad of disciplines, including genetics, epidemiology, and neurochemistry. New insights are gained as seemingly unrelated fields such as neuroimaging and computer science fruitfully interact and provide us with a better understanding of movement control and its disorders.

Against this backdrop, the practicing clinician continues to seek guidance when confronted with the typical or, not infrequently, the atypical patient with a movement disorder. As in the previous edition, we hope to meet this need with the current text. After the first edition was published,

we received much warm encouragement as well as many thoughtful and cogent ideas for improvement. We hope we have made good use of this input in preparing the second edition. Most of our original contributors have been kind enough to return, and there are some outstanding new additions as well. Many chapters have been updated and freshened, and some fascinating new ones have been added. We are pleased with the result and hope the reader will enjoy using the book as much as we enjoyed preparing it.

ABJ
RRY

Involuntary Movements: An Overview

ASHA KISHORE DONALD B. CALNE

INTRODUCTION

The term *extrapyramidal disease* is associated with disordered function in the basal ganglia or substantia nigra. Such diseases are characterized by the occurrence of involuntary movements. As the anatomic site of origin of involuntary movements is not known, the term *movement disorders* has been coined for diseases characterized by excessive and abnormal movements occurring in a conscious patient.

The terminology employed to describe the various patterns of involuntary movement is complex. Many diseases are associated with more than one type of abnormal movement. Scoring protocols have been devised to evaluate the severity of involuntary movements, and videotape recording has proved invaluable for such assessment. Here, we shall provide a brief descriptive comment on the various forms of involuntary movement and the terms employed to describe them. The characteristics that allow separation of the different types of involuntary movement are distribution, velocity, rhythmicity, amplitude, relation to activity/posture, and suppressibility.

Dyskinesia

This term can be applied to any type of involuntary movement. It is most frequently employed for the rather complex choreatic and dystonic movements that occur after prolonged treatment with neuroleptics (tardive dyskinesia) and the similar movements caused by L-dopa in patients with idiopathic parkinsonism. However, the term *dyskinesia* could be employed for any form of tremor, chorea, ballism, dystonia, tic, or myoclonus (or any combination of these).

Tremor

Tremor is a repetitive rhythmic movement that is consistent in time and space. The most common cause is essential tremor, followed by idiopathic parkinsonism. Sometimes a qualifying descriptive term is added (resting tremor, action tremor, postural tremor).

Chorea

Chorea is a quick, irregular, and predominantly distal involuntary movement. The term *semipurposive* has been used to facilitate its identification. The word *chorea* derives from the Greek word for dance, and often the movements resemble dancing gestures of the limbs.

Ballism

Ballism is proximal, high amplitude movement that is related to chorea: as patients recover from a stroke that has caused ballism, they often go through a stage of chorea. The word *ballism* implies coarse, high-velocity displacement; the root is the same as that for "ballistics."

Dystonia

Dystonia is characterized by more sustained spasms of contraction than other involuntary movements. Spasms may last many seconds at a time. If a joint will allow twisting, this is commonly seen (torsion dystonia). There are often fast components superimposed on the slower involuntary movement. The commonest form of idiopathic dystonia is spasmodic torticollis. Between muscle spasms, muscle tone is normal.

Myoclonus

Myoclonus is a term applied to sudden fast movements, generally repeated in the same portion of the body. Sometimes myoclonus is regularly repetitive and may resemble tremor; this is particularly likely when myoclonus is precipitated by voluntary movement (action myoclonus). Distinction between high-amplitude action tremor and low-amplitude rhythmic myoclonus may be difficult. Indeed, the separation may be more semantic than substantive.

Tic

Tic is a quick movement that is generally repeated in space (same muscle groups) but is irregular in time. The characteristic feature of tic is that the movement is usually preceded by an urge to move, and it can be suppressed for a short time (about 30–60 s) by voluntary effort.

Athetosis

Athetosis is a term that is now seldom used. It was employed to describe slow writhing movements. For a while, the term *athetotic dystonia* was in vogue, but now such movements are generally referred to as dystonia.

GENERAL FEATURES OF INVOLUNTARY MOVEMENTS

The advent of drugs that are agonists or antagonists of dopamine receptors has increased our understanding of involuntary movement. It is quite remarkable that every category of involuntary movement can occur as the result of manipulation of dopamine receptors. This observation strengthens the linkage between involuntary movements and the basal ganglia, an association that was originally proposed on the basis of meticulous clinicopathologic correlation.

All involuntary movements are subject to modulation by the level of excitement or relaxation of the patient. Involuntary movements are worse in an anxious patient, and they disappear during sleep (with the exception of certain forms of myoclonus).

THE MOST COMMON CAUSES OF INVOLUNTARY MOVEMENT

The most common disorder associated with abnormal movements is essential tremor. Some 50% of cases have a genetic origin, and such patients are designated as having "familial tremor." Idiopathic parkinsonism is the next most frequent cause of involuntary movement. Often the tremor is associated with chorea or dystonia (or both) induced by treatment with L-dopa.

Tardive dyskinesia is a common consequence of neuroleptic therapy. The movements can take any form, chorea and dystonia being the most common.

Focal dystonias are now recognized to be far more frequent than was previously thought, particularly spasmodic torticollis. The cause of focal dystonia is not known in most patients, but occasionally a primary cause can be found such as an arteriovenous malformation or exposure to a neuroleptic.

Huntington's disease is characterized by chorea, dystonia, and dementia. When symptoms start in children, presentation often resembles a parkinsonian syndrome. Genetic testing is now available for Huntington's disease and several other movement disorders such as idiopathic torsion dystonia, dentatorubropallidoluysian atrophy, and dopa-responsive dystonia.

There are many other diseases that produce involuntary movements, but they are unusual outside a movement disorder clinic. As a group, the movement disorders are a particularly rewarding challenge for the neurologist. Both diagnosis and management can exercise the clinician's skills, and the postmortem brain is a continuing source of enlightenment for the neurobiologist.

Disorders of Movement Associated with Drugs

Drug-Induced Dyskinesias: An Overview

Lucinda G. Miller   Joseph Jankovic

INTRODUCTION

The term *dyskinesia* describes any abnormal involuntary movement, irrespective of etiology. It is commonly used in the context of drug-induced repetitive and stereotypic orofacial movement that persists even after the offending drug has been stopped; hence the term *tardive dyskinesia* (TD). While most drug-induced dyskinesias occur in a form of stereotypy, defined as a repetitive, coordinated, seemingly purposeful movement, other drug-induced dyskinesias are manifested by dystonia, chorea, tics, myoclonus, tremor, and miscellaneous involuntary movements (1). Orofacial stereotypy is the most typical presentation of TD, but repetitive orofacial movements can also occur spontaneously, as in edentulous elderly individuals (2–6). This review will focus on drug-induced dyskinesias.

Most drug-induced movement disorders are caused by dopamine receptor blocking drugs, also known as neuroleptics. The term *neuroleptic* which literally means "that which takes the neuron," was coined by Deniker (7) to denote a class of "major tranquilizers." The use of the word has broadened to include antipsychotic and antiemetic drugs that block dopamine receptors.

Involuntary buccolingual masticatory movements (e.g., chewing, puckering, smacking, "fly-catching" movements of the tongue) are the most recognized manifestations of TD. Choreic movements of the fingers, hands, arms and feet also occur in TD (8). In respiratory dyskinesias, the diaphragm and chest muscles are involved resulting in noisy and difficult breathing (9). Dyskinesia may also involve the abdominal and pelvic muscles producing truncal or pelvic rocking movements ("copulatory" dyskinesia). Other forms of TD include tardive dystonia (10–14), tardive tourettism (11,15,17–22), tardive myoclonus (23,24), tardive akathisia (25), and tardive tremor (26). Parkinsonism may also result

from the same drugs that cause the hyperkinetic movement disorders, and the two types of movement disorders can coexist (27,28).

TD is the most recognized complication of neuroleptic therapy, but neuroleptic drugs can produce a variety of movement disorders. Acute dystonia, a sustained twisting movement, often occurs immediately after drug exposure (29). This acute dystonic reaction usually resolves spontaneously, but tardive dystonia can occur and persist as a permanent complication of neuroleptics (10–13). Akathisia, a feeling of restlessness, often presents within three months of neuroleptic use but may persist as tardive akathisia after the offending drug is stopped (30). Ninety percent of the patients with drug-induced parkinsonism (DIP) have the onset of symptoms within three months of initiation of neuroleptic treatment (31,32). Tardive dystonia and TD usually present after months to years of neuroleptic therapy (10,33).

Since the recognition of the predominant phenomenology of the movement disorder is critical to correct categorization, it will be discussed first. The pharmacology of specific drugs causing movement disorders and treatment of drug-induced movement disorders will be reviewed in the second half.

HISTORICAL BACKGROUND

With the introduction in 1952 of chlorpromazine (Thorazine; Smith, Kline and French Laboratories) came a dramatic improvement in the care of psychiatric patients. Effective outpatient care became possible, lessening the burden of inpatient admissions. In 1956, however, an emergence of abnormal movements as a complication of neuroleptic therapy was first documented (34). It is likely that movement disorders were seen earlier but were not recognized as drug-induced. For example, akathisia may have been confused with a worsening of the psychiatric condition leading to an increase in the dose of the neuroleptic. Neuroleptic-induced dyskinesias may have been also attributed to spontaneous dyskinesias (2). With this confusion, many years passed before TD became recognized as an adverse effect of neuroleptic use. It was not until 1964 that Faurbye et al described the movement disorders associated with antipsychotic use as TD (35). Today, the association of TD with neuroleptic use is well-recognized. It has been estimated that 10% to 20% of patients exposed to neuroleptics will develop some form of TD (36).

DIAGNOSIS

Drug-induced movement disorders can be categorized according to their phenomenology and whether they are acute or chronic. The following discussion is organized according to this classification with a clinical description of each of the movement disorders and the relevant epidemiologic data.

Acute Dystonia

Acute dystonic reactions are sustained, repetitive, patterned, muscle spasms resulting in twisting, squeezing, pulling, and often painful posturing. Oculogyric crisis, spasmodic torticollis, retrocollis, trismus, and blepharospasm are examples of focal dystonia (29). Children and young adults seem to be more commonly affected in the trunk region resulting in opisthotonos, scoliosis, trunk-flexion, writhing movements, and dystonic gait (37). These trunk movements are often accompanied by arm extensions. Dystonias have been postulated to correlate with falling plasma concentrations of the offending drug possibly resulting in a disruption of the normal dopamine-acetylcholine balance in the striatum (38). The symptoms may occur within hours after administration of the offending drug and may be the first extrapyramidal side effect encountered with the neuroleptic. Fifty percent occur within 48 hours and 90% within five days of drug treatment (30). In a study of 1,152 psychiatric patients, the highest incidence of dystonia was associated with haloperidol and the long-acting injectable fluphenazines (39). Overall, acute dystonias have been estimated to occur in 2.3% of patients exposed to phenothiazines (30).

Acute and Tardive Akathisia

Akathisia may occur within the first three months of neuroleptic therapy and may persist as tardive akathisia even when the offending drug is stopped. It is characterized by a subjective feeling of restlessness accompanied by motor stereotypies (40). The restlessness has been described using such phrases as "nervousness," "all wound up like a spring," "unable to feel comfortable in any position," "rowdy-like," "irritable," "like jumping out of my skin," and "heebies-

jeebies" (41). Patients will engage in seemingly purposeless activity such as picking at clothes, folding and unfolding of arms, shifting of weight, and rocking. Leg movements may include crossing and uncrossing, abduction and adduction, pumping legs up and down while sitting, spontaneously rising from chair, pacing, body rocking, and marching in place. Unfortunately this symptomatology is sometimes mistaken for a worsening of the psychosis or anxiety and has led to an increase in the dose of the neuroleptic, with eventual exacerbation of the restlessness (42).

Because akathisia is often not recognized, particularly at onset, the true incidence of this movement disorder in neuroleptic-treated patients is unknown. Haloperidol when given as a 5-mg test dose was associated with akathisia within the first six hours in 40% of 44 schizophrenic patients (43). By the seventh day of treatment, 76% of the patients had experienced akathisia. In the same study, 20% of 67 patients experienced akathisia 12 hours after exposure to thiothixene (43). During the ensuing four weeks the cumulative percentage rose to 63%.

Akathisia can be seen in patients with idiopathic Parkinson's disease (PD). It has long been believed that akathisia in this population is an expression of an urge to relieve discomfort from parkinsonian rigidity and bradykinesia. In a study of 100 patients though, 26% experienced an inability to sit still unrelated to the PD and was considered a state of true akathisia (44). Akathisia was found to be more frequent in patients with an akinetic-rigid form of PD versus those with predominant tremor. Because akathisia occurs so frequently and has led to suicide, its appearance should not be considered trivial (45).

Akathisia may be a forerunner of TD, particularly if it persists despite a decrease in the dose of the offending medication (1,25,46,47). Akathisia may not only herald the development of TD, but may be one of the tardive syndromes (25). Thus, akathisia may be both an early (acute) and late (chronic, tardive) phenomenon associated with the use of dopamine receptor antagonists.

Parkinsonism

Drug-induced parkinsonism (DIP) mimics PD in all the cardinal neurologic signs such as rigidity, akinesia, tremor, and postural abnormalities (31,32). Bradykinesia is the most common and sometimes the only symptom of DIP, seen in up to 80% of patients with DIP. Twenty-five percent of patients with DIP could not walk upon initial presentation, 50% had urinary incontinence, and 80% had reduction of arm swing on walking (48). In contrast, only 10% of patients with PD could not walk upon presentation with similar percentages for the other two parameters (48). While DIP and PD share some clinical features, the two movement disorders can be distinguished by the history of drug exposure in relationship to the onset of symptoms, age at onset, duration of symptoms, nature of tremor, bilateral versus unilateral, or asymmetrical signs and response to anticholinergics

(Table 2.1) (49). DIP typically occurs precipitously within three months of therapy whereas the onset of PD is insidious and delayed. DIP can occur at any age while most patients with PD are older than 50 years (49). The pill-rolling resting tremor common to PD is not usually seen in DIP (37). High-frequency action tremor is common to both phenotypes. DIP tends to be symmetric in its presentation whereas PD usually begins in an asymmetric fashion (49). DIP responds favorably to anticholinergic therapy; patients with PD usually require dopamine agonist therapy in addition to anticholinergic therapy (49).

DIP occurs in 10% to 15% of the patients treated with neuroleptics, but the frequency of this adverse effect varies widely depending on the population studied, drug and dosage of neuroleptics, and other factors (37). In one study, 66% of the patients with DIP recovered after an average of seven weeks following drug discontinuation (48). DIP is usually a transient phenomenon, resolving upon cessation of neuroleptic therapy unless there is an underlying disorder. In one report, 11% of patients who recovered from an initial bout of DIP later developed PD suggesting an underlying pathologic dysfunction (32,50). It is not known how many patients with reversible DIP have underlying PD, but subclinical PD may be an important risk factor for DIP.

Tardive Dyskinesia

The American Psychiatric Association Task Force defines tardive dyskinesias as abnormal involuntary movement resulting from treatment with a neuroleptic drug for three months in a patient with no other identifiable cause for movement disorders (51). However, we have seen patients with persistent dyskinesia, usually dystonia, after a shorter period of treatment (10). Since stereotypic movements usually predominate, the term *tardive stereotypy* is more appropriate than the less specific term *tardive dyskinesia*. Involuntary mouthing, sucking, chewing, and licking movements comprise the typical buccal–lingual masticatory syndrome (Figure 2.1). The oral movements may worsen under emotional stress but disappear during sleep (52). In some cases, stereotypy can be combined with other movement disorders, such as chorea and dystonia. Choreoathetosis, slow choreic movements, may occur alone or be superimposed on dystonic posturing. Such movements may involve

the fingers, hands, arms, and feet. Respiratory dyskinesias involving diaphragmatic and chest muscles have also been reported and, in rare cases, may be life-threatening (46, 53–55).

TD is often a persistent disorder, but spontaneous remissions are frequently encountered, particularly in the younger population. An inverse correlation between rates of spontaneous remission and age has been noted (56). Patients younger than 60 years have a threefold greater chance of

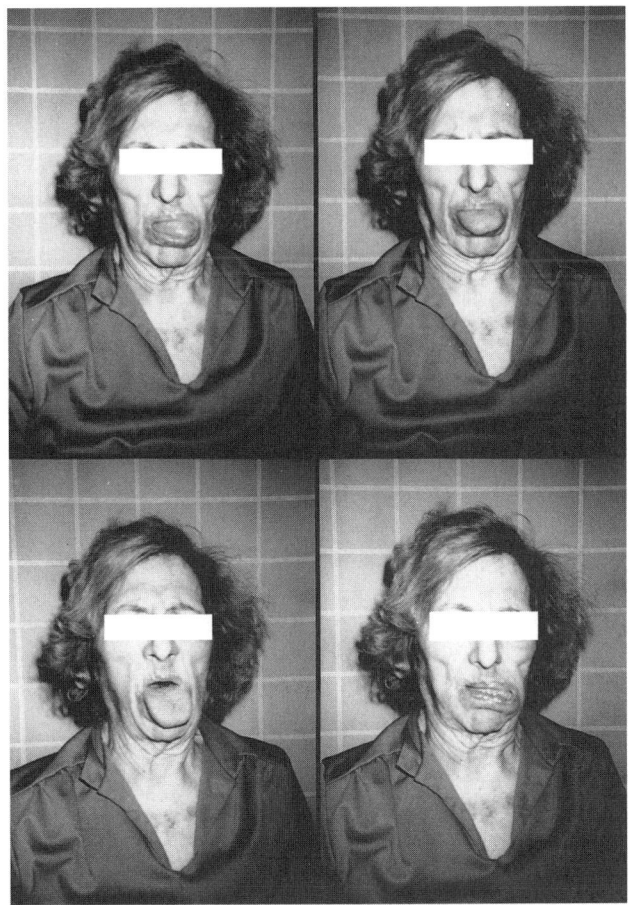

FIGURE 2.1 *A psychotic woman treated with numerous neuroleptic drugs for at least 15 years developed typical orofacial–buccolingual TD.*

Table 2.1 Differentiation of Parkinsonian Disorders

Criteria	Parkinson's Disease	Drug-Induced Parkinsonism
Prior neuroleptic exposure	No	Yes, symptoms often start within 3 months of therapy
Age at onset (years)	>50	Any age
Natural course	Progressive	Usually resolves within a few days to months after stopping the offending drug
Tremor	4–5 Hz rest tremor (supination–pronation)	Action–postural tremor, rapid (>5 Hz) rest tremor
Distribution of symptoms at onset	Asymmetric	Symmetric
Response to pharmacologic therapy	Usually requires dopaminergic therapy	Favorable response with anticholinergics and amantadine

improving as compared with older patients (42). In a study of 13 psychiatric patients with TD, over half (53.8%) remitted during follow-up (mean follow-up: 1.6 years). The group's average age at onset was 62 years (range: 53–79) (11). Twenty-seven psychiatric patients were studied serially over a five-year period to determine if adjusting or eliminating the neuroleptic dose could substantially affect the long-term prognosis of TD (57). The majority of the patients improved by more than 50% with 29.6% (n = 8) experiencing total resolution of TD.

TD may be combined with other movement disorders, including parkinsonism. In a study of 132 psychiatric patients, 23 (17.4%) had coexistent TD and parkinsonism (25). In another study of 46 patients with TD, 15 (33%) had concurrent parkinsonism (28). In this series, patients with parkinsonism associated with TD had a later age of onset of TD (seventh or eighth decade) than those patients who experienced TD alone (mean age of onset: 54 years) (28). The coexistence of TD and parkinsonism seems to be an expression of opposite pharmacologic mechanisms, where parkinsonism is a consequence of dopamine depletion and TD reflects an excessive response to dopamine. It has been explained in terms of regional differences. For example, postsynaptic receptor supersensitivity in one region of the basal ganglia may be expressed as TD while parkinsonian symptoms may appear consequent to dopamine depletion in another area (28).

Tardive Tremor

Tardive tremor is a relatively rare form of TD (26). This rhythmic movement is distinguishable from the more common stereotypy in that it consists of an oscillatory movement rather than coordinated, seemingly purposeful movement seen in tardive stereotypy. Tardive tremor differs from tremor observed in patients with Parkinson's disease in that it is predominantly postural and kinetic and it is not necessarily accompanied by other parkinsonian signs. Tardive tremor does not respond to therapy conventionally used for essential tremor or Parkinson's disease but rather improves within 30 to 60 minutes of tetrabenazine administration (26). In contrast, tetrabenazine would be expected to exacerbate parkinsonian tremor. In the absence of other etiologies for tremor, such as hyperthyroidism, the diagnosis of tardive tremor should be considered.

Tardive Dystonia

Tardive dystonia is a persistent dystonic movement disorder and therefore it differs from acute transient dystonic reaction (10–13). Criteria for its diagnosis include the presence of chronic dystonia, prior or concurrent neuroleptic use, exclusion of known causes of secondary dystonia, and a negative family history for dystonia (12). Characterized by sustained, patterned, slow or rapid twisting movements involving the face, neck, trunk, or limbs, tardive dystonia may occur after only three days of antipsychotic treatment, but usually it follows months of neuroleptic therapy (Figure 2.2) (13). The face and neck are the most frequently affected regions at onset and are also most frequently involved at the time of maximum severity of illness (13). Nearly half of the patients with neck involvement displayed retrocollis (Figure 2.3). The dystonic movements usually subside during sleep and are often relieved by tactile maneuvers, referred to as sensory tricks or geste antagonistique (13). The dystonic movements may be superimposed on stereotypic rapid jerking movements of TD. Coexistent TD was seen in 14 (21%) of 67 patients with tardive dystonia (13).

Because of resemblance to typical tardive dystonia, idiopathic dystonia with blepharospasm-oromandibular dystonia (Meige's syndrome) is frequently misdiagnosed as tardive dystonia, even though there is no history of neuroleptic exposure (58,59). Although there is no universal agreement, most authorities believe that if there is no history of neuroleptic use for at least six months prior to the onset of the movement disorder, then it could not be considered "drug-induced" (Table 2.2) (13). Tardive dystonia has been noted in 1.5% (5 of 331) of patients hospitalized in a psychiatric hospital (60). However, in another study, 21% of 125 patients in a Veterans Administration psychiatric facility had tardive dystonia (61). Mental retardation and electroconvulsive therapy were identified as risk factors for this movement disorder (60).

Tardive dystonia, frequently more disabling than classic TD, may be more persistent (12). In a study of nine psychiatric patients with tardive dystonia examined for an averaged follow-up period of 2.5 years (range: 4 months to 8 years), no spontaneous remissions were encountered (11). In other studies, five (12%) of 42 patients and five of 67 (7.5%) experienced spontaneous remission of tardive dystonia, respectively. This occurred within 2.4 years from onset

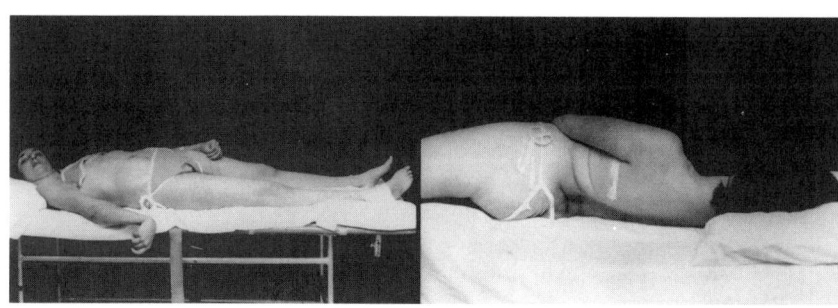

FIGURE 2.2   *A young schizoprenic woman with generalized tardive dystonia producing dystonic flexion of hand (left) and opisthotonic trunkal extension (right).*

(range: 1 to 4 years) (10). Thus, unlike idiopathic torsion dystonia, tardive dystonia can remit but the remission rate is much less than the 25% to 57% rate noted with TD (11,13,61,62).

Tardive Tourettism

Gilles de la Tourette syndrome (TS) is a neurobehavioral disorder characterized by motor and phonic tics and a variety of behavioral problems. Motor tics are coordinated involuntary movements occurring in patterned sequences in a spontaneous, unpredictable, abrupt, and transient manner (63). Involuntary vocalizations, repetition of words as phrases (echolalia), use of obscenities (coprolalia), and mimicking of gestures (echopraxia) often occur in the patient with TS (63). Obsessive–compulsive behavior, sleep disturbance, and an attention deficit with hyperactivity are additional manifestations of this disorder (64). Dopamine receptor supersensitivity as evidenced by low cerebrospinal fluid homovanillic acid and a favorable response to dopamine blocking and depleting drugs has been suggested as the underlying pathophysiology for TS (65).

Tardive tourettism has been recognized as one of the acquired tourettisms (15–17). Patients with tardive tourettism display all the classic symptoms of TS. Unlike TS,

however, which usually manifests between 2 and 15 years of age, tardive tourettism may not occur until later in adulthood (17).

The neuropharmacology underlying tardive tourettism parallels that of TD and idiopathic TS (17). All three disorders may represent different expressions of supersensitive dopamine receptors, involving different dopaminergic pathways. Furthermore, TD and tardive dystonia may occur as complications of neuroleptic therapy in patients with idiopathic TS (Figure 2.4) (66).

Antipsychotics are the principal drugs associated with tardive tourettism. Klawans et al described a 28-year-old schizophrenic woman treated with chlorpromazine for six years (18). One month after stopping chlorpromazine, she developed tic-like symptoms consistent with TS. A second case was reported in 1981 in a 16-year-old man who developed spontaneous vocalizations (hissing, guttural, and barking sounds) two weeks after discontinuing haloperidol (9). Eight additional patients who developed tardive tourettism following 2 to 20 years of neuroleptic use have since been reported (15,17,20,21). In two of these cases, tourettism developed after exposure to haloperidol and thioridazine for two weeks, but these patients had a previous history of motor and phonic tics following stimulant therapy (20). A 65-year-old man with TD consequent to thioridazine and perphenazine therapy experienced relief from TD after discontinuation of the neuroleptics only to be

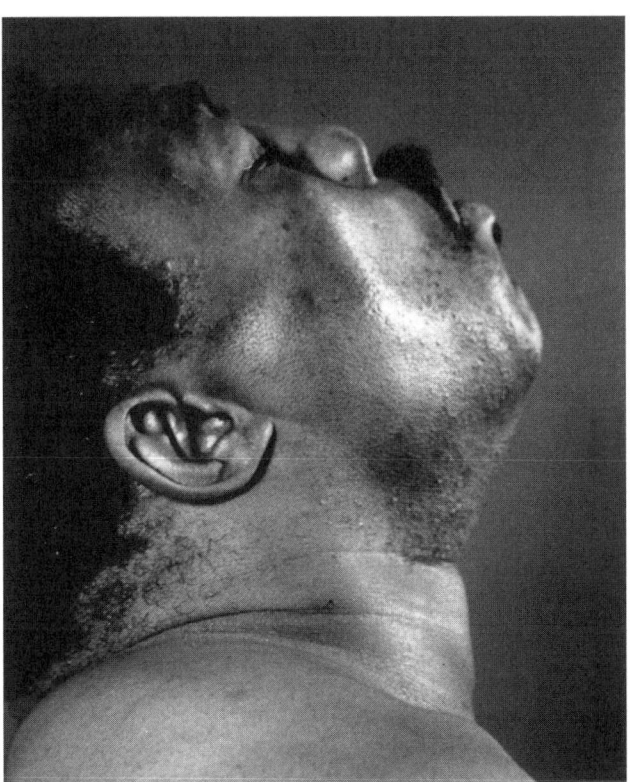

FIGURE 2.3   *A schizophrenic man with tardive retrocollis. As a result of tardive cervical dystonia and hypertrophy of cervical muscles, his neck size increased from 15.5 to 18.5 inches in less than three months.*

Table 2.2   Differential Diagnosis of Cranial–Cervical Dystonia (Meige's Syndrome) Versus TD

Clinical Features	Cranial–Cervical Dystonia	TD
Blepharospasm	+	−
Oromandibular–cervical dystonia	+	−
Axial-limb dystonia	+	−
Stereotyped repetitive movements	−	+
Photophobia	+	−
Respiratory dyskinesias	+	+
Vocalizations	+/−	−
Improvements with "tricks"	+	−
Movements are of major concern to the patient	+	−
Akathisia	+	−
Essential tremor	+	−
Spasmodic dysphonia	+	−
Positive family history	+/−	−
History of antipsychotic medications	−	+
Improvement with antipsychotic medications (haloperidol)	+/−	+
Improvement with apomorphine/lisuride	+/−	−
Improvement with physostigmine	−	+
Improvement with anticholinergics	+/−	−
Improvement with tetrabenazine	+/−	+

+ = often present; − = absent or seldom present.

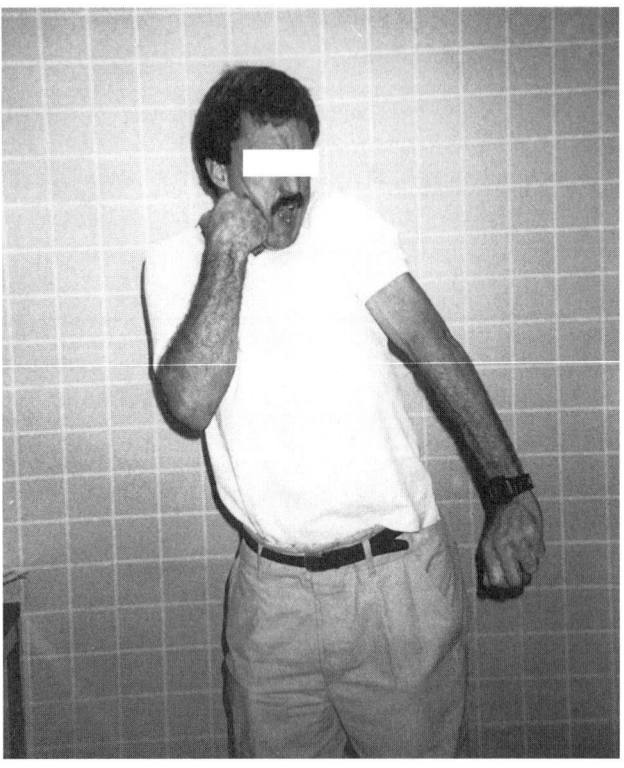

FIGURE 2.4   *A young man with Tourette's syndrome and tardive dystonia producing torticollis, left arm extension, and right arm flexion.*

replaced by tardive tourettism (22). It is possible that these patients have subclinical TS, which is "unmasked" by neuroleptic withdrawal.

The occurrence of tardive tourettism following neuroleptic therapy raises important concerns about the use of neuroleptics for idiopathic TS. Additionally, the decision to use these drugs in the treatment of TS must be carefully weighed against the potential complications, including tardive dystonia and TD (66).

Tardive Myoclonus

Myoclonus, a jerk-like contraction of muscle groups, may be rhythmic or arrhythmic, arising from cortical, subcortical (e.g., brainstem reticular formation), and spinal cord structures (67). Myoclonus must be differentiated from other movement disorders. Tics differ from myoclonus in that tics can be voluntarily controlled and are more complex movements. Dystonic contractions are more prolonged and often twisting whereas myoclonic jerks are brief and simple (68). Tremors are oscillatory, movements that differentiate them from rhythmic myoclonus which are secondary to repetitive agonist muscle contractions (68). Myoclonus differs from chorea in that chorea is a random flow of brief contractions. Thus, late-onset (tardive) myoclonus represents

another distinct movement disorder complicating neuroleptic therapy.

Myoclonus associated with a prolonged course of antipsychotic medications has been described (24). In one study of drug-induced myoclonus, 32 (24%) of 133 patients who had taken antipsychotics for more than three months developed postural myoclonus (23). These myoclonic jerks occurred in 34% of the 73 male patients and in 13% of the 60 female patients. However, the brief description of the movement disorder was insufficient to be certain that the involuntary movements were truly myoclonic. One of the authors (Jankovic) described a 46-year-old psychotic woman who, after receiving chlorpromazine and thioridazine for 30 years and loxapine for seven months, developed persistent myoclonus five months after discontinuation of therapy (24). The jerk-like, rhythmic extension head movements recurred one to two times per second.

Neuroleptic Malignant Syndrome

Neuroleptic malignant syndrome (NMS), first described by Delay & Denker in 1968, is believed to be a consequence of impaired hypothalamic and striatal dopamine transmission or sudden withdrawal from dopamine therapy (69–71). NMS is characterized by hyperpyrexia, muscular rigidity, autonomic dysfunction, and alterations in consciousness (71,72). Parkinsonism is the most common movement disorder but lead-pipe rigidity, trismus, choreiform movements, and opisthotonos may be present as well (73,74). Altered mental status, ranging from confusion to coma occurs in nearly three-fourths of patients affected (74). The most serious complication of NMS is rhabdomyolysis (75). Fatalities occur in 20% of the cases primarily due to respiratory failure, renal failure, arrhythmias, or cardiovascular collapse (70). Persistent neurologic sequela for those who survive include parkinsonism, dyskinesia, dementia, and ataxia (74). NMS thus represents another consequence of neuroleptic therapy involving involuntary movement disorders.

Believed to be a rare event affecting 0.5% to 1.0% of patients exposed to neuroleptics, recent estimates demonstrate a prevalence rate of 1.4% to 2.4% (72,76). Ten percent of patients will develop NMS within 24 hours of receiving the first dose while 90% (n = 47) have been shown in one study to develop NMS within two weeks of initiating neuroleptic treatment or increasing the dose (74). For those 80% of patients who are to survive, NMS usually resolves within 5 to 10 days after discontinuing therapy but symptoms have been known to persist for three to eight weeks (77–79). NMS occurs more frequently in men, young patients, and those patients with affective disorders (80). In one study, men constituted 68% (n = 32) and women 32% (n = 15) of cases (75). Renal insufficiency may represent an additional risk factor (81). A genetic predisposition to NMS has not yet been reported although malignant hyperthermia appears to be inherited (74).

Butyrophenones, phenothiazines, and thioxanthines in therapeutic doses resulting in nontoxic blood levels are most often implicated in the pathogenesis of NMS (70,71). Haloperidol and fluphenazine are the most commonly cited drugs (perhaps reflecting their increased use) (70). In one review, haloperidol accounted for 63% of NMS cases, fluphenazine 22%, and chlorpromazine 19% (74). Of 52 patients experiencing NMS, 60% (n = 31) received single drug therapy while 40% (n = 21) received combination neuroleptic therapy (74). Although usually thought of in context of antipsychotic use, NMS may also occur following use of droperidol and metoclopramide for postoperative or diabetic-associated nausea (81,82). It has also been reported as a consequence of cocaine and ecstasy abuse (83,84).

EPIDEMIOLOGY

Epidemiologic studies of drug-induced movement disorders are difficult to interpret largely because of nosologic and methodologic problems. The term *extrapyramidal syndrome* or *EPS* has been used in the psychiatric literature to designate any of the drug-induced movement disorders, and in some studies little or no attempt was made to separate the different disorders. Until a specific biologic marker is identified that reliably differentiates the types of drug-induced movement disorders, the diagnosis of the various movement disorders will depend on the clinical recognition of the distinguishing phenomenology (85). Thus, TD may include any or a combination of the following syndromes: tardive stereotypy, tardive tremor, tardive dystonia, tardive chorea, tardive tics, and tardive myoclonus (11,24,85).

Because orofacial dyskinesia is the most typical form of TD, any study of the prevalence of TD must take into account the occurrence of orofacial dyskinesia in a general population never treated with neuroleptics. The estimates of frequency of spontaneous orofacial dyskinesias range from 0.22% to 38% depending on the population studied (2–4,86–88).

Elderly women seem to have increased risk for developing drug-induced dyskinesias (36). The cumulative annual incidence of TD among psychiatric outpatients averaging 65.5 years old treated with relatively low daily doses (average: 150 mg of chlorpromazine equivalent) of neuroleptics is 26.1% (five to six times that of younger adults) (89). In a study of 270 elderly subjects, of which one-fourth had movement disorders, 27% were women while 12% were men (36). In our study of 125 patients with drug-induced movement disorders, we found a 4:1 female preponderance for all diagnoses (TD, parkinsonism, akathisia, tremor) with only tardive dystonia exhibiting no gender predilection (90).

Spontaneous remissions are more likely to occur in younger patients. Patients with TD starting before age 60 years improved three times more often than older patients

(91). The older the patient when first started on the neuroleptic, the sooner he or she is likely to develop TD (92). Furthermore, patients with affective disorder seem to develop TD at a younger age than patients with other psychiatric problems (93).

While age has been associated with an increased risk for movement disorders, youth does not necessarily confer protection (94). Three of 41 children (7.3%) with psychiatric disorders exposed to neuroleptic therapy developed tardive dyskinesia while 13 of 38 mentally retarded children (34%) developed tardive dyskinesia following neuroleptic exposure (94,95).

MANAGEMENT

Clinical management of drug-induced movement disorders, in particular TD, has remained a challenging problem. Numerous approaches to medical management have been tried with varying degrees of success (Table 2.3). Use of a neuroleptic to block dopamine receptors as a symptomatic treatment of TD should be reserved for only severe, disabling, or life-threatening cases (e.g., respiratory dyskinesias). Modulation of the other neurotransmitter systems may prove successful. Stimulation of the GABAergic system with baclofen has resulted in moderate improvement of inpatients maintained on neuroleptics but was ineffective when the neuroleptic was withdrawn (96,97). Gamma-vinyl-GABA, believed to increase GABA activity by inhibiting GABA transaminase, has been reported to relieve symptoms of TD (98). Similarly, sodium valproate is thought to inhibit GABA transaminase, but its benefit in TD has not been consistent (99,100). In one report, clonidine in doses ranging from 0.15 to 0.45 mg/day resulted in moderate improvement of TD in 75% of patients treated and in full resolution in 50% of patients (101). If confirmed this would suggest that alpha-noradrenergic pathways are involved in the pathogenesis of TD. Despite earlier reports of potential benefit, manipulation of the cholinergic system has not been successful in the treatment of TD (102,103).

Tetrabenazine has demonstrated therapeutic value in the treatment of TD (104–107). Tetrabenazine is a presynaptic monoamine depleting agent as well as a postsynaptic dopamine receptor blocker (107,108). Improvement was noted in a double-blind study of 13 patients administered a maximum dose of 200 mg/day (107). In a long-term open trial of 400 patients with a variety of hyperkinetic movement disorders, tetrabenazine was found most effective in patients with TD (105,108). Because tetrabenazine is not readily available in the U.S., reserpine, which has similar pharmacologic action, may be a useful alternative (105).

Additional modes of therapy have been tried for other movement disorders. Diphenhydramine's antidystonic effectiveness is attributed to its antihistamine properties (110,111). Intrathecal baclofen infused at initial doses of

Table 2.3   Drugs Reported Effective in the Treatment of Tardive Dyskinesias

Dopamine antagonists
    Phenothiazines
    Butyrophenones
    Substituted benzamides (e.g., metoclopramide)
    Pimozide
    Papaverine
    D_2 receptor blockers (e.g., sulpiride, tiapride)
    Estrogens
Dopamine agonists
    Amantadine
    Apomorphine
    Bromocriptine
    Melanocyte-stimulating-hormone inhibiting factor
Blockers of catecholamine synthesis
    Methyldopa
    Alpha-methyltyrosine
    Dopamine-beta-hydroxylase inhibitors (e.g., fusaric acid, disulfiram)
Blockers of catecholamine release
    Lithium
Gamma-aminobutyric acid agonists
    Valproate
    Baclofen
    Gamma-vinyl-GABA
    Benzodiazepines
Antiseritonin agents
    Cyproheptadine
Endorphin modulation of dopaminergic system
    Opiate
Alpha-adrenergic agents
    Clonidine
Beta-adrenergic agents
    Propranolol
Cholinergic agents
    Deanol
    Physostigmine
    Choline
    Lecithin
Dibenzodiazepine
    Clozapine
Catecholamine-depleting agents
    Tetrabenazine
    Reserpine

Modified from Jankovic J. Drug-induced and other orofacial-cervical dyskinesias. Ann Intern Med 1981;94:788–793.

4 mcg/mL titrated to obtain optimal control may prove useful for intractable cases of dystonia (112). Milacemide, a prodrug of glycine, did not benefit 10 patients with myoclonus and other intractable movement disorders (e.g., dystonia), despite doses of 4,800 mg/day (113). Iron supplementation for the treatment of akathisia has been suggested based on the observation of iron deficiency in patients with akathisia (114). However, neuroleptics chelate iron, mobiliz-

ing it from peripheral stores and depositing it in the basal ganglia resulting in TD (114). It is doubtful whether peripheral levels of iron in any way reflect central iron stores, hence the rationale for iron supplementation based on lower serum levels is relatively weak and much more work must be completed before such a therapeutic intervention can be recommended for akathisia (114). Additionally, such therapy may theoretically contribute to the onset of TD since iron may increase oxidative stress and as such may accelerate neuronal damage (115). Systemic administration of iron, however, probably does not affect brain concentrations.

Stereotactic thalamotomy has been used for selected cases of dystonia; modest improvements associated with this procedure suggest the primary mechanism underlying dystonia is not hyperactivity of thalamocortical connections (116).

Botulinum toxin has proven successful for patients with a wide variety of movement disorders including focal dystonia, palatal myoclonus, tremor, and tics (117). Botulinum toxin exerts chemodenervation at the neuromuscular junction by binding to presynaptic cholinergic terminals. It serves as a zinc endopeptidase, cleaving various proteins essential for the normal docking of the presynaptic acetylcholine vesicles with the presynaptic membrane (118,119). This process is reversed within three to four months as reinnervation occurs. This correlates with observable clinical effects and duration of benefit (120,121). The dose employed varies with the affected muscle groups. Botulinum toxin 2.5 units may suffice for incomitant strabismus but up to 700 units may be required for spasmodic torticollis (122). Immunoresistance may develop to botulinum toxin injections paralleling the presence of botulinum toxin antibodies (123,124). These patients may benefit from treatment with alternative serotypes (e.g., botulinum toxin type F injections instead of type A).

PREVENTION

Because of lack of uniformly effective treatment for TD, the best approach is prevention. An important focus of current research is to identify risk factors for the development of TD and other drug-induced movement disorders (125). Although awareness of risk factors should help identify certain populations at risk (e.g., the elderly for drug-induced parkinsonism or women for TD) it is presently impossible to predict with certainty if a specific individual will develop a movement disorder upon exposure to a particular neuroleptic.

Primary prevention should include reducing neuroleptic drug exposure as much as clinically possible (126). Whenever possible, non-neuroleptic drugs should be used for nausea, psychiatric problems, and other disorders for which neuroleptics are frequently selected. Early diagnosis of the drug-induced movement disorder and prompt intervention may reverse what was once thought an irreversible condition (127–129). Of utmost importance are educational methods to alert physicians to the occurrence of drug-induced movement disorders and their early detection. The medical and legal concerns regarding drug-induced movement disorders should encourage each prescribing physician to learn about the potential extrapyramidal effects of each drug and to learn to recognize the early signs of the drug-induced movement disorders so that appropriate action can be taken.

Early recognition of the disorder and discontinuation of the offending agent may prevent the development of the full syndrome. In some cases this may cause transient exacerbation of the movement disorder in addition to re-emergence of the original disorder for which the drug was prescribed. If the original disorder is psychosis, alternative antipsychotics are now available that seem to have the same therapeutic efficacy as the typical antipsychotics but with a lower risk for development of TD. One such drug, clozapine, has been used effectively in the treatment of schizophrenia, but the risk of potentially fatal agranulocytosis and a high cost of the drug and frequent monitoring make it difficult for many patients to fully benefit from this drug (130–132). Although the atypical antipsychotic drugs appear to carry a lower risk for persistent neuroleptic-induced movement disorder (NIMD), it is doubtful that these drugs can be used safely and effectively in the treatment of TD (132). While concomitant use of anticholinergic drugs may reduce the risk of neuroleptic induced-adverse drug reactions (ADRs) (133), anticholinergic therapy could, at least theoretically, increase the risk of subsequent TD.

DRUGS ASSOCIATED WITH MOVEMENT DISORDERS

Below is a partial list of drugs known to cause or exacerbate drug-induced movement disorders. A review of the patient's drug history constitutes the first step in management.

Dopamine Antagonists

Antipsychotics
Phenothiazines, thioxanthenes, butyrophenones, and other heterocyclic compounds such as loxapine, molindone, and pimozide are antipsychotics currently marketed in the United States (134). Antipsychotics were first recognized as inducers of TD in the 1960s. Attempts have been made to correlate drug potency on specific neuronal systems with the increased incidence of movement disorders (134,135). Of the antipsychotics used in the United States, thiothixene has been shown to possess the highest affinity for binding to postsynaptic dopamine (D_2) receptors whereas promazine has the lowest affinity (136). Thioridazine and haloperidol have been shown to be similar in their dopamine-blocking ability within the limbic system (137). Although thioridazine has been reported to be less active on striatal dopamine

receptors, another study showed no difference in 3H-spiperone binding of accumbens and putamen dopamine receptors for the two agents (138). The relative rarity of thioridazine-induced parkinsonism has been attributed to its anticholinergic properties (138,139), but the anticholinergic property may promote the occurrence of TD. In our series of 125 patients, although not an epidemiologic study, thioridazine was second only to haloperidol among all the drugs causing movement disorders (90). Thioridazine-induced parkinsonism occurred in only nine patients.

Neuroleptics exert a pharmacologic effect on more than one neurotransmitter within the brain and, therefore, it is difficult to ascribe a particular movement disorder to the drug's effect on any one neurotransmitter system (140). In a study of 15 neuroleptics in rats, all drugs blocked dopamine receptors in the corpus striatum whereas norepinephrine was blocked to varying degrees by the neuroleptics; pimozide blocked only dopamine with no effect on norepinephrine levels; fluphenazine, haloperidol, and perphenazine blocked dopamine with only small effects on norepinephrine receptors; chlorpromazine, thioridazine, and chlorprothixene blocked beta receptors more evenly (140). In another study of 17 neuroleptics, it was noted that neuroleptics have a greater affinity for dopamine D_2 receptor sites than for muscarinic acetylcholine, histamine H_1, alpha$_1$-adrenergic$_2$ or alpha$_2$-adrenergic receptors (136). Although this data may prove helpful in minimizing certain adverse effects (e.g., hypotension), it does not help in predicting the risk of movement disorders. Thus, despite differing chemical structures and receptor binding characteristics, there is no compelling evidence that any single class of drug has a greater propensity to cause dyskinesias (135).

A relationship between serum levels of antipsychotics and the incidence of TD has been difficult to establish. Higher ratio of serum concentrations to daily dose was found in patients with TD versus controls (141–143). If a dose–response relationship does exist as related to serum levels, the relationship may not necessarily be linear (144).

Attempts have been made to correlate dose and duration of antipsychotic therapy to the severity of TD. Of 56 studies on TD, 18 addressed the possible correlation between cumulative drug dose and occurrence of TD (36). Only four studies could demonstrate a positive relationship. Kane and Smith identified six studies showing that increased duration of neuroleptic exposure increased the risk of TD (36). However, no significant relationship between duration of treatment and the occurrence of TD was found in 15 other studies (36). Positive correlation between dose, duration of treatment, and TD is yet to be substantiated by a well-designed prospective study.

Drug holidays from antipsychotic use have been advocated by some to allow assessment for evidence of TD and to afford protection from long-term deleterious effects of these agents (51). Although drug-free intervals decreased the prevalence of TD in individuals taking piperazine phenothiazines (e.g., trifluoperazine) and butyrophenones (e.g., haloperidol) (145), other studies showed up to five 2-month drug interruptions increased the risk for persistent TD (146). Consequently, intermittent neuroleptic withdrawal as a means of preventing TD and other drug-induced movement disorders cannot be recommended.

Some studies have suggested that diabetics are more likely to develop TD than nondiabetics. In a study of 38 neuroleptic-treated diabetics, 38 neuroleptic-treated nondiabetics, and 38 diabetic controls, it was found that neuroleptic-treated diabetics had a significantly higher prevalence of TD (Wilcoxon's test, $p < 0.01$) (147). Hyperglycemia has been found in animal studies to reduce dopamine transmission and increase dopamine postsynaptic receptor sensitivity (148). Microvascular and macrovascular damage secondary to chronic hyperglycemia may predispose diabetic patients to further cellular injury imposed by neuroleptics. More studies, however, are needed before the mechanism by which diabetes increases the risk of TD is understood.

The risk of developing TD seems to be lower with the new atypical antipsychotics such as clozapine. There have been reports of TD following clozapine use, but the risk appears minimal (149,150). In one study of 28 patients, two developed mild TD according to the Simpson Dyskinesia Scale following nine years of clozapine administration (150). The authors, however, were unable to rule out preexisting TD in these patients. In the other two-case report, one patient had worsening of preexisting TD when administered clozapine while the other patient developed TD two years after beginning clozapine (149). Hence, these two reports do not provide compelling undisputable evidence of a causal relationship.

Clozapine has a higher affinity for D_1 and lower affinity for D_2 receptors than conventional antipsychotics, translating into fewer movement disorders associated with its use (151). In fact, clozapine (625 mg/day) has afforded four years of relief to a patient with severe axial tardive dystonia (152). Another patient, 45 years old, developed severe torsion truncal movements, left torticollis, and axial dystonia secondary to neuroleptics responsive only to clozapine (450 mg/day) (153). Similarly, clozapine has been found useful in decreasing dyskinesias experienced by patients with PD (154). Improvements are statistically apparent at 75 mg/day. Improvement has also been noted in patients with TD (155). When compared to patients receiving haloperidol, clozapine produced significantly greater improvement in motor symptoms at 12 months ($p < 0.001$). Optimism should be tempered by the observation that clozapine has been associated with dystonia, akathisia, and myoclonus (156,157). One patient, a 51-year-old schizophrenic female patient, developed acute dyskinesia four hours after her first parenteral drug administration (158). In another study of 29 patients in a state hospital, 6.8% (n = 2) were rated as having akathisia according to the Barnes Rating Scale for Drug-Induced Akathisia (159). Five patients have been reported to suffer myoclonus secondary to clozapine (157). All symptoms improved following clozapine discontinuation, dose reduction, or administration of concomitant carbamazepine. Hence, while clozapine represents a substantial improvement in terms of movement disorders as compared to conventional neuroleptics, the drug is not without risk of inducing selected movement disorders.

Risperidone, another atypical antipsychotic, has not yet been associated with TD (160). In a randomized, double-blind trial of risperidone versus haloperidol in 36 schizophrenic patients, risperidone did not differ from placebo but was significantly less than haloperidol on assessment scales of extrapyramidal side effects (161). In fact, in another randomized, double-blind study of risperidone versus haloperidol (n = 44), consumption of antiparkinsonian medication was 10 times lower with risperidone (162). Yet in another report of six patients with psychosis, five experienced intolerable exacerbations of parkinsonism requiring nursing home placement for one patient (163). Four of the patients subsequently did well on clozapine. In a study of 10 chronic schizophrenic patients with TD, risperidone up to 6 mg/day for one month did not affect TD (164). Contrary to this report is a study of 11 elderly hospitalized patients with schizophrenia, schizoaffective disorder, bipolar disorder, or senile dementia treated with risperidone (165). Four of these patients who had preexisting TD found those symptoms decreased in response to risperidone treatment. This concurs with a double-blind, multicenter trial of 135 hospitalized chronic schizophrenic patients where risperidone (6–16 mg/day) showed significantly ($p < 0.05$) lower dyskinetic scores than those receiving placebo or haloperidol (166). Preliminary evidence suggests risperidone offers a safe alternative to typical neuroleptics with a significantly lower incidence of drug-induced movement disorders (167).

Newer atypical antipsychotics are on the horizon that hold promise of comparative efficacy but with fewer movement disorders than conventional antipsychotics. These include remoxipride, melperone, and seroquel (168). At doses of 150 to 600 mg/day, remoxipride significantly reduced the dyskinesia score 44% without increasing parkinsonism (n = 8) (169). However, remoxipride has been associated with dystonia and neuroleptic malignant syndrome (170–173). Similarly, melperone has also been associated with dystonia (172,173). No movement disorders have yet been associated with seroquel but it is in the early stages of development (174). These newer antipsychotics potentially will have a less, albeit not absent, incidence of movement disorders associated with their use.

Sulpiride is a substituted benzamide with selective dopamine D_2 receptor antagonist properties used as an antipsychotic and antidepressant (134). Initially it was claimed that this drug was devoid of extrapyramidal effects, however, this has been disproven. A 37-year-old man developed persistent segmental dystonia within two months of starting sulpiride (175). Tardive akathisia, orolingual dyskinesia, and parkinsonism developed in a 56-year-old woman after withdrawal from sulpiride that had been administered for 10 years (176). Other reports establishing an association between TD, tardive akathisia, and sulpiride have also been documented (177–179). Hence, the clinician needs to exercise skepticism and caution when new dopamine antagonists are marketed with claims of no association with movement disorders.

Metoclopramide

Metoclopramide, a D_2 receptor antagonist, has been used in the treatment of esophageal reflux, dyspepsia, gastroparesis, and chemotherapy-induced emesis (180). Its use has been associated with TD, drug-induced parkinsonism, akathisia, and dystonia (90,182–190). Although it has been suggested that respiratory and copulatory dyskinesias are more common in metoclopramide-treated patients than those receiving other neuroleptics, no formal comparison study has been performed (191). In a study of 104 patients, metoclopramide-treated diabetics seemed to have a greater severity of TD than metoclopramide-treated nondiabetics, but this difference did not reach statistical significance (192).

The mean duration of metoclopramide treatment before the onset of TD is typically 14 months (182), but the movement disorder has occurred as early as three days after discontinuation of a four-day course of intravenous administration of 700 mg in a cancer patient previously exposed to metoclopramide (183). In a series of 10 patients, metoclopramide-induced parkinsonism developed after administration of the drug from two months to two years (185). Yamamoto et al recently described a typical scenario where an elderly patient who after receiving metoclopramide 30 mg/day for gastritis for nine months, developed severe gait disturbance, dysarthria, orlingual dyskinesia, and neck rigidity consistent with parkinsonism and TD (184). Nine days following discontinuation of metoclopramide, the parkinsonism resolved but the orolingual dyskinesia continued. Thus while metoclopramide-associated TD may be permanent, drug-induced parkinsonism usually resolves after the drug is stopped. In our series of 125 patients with drug-induced movement disorders seen in the Movement Disorders Clinic, 10 were related to metoclopramide use; 6 had TD, 3 parkinsonism, and 1 tardive dystonia (90).

Akathisia has been reported in up to 20% of patients exposed to metoclopramide (186–188). Motor restlessness has occurred following three to four months of treatment with 10 mg three to four times a day orally (186). It is often accompanied by anxiety, panic attacks, insomnia, and weight loss. Metoclopramide-induced akathisia may persist several years after cessation of the drug therapy.

Metoclopramide is one of the most under-recognized causes of drug-induced dyskinesias. In one study, metoclo-pramide was continued for an average of six months after the onset of abnormal movements in 81% (n = 15) of patients (193). This reflects a lack of recognition of metoclopramide as an etiologic agent of dyskinesias and translates into increased and continuing disability for affected patients. In most cases, alternative therapies with less potent drugs for a shorter duration would have sufficed to control the gastrointestinal symptoms.

Dopamine Agonists

Levodopa

Levodopa (L-dopa)-induced dyskinesia is beyond the scope of this chapter and the reader is referred to some recent reviews (194–196). Similar to TD, stereotypy, chorea, and dystonia are the most common hyperkinesias associated with L-dopa therapy for PD (197). In contrast to TD, however, these hyperkinetic movement disorders are dose-dependent and they disappear with reduction in levodopa dosage. In a study of the therapeutic results and survival of 100 parkinsonian patients treated with L-dopa, movement disorders were experienced in nearly half of the patients (197). About 10% of the patients may experience dystonic posturing such as oromandibular dystonia, torticollis, foot inversion, supination of the hands, or flexion or extension of the toes (199,200). These dyskinesias typically occur at the time of maximum improvement of the parkinsonian symptoms corresponding with a peak level of L-dopa and may last from several minutes up to one to two hours (199,201). Dyskinesias can be diminished by decreasing the amount of the individual dose but administering it more frequently, thus avoiding excessive peaks in L-dopa plasma levels (199). Alternatively, a controlled-release preparation of L-dopa/carbidopa may be tried to maintain stable drug levels (202). These drugs, however, prolong plasma and brain levels and in patients who already experience L-dopa-induced dyskinesias, these may be exacerbated with the long-acting preparations of levodopa. Periodic L-dopa withdrawal for at least a week has been advocated by some, but not all, to restore responsiveness to L-dopa in patients who no longer show any improvement or who have undesirable side effects even at relatively low doses (203). About half of patients need less L-dopa after the "drug holiday" thus diminishing dyskinesias and other, particularly psychiatric, side effects (204). In a study of 28 patients however, a 10-day "holiday" did not affect disease progression or severity, capacity for daily living activities, or the total amount of dopamine agonists used (205,206).

Onset and end-of-dose dyskinesias, usually dystonias, have also been described following L-dopa therapy (207). These dyskinesias typically last 30 to 60 minutes (208). Unlike peak-dose dyskinesia, they may be relieved by increasing the daily dosage of L-dopa (207).

Although neuroleptic-induced and levodopa-associated dyskinesias appear to have a common pathophysiology, both resulting from enhanced dopaminergic transmission, differences do exist. While neuroleptic-induced TDs occur after long-term neuroleptic therapy, L-dopa-induced dyskinesia can occur within minutes after ingestion. The risk of TD increases in older patients while L-dopa-induced dyskinesia seems more common in young-onset PD (209). These two types of dyskinesias respond differently to GABAergic therapy suggesting dissimilar pathophysiologic substrates. Progabide, a specific gamma-aminobutyric acid (GABA) receptor agonist, produced no change in the severity of dyskinesia when administered to patients with L-dopa-induced dyskinesias (210). Conversely, patients with TD demonstrated a good-to-excellent response after receiving progabide. In contrast, L-dopa-induced dystonia often responds to baclofen, a GABA-B receptor agonist, but this drug rarely has any beneficial effect in patients with tardive syndromes.

Central Nervous System Stimulants

Central nervous system (CNS) stimulants, including methylphenidate, dextroamphetamine, pemoline, and ephedrine, due to their ability to increase dopamine and norepinephrine activity, have been associated with various hyperkinesias, most notably tic-like movement disorders and TS (211–214).

Amphetamine

Amphetamine, a sympathomimetic amine with CNS stimulant activity, has been shown to reduce brain serotonin and to increase the release of endogenous norepinephrine and dopamine within the brain (215,216). Progressive downregulation of dopamine autoreceptors following exposure to amphetamine may result in an enhanced response to dopamine agonists due to dopamine supersensitivity (217). Dyskinesias have been reported in patients following chronic amphetamine abuse and when used for hyperactivity or narcolepsy. Choreoathetoid movements of facial muscles, body, arms, and legs have been observed during use and during abstinence (218,219).

Methylphenidate

CNS stimulants such as methylphenidate increase dopamine and norepinephrine activity and have been associated with tic-like movement disorders and exacerbations of TS (211–214). Denckla et al reported that 1.3% of 1520 patients exposed to methylphenidate developed tics (220). More than 50% of pediatric patients with TS manifest attention-deficit disorder (ADD) with hyperactivity (221,222). Proper or improper use of CNS stimulants in these children may precipitate tics even after the CNS stimulants are withdrawn (211–214,221–225). However, judicious use of CNS stimulants in TS patients with ADD and attention-deficit/hyperactivity disorder (ADHD) may improve attention without necessarily exacerbating TS, as was noted in 72% of 39 patients in one study (212).

Pemoline

Pemoline, which is structurally dissimilar from amphetamines and methylphenidate, has also been associated with TS (226). In one case, a 10-year-old boy, previously treated with methylphenidate and thioridazine for hyperactivity, received pemoline 37.5 mg daily (226). Within three months he developed a tic disorder that resolved within two weeks of discontinuation of the pemoline. Upon rechallenge with pemoline, the tics reappeared. The degree to which prior therapy with methylphenidate and thioridazine predisposed this patient to a movement disorder is unknown. Reversible pemoline-induced chorea and TS has also been reported following an overdose of pemoline 400 mg and procyclidine 200 mg in a 52-year-old man with a psychiatric disorder (227). This patient too had previous exposure to a medication that may have predisposed him to the development of movement disorders (fluphenazine).

Not all patients with TS exposed to stimulants will experience a change in their movement disorder. In 39 patients with preexisting tics, 26 (67%) experienced no change and 2 experienced a decrease in their tics when exposed to stimulants, whereas 11 experienced increased tics (212). In another report, 15 (42%) of 32 patients with TS did not experience exacerbations of their movement disorder when exposed to either methylphenidate, dextroamphetamine, imipramine, chlorpheniramine, or methamphetamine (213). Thus it would be imprudent to deny all patients with TS and hyperactivity the benefit of stimulant therapy. Twenty-two (46%) of 48 patients with TS experienced behavior improvement while on stimulant therapy and of these 22 nearly 60% (n = 13) had no increase in tics (212). Thus a cautious approach to stimulant therapy in patients with TS should be adopted.

Whether stimulants cause or exacerbate tics in a patient with previously unexpressed TS is yet unresolved. Further studies are needed (228).

Cocaine

Cocaine, a local anesthetic, has found widespread abuse due to its CNS stimulant properties (229). Chronic cocaine use with its attendant dopamine deficiency has been speculated to cause dopamine receptor supersensitivity; thus we may expect to see an increase in movement disorders in the drug-abuser population (230). Dopamine depletion has been cited as the most important pharmacologic mechanism of cocaine dependency (230). Consequently, bromocriptine, a dopamine agonist, and amantadine have been found useful in reducing cocaine craving and other withdrawal symptoms for the patient initiating abstinence (230). Cocaine has been noted to exacerbate movement disorders that have been quiescent for years. A 24-year-old man had been diagnosed with TS at age eight which went into remission at puberty (231). This remission continued until age 20, when the motor tics resumed following six months of regularly snorting cocaine. Similarly, reemergence of movement disorders occurred in a 31-year-old woman with idiopathic dystonia and essential-like tremor and in a 30-year-old man with tardive dystonia following cocaine ingestion by snorting (231). Hence, cocaine has been identified as a risk factor for movement disorders (232,233).

Norpseudoephedrine

Norpseudoephedrine (NPE) is an over-the-counter appetite suppressant that has been associated with persistent movement disorders. A 43-year-old woman took NPE 30 mg/day for nine months and developed dystonic symptoms with increasing retrocollis and spasmodic torticollis to the right (234). She discontinued NPE after an additional three months. Despite discontinuation of NPE, symptoms persisted for one year necessitating botulinum toxin therapy. Progressive cranial dystonia affecting facial, cervical, and pharyngeal muscles occurred in a 55-year-old woman who ingested 3150 mg NPE over three months (234). Symptoms began after six months of NPE therapy and persisted for 15 years despite NPE discontinuation. Structurally related to amphetamine derivative, NPE shows comparable neuropharmacological effects on the noradrenergic and dopaminergic systems.

Ecstasy

3,4-Methylenedioxymethamphetamine (MDMA), also known as "Ecstasy," is a popular recreational drug abused for its stimulant properties. A 19-year-old woman with overlapping symptoms of neuroleptic malignant syndrome (NMS) and serotonin syndrome after a single exposure to MDMA has been described and is representative of the approximate 15 other cases reported in the literature (84). This female college student presented with acute confusional state following a day of skiing when she and several of her friends had taken one tablet of "Ecstasy." Within 15 minutes of taking the drug, she became nauseated and vomited. She was disoriented and somnolent, experiencing diarrhea enroute to the emergency room. Upon arrival she was tachycardiac, drowsy, but responsive to pain and her pupils were dilated. Urine toxicity screen was positive only for amphetamine. Her lactate dehydrogenase (LD) was elevated to 1060 (IU/L) and creatinine phosphokinase (CK) to 3960 U/L. While being transferred to the hospital, she had a generalized seizure. Upon hospitalization her laboratory values further increased with aspartate aminotransferase (AST) to 136 IU/L (normal: 5 to 30), LD 1273 IL/L (normal: 287 to 580), and CD to 6357 IU/L (normal: 35 to 230). EEG showed grade III, diffuse dysrhythmia, and very severe delta grade I slowing and disorganization of background activity, suggesting severe and diffuse cortical dysfunction. The patient was diagnosed with possible NMS and rhabdomyolysis. Following gastric lavage with charcoal and sorbitol and treatment with intravenous (IV) fluids, bromocriptine (up to 30 mg/day) and IV dantrolene sodium (900 mg/day), she improved. She became oriented four days after admission and was discharged 11 days later. When evaluated at the Movement Disorders Clinic 10 days after her discharge, she was noted to have bilateral, mild postural tremor. Previously reported cases similar to this patient have presented with alterations in mental status, convulsions, hyperthermia, hypo- or hypertension tachycardia, mydriasis, rigidity, coagulopathy, and rhabdomyolysis.

Characteristic of this MDMA syndrome is the rapid onset of symptoms with a latency of 15 minutes to six hours following drug ingestion. Symptom severity and outcome do not seem to be correlated with dose. Animal studies have shown that MDMA causes an acute release of 5-hydroxytryptamine (5-HT) from central serotonergic nerve terminals within minutes after drug ingestion, maximizing one to three hours later (235–237). Since MDMA's more pronounced effect is on the serotonergic rather than the dopaminergic system, the syndrome is more likely serotonin syndrome than NMS. This syndrome can prove fatal.

Other Drugs

Drug-induced movement disorders have been described with other medications but the association is not nearly as clearly defined or well-established as that with phenothiazines, butyrophenones, or substituted benzamides. Typically, anecdotal reports, often with various confounding factors present, constitute the basis for the presumed association.

Lithium

Lithium, an antimanic drug, increases norepinephrine reuptake and increases serotonin receptor sensitivity believed to contribute to its mood stabilizing effects (134). Lithium-induced tremor is well recognized but dyskinesias have rarely been seen in this psychiatric population, although it has been reported in some patients with Parkinson's disease (238). In five patients reported, the dyskinesias were characterized orofacial dyskinesias, choreoathetosis, hemiballismus, and dystonias (238). Lithium-induced dyskinesias have also been reported following concurrent use with the MAO inhibitor, tranylcypromine, in two patients with bipolar affective disorder (239). Lithium reportedly reinduced dyskinesia that had been quiescent for years in a patient previously treated with neuroleptics (240). In a study of 110 stable outpatients with bipolar disorder receiving lithium, 20.8% were noted to experience tremor, 7.7% had parkinsonism, 4.6% encountered akathisia, 3.8% had dystonia, and TD was present in 9.2% (241).

Lithium, because of its antidopaminergic effect, has been used successfully in the treatment for TD, helping to substantiate the finding that chronic lithium treatment reduces the number of dopamine receptors thereby preventing dopamine receptor supersensitivity (242). Lithium may have weak neuroleptic-like activity that may explain its ability to both alleviate and cause TD (243). When combined with tetrabenazine, lithium often enhances the anti-TD effects (108).

Antidepressants

Tricyclic antidepressants, by inhibiting the reuptake at nerve terminals of the neurotransmitters, particularly norepinephrine and serotonin, relieve depression (134). Case reports have described an association between tricyclic antidepressants, particularly amitriptyline and amoxapine, and TD (244–247). Some antidepressants, such as amoxapine, have additional dopamine blocking ability, which may account for the movement disorders associated with it. The aliphatic side chain of the tricyclic antidepressants confers anticholinergic properties perhaps triggering or exacerbating TD in a susceptible individual, but there has been no convincing cases reported of tricyclic-induced TD without confounding variables. In a systematic analysis of 50 patients receiving antidepressant therapy, 6% developed TD (248). However, in a depressed population it is difficult to exclude prior or concurrent treatment with antipsychotics. Additionally, the depressive state itself has been associated with dyskinesias (249). Unlike TD, which usually occurs after at least three months of therapy and usually persists, the rare hyperkinesia associated with tricyclic antidepressants has been reported to occur within two months of therapy and it usually disappears upon reducing the dose or discontinuation (248).

Akathisia has been reported with tricyclic antidepressants (250–251). Whereas neuroleptic-induced akathisia is common, akathisia associated with antidepressants is very rare and may be due to "contamination" of the patient with antipsychotics.

Trazodone, a novel nontricyclic compound, is a selective inhibitor of serotonin reuptake (252). It has been reported to induce parkinsonism (253). A 74-year-old woman received trazodone 300 mg/day for reactive depression. Within three months she began to experience parkinsonian symptoms. When examined seven months later, she had resting tremor and bilateral cogwheel rigidity. Within two months of stopping trazodone she began to note gradual improvement in symptoms, which completely remitted by 14 months. Similarly, a 65-year-old woman displayed choreic and myoclonic symptoms after receiving high doses of trazodone (600 mg/day) (254). With a reduction of the dose to 400 mg/day and administration of lithium, the parkinsonian symptoms resolved. Myoclonus and tremor was also reported after five weeks of trazodone therapy (300 mg/day) in a 38-year-old woman (255). Within a week of stopping trazodone, her symptoms subsided. This finding supports a role of serotonin in the pathogenesis of myoclonus. Myoclonus, however, is usually associated with a decrease in serotonin and it improves with 5-hydroxyl-L-tryptophan, a serotonin precursor.

Myoclonus has also been reported with other antidepressants (256,257). Nearly one-third (31%) of 98 patients receiving antidepressants experienced myoclonus that was reversible upon drug discontinuation (256). Closer examination of some of the patients with myoclonus leads one to question the relevance of the serotonin hypothesis to drug-induced myoclonus because maprotiline, a specific inhibitor of norepinephrine reuptake in the CNS, has no known effect on serotonin (256,257). In one patient, however, maprotiline did induce myoclonus whereas trazodone did not, arguing against serotonin involvement in this case.

Mianserin has been associated with involuntary movement disorders in patients with preexisting brain dysfunction (258,259). In one such case, a 69-year-old woman experienced re-emergence of facial grimacing, mouth and eye tics, and inarticulate vocal sounds (diagnosed as partial and transitory TS) when she began mianserin 30 mg/day (259). This occurred after 33 years of absence of these movements. She was also taking ranitidine and cisapride for reflux esophagitis. Her CT scan showed slight central and cortical atrophy. The movements completely resolved within a few weeks after discontinuation of mianserin. While confounding factors exist such as depression and intake of a histamine antagonist and cisapride, mianserin should be used with extreme caution in patients with preexisting brain dysfunction and with a history of involuntary movements.

Serotonin-specific reuptake inhibitors (SSRI) have also been associated with movement disorders. SSRIs preferentially increase synaptic availability of serotonin, which is known to modulate dopamine transmission. The acute effect of SSRI administration is increased serotonin in the synaptic cleft with a resultant reduction in dopamine transmission (260). Hence, fluoxetine has been associated with akathisia and dyskinesia and fluvoxamine has been reported to cause dyskinesias (261–266). Five patients averaging 21 years old (range: 18 to 35) experienced akathisia within five days of starting treatment with fluoxetine, with one case occurring within 12 hours (263). Symptoms continued for more than one year in one patient who continued fluoxetine treatment suggesting tolerance does not develop to this side effect. An 88-year-old woman developed buccolingual dyskinesia characterized by repetitive involuntary mouth opening, tongue protrusion with "flycatcher" tongue movements, after 35 days of fluoxetine therapy (261). Within one day of dyskinesia's onset, fluoxetine was discontinued with prompt movement resolution over six days paralleling the seven-to-nine-day half-life of norfluoxetine, the active metabolite. Blepharospasm, lip protrusion, and bruxism were reported in a 38-year-old woman after two months of therapy with fluvoxamine for obsessive-compulsive disorder that resolved within one day of discontinuation (262). Movement disorders have not yet been described with paroxetine and sertraline. Given the experience with fluoxetine and fluvoxamine, SSRIs may not be a suitable alternative for patients experiencing movement disorders secondary to tricyclic antidepressant administration.

Benzodiazepines

Benzodiazepines, due to their calming effects on reticular formation and the limbic system and due to potentiation of gamma-aminobutyric acid (GABA), provide antianxiety, hypnotic, and anticonvulsant effects (134). An association between TD and exposure to lorazepam, diazepam, and flurazepam is not clearly defined due to concurrent therapy with other drugs associated with TD (tricyclic antidepressants, sulpiride) (267,268). In each of these case reports, however, the dyskinesias resumed upon rechallenge with the benzodiazepine. The relationship between benzodiazepines and drug-induced movement disorders currently is speculative and unsubstantiated.

Antihistamines

Antihistamines competitively antagonize histamine at the H1 receptor and provide relief from rhinitis and allergic conditions. The anticholinergic side chain common to both benzodiazepines and antihistamines may precipitate the dopamine–cholinergic imbalance resulting in dyskinesias. Case reports provide the documentation thus far of an association between movement disorders and antihistamines. A 50-year-old woman with chronic schizophrenia had been treated for 20 years with various antipsychotics finally becoming stabilized on haloperidol with no neurologic sequela (269). After ingesting six tablets of diphenhydramine 25 mg, she experienced TD which included involuntary respiratory movements and repetitive blinking. Diphenhydramine was discontinued. The movement disorder subsided within three days. Brompheniramine and chlorpheniramine have also been implicated in some cases of TD but in each case an additional potentially offending agent (fluphenazine and chlordiazepoxide, respectively) was taken, obscuring the exact relationship (270).

Calcium Channel Blockers

Calcium channel blockers inhibit the movement of calcium ions across cell membranes thereby conferring antiarrhythmic, antihypertensive, and antianginal effects (271). Nifedipine, verapamil, and diltiazem are presently available in the United States while cinnarazine and flunarizine are available elsewhere. Cinnarazine and flunarizine, selective calcium channel blockers used to treat and prevent vertigo, caused extrapyramidal side effects (272–274). In 15 patients with extrapyramidal reactions to these drugs, parkinsonism was experienced by 11 and orofacial tremor, acute dystonic reaction, acute akathisia, and persistent akathisia were seen in one patient each (272). Several patients, however, had depression that may have predisposed them to extrapyramidal disorders (152). Akathisia was noted in a 62-year-old man after a three-day therapy with diltiazem at 30 mg per day (275). The akathisia resolved within 24 hours after diltiazem was stopped, but when the patient was rechallenged with the drug two months later, akathisia recurred. Diltiazem-induced akathisia was also described in another patient (276). In contrast, diltiazem in doses up to 360 mg daily has been reported to be useful in the treatment of TD (273). Verapamil, another calcium channel blocker, has been considered palliative for TD and myoclonic tardive dystonia (277,278). Thus the role of calcium channel blockers in the

pathophysiology of movement disorders is unclear at this time.

Phenytoin

Phenytoin is a hydantoin anticonvulsant whose ability to promote sodium efflux stabilizes the neuron membrane against hyperexcitability (279). Phenytoin has been infrequently associated with movement disorders both of the choreatic and dystonic nature (280–283). Usually thought of as a manifestation of toxicity, it has also been noted when phenytoin is present in normal serum concentrations (283–285). Phenytoin has also been reported to exacerbate existing TD, which returned to baseline following discontinuation of phenytoin (286). Although patients of all ages have been affected, 50% of reported cases occurred in patients less than 20 years old (287).

Nausieda noted phenytoin-associated dyskinesias present as orolingual dyskinesias in patients previously exposed to neuroleptics, as hemichorea in patients with contralateral structural lesions, and as generalized chorea in patients with corpus striatum lesions or a history of Sydenham's chorea (288). Morement disorders can manifest insidiously or acutely as in the case of toxicity (281,284). If movement disorders occur despite normal total phenytoin levels, free levels should be checked, especially if the patient is receiving concomitant therapy with other drugs (e.g., valproic acid, phenobarbital) known to increase free phenytoin levels.

The mechanism of phenytoin-induced movement disorders is unknown. Dopamine antagonist properties of phenytoin have been proposed (289). Phenytoin, acting as a central anticholinergic agent and stimulant of serotonin, has also been proposed as the basis for alteration of neurotransmitters resulting in movement disorders (281). In an excellent review of clinical and experimental studies of phenytoin-induced movement disorders, underlying pathologic changes in the basal ganglia are suggested as the mechanism (288). Phenytoin may have dopamine antagonist properties causing dyskinesia in toxic levels (290). A patient having experienced lip smacking, tongue protrusions, and dystonic posturing of the head and neck at 300 mg/day, experienced disappearance of all symptoms when the dose was reduced to 100 mg/day (290). Thus the phenomenon may be dose-sensitive.

Carbamazepine

Carbamazepine, a tricyclic antidepressant employed as an anticonvulsant, has been implicated in drug-induced movement disorders (291,292). Akathisia was experienced by a 38-year-old man after receiving 1 g/day. When his dose was lowered to 600 mg/day, the patient's mood was controlled and motor restlessness was minimal (292). However, the patient had previously taken two phenothiazine antipsychotics, several tricyclic antidepressants, benzodiazepines, and lithium, all of which obscured the exact cause of the akathisia.

Dyskinesia has also been reported following carbamazepine therapy (291–293). The cause–effect relationship is less clearly defined after considering the patient had other factors potentially contributing to tardive dyskinesia—depression, amoxapine, phenytoin, and antihistamine use (293).

Carbamazepine-induced tics have also been reported. It appears that carbamazepine precipitates or exacerbates underlying TS (294,295), but it has also been reported to elicit facial motor tics in the absence of underlying major neurologic deficits or clinical drug intoxication (296). In the latter, all three children had carbamazepine blood levels within the normal range. Carbamazepine was continued at the same or higher dose with tic abatement spontaneously in less than six months. Hence, this movement disorder may be transient and may not necessarily require drug discontinuation.

Carbamazepine, 1,600 mg/day, has been helpful in suppressing dyskinesias in a patient suffering from schizoaffective psychosis (297). However, in a study treating TD in 11 schizophrenic patients, excluding those patients with affective psychosis, no beneficial effect was found with carbamazepine (298).

Felbamate

Felbamate, a recently approved antiepileptic, is indicated as monotherapy or adjunctive therapy for partial seizures with and without secondary generalization in adults and as adjunctive therapy for partial and primary generalized seizures in children with Lennox-Gastaut syndrome. Two cases of involuntary movement disorders occurring in children have been reported (299). A marked choreoathetoid dystonic reaction occurred in a 13-year-old boy after three days of receiving felbamate but resolved upon drug discontinuation. A dystonic reaction was noted in a two-month-old boy after receiving felbamate 24 mg/kg/day escalated to 41 mg/kg by the fourth day (299). The patient was also receiving phenytoin but the unbound phenytoin level was only 0.7 mcg/mL. The movement disorder resolved within 36 hours of discontinuing felbamate therapy. Because the clinical use of felbamate is now discouraged owing to potentially serious side effects (aplastic anemia, acute renal failure), it is unlikely that felbamate-induced movement disorders will be seen frequently in the future.

Gabapentin

Gabapentin is an antiepileptic recently marketed in the United Kingdom (300). When used as add-on therapy in patients with refractory partial seizures over a 12-week period, 35% to 71% of patients experienced a 50% or greater reduction in seizure frequency (301). In the 225 patient-years of this study, tremor was reported in greater than 10% of patients, hence caution is advised.

Alcohol

Chronic heavy alcohol intake may lead to dopamine receptor supersensitivity (302). In the early abstinence stage from alcohol, increased central dopamine sensitivity results in a lower threshold for psychotic symptoms and neuroleptic-induced extrapyramidal symptoms (303). Mullin et al first described a syndrome of choreoathetosis in 12 patients undergoing alcohol withdrawal (304). These patients had no gross liver disease, no history of phenothiazine use, and no abnormalities in thiamine, nicotinic acid, magnesium, or vitamin B12 levels (304). Transient choreiform dyskinesias have also been observed in three chronic alcoholics undergoing withdrawal (302).

Parkinsonism has also been associated with alcohol use. Experienced as a component of alcohol withdrawal, this transient basal ganglia dysfunction is distinct from movement disorders occurring secondary to hepatolenticular degeneration seen in some chronic alcoholics (305). In a typical case, a 60-year-old man experienced severe acute parkinsonism after discontinuing chronic alcohol intake (306). Without specific therapy, he had completely recovered within three months. It has been suggested that alcohol increases lipid peroxidation of cell membranes increasing nigral cell death hence predisposing the patients to parkinsonism (307,308), yet long-term follow-up suggests that acute presentation of parkinsonism during alcohol withdrawal does not translate into future PD. In a study following three alcoholic patients, all exceeding the age of 50, no evidence of parkinsonism was seen 9 to 11 years after their initial acute presentation (309). This funding suggests transient reduction in dopamine transmission secondary to alcohol withdrawal does not necessarily mean these patients will eventually develop PD. Hence, alcohol withdrawal parkinsonism is thought to be a completely reversible abnormality in nigrostriatal dopamine transmission.

Methyldopa

Methyldopa exerts its hypotensive effect via its conversion within the central nervous system to alpha-methyl-norepinephrine, a potent alpha-adrenergic agonist (310). Choreic movements developed after 25 days of methyldopa therapy when the dose was increased from 1/day to 1.5/day in a 59-year-old hypertensive patient (311). Within 24 hours of discontinuation, the dyskinesia markedly abated. Because methyldopa interferes with the metabolism of 5-hydroxytryptophan to serotonin, it has been proposed that serotonergic mechanisms were involved (311). Methyldopa may also act as a false neurotransmitter and as such can cause symptoms of parkinsonism (311). This extrapyramidal effect, however, must be rare with methyldopa, accounting for the paucity of reports.

Meperidine and Related Compounds

Meperidine, structurally dissimilar from morphine, is a narcotic analgesic that binds to opioid receptors (312). Meperidine has been reported to produce parkinsonian symptoms (313). A 72-year-old man received 4,000 mg of meperidine over nine days for postoperative pain. He developed a shuffling walk that persisted despite discontinuation of meperidine. His condition progressed to include hypomimia, rigidity, and a resting tremor. The patient had never received phenothiazines or butyrophenones. He improved dramatically on carbidopa-levodopa (Sinemet CR) 25/100 four times a day. After two months of therapy, he was symptom-free. The Sinemet CR was stopped and the patient has remained free of PD. It has been suggested that this meperidine-induced disorder may in part be related to the formation of 1-methyl-4-phenyl-1,2,5,6-tetrahydropyridine (MPTP), a known neurotoxin that causes parkinsonism in humans and animals after it is oxidized and taken up by the dopaminergic neurons in the substantia nigra (314–318).

MPTP has resulted in severe parkinsonism in patients following both intravenous and intranasal exposure (316–318). A 37-year-old industrial chemist utilizing MPTP as a synthetic intermediate developed parkinsonism without ingestion (320). MPTP is metabolized by monoamine oxidase type B to 1-methyl-4-phenylpyridine (MPP+), which selectively damages dopaminergic neurons in the substantia nigra (221,322). MPTP when administered systemically can produce parkinsonism in humans and in experimental animals.

It is especially important to avoid employing selegiline (deprenyl; Eldepryl) to treat parkinsonism secondary to meperidine. Because selegiline is a monoamine oxidase (MAO) type B inhibitor, stupor, muscular rigidity, severe agitation, and elevated temperature may result if given concomitantly with meperidine. This is considered a life-threatening interaction (324).

Buspirone

Buspirone is a nonbenzodiazepine anxiolytic whose potential to induce movement disorders should be closely monitored. Buspirone's mechanism of action is unknown but it has been shown to influence serotonergic, noradrenergic, cholinergic, and dopaminergic activity in the brain with its prominent effect on dopaminergic transmission (325,326). Buspirone exhibits both agonist and antagonist effects on the dopaminergic system (326,327). It increases the firing rate of dopaminergic neurons and blocks inhibition produced by dopamine agonists (327). The autoreceptor blockade reduces feedback inhibition producing a sustained increase in dopaminergic activity (328). Striatal dopamine synthesis and metabolism are increased 400% (329). The drug has minimal agonist activity on the postsynaptic receptors (329). In the hypothalamus, dopamine agonist activity predominates resulting in a surge of growth hormone, and in the pituitary gland, dopamine antagonism predominates resulting in increase in prolactin levels (330). Because autoreceptor blockade induced by buspirone reduces feedback inhibition, it was hoped that it would prove beneficial in patients with Parkinson's disease. Beneficial effect from buspirone, however, could not be demonstrated in a study of 11 parkinsonian patients treated for 10 weeks at a dose of 50 to 70 mg/day. Two of six patients treated for an additional 3 to 11 weeks at increased doses (65 to 100 mg/day) experienced a mild worsening of parkinsonian symptoms

(327). In fact, in a study of 16 outpatients with Parkinson's disease, a significant worsening of disability scores was noted as doses approached 100 mg/day (331). Inner tension and restlessness were described in seven patients (44%) (but was not referred to as akathisia) (331). Buspirone, in conventional doses, has been associated with orofacial dyskinesia, dystonia, akathisia, and myoclonus (332–335). A 45-year-old man receiving buspirone 40 mg per day for anxiety developed bruxisms and rapidly jerking neck movements with sustained head posturing after three months (334). He had received chlorpromazine 50 mg/day for a few days without incident two years before receiving buspirone. Despite interventions with baclofen and trihexyphenidyl, the involuntary movements have persisted. Another patient receiving 30 mg/day for six weeks developed exacerbation of preexisting spasmodic torticollis and TD in addition to onset of involuntary phonations (336). These cases highlight the potential persistent nature of movement disorders observed secondary to buspirone and also notes prior neuroleptic use that causes cellular damage that may set the stage for future movement disorders.

Methysergide

Methysergide, a semisynthetic ergot derivative, is indicated in the treatment of vascular headaches. It blocks the effects of serotonin and has been shown to be a dopamine antagonist while its metabolite, methergine, is a dopamine agonist (337). A 35-year-old man treated with methysergide, 2 mg twice daily for vascular headaches, experienced akathisia (338). The patient had never taken neuroleptic drugs but had been previously treated with amitriptyline and verapamil for the headaches. Akathisia remitted following discontinuation of methysergide but reappeared following rechallenge. Understanding the pharmacologic basis for the akathisia in this case is difficult, recognizing that methysergide and its metabolite expose the patient to both dopamine agonism and antagonism. Perhaps antagonism predominates, which explains the clinical presentation of akathisia. Surveillance is advocated for extrapyramidal syndromes with methysergide and other mixed dopamine agonists/antagonists (e.g., buspirone).

Oral Contraceptives

Oral contraceptives, usually containing an estrogen (e.g., ethinyl estradiol) and a progestin (e.g., norethindrone) have been associated with movement disorders, typically chorea. First described by Fernando in 1966, numerous reports have since been documented (339–345). Oral contraceptives create a hormonal milieu referred to as "pseudo-pregnancy," leading some to link chorea gravidarum to oral contraceptive-induced chorea (339,346). Some reviews, however, suggest that chorea presents in women with previous basal ganglia abnormalities and it is unlikely to occur in normal individuals (347). It has also been proposed that ischemic lesions of the basal ganglia consistent with the cardiovascular side effects of oral contraceptives contribute to the onset of chorea (342).

Unilateral or asymmetric abnormal movements usually present one to three months after initiating oral contraceptives and typically resolve one to two months after discontinuation of the medication (340). Subsequent pregnancy may or may not be complicated by chorea (341,343). This reflects a similar pattern seen in patients with chorea gravidarum, which is usually experienced by primiparous women and may not recur in subsequent pregnancies (346). A 28-year-old nulliparous woman developed a paraballistic syndrome with choreatic features following four months of oral contraceptive therapy (347). A few days after discontinuing the oral contraceptive, the paraballistic movements decreased and were replaced by choreatic movements, which then resolved within two weeks. One year later, she gave birth to a healthy child having experienced no abnormal involuntary movements during pregnancy.

Although the mechanism underlying this phenomenon is not known, enhanced central dopaminergic activity is thought to be involved (341). No particular oral contraceptive combination has been consistently implicated with the hormone-related movement disorders (341).

Histamine-2 Antagonists

Cimetidine, ranitidine, and famotidine are competitive inhibitors of histamine H_2-receptors, devoid of anticholinergic properties, used in the management of peptic ulcer disease. These drugs have no known effect on dopaminergic pathways yet cimetidine has been implicated in four reports of extrapyramidal reactions (348–351). In 1982, cimetidine was first associated with restlessness, tremor, cogwheel rigidity, and orofacial dyskinesia in a 72-year-old man following three and one-half weeks of therapy with cimetidine (348). Within three weeks of discontinuation of the cimetidine, the tremor resolved and the rigidity slowly improved. This temporal relationship, however, was complicated by the patient's history of preexisting cerebral vascular disease and dementia thus obscuring an exact cause–effect relationship. Also in 1982, a 72-year-old woman was reported who developed chorea following 11 months of therapy with cimetidine, 300 mg four times daily (349). Within a week of discontinuing the cimetidine, the abnormal movements resolved but reappeared when rechallenged with cimetidine. More recently, cimetidine reportedly induced an acute dystonic reaction in a 20-year-old woman following five 300 mg doses of oral cimetidine (350). The patient presented with sudden onset of right-sided mandibular pain, trismus, dysphonia, and an involuntary turning of her right foot. She was given 50 mg of diphenhydramine HCl IV with immediate resolvement of the oromandibular dystonia and marked improvement in phonation. She was discharged on oral diphenhydramine and at 48 hour follow-up presented with no neurologic abnormalities. The patient's medical history was significant only for a patent foramen ovale that was corrected surgically in childhood and peptic ulcer disease for which she received H_2 antagonists. She was on no other medications

except oral contraceptives, which she had taken for more than a year. Thus, in this case, the oral contraceptives may have predisposed the patient to drug-induced movement disorder with the cimetidine precipitating the extrapyramidal event rather than being singularly responsible for it.

Restless leg syndrome secondary to cimetidine therapy was reported in a 65-year-old woman receiving 300 mg four times a day for 10 years for esophageal reflux (351). Clonazepam, propranolol, and acetaminophen with codeine afforded relief of the restlessness. Chorea and dystonia have also been reported with ranitidine (352,353). Interestingly, a 76-year-old woman experienced dyskinesia following an initial exposure to ranitidine and after cimetidine rechallenge. Initially she experienced bilateral choreiform movements of the face, mouth, neck, and arms after two months of oral ranitidine 150 mg twice daily. Within one month of discontinuation, the movement disorders resolved. One month later she was started on cimetidine 400 mg twice daily and within five days developed chorea again with a similar distribution but with larger movements. The movements resolved within three days of stopping cimetidine. Six months later she remains free of involuntary movements. This case suggests the pharmacology underlying cimetidine-induced movement disorders is shared with other H_2 antagonists. In furtherance of this notion, ranitidine alone has caused dyskinesias. A 72-year-old man experienced dystonia following seven days of intravenous ranitidine therapy (352). All symptoms resolved within one week of discontinuation of ranitidine but recurred within 24 hours of rechallenge.

Based on the anecdotal reports of cimetidine- and ranitidine-associated movement disorders documented thus far and the absence of such reports with famotidine and nizatidine, it is not possible to establish a cause and effect relationship between drug-induced movement disorders and H_2 antagonists. It would, however, be prudent to exercise caution when prescribing H_2 antagonists in combination with drugs known to be associated with drug-induced movement disorders (e.g., phenothiazines, butyrophenones, and benzamides).

Etretinate

Etretinate is an aromatic retinoic acid derivative used for severe recalcitrant psoriasis and other dyskeratoses (354). A syndrome of axial muscle rigidity following two weeks to three months of etretinate therapy 0.3 to 1.0 mg/kg/day has been described in three patients (355). Distinctive features include rigidity of proximal leg and axial muscles, impairment of anteflexion at the waist, and severe impairment of lateral flexion of both the waist and neck. Two of the patients responded satisfactorily to L-dopa. The third patient continued etretinate 0.6 mg/kg/day and stiffness persisted but he has not sought further treatment. Extraspinal tendon and ligament calcification has previously been reported in 38 patients treated with etretinate (356). Radiographs of the spine and hips of the three patients reported revealed small bone protuberances arising from several lumbar vertebral bodies and evidence of skeletal hypertosis, which it was felt were unrelated to the symptoms (355). Instead, it was theorized that the syndrome was of CNS origin, possibly involving a catecholaminergic pathway explaining the favorable response to L-dopa (355). Axial muscle rigidity has not yet been reported with isotretinoin, a related retinoid.

Monoamine Depletors

Reserpine and tetrabenazine are presynaptic monoamine depleting agents found to depress dopamine levels (357–359). Tetrabenazine differs from reserpine in that its inhibition of amine reuptake is reversible, rapid in onset, and of short duration (359–361). Additionally, tetrabenazine has been found to have pharmacologic properties typical of a dopamine receptor antagonist (108). Consequent to these properties, both reserpine and tetrabenazine have been associated with parkinsonism; parkinsonism may occur after only one week of therapy with 200 mg/day tetrabenazine (109,362). This dopamine-depleting property, however, has proven advantageous in the treatment of TD (106,108).

BASIC SCIENCE

Attempts to explain the pathophysiology of drug-induced movement disorders in terms of imbalance between the dopaminergic and cholinergic systems within the basal ganglia is an oversimplification at best. Chronic dopamine receptor blockade by neuroleptics may indeed result in dopamine receptor supersensitivity, as demonstrated by higher affinity of the dopamine receptors for ligand binding (37). In one study, exposure to haloperidol has resulted in a 60% increase in binding sites and a ninefold increase in the affinity constant in the caudate-putamen (363).

The effects of the dopamine system may be counterbalanced by the cholinergic system such that anticholinergic drugs exacerbate TD while cholinergic drugs, in a limited fashion, partially alleviate TD (37,364). The influence of striatal cholinergic function on the induction of TD, however, has recently been questioned in view of comparative data between haloperidol and clozapine (365). Haloperidol, which is associated with a high prevalence of TD, had similar effects on striatal choline acetyltransferase activity and 3H quinuclidinyl benzilate binding as clozapine, which is not associated with drug-induced movement disorders (365).

Because there is no accurate animal model of TD, neuropharmacologic studies to better define the dopamine–choline relationship in TD have been frustrated (8). In contrast to usually persistent TD, the experimental models show only transient pharmacologic and behavioral changes and the movement disorder in the animal must be pharmacologically induced as opposed to spontaneous movements in TD. Within days to weeks following discontinuation,

this chemical phenomenon disappears (34). Thus the dopamine–choline imbalance theory based on the current animal model does not completely, or accurately, explain the pathophysiology underlying TD.

Perhaps the initial dopamine–cholinergic imbalance triggers damage in the modulating systems that contributes to the persistent nature of TD long after the dopamine–cholinergic imbalance has been corrected. Most notably, gamma-amino-butyric acid (GABA) and noradrenergic neurotransmitters may be involved in the modulating systems that regulate feedback mechanisms, but other presently unknown neurotransmitters may be involved as well (366–368). The GABA hypothesis contends that decreased GABA function in the medial segment of pallidus and in the zona reticulata of substantia nigra is associated with dyskinesias (369). The neuroleptic-induced decrease in GABA activity would then be consistent with the development of TD (367).

It has also been theorized that because chronic neuroleptic exposure resulting in dopamine antagonism results in abnormally high rates of subthalamic nucleus discharges, a functional lesion of the globus pallidus results secondary to glutamate-mediated excitatory neurotoxicity (370). This would explain the decreased levels of glutamate decarboxylase (GAD), the synthetic enzyme for GABA, in the globus pallidus and subthalamic nucleus noted in Cebus monkeys receiving chronic neuroleptic treatment (371).

Following withdrawal from chronic blockade of dopamine receptors with haloperidol in rats, there is an increased sensitivity of postreceptor coupling mechanisms with a selective increase in sensitivity of adenylate cyclase to stimulation by calmodulin (367). Modulation of calmodulin activity by calcium channel blockers may explain the ability of these agents to both induce and alleviate movement disorders. Additionally, patients with TD have significantly higher norepinephrine concentrations in the cerebrospinal fluid than patients with spontaneous dyskinesias or no dyskinesias (368).

Free radical destruction of dopamine neurons, GABAergic neurons, and neurons in other neurotransmitter systems is gaining acceptance among the experts as one of the best explanations for the underlying pathophysiology of drug-induced movement disorders. Neuroleptics, due to their lipophilicity, become incorporated into cell membranes where they produce free radicals that evoke structural changes (372,373). Patients receiving phenothiazines have higher cerebrospinal fluid concentrations of lipid peroxidation products than control subjects matched for age and sex (374). Alpha tocopherol (vitamin E), an antioxidant, has been shown to prevent tissue damage due to peroxidation reactions (375). Fifteen patients administered alpha-tocopherol, 400 IU to 1,200 IU daily, had a mean reduction of 43% in Abnormal Involuntary Movement Scale (AIMS) scores with seven patients experiencing more than a 50% reduction in dyskinesia (376). Eleven patients receiving vitamin E up to 1,200 IU daily in a double-blind, placebo-controlled study for 12 weeks experienced a 36% improvement as measured by AIMS (377). However, in a study of 21 patients administered 1,600 IU of vitamin E in double-blind, placebo-controlled, crossover fashion, vitamin E had minor beneficial effects (18.5% reduction in TD movements) for only the group of patients who had had TD for five years or less (378). Preliminary studies in rats indicate selenium exerts a neuroprotective effect related to reduced free radical production (379). The premise of free radical-induced alterations in the catecholaminergic and GABAergic system may more completely explain the pathophysiology of drug-induced movement disorders and certainly warrants further investigation. However, until more conclusive data are available, it is not possible yet to advocate concurrent administration of vitamin E or selenium with neuroleptics as an approach to decrease the incidence of drug-induced movement disorders.

The pharmacology of TD and other drug-induced movement disorders is still poorly understood. Besides the obvious involvement of the dopaminergic system, other neurotransmitters and neuromodulators may be involved. There may be undiscovered neuropeptides or unknown interrelationships between known neuropeptides that preclude effective treatment of TD.

SUMMARY

Although extrapyramidal side effects such as TD and drug-induced parkinsonism have been recognized in association with neuroleptic use for approximately 30 years, diagnostic inaccuracies have precluded accurate assessment of epidemiology. Neuroleptics such as the phenothiazines, butyrophenones, and benzamides are well-recognized as causing movement disorders. Less clearly defined are the reports of movement disorders with lithium, tricyclic antidepressants, benzodiazepines, antihistamines, calcium channel blockers, phenytoin, carbamazepine, methyldopa, oral contraceptives, cimetidine, and methysergide. The status of buspirone in this regard is unknown. Not only have dopamine antagonists been implicated in causing movement disorders, L-dopa, dopamine agonists, and CNS stimulants also produce dyskinesias, presumably by a different mechanism (Table 2.4).

Prevention is the best "treatment" for TD and the other drug-induced movement disorders. When treatment is required, the use of monoamine depleters such as reserpine and tetrabenazine may be the best approach.

Table 2.4   Drug-Induced Movement Disorders

Movement Disorders	Drug
Accentuated physiologic tremor	Epinephrine, isoproterenol, caffeine, theophylline, lithium, tricyclic antidepressants, thyroid hormone, hypoglycemic agents, sodium valproate, nicotinic acid, cyclosporine
Cerebellar ataxia and tremor	Phenytoin, barbiturates, lithium, 5-fluorouracil, cimetidine–triazolam interaction
Chorea-dyskinesia	Neuroleptics, L-dopa, bromocriptine, phenytoin, ethosuximide, carbamazepine, oral contraceptives, chloroquine, antidepressants, metoclopramide, lithium, benzodiazepines, antihistamines, calcium channel blockers, cocaine, methyldopa, cimetidine
Dystonia	Neuroleptics, L-dopa, bromocriptine, lithium, metoclopramide, carbamazepine, cimetidine, chlorzoxazone, calcium channel blockers
Myoclonus and tics	Neuroleptics, amphetamines, methylphenidate, fenfluramine, L-dopa, bromocriptine, antidepressants, pemoline, cocaine
Parkinsonism	Neuroleptics, reserpine, tetrabenazine, methyldopa, α-methyltyrosine, lithium, diazoxide, physostigmine, metoclopramide, trazodone, meperidine, etretinate, cimetidine, cinnarizine, flunarizine
Akathisia	Neuroleptics, reserpine, tetrabenazine, metoclopramide, antidepressants, calcium channel blockers, buspirone, methysergide, cimetidine

Modified from Jankovic J, Casabona J. Coexistent tardive dyskinesia and parkinsonism. Clin Neuropharmacol 1987;10:511–521.

REFERENCES

1. Jankovic J. Tardive syndromes and other drug-induced movement disorders. Clin Neuropharmacol 1995;18:197–214.
2. Bourgeois M, Bouilh P, Tignol J, et al. Spontaneous dyskinesias versus neuroleptic-induced dyskinesias in 270 elderly subjects. J Nerv Ment Dis 1980;168:177–178.
3. Varga E, Sugerman AA, Varga V, et al. Prevalence of spontaneous oral dyskinesia in the elderly. Am J Psychiatry 1982;130:329–331.
4. Delwaide PJ, Desseilles M. Spontaneous bucco-linguofacial dyskinesia in the elderly. Acta Neurol Scand 1977;56:256–262.
5. Koller WC. Idiopathic orofacial dyskinesia. In: Jankovic J, Tolosa E, eds. Advances in neurology. Vol. 49. Facial dyskinesias. New York: Raven, 1988:177–183.
6. D'Allesandro R, Benassi G, Christin E, et al. The prevalence of lingual-facial-buccal dyskinesias in the elderly. Neurology 1986;36:1350–1351.
7. Deniker K. Introduction to neuroleptic chemotherapy into psychiatry. In: Ayd FJ Jr, Blackwell B, eds. Discoveries in biological psychiatry. Philadelphia: JB Lippincott, 1970:155–164.
8. Klawans HL, Tanner CM, Goetz CG. Epidemiology and pathophysiology of tardive dyskinesias. In: Jankovic J, Tolosa E, eds. Advances in neurology. Vol 49. Facial dyskinesias, 1988:185–187.
9. Chiang E, Pitts WM Jr., Rodriguez-Garcia M. Respiratory dyskinesia: review and case reports. J Clin Psychiatry 1985;46:232–234.
10. Burke RE, Fahn S, Jankovic J, et al. Tardive dystonia: late-onset and persistent dystonia caused by antipsychotic drugs. Neurology 1982;32:1334–1346.
11. Gimenez-Roldan S, Mateo D, Bartholome P. Tardive dystonia and severe tardive dyskinesia. Acta Psychiatr Scand 1985;71:488–494.
12. Kang UJ, Burke RE, Fahn F. Natural history and treatment of tardive dystonia. Mov Disord 1986;1:193–208.
13. Burke RE, Kang UJ. Tardive dystonia: clinical aspects and treatment. In: Jankovic J, Tolosa E, eds. Advances in neurology. Vol 49. Facial dyskinesias. New York: Raven, 1988:199–210.
14. Keegan DC, Rajput AH. Drug induced dystonia tarda: treatment with levodopa. Dis Nerv Syst 1973;38:167–169.
15. Fog R, Pakkenberg H, Reqeur L, et al. "Tardive" tourette syndrome in relation to long-term neuroleptic treatment of multiple tics. In: Friedhoff AJ,

Chase TN, eds. Advances in Neurology. Vol. 35. Gilles de la Tourette syndrome. New York: Raven, 1982:419–421.

16. Sacks OW. Acquired tourettism in adult life. In: Friedhoff AJ, Chase TN, eds. Advances in Neurology. Vol. 35. Gilles de la Tourette syndrome. New York: Raven, 1982:89–92.

17. Stahl SM. Tardive Tourette's syndrome in an autistic patient after long-term neuroleptic administration. Am J Psychiatry 1980;137:1267–1269.

18. Klawans HL, Falk DA, Nausieda PA, et al. Gilles de la Tourette syndrome after longer-term chlorpromazine therapy. Neurology 1978;28:1064–1065.

19. Singer WD. Transient Gilles de la Tourette Syndrome after chronic neuroleptic withdrawal. Dev Med Child Neurol 1981;23:518–530.

20. Gualtieri CT, Patterson DR. Neuroleptic-induced tics in two hyperactive children. Am J Psychiatry 1986;143:1176–1177.

21. Klawans HL, Nausieda PA, Goetz CC, et al. Tourette-like symptoms following chronic neuroleptic therapy. In: Friedhoff AJ, Chase TN, eds. Advances in Neurology. Vol. 35. Gilles de la Tourette syndrome. New York: Raven, 1982:415–418.

22. DeVeaugh-Geiss J. Tardive Tourette syndrome. Neurology 1980;30:562–563.

23. Tominaga H, Fukuzako H, Izumi K, et al. Tardive myoclonus. Lancet 1987;1:322.

24. Little JT, Jankovic J. Tardive myoclonus: a case report. Mov Disord 1987;2:307–311.

25. Braude WM, Barnes TRE. Late-onset akathisia—an indicant of covert dyskinesia: two case reports. Am J Psychiatry 1983;140:611–612.

26. Stacy M, Jankovic J. Tardive tremor. Mov Disord 1992;7:53–57.

27. Richardson MA, Craig TJ. The coexistence of parkinsonism-like symptoms and tardive dyskinesia. Am J Psychiatry 1982;139:341–343.

28. Jankovic J, Casabona J. Coexistent tardive dyskinesia and parkinsonism. Clin Neuropharmacol 1987;10:511–521.

29. Jankovic J, Fahn S. Dystonic syndromes. In: Jankovic J, Tolosa E, eds. Parkinson's disease and movement disorders. 2nd ed. Baltimore: Williams and Wilkins, 1993:337–374.

30. Ayd FJ. A survey of drug-induced extrapyramidal reactions. JAMA 1961;175:1054–1060.

31. Klawans HL, Bergen D, Bruyn GW. Prolonged drug-induced parkinsonism. Contin Neurol 1973;35:368–377.

32. Rajput AH, Rozdilsky B, Hornykiewicz O, et al. Reversible drug-induced parkinsonism: clinicopathologic study of two cases. Arch Neurol 1982;39:644–646.

33. Gotez CG. Diagnosis of tardive dyskinesia. Clin Neuropharmacol 1983;6:101–107.

34. Hall RA, Jackson RB, Swain JM. Neurotoxic reactions resulting from chlorpromazine administration. JAMA 1956;161:214–218.

35. Faurbye A, Rasch RJ, Petersen PB, et al. Neurological symptoms in pharmacotherapy of psychosis. Acta Psychiatr Scand 1964;40:10–27.

36. Kane JM, Smith JM. Tardive dyskinesia: prevalence and risk factors, 1959 to 1979. Arch Gen Psychiatry 1982;39:474–481.

37. Tarsy D. Neuroleptic-induced extrapyramidal reactions: classification, description, and diagnosis. Clin Neuropharmacol 1983;6(suppl 1):S9–S26.

38. Garver DC, Davis JM, Dekirmenjian H, et al. Dystonic reactions following neuroleptics: time course and proposed mechanism. Psychopharmacology 1976;47:199–201.

39. Swett C. Drug-induced dystonia. Am J Psychiatry 1975;132:532–534.

40. Lang AE. Akathisia and the restless leg syndrome. In: Jankovic J, Tolosa E, eds. Parkinson's disease and movement disorders. Baltimore: Urban and Schwarzenberg Medical, 1988.

41. VanPutten T, Marder SR. Behavioral toxicity of antipsychotic drugs. J Clin Psychiatry 1987;48(suppl 9):13–19.

42. Munetz MR, Carnes CL. Distinguishing akathisia and tardive dyskinesia: a review of the literature. J Clin Psychopharmacol 1983;3:343–350.

43. VanPutten T, May PRA, Marder SR. Akathisia with haloperidol and thiothixene. Arch Gen Psychiatry 1984;41:1036–1039.

44. Lang AE, Johnson K. Akathisia in idiopathic Parkinson's disease. Neurology 1987;37:477–481.

45. Drake RE, Ehrlich J. Suicide attempts associated with akathisia. Am J Psychiatry 1985;142:499–501.

46. Goswami U, Channabasavanna SM. Is akathisia a forerunner of tardive dyskinesia? Clin Neurol Neurosurg 1984;86:107–111.

47. Barnes TRE, Braude WM. Persistent akathisia associated with early tardive dyskinesia. Postgrad Med J 1984;60:359–361.

48. Stephen PJ, Williamson J. Drug-induced parkinsonism in the elderly. Lancet 1984;2:1082–1083.

49. Hausner RS. Neuroleptic-induced parkinsonism and Parkinson's disease: differential diagnosis and treatment. J Clin Psychiatry 1983;44:13–16.

50. Peabody CA, Warner D, Whiteford HA. Neuroleptics and the elderly. J Am Geriatr Soc 1987;35:233–238.

51. Baldessarini RJ, Cole JO, Davis JM, et al. Tardive dyskinesia: summary of a Task Force Report of the American Psychiatric Association. Am J Psychiatry 1980;137:1163–1172.

52. Schiele BC, Gallant D, Simpson G, et al. Neurologic syndromes associated with antipsychotic drug use. N Engl J Med 1973;289:20–23.

53. Goswami U. On the lethality of acute respiratory component of tardive dyskinesia. Clin Neurol Neurosurg 1985;87:99–102.

54. Faheem AD. Respiratory dyskinesias and dysarthria from prolonged neuroleptic use: tardive dyskinesia? Am J Psychiatry 182;139:517–518.

55. Wilcox PG, Bassett A, Jones B, Fleetham JA. Respiratory dysrhythmias in patients with tardive dyskinesia. Chest 1994;105:203–207.

56. Smith JM, Baldessarini RJ. Changes in prevalence, severity, and recovery in tardive dyskinesia with age. Arch Gen Psychiatry 1980;37:1368–1373.

57. Casey DE. Tardive dyskinesia; reversible and irreversible. In: Casey DE, Chase TN, Christensen AV, et al, eds. Dyskinesia: research and treatment. New York: Springer-Verlag 1985:88–97.

58. Jankovic J. Etiology and differential diagnosis of blepharospasm and oromandibular dystonia. In: Jankovic J, Tolosa E, ed. Advances in neurology. Vol. 49. Facial dyskinesias. New York: Raven, 1988:103–116.

59. Jankovic J. Cranial-cervical dyskinesias. In: Appel S, ed. Current neurology. Vol. 6. Chicago: Year Book Medical, 1986:153–176.

60. Friedman JH, Kucharski LT, Wagner RL. Tardive dystonia in a psychiatric hospital. J Neurol Neurosurg Psychiatry 1987;50:801–803.

61. Sethi KD, Hess DC. Prevalence of tardive dystonia. Neurology 1988;38(suppl 1):285.

62. Marsden CD, Harrison MJG. Idiopathic torsion dystonia; a review of 42 patients. Brain 1974;97:793–810.

63. Jankovic J, Fahn J. The phenomenology of tics. Mov Disord 1986;1:17–26.

64. Shapiro AK, Shapiro ED, Bruun RD, et al. Gilles de la Tourette syndrome. New York, Raven, 1978.

65. Jankovic J. The neurology of tics. In: Marsden CD, Fahn S, eds. Movement disorders 2. London: Butterworth, 1987:383–405.

66. Singh S, Jankovic J. Tardive dystonia in patients with Tourette's syndrome. Mov Disord 1988;3:274–280.

67. Patel V, Jankovic J. Myoclonus. In: Appel S, ed., Current neurology. Vol. 8. Chicago: Year Book Medical, 1988;8:77–106.

68. Jankovic J, Pardo R. Segmental myoclonus: clinical and pharmacologic study. Arch Neurol 1986;43:1025–1031.

69. Delay J, Demker D. Drug-induced extrapyramidal syndromes. In: Vinken PS, Bruyn TW, eds. Handbook of clinical neurology: diseases of the basal ganglia. Amsterdam: North Holland 1968:248–266.

70. Martin ML, Lucid EJ, Walker RW. Neuroleptic malignant syndrome. Am Emerg Med 1985;14:354–358.

71. Hashimoto A, Sherman CB, Jeffrey WH. Neuroleptic malignant syndrome and dopaminergic blockade. Arch Intern Med 1984;144:629–630.

72. Buckley PF, Hutchinson M. Neuroleptic malignant syndrome. J Neurol Neurosurg Psychiatry 1995;58:271–273.

73. Pope HG, Keck PE, McElroy SL. Frequency and presentation of neuroleptic malignant syndrome in a large psychiatric hospital. Am J Psychiatry 1986;143:1227–1233.

74. Jurlan R, Hamill R, Shoulson I. Neuroleptic malignant syndrome. Clin Neuropharmacol 1984;7:109–120.

75. Levenson J. Neuroleptic malignant syndrome. Am J Psychiatry 1985;142:1137–1145.

76. Addonizio G, Susman VL, Roth SD. Symptoms of neuroleptic malignant syndrome in 82 consecutive inpatients. Am J Psychiatry 1986;143:1587–1590.

77. Greenberg LB, Gujavarty K. The neuroleptic malignant syndrome: review and report of three cases. Compr Psychiatry 1985;26:63–70.

78. Jee A. Neuroleptic malignant syndrome and tardive dyskinesia. Br J Psychiatry 1987;150:880.

79. Moore A, O'Donohoe NV, Monaghan H. Neuroleptic malignant syndrome. Arch Dis Child 1986;61:793–795.

80. Sternberg DE. Neuroleptic malignant syndrome: the pendulum swings. Am J Psychiatry 1986;143:1273–1275.

81. Friedman LS, Weinrauch LA, D'Elia JA. Metoclopramide-induced neuroleptic malignant syndrome. Arch Intern Med 1987;147:1495–1497.

82. Patel P, Bristow G. Postoperative neuroleptic malignant syndrome: a case report. Can J Anaesth 1987;34:515–518.

83. Kosten TR, Kleber HD. Sudden death in cocaine abusers: relation to neuroleptic malignant syndrome. Lancet 1987;1:1198–1199.

84. Demirkiran M, Jankovic J, Dean JM. Ecstasy intoxication: an overlap between serotonin syndrome and neuroleptic malignant syndrome. Clin Neuropharmacol 1996;19:157–164.

85. Stacy M, Cardoso F, Jankovic J. Tardive stereotypy and other movement disorders in tardive dyskinesia. Neurology 1993;43:937–941.

86. Varga E, Sugerman A, Varga V, et al. Prevalence of spontaneous oral dyskinesia in the elderly. Am J Psychiatry 1982;239:329–331.

87. Green BH, Dewey ME, Copeland JRM, et al. Prospective data on the prevalence of abnormal involuntary movements among elderly people living in the community. Acta Psychiatr Scand 1993;87:418–421.

88. Lewis IK, Hanlon JT, Hobbins MJ, Beck JD. Use of medications with potential oral adverse drug reactions in community-dwelling elderly. Spec Care Dentistry 1993;13:171–176.

89. Jeste DV, Caliguiri MP, Paulsen JS, et al. Risk of tardive dyskinesia in older patients: a prospective longitudinal study of 266 outpatients. Arch Gen Psychiatry 1995;52:756–765.

90. Miller LG, Jankovic J. Neurologic approach to drug-induced movement disorders in 125 patients. South Med J 1990;83:525–532.

91. Smith JM, Baldessarini RJ. Changes in prevalence, severity, and recovery in tardive dyskinesia with age. Arch Gen Psychiatry 1980;37:1368–1373.

92. Chouinard G, Annablie L, Ross-Chouinard A, et al. Factors related to tardive dyskinesia. Am J Psychiatry 1979;136:79–83.

93. Yassa R, Chadirian AM, Schwart G. Prevalence of tardive dyskinesia in affective disorder patients. J Clin Psychiatry 183;44:410–412.

94. Gualtieri CT, Quade D, Hicks RE, et al. Tardive dyskinesia and other clinical consequences of neuroleptic treatment in children and adolescents. Am J Psychiatry 1984;141:20–23.

95. Gualtieri CT, Schroeder SR, Hicks RE, et al. Tardive dyskinesia in young mentally retarded individuals. Arch Gen Psychiatry 1986;43:335–340.

96. Klawans HL, Goetz CG, Tanner CM, et al. Baclofen and tardive dyskinesia (abstract). Neurology 1981;31(suppl):78–79.

97. Stewart RM, Rollins J, Beckham B, et al. Baclofen in tardive dyskinesia patients maintained on neuroleptics. Clin Neuropharmacol 1982;4:365–373.

98. Tell GP, Shecter PJ, Koch-Weser J, et al. Effects of gamma vinyl GABA (letter). N Engl J Med 1981;302:581–582.

99. Linnoila M, Viukar M, Hietala O. Effect of sodium valproate on tardive dyskinesia. Br J Psychiatry 1976;129:114–119.

100. Nair NPV, Lal S, Schwartz G, et al. Effects of sodium valproate and baclofen in tardive dyskinesia: clinical and neuroendocrine studies. In: Cattabeni F, Racogni G, Spano PF, Costa E, eds. Long-term effects of neuroleptics. New York: Raven, 1980:437–441.

101. Nishikawa T, Tanaka M, Tsuda A, et al. Clonidine therapy for tardive dyskinesia and related syndromes. Clin Neuropharmacol 1984;7:239–245.

102. Klawans HL, Topel JL, Bergen D. Deanol in the treatment of levodopa-induced dyskinesias. Neurology 1975;25:290–293.

103. Growdon JH. Choline, lecithin, and tardive dyskinesia. Adv Neurol 1979;24:387–394.

104. Godwin-Austen RB, Clark T. Persistent phenothiazine dyskinesia treated with tetrabenazine. Br Med J 1971;4:25–26.

105. Lang AE, Marsden CD. Alphamethylparatyrosine and tetrabenazine in movement disorders. Clin Neuropharmacol 1982;5:375–387.

106. Jankovic J, Orman J. Tetrabenazine therapy of dystonia, chorea, tics and other dyskinesias. Neurology 1988;38:391–394.

107. Asher SW, Aminoff MJ. Tetrabenazine and movement disorders. Neurology 1981;31:1051–1054.

108. Jankovic J, Beach J. Long-term effects of tetrabenazine in hyperkinetic movement disorders. Neurology 1997;48:358–362.

109. Jankovic J. Treatment of hyperkinetic movement disorders with tetrabenazine: a double-blind crossover study. Ann Neurol 1982;11:41–47.

110. Truong DD, Sandroni P, van der Noort S, Matsumoto RR. Diphenhydramine is effective in the treatment of idiopathic dystonia. Arch Neurol 1995;52:405–407.

111. Vant Groenewout JL, Stone MR, Vo VN, et al. Evidence for the involvement of histamine in the antidystonic effects of diphenhydramine. Exper Neurol 1995;134:253–260.

112. Narayan RK, Loubser PG, Jankovic J, et al. Intrathecal baclofen for intractable axial dystonia. Neurology 1991;41:1141–1142.

113. Gordon MF, Diaz-Olivo R, Hunt AL, Fahn S. Therapeutic trial of milacemide in patients with myoclonus and other intractable movements disorders. Mov Disord 1993;8:484–488.

114. Gold R, Lenox RH. Is there a rationale for iron supplementation in the treatment of akathisia? A review of the evidence. J Clin Psychiatry 1995;56:476–483.

115. Sachdev P. Neuroleptic-induced movement disorders and body iron status. Prog Neuro-Psychopharmacol Biol Psychiatry 1992;16:647–653.

116. Cardoso F, Jankovic J, Grossman RG, Hamilton WJ. Outcome after stereotactic thalamotomy for dystonia and hemiballismus. Neurosurgery 1995;36:501–508.

117. Jankovic J. Botulinum toxin in movement disorders. Curr Opin Neurol 1994;7:358–366.

118. Schiavo G, Benfanati F, Poulain B, et al. Tetanus and botulinum B neurotoxins block neurotransmitter release by proteolytic cleavage of synaptobrevin. Nature 1992;359:832–835.

119. Jankovic J, Brin F. Therapeutic uses of botulinum toxin. N Engl J Med 1992;324:1186–1194.

120. Jankovic J. Botulinum toxin in the treatment of dystonic tics. Mov Disord 1994;9:347–349.

121. Jankovic J, Schwartz K. Use of botulinum toxin in the treatment of hand dystonia. J Hand Surg 1993;18A:883–887.

122. Williams A. Consensus statement for the management of focal dystonias. Br J Hosp Med 1994;50:655–659.

123. Jankovic J, Schwartz K. Response and immunoresistance to botulinum toxin injections. Neurology 1995;45:1743–1746.

124. Borodic GE, Johnson E, Goodnough M, Schantz E. Botulinum toxin therapy, immunologic resistance and problems with available materials. Neurology 1996;46:26–29.

125. Jankovic J. Treatment of hyperkinetic movement disorders with tetrabenazine: a double-blind crossover study. Ann Neurol 1982;11:41–47.

126. VanPutten T. Vulnerability to extrapyramidal side effects. Clin Neuropharmacol 1983;6(suppl 1):s27–34.

127. Gardos G, Cole JO. Overview: public health issues in tardive dyskinesia. Am J Psychiatry 1980;137:776–781.

128. Quitkin F, Rifkin A, Gochfeld L, et al. Tardive dyskinesia: are first signs reversible? Am J Psychiatry 1977;134:84–87.

129. Klawans HL, Tanner CM, Barr A. The reversibility of "permanent" tardive dyskinesia. Clin Neuropharmacol 1984;7:153–159.

130. Kane J, Honigfeld G, Singer J, et al. Clozapine for the treatment-resistant schizophrenic. Arch Gen Psychiatry 1988;45:789–796.

131. Marder SR, Van Putten T. Who should receive clozapine? Arch Gen Psychiatry 1988;45:865–867.

132. Lieberman JA, Saltz BL, Johns CA, et al. Clozapine effects on tardive dyskinesia. Psychopharmacol Bull 1989;25:57–62.

133. Arana GW, Goff DC, Baldessarini RJ, Keepers GA. Efficacy of anticholinergic prophylaxis for neuroleptic-induced acute dystonia. Am J Psychiatry 1988;145:993–996.

134. Baldessarini RJ. Drugs and the treatment of psychiatric disorders. In: Gilman AG, Goodman LS, Rall TW, Murad F. The pharmacologic basis of therapeutics. New York: Macmillan Publishing, 1985:387–445.

135. Burke RE. Tardive dyskinesia: current clinical issues. Neurology 1984;34:1348–1353.

136. Richelson E. Neuroleptic affinities for human brain receptors and their use in predicting adverse effects. J Clin Psychiatry 1984;45:331–336.

137. Borison RL, Fields JZ, Diamond BI. Site specific blockade of dopamine receptors by neuroleptic agents in human brain. Neuropharmacol 1981;20:1321–1322.

138. Reynolds GP, Cowey L, Rossor MN, et al. Thioridazine is not specific for limbic dopamine receptors. Lancet 1982;2:499–500.

139. Snyder S, Greenberg D, Yamamura HI. Antischizophrenic drugs and brain cholinergic receptors: affinity for muscarinic sites predicts extrapyramidal effects. Arch Gen Psychiatry 1974;31:58–61.

140. Anden NE, Butcher SG, Corrodi H, et al. Receptor activity and turnover of dopamine and noradrenalin after neuroleptics. Eur J Pharmacol 1970;11:303–314.

141. Jeste DV, Linnoila M, Wagner R, et al. Serum neuroleptic concentrations and tardive dyskinesia. Psychopharmacology 1982;76:377–378.

142. Jeste DV, Rosenblatt JE, Wagner RL, et al. High serum neuroleptic levels in tardive dyskinesia? N Engl J Med 1979;300:1184.

143. Hansen LB, Larsen NE, Vestergard P. Plasma levels of perphenazine (Trilafon^R) related to development of extrapyramidal side effects. Psychopharmacology 1981;74:306–309.

144. Kane JM. Antipsychotic drug side effects: their relationship to dose. J Clin Psychiatry 1985;46:16–21.

145. Jus A, Pineau R, Lachance R, et al. Epidemiology of tardive dyskinesia: Part II. Dis Nerv Sys 1976;37:257–261.

146. Jeste DV, Potkin SG, Sinha S, et al. Tardive dyskinesia—reversible and persistent. Arch Gen Psychiatry 1979;36:585–590.

147. Ganzini L, Heintz RT, Hoffman WF, Casey DE. The prevalence of tardive dyskinesia in neuroleptic-treated diabetics. Arch Gen Psychiatry 1991;48:259–263.

148. Saller CF, Chiodo LA. Glucose suppresses basal firing and haloperidol-induced increases in the firing rate of central dopaminergic neurons. Science 1980;210:1269–1271.

149. Dave M. Clozapine-related tardive dyskinesia. Biol Psychiatry 1994;35:886–887.

150. Kane JM, Woerner MG, Pollack S, et al. Does clozapine cause tardive dyskinesia? J Clin Psychiatry 1993;54:327–330.

151. Meltzer HY. An overview of the mechanism of action of clozapine. J Clin Psychiatry 1994;55(suppl B):47–52.

152. Trugman JM, Leadbetter R, Zalis ME, et al. Treatment of severe axial tardive dystonia with clozapine: case report and hypothesis. Mov Disord 1994;9:441–446.

153. Wolf ME, Moxnaim AD. Improvement of axial dystonia with the administration of clozapine: case report and hypothesis. Mov Disorder 1994;9:441–446.

154. Bennett JP Jr, Landow ER, Dietrich S, Schuh LA. Suppression of dyskinesias in advanced Parkinson's disease: moderate daily clozapine doses provide long-term dyskinesia reduction. Mov Disord 1994;9:409–414.

155. Tamminga CA, Thaker GK, Moran M, Kakigi T, Gao SM. Clozapine in tardive dyskinesia: observations from human and animal model studies. J Clin Psychiatry 1994;55(suppl B):102–106.

156. Worrall R, Wilson A, Cullen M. Dystonia and drug-induced hepatitis in a patient treated with clozapine. Am J Psychiatry 1995;152:647–648.

157. Bak TH, Bauer M, Schaub RT, et al. Myoclonus in patients treated with clozapine: a case series. J Clin Psychiatry 1995;56:418–422.

158. Heim M, Rhein C. Early dyskinesia with administration of clozapine. Nervenarzt 1994;65:486–487.

159. Chengappa KN, Shelton MD, Baker RW, et al. The prevalence of akathisia in patients receiving stable doses of clozapine. J Clin Psychiatry 1994;55:142–145.

160. Cohen LJ. Risperidone: Pharmacotherapy 1994;14:253–265.

161. Borison RL, Pthiraja AP, Diamond BI, Meibach RL. Risperidone: clinical safety and efficacy in schizophrenia. Psychopharmacol Bull 1992;28:213–218.

162. Claus A, Bollen J, DeCuyper H, et al. Risperidone versus haloperidol in the treatment of chronic schizophrenic inpatients: a multicentre double-blind comparative study. Acta Psychiatr Scand 1992;85:295–305.

163. Rich SS, Friedman JH, Oh BR. Risperidone versus clozapine in the treatment of psychosis in six patients with Parkinson's disease and other akinetic syndromes. J Clin Psychiatry 1995;56:556–559.

164. Meco G, Bedin L, Bonifati V, Sonsini U. Risperidone in the treatment of chronic schizophrenia with tardive dyskinesia. Curr Ther Res 1989;46:876–883.

165. Madhusoodanan S, Blenner R, Araujo L, Abazo A. Efficacy of risperidone treatment for psychosis with schizophrenia, schizoaffective disorder, bipolar disorder or senile dementia in 11 geriatric patients: a case series. J Clin Psychiatry 1995;56:514–518.

166. Chouinard G. Effects of risperidone in tardive dyskinesia: an analysis of the Canadian multicenter risperidone study. J Clin Psychopharmacol 1995;15:365–374.

167. Owens DG. Extrapyramidal side effects and tolerability of risperidone: a review. J Clin Psychiatry 1994;55(suppl):29–35.

168. Meltzer HY, Lee MA, Ranjan R. Recent advances in the pharmacotherapy of schizophrenia. Acta Psychiatr Scand 1994;384(suppl):95–101.

169. Andersson U, Haggstrom JE, Nilsson MI, Widerlov E. Remoxipride, a selective D2 receptor antagonist in tardive dyskinesia. Psychopharmacol 1988;94:167–171.

170. Keks N, McGrath J, Lambert T, et al. The Australian multicenter double-blind comparative study of remoxipride and thioridazine in schizophrenia. Acta Psychiatr Scand 1994;90:356–365.

171. Kopenen JH, Lepola UM, Leinonen EV. Neuroleptic malignant syndrome during remoxipride treatment. A case report. Eur Neuropsychopharmacol 1993;3:517–519.

172. Casey DE. Serotonergic and dopaminergic aspects of neuroleptic-induced extrapyramidal syndromes in nonhuman primates. Psychopharmacol 1993;112(suppl):s55–s59.

173. Casey DE. Extrapyramidal syndromes in nonhuman primates: typical and atypical neuroleptics. Psychopharmacol Bull 1991;27:47–50.

174. Wetzel H, Szeged A, Hain C, et al. Seroquel (ICI 204 636), a putative "atypical" antipsychotic in schizophrenia with positive symptomatology: results of an open clinical trial and changes of neuroendocrinological and EEG parameters. Psychopharmacology 1995;119:231–238.

175. Miller LG, Jankovic J. Sulpiride-induced tardive dystonia. Mov Disord 1990;5:83–84.

176. deMunain AL, Poza JJ, Gorospe A, et al. Tardive akathisia due to sulpiride. Clin Neuropharmacol 1994;17:481–483.

177. Gerlach J, Casey DE. Sulpiride in tardive dyskinesia. Act Psychiatr Scand 1984;311(suppl):93–102.

178. Sandyk R. Tardive dyskinesia induced by sulpiride in a patient with hypothyroidism. Clin Neuropharmacol 1986;9:100–101.

179. Lopez deMunain A, Poza JJ, Gorospe A, et al. Tardive akathisia due to sulpiride. Clin Neuropharmacol 1994;17:481–483.

180. Harrington RA, Hamilton DW, Grogden RH, et al. Metoclopramide: an updated review of its pharmacologic properties and clinical use. Drugs 1983;25:451–494.

181. Hassan MN, Reches A, Kuhn C, et al. Pharmacologic evaluation of dopaminergic receptor blockade by metoclopramide. Clin Neuropharmacol 1986;9:71–78.

182. Wiholm BE, Mortimer O, Boethius G, et al. Tardive dyskinesia associated with metoclopramide. Br Med J 1984;288:545–547.

183. Breitbart W. Tardive dyskinesia associated with high-dose intravenous metoclopramide. N Engl J Med 1986;315:518–519.

184. Yamamoto M, Ujike H, Ogawa N. Metoclopramide-induced parkinsonism. Clin Neuropharmacol 1987;10:287–289.

185. Indo T, Ando K. Metoclopramide-induced parkinsonism: clinical characteristics of ten cases. Arch Neurol 1982;39:494–496.

186. Jungmann E, Schofflang C. Akathisia and metoclopramide. Lancet 1982;2:221.

187. Shearer RM, Bownes IT, Curran P. Tardive akathisia and agitated depression during metoclopramide therapy. Acta Psychiatr Scand 1984;70:428–431.

188. Strum SB, McDermed JE, Opfell RW, et al. Intravenous metoclopramide: an effective antiemetic in cancer chemotherapy. JAMA 1982;247:2683–2686.

189. Robinson OPW. Metoclopramide-side effects and safety. Postgrad Med J 1973;49:77–80.

190. Kris MG, Tyson LB, Gralla RJ, et al. Extrapyramidal reactions with high-dose metoclopramide. N Engl J Med 1983;309:433.

191. Lang AE. Clinical differences between metoclopramide- and antipsychotic-induced tardive dyskinesias. Can J Neurol Sci 1990;17:137–139.

192. Ganzini L, Casey DE, Hoffman WF, McCall AL. The prevalence of metoclopramide-induced tardive dyskinesia and acute extrapyramidal movement disorders. Arch Intern Med 1993;153:1469–1475.

193. Miller LG, Jankovic J. Metoclopramide-induced movement disorders: clinical findings with a review of the literature. Arch Intern Med 1989;149:2486–2492.

194. Luquin MR, Scipioni O, Vaamonde J, et al. Levodopa-induced dyskinesias in Parkinson's disease: clinical and pharmacological classification. Mov Disord 1992;7:117–124.

195. Marconi R, Lefebvre-Caparros D, Bonnet A-M, et al. Levodopa-induced dyskinesia in Parkinson's disease: phenomenology and pathophysiology. Mov Disord 1994;9:2–12.

196. Nutt JG, Holford NHG. The response to levodopa in Parkinson's disease: Imposing pharmacological law and order. Ann Neurol 1996;39:561–573.

197. Fahn S. "On-off" phenomenon with levodopa therapy in parkinsonism. Neurology 1974;24:431–441.

198. Sweet RD, McDowell FH. Five years' treatment of Parkinson's disease with levodopa. Ann Intern Med 1975;83:456–463.

199. Jankovic J. Management of motor side effects of chronic levodopa therapy. Clin Neuropharmacol 1982;5(Suppl 1):s19–s28.

200. Poewe WH, Lees AJ, Stern GM. Low-dose L-dopa therapy in Parkinsons' disease. A 6 year follow-up. Neurology 1986;36:1528–1530.

201. Muenter MD, Tyce GM. L-dopa therapy of Parkinson disease: plasma L-dopa concentration, therapeutic response and side effects. Mayo Clin Proc 1971;46:231–239.

202. Cedarbaum JM, Breck L, Kutt H, et al. Controlled-release levodopa/carbidopa. II. Sinemet CR4 treatment of response fluctuations in Parkinson's disease. Neurology 1987;37:1607–1612.

203. Direnfeld LK, Feldman RG, Alexander MP, et al. Is L-dopa drugs holiday useful? Neurology 1980;30:785–788.

204. Weiner WJ, Koller WC, Perlik S, et al. Drug holiday and management of Parkinson disease. Neurology 1980;30:1257–1261.

205. Mayeux R, Stein Y, Mulveyk, et al. Reappraisal of temporary levodopa withdrawal ("drug holiday") in Parkinson's Disease. N Engl J Med 1985;313:724–728.

206. Kurlan R, Tanner CM, Goetz C, et al. Levodopa drug holiday versus drug dosage reduction in Parkinson's disease. Clin Neuropharmacol 1994;17:117–127.

207. Lhermitte F, Agid Y, Signoret JL. Onset and end-of-dose levodopa-induced dyskinesias. Arch Neurol 1978;35:261–263.

208. Barbeau A. Diphasic dyskinesia during levodopa therapy. Lancet 1975;1:756.

209. Quinn N, Critchley P, Marsden CD. Young onset Parkinson's Disease. Mov Disord 1987;2:73–91.

210. Ziegler M, Fournier V, Bathien H, et al. Therapeutic response to progabide in neuroleptic- and L-dopa-induced dyskinesias. Clin Neuropharmacol 1987;10:238–246.

211. Sleator EK. Deleterious effects of drugs used for hyperactivity on patients with Gilles de la Tourette Syndrome. Clin Pediatr 1980;19:453–454.

212. Erenberg G, Cruse RP, Rothner AD. Gilles de la Tourette's syndrome: effect of stimulant drugs. Neurology 1985;35:1346–1348.

213. Golden GS. The effect of central nervous system stimulants on Tourette syndrome. Ann Neurol 1977;2:69–70.

214. Lowe TL, Cohen DJ, Dettor J, et al. Stimulant medications precipitate Tourette's syndrome. JAMA 1982;247:1729–1731.

215. Stevanka LR, Sanders-Bush E. Long-term reduction of brain serotonin by p-chloroamphetamine: effects of inducers and inhibitors of drug metabolism. J Pharmacol Exp Ther 1978;206:460–467.

216. Arnold EB, Molinoff PB, Rutledge CO. The release of endogenous norepinephrine and dopamine from cerebral cortex by amphetamine. J Pharmacol Exp Ther 1977;202:544–557.

217. Antelman SM, Chiodo LA. Dopamine autoreceptor subsensitivity: a mechanism common to the treatment of depression and the induction of amphetamine psychosis? Biol Psychiatr 1981;17:717–727.

218. Lundh H, Tunving K. An extrapyramidal choreiform syndrome caused by amphetamine addiction. J Neurol Neurosurg Psychiatry 1981;44:728–730.

219. Mattson RH, Calverley JR. Dextroamphetamine sulfate-induced dyskinesias. JAMA 1968;204:400–402.

220. Denckla MB, Bemporad JR, MacKay MC. Tics following methylphenidate administrations: a report of 20 cases. JAMA 1976;235:1349–1351.

221. Golden GS. Tourette syndrome: the pediatric perspective. Am J Dis Child 1977;131:531–534.

222. Shapiro E, Shapiro AK. Tic disorders. JAMA 1981;245:1583–1585.

223. Golden GS. Gilles de la Tourette's syndrome following methylphenidate administration. Dev Med Child Neurol 1974;16:76–78.

224. Pollack MA, Cohen NL, Friedhoff AJ. Gilles de la Tourette's syndrome: familiar occurrence and precipitation by methylphenidate therapy. Arch Neurol 1977;34:630–632.

225. Bremness AB, Sverd J. Methylphenidate-induced Tourette syndrome: case report. Am J Psychiatry 1979;136:1334–1335.

226. Mitchell E, Matthews KL. Gilles de la Tourette's disorder associated with pemoline. Am J Psychiatry 1980;137:1618–1619.

227. Bonthala CM, West A. Pemoline-induced chorea and Gilles de la Tourette's syndrome. Br J Psychiatry 1983;143:300–302.

228. Shapiro AK, Shapiro E. Do stimulants provoke, cause, or exacerbate tics and Tourette's syndrome? Compr Psychiatry 1981;22:265–273.

229. Ritchie JM, Greene NM. Local anesthetics. In: Gilman AG, Goodman LS, Rall TW, Murad F, eds. The pharmacologic basis of therapeutics. New York: Macmillan, 1985:302–321.

230. Tennant FS, Sagherian AA. Double-blind comparison of amantadine and bromocriptine for ambulatory withdrawal from cocaine dependence. Arch Intern Med 1987;147:109–112.

231. Cardoso FEC, Jankovic J. Cocaine-related movement disorders. Mov Disord 1993;8:175–178.

232. Farrell PE, Diehl AK. Acute dystonic reaction to crack cocaine. Ann Emerg Med 1991;20:322.

233. Hegarty AM, Lipton RB, Merriam AE, Freeman K. Cocaine as a risk factor for acute dystonic reactions. Neurology 1991;41:1670–1672.

234. Thiel A, Dressler D. Dyskinesias possibly induced by norpseudoephedrine. J Neurol 1994;241:167–169.

235. Battaglia G, Zackzek R, DeSouza EB. MDMA effects in brain: pharmacologic profile and evidence of neurotoxicity from neurochemical and autoradiographic studies in MDMA. In: Peroutka SJ, ed. Ecstasy and/or human neurotoxin. Norwell, MA: Kluwer Academic, 1989:171–199.

236. Schmidt CJ, Wu L, Lovenberg W. Methylenedioxymethamphetamine: a potentially neurotoxic amphetamine analog. Eur J Pharmacol 1986;124:175–178.

237. Stone DM, Stahl DC, Hanson GR, Gibb JW. The effects of 3,4 methylenedioxy-methamphetamine (MDMA) and 3,4-methylenedioxyamphetamine (MDA) on monoaminergic systems in the rat brain. Eur J Pharmacol 1986;128:41–48.

238. Coffey CE, Ross DR, Massey EY, et al. Dyskinesias associated with lithium therapy in parkinsonism. Clin Neuropharmacol 1984;7:223–229.

239. Stancer HC. Tardive dyskinesia not associated with neuroleptics. Am J Psychiatry 1979;136:727.

240. Beitman BD. Tardive dyskinesia reinduced by lithium carbonate. Am J Psychiatry 1978;135:1229–1230.

241. Ghadirian AM, Annable L, Belanger MC, Chouinard G. A cross-sectional study of parkinsonism and tardive dyskinesia in lithium treated affective disordered patients. J Clin Psychiatry 1996;57:22–28.

242. Lozovsky D, Saller CF, Kopin IJ. Lithium and the prevention of dopamine receptor supersensitivity in diabetic rats. Am J Psychiatry 1983;140:613–614.

243. Reda FA, Escobar JI, Scanlan JM. Lithium carbonate in the treatment of tardive dyskinesia. Am J Psychiatry 1975;132:560–562.

244. Fann WE, Sullivan JL, Richman BW. Dyskinesias associated with tricyclic antidepressants. Br J Psychiatry 1976;128:490–493.

245. Koller WC, Musa MN. Amitriptyline-induced abnormal movements. Neurology 1985;35:1086.

246. Woogen S, Graham J, Angrist B. A tardive dyskinesia-like syndrome after amitriptyline treatment. J Clin Psychopharmacol 1981;1:34–36.

247. Lapierre YD, Anderson K. Dyskinesia associated with amoxapine antidepressant therapy: a case report. Am J Psychiatry 193;140:493–494.

248. Yassa R, Camille Y, Belzile L. Tardive dyskinesia in the course of antidepressant therapy: a prevalence study and review of the literature. J Clin Psychopharmacol 1987;7:243–246.

249. Sachdev P. Depression-dependent exacerbation of tardive dyskinesia. Br J Psychiatry 1989;155:253–255.

250. Ross DR, Walker JI, Peterson J. Akathisia induced by amoxapine. Am J Psychiatry 1983;140:115–116.

251. Zubenko GS, Cohen BM, Lipinski JF. Antidepressant-related akathisia. J Clin Psychopharmacol 1987;7:254–257.

252. Blackwell B. Newer antidepressant drugs. In: Meltzer HY, ed. Psychopharmacology: the third generation of progress. New York: Raven, 1987:1041–1049.

253. Albanese A, Rossi P, Altavista MC. Can trazodone induce parkinsonism? Clin Neuropharmacol 1988;11:1180–1182.

254. DeMuth GW, Breslow RE, Drescher J. The elicitation of a movement disorder by trazodone: case report. J Clin Psychiatry 1985;46:535–536.

255. Patel HC, Bruza D, Yerogani V. Myoclonus with trazodone. J Clin Psychopharmacol 1988;8:152.

256. Garvey MJ, Tollefson GD. Occurrence of myoclonus in patients treated with cyclic antidepressants. Arch Gen Psychiatry 1987;44:269–272.

257. DeCastro RM. Antidepressants and myoclonus: case report. J Clin Psychiatry 1985;46:284–287.

258. Otani K, Kaneko S, Fukushima Y, Kubota S. Involuntary movements associated with mianserin treatment. A case report. Br J Psychiatry 1989;154:113–114.

259. Bjorksten KS, Walinder J. Does mianserin induce involuntary movements in brain damaged patients? Int Clin Psychopharmacol 1993;8:203–204.

260. Sachdev P. Serotonin and drug-induced movement disorders. Aust N Z J Psychiatry 1994;28:695–696.

261. Mander AG, McCausland B, Workman B, et al. Fluoxetine-induced dyskinesia. Aust N Z J Psychiatry 1994;28:328–330.

262. Arya DK, Szabadie E. Dyskinesia associated with fluvoxamine. J Clin Psychopharmacol 1993;13:365–366.

263. Lipinski JF, Mallya G, Zimmerman P, Pope HG. Fluoxetine-induced akathisia: clinical and theoretical implications. J Clin Psychiatry 1989;50:339–342.

264. Falcon BA, Liebowitz R. Fluoxetine and extrapyramidal symptoms in CNS lupus. J Clin Psychopharmacol 1991;11:147–148.

265. Tate JL. Extrapyramidal symptoms in a patient taking haloperidol and fluoxetine. Am J Psychiatry 1989;146:399–400.

266. Brod TM. Fluoxetine and extrapyramidal side-effects. Am J Psychiatry 1989;146:1353.

267. Kaplan SR, Murkofsky C. Oral-buccal dyskinesia symptoms associated with low-dose benzodiazepine treatment. Am J Psychiatry 1978;135:1558–1559.

268. Sandyk R. Orofacial dyskinesias associated with lorazepam therapy. Clin Pharm 1986;5:419–421.

269. Janet B, Lal S. Tardive dyskinesia uncovered after ingestion of Sominex^R, an over-the-counter drug. Can J Psychiatry 1985;30:370–371.

270. Thach BT, Chase TN, Bosma JF. Oral facial dyskinesia associated with prolonged use of antihistaminic decongestants. N Engl J Med 1975;293:486–487.

271. Needleman P, Corr PB, Johnson EM. Drugs used for the treatment of angina, organic nitrates, calcium channel blockers, and beta-adrenergic antagonists. In: Gilman AG, Goodman LS, Rall TW, Murad F, eds. The pharmacologic basis of therapeutics. New York: Macmillan, 1985:806–826.

272. Micheli F, Paradal MF, Gatto M, et al. Flunarizine and cinnarizine-induced extrapyramidal reactions. Neurology 1987;37:881–884.

273. Ross JL, Mackenzie TB, Hanson DR, et al. Diltiazem for tardive dyskinesia. Lancet 1987;1:268.

274. Brink DD. Diltiazem and hyperactivity. Ann Intern Med 1984;100:459–460.

275. Yassa R, Schwartz G. Depression as a predictor in the development of tardive dyskinesia. Biol Psychiatry 1984;19:441–444.

276. Jacobs MB. Diltiazem and akathisia. Ann Intern Med 1983;99:794–795.

277. Barrow N, Childs A. An anti-tardive dyskinesia effect of verapamil. Am J Psychiatry 1986;143:1485.

278. Abad V, Ovsiew F. Treatment of persistent myoclonic tardive dystonia with verapamil. Br J Psychiatry 1993;162:554–556.

279. Rall TW, Schleifer LS. Drugs effective in the therapy of the epilepsies. In: Gilman AG, Goodman LS, Rall TW, Murad F, eds. The pharmacologic basis of therapeutics. New York: Macmillan, 1985:446–472.

280. Luhdorf K, Lund M. Phenytoin-induced hyperkinesia. Epilepsia 1977;18:409–415.

281. Chalhub EG, Devivo DC, Volpe JJ. Phenytoin-induced dystonia and choreoathetosis in two retarded epileptic children. Neurology 1976;26:494–498.

282. Corey A, Koller W. Phenytoin-induced dystonia. Ann Neurol 1983;14:92–93.

283. Rasmussen S, Kristensen M. Choreoathetosis during phenytoin treatment. Acta Med Scand 1977;201:239–241.

284. Koolker JC, Sumi SM. Movement disorder as a manifestation of diphenylhydantoin intoxication. Neurology 1974;24:68–71.

285. McLellan DL, Swash M. Choreoathetosis and encephalopathy induced by phenytoin. Br Med J 1974;2:204–205.

286. DeVeaugh-Geiss J. Aggravation of tardive dyskinesia by phenytoin. N Engl J Med 1978;298:457–458.

287. Harrison MB, Lyons GR, Landow ER. Phenytoin and dyskinesias: a report of two cases and review of the literature. Mov Disord 1993;8:19–27.

288. Nausieda PA, Koller WC, Weiner WJ, et al. Clinical and experimental studies of phenytoin-induced hyperkinesias. J Neurol Transmission 1979;45:291–305.

289. Chadwick D, Reynolds EH, Marsden CD. Anticonvulsant-induced dyskinesias: a comparison with dyskinesias induced by neuroleptics. J Neurol Neurosurg Psychiatry 1976;39:1210–1218.

290. Chadwick D, Reynolds EH, Marsden CD. Anticonvulsant-induced dyskinesias: a comparison with dyskinesias induced by neuroleptics. J Neurol Neurosurg Psychiatry 1976;39:1210–1218.

291. Joyce R, Gunderson C. Carbamazepine-induced orofacial dyskinesia. Neurology 1980;30:1333–1334.

292. Schwartz G, Gosenfeld L, Gilderman A, et al. Akathisia associated with carbamazepine therapy. Am J Psychiatry 1986;143:1190–1191.

293. McMahon T. Dyskinesia associated with amoxapine withdrawal and use of carbamazepine and antihistamines. Psychosomatics 1986;27:145–148.

294. Neglia JP, Glazen DG, Zion TE. Tics and vocalizations in children treated with carbamazepine. Pediatrics 1984;73:841–844.

295. Kurlan R, Kersun J, Behr J, et al. Carbamazepine-induced tics. Clin Neuropharmacol 1989;12:298–302.

296. Robertson PL, Garofalo EA. Silverstein FS, Komarynski MA. Carbamazepine-induced tics. Epilepsia 1993;34:965–968.

297. Cutler NR, Post RM. State-related cyclical dyskinesias in manic-depressive illness. J Clin Psychopharmacol 1982;2:350–354.

298. Perenyi A, Sztaniszlav D. Carbamazepine in tardive dyskinesia. Psychopharmacol Bull 1985;21:345–346.

299. Kerrick JM, Kelley BJ, Maister BH, et al. Involuntary movement disorders associated with felbamate. Neurology 1995;45:185–187.

300. Patsalos RN, Sander JW. Newer antiepileptic drugs. Toward an improved risk-benefit ratio. Drug Saf 1994;11:37–67.

301. US Gabapentin Study Group. The long-term safety and efficacy of gabapentin (Neurontin) as add-on therapy in drug-resistant partial epilepsy. Epilepsy Res 1994;18:67–73.

302. Fornazzari L, Carlen PL. Transient choreiform dyskinesias during alcohol withdrawal. Can J Neurol Sci 1982;9:89–90.

303. Balldin J, Alling C, Gottfries CG, et al. Changes in dopamine receptor sensitivity in humans after heavy alcohol intake. Psychopharmacology 1985;86:142–146.

304. Mullin PJ, Kershaw PW, Bolt JWM. Choreoathetotic movement disorder in alcoholism. Br Med J 1970;4:278–281.

305. Neiman J, Lang AE, Fornazzari L, Carlen PL. Movement disorders in alcoholism: a review. Neurology 1990;40:741–746.

306. Luijckx GJ, Nieuwhof C, Troost J, Weber WE. Parkinsonism in alcohol withdrawal: case report and review of the literature. Clin Neurol Neurosurg 1995;97:336–339.

307. Corsini GU, Zuddas A, Bonuccelli U, et al. 1-Methyl-4-phenyl-1,2,3,6-tetrahydropyridine (MPTP) neurotoxicity in mice is enhanced by ethanol or acetaldehyde. Life Sci 1987;40:827–832.

308. Neimann J, Borg S, Wahlund LO. Parkinsonism and dyskinesia during ethanol withdrawal. Br J Addict 1988;83:437–439.

309. Shandling M, Carlen PL, Lang AE. Parkinsonism in alcohol withdrawal: a follow-up study. Mov Disord 1990;5:36–39.

310. Rudd P, Blaschke TF. Antihypertensive agents and the drug therapy of hypertension. In: Gilman AG, Goodman LS, Rall TW, Murad F, eds. The pharmacologic basis of therapeutics. New York: Macmillan, 1985:784–805.

311. Yamadori A, Albert ML. Involuntary movement disorder caused by methyldopa. N Engl J Med 1972;286:610.

312. Jaffee JH, Martin WR. Opioid analgesics and antagonists. In: Gilman AG, Goodman L, Rall TW, Murad F, eds. The pharmacologic basis of therapeutics. New York: Macmillan, 1985:491–531.

313. Lieberman AN, Goldstein M. Reversible parkinsonism related to meperidine. N Engl J Med 1984;312:509–510.

314. Eldridge R, Rocca WA. The clinical syndrome of striatal dopamine deficiency: parkinsonism induced by MPTP. N Engl J Med 1985;313:1159–1160.

315. Langston JW, Ballard P, Tetrud JW, et al. Chronic parkinsonism in humans due to a product of meperidine-analog synthesis. Science 1983;219:979–980.

316. Davis GC, Williams AC, Markey SP, et al. Chronic parkinsonism secondary to intravenous injection of meperidine analogues. Psychiatry Res 1979;1:249–254.

317. Langston JW, Ballard P. Parkinsonism induced by 1-methyl-4-phenyl-1,2,3,6-tetrahydropyridine (MPTP): implications for treatment and the pathogenesis of Parkinson's disease. Can J Neurol Sci 1984;11:160–165.

318. Langston JW. MPTP Neurotoxicity: an overview and characterization of phases of toxicity. Life Sci 1985;36:201–206.

319. Wright JM, Wall RA, Perry TL, et al. Chronic parkinsonism secondary to intranasal administration of a product of meperidine-analogue synthesis. N Engl J Med 1984;310:325.

320. Langston JW, Ballard PA. Parkinson's disease in a chemist walking with MPTP. N Engl J Med 1983;309:310.

321. Snyder SH, D'Amato RJ. MPTP: a neurotoxin relevant to the pathophysiology of Parkinson's disease. Neurology 1986;36:250–258.

322. Langston JW. MPTP: The promise of a new neurotoxin. In: Marsden CD, Fahn S, eds. Movement disorders 2. Boston: Butterworth, 1987:73–90.

323. Calne DB, Langston JW, Martin WR, et al. Observations relating to the cause of Parkinson's disease. PET scans after MPTP. Nature 1985;317:246–248.

324. Zornberg GL, Bodkin JA, Cohen BM. Severe adverse interaction between pethidine and selegiline. Lancet 1991;337:246.

325. Dommissee CS, Devane CL. Buspirone: a new type of anxiolytic. Drug Intell Clin Pharm 1985;19:624–628.

326. Taylor DP, Riblet LA, Stanton HC, et al. Dopamine and anti-anxiety activity. Pharmacology Biochem Behav 1982;17(suppl 1):25–35.

327. Hammerstad JP, Carter J, Nutt JG, et al. Buspirone in Parkinson's disease. Clin Neuropharmacol 1986;9:556–560.

328. Weintraub M, Standish R. Buspirone: a chemically and pharmacologically distinct anti-anxiety agent. Hosp Form 1984;19:203–207.

329. McMiller BA, Matthews RT, Sanghera MK, et al. Dopamine receptor antagonism by the novel anti-anxiety drug buspirone. J Neuroscience 1982;3:733–738.

330. Goldberg HL. Buspirone hydrochloride: a unique new anxiolytic agent: pharmacokinetics, clinical pharmacology, abuse potential and clinical efficacy. Pharmacother 1983;4:315–324.

331. Ludwig CL, Weingerger DR, Bruno G, et al. Buspirone, Parkinson's disease and the locus ceruleus. Clin Neuropharmacol 1986;9:373–378.

332. Strauss A. Oral dyskinesia associated with buspirone use in an elderly woman. J Clin Psychiatry 1988;49:322–323.

333. Patterson JF. Akathisia associated with buspirone. J Clin Psychopharmacol 1988;8:296–297.

334. Boylan K. Persistent dystonia associated with buspirone. Neurology 1990;40:1904.

335. Ritchie EC, Bridenbaugh RH, Jabbari B. Acute generalized myoclonus following buspirone administration. J Clin Psychiatry 1988;49:242–243.

336. LeWitt PA, Walters A, Hening W, McHale D. Persistent movement disorders induced by buspirone. Mov Disord 1993;8:331–334.

337. Lamberts SW, MacLeod RM. The interaction of the serotonergic and dopaminergic systems on prolactin secretion in the rat. Endocrinology 1978;103:287–295.

338. Bernick C. Methysergide-induced akathisia. Clin Neuropharmacol 1988;11:87–89.

339. Fernando SJM, Chir B. An attack of chorea complicating oral contraceptive therapy. Practitioner 1966;197:210–211.

340. Gamboa ET, Isaacs G, Harter DH. Chorea associated with oral contraceptive therapy. Arch Neurol 1971;25:112–114.

341. Nausieda PA, Koller WC, Weiner WJ, et al. Chorea induced by oral contraceptives. Neurology 1979;29:1605–1609.

342. Pulsinelli WA, Hamill RW. Chorea complicating oral contraceptive therapy: case report and review of the literature Am J Med 1978;65:557–559.

343. Green PM. Chorea induced by oral contraceptives. Neurology 1980;30:1131–1132.

344. Dove DJ. Chorea associated with oral contraceptive therapy. Am J Obstet Gynecol 1980;137:740–742.

345. Wadlington WB, Erlendson LW, Burr LM. Chorea associated with the use of oral contraceptives: report of a case and review of the literature. Clin Pediatr 1981;20:804–806.

346. Willson P, Preece A. Chorea gravidarum. Arch Intern Med 1932;49:524.

347. Driesen JJM, Wolters EC. Oral contraceptive-induced paraballism. Clin Neurol Neurosurg 1987;89:49–51.

348. Handler CE, Besse C, Wilson AO. Extrapyramidal and cerebellar syndrome with encephalopathy associated with cimetidine. Postgrad Med J 1982;58:527–528.

349. Romisher S, Feller R, Dougherty J, et al. Tagamet^R-induced acute dystonia. Ann Emerg Med 1987;16:1162–1164.

350. Kushner MJ. Chorea and cimetidine. Ann Intern Med 1982;96:126.

351. O'Sullivan RL, Greenberg DB. H₂ antagonists, restless leg syndrome and movement disorders. Psychosomatics 1993;34:530–532.

352. Davis BJ, Aul EA, Granner MA, Rodnitzky RL. Ranitidine-induced cranial dystonia. Clin Neuropharmacol 1994;17:489–491.

353. Lehmann AB. Reversible chorea due to ranitidine and cimetidine. Lancet 1988;2:158.

354. Ward A, Brogden RN, Heel RC, et al. Etretinate: a review of its pharmacological properties and therapeutic efficacy in psoriasis and other skin disorders. Drugs 1983;26:9–43.

355. Albin RL, Silverman AK, Ellis EN, et al. A new syndrome of axial muscle rigidity associated with etretinate therapy. Mov Disord 1988;3:70–76.

356. DiGiovanna JJ, Helfgott RK, Gerber LH, et al. Extraspinal tendon and ligament calcification associated with long-term therapy with etretinate. N Engl J Med 1986;315:1177–1182.

357. Casey DE. Tardive dyskinesia. In: Meltzer HY, ed. Psychopharmacology: the third generation of progress. New York: Raven, 1987:1416–1419.

358. Carlsson A. Monoamines of the central nervous system: a historical perspective. In: Meltzer HY, ed. Psychopharmacology: the third generation of progress. New York: Raven, 1987:39–48.

359. Ross SB, Renyi AL. In vitro inhibition of 3H–noradrenaline uptake by reserpine and tetrabenazine in mouse cerebral cortex tissues. Acta Pharmacol Toxicol 1966;24:73–88.

360. Pletscher A, Brossi A, Gey KF. Benzoquinolizine derivatives: a new case of monoamine decreasing drugs with psychotropic action. Int Rev Neurobiol 1962;4:275–306.

361. Tomlinson DR. The mode of action of tetrabenazine on peripheral noradrenergic neurons. Br J Pharmacol 1977;61:339–344.

362. Rushkevich IUE. Age characteristics of the development of a reserpine model of parkinsonism in rats. Bull Eksp Biol Med 1987;104:654–657.

363. Hitri A, Weiner WJ, Barison RL, et al. Dopamine binding following prolonged haloperidol treatment. Ann Neurol 1978;3:134–140.

364. Alphs LD, Davis JM. Cholinergic treatments for tardive dyskinesia. Mod Probl Pharmacopsychiatry 1983;21:168–186.

365. Rupniak NMJ, Briggs RS, Petersen MM, et al. Differential alterations in striatal acetylcholine function in rats during 12 months' continuous administration of haloperidol, sulpiride or clozapine. Clin Neuropharmacol 1986;9:282–292.

366. Coward DM. Classical and nonclassical neuroleptics induce supersensitivity of nigral GABAergic mechanism induce supersensitivity of nigral GABAergic mechanisms in the rat. Psychopharmacology 1982;78:180.

367. Treisman GJ, Muirhead N, Gnegy ME. Increased sensitivity of adenylate cyclase activity in the striatum of the rat to calmodulin and GppNHp after chronic treatment with haloperidol. Neuropharmacology 1986;25:587–595.

368. Jeste DV, Doongaji DR, Linnoila M. Elevated cerebrospinal fluid noradrenaline in tardive dyskinesia. Br J Psychiatry 1984;144:177–180.

369. Scheel-Kruger T, Annt J. New aspects of the role of dopamine, acetylcholine and GABA in the development of tardive dyskinesia. In: Casey DE, Chase T, Christensen AV, Gerlach J, eds. Dyskinesia: research and treatment. Berlin: Springer-Verlag, 1995:46–59.

370. DeKeyser J. Excitotoxic mechanisms may be involved in the pathophysiology of tardive dyskinesia. Clin Neuropharmacol 1991;14:565–568.

371. Mitchell IJ, Crossman AR, Liminga U, et al. Regional changes in 2-deoxy-glucose uptake associated with neuroleptic-induced tardive dyskinesia in the Cebus monkey. Mov Disord 1992;7:32–37.

372. Cadet JL, Lohr JB, Jeste DV. Free radicals and tardive dyskinesia. Trends Neurosci 1986;9:107–108.

373. Cadet JL, Kahler LA. Free radical mechanisms in schizophrenia and tardive dyskinesia. Neuroscience Biobehav Rev 1994;18:457–467.

374. Pall HS, Blake DR, Williams AC, et al. Evidence of enhanced lipid perioxidation in the cerebrospinal fluid of patients taking phenothiazines. Lancet 1987;2:596–599.

375. Cadenas E, Ginsberg M, Rabe U, et al. Evaluation of alpha-tocopherol antioxidant activity in microsomal lipid perioxidation as detected by low level chemiluminescence. Biochem J 1984;223:755–759.

376. Lohr JB, Cadet JL, Lohr MA, et al. Alpha-tocopherol in tardive dyskinesia. Lancet 1987;2:913–914.

377. Dabiri LM, Pasta D, Darby JK, Mosbacher D. Effectiveness of vitamin E for treatment of long-term tardive dyskinesia. Am J Psychiatry 1994;151:925–926.

378. Egan MF, Hyde TM, Albers GW, et al. Treatment of tardive dyskinesia with vitamin E. Am J Psychiatry 1992;149:773–777.

379. Al-Deeb S, Al-Moutaery K, Bruyn GW, Tariq BM. Neuroprotective effect of selenium: iminodipropionitrite-induced toxicity. J Psychiatry Neurosci 1995;20:189–192.

380. Jankovic J. Drug-induced and other orofacial-cervical dyskinesias. Ann Intern Med 1981;94:788–793.

Tardive Dyskinesia

JOHN M. KANE

INTRODUCTION

The introduction of effective medications for the treatment of schizophrenia and other psychoses remains a major advance in twentieth-century medicine. The value of antipsychotic agents in both the acute and long-term treatment of schizophrenia has been established in numerous placebo-controlled, double-blind trials (1,2). However, these drugs are also capable of producing a variety of adverse effects among the most common of which are neurologic (3).

These chemicals were initially labeled "neuroleptic" because of their tendency to produce acute extrapyramidal side effects, and initially some clinicians and investigators felt this was an essential characteristic of a drug that would have therapeutic activity in the treatment of schizophrenia. Since that time the association between "neuroleptic" effect and clinical efficacy has been largely, though not completely, abandoned.

Within five years after the introduction of antipsychotic drugs, Schonecker (4) described the occurrence of tardive dyskinesia (TD) as an involuntary movement disorder characterized by a variable mixture of the following: orofacial and lingual dyskinesia, tics, grimacing, truncal or axial muscle involvement, chorea, athetosis, and dystonias. Speech and respiration may also be affected. Since the early description of this syndrome in the late 1950s, there have been numerous prevalence surveys in various populations (5,6). Prevalence estimates have varied enormously and a variety of methodologic problems have made it difficult to establish estimates of true prevalence with any degree of confidence.

There are no reliable and well-validated strategies for identifying a true case of TD, and a variety of neuromedical conditions may produce abnormal involuntary move-ments that may be difficult to distinguish from TD. There continues to be some controversy as to what extent antipsychotic drug treatment is necessary or sufficient to produce abnormal involuntary movements in some psychiatric patients (7).

The existence of so-called spontaneous dyskinesias has been suggested and some investigators have proposed that the schizophrenic illness itself may result in such disorders of movement without any exposure to antipsychotic drugs (7).

Though this remains a difficult issue to address methodologically (as most individuals with diagnosed cases of schizophrenia have at least some exposure to neuroleptics), there are several lines of evidence that implicate antipsychotic drugs as playing an important role in either producing or precipitating abnormal involuntary movements. First, in those studies that have compared drug-treated and drug-naive patients, the overwhelming majority find a significantly higher prevalence of abnormal movements among drug-treated populations (5,6). Second, those prospective studies that have been conducted indicate an increasing cumulative incidence of TD with increasing durations of drug exposure (8–12). And third, the likelihood of TD improving or remitting completely is substantially increased when antipsychotic drugs are discontinued or reduced in dosage.

In addition, many reviews have concluded that the prevalence of TD has increased over the last two decades, which might result from the fact that an increasing number of patients have been exposed to neuroleptics for longer intervals, as their widespread clinical use only dates back 25 to 30 years. It is important to note that reported rates of spontaneous dyskinesia have also increased during this time, suggesting that increased diagnostic sensitivity may have contributed to an apparent increase in prevalence. It is certainly possible that both a true increase and a further perceived increase have occurred simultaneously.

Other findings that bear upon the role of antipsychotic drugs in the development of TD include the fact that abnormal involuntary movements that appear similar to TD are rarely seen in untreated, first-episode schizophrenics (J. Lieberman and J. Kane, unpublished data) and that patients with a variety of other psychiatric conditions as well as nonpsychiatric patients have developed TD when chronically treated with antipsychotic medication (13). It would be safe to conclude that the epidemiologic data implicating neuroleptic drugs as playing a major role in the development of TD is compelling.

DIAGNOSIS

The most common clinical presentation of TD involves the buccolingual masticatory syndrome. Patients may exhibit lip smacking, tongue movements, and chewing as well as grimacing or other movements involving facial muscles. TD may also involve the neck, axial, and extremity musculature as well. Tardive dystonia occurs much less frequently but has been reported particularly in patients who are not schizophrenic, but who are treated with neuroleptics.

Disorders of movement in patients with schizophrenia were described in the preneuroleptic era and considerable controversy has surrounded the question of whether dyskinesias such as chorea and athetosis occur "spontaneously" in patients with schizophrenia or whether these movements are more appropriately characterized as "mannerism" or "stereotypies."

As Marsden et al have emphasized (14), confusion in the use of descriptive terminology has been a consistent problem in this area. In addition, a variety of neurologic conditions that are capable of producing abnormal movements may also be associated with dementias or schizophreniform psychoses. The extent to which these conditions may have been included in the preneuroleptic descriptions of movement disorders in "schizophrenic" patients is obviously impossible to ascertain.

One critical step for any physician prescribing neuroleptic drugs for a patient, particularly for the first time, is to carefully examine the patient for preexisting abnormal movements and to take a complete medical and neurologic history. The documentation of the resulting information can prove extremely useful in the differential diagnosis of any movements that might subsequently occur. In addition, patients should be regularly examined by a physician (or other trained professional) to identify the occurrence of abnormal movements so that their nature and mode of onset can be documented.

If abnormal movements do occur in the context of neuroleptic drug treatment, we have proposed diagnostic criteria to help facilitate communication between investigators, but this framework might be useful in helping to document clinical impressions as well (15).

There are no definitive tests for establishing a diagnosis of TD and as indicated a variety of neuromedical conditions may produce abnormal movements that might be mistaken for TD.

In order to rule out other etiologies, a variety of clinical laboratory or other procedures can be helpful. Although we would in no way minimize the importance of identifying other causes of abnormal movements, it should be recognized that in the overwhelming majority of cases no alternative etiology will be identified (16).

MANAGEMENT

The management of TD depends to a great extent on the nature of the psychiatric condition for which neuroleptic drugs were initially prescribed. If the patient has an illness other than schizophrenia and can be treated with an effective alternative to neuroleptic drugs, then discontinuation of the neuroleptic drug is clearly indicated. In the case of patients with schizophrenia or other psychosis for which efficacious alternative treatments are not available, the management of TD becomes much more complicated.

No proven safe and effective treatments for TD have been established and the single most desirable management strategy is neuroleptic drug discontinuation. In patients with schizophrenia, the treatment of the psychiatric illness must be considered in conjunction with the management of TD. It is beyond the scope of this chapter to review the role of neuroleptic medication in the treatment of schizophrenia, but these agents remain the mainstay of medical management for this illness. In individuals who have well-diagnosed schizophrenia and have experienced two or more psychotic episodes, the risk of psychotic relapse in the year following neuroleptic drug discontinuation is greater than 50% (17); therefore, the management of TD must be approached in this context. In recent years it has also become clearer that TD is not always progressive in severity and that in a substantial proportion of patients some improvement may occur even with continued neuroleptic treatment, particularly if the dosage of the neuroleptic can be reduced. Many cases appear to reach a stable plateau of intensity at the mild level and this too must be considered in evaluating the relative risks and benefits of continued neuroleptic treatment. At the same time, the likelihood of some degree of persistence probably increases as neuroleptic drugs are continued for longer intervals after the development of TD. In addition, although severe and disabling cases represent the minority of patients with TD, these severe subtypes do occur and at present we are unable to identify those cases most likely to progress to this stage. Therefore, caution is advisable in all patients. A clear documentation of the clinical data and judgment process should be available in the medical record as well as a statement that informed consent has been obtained from the patient (and significant others when appropriate).

In terms of treatments specifically directed toward TD, an extensive series of compounds have been tested (with varying degrees of methodologic rigor) and in general none has been found to have consistent reproducible therapeutic activity (18). As some agents (e.g., neuroleptic drugs themselves) are capable of suppressing or masking the condition, it is critical to discriminate this effect from a true therapeutic effect by examining the course of the dyskinesia once the experimental treatment agent has been discontinued. In the case of neuroleptic drugs, one would expect to see a rebound in severity or a re-emergence of involuntary movements.

Treatment strategies have been largely influenced by theories of pathophysiology with major emphasis having been placed on the dopamine receptor supersensitivity hypothesis. The assumption that a reduction in dopaminergic activity would lead to a reduction in abnormal movements suggests the potential "therapeutic" effect of dopamine receptor antagonists (neuroleptics), dopamine depletors (reserpine, tretrabenazine), or a downregulation strategy employing dopamine agonists (L-dopa or bromocriptine). Alternatively, increasing cholinergic activity with putative cholinergic agonists (choline, lecithin) or cholinesterase inhibitors (physostigmine) should also improve TD if this theory is relevant. More recently a gamma-aminobutyric acid (GABA) deficiency hypothesis has fostered the use of putative GABA agonists (gamma-vinyl GABA, benzodiazepines, progabide). In general, response to pharmacologic agents in TD is very heterogeneous, suggesting that current pathophysiologic hypotheses are overly simplistic, that the condition is heterogeneous, or that the compounds available are inadequate to achieve the specific neurochemical effects desired. (It is likely that all three are true.)

The inconsistent and unimpressive results from most therapeutic trials may also be due in part to a variety of methodologic problems. Many studies are small and uncontrolled, and may not necessarily include those patients most likely to respond to a relatively short-term treatment (e.g., duration of TD may be an important determinant of potential treatment response).

The basic therapeutic strategy depends largely on the nature and severity of the dyskinesia as well as the underlying condition for which neuroleptic drugs were initially prescribed. In a patient for whom neuroleptic drug discontinuation is feasible, this is the ideal strategy. If a patient requires neuroleptic treatment, then dosage reduction to the extent possible is highly desirable. In severe or disabling forms of the condition, an experimental treatment may be called for; however, at this point there are not sufficient data to suggest a specific order of experimental treatments.

There has been considerable controversy as to whether a specific neuroleptic or neuroleptic class is indicated for those patients who have developed TD but require continued neuroleptic administration. Our impression is that among drugs currently marketed in the United States there are no established differences. (Such differences may exist, but they have not been established in well-designed, well-controlled clinical trials.) Clozapine may prove to be an exception in

that the incidence of TD (if any) appears to be considerably lower with this compound (J. Kane, unpublished data) and this might make it an appropriate antipsychotic drug for patients with TD (but the apparent increased risk of agranulocytosis must also be considered).

RISK FACTORS

Given the lack of effective treatments for TD, prevention remains an important goal. Considerable effort has gone into the identification of risk factors or individual characteristics that might predispose specific patients to the development of TD. In general, this is an area plagued with methodologic pitfalls, but some conclusions are possible. Increasing age appears to substantially increase the risk of TD (given the same degree of neuroleptic exposure). In addition, increasing degree of severity and persistence are found among older individuals.

Although some investigators have suggested that abnormal involuntary movements are also seen relatively frequently among older individuals who have not been treated with neuroleptics, in our experience if one focuses on healthy elderly subjects the prevalence of abnormal movements is quite low (16,19). On the other hand, if patients with a variety of neuromedical illnesses requiring inpatient treatment or chronic nursing care are examined, the prevalence of abnormal movements is much higher (16). The highest rates by far, however, are found among elderly individuals who have also been treated with neuroleptic drugs.

Female gender has also been associated with higher prevalence rates of TD, but this association is seen primarily in the fifth through seventh decade suggesting the possibility that endocrine changes associated with menopause may play a role; however, no definitive pathophysiologic explanation has been established.

Psychiatric diagnosis is difficult to study as a risk factor, but several reports do suggest a higher incidence, increased severity, and possibly greater degrees of persistence of TD among patients with affective illness who are treated with neuroleptic drugs (20,21). As previously discussed, this would certainly argue that TD is not a manifestation of schizophrenia mistakenly attributed to neuroleptic drugs. In addition, this association might provide an important clue to factors producing individual vulnerability, as it is assumed that affective illness and schizophrenia have different neurochemical substrates. This association should also be the basis to urge clinicians to be very cautious in using neuroleptic drugs to treat nonpsychotic conditions that may be responsive to other pharmacologic therapies.

Data from our ongoing prospective study (8) suggest that patients who develop clinically significant acute parkinsonian side effects are also more likely to subsequently develop TD. This association may have implications for further understanding of pathophysiology and identification of individuals at particular risk.

Duration of neuroleptic treatment and cumulative dosage contribute to the risk of TD, but this association has been difficult to document in cross-sectional prevalence surveys with retrospective assessment of drug history. The increasing incidence with increasing years of neuroleptic exposure supports this as a factor, and studies that involve random assignment to different guaranteed dosage levels of neuroleptic medication also suggest that dosage is important (22). Given the fact that not all patients have the same vulnerability to TD and that there are also enormous individual differences in compliance as well as absorption and metabolism of neuroleptic drugs, it is not surprising that the association between neuroleptic dose and/or duration of neuroleptic treatment and TD risk has been difficult to demonstrate with the methodology that has generally been employed.

CENTRAL NERVOUS SYSTEM DYSFUNCTION

Although it is assumed that schizophrenia and many other mental disorders are due to central nervous system dysfunction the question has been asked as to whether or not those patients with demonstrable "organic" findings may be more vulnerable to TD than those without such objective findings. In general, the methodology employed in exploring this association has varied enormously and has included measures such as history of epilepsy, alcoholism, leucotomy, electroencephalography, computerized tomography, and neuropsychologic testing. Although there is relatively little consistency in results, some studies do suggest an association and this is an area requiring further research.

SCHIZOPHRENIA SUBTYPES AND TD

It has been suggested that patients with so-called negative symptoms (e.g., emotional withdrawal, blunted affect, poverty of speech, psychomotor retardation) are more likely to manifest abnormal movements both with and without chronic exposure to neuroleptics (23). Although several studies have reported such an association, here too a variety of methodologic concerns prevent firm conclusions. For example, the differentiation of negative symptoms such as blunted affect and motor retardation from the neurologic effects of antipsychotic drugs (akinesia) is not always given adequate attention, and if drug-induced parkinsonism is evidence of increased vulnerability to TD, then this relationship might involve other factors as well.

PATHOPHYSIOLOGY

Involvement of dopaminergic systems in TD has been assumed on the basis of a variety of observations:

1. the epidemiologic data implicating dopamine receptor antagonists in the etiology of TD is compelling;
2. the fact that increasing dosages of neuroleptic drugs may suppress some manifestations of TD and decreasing doses may produce exacerbation;

3. many aspects of TD symptomatology can be produced in patients with Parkinson's disease by the administration of L-dopa; and
4. administration of dopamine agonists to patients with TD can in some cases cause an increase in symptoms.

All of these observations suggest that an increase in dopamine receptor sensitivity is playing some role in the pathophysiology of TD. Animal experiments have supported the notion that chronic administration of dopamine receptor antagonists, by depriving receptors of their usual level of stimulation, can create a situation analogous to denervation postsynaptic receptor supersensitivity (24).

The question remains, however, as to what extent this phenomenon accounts for the development of clinical TD. In animals, all typical neuroleptic drugs are capable of producing dopamine receptor hypersensitivity as measured by increased stereotypic response to dopamine agonists such as apomorphine or increase in receptor binding sites for dopamine type 2 (D_2) ligands (in vitro). In humans, however, not all patients exposed to these drugs in equal amounts for equal intervals develop TD. It is also important to note that the dopamine receptor hypersensitivity that can be produced in animals occurs in a matter of weeks; on the other hand, the clinical condition in humans is usually not apparent for months or years.

Chronic neuroleptic treatment may affect a variety of neurochemical systems other than dopaminergic ones, for example, acetylcholine, serotonin, and alpha-adrenergic systems. In addition, GABAergic and peptidergic neurons are affected by and may affect dopaminergic function in specific brain areas such as the basal ganglia. The extent to which alterations in these other systems may be involved in the development of clinical TD is of enormous importance. Gunne et al (25) reported a decrease in glutamic acid decarboxylase activity in postmortem tissue from the substantia nigra in monkeys who had developed TD symptoms after chronic neuroleptic treatment but not in those monkeys who had not exhibited that type of abnormal involuntary movement.

The fact that evidence implicating dopamine receptor hypersensitivity has involved D_2 receptors is also important when considering the observation that some "atypical" neuroleptics have not been associated with the development of TD (i.e., clozapine). It has been suggested that dopamine type 1 (D_1) receptor effects may be important in modulating D_2 receptor function and that the balance of D_1 and D_2 effects within a particular drug may determine its propensity to produce TD (26).

There remain many unanswered questions regarding the pathophysiology of TD and it is also important to consider that TD (much like the diseases for which neuroleptic drugs are used to treat) is a heterogeneous condition. Those studies (27) utilizing pharmacologic probes in patients with clinical TD suggest that response is not consistent across patients suggesting that an all-encompassing neurochemical hypothesis may be unrealistic.

PREVENTION

Given the fact that there are no proven safe and effective treatments for TD, prevention remains a critical goal. Clearly, neuroleptic drugs should be reserved for those clinical indications where no other equally effective but less toxic treatments are available. In addition, for those patients who do receive a course of neuroleptic treatment, there should be adequate evidence (and documentation) of clinical benefit and ongoing evaluation of need and benefit. It is important that all patients be examined for the presence of abnormal involuntary movements before the introduction of neuroleptic drugs in order to ensure recognition and documentation of any preexisting movement disorders. When neuroleptic drugs are indicated, they should be employed in the lowest dose and for the shortest duration possible (though certainly many schizophrenic patients require continuous neuroleptic treatment). Dosage requirements may vary between individuals and even for a given individual depending upon the phase of the illness. In recent years we have seen the introduction of various dosage reduction strategies for the long-term use of neuroleptics, and in a subgroup of patients very low doses of neuroleptic drugs may be sufficiently effective in preventing major psychotic relapse. A variety of factors may, however, influence the success of such strategies and clinicians (and patients) should be informed as to the potential benefits and risks.

Given the importance of advancing age, particular caution should be employed when utilizing these drugs in elderly populations. This is all the more important since the role of neuroleptics in many aspects of geriatric psychiatry has not been well studied. Preliminary data from our ongoing prospective study of TD development in the elderly (28) suggests that the incidence of TD may be fourfold to fivefold greater among elderly patients as compared with younger adults given the same duration of treatment.

It is also critical that neuroleptic-treated patients be examined at regular intervals for the presence of abnormal movements as the outcome of TD, once it develops, may be influenced by the promptness with which neuroleptic drugs are discontinued or dosage reduced.

Given our current state of knowledge, it is inevitable that some individuals will develop TD even with our best efforts at prevention. It is important that patients and their families be informed as to the potential benefits and risks of long-term neuroleptic treatment and that this process be documented in the medical records and periodically reviewed and repeated.

ACKNOWLEDGMENTS

This research was supported by NIMH grants MH-31776; MH-32369; MH-40015; MH-41960 and contract 278-81-0032.

REFERENCES

1. Klein DF, Davis JM. Diagnosis and Drug Treatment of Psychiatric Disorders. Baltimore: Williams & Wilkins, 1969.
2. Davis JM, Schaffer CB, Killian GA, Kinard C, Chan C. Important issues in the drug treatment of schizophrenia. Schizophr Bull 1980;6:70–87.
3. Marsden CD, Tarsy D, Baldessarini RJ. Spontaneous and drug induced movement disorders in psychotic patients. In: Benson DF, Bloomer D, eds. Psychiatric Aspects of Neurologic Disease. New York: Grune & Stratton, 1975:219–266.
4. Schonecker M. Ein eigentumliches Syndrom im oralen Bereich bei Megaphen Applikation. Nervenarzt 1957;28:35.
5. Jeste DV, Wyatt RJ. Understanding and Treating Tardive Dyskinesia. New York: Guilford, 1982.
6. Kane JM, Smith JM. Tardive dyskinesia: prevalence and risk factors, 1959 to 1979. Arch Gen Psychiatry 1982;39:473–481.
7. Owens DGC, Johnstone EC, Frith CD. Spontaneous involuntary disorders of movement: their prevalence, severity and distribution in chronic schizophrenics with and without treatment with neuroleptics. Arch Gen Psychiatry 1982;39:452–461.
8. Kane JM, Woerner M, Weinhold P, et al. Incidence of tardive dyskinesia: five-year data from a prospective study. Psychopharmacol Bull 1984;20:39–40.
9. Barron ET, McCreadie RG. One year follow-up of tardive dyskinesia. Br J Psychiatry 1983;143:423–424.
10. Yassa R, Nair V, Schwartz G. Tardive dyskinesia: a two year follow-up study. Psychosomatics 1984;25:852–855.
11. Chouinard G, Annable L, Mercier R, Ross-Chouinard A. A five year follow-up study of tardive dyskinesia. Psychopharmacol Bull 1986;22:259–263.
12. Barnes TRE, Kidger T, Gore SM. Tardive dyskinesia: a three year follow-up study. Psychol Med 1983;13:71–81.
13. Kane JM, Struve FA, Weinhold P, Woerner M. Strategy for the study of patients at high risk for tardive dyskinesia. Am J Psychiatry 1980;137:1265–1267.
14. Marsden CD. Is tardive dyskinesia a unique disorder? In: Casey DE, Chase TN, Christensen AV, Gerlach J, eds. Dyskinesia: Research and Treatment. Berlin: Springer-Verlag, 1985:64–71.
15. Schooler NR, Kane JM. Research diagnoses for tardive dyskinesia. Arch Gen Psychiatry 1982;39:486–487.
16. Woerner M, Kane JM, Lieberman JA, et al. The prevalence of tardive dyskinesia. J Clin Psychopharmacol 1991;11:34–42.
17. Kane JM, Lieberman J. Maintenance pharmacotherapy in schizophrenia. In: Meltzer HY, ed. Psychopharmacology: The Third Generation of Progress. New York: Raven, 1987:1103–1109.
18. Jeste DV, Wyatt RJ. Therapeutic strategies against tardive dyskinesia. Arch Gen Psychiatry 1982;39:803–816.
19. Kane JM, Weinhold P, Kinon B, et al. Prevalence of abnormal involuntary movements ("spontaneous dyskinesias") in the normal elderly. Psychopharmacology 1982;77:105–108.
20. Davis K, Berger P, Hollister L. Tardive dyskinesia and depressive illness. Psychopharmacol Comm 1976;2:125.
21. Rosenbaum AH, Niven RG, Hansen HP, Swanson DW. Tardive dyskinesia: relationship with primary affective disorders. Dis Nerv Syst 1977;38:423–426.
22. Kane JM, Rifkin A, Woerner M, et al. Low-dose neuroleptic treatment of outpatient schizophrenics. Arch Gen Psychiatry 1983;40:893–896.
23. Barnes TRE. Tardive dyskinesia: risk factors, pathophysiology and treatment. In: Granuille-Grossman K. Recent Advances in Clinical Psychiatry. London: Churchill Livingstone, 1988:185–207.
24. Jenner P, Marsden CD. Neuroleptic induced tardive dyskinesia. Acta Psychiatr Belg 1987;87:566–598.
25. Gunne L-M, Haggstrom JE, Sjoquist B. Association with persistent neuroleptic-induced dyskinesia of regional changes in brain GABA synthesis. Nature 1984;309:347–349.
26. Christensen AV, Arnt J, Svendsen O. Pharmacological differentiation of dopamine D-1 and D-2 antagonists after single and repeated administration. In: Casey DE, Chase TN, Christensen AV, Gerlach J, eds. Dyskinesia: Research and Treatment. Berlin: Springer-Verlag, 1985:182–190.
27. Lieberman JA, Pollack S, Lesser M, Kane J. Pharmacologic characterization of tardive dyskinesia. J Clin Psychopharmacol 1988;8:254–260.
28. Saltz BL, Kane JM, Woerner MG, et al. Prospective study of TD in the elderly. JAMA 1991;266:2402–2406.

Severe Tardive Dyskinesia

George Gardos   Jonathan O. Cole

INTRODUCTION

Tardive dyskinesia (TD) has emerged as the principal risk of long-term neuroleptic (NL) therapy by virtue of its considerable prevalence (see previous chapter), its potential for progression to severe and incapacitating degrees, and its occasional irreversibility. In one of the early reports of TD, for instance, Hunter et al (1) provide vivid clinical vignettes of chronic NL-treated patients with continuous grimacing, writhing of the tongue, and jaw and lip movements, together with speech and respiratory dyskinesia and distress over the continual movements. Until recently, studies of severe TD involving cohorts of afflicted patients have been unavailable because, fortunately, severe dyskinesia seemed rare enough for only tertiary referral centers to have accumulated sufficient numbers of cases. More recently, several review articles of severe TD have appeared (2–6). The focus of this chapter is on severe choreoathetoid dyskinesia. Tardive dystonia and tardive akathisia, which often coexist with and at times overshadow choreoathetoid movements in terms of greater incapacitation and/or distress, are dealt with in separate chapters of this volume.

EPIDEMIOLOGY

The best prevalence estimates of severe dyskinesia are provided by a handful of studies that report separate figures for varying levels of TD severity. Integrating data from these studies is hampered by the widely varying criteria of what constitutes severe TD.

Brandon et al (7) found 14 patients (1.5%) with severe facial dyskinesia (global ratings) in a cohort of 910 chronic hospitalized patients. Edwards (8) reported a 12.2% (16 of 131) prevalence of severe oral dyskinesia by global ratings in a cohort of elderly hospitalized female patients. Gibson (9) assessed buccolingual masticatory movements in 374 outpatients receiving depot fluphenazine or flupenthixol over three years. The number of patients rated as severe remained constant at six (2.6%) throughout the study. Smith et al (10) defined severe TD as a score of 4 (severe) on any one of the Abnormal Involuntary Movements Scale (AIMS) items (11). Examination of 377 inpatients yielded a 6.8% prevalence of severe TD. Asnis et al (12) also employed AIMS but classified patients on the basis of minimal, mild, and moderate impairment. In a cohort of 69 outpatients, 4.3% showed moderate impairment. Wojcik et al (13) rated 210 inpatients and outpatients on AIMS. Using global severity ratings, two (1%) patients showed severe dyskinesia. McCreadie et al (14) examined 117 schizophrenic inpatients and outpatients using AIMS and found 1% with severe dyskinesia. Barnes et al (15) used percent time that dyskinesia was present as their severity criterion and found 10 of 88 (11.4%) severe TD among NL-treated inpatients and outpatients. Guy et al (16) reported a 1.9% prevalence of moderate or severe TD (AIMS global) in 739 chronic schizophrenics participating in an international survey. In the absence of uniform definition for severe TD, the best guess is that the prevalence in chronic NL-treated patients is likely to be in the 1% to 5% range. As the papers reviewed above included cases of tardive dystonia and akathisia, as well as severe choreoathetoid dyskinesia, the true prevalence of only the latter is considerably lower and probably closer to the 1% value. With the increasing clinical use of atypical NL such as risperidone and clozapine during the 1990s, these prevalence figures may be further reduced in future studies.

Individual vulnerability to developing severe TD may be approached by looking for association between patient characteristics and severe choreoathetosis. Age has been consistently associated with severity of TD in prevalence studies

(17). Older age was found to correlate with severe choreoathetoid dyskinesia but not with tardive dystonia (3,4). Brandon et al (7) found that of 14 patients with severe facial dyskinesia, only two were under 50 years and most were between 60 and 70 years of age. Female gender, an often reported but not clearly demonstrated risk factor of TD development (18), has been found to be associated with severe choreoathetoid dyskinesia in two studies (3,10). Diagnosis of affective disorder was found in the majority of severe dyskinesia patients (both choreoathetoid and dystonic) in the series by Gardos et al (4). Organic brain disease has also been proposed as a risk factor for severe orofacial dyskinesia (7,8,19). NL exposure has not been a readily identifiable risk factor. Gualtieri et al (20) found a significant correlation between cumulative NL dose and the development of severe TD in young mentally retarded individuals, and Crane (21) obtained positive correlations between cumulative NL dosage and TD duration and severity. Neither NL duration nor NL dosage, however, was found to be associated with severe TD in other published series of mostly adult psychiatric patients (2,3,7,15). Lithium treatment at onset of dyskinesia was associated with subsequent mild rather than severe TD (2), suggesting a possible protection by lithium against developing severe TD. However, Mann et al (22) described a case of severe dyskinesia developing rapidly after haloperidol was added to maintenance lithium treatment in a bipolar male patient. Other treatment variables such as electroconvulsive therapy, antiparkinsonian drugs, or duration of hospitalization have not been associated with severe TD (2,7).

CLINICAL FEATURES

Severe choreoathetoid dyskinesia differs from the milder forms, principally by the frequency and amplitude of the abnormal movements. Orofacial dyskinesia, mostly involving the tongue, jaw, and lips, is the most common manifestation of both mild and severe dyskinesia, while extremity and truncal dyskinesias are rarer (7,8,16). Moderate to severe dyskinesia of the upper limb occurred almost twice as frequently as lower limb dyskinesia in one study (16). Some cases of severe dyskinesia described in the literature consist of generalized choreoathetosis of the face, trunk, and all four limbs (4,22,23). Many instances of severe dyskinesia in addition to choreoathetoid movements include dystonic spasms (24–26), parkinsonism (27), and akathisia (7,28). Severe TD has also been reported in association with Tourette's syndrome (29) and with the NL malignant syndrome (30). From these reports, one may surmise that severe choreoathetoid dyskinesia may frequently coexist with other forms of dyskinesia.

Subjective distress appears to be a common accompaniment of severe dyskinesia. In the study by Wojcik et al (13), 9 of 37 TD patients (24.5%) complained of mild to moderate distress from their movements. Smith et al (31) report that of their 113 patients with a rating of "3" (moderate)

on any one AIMS item, only nine (8%) were aware of their TD symptoms and only four (3.5%) expressed any degree of distress. Guy et al (16) report higher figures: approximately 50% of patients satisfying research diagnostic criteria had some degree of awareness. Case reports vividly illustrate the anguish individual patients suffer from their severe movement disorder (26,32). Suicidal ideation may result from distress over the persisting severe dyskinesia and successful suicides have been reported (2,5,24). However, the relative contribution to suicidality of factors such as type of dyskinesia (choreoathetoid versus dystonic or akathisia) and the role of the underlying psychiatric disorder, often an affective illness with a sizeable suicide potential, is not easy to disentangle.

Mild TD rarely leads to complications. The same is not true for severe dyskinesia that may interfere with basic everyday functions depending on which body areas are involved. Wojcik et al (13) reported that 4 of 37 TD patients have shown mild to moderate incapacitation by their movements. Guy et al (16) found 11% of TD patients by research diagnostic criteria (33) to have been rated moderately or severely incapacitated. Catatonic schizophrenics with mannerisms had the highest prevalence of moderate or severe TD and the highest percentage of incapacity (16).

Severe oral dyskinesia may give rise to a variety of functional impairments. Constant tongue movements may loosen both natural and artificial teeth (5). Dysphagia may result from the forward thrust of the tongue during swallowing (34). Abnormal articulation in the form of muffled or indistinct speech is frequently observed in patients with severe TD (25,33,35). Lingual dyskinesia disrupting the normal positioning and movement of the tongue appears to be the basis for the dysarthria.

Respiratory dyskinesia is not uncommon. Yassa and Lal (36) reported respiratory irregularities in 8 of 108 TD patients (7.4%), the majority with an organic mental disorder. Weiner et al (37) and Ayd (38) described the prominent features as (a) shortness of breath at rest; (b) irregular breathing pattern; (c) involuntary grunting and gasping noises; (d) presence of marked facial and lingual dyskinesia; and (e) normal physical and laboratory tests (except for respiratory alkalosis). The abnormal respiration becomes worse during stress and improves during sleep (39).

Gastrointestinal complications of severe TD have been described by Yassa and Jones (5). Disturbance of the gag reflex as a result of TD and the use of anticholinergic drugs was reported by Craig et al (40). In addition to dysphagia due to lingual dyskinesia, disruption of the normal activity of the esophagus by TD led to severely impaired nutrition requiring gastrostomy in one patient (5). Vomiting after meals, episodes of retching, weight loss, aerophagia, and distention of the abdominal wall were observed in a patient where TD became a life-threatening illness (23). The authors treated one case where frequent gagging and choking led to severe eating difficulties and weight loss. However, weight loss is not a frequent complication of TD even when severe (41).

Abnormal gait as part of severe dyskinesia is cited in case reports (5,28,29). Simpson and Shrivastava (42) described the different gaits observed in 42 patients with at least moderately severe TD. Wide gait with a wide arm swing and unsteadiness was seen in seven patients, and spastic gait with the dragging of one foot was seen in two. Another nine patients showed abnormal gaits that were not typical of any described neurologic gait.

A more general impairment of instrumental functioning may result from the overall severity of the movement disorder. Occupational impairment is stressed by Yassa and Jones (5). Difficulties in performing work tasks due to TD need to be distinguished from the psychiatric illness and other NL side effects. Nevertheless, severe TD involving the trunk and upper and lower extremities often interferes with functioning in jobs requiring stamina, coordination of several muscle groups, or manual dexterity. Social embarrassment is frequently observed in patients with severe TD (5). Some patients are distressed by being stared at in public and are reluctant to leave home. The social stigmatization of TD as distinct from mental illness has been referred to (5).

Increased mortality due to TD has been suggested (43), but has not been substantiated (44,45).

COURSE AND OUTCOME

The onset of severe dyskinesia is in many instances rapid, at least in comparison with the usually slow insidious onset of typical cases of mild TD (2). Rapid onset of severe TD was also described in a lithium-treated bipolar patient after brief exposure to haloperidol (22).

The course and outcome of severe TD vary considerably. Every possible outcome from significant remission to unrelenting constant motion has been encountered. In our series (4), after an average of 62 months of observation, two of seven patients with severe choreoathetosis improved significantly, three changed little, and two became worse. However, one of the deteriorated patients subsequently showed a reversal and is now improved over baseline. Five of the seven patients had to remain on NL for treatment of their psychiatric disorder. Gimenez-Roldan et al (3) obtained better results in their 13 severe dyskinetic patients. In more than half (53.8%), the dyskinesia proved to be reversible while 61.5% of patients were successfully withdrawn from NL. Itoh and Yagi (46) reported better long-term outcome in patients with longer (more than eight years) than shorter term dyskinesia. Irreversibility, therefore, is not an inevitable consequence of either severe or of long-lasting TD.

TREATMENT OF SEVERE DYSKINESIA

The clinical management of patients with severe choreoathetoid dyskinesia is complex and challenging. Whereas most patients with mild TD only require periodic assessment for TD to ensure that no significant progression of the dyskinesia has occurred, severe dyskinesia calls for intervention to attempt to reduce the incapacitation and distress caused by the movement disorder. Having to treat concurrently the underlying psychiatric disorder (schizophrenia, affective disorder, organic brain disorder, etc.) places constraints on therapeutic approaches. For example, NL withdrawal, which intuitively appears the best strategy by virtue of removing the presumed causative agent, is not always feasible in the presence of an active psychotic illness (47). Furthermore, NL withdrawal tends to aggravate severe dyskinesia to an unacceptable and dangerous level, making urgent intervention usually in the form of reinstitution of NL drugs the only feasible procedure (23,24,26,48). Gradual withdrawal of NL with slow dose tapering is clinically more attractive, but whether the withdrawal is sudden or gradual, the results tend to be variable. Edwards (8) withdrew phenothiazines from 34 patients with moderate to severe oral dyskinesia. Of the 19 patients who were able to stay off NL, only one showed improvement after 10 to 12 months, while in five the dyskinesia became more severe. In our series of seven patients with severe choreoathetoid dyskinesia, one of the two patients who could be kept off NL improved (4). Itoh and Yagi (46) attempted to withdraw NL from 19 patients with persistent severe dyskinesia and found that "reinstitution of neuroleptic therapy was inevitable intermittently." At the same time, some of their cases showed marked remission of TD symptoms following NL discontinuation. Gimenez-Roldan et al (3) found that over half their severe choreoathetoid cases proved reversible after NL discontinuation.

Suppression of dyskinesia by NL is often effective, at least temporarily (23,24,26,48). Breakthrough of dyskinesia is theoretically possible, but we found no evidence of clinically obvious breakthrough of TD during an average 62 months of observation (4). A potential problem with using NL to suppress dyskinesia is the risk of inducing significant parkinsonian side effects (4,24,27,48). The tug-of-war between severe TD and severe parkinsonism at times becomes a most unappealing and unavoidable therapeutic dilemma: adjusting NL doses to a level that leaves both TD and parkinsonian symptoms obvious but tolerable is often the best compromise. NL suppression together with reserpine therapy was employed in a severe TD patient resulting in partial improvement (25).

Specific pharmacotherapy for severe choreoathetoid TD is practically nonexistent. Lennox et al (49) reported modest benefit from low-dose bromocriptine (0.75 to 7.5 mg) with NL in 12 patients with moderate to severe TD. This therapeutic effect was ascribed to the activity of bromocriptine at presynaptic dopaminergic receptor sites in the nigrostriatal system. Diltiazem, a calcium channel blocker, was found to be immediately effective in doses up to 360 mg daily in three patients with severe choreoathetoid TD (50). In general, drug treatment strategies for severe TD are not different from treating milder forms of TD. Reviews of TD treatment (51,52) emphasize the unsatisfactory and heterogeneous results of treatment trials with a variety of agents. We have achieved modest success with empirical and not always entirely rational combinations of low-dose NL, lithium, antiparkinsonian drugs, and benzodiazepines (4).

Atypical neuroleptics are recently introduced antipsychotic drugs with low propensity to cause parkinsonism and with marked efficacy for positive, negative, and disorganization symptoms of schizophrenia (53). Clozapine, a dibenzodiazepine derivative, is an effective antipsychotic with several unusual properties. It has low affinities for the D_1 and D_2 receptors and high affinity for the D_4 dopamine receptor (54). Clozapine was found to reduce TD in clinical studies and, furthermore, clozapine-treated patients failed to show the rebound increase in dyskinesia after drug withdrawal (55,56). Risperidone is an antipsychotic with potent central 5-HT2 antagonism at low doses and marked dopamine D_2 receptor antagonism at high doses (57). A double-blind, multicenter study found risperidone at the optimal dose of 6 mg/day to have been significantly more effective than haloperidol in reducing TD (57). Despite the apparent antidyskinetic effect, the role of risperidone in the treatment of TD, and especially in severe TD, remains to be established.

Vitamin E is a lipid-soluble antioxidant. It effectively reduced TD in several controlled studies (58–61). Best results were obtained at 1,600 IU/day and when treatment was continued beyond eight weeks (61). Vitamin E appears safe and well tolerated but whether it can benefit severe TD remains to be demonstrated.

REFERENCES

1. Hunter R, Earl CJ, Thornicroft S. An apparently irreversible syndrome of abnormal movements following phenothiazine medication. Proc R Soc Med 1964;57:24–28.
2. Gardos G, Cole JO, Schniebolk S, Salomon M. Comparison of severe and mild tardive dyskinesia: implications for etiology. J Clin Psychiatry 1987;48:359–362.
3. Gimenez-Roldan S, Mateo D, Bartolome P. Tardive dystonia and severe tardive dyskinesia. Acta Psychiatr Scand 1985;71:488–494.
4. Gardos G, Cole JO, Salomon M, Schniebolk S. Clinical forms of severe tardive dyskinesia. Am J Psychiatry 1987;144:895–902.
5. Yassa R, Jones BD. Complications of tardive dyskinesia: a review. Psychosomatics 1985;26:305–313.
6. Gardos G, Cole JO. The prognosis of tardive dyskinesia. J Clin Psychiatry 1983;44:177–179.
7. Brandon S, McClelland HA, Protheroe C. A study of facial dyskinesia, in a mental hospital population. Br J Psychiatry 1971;118:171–184.
8. Edwards H. The significance of brain damage in persistent oral dyskinesia. Br J Psychiatry 1970;116:271–275.
9. Gibson AC. Depot injections and tardive dyskinesia. Br J Psychiatry 1978;132:261–265.
10. Smith JM, Kucharski LT, Oswald WT, Waterman LJ. Tardive dyskinesia: effect of age, sex and criterion level of symptomatology on prevalence estimates. Psychopharmacol Bull 1979;15:69–71.
11. Guy W. ECDEU Assessment Manual for Psychopharmacology. Washington DC: US Department of Health, Education and Welfare, 1976:534–537.
12. Asnis GM, Leopold MA, Duvoisin RC, Schwartz AH. A survey of tardive dyskinesia in psychiatric outpatients. Am J Psychiatry 1977;134:1367–1370.
13. Wojcik JD, Gelenberg AJ, LaBrie RA, Mieske M. Prevalence of tardive dyskinesia in an outpatient population. Compr Psychiatry 1980;21:370–380.
14. McCreadie G, Barron ET, Winslow GS. The Nithsdale schizophrenia survey: II. Abnormal movements. Br J Psychiatry 1982;140:587–590.
15. Barnes TRE, Kidger T, Gore SM. Tardive dyskinesia: a 3-year follow-up study. Psychol Med 1983;13:71–81.
16. Guy W, Ban TA, Wilson WH. The prevalence of abnormal involuntary movements among chronic schizophrenics. Int Clin Psychopharmacol 1986;1:134–144.
17. Smith JM, Baldessarini RJ. Changes in prevalence, severity and recovery of tardive dyskinesia with age. Arch Gen Psychiatry 1980;37:1368–1373.
18. Kane JM, Smith JM. Tardive dyskinesia prevalence and risk factors: 1959 to 1979. Arch Gen Psychiatry 1982;39:473–481.
19. Waddington JL, Youssef HA, Dolphin C, Kinsella A. Cognitive dysfunction, negative symptoms, and tardive dyskinesia in schizophrenia. Arch Gen Psychiatry 1987;44:907–912.
20. Gualtieri CT, Schroeder SR, Hicks RE, Quade D. Tardive dyskinesia in young mentally retarded individuals. Arch Gen Psychiatry 1986;43:335–340.
21. Crane GE. Risks of long-term therapy with neuroleptic drugs. In: Sedval G, Uunäs B, Zotterman Y, eds. Antipsychotic drugs, pharmacodynamics and pharmacokinetics. Oxford: Pergamon, 1976:411–419.
22. Mann SC, Greenstein RA, Eilers R. Early onset of severe dyskinesia following lithium–haloperidol treatment. Am J Psychiatry 1983;140:1385–1386.
23. Casey DE, Rabins P. Tardive dyskinesia as a life-threatening illness. Am J Psychiatry 1978;135:486–488.
24. Tarsy D, Granacher R, Bralower M. Tardive dyskinesia in young adults. Am J Psychiatry 1977;134:1032–1034.
25. Nasrallah HA, Pappas NJ, Crowe RB. Oculogyric dystonia in tardive dyskinesia. Am J Psychiatry 1980;137:850–851.
26. McLean P, Casey DE. Tardive dyskinesia in an adolescent. Am J Psychiatry 1978;135:969–971.
27. Bitton V, Melamed E. Coexistence of severe parkinsonism and tardive dyskinesia as side effects of neuroleptic therapy. J Clin Psychiatry 1984;45:28–30.
28. Chouinard G, Bradwejn J. Reversible and irreversible tardive dyskinesia: a case report. Am J Psychiatry 1982;139:360–362.
29. Caine ED, Margolin DI, Brown GI, Ebert MH. Gilles de la Tourette's syndrome, tardive dyskinesia, and psychosis in an adolescent. Am J Psychiatry 1978;135:241–243.
30. Haggerty JJ Jr, Bentsen BS, Gillette GM. Neuroleptic malignant syndrome superimposed on tardive dyskinesia. Br J Psychiatry 1987;150:104–105.
31. Smith JM, Kucharski LT, Oswald WT, Waterman LJ. A systematic investigation of tardive dyskinesia in inpatients. Am J Psychiatry 1979;136:918–922.
32. Evans JH. Persistent oral dyskinesia in treatment with phenothiazine derivatives. Lancet 1965;i:458–460.
33. Schooler N, Kane JM. Research diagnoses for tardive dyskinesia (RD-TD). Arch Gen Psychiatry 1982;39:486–487.
34. Massengill R, Nashold B. A swallowing disorder denoted in tardive dyskinesia patients. Acta Otolaryngol 1969;68:457–458.
35. Faheem AD, Brightwell DB, Burton GC, Struss A. Respiratory dyskinesia and dysarthria from prolonged neuroleptic use: tardive dyskinesia? Am J Psychiatry 1982;139:517–518.
36. Yassa R, Lal S. Respiratory irregularity and tardive dyskinesia. A prevalence study. Acta Psychiatr Scand 1986;73:506–510.
37. Weiner WJ, Goetz CG, Nausieda PA, et al. Respiratory dyskinesias: extrapyramidal dysfunction and dyspnea. Ann Intern Med 1978;88:327–331.
38. Ayd FJ, ed. Respiratory dyskinesias in patients with neuroleptic-induced extrapyramidal reactions. Int Drug Ther Newsl 1979;14:1–4.
39. Greenberg DB, Murray GB. Hyperventilation as a variant of tardive dyskinesia. J Clin Psychiatry 1981;42:401–403.
40. Craig TJ, Richardson MA, Back NM, et al. Impairment of swallowing, tardive dyskinesia and anticholinergic use. Psychopharmacol Bull 1982;18:84–86.
41. Johnson GS, Hunt GE, Rey JM. Tardive dyskinesia and body weight in psychiatric outpatients. Am J Psychiatry 1981;138:1398.
42. Simpson GM, Shrivastava RK. Abnormal gaits in tardive dyskinesia. Am J Psychiatry 1978;135:865.
43. Mehta D, Mallya A, Volavka J. Mortality of patients with tardive dyskinesia. Am J Psychiatry 1978;135:371–372.
44. Kucharski IT, Smith JM, Dunn DD. Mortality and tardive dyskinesia. Am J Psychiatry 1979;136:1228.
45. Yassa R, Mohelsky H, Dimitry R, Schwartz G. Mortality rate in tardive dyskinesia. Am J Psychiatry 1984;141:1018–1019.
46. Itoh H, Yagi G. Reversibility of tardive dyskinesia. Folia Psychiatr Neurol Jpn 1979;33:43–54.
47. Casey DE, Toenniessen LM. Neuroleptic treatment in tardive dyskinesia: can it be developed into a clinical strategy for long-term treatment? In: Bannet J,

Belmaker RH, eds. Modern problems in pharmacopsychiatry, vol. 21, New Directions in Tardive Dyskinesia Research. Basel: S. Karger, 1983:65–86.

48. Gilbert MM. Haloperidol in severe facial dyskinesia. Dis Nerv Syst 1969;30:481–482.

49. Lenox RH, Weaver LA, Saran BM. Tardive dyskinesia: clinical and neuroendocrine response to low dose bromocriptine. J Clin Psychopharmacol 1985;5:286–292.

50. Ross JL, Mackenzie TB, Hanson DR, Charles CR. Diltiazem for tardive dyskinesia. Lancet 1987;i:268.

51. Jeste DV, Wyatt RJ. Treatment of tardive dyskinesia: review of the literature. In: Jeste DV, Wyatt RJ, eds. Understanding and treating tardive dyskinesia. New York: Guilford, 1982:215–288.

52. Simpson GM, Pi EH, Sramek JJ. An update on tardive dyskinesia. Hosp Comm Psychiatry 1986;37:362–369.

53. Meltzer HY. Clozapine and other atypical neuroleptics, efficacy, side effects, optimal utilization. Clin Psychiatry Monogr 1994;12(2):38–42.

54. Baldessarini RJ, Frankenburg FR. Clozapine—a novel antipsychotic agent. N Engl J Med 1991;325:746–754.

55. Tamminga CA, Thaker GK, Moran M, Kakigi T, Gao XM. Clozapine in tardive dyskinesia: observations from human and animal model studies. J Clin Psychiatry 1996;55(9 suppl B):102–106.

56. Lieberman JA, Saltz BL, Johns CA, Pollack S, Borenstein M, Kane JM. The effects of clozapine on tardive dyskinesia. Br J Psychiatry 1991;158:503–510.

57. Chouinard G, Jones B, Remington G, et al. A Canadian multicenter placebo-controlled study of fixed doses of risperidone and haloperidol in the treatment of chronic schizophrenic patients. J Clin Psychopharmacol 1993;13:25–40.

58. Lohr B, Cadet JL, Lohr MA, et al. Vitamin E in the treatment of tardive dyskinesia: the possible involvement of free radical mechanisms. Schizophr Bull 1988;14:291–296.

59. Elkashef AM, Ruskin PE, Bacher N, Barrett D. Vitamin E in the treatment of tardive dyskinesia. Am J Psychiatry 1990;147:505–509.

60. Egan MF, Hyde TM, Albers GW, et al. Treatment of tardive dyskinesia with vitamin E. Am J Psychiatry 1992;149:773–777.

61. Adler LA, Peselow E, Rosenthal M, et al. Vitamin E treatment of tardive dyskinesia. Biol Psychiatry 1992;31:160A.

Medicolegal Issues Regarding Tardive Dyskinesia

Thomas G. Gutheil   Roderick W. Pettis

INTRODUCTION

Tardive dyskinesia (TD) clearly represents the "bad news" complement to the "good news" offered to psychiatry when antipsychotic medications were first discovered and used in the 1950s. Phenothiazines (and similar drugs in other chemical categories) proved startlingly successful in ameliorating symptoms of schizophrenia and other psychoses and in permitting countless numbers of patients (often for the first time in their lives) to live outside institutions, which led to highly appropriate therapeutic enthusiasm for clinicians and relief for patients and their families. So dramatic was the efficacy of these new agents that understandable resistance and reluctance characterized the slow acknowledgment of the relevance of an old axiom: "There is no such thing as a free lunch," or in this case, as a medication without side effects.

In the wake of growing clinical awareness of the appearance of this disabling and lasting condition, concern with litigation based on TD has grown among psychiatrists (1–5). While TD litigation had been described as the "malpractice area of the 1980s," surprisingly this subject area for feared civil suits has not thus far materialized, and a review of the cases and the outcomes reveals several other curiosities. We begin our discussion of this subject with examination of some of these puzzles.

One of the largest awards in the recent history of psychiatric malpractice litigation flowed from a TD suit (6), yet this suit has very little to do with common psychiatric practice and contains few useful lessons for the clinician. The case involved treatment of a retarded person with phenothiazines under dubious indications with highly questionable informed consent, in the context of an institution where the general level of care appeared quite low in all parameters. Another suit, in Ohio, settled for $800,000 on the basis of an allegation of failure to obtain informed consent (7). Many other cases have failed on procedural issues such as bringing suit after the statute of limitations had expired. Thus, it remains unclear whether bad care itself, rather than TD, is the true or latent subject of the cases.

Despite the slowly growing number of malpractice suits for drug-related issues, it is safe to say that there has not yet been a good (that is, heuristically useful or instructive) liability suit about TD. While it is, of course, not the court's problem to generate good teaching cases nor to teach clinicians about their practice, one can yet hope for illuminating judicial opinions. From such data we may often glean valuable insights into how psychiatry is viewed by the profession of law, which can only benefit those clinicians who wish to inform their practice with such understanding. No case has as yet dealt squarely with the inescapable core issue that lies at the heart of the TD problem. That is, no case to date has looked at 1) a diagnostically clear case of schizophrenia, convincingly defined by research criteria or similar solid standard; 2) where antipsychotics were clearly indicated based on recognized disease-specific symptomatology likely to respond to such treatment; 3) where TD developed and was identified at least relatively early; 4) where some reasonable semblance of informed consent was negotiated; 5) where a careful risk–benefit analysis of the issue was performed, balancing the value of antipsychotics in freedom from symptoms or from consequent hospitalization against the harm of TD; and 6) where suit was brought for the harm of TD.

What cases there have been thus far have focused on egregious failures of clinical judgment, lack of informed consent, ill-defined indications for use of medication, bad care, or other clear deviations from standards of good psychiatric practice.

It may also be surprising to realize that, although maximum fuss may be made over TD and maximum fear may preoccupy physicians, this particular side effect has no essentially different valence from any other side effect, allergic response, or bad reaction in the medicolegal area. It probably looms larger than it deserves in clinicians' minds in part because TD was so emphatically stressed by legal advocates in right-to-refuse-treatment litigation, where the risk of TD was cited as the ultimate objection to involuntary medication treatment of psychiatric patients. As a result, what little the law knows about psychopharmacology includes TD as the "horrible example" of unchecked enthusiasm for treatment.

Finally, with regard to informed consent, many clinicians find it hard to believe that even a patient who has already developed TD may yet consent, if competent, to continue on the medications for their perceived benefits despite the risk of worsening of the condition. Conversely, the competent patient troubled by TD can elect to stop medications and risk the relapse of illness. Here the national awareness of patients' rights, as well as judicial endorsement of patients' autonomy in decisions about treatment, clearly supports this view.

The flood of suits anticipated in the 1990s has failed to materialize. This may perhaps be due in part to increasing prescription of newer antipsychotic medications, such as clozapine and risperidone, in which the risk of TD is lower when compared with older antipsychotics. Despite the increased margin of safety with these new antipsychotics, however, the risk of TD has not been eliminated. In any event, the principles offered in this chapter attempt to provide guidelines for effective risk management.

FUNDAMENTALS OF LIABILITY

In order to place the above introductory summary into context, a brief introduction to the principles of liability may be in order. In a malpractice case, four elements must be proven by the plaintiff (patient) by a preponderance of the evidence (8). First, a duty must exist in the form of a doctor–patient relationship; in this instance, the physician who evaluated the patient and prescribed the medication would be the bearer of that duty. Second, that duty must have been breached by negligence, that is, by deviation from the standard of care as established by the "average reasonable practitioner" of that specialty (the precise wording of this standard may vary among jurisdictions). Third, damages must have ensued in the form of harms suffered by the patient; here, the disfigurement, social stigma, impaired physical functioning, or change in employability might represent the alleged harm in question. Finally, the plaintiff must demonstrate a direct causal link between the negligence alleged and the damages. The appearance of TD would be alleged to flow causally from some negligence on the part of the physician.

While, as noted above, a "good" case on this matter has not been tried as yet, the allegations in a TD malpractice case would likely cover some or all of the following: 1) the assessment of the patient was faulty and the indications for prescribing these medications incorrectly identified; 2) the prescribing practices were wrong and excessive dosage amounts, or excessive length of prescribing, were employed; 3) inadequate monitoring was employed in the form of Abnormal Involuntary Movements Scale (AIMS) testing (or similar check); drug holidays (controversial as to efficacy); periodic trials off all medications; and the like; 4) the risk–benefit decision for prescription of antipsychotics was improperly assessed in the case at hand, either at the outset of the case or at the time of the first appearance of TD; and 5) informed consent was not obtained or was inadequately obtained, or the patient was not really competent to consent to the treatment risks.

VIVIDNESS, VISIBILITY, AND RISK-AVERSION

While the point has been made above that TD is no different from any other side effect or bad reaction that might follow in the wake of psychopharmacologic treatment, there are some contextual factors specific to TD that have an impact on liability.

The effects of TD are grossly visible; that is, a judge and/or jury can literally see this phenomenon in action. It has been suggested (9,10) that TD can become for these decisionmakers a concrete embodiment of the stigma of being mentally ill. Indeed, this visible sign may appear to a jury to be more damaging than its alternative—untreated mental illness—which, while unpleasant to patients and families, may nevertheless not evoke the emotional response of a disfiguring side effect.

Because of this visibility, TD can often be demonstrated to the jury in a direct visual way as the risk in question. In contrast, it is not possible to demonstrate with equal vividness an abstraction such as "ten years without requiring rehospitalization"—the benefit side of the equation. Phenothiazine maintenance thus shares, with other prophylactic measures (such as vaccination), the quality that the reward for success is that nothing happens: a reassuring result, but an insufficiently dramatic one, perhaps, with which to impress a jury.

For the plaintiff's case, the concreteness of the "risk" side may be buttressed by the tendency of the courts to be risk-aversive, that is, they have historically paid attention to the harms to be avoided rather than the benefits to be obtained. No one, after all, sues for a benefit gained. Thus, the law is fundamentally more attuned to the risk side of the risk–benefit decision intrinsic to all prescribing of medication. For antipsychotic medications, one risk is TD.

INFORMED CONSENT

Informed consent is often a problematic issue for clinicians, who may see it as a legalistic minefield, a burdensome but empty exercise in paperwork, or an opportunity to give patients bad news so that they refuse needed treatment. Fears about consent issues may be fanned by the clinician's awareness that informed consent is almost universally recognized as a part of the standard of care; thus, failure to obtain informed consent may represent malpractice.

In reality, informed consent is probably the most effective liability preventative as well as an alliance builder, decreasing either the likelihood of litigation itself or a finding against the physician if a suit does come about (11). In the service of this goal, informed consent should be viewed not as a "hurdle" to be cleared or a form to be signed but as an ongoing dialogue between doctor and patient, where exploration of the effects of the medication, positive and negative, and their implications may take place candidly at any point during treatment.

Some useful points about informed consent have been made elsewhere (8,12,13) and will not be repeated here. Several key reminders, however, should be emphasized. First, informed consent consists of three elements: information, voluntary, and competence. The information in the present context is the expected benefits of antipsychotic medication and the potential risk of TD (as well as of other side effects, of course). Voluntary refers to the patient's willing decision to take the medication; forced, emergency, or court-ordered medication are examples of nonvoluntary treatment. The test of voluntary, moreover, is whether the patient can withdraw consent. Finally, competence refers to the patient's capacity to weigh the risks and benefits of treatment in a realistic manner and to make a reasonable decision about treatment (8).

It is important for the treating psychiatrist to recall that a competent patient—even one who has begun to develop early tardive dyskinesia—can yet consent to ongoing neuroleptic treatment and potential worsening of that condition if the patient's preference for freedom from psychotic symptoms outweighs the risk of TD. In a complementary fashion, the competent patient concerned about TD may elect to stop taking antipsychotics even at the risk of relapse, rehospitalization, or other serious negative outcomes. As should be implicit from these examples, however, the critical factors in such choices are the patient's reliable competence and an accurate assessment by patient and doctor of the true risk–benefit picture.

A clinician who "inherits" a patient who has been on antipsychotic medication chronically should not assume that the patient's informed consent has already been obtained. The only safe approach is to renegotiate or establish informed consent oneself when beginning to care for such a patient.

The importance of documentation must be underscored. It should include the clinician's risk–benefit analysis regarding treatment and observations about the presence or absence of emerging symptoms. Such documentation should also summarize the content of the discussion between the clinician and the patient. Documentation of consultation with colleagues adds an extra measure of protection should

litigation result, as it supports the assertion that treatment was commensurate with the relevant standard of care.

Physicians often worry about the value of discussing the risks of TD when starting antipsychotics on newly admitted, grossly psychotic patients, who may be given antipsychotics for relatively short periods of time. One approach to this area of ambiguity may be to inform the patient of the short-term risks (extrapyramidal syndrome [EPS], hypotension, etc.). After the patient's condition has stabilized, if long-term prescription is contemplated, the longer term risk–benefit picture can be explored. Some clinicians repeat the entire informed consent discussion at discharge because 1) that is a time of likely patient competence and 2) that threshold heralds a reassessment, not only of the risks and benefits of medication, but of a new context for treatment as well.

Finally, as a liability preventative, informed consent establishes the climate between doctor and patient that militates against litigation. The patient who experiences a side effect and notes, "Ah, yes, there is that muscle stiffness the doctor warned me I might feel," is in a completely different frame of mind regarding litigation from the patient whose response more closely resembles, "My God! What is the doctor doing to my body?" The surprise in the latter scenario is not uncommonly the emotional wellspring of a malpractice suit; the former scenario strengthens the therapeutic alliance by confirming the doctor's knowledge of his or her craft. In this instance as well, the patient becomes a partner in helping to alert the clinician to other potentially serious side effects such as dystonic reactions and neuroleptic malignant syndrome.

In the event of litigation despite this relationship, when informed consent has been properly negotiated, the physician still benefits from the protection of having used reasonable judgment in the treatment decision, and the patient shares in responsibility for the decisionmaking as an active participant.

Liability Prevention

In practical terms, as described elsewhere in this book, lowest doses, shortest courses of treatment, regular monitoring (e.g., with AIMS), and repeated active efforts to stop medications should be the cornerstones of neuroleptic prescription.

The "twin pillars" of liability prevention (8) are documentation and consultation. Being able to provide documentation, from a liability standpoint, coheres with the concrete thinking of the courts: If you did not write it, it did not happen. It is essential to document the following: 1) the indications for neuroleptic treatment; 2) the risk–benefit analysis of such treatment (expected benefits versus TD); 3) the patient's competence to consent to treatment (if the patient is incompetent, depending on jurisdiction, a guardian or a judge may have to make the decision on behalf of the patient (8); and 4) the informed consent process, including explicit information given to the patient about the possibility, irreversibility, and consequences of TD.

Consultation has two major liability prevention effects. First, it brings the clinician into contact with the standard of care: If two reasonable clinicians feel that the use of antipsychotics is reasonable, it is many times more difficult for the plaintiff to assert that it is unreasonable. More importantly, perhaps, consultation reveals the practitioner to be one who seeks second opinions by submitting clinical judgment to the scrutiny of a peer—a habit that reveals that clinician's high standards of practice.

Consultation may be of particular benefit when the indications for neuroleptic use are muddy or uncertain; where the patient's competence is in doubt; or where the risk–benefit ratio is unclear or controversial.

CONCLUSION

It is helpful and somewhat surprising to note that a recent review of cases in this area reveals 1) that the flood of TD litigation has not occurred and 2) that there are as yet no cases instructive on the issue of the court's view of the risk and benefits of antipsychotic medications in the context of care that clearly meets the standard in all regards.

This chapter can serve only as a brief summary of the complex issue of the medicolegal aspects of TD. The authors hope however, that the suggestions here may diminish clinicians' fears about liability for this regrettable outcome and replace those fears with the encouragement that comes from a coherent and effective strategy to approach the problems for the patients' benefit.

REFERENCES

1. Wettstein RM. Tardive dyskinesia and malpractice. Behav Sci and the Law 1983;1:85–107.
2. Taubs S. Tardive dyskinesia: medical facts and legal fictions. St. Louis L.J. 1986;930:833–873.
3. Gaultieri CT, Sprague RL, Cole JO. Tardive dyskinesia litigation and the dilemmas of neuroleptic treatment. J Psychiatry Law 1986;1:187–206.
4. Mills MJ, Norquist AS, Shelton RC, et al. Consent and liability with neuroleptics: the problem of tardive dyskinesia. Int J Law Psychiatry 1986;9:243–252.
5. Appelbaum PS, Schaffer K, Meisel A. Responsibility and compensation for tardive dyskinesia. Am J Psychiatry 1985;142:806–810.
6. *Clites v. Iowa*, 322 N.W.2d 917 (1982).
7. *Snider v. Harding* (settled August 1988), LRP Publication No. 34665.
8. Appelbaum PS, Gutheil TG. Clinical Handbook of Psychiatry and the Law. 2nd ed. Baltimore: Williams & Wilkins, 1991.
9. Gutheil TG. Medicolegal psychopharmacology. In: Gelenberg A, Bassuk E, eds. The practitioner's guide to psychoactive drugs. 4th ed. New York: Plenum, 1997:501–511.
10. Gutheil TG. Liability issues and malpractice prevention. In: Shader RI, Tupin J, Harnett D, eds. Handbook of clinical psychopharmacology, 2nd ed. New York: Jason Aronson, 1988:439–453.
11. Gutheil TG, Bursztajn H, Brodsky A. Malpractice prevention through the sharing of uncertainty: informed consent and the therapeutic alliance. N Engl J Med 1984;311:49–51.
12. Appelbaum PS, Lidz CW, Meisel A. Informed Consent. New York: Oxford University, 1987.
13. Lidz CW, Meisel A, Zerubavel E, et al. Informed Consent: a study of decision making in psychiatry. New York: Guilford, 1984.

Risk Factors in Tardive Dyskinesia and Supersensitivity Psychosis

Guy Chouinard   Lawrence Annable

INTRODUCTION

Long-term administration of antipsychotics is currently the most efficacious treatment for chronic schizophrenia. This type of treatment, however, is not without serious risk for the central nervous system, particularly for the neostriatum (tardive dyskinesia) and for the mesolimbic regions (supersensitivity psychosis).

TARDIVE DYSKINESIA

Tardive dyskinesia (TD), a neuroleptic-induced extrapyramidal hyperkinetic syndrome (1–3), becomes potentially irreversible after the age of 40. It is characterized by involuntary, repetitive, and purposeless movements that vary in localization and form. The clinical manifestations involve eight main areas: tongue, jaw, cheek–lips, trunk, upper and lower extremities, face, and respiratory system. The most common manifestation is the buccofaciolingual masticatory syndrome that involves the muscles of the mouth, tongue, lips, cheeks, and jaws, and manifests itself by lateral jaw movements or tongue movements within the oral cavity, protrusion or torsion of the tongue, and slow lateral movements of the tongue. The syndrome also includes choreoathetoid movement of upper and lower extremities and of the trunk.

Early studies reported a prevalence of tardive dyskinesia of 2% to 15% in neuroleptic-treated patients (4). In 1980 the Task Force of the American Psychiatric Association estimated the prevalence in patients at risk to be at least 10% to 20%, and 40% in elderly patients (5). The prevalence had been progressively rising and reached 25% during the period 1976 to 1981 (6). In 1982, Kane and Smith reviewed 65 studies with an average prevalence of 20% in neuroleptic-treated patients compared with 5% showing dyskinesia-like

movements in untreated patients (4). More recent estimates (7–16) from 1981 to 1986 have been even higher with an average prevalence of 30%. In contrast, the prevalence of spontaneous dyskinesia in healthy elderly volunteers was found to be 1.2% (12), 1.5% (17), and in a geriatric medical population to be 4.8% (12). Also, in a series of studies conducted in Turkey in chronic schizophrenic patients who were treated with minimal doses of neuroleptics, Crane (1,2) was able to distinguish between tardive dyskinesia and schizophrenic stereotypies, thus showing that even though schizophrenics may have abnormal movements, these could be differentiated from tardive dyskinesia.

Concerning risk factors, there is agreement that tardive dyskinesia is more prevalent in elderly patients (4,6–8,18,19). Other risk factors that have been reported are a) total exposure to neuroleptics (8,19), b) neuroleptic treatment of affective disorder (20), and c) fluphenazine (12,15,18,21–23).

SUPERSENSITIVITY PSYCHOSIS

We have previously reported another long-term side effect of antipsychotic and neuroleptic treatment that we called "supersensitivity psychosis" (24,25). Receptor changes in the dopaminergic pathways of the mesolimbic (26) dopaminergic regions of the brain could explain the disorder in the same way that changes in the neostriatum are thought to be responsible for tardive dyskinesia.

There are difficulties associated with the diagnosis of supersensitivity psychosis (27). The symptoms of the latter are nearly the same as the disease process itself, the distinctions being that only positive symptoms of schizophrenia are exhibited, that the symptoms fluctuate according to the masking effect of increased antipsychotic and/or neuroleptic dose or unmasking effect of decreased dose, and that relapses occur more rapidly than would be expected from the normal course of the illness. In this respect, perhaps it is worth mentioning that the symptoms of tardive dyskinesia have also been mistaken for mannerisms of schizophrenia, hyperkinetic parkinsonian side effects (akathisia or tremors), and senile choreic movements.

As with tardive dyskinesia, clinical symptoms of supersensitivity psychosis are masked by antipsychotics and neuroleptics. As most antipsychotics and neuroleptics currently available have prolonged brain half-lives, recognition of the disorder is difficult. One would predict that metaclopramide, a short-acting dopamine receptor blocking agent, when given in doses effective in treating schizophrenia, would give clear evidence of supersensitivity relapse upon abrupt withdrawal. Cases of supersensitivity psychosis have been reported following withdrawal of clozapine (28,29), a drug with a short half-life and a greater affinity for mesolimbic than striatal dopamine receptors. Other cases have been reported following withdrawal of neuroleptics in manic–depressive illness (30,31), and reserpine (32).

The disorder may be less readily apparent in inpatient populations because, like tardive dyskinesia, supersensitivity psychosis is identified most readily in patients under increased vigilance and stress. Tardive dyskinetic symptoms are exacerbated during periods of increased concentration or anxiety. Similarly, the most potent stressors for supersensitivity psychosis are the normal activities of the patient's life, which are difficult to recreate in a hospital setting.

Given the difficulties in diagnosing supersensitivity psychosis, we carried out a survey of the disorder in an outpatient population for which conditions of treatment optimized the possibility of observing its presence. At the same time, we carried out a five-year follow-up study of tardive dyskinesia (33).

TARDIVE DYSKINESIA AND SUPERSENSITIVITY PSYCHOSIS

We carried out a cross-sectional survey of supersensitivity psychosis in 224 schizophrenic outpatients chronically maintained on neuroleptic treatment. The patients studied attended an outpatient clinic in which all patients have a diagnosis of schizophrenia according to the research diagnostic criteria (35). Within the clinic, pharmacotherapy was under strict control and the drug treatment was standardized (single neuroleptic, one antiparkinsonian, no antidepressant, no mood stabilizers, no benzodiazepines (18,34)). Medication was reviewed each time the patient came to the clinic.

Patients were rated during their regular visit to the clinic by the author (G.C.) who had been in charge of their treatment for the last 10 years. The following ratings were carried out:

1. clinical global impression (CGI) of the presence of supersensitivity psychosis, rated on a 3-point rating scale (0 = absent; 1 = doubtful or borderline; 2 =

definite). Even though the following scale of supersensitivity psychosis was not systematically used (Table 6.1), the same criteria were guiding the rater to make the diagnosis. Borderline cases were classified as such if:

(a) a patient had developed definite drug tolerance but no definite relapse when medication was decreased or if medication was never decreased sufficiently to assess withdrawal; and

(b) patients had showed definite relapse upon decrease or discontinuation of medication, but the relapse occurred shortly after 6 weeks for oral medication or 3 months for depot injectable neuroleptics.

2. CGI of therapeutic response to treatment, rated on a 5-point rating scale (1 = marked improvement and 5 = worse); and

3. CGI of overall severity of illness, rated on a 7-point rating scale (1 = normal and 7 = extremely ill).

Independently, patients underwent an extrapyramidal symptom assessment, using a standardized examination procedure for parkinsonian symptoms and tardive dyskinesia, and were rated on the extrapyramidal symptom rating scale (ESRS) by a neurologist (AR-C) (36,37). Blood was drawn for determination of plasma prolactin concentration and was analyzed for neuroleptic activity using a neuroleptic radioreceptor assay (38–40).

A total of 224 patients (113 men and 111 women) were evaluated. Women tended to be older (48.4 ± 11) but required a lower neuroleptic maintenance dose (454 + 552 chlorpromazine (CPZ) units) (41) than men (age: 41.9 + 10.9, 706 + 885 CPZ units). Regarding the length of neuroleptic treatment, the groups did not differ significantly (men: 12.7 ± 6.3 years, women: 14.9 ± 5.8 years). The prevalence of tardive dyskinesia, using the research diagnostic criteria of Schooler and Kane (42) (which require presence of at least "moderate" dyskinetic movements in one or more body areas or at least "mild" dyskinetic movements in two or more body areas) was 45%. The prevalence of definite cases of supersensitivity psychosis (22%) was about one-half that of tardive dyskinesia (45%) and did not vary with gender. If borderline cases of supersensitivity are included, the prevalence found is 43%.

Table 6.2 compares the age and neuroleptic dosage of patients with and without supersensitivity psychosis and tardive dyskinesia. Patients with supersensitivity psychosis were receiving a larger mean neuroleptic dose than patients without this syndrome (t = 4.07, $p < 0.001$), but there was no difference with respect to mean age. Patients with tardive dyskinesia, on the other hand, tended to be older than patients without tardive dyskinesia (t = 4.05, $p < 0.001$), but there was no difference with respect to mean neuroleptic dose.

Patients receiving low-potency neuroleptics tended to have different characteristics from those receiving high-

Table 6.1 Research Diagnostic Criteria for Supersensitivity Psychosis

1 Date (MM DD YY)	1 2 3 4 5 6		
2 Visit	7 8 9		
3 Mark 1 if evaluation off schedule	10		
4 Subject No.	11 12 13		
5 Sex (M = 1, F = 2)	14		
6 Evaluator	15 16		
7 Project	17 18 19 20		
I Does the patient have a history of receiving neuroleptics or antipsychotics for at *least 3 months*?	0	1	21
	No	Yes	
II *Major criteria*: at least *one* must be present			
1 Has the patient's medication been decreased or discontinued within the last 5 years? If yes, rate if any decrease or discontinuation induced a reappearance of psychotic symptoms (relapse), occurring: (a) within 6 weeks for oral medication; or (b) within 3 months for i.m. depot medication	0	1	22
	No	Yes	
2 Has patient shown greater frequency of relapses (acute psychotic exacerbation) since he/she is on continuous neuroleptic treatment?	0	1	23
	No	Yes	
3 Has patient shown tolerance to the antipsychotic effect of the neuroleptic (absolute increase of 20% or more in dose during the last 5 years)?	0	1	24
	No	Yes	
4 Has patient shown extreme tolerance: worsening of psychosis whenever dosages are increased, without presence of significant parkinsonian symptoms?	0	1	25
	No	Yes	
5 Psychotic symptoms upon decrease of medication were: (a) not previously seen (new schizophrenic symptoms); or (b) are of greater severity	0	1	26
	No	Yes	
6 Has patient shown psychotic relapse upon sudden decrease (≥10%) of medication but not if same decrease is gradual (≤10%)?	0	1	27
	No	Yes	
7 Presence of drug tolerance in the past but presently treated with high doses of neuroleptics on at least a b.i.d. regimen	0		28
	No	Yes	
III *Minor criteria*: at least *one* must be present, if only one of the major criteria is present			
1 Is tardive dyskinesia present? (a standard examination must be used)	0	1	29
	No	Yes	
2 Is there rapid improvement (within 1 week) of psychotic symptoms when the effective neuroleptic dose is increased after a decrease or discontinuation of medication?	0	1	30
	No	Yes	
3 Has patient shown clear exacerbation of psychotic symptoms by stress?	0	1	31
	No	Yes	
4 If patient is treated with i.m. long-acting medication only, has there been appearance of psychotic symptoms at the end of the injection interval?	0	1	32
	No	Yes	
5 Does patient have high levels of prolactin or neuroleptic activity? (twice the normal range—at least once within the last 2 years)	0	1	33
	No	Yes	
IV *Exclusion criteria*: both must be absent			
1 Is patient in his/her first acute phase of the illness? (If yes, the patient cannot be rated at this time)	0	1	34
	No	Yes	
2 Does patient have a continued severe psychotic illness which did not respond to neuroleptic treatment? (If *yes*, the patient cannot be rated at this time)	0	1	35
	No	Yes	
V Does patient meet diagnostic criteria for supersensitivity psychosis? If yes, which subtype?	0	1	
	No	Yes	
1 Stage I. Withdrawal type: reversible—when only major criteria #1 and/or #6 are present (no other major criteria present)	1		
	Yes		

Table 6.1   Continued

2 Stage II. Tardive type:	2		
IIA—masked and mostly reversible	Yes		
—when major criteria #3 is present without any other major criteria			
IIB—masked and mostly irreversible	3		
—when the only major criterion present is #7	Yes		36
IIC—overt and mostly irreversible			
—when major criterion for no. 1 is present with any other major criteria (other than #6)	4		
	Yes		
3 Stage III. Severe type: when major criteria #4 is present	5		
VI *Was medication decreased or discontinued?*			
If yes, specify as follows:			
1 <25%	0	1	
	No	Yes	
2 25–50%	0	1	
	No	Yes	37
3 >50%	0	1	
	No	Yes	
4 Complete discontinuation	0	1	
	No	Yes	
VII *Type of medication*			
Is patient on:			
1 oral medication?	0	1	
	No	Yes	
2 i.m. (depot)?	0	1	
	No	Yes	38
3 both?	0	1	
	No	Yes	

Table 6.2   Characteristics of Patients With and Without Supersensitivity Psychosis (Definite), and Tardive Dyskinesia (Research Diagnostic Criteria): Mean (SD)

	Supersensitivity Psychosis		Tardive Dyskinesia	
	Present (n = 50)	**Absent** (n = 174)	**Present** (n = 101)	**Absent** (n = 124)
Age (years)	44 (12)	46 (14)	48 (11)[a]	42 (11)
Neuroleptic dose (mg/day CPZ units)	940 (1,002)[b]	472 (614)	625 (854)	526 (632)

[a] Statistically significant ($p < 0.001$) difference in mean age between patients with and without tardive dyskinesia.
[b] Statistically significant ($p < 0.01$) difference in mean neuroleptic dose between patients with and without supersensitivity psychosis.

potency neuroleptics and were considered as a separate group. Table 6.3 shows the results for different variables according to the rating given for supersensitivity psychosis in patients receiving high-potency neuroleptics only. Patients with a definite diagnosis of supersensitivity psychosis were receiving significantly greater neuroleptic doses (t = 4.35, $p < 0.001$) and had significantly higher prolactin levels (men: t = 1.68, $p < 0.10$, women: t = 2.38, $p < 0.05$) than those without supersensitivity psychosis. There was also a nonsignificant trend for higher neuroleptic radioreceptor assay levels in patients with supersensitivity psychosis than

those without the disorder (these were measured in 71 patients only so there was less statistic power to detect differences).

Table 6.4 shows similar results for patients receiving low-potency neuroleptics. Although the numbers of subjects in this group are small the same trend for increasing neuroleptic dose and radioreceptor assay levels is present in patients with supersensitivity psychosis. In general, patients treated with low-potency drugs tended to be older and have more tardive dyskinesia than the high-potency group.

T a b l e 6 . 3 Supersensitivity Psychosis, Tardive Dyskinesia, and Patient Characteristics: Patients Treated with High-Potency Neuroleptics (*n* = 191)

	Mean (SD) Supersensitivity Psychosis			
	Not Present 0 (*n* = 93)	Borderline 1 (*n* = 39)	Definite 2 (*n* = 45)	Not Assessable 3 (*n* = 14)
Age	44.5 (11.4)	42.2 (12.1)	43.4 (11.5)	46.5 (8.7)
Neuroleptic dose (CPZ units)	339 (473)	699 (810)	913 (917)[b]	421 (271)
Neuroleptic—RRA level[a]	14.2 (31.8)	15.3 (16.5)	23.5 (35.9)	6.2 (5.9)
CGI of therapeutic effect	1.5 (0.6)	1.5 (0.7)	1.5 (0.5)	1.1 (0.4)
CGI of severity of illness	4.4 (0.9)	4.4 (1.0)	4.7 (1.2)[c]	4.6 (0.6)
Prolactin female (ng/mL)	33.2 (25.6)	42.5 (33.8)	52.5 (38.1)[d]	44.7 (38.1)
Prolactin male (ng/mL)	17.8 (11.4)	21.6 (14.6)	23.5 (16.1)[c]	16.4 (9.6)
Tardive dyskinesia (research criteria)	45.2%	33.3%	42.2%	50.0%

[a] Measured in 99 subjects only, classified according to supersensitivity psychosis as follows: not present *n* = 43; borderline *n* = 19; definite *n* = 28; not assessed *n* = 9.
[b,c,d] Significantly different (*p* < 0.001, *p* < 0.05, and *p* < 0.10, respectively) from corresponding mean value for patients without supersensitivity psychosis (*t*-test).

T a b l e 6 . 4 Supersensitivity Psychosis Rating, Tardive Dyskinesia, and Patient Characteristics: Patients Treated with Low-Potency Neuroleptic (*n* = 33)

	Mean (SD) Supersensitivity Psychosis			
	Not Present 0 (*n* = 14)	Borderline 1 (*n* = 8)	Definite 2 (*n* = 5)	Not Assessable 3 (*n* = 6)
Age	52.9 (9.8)	50.3 (8.9)	52.8 (10.0)	52.8 (10.3)
Neuroleptic dose (CPZ units)	216 (169)	681 (684)	1190 (1,718)	725 (1,483)
Neuroleptic—RRA level*	13.1 (6.9)	34.3 (24.6)	41.9 (63.0)	55.1 (0.4)
CGI of therapeutic effect	1.1 (0.3)	1.3 (0.5)	1.8 (0.8)	1.8 (0.8)
CGI of severity of illness	4.0 (0.8)	4.5 (0.8)	4.4 (0.5)	3.3 (0.8)
Prolactin level (ng/mL)	21.2 (23.3)	24.5 (25.6)	19.3 (10.5)	21.4 (14.3)
Tardive dyskinesia (research criteria)	50.0%	50.0%	60.0%	83.3%

* Measured in 14 patients only, classified according to supersensitivity psychosis as follows: not present *n* = 6; borderline *n* = 3; definite *n* = 3; not assessed *n* = 2.

When we compare patients with supersensitivity psychosis and those without the syndrome with respect to schizophrenic prognosis, there was a tendency (*p* < 0.1) (χ^2 = 3.12, Yates' correction applied in patients treated with high-potency neuroleptics) for supersensitivity psychosis to be more frequent in patients diagnosed as "good prognosis" (atypical, schizophreniform, paranoid subtype) (37 of 44) than in those diagnosed as "poor prognosis" (other subtypes; 62 of 91).

DISCUSSION

The prevalence of tardive dyskinesia meeting the Schooler and Kane research criteria (42) in these schizophrenic outpatients was 45%, about twice that of diagnosed cases of supersensitivity psychosis, 22%. We have elsewhere reported (34) that over a five-year period the annual incidence rate of tardive dyskinesia corrected for remissions in these patients was 2.9%, similar to that reported by Kane et al (43) from a prospective study of tardive dyskinesia development. Thus, our patients would be comparable with those included in Kane's prospective study, regarding their vulnerability to tardive dyskinesia.

A diagnosis of supersensitivity psychosis was associated with a higher maintenance dose of neuroleptics, high prolactin levels, and a "good" schizophrenic prognosis.

Thus, our results suggest that the use of low doses of antipsychotics and neuroleptics whenever feasible will decrease the incidence of supersensitivity psychosis, while it may not necessarily affect the incidence of overt cases of tardive dyskinesia. No relationship was seen, however, between tardive dyskinesia and supersensitivity psychosis. The trend for a higher dose and prolactin level to be seen in patients with supersensitivity psychosis may reflect the development of dopamine supersensitivity in areas of the brain responsible for the appearance of psychotic symptoms. The latter would necessitate increased neuroleptic dosage to maintain clinical improvement. Of course, it could be argued that one of the features used to make the diagnosis was evidence of drug tolerance. However, not all patients were diagnosed based on the presence of this feature and drug tolerance was defined as the need for dosage increases over time after a patient had been stable on a lower dose, and not simply the presence of a large absolute dose of neuroleptic unchanged from the dose needed to control a previous acute relapse of the illness. Thus these indirect measures of increased dopaminergic antagonist activity in patients diagnosed as having supersensitivity psychosis do provide some measure of support for the diagnosis.

That patients with good prognosis schizophrenia show a tendency toward greater susceptibility to supersensitivity psychosis could explain the lack of correlation with tardive dyskinesia. That syndrome is more often seen in poor prognosis patients (18) and a different susceptibility based on prognosis could obscure any relationship between these two supersensitivity disorders in an individual patient. In an earlier study carried out with chronically hospitalized inpatients having poor prognosis schizophrenia, we found an association between tardive dyskinesia and supersensitivity psychosis. But, in this outpatient study including both poor and good prognosis patients, such a relationship was not found.

It should be mentioned that the great majority of patients included in this study were receiving fluphenazine, given either orally or in the long-acting injectable form (decanoate or enanthate). Thus the role of fluphenazine cannot be assessed. Further cross-sectional studies involving neuroleptics with more selective dopamine type 2 (D_2) receptor blocking properties (greater D_2/D_1 ratios than phenothiazines or thioxanthenes) are now under way with the same group of patients. It has been our clinical experience that fluphenazine treatment (oral or depot injection) leads to a somewhat greater incidence of supersensitivity psychosis as opposed to the more selective D_2 receptor, such as haloperidol (20%).

CONCLUSION

Table 6.5 summarizes our findings from two epidemiologic studies conducted in tardive dyskinesia (18,34) and one in supersensitivity psychosis (33). Risk factors associated with tardive dyskinesia have been better documented and several of them have become accepted. Increased age has become a widely accepted factor; after age, presence of affective disorder is considered to increase the risk by twofold; finally, the presence of a history of brain damage appears to lead

Table 6.5 Risk Factors (Host and Drug) for Tardive Dyskinesia and Supersensitivity Psychosis

	Tardive Dyskinesia	Supersensitivity Psychosis
Host factors	Age[+++] Poor prognosis[+] Affective disorder[+++] Organic syndrome[++]	Good prognosis schizophrenia[++]
Drug factors	Duration of neuroleptic treatment[++]	High doses of medication[+++] Short half-life[++]
	Unselective dopamine blockers (low-potency neuroleptics)[++]	
	Unselective D_2 blockers (fluphenazine)[+]	

Relative importance indicated by the number of [+] signs.

to an increased severity of tardive dyskinesia. Also listed in Table 6.5 is the presence of poor prognosis schizophrenia. Even though we found it consistently in our own studies, more studies will be needed to establish its importance. In contrast, for supersensitivity psychosis, in this preliminary analysis of the results, we found that good prognosis schizophrenia tended to be associated with its presence. On the other hand, regarding drug factor, high doses of neuroleptic associated with high levels of prolactin and high neuroleptic levels (radioreceptor assay, RRA) strongly suggest its association with the syndrome. In contrast, no specific drug factor has been well-established to predict the presence of tardive dyskinesia, but some drug factors have been suggested to be of importance.

REFERENCES

1. Crane GE. Dyskinesia and neuroleptics. Arch Gen Psychiatry 1968;19:700–703.
2. Crane GE. Persistent dyskinesia. Br J Psychiatry 1973;122:395–405.
3. American College of Neuropsychopharmacology—Food and Drug Administration Task Force. Neurological syndromes associated with antipsychotic drug use. Arch Gen Psychiatry 1973;28:463–466.
4. Kane JM, Smith JM. Tardive dyskinesia. Prevalence and risk factors, 1959 to 1979. Arch Gen Psychiatry 1982;39:473–481.
5. American Psychiatric Association. Tardive Dyskinesia: Summary of a Task Force Report of the American Psychiatric Association. Am J Psychiatry 1980;137:1163–1172.
6. Jeste DV, Wyatt RJ. Changing epidemiology of tardive dyskinesia: an overview. Am J Psychiatry 1981;138:297–309.
7. Barnes TRE, Kidger T, Gore SM. Tardive dyskinesia: a 3-year follow-up study. Psychol Med 1983;13:71–81.
8. Richardson MA, Pass R, Craig TJ, Vickers E. Factors influencing the prevalence and severity of tardive dyskinesia. Psychopharmacol Bull 1984;20:33–38.
9. Waddington JL. Tardive dyskinesia, fluphenazine decanoate, and haloperidol (letter). Am J Psychiatry 1982;139:703–704.
10. Kane JM, Woerner M, Lieberman J, et al. The prevalence of tardive dyskinesia. Psychopharmacol Bull 1985;21:136–139.
11. Chouinard G, Annable L, Ross-Chouinard A. Supersensitivity psychosis and tardive dyskinesia: a survey in schizophrenic outpatients. Psychopharmacol Bull 1986;22:891–896.

12. Ezrin-Waters C, Seeman MV, Seeman P. Tardive dyskinesia in schizophrenic outpatients: prevalence and significant variables. J Clin Psychiatry 1981;42:16–22.

13. Guy W, Ban TA, Wilson WH. The prevalence of abnormal involuntary movements among chronic schizophrenics. Int Clin Psychopharmacol 1986;1:134–144.

14. Williams R, Naya A, Dalby JT. Tardive dyskinesia in outpatient schizophrenics treated with depot phenothiazines (letter). J Clin Psychopharmacol 1986;6:318–319.

15. Morgenstern H, Glazer WM, Gibowski LD, Holmberg S. Predictors of tardive dyskinesia: results of a cross-sectional study in an outpatient population. J Chronic Dis 1987;40:319–327.

16. Holden TJ. Tardive dyskinesia in long-term hospitalised Zulu psychiatric patients. S Afr Med J 1987;71:88–90.

17. D'Alessandro R, Benassi G, Cristina E, Gallassi R, Manzaroli D. The prevalence of lingual–facial–buccal dyskinesias in the elderly. Neurology 1986;36:1350–1351.

18. Chouinard G, Annable L, Ross-Chouinard A, Nestoros JN. Factors related to tardive dyskinesia. Am J Psychiatry 1979;136:79–83.

19. Kane JM, Woerner M, Weinhold P, Wegner J, Kinon B. Incidence of tardive dyskinesia: five-year data from a prospective study. Psychopharmacol Bull 1984;20:39–40.

20. Kane JM, Woerner M, Borenstein M, Wegner J, Lieberman J. Integrating incidence and prevalence of tardive dyskinesia. Psychopharmacol Bull 1986;22:254–258.

21. Mukherjee S, Rosen AM, Cardenas C, Varia V, Olarte S. Tardive dyskinesia in psychiatric outpatients. Arch Gen Psychiatry 1982;39:466–469.

22. Gardos G, Cole JO, La Brie RA. Drug variables in the etiology of tardive dyskinesia–application of discriminant function analysis. Prog Neuropsychopharmacol 1977;1:147–154.

23. Smith RC, Strizich M, Klass D. Drug history and tardive dyskinesia. Am J Psychiatry 1978;135:1402–1403.

24. Chouinard G, Jones BD, Annable L. Neuroleptic-induced supersensitivity psychosis. Am J Psychiatry 1978;135:1409–1410.

25. Chouinard G, Jones BD. Neuroleptic-induced supersensitivity psychosis: Clinical and pharmacologic characteristics. Am J Psychiatry 1980;137:16–21.

26. Davis KL, Rosenberg GS. Is there a limbic system equivalent of tardive dyskinesia? Biol Psychiatry 1979;14:699.

27. Chouinard G, Jones BD. Neuroleptic-induced supersensitivity psychosis, the hump course and tardive dyskinesia. J Clin Psychopharmacol 1982;2:143–144.

28. Ekholm B, Eriksson K, Lindstrom LHH. Supersensitivity psychosis in schizophrenic patients after sudden clozapine withdrawal. Psychopharmacology 1984;83:293–294.

29. Perenyi A, Kuncz E, Bagdy G. Early relapse after sudden withdrawal or dose reduction of clozapine. Psychopharmacology 1985;86:244.

30. Witschy JK, Malone GL, Holden LD. Psychosis after neuroleptic withdrawal in a manic-depressive patient. Am J Psychiatry 1984;141:105–106.

31. Steiner W, Laporta M, Chouinard G. Neuroleptic-induced supersensitivity psychosis in patients with bipolar affective disorder. Acta Psychiatr Scand 1990;81:437–444.

32. Kent TA, Wilber RD. Reserpine withdrawal psychosis: the possible role of denervation supersensitivity of receptors. J Nerv Ment Dis 1982;170:502–504.

33. Chouinard G, Annable L, Ross-Chouinard A. Neuroleptic-induced psychological supersensitivity syndromes: are these syndromes myth or reality? Psychopharmacol Bull 1986;3:891–896.

34. Chouinard G, Annable L, Ross-Chouinard A, Mercier P. A five-year prospective longitudinal study of tardive dyskinesia: factors predicting appearance of new cases. J Clin Psychopharmacol 1988;8:215–269.

35. Spitzer RL, Endicott J, Robins E. Research diagnostic criteria. 3rd ed. New York: Biometrics Research, 1977.

36. Chouinard G, Annable L, Ross-Chouinard A, Kropsky M. Ethopropazine and benztropine in neuroleptic-induced parkinsonism. J Clin Psychiatry 1979;40:147–152.

37. Chouinard G, Ross-Chouinard A, Annable L, Jones BD. Extrapyramidal symptom rating scale. Can J Neurol Sci 1980;7:233.

38. Creese I, Snyder SH. A simple and sensitive radioreceptor assay for antischizophrenic drugs in blood. Nature 1977;270:180–182.

39. Lader SR. A radioreceptor assay for neuroleptic drugs in plasma. J Immunoassay 1980;2:57–75.

40. Cohen BM, Herschel M, Miller E, et al. Radioreceptor assay of haloperidol tissue levels in the rat. Neuropharmacology 1980;9:663–668.

41. Davis JM. Antipsychotic drugs. In: Freedman AM, Kaplan HI, Sadock BJ, eds. Comprehensive textbook of psychiatry. 3rd ed., vol. 3. Baltimore: Williams & Wilkins, 1980:2257–2289.

42. Schooler NR, Kane JM. Research diagnoses for tardive dyskinesia. Arch Gen Psychiatry 1982;39:486–487.

43. Kane JM, Woerner M, Weinhold P, et al. A prospective study of tardive dyskinesia development: preliminary results. J Clin Psychopharmacol 1982;2:345–349.

Drug-Induced Parkinsonism and Concomitant Tardive Dyskinesia

GEORGE GARDOS   JONATHAN O. COLE

INTRODUCTION

The introduction of the neuroleptic (NL) antipsychotic drugs quickly led to the recognition of not only their therapeutic properties but their troublesome side effects as well. All classic NLs such as phenothiazines, thioxanthenes, and butyrophenones commonly induce extrapyramidal symptoms (EPS) of tremor, rigidity, and bradykinesia that resemble Parkinson's disease. The frequent occurrence of drug-induced EPS was documented as early as 1961 by Ayd, who found a 15.4% prevalence of EPS (including akathisia and acute dystonia as well as drug-induced parkinsonism (DIP)) in a survey of 3775 patients treated with NL (1). The apparent reversibility of DIP and its effective treatment with antiparkinsonian drugs might be the major reasons why this easily recognizable and common side effect has been rarely considered a major clinical problem. In fact, for a time the production of a minimal degree of parkinsonism ("the NL threshold") (2) was aimed for during NL therapy as the *sine qua non* of antipsychotic efficacy. This notion of a "NL threshold" was later abandoned, however, because of evidence that DIP was neither necessary nor sufficient for antipsychotic effect.

Tardive dyskinesia (TD), in contrast to DIP, may be credited with the dubious distinction of being by far the most extensively covered NL side effect in the literature. The TD syndrome consists mainly of choreoathetoid movements of the face, trunk, and extremities, and of tics and grimaces. Vermicular and undulating movements of protrusion of the tongue, chewing, and puckering or pouting of the lip are typical features of oral dyskinesia. Following the early clinical descriptions published in the late 1950s, there has been a burgeoning literature on TD growing at an almost exponential rate. The potential irreversibility, rising prevalence (3) (as compared with DIP, which may be a decreasing inci-

dence according to Ayd's second survey from 1981 (4)), and the lack of effective treatment have combined to make TD a unique and portentous NL side effect. However, the notion of DIP as a benign and TD as a malignant complication of NL treatment is as simplistic as it is inaccurate. There is a great deal of variability in the severity of symptoms and in the course and prognosis of patients with either TD or DIP.

The focus of this chapter is on the relative prevalence, pathophysiology, clinical impact, and management of these two NL-related EPS, when occurring together.

PREVALENCE OF CONCOMITANT DIP AND TD

The assumption of contrasting pathophysiology responsible for DIP and TD, namely, striatal dopamine (DA) deficiency and overactivity, respectively, leads one to expect that these two conditions might be mutually exclusive and therefore not found in the same patient. This assumption has been proven wrong. There are numerous methodologically adequate published studies comparing DIP and TD in the same population. In what is probably the earliest publication devoted to this topic, Fann and Lake described three patients on long-term phenothiazines who demonstrated typical DIP as well as buccofaciolingual dyskinesia (5). Treatment of these patients with antiparkinsonian drugs resulted in an increase of TD severity and a decrease in DIP in line with the DA deficiency/excess hypothesis. Although not the focus of their research, other investigators had previously made mention of the coexistence of DIP and TD (6–8). Attempts to estimate how frequently these two syndromes are observed together may be gauged from epidemiologic studies in which TD and DIP were concurrently assessed. Table 7.1 summarizes the relevant research data.

Table 7.1   Studies of Concurrent DIP and TD Prevalence

Author	Year	n	Condition	Measures	TD%	DIP%	Other Findings
Demars (9)	1966	371	Chronic IP	Clinical judgment	7.0	8.6	DIP and facial dyskinesia were mostly mild and not necessarily irreversible
Degkwitz and Wenzel (6)	1967	1,291	IP	Clinical judgment	15.9	16.5	19.2% coexistent TD and DIP
Crane (8)	1972	180	IP	Clinical judgment	24.4	28.3	4.5% patients with coexistent TD and DIP. Neuroleptic decrease resulted in decreasing DIP and increasing TD
Chouinard et al (10)	1979	261	Schiz. OP	AIMS, ESRS	30.7	65.5	Inverse relationship between TD and DIP
Chouinard et al (11)	1986	169	5-year FU of above	AIMS, ESRS	44.0	72.0	TD and DIP "were commonly present simultaneously." Change in DIP was best predictor of TD development
Wojcik et al (12)	1980	210	Mostly OP	AIMS, TAKE	17.6	—	TD patients had significantly more bradykinesia ($p = 0.005$) and rigidity ($p = 0.0001$) than patients without TD
McCreadie et al (13)	1982	133	Schiz.	AIMS, TAKE	31.0	31.0	9% with coexistent TD and DIP. DIP patients more aware of side effects than TD patients.
Mukherjee et al (14)	1982	153	OP	AIMS, S-A	30.7	12.4	Positive correlation between TD and DIP ($p = <0.0001$)
Wolf et al (15)	1983	88	Male IP	ADS	56.8	38.4	27.3% coexistent TD and DIP, significant positive correlation ($p = 0.95, p < 0.0001$) between S-A and ADS scores in 7 patients followed longitudinally
Toenniessen et al (16)	1985	57	IP > 55 years old	AIMS, Global DIP	49.0	51.0	Significant negative correlation between TD and DIP
Casey et al (17)	1986	33	Elderly IP (FU Study)	AIMS, Gerlach Scale	27.0% decrease in scores	34.0% increase in scores	TD and DIP changed reciprocally over several years. The large majority of patients had coexistent TD and DIP
Richardson et al (18)	1986	301	IP	ADS, S-A	30.0	15.0	24% coexistent TD and DIP, higher in older patients and with longer treatment duration
Kolakowska et al (19)	1986	91	Schizophrenic (77) and schizo-affective (14) patients	AIMS, S-A	25.3	38.4	DIP more common in TD pts (56.8%) than among dose-matched non-TD subjects (28.8%)
Richardson et al (20)	1987	41	Child IP on NL	AIMS, ADS, S-A	12.0	42.0	DIP associated with higher TD score ($p < 0.05$)
Kucharski et al (21)	1987	331	IP	AIMS, REPS	32.1	26.8	TD and DIP inversely related. 27 (8.2%) patients with coexistent TD and DIP more impaired on memory test corrected for age differences

T a b l e   7 . 1   Continued

Author	Year	n	Condition	Measures	TD%	DIP%	Other Findings
Binder et al (22)	1987	126	IP	AIMS, Global DIP	20.6	40.5	All patients on antiparkinsonian drugs, TD more prevalent with higher NL doses
Gardos et al (23)	1987	100	Mostly OP with early TD	AIMS, S-A	—	23.0	Longitudinal study of early TD. DIP more frequent in unipolar depression ($p = 0.05$), less frequent in bipolar depression ($p = 0.05$), S-A did not correlate significantly with AIMS
Hansen et al (24)	1988	66	IP with TD	AIMS, St. Hans	—	56.0	Risk factors for DIP in TD patients similar to no-TD patients: older age recent use of NL. TD severity, fewer years of past NL
Perenyi et al (25)	1988	241	OP (5-year FU)	AIMS, S-A	17.0% increase in AIMS scores	72.0% increase in S-A scores	TD and DIP changes did not correlate significantly
Yassa and Nair (26)	1988	315	Chronic IP	Smith TD = DIP scales	TD% 32.4	DIP% 12.7	3.8% had coexistent TD & DIP. Age and affecting disorders risk factors for both TD & DIP

IP, inpatients; Schiz., schizophrenics; AIMS, Abnormal Involuntary Movements Scale (27); S-A, Simpson-Angus Scale (28); OP, outpatients; NL, neuroleptic; TAKE, targeting abnormal kinetic effects (12); ESRS, Extrapyramidal Rating Scale (29); ADS, abbreviated Simpson dyskinesia scale (31); FU, follow-up; REPS, Reversible EPS Scale (21); St. Hans, St. Hans Rating Scale for EPS (30).

One of the obvious problems comparing the studies is the heterogeneity of the populations and of the measures employed. Even though the Abnormal Involuntary Movement Scale (AIMS) was used to assess TD in the majority of studies, the diverse criteria chosen from rating scores to define a TD case makes comparing TD prevalence rates difficult. Even less consistency was seen in the assessment of DIP prevalence. Various rating scales were employed and the definition of a case of DIP based on scores seemed arbitrary. The published prevalence rates are therefore at best a rough guide as to the frequency and severity of TD and DIP. Since in the majority of studies DIP rates exceeded TD prevalence, the data suggest that DIP might be as common, and possibly more so, than TD. The actual prevalence rates of simultaneously observed TD and DIP varied considerably, which is hardly surprising because the lack of uniform criteria for defining TD and DIP cases increases the variability even more for their joint occurrence. The reported joint prevalence rates ranged from 5.5% to 27.3%, which could be an underestimate of the true prevalence. Casey et al (17) did not give prevalence estimates but found that the majority of their patients about 65 years old had both disorders, and Chouinard et al (11) also found the two disorders to frequently occur together. In a study of TD patients by Hansen et al, the prevalence of DIP was as high as 56% (24).

A different statistical approach to the phenomenon of coexisting TD and DIP is to calculate their correlation coefficients. Several authors reported correlations of scores or of changes in TD and DIP over time. The findings are, however, equivocal. Some studies reported negative correlations between TD and DIP—higher TD scores being associated with lower DIP scores and vice versa (10,16) or increase in one accompanied by decrease in the other (8,17). Other studies found positive correlations (12,14,20). The data provide no clear support either for the notion that DIP and TD are opposites or for the view of their frequent coexistence. The best interpretation of the data is that DIP and TD are overlapping phenomena.

The data presented in Table 7.1 focuses on TD and DIP rates and only peripherally touches on factors associated with these syndromes such as age, gender, diagnosis, and NL variables. The interaction of these variables is complex and may be assumed to influence TD and DIP prevalence. For instance, men and women show different age-related changes in TD and DIP in association with changing levels of relevant hormones and monoamines (e.g., estrogens, monoamine oxidase) (18). Extensive discussion of these relationships is beyond the scope of this chapter. Overall, the factors found in a study to be related to TD tended not to be the same as those featured in the development of DIP. Another interesting observation is the apparently high rate of DIP despite antiparkinsonian drug therapy. For instance in the Japanese survey by Binder et al, the 40.5% DIP rate was observed with all patients being on antiparkinsonian drugs (22). Treatment-resistant DIP was also observed in our Hungarian cohort (25) as well as in American patients (8,32).

PATHOPHYSIOLOGIC MECHANISMS

The original DA deficiency/excess hypothesis postulated that DIP and TD represented opposite pathophysiologic states and were, therefore, mutually exclusive and not expected to occur in the same patient at the same time. With the emergence of convincing data of the coexistence of TD and DIP in carrying proportions of NL-treated patients, the hypothesis had to be modified and expanded.

DIP is a Forerunner of TD

Epidemiologic data suggest that DIP observed early in NL therapy may lead to subsequent TD development. The bulk of the data is derived from TD prevalence studies in which TD status was associated with DIP, the latter often assessed retrospectively (6,7,10,11,33,34). These data are greatly strengthened by the prospective study of TD development by Kane et al, which also shows a statistically significant association between DIP and subsequent TD (35,36). The different symptom components of DIP are not associated equally with TD development. Chouinard et al (10,11) believe that the hyperkinetic symptoms of tremor and akathisia are principally the precursors of TD, while Gerlach lays emphasis on bradykinesia as the most relevant parkinsonian symptom for TD development (33). Following NL drug discontinuation, Crane (8) observed TD developing in some patients who showed tremor and/or bradykinesia while still on NL. The pathogenetic connection implicating DIP in the development of TD was elegantly spelled out by Gerlach (33) in the following hypothesis: the pathophysiology of involuntary hyperkinesia in NL-treated psychiatric patients may consist of a primary DA deficiency (pharmacologic or structural) and a secondary relative hyperactivity in the dopaminergic system ("DA hypersensitivity"). Although this hypothesis does not directly account for concomitant TD and DIP, it appears to be a useful explanatory concept for the topographic differences in the formulations that follow.

DIP and TD are Different Manifestations of the Same Underlying Vulnerability

The susceptibility of the neostriatum to altered function was proposed as the mechanism leading to both DIP and TD following NL treatment (5,18). Hansen et al (24) found similar risk factors for DIP occurring in TD as well as in non-TD patients. Chouinard et al (11) suggested that vulnerability to DIP and TD increased with advancing age

because of decreasing DA synthesis. They cite data where DIP and TD were more commonly seen together at the five-year follow-up than at baseline (11). The notion of age-related joint vulnerability is by itself not a sufficient explanation for concomitant TD and DIP, but it may be regarded as a factor tending to increase their coexistence, especially in the elderly.

Topographic Differences

The idea that different NL side effects occurring simultaneously might reflect different neuropharmacologic events at different locations of the neostriatum is intuitively appealing. Crane (38) proposed that "different types of biochemical imbalance in the affected areas of the CNS" account for TD and DIP occurring at different times or simutaneously at different body areas. Different anatomic areas in the striatum underlying EPS of the face and of the upper extremities was the explanation offered for the association of orofacial dyskinesia and parkinsonian tremor found by Hansen et al (39). Gerlach suggested that a topographic organization of the neostriatum could explain the localization of TD primarily in the orofacial region (37,40). By contrast, the topographic distribution of parkinsonism is more generalized. The gradual shift of the predominance of choreoathetoid movements from the extremities in younger patients to the orofacial region of the elderly may be based on age-related changes in the oral somatotropic region of the basal ganglia (37,40). However, Brown and White (41) found that in TD subjects limb-truncal scores correlated negatively with Mini Mental State examination scores and positively with negative schizophrenic symptoms, while orofacial scores correlated only with negative symptoms, suggesting more cognitive impairment in patients with truncal and limb dyskinesia.

The different EPS observed simultaneously in different body regions may reflect different DA mechanisms (13,39). The old theory of DA deficiency/excess is being reformulated with new research on multiple DA receptors. The presence of DA type 1 and 2 (D_1 and D_2) receptors in the striatum is now generally accepted (42). Animal data provide evidence that D_1 and D_2 receptors are related to different neuronal pathways and that they are not only pharmacologically but functionally distinct (43). The topographic differences involved in concomitant DIP and TD could, therefore, be explained on the basis of the different properties of DA receptor types: blockage of one DA receptor type might mediate DIP, while stimulation of another could be involved in TD development (44).

Effect of Psychotropic Drugs

Certain psychopharmacologic agents may contribute to simultaneous DIP and TD. Wojcik et al (12) suggested, for instance, that antiparkinsonian drugs when prescribed for DIP induce or aggravate orofacial TD, while the trunk and extremities may retain varying degrees of parkinsonian manifestations. Fann and Lake offered similar speculations with regard to NL with anticholinergic potency: the anti-DA effects of the drug may promote DIP, while the anticholinergic effects increase TD potential (5). These explanations are consistent with topographic differences in the striatum as described above, but emphasize the differential impact on EPS of compounds affecting the cholinergic system. Owing to the complexity of the interaction of neurotransmitters, the traditional emphasis on the DA/acetylcholine balance is almost certainly an oversimplification. A scheme based on the heterogeneous organization of the striatum with complex balance between various DA, cholinergic, and gamma-aminobutyric acid (GABA)-ergic systems may be a more appropriate model for explaining the diverse extrapyramidal effects of NL (45).

In recent years the atypical neuroleptics risperidone and clozapine have become widely used in the treatment of schizophrenia (46) and other psychotic disorders. These compounds produce DIP less frequently than traditional NLs and may also be associated with less TD development. The lower prevalence of coexistent TD and DIP during treatment with atypical NLs needs to be demonstrated in new studies.

MANAGEMENT OF CONCOMITANT DIP AND TD

Both conditions are common NL side effects and usually occur in the presence of serious psychotic disorder. The optimal strategy of managing simultaneous DIP and TD, therefore, has to take into account the need to treat the psychosis as well. Discontinuation of NL, even if it were effective for DIP and TD symptoms, is rarely feasible in schizophrenics because of the high likelihood of psychotic decompensation (47), although patients belonging to other diagnostic categories may fare better without NL. Another key principle of management is based on the recognition that DIP and TD are often linked and "share reciprocally functioning or dysfunctioning mechanisms" (17).

The inverse functional relationship has also been stressed by other investigators (10,14,16). The corollary of the negative association is the expectation that any intervention that helps one disorder will aggravate the other. Antiparkinsonian drugs ameliorate DIP while tending to worsen the manifestations of TD (5,33,37,45,48). Attempted pharmacotherapy of TD with anti-DA, cholinergic, and GABAergic compounds, on the other hand, tend to exacerbate parkinsonian symptoms (33,44,48). The practicing clinician is thus often caught on the horns of dilemma: the obvious interventions of NL withdrawal, antiparkinsonian drugs, and anti-DA treatments may be therapeutic for some symptoms but may worsen others. However, it is possible to devise strategies to handle most clinical situations in which DIP, TD, and a psychotic illness all need to be managed. Two treatment principles are briefly discussed here.

Side effects causing distress and functional disturbance need primary attention. TD in some instances may be highly visible, yet the concomitant DIP may be more distressing and incapacitating. Treatment with antiparkinsonian drugs is likely to relieve the DIP-related complaints, although at the likely expense of aggravating TD. If TD rather than DIP is the more distressing condition, the rational treatment approach would aim at reducing TD severity, even though DIP may worsen as a result.

Rare but serious clinical situations arise when severe TD or severe DIP alternate depending on which syndrome is being treated pharmacologically. Case reports illustrate the difficulties encountered in managing such difficult patients (5,44,48,49). For example, Bitton and Melamed describe two patients afflicted with severe and distressing TD who also showed evidence of DIP (44). NL treatment suppressed the former but greatly exacerbated the latter, while L-dopa/carbidopa treatment tended to control DIP but precipitated severe choreoathetosis. Judicious pharmacotherapy with compounds affecting the major relevant and known neurotransmitters (DA, acetylcholine, GABA) that provide reasonable control of the major symptoms is a desirable but not easily attainable clinical goal.

Whenever possible, decreasing NL exposure should be considered. The only treatment intervention that is likely to favorably affect both DIP and TD in the long run is NL dose reduction or NL discontinuation. A stepwise, slow, gradual dose-tapering is often feasible clinically, as symptom exacerbation is usually slow to commence and NL dose adjustment upward can be readily undertaken to prevent full relapse. A variety of low-dose strategies have recently been developed, all of which substantially reduce NL exposure (50). Complete NL discontinuation may be feasible in patients with affective illness or other nonschizophrenic patients. Following NL discontinuation, DIP is likely to remit promptly. TD, on the other hand, may get worse temporarily, but is likely to improve eventually (51,52,57).

An alternative approach to reducing NL exposure is to substitute for NL a drug with little or no propensity to induce EPS. The atypical NLs may be suitable candidates. There is accumulating evidence, for instance, that clozapine and benzamide compounds may beneficially influence already manifest TD and may prevent the development of TD while causing less DIP and classic NLs (53,54). The availability of risperidone and the imminent appearance on the market of other new atypical NLs will very likely reduce the incidence of all the major neuroleptic side effects.

REFERENCES

1. Ayd FJ Jr. A survey of drug-induced extrapyramidal reactions. JAMA 1961;75:1054–1060.
2. Haase HJ. The action of neuroleptic drugs. Chicago: Year Book Medical, 1965.
3. Jeste DV, Wyatt RJ. Changing epidemiology of tardive dyskinesia: an overview. Am J Psychiatry 1981;138:297–308.
4. Ayd FJ Jr. Drug-induced parkinsonism: a follow-up. Int Drug Ther Newl 1987;22:9–10.

5. Fann WE, Lake RL. On the coexistence of parkinsonism and tardive dyskinesia. Dis Nerv Sys 1974;35:324–326.

6. Degkwitz R, Wenzel W. Persistent extrapyramidal side effects after long-term application of neuroleptics. In: Brill H, ed. Neuropsychopharmacology. New York: Excerpta Medica, 1967:608–615.

7. Crane GE. Persistence of neurological symptoms due to neuroleptic drugs. Am J Psychiatry 1971;127:1407–1410.

8. Crane GE. Pseudoparkinsonism and tardive dyskinesia. Arch Neurol 1972;27:426–430.

9. Demars JPCA. Neuromuscular effects of long-term phenothiazine medication, electroconvulsive therapy and leucotomy. J Nerv Ment Dis 1966;143:73–79.

10. Chouinard G, Annable L, Ross-Chouinard A, Nestoros JN. Factors related to tardive dyskinesia. Am J Psychiatry 1979;136:79–83.

11. Chouinard G, Annable L, Mercier P, Ross-Chouinard A. A five-year follow-up study of tardive dyskinesia. Psychopharmacol Bull 1986;22:259–263.

12. Wojcik JD, Gelenberg AJ, LaBrie RA, Mieske M. Prevalence of tardive dyskinesia in an outpatient population. Compr Psychiatry 1980;21:370–380.

13. McCreadie RG, Barron ET, Winslow GS. The Nithsdale schizophrenia survey: II. Abnormal movements. Br J Psychiatry 1982;140:587–590.

14. Mukherjee S, Rosen AM, Cardenas C, Varia V, Alarte S. Tardive dyskinesia in psychiatric outpatients. Arch Gen Psychiatry 1982;39:466–469.

15. Wolf ME, Chevesich J, Lehrer E, Mosnaim AD. The clinical association of tardive dyskinesia and drug-induced parkinsonism. Biol Psychiatry 1983;18:1181–1188.

16. Toenniessen LM, Casey DE, McFarland BH. Tardive dyskinesia in the aged. Arch Gen Psychiatry 1985;42:278–284.

17. Casey DE, Poulsen VJ, Meidahl B, Gerlach J. Neuroleptic-induced tardive dyskinesia and parkinsonism: changes during several years of continuing treatment. Psychopharmacol Bull 1986;22:250–253.

18. Richardson MA, Pass R, Craig TJ. The coexistence of parkinsonism-like symptoms and tardive dyskinesia—revisited. In: Shagass C, Josiassen RC, Bridger WH, et al, eds. Biological psychiatry. Vol. 17. New York: Elsevier, 1986.

19. Kolakowska T, Williams AO, Ardern M, Reveley MA. Tardive dyskinesia in schizophrenics under 60 years of age. Biol Psychiatry 1986;21:161–169.

20. Richardson MA, Haugland G, Summers I, et al. Associations: neuroleptic use and side effects in child psychiatric patients. Presented at the 140th Annual Meeting of the American Psychiatric Association, Washington, 1987.

21. Kucharski LT, Wagner RL, Friedman JH. An investigation of the coexistence of abnormal involuntary movements, parkinsonism, and akathisia in chronic psychiatric inpatients. Psychopharmacol Bull 1987;23:215–217.

22. Binder RL, Kazamatsuri H, Nishimura T, McNeil DE. Tardive dyskinesia and neuroleptic-induced parkinsonism in Japan. Am J Psychiatry 1987;144:1494–1496.

23. Gardos G, Cole JO, Haskell DS, et al. Neuroleptic-induced parkinsonian symptoms at different stages of TD development. Poster presented at Society of Biological Psychiatry Annual Meeting, Chicago, May 9, 1987.

24. Hansen TE, Brown WL, Weigel RM, Casey ED. Risk factors for drug-induced parkinsonism in tardive dyskinesia patients. J Clin Psychiatry 1988;49:139–141.

25. Perenyi A, Gardos G, Samu I, Kallos M, Cole JO. Changes in extrapyramidal symptoms following antiparkinson drug withdrawal. Clin Neuropharmacol 1983;6:55–61.

26. Yassa R, Nair V. The association of tardive dyskinesia and pseudoparkinsonism. Prog Neuro-Psychopharmacol & Biol Psychiatry 1988;12:909–914.

27. Guy W. ECDEU assessment manual for psychopharmacology. US Department of Health Education and Welfare Publication 76-228, 1986:534–537.

28. Simpson GM, Angus JWS. A rating scale for extrapyramidal effects. Acta Psychiatr Scand 1970;46(suppl 212):11.

29. Chouinard G, Annable L, Ross-Chouinard A. A double-blind controlled study of fluphenazine decanoate and enathate in the maintenance treatment of schizophrenic outpatients. In: Ayd FS Jr, ed. Depot fluphenazines: twelve years' experience. Baltimore: Ayd Medical Communications, 1978.

30. Gerlach J. Tardive dyskinesia. Dan Med Bull 1979;26:209–244.

31. Simpson GM, Klee JH, Zoubok B, Gardos G, Cole JO. A rating scale for tardive dyskinesia. Am J Psychiatry 1982;139:341–343.

32. Richardson MA, Craig TJ. The coexistence of parkinsonism-like symptoms and tardive dyskinesia. Am J Psychiatry 1982;139:341–343.

33. Gerlach J, Thorsen K. The movement pattern of oral tardive dyskinesia in relation to anticholinergic and antidopaminergic treatment. Int Pharmacopsychiatry 1976;11:1–7.

34. DeVeaugh Geiss J. Epidemiology of tardive dyskinesia. In: DeVeaugh Geiss J, ed. Tardive dyskinesia and related involuntary movement disorders. Boston: John Wright, PSG Inc., 1982.

35. Kane JM, Woerner M, Weinhold P, et al. A prospective study of tardive dyskinesia development: preliminary results. J Clin Psychopharmacol 1982;2:345–349.

36. Kane JM, Woerner M, Borenstein M, et al. Integrating incidence and prevalence of tardive dyskinesia. Psychopharmacol Bull 1986;222:254–258.

37. Gerlach J. Relationship between tardive dyskinesia. L-dopa-induced hyperkinesia and parkinsonism. Psychopharmacology 1977;51:259–263.

38. Crane GE. Tardive dyskinesia: a review. Neuropsychopharmacology. Excerpta Medica Intern Congress Series No. 359, Amsterdam, 1974.

39. Hansen TE, Glazer WM, Moore DC. Tremor and tardive dyskinesia. J Clin Psychiatry 1986;47:461–464.

40. Gerlach J. Pathophysiological mechanisms underlying tardive dyskinesia. In: Casey DE, Chase TN, Christensen AV, Gerlach J, eds. Dyskinesia: research and treatment. Berlin: Springer-Verlag, 1985:98–103.

41. Brown KW, White T. The influence of topography on the cognitive and psychopathological effects of tardive dyskinesia. Am J Psychiatry 1992;149:1385–1389.

42. Seeman P. Brain dopamine receptors. Pharmacol Rev 1980;32:229–313.

43. Ungerstedt V, Herrera-Marschitz M, Stahle L, et al. Functional classification of different dopamine receptors. In: Casey DE, Chase TN, Christensen AV, Gerlach J, eds. Dyskinesia: research and treatment. Berlin: Springer-Verlag, 1985:19–30.

44. Bitton V, Melamed E. Coexistence of severe parkinsonism and tardive dyskinesia as side effects of neuroleptic therapy. J Clin Psychiatry 1984;45:28–30.

45. Scheel-Kruger J, Arnt J. New aspects on the role of dopamine, acetylcholine, and GABA in the development of tardive dyskinesia. In: Casey DE, Chase TN, Christensen AV, Gerlach J, eds. Dyskinesia: research and treatment. Berlin: Springer-Verlag, 1985:46–57.

46. Kane JM. Schizophrenia. N Engl J Med 1996;334:34–41.

47. Davis JM. Overview: maintenance therapy in psychiatry. I. Schizophrenia. Am J Psychiatry 1975;132:1237–1245.

48. DeFraites EG Jr, David KL, Berger PA. Coexisting tardive dyskinesia and parkinsonism: A case report. Biol Psychiatry 1977;12:267–272.

49. Greil W, Haag H, Rossnagl G, Ruther E. Effect of anticholinergics on tardive dyskinesia. A controlled discontinuation study. Br J Psychiatry 1984;145:304–310.

50. Kane JM, Lieberman JA. Maintenance pharmacotherapy in schizophrenia. In: Meltzer HY, ed. Psychopharmacology: the third generation of progress. New York: Raven, 1987:1103–1109.

51. Gardos G, Cole JO. The prognosis of tardive dyskinesia. J Clin Psychiatry 1983;44:177–179.

52. Casey DE, Toenniessen LM. Neuroleptic treatment in tardive dyskinesia: can it be developed into a clinical strategy for long-term treatment? In: Bennet J, Belmaker RH, eds. Modern problems in pharmacopsychiatry. Vol. 21, New Directions in Tardive Dyskinesia Research. Basel: Karger, 1983:65–79.

53. Pi EH, Simpson GM. Atypical neuroleptics: clozapine and the benzamides in the prevention and treatment of tardive dyskinesia. In: Bennet J, Belmaker RH, eds. Modern Problems in Pharmacopsychiatry. Vol. 21, New Directions in Tardive Dyskinesia Research. Basel: Karger, 1983:80–86.

54. Claghorn J, Honigfeld G, Abuzzahab FS, et al. The risks and benefits of clozapine versus chlorpromazine. J Clin Psychopharmacol 1987;7:377–384.

Paradoxical Tardive Dyskinesia

DANIEL E. CASEY

INTRODUCTION

The initial proposals for understanding "paradoxical tardive dyskinesia" as a subtype of tardive dyskinesia occurred in the mid-1970s (1–3). They were prompted by the observation of atypical or paradoxical responses to drug treatment that contrasted with the responses usually seen in tardive dyskinesia. A series of brief reports and articles soon confirmed these findings (4–8).

Retrospective analyses of tardive dyskinesia drug treatment studies also frequently identified specific patients with responses that were atypical from the larger group of patients in the study. These patients, described both before and after the concept of paradoxical tardive dyskinesia was proposed, quite probably represented examples of this atypical syndrome but were not recognized as such. Other phrases that have been used to describe patients associated with paradoxical tardive dyskinesia include "initial hyperkinesia," "primary hyperkinesia," "paradoxical dyskinesia," and "hypercholinergic dyskinesia" (1,5,8).

DIAGNOSIS

Clinical Description

Both paradoxical tardive dyskinesia and typical tardive dyskinesia are characterized by involuntary, hyperkinetic abnormal movements that primarily involve the orofacial region but may also include chloreoathetoid symptoms in the limbs and trunk. Often, it is not possible to differentiate these two syndromes solely on the basis of clinical phenomenology. In some cases, however, a distinguishing feature of paradoxical tardive dyskinesia is the more stereotyped and repetitive nature of the dyskinetic symptoms. Occasionally this stereotyped component is so prominent that it may be difficult to distinguish the symptoms from akathisia.

Epidemiology

The true prevalence of paradoxical tardive dyskinesia is unknown because of the limited research in this area. Initial reports suggested it may occur in 25% to 50% of patients who appear to have typical tardive dyskinesia (1,3,7). The few subsequent reports suggested the disorder is less common. Perhaps a realistic estimate of the frequency of paradoxical tardive dyskinesia is 10% of those patients who appear to have typical tardive dyskinesia.

Risk Factors

Risk factors for paradoxical tardive dyskinesia are only hinted at in the literature. Younger patients (under 55 years) are the most frequently described subjects, although there is no particular reason to suspect that paradoxical tardive dyskinesia cannot occur in older patients. Both high- and low-potency neuroleptics have been associated with this syndrome, although there are somewhat more reports implicating the high-potency compounds. Most cases are associated with moderate drug dosage. Temporal aspects of paradoxical tardive dyskinesia are also unclear. The syndrome can occur at any time during neuroleptic therapy. However, its appearance early (days to weeks) after starting a course of neuroleptic treatment helps distinguish it from the much later onset tardive dyskinesia.

Differential Diagnosis

The most important syndrome to distinguish from paradoxical tardive dyskinesia is tardive dyskinesia (9). This is often impossible on the basis of clinical symptoms alone because these symptoms are often identical. The intervention strategies described below can assist in the differential diagnosis. It is also important to differentiate stereotypic behavior that is due to psychotic conditions. A distinguishing difference in these two syndromes is the frequent decrease in stereotypic behavior with neuroleptic administration, which is opposite to the increase seen in paradoxical tardive dyskinesia.

A very challenging clinical situation is to separate paradoxical tardive dyskinesia from other neuroleptic drug-induced acute extrapyramidal syndromes, such as dystonia, parkinsonism, and particularly akathisia. Frequently, the stereotyped repetitive symptoms of paradoxical tardive dyskinesia look very similar to the repetitive movements of akathisia. Indeed, some of the cases in the literature sound as though they are misdiagnoses of akathisia rather than the separate syndrome of paradoxical tardive dyskinesia. Alternatively, it may be that these are actually separate syndromes that coexist. If so, it is extremely difficult to accurately attribute specific symptoms to specific types of extrapyramidal syndrome subtypes.

MANAGEMENT

There are two strategies for managing paradoxical tardive dyskinesia. The first approach is to reduce or discontinue neuroleptic drugs. This should lead to a decrease or resolution of the dyskinetic symptoms. The time course of improvement may range from a few days to a few weeks before discernible changes occur. If no symptom alteration is noted with a dose decrease, it may be necessary to further decrease or even to discontinue the neuroleptic before a substantial symptom amelioration occurs. Conversely, an increase in the neuroleptic dose will often lead to an increase in paradoxical tardive dyskinetic symptoms. These responses in paradoxical tardive dyskinesia are opposite to those responses associated with classical tardive dyskinesia but are characteristic of responses to acute extrapyramidal syndromes.

The second treatment approach involves the use of anticholinergic, antiparkinson drugs. If it is not clinically feasible to decrease or discontinue the neuroleptic drug because of existing psychosis or the fear of exacerbating recently controlled psychotic symptoms, it may be worthwhile to add anticholinergic drugs. In this case, increasing the anticholinergic agents should lead to a decrease in paradoxical tardive dyskinesia. The time course for response is again within a few days to a few weeks. The initial anticholinergic dose may be insufficient, so a full clinical course spanning the appropriate therapeutic dose range is indicated. Decreasing anticholinergic agents usually leads to no change or an increase in symptoms.

The response to other psychotropic drugs that have been used in other extrapyramidal syndromes is unstudied. It is not known whether agents such as beta-adrenergic blockers or benzodiazepines will have an effect on paradoxical tardive dyskinesia.

BASIC SCIENCE

There is no direct evidence available to explain the underlying pathophysiology of paradoxical tardive dyskinesia. The clinical response to drug intervention is opposite to the typical responses seen in classical tardive dyskinesia. This characterization by clinical pharmacology, however, does not necessarily provide a clear understanding of the pathophysiology since the cause of tardive dyskinesia is unknown (10). While it is frequently stated that tardive dyskinesia is due to dopaminergic receptor hypersensitivity, there is no direct evidence supporting this hypothesis and there are many findings that are not compatible with this explanation (10).

The pharmacologic responses of paradoxical tardive dyskinesia are similar to those seen with other acute extrapyramidal syndromes. These are associated with the initiation and continuation of dopamine receptor blockade induced by the continuous use of neuroleptic drugs. As with the acute extrapyramidal syndromes of dystonia, parkinsonism, and akathisia, paradoxical tardive dyskinesia also responds to anticholinergic agents. The response to these anticholinergic drugs has led to the proposal that paradoxical tardive dyskinesia is due to a hypercholinergic dysfunction (1). While this description may be correct, it does not necessarily mean that either dopamine receptor blockade or the resultant relative cholinergic hyperactivity is the primary underlying pathophysiology. These neurotransmitter alterations may only be involved somewhere in the pathway of multiple neurotransmitter imbalances that underlie the acute extrapyramidal syndromes and/or typical tardive dyskinesia.

In summary, paradoxical tardive dyskinesia is phenomenologically similar to tardive dyskinesia but may also share some symptom characteristics in common with other acute extrapyramidal syndromes. Paradoxical tardive dyskinesia is seldom reported, although it probably occurs more often than is reflected in the literature. Perhaps up to 10% of the patients who appear to have classical tardive dyskinesia actually have paradoxical tardive dyskinesia. Unfortunately, accurate estimates of prevalence are limited because of the sparse literature.

Paradoxical tardive dyskinesia is reported more often in patients under 55 years old and is more frequently associated with the high-potency neuroleptics. No particular drug dose appears as a special risk factor, and symptoms may occur at any time during neuroleptic treatment. The differential diagnosis includes tardive dyskinesia, stereotypies of psychosis, and other acute extrapyramidal syndromes. There are no laboratory assessments to aid in the diagnosis of paradoxical tardive dyskinesia. Management strategies include decreasing or discontinuing neuroleptics and/or using anticholinergic agents. The underlying pathophysiology of this disorder is unknown, although it is pharmacologically characterized as an acute extrapyramidal syndrome. More research is required to better understand this perplexing dyskinesia.

ACKNOWLEDGMENTS

This work was supported in part by funds from the Veterans Affairs Research Program, NIMH Grant MH 36657, and core grant RP00163. The typescript was prepared by Crystal Berger.

REFERENCES

1. Gerlach J, Reisby N, Randrup A. Dopaminergic hypersensitivity and cholinergic hypofunction in the pathophysiology of tardive dyskinesia. Psychopaharmacology 1974;34:21–35.
2. Casey DE. Tardive dyskinesia: are there new subtypes? N Engl J Med 1976;295:1078.
3. Casey DE, Denney D. Pharmacological characterization of tardive dyskinesia. Psychopharmacology 1977;54:1–8.
4. Granacher R, Baldessarini R, Cole JO. Deanol for tardive dyskinesia (letter). N Engl J Med 1975;292:926–927.
5. Gerlach J. Tardive dyskinesia. Dan Med Bull 1977;26:209–245.
6. Glazer W, Moore D. The diagnosis of rapid abnormal involuntary movements associated with fluphenazine deconoate. J Nerv Ment Dis 1980;168(7):439–441.
7. Moore DC, Bowers MB. Identification of subgroup of tardive dyskinesia patients by pharmacologic probes. Am J Psychiatry 1980;137(10):1202–1205.
8. Gerlach J, Korsgaard S. Classification of abnormal involuntary movements in psychiatric patients. Neuropsychiat Clin 1983;2:201–208.
9. Casey DE. The differential diagnosis of tardive dyskinesia. Acta Psychiatr Scand 1981;63(suppl 291):71–87.
10. Casey DE. Tardive dyskinesia. In: Meltzer HY, ed. Psychopharmacology: the third genereration of progress. New York: Raven, 1987:1411–1419.

Chapter

9

Neuroleptic-Induced Pseudoparkinsonism

DAVID N. OSSER

INTRODUCTION

Since the first edition of this book, the diagnosis and treatment of neuroleptic-induced pseudoparkinsonism (NP) have become of less concern. With the current availability of risperidone, olanzapine, and quetiapine, new antipsychotics associated with decreased NP, and the anticipation of additional similar agents in the near future, clinical and basic research on NP has declined. During the same period, however, we have seen an increase in the influence of managed care on the availability and usage of medications by prescribing clinicians. Owing to cost considerations, the older neuroleptics are still being advocated and sometimes required for first-line use. In addition, practice guidelines endorsed by some prominent experts still encourage routine use of the standard, typical, NP-producing antipsychotics (1). Hence, a thorough familiarity with their side effects and their clinical implications continues to be essential for the prescribing clinician.

A few historical observations may be of interest. When chlorpromazine was first used in manic and schizophrenic patients in 1952, it was noted to be particularly effective in reducing excitement but often the patients developed symptoms resembling Parkinson's disease, such as motor retardation, a wooden facial expression, and an unsteady gait (2). In a review of the history of neuroleptic-induced extrapyramidal symptoms (EPS), Rifkin recalls that some early investigators assumed that this neurologic slowing was the cause of the patients' reduced excitement (3). This notion was not supported by subsequent observations, such as the fact that antiparkinsonian drugs reduced EPS while generally not reducing the improvement in psychosis, and that some drugs developed later, such as clozapine, were effective antipsychotics but caused practically no EPS (4). Hence, the parkinsonian syndrome came to be understood as a common but

undesirable neurologic side effect of "typical" neuroleptics such as chlorpromazine and haloperidol.

Ayd's two surveys of EPS (1961, 1981) involving 8,775 patients helped establish the phenomenology of NP (5,6). He and others (7,8) considered its essential features of tremor and rigidity to be quite similar to those of Parkinson's disease.

In this chapter, the focus is on the diagnosis and treatment of NP and on the use of mild NP as a potential marker for the minimally effective antipsychotic dose of a typical neuroleptic. The latter may have applicability in the treatment of acutely psychotic patients (9,10). At the conclusion, reference will also be made to the use of this marker in the assessment and treatment of patients with neuroleptic-resistant psychoses.

DIAGNOSIS

Symptoms of NP in the past were regarded as being the last to appear of the three main types of EPS (dystonia, akathisia, and pseudoparkinsonism) that occur after treatment is commenced with a typical neuroleptic (5,6). In the Ayd surveys, 90% of cases of pseudoparkinsonism occurred within the first 72 days. However, Ayd only recorded cases of moderate to severe NP, as indicated by the finding of a total incidence of only 15% (5). Efforts to define the more common, milder spectrum of NP have been frustrated by the difficulty in distinguishing mild akinesia from negative and catatonic schizophrenic symptoms or the motor retardation of depression in schizophrenia (11). Despite these problems, it seems quite clear now that the large majority of patients treated with therapeutic doses of typical neuroleptics will show some signs of mild parkinsonism within the first few days of treatment if a careful examination is performed (9). Some patients, however, are at greater risk for more severe

NP at low doses. These risk factors include female sex (2:1 over males in all age groups except under 10 and over 80), increased age, children and adolescents (12), hyperthyroidism (13), family history of Parkinson's disease, family history of affective disorder (5), and Asian ethnicity (14).

Parkinsonian Tremor

Parkinsonian tremor is perhaps the most easily recognized sign of NP, but it tends to occur in patients with moderate to severe symptoms (15) and therefore is not particularly useful for identifying early and subtle cases. In contrast, patients with Parkinson's disease most often present initially with tremor (16). The tremor is a regular, rhythmic, 4 to 8 per second (Hz) oscillation noted most often in the extremities, fingers, jaw, mouth, tongue, and lips. Tremor of the lips has been termed the "Rabbit syndrome," and although it may be confused with tardive dyskinesia because of the location, it is in all respects a typical parkinsonian tremor (8,17). The tremors of NP and Parkinson's disease have both been described as occurring asymmetrically, with greater effect noted on the right side (18). They occur characteristically when the affected body part is at rest and disappear temporarily with voluntary movement.

To examine for this tremor, the patient is observed with hands hanging unsupported between or in front of the legs. Also, the tongue is examined at rest in the floor of the mouth. The tremor is reduced or stops on initiation of movement. Tardive dyskinesia is also a resting tremor and it may be observed during this examination of resting body parts (19), but the choreiform and athetoid movements of this disorder should be sufficiently different in appearance from NP so that there will be no confusion between the two. Action tremors may also be noted as the patient initiates an activity during the examination. Such tremors are extremely common in psychiatric patients and are often caused by high doses of the neuroleptic itself (15), or they may be physiologic or essential tremors amplified by other drugs, caffeine, alcohol withdrawal, or other medical conditions (15,20). Most are moderately rapid (8 to 12 Hz) and of small amplitude and so should be easily distinguished from the parkinsonian variety, although with increased age they may get slower and eventually assume the same frequency as the tremor of NP. They should still be recognizable as different from NP by the action occurrence, lack of accompanying bradykinesia or rigidity (to be described), and frequent presentation in the head as a whole or in the voice (21).

Even if a parkinsonian tremor is not visually observed, there may be objective, easily elicited palpable evidence of this tremor in the form of *cogwheel rigidity*. Cogwheeling is a ratchety pattern of resistance and relaxation noted by an examiner when a limb or joint with an underlying parkinsonian tremor is passively manipulated. It may be felt if the patient does not attempt voluntary movement at the joint,

but it may disappear if the patient does move the joint, thereby recruiting the more dominant pyramidal tract influence on the muscles. Studies (9,10) have shown that the incidence of this sign in patients on clinical doses of a typical, high-potency neuroleptic is over 90% if the patient is carefully examined. It is often present even if the patient is on an antiparkinsonian agent such as benztropine (22).

The evaluation of cogwheeling is complicated by the fact that metabolic or essential tremors are also associated with cogwheel rigidity. The cogwheeling from this kind of underlying tremor feels distinctly different from parkinsonian cogwheeling, however. Robert Stowe, of the Department of Neurology at Boston's Beth Israel Hospital, has suggested that the cogwheeling of metabolic or essential tremors is rapid, fine, ripple-like, and fluttery, whereas parkinsonian cogwheeling is slower, more coarse, and more ratchety, in keeping with the slower frequency of the underlying tremor. With experience it seems possible to feel the difference between these two common kinds of cogwheeling, but objective proof that they can be reliably differentiated is lacking.

A thorough examination for cogwheeling should include passive extension, flexion, and rotation at the wrist while the patient is performing some task with the other arm that requires concentration, such as writing his name in the air with the index finger or performing dysdiadokokinetic alternating hand movements on the knee. Both wrists should be checked in this manner. Parkinsonian tremors and associated cogwheeling are said to be more evident in distal as opposed to proximal joints (e.g., wrist versus elbow).

A brief description of how to place highly psychotic or paranoid patients at ease so as to examine for NP and other neurologic symptoms might be useful at this point. First, the examiner initiates a brief inquiry into the patient's subjective experience of medication side effects. Then, the patient is asked to extend his arms while the examiner observes at a distance for action tremors. Similarly, the arms are observed hanging unsupported. Next, as final preparation for the physical contact that the examiner will soon begin, the patient is asked if he is right-handed or left-handed. Then the examiner asks the patient if he may now check his right arm and wrist for signs of stiffness. If the arm is held rigidly by the patient at first, the examiner verbally encourages him to relax and shakes the arm gently for a few seconds. It is rare that a patient will be uncooperative with this procedure.

Akinesia

Akinesia or bradykinesia (slowness of movement), the second major clinical feature of NP, is defined as a toxic behavioral state of diminished spontaneity, masked facial expression, absent arm swing, rigid and flexed posture, tiredness, emotional blunting, and poor social adjustment (23,24).

By this definition, it too seems to occur to some degree in most patients treated with a neuroleptic, especially when the high potency agents are used (25). It also can occur to severe degrees, causing gait and posture disturbances and drooling. When akinesia is suspected, the presence of cogwheel rigidity may again provide confirmatory evidence of NP. McEvoy et al (9,10) consider cogwheeling to be the "primary criterion" of hypokinesia, and Goetz and Klawans (8) also state that cogwheeling is useful in the differential diagnosis of akinesia, although they cite their experience that any parkinsonian feature can rarely occur without the others.

Patients with akinesia may also display a pattern of waxy or lead-pipe resistance to passive movement of the limbs. This "catatonic rigidity" is also a common side effect of neuroleptics, but it is not as diagnostically specific for NP as cogwheeling since catatonia is frequently seen in unmedicated psychotic patients (26). Other probable synonyms in the literature for this rigidity include "gegenhalten" (16) and "generalized rigidity." Catatonia may be part of the negative symptom dimension in schizophrenia, and it is also frequently seen in patients with mania (27).

Other reportedly useful correlates of subtle akinesia include a subjective sense of drowsiness (in 88% versus 18% of controls) persisting 12 hours after ingestion of a bedtime dose of neuroleptic (28) and a very low frequency of spontaneous leg crossing when seated, seen in 80% versus 10% of controls (29).

Differential Diagnosis

The differential diagnosis of NP includes primary parkinsonism (or a predisposition to it) coexisting with a psychotic disorder in the same patient (30). This should not be common, given the 0.1% to 0.15% prevalence of parkinsonism in the general population (16) and the 1.0% prevalence in patients over 60 years of age (31). A 20-year follow-up of 200 NP patients from Ayd's first survey revealed that 3% developed apparent primary parkinsonism within five years after neuroleptics were stopped (6). This certainly seems to exceed the expected chance occurrence rate, but Ayd only recorded moderate to severe cases of NP in his survey and this may have resulted in a selection for unusually susceptible individuals. Some of these represent cases of neuroleptic-induced persistent parkinsonism, which may be a form of tardive dyskinesia (32,33). In one report, a series of such cases did not respond well to levodopa therapy (34).

Recent studies have demonstrated that mild bradykinesia is frequently present in patients with schizophrenia who are first-episode and neuroleptic-naive. In three studies involving 134 patients, 18% to 24% had some parkinsonian rigidity or bradykinesia (35–37). These patients seem to be at higher risk for developing NP when treated with a neuroleptic and their psychoses were less responsive to this treatment (37). Baseline evaluation for this parkinsonism would appear useful for determining how much subsequently detected parkinsonism is due to the neuroleptic.

These data regarding first-onset patients also suggest that parkinsonian signs may be linked in some fundamental manner to the "primary negative symptoms" of schizophrenia—slowed movements, restricted range of affect, and decreased spontaneity and motivation—that have been associated with persistent disability (38). "Secondary" negative symptoms are presumed to be due to NP and may respond to antiparkinsonian drug treatment or may improve with use of antipsychotics lacking NP side effects. However, distinguishing with certainty which negative symptoms are primary or secondary in a medicated patient may not be possible.

Some commonly prescribed drugs can cause parkinsonism-like symptoms. Lithium, which is well known for producing a nonparkinsonian action-type tremor, is associated with cogwheel rigidity, although studies vary widely in the frequency with which this is observed, from 5% to 75% (39). The wide differences in reported incidence of cogwheeling may partly be due to residual effects from previous neuroleptic use in some of the patients studied (40). Alternatively, it may reflect differences in examination technique: if distraction (as described earlier) is routinely employed, a much higher rate of detection of cogwheeling would be expected. We suspect that this cogwheeling is not parkinsonian but is the fine, "fluttery" type described earlier as being associated with metabolic tremors. Thus for patients on combined therapy with lithium and neuroleptics, cogwheeling cannot be assumed to be derived from neuroleptic activity. Notably, those lithium patients described in the literature who had cogwheeling did not seem to have any detectable akinesia (22).

Selective serotonin reuptake inhibitor antidepressants have been associated with rare reports of parkinsonism (41), which may be due to serotonin-mediated mechanisms in susceptible individuals (42). However, fluoxetine did not aggravate symptoms of Parkinson's disease in a series of 14 patients (43).

Metoclopramide (44), amoxapine, reserpine, and prochlorperazine are four drugs whose known neuroleptic effects are sometimes overlooked and therefore they may seem to be associated with unexpected NP. Tricyclic antidepressants have also been reported to occasionally produce parkinsonian tremor. Goetz and Klawans (8) question these reports and state that all cases they have observed were action tremors and none were the tremors at rest of parkinsonism. Probably any such tremor on a tricyclic alone would be extremely rare.

MANAGEMENT

Treatment strategies for NP include dosage reduction, use of adjunctive symptomatic treatments, and substitution of "atypical" (that is, low parkinsonism-inducing) antipsychotics (45). Management of NP in patients on long-acting injectable neuroleptics with dosage reduction is especially important. These individuals usually have a history of noncompliance with oral medication. If they are noncompliant with their oral antiparkinsonian medication, they develop even worse NP and akathisia, and may then be even more reluctant to accept oral antipsychotic therapy. The ideal approach would be to initiate with the lowest possible dose of injectable medication because subsequent lowering of an initially high dose will result in a significant number of relapses (46,47). It would be a testable hypothesis that the better candidates for dosage reduction without danger of relapse would be patients who manifest moderate or greater NP. They may have some room to go down on side effects without substantial loss of therapeutic effects.

The patient with moderate or greater NP and marginally controlled aggressive behavior presents a clinical dilemma, however. Clearly, there is a risk of further decompensation if the dose is lowered. The clinician would probably be inclined to actually increase the dose if it were not for the considerable toxicity already present. If immediate exacerbation of psychosis occurs when the dose is lowered slightly, this may exemplify rebound "supersensitivity" psychosis (48). Other patients who decompensate when the dose is lowered might be neuroleptic nonresponders whose apparent improvement so far is due to nonspecific sedation, milieu factors, or to physical restraint of the patient by neuroleptic-induced akinesia. Despite the risk of decompensation, it may be reasonable to try to avoid the high risk of tardive dyskinesia associated with more persistent NP (49), which especially applies if the patient is affectively ill (50). Addition of anticonvulsants (e.g., carbamazepine, valproic acid, or clonazepam) may make it easier to lower the neuroleptic and may help the psychosis as well (51,52).

As noted earlier, NP symptoms sometimes increase when neuroleptics are withdrawn (33). It is also commonly observed that NP symptoms may disappear at high doses of high-potency neuroleptics. Taken together, these observations suggest that clinicians should be prepared to find a "window" dose–response relationship for NP as high-potency neuroleptic dosage is changed. This may be the net effect of dose-related interactions with presynaptic and postsynaptic dopamine and serotonin receptors. It also may involve the induction of homeostatic changes (53).

Adjunctive drug treatments for NP are employed routinely. However, they have significant adverse effects that limit their usefulness, especially in patients with severe NP. Thus, initial reduction of neuroleptic dosage may be critical to achieving the optimal cost-to-benefit ratio from neuroleptics. Knowledge of the pharmacokinetics of antiparkinsonians can help optimize their usefulness. Benztropine's half-life is not known but it appears to be quite long, judging by its common successful usage on a once or twice daily basis. In one withdrawal study, its effects seemed

to persist on average about twice as long as other antiparkinsonians (54). By contrast, trihexyphenidyl's known four-hour half-life (55) suggests that a twice daily dosage may be insufficient for many patients to maintain control over symptoms. With both drugs, the frequent practice of giving the entire daily dose at bedtime results in many patients' being quite uncomfortable by late afternoon the next day. Thus, the schedule of administration of these agents may be critical to maximizing their benefits.

Amantadine has received some support as a potentially superior antiparkinsonian agent because of its much lower incidence of memory loss and other central as well as peripheral anticholinergic side effects compared to the antimuscarinic agents (56,57). However, these studies used a relatively large dose of the latter compared to the amantadine (e.g., 2 mg of benztropine being considered equal to 100 mg of amantadine, whereas 1 mg would have been the correct equivalence). In another comparative study, stabilized psychotic patients were blindly switched to amantadine or benztropine from their maintenance antiparkinsonian agent. They frequently developed more severe NP on amantadine (58). Another concern with amantadine is that it may occasionally exacerbate schizophrenic symptoms, perhaps because of its dopamine agonist properties (59). There was also a report of a fatality in a 34-year-old man who overdosed on twenty 100-mg tablets (60). However, a recent study comparing amantadine to biperiden, another widely used treatment for NP, found equal efficacy (61). Overall, amantadine may well have fewer side effects and, rather than considering it only a second line agent for severe or refractory symptoms, it perhaps deserves to be tried more often especially in milder cases of NP or following dosage reduction. This particularly applies to the elderly patient.

Early clinical (62) and animal model studies (53,63) suggested that tolerance to NP developed and that after several months the antiparkinsonian agents could usually be stopped. However, it has become clear that for most patients maintained on typical doses of neuroleptics, the antiparkinsonian agents cannot be withdrawn without eventual (in up to four weeks) recurrence of uncomfortable NP and/or rebound dysphoria (54,64). Despite this, periodic attempts to remove these agents still seem justified, especially if the antiparkinsonian was originally begun prophylactically and the patient never developed obvious NP.

Besides dosage reduction and adjunctive medication, the predominant strategy today for dealing with NP is switching to an antipsychotic with a low incidence of these side effects. In the past, the older neuroleptics thioridazine or mesoridazine (the latter an active metabolite of thioridazine) were considered to have the least NP and were often employed for this purpose. They are sometimes better tolerated overall. Mesoridazine might occasionally have slightly superior efficacy as well (65–67). Slightly superior efficacy is also claimed for the newest antipsychotics: risperidone, olanzapine, and quetiapine, at least for secondary negative symptoms that may be related to NP and other EPS (68–70). The new antipsychotics have become the routine choices today for patients who are sensitive to NP. All show placebo-level or better frequency of NP in their optimal dose ranges, with some increase of NP above placebo level in the upper range of approved dosage for risperidone and olanzapine. It should be noted that "placebo level" frequencies of NP in these studies are 10% to 20%. This is due to the incomplete washout of previous typical neuroleptics prior to the double-blind phase. The real incidence of NP with low to moderate doses of the three new agents in drug-naive patients is unclear; it is probably significantly greater than zero. It does appear that quetiapine has significantly less NP than the others (70).

Clozapine, by contrast, causes practically no NP or tardive dyskinesia. It also clearly provides superior efficacy in patients resistant to typical neuroleptics. In the now-classic multicenter, controlled study by Kane et al of 268 chronically psychotic patients who had failed on several neuroleptics (including an especially good trial of haloperidol during the lead-in phase of the study), clozapine produced significant improvement in 30% versus only 4% in a control group given chlorpromazine (71). Clozapine is indicated for patients whose response has been unsatisfactory to at least two adequate trials of the other antipsychotics. It may also be used in patients who get severe NP and other EPS from all neuroleptics or who have severe tardive dyskinesia.

CLINICAL APPLICATIONS OF BASIC SCIENCE

It is thought that NP results from dopamine-type 2 (D_2) receptor blockade in the corpus striatum (a part of the extrapyramidal motor system), and it has been proposed that antipsychotic effects derive from blockade of similar D_2 receptors in the limbic nuclei and areas of the prefrontal cortex that have been associated with emotional behavior (72). Typical neuroleptics block D_2 receptors simultaneously and with equal affinity in both systems (73,74), although there are differences among them in the effects on other neurotransmitter systems, such as those involving serotonin, norepinephrine, acetylcholine, gamma-amino butyric acid, and various peptides. These neurotransmitters may interact with dopaminergic transmission and affect the expression of clinical NP (75). This probably contributes to the low incidence of parkinsonism with clozapine and some of the newer antipsychotics.

In rat brain, typical neuroleptics produce an immediate postsynaptic D_2 receptor blockade and then gradually, over the course of several weeks, the presynaptic striatal and ventral tegmental (limbic) neurons stop firing (76). This "depolarization block" could be the neurophysiological correlate of both the NP and the antipsychotic effects of typical neuroleptics, with the two occurring simultaneously (77). If

this is so, clinical overlap of NP and antipsychotic effects might be expected to occur with these neuroleptics. McEvoy (10) suggested that even minimal NP could reflect the early induction of depolarization block in striatal and limbic neurons and could predict ultimate occurrence of antipsychotic effect over the next several weeks in patients who are capable of an antipsychotic response to neuroleptics. This corresponds to the common clinical experience that once an adequate antipsychotic dose is achieved, patients usually proceed gradually to improvement without need for further increase in dose.

Positron emission tomography (PET) studies have refined these concepts. Blockade of striatal D_2 receptors with receptor occupancy above 80% using typical neuroleptics such as haloperidol produces potent NP and antipsychotic effects simultaneously (78). At occupancies of 50% to 80%, however, the NP effect is minimal but strong antipsychotic effects still occur (79). The dosage of oral haloperidol that produces 50% to 80% occupancy of D_2 receptors is 2–4 mg per day, particularly for first-episode patients. This appears to be the dose (or equivalent dose with other neuroleptics) that clinicians should use to initiate treatment with psychotic patients when using the typical neuroleptics in order to maximize benefits while minimizing NP. Other neurobiological lines of evidence support the dosage of 2–4 mg per day (80,81).

A variety of clinical reviews have also emphasized that more modest doses of standard neuroleptics, by comparison with the higher doses typically used, are both more effective and produce decreased EPS including NP (82,83). Routine use of a low dose is not, however, a sufficient strategy: the reviews make it clear that in prospective studies with fixed low doses, more treatment failures or relapses occur along with the benefit of less NP. Perhaps the best way of determining the ideal dose for any individual patient is to utilize the "neuroleptic threshold" approach; this involves finding the dose that produces minimal but clinically detectable NP. It is a dose that can be expected to produce substantial and close to maximal antipsychotic effects while by definition keeping NP to a minimum (84,85).

McEvoy et al (9,10,85–87) have provided support for utilizing this technique. Somewhat similar investigations with perphenazine have also been reported (88). Using haloperidol, McEvoy's group used a simple rating instrument (9) for the presence of NP that emphasizes a clinical examination for cogwheel rigidity from which the one described earlier in this chapter was adapted. With acute treatment, they checked for NP daily as haloperidol, started at 2 mg per day, was increased by 2 mg every other day (9). A neuroleptic threshold was identified in 44 of 47 patients (94%) at a median dose of 4 mg per day (most were between 0.5 and 10.0 mg per day). The rate of moderate or better response for patients at neuroleptic threshold, who had a history of five or fewer previous hospitalizations, was 82% (27 of 33 patients). The results with patients who had more than five previous admissions were that only 33% improved (three of nine patients). Fairly small amounts of lorazepam was used as an adjunctive sedative medication when needed (McEvoy JP, personal communication).

A more rigorous test of this approach occurred in a double-blind study published in 1991 (86). A total of 91 patients treated at neuroleptic threshold dosage of haloperidol for two weeks were then randomly assigned to either an increase in dose to 10–20 mg per day as tolerated, or continued at the original neuroleptic threshold dose for two more weeks. The patients given more neuroleptic had only slightly more antipsychotic benefit (the only difference was on the Suspiciousness Factor of the Brief Psychiatric Rating Scale), but they more frequently developed severe NP compared to the control group. Another finding was that there was no loss of the initial response in the responders in the threshold group during this second phase of the study, as they were continued on this low dose.

The most recent study from McEvoy and colleagues tested whether moving below the neuroleptic threshold dose will result in loss of efficacy (87). Sixty acutely psychotic patients were titrated to a neuroleptic threshold dose of haloperidol over a two-week period (mean of 4.3 mg per day). They were then randomly assigned to four more weeks of treatment with either the same dose, one-third that dose (1.6 mg), or triple that dose (14.3 mg). All patients received benztropine after randomization to prevent dystonia in those who might be susceptible to it. The results were that patients who were randomized to move to the lower dose did not improve over the next four weeks, and if there had been any improvement during the two-week neuroleptic threshold identification phase, this was rapidly lost. Patients who continued on the neuroleptic threshold dose improved significantly and so did the patients on triple dosage. As in the earlier controlled study, the high-dose group improved a bit more than the threshold dose group (about 0.2 on the Clinical Global Impression) but at the cost of more NP and other side effects.

In conclusion, the neuroleptic threshold dose appears to be the best dose for the initial treatment of first-onset or recently relapsed schizophrenic patients. The caveat should be added that if improvement occurs without the clinician noting any NP, the dose need not be increased further: the patient could be at D_2 receptor occupancy in the 50% to 60% range, which is enough to produce substantial antipsychotic effect but with low, clinically undetectable levels of NP (79). It is important to keep in mind, however, that the improvement could be from nonspecific factors such as hospitalization (89). Further, NP might not become detectable until several weeks of treatment have occurred, during the time in which depolarization block may be presumed to be gradually developing in more and more nigrostriatal neurons. Therefore, it might be of interest to recheck for neuroleptic threshold parkinsonism a few weeks later to see if it has appeared.

Finally, it may be noted that the neuroleptic threshold examination for NP may be useful (in combination with other information) in identifying subgroups of neuroleptic resistant patients, suggesting reasons for their poor response, and indicating possible treatments (90–92). This subject is beyond the scope of this chapter, but the reader is encouraged to consult the indicated references.

REFERENCES

1. McEvoy JP, Weiden PJ, Smith TE, et al, eds. The expert consensus guideline series: treatment of schizophrenia. J Clin Psychiatry 1996;57[suppl 12B]:1–58.
2. Delay D, Deniker P, Harl JM. Utilisation en therapeutique psychiatrique d'une phenothiazine d'action centrale elective. Ann Med Psychol 1952;110:112–117.
3. Rifkin A. Extrapyramidal side effects: a historical perspective. J Clin Psychiatry 1987;48(suppl 9):3–6.
4. Ayd FJ Jr. Clozapine: a unique new neuroleptic. Int Drug Ther Newslett 1974;2,3:1–12.
5. Ayd FJ Jr. A survey of drug-induced extrapyramidal reactions. JAMA 1961;75:1054–1060.
6. Ayd FJ Jr. Early-onset neuroleptic-induced extrapyramidal reactions: a second survey 1961–1981. In: Coyle JT, Enna SJ, eds. Neuroleptics: neurochemical, behavioral, and clinical perspectives. New York: Raven, 1983:75–92.
7. Greenblatt DJ, Shader RI, DiMascio A. Extrapyramidal effects. In: Shader RI, DiMascio A, eds. Psychotropic drug side effects. Baltimore: Williams and Wilkins, 1970:92–106.
8. Goetz CG, Klawans HL. Drug-induced extrapyramidal disorders—a neuropsychiatric interface. J Clin Psychopharmacol 1981;1:297–303.
9. McEvoy JP, Stiller RL, Farr R. Plasma haloperidol levels drawn at neuroleptic threshold doses: a pilot study. J Clin Psychopharmacol 1986;6:133–138.
10. McEvoy JP. The neuroleptic threshold as a marker of minimum effective neuroleptic dose. Compr Psychiatry 1986;27:327–335.
11. Prosser ES, Csernansky JG, Kaplan J, Thiemann S, Becker TJ, Hollister LE. Depression, parkinsonian symptoms, and negative symptoms in schizophrenics treated with neuroleptics. J Nerv Ment Dis 1987;175:100–105.
12. Baldessarini RJ, Teicher MH. Dosing of antipsychotic agents in pediatric populations. J Child Adol Psychopharmacol 1995;5:1–4.
13. Witschy JK. Extrapyramidal reaction to fluphenazine potentiated by thyrotoxicosis. Am J Psychiatry 1981;138:246–247.
14. Lim K-M, Poland RE. Ethnicity, culture, and psychopathology. In: Bloom FE, Kupfer DJ, eds. Psychopharmacology: the fourth generation of progress. New York: Raven, 1995:1907–1917.
15. Young RR, Shahani BT. Pharmacology of tremor. In: Klawans HL, ed. Clinical neuropharmacology. Vol. 4. New York: Raven, 1979:139–155.
16. Yahr MD. Parkinsonism. In: Rowland LP, ed. Merritt's textbook of neurology. Philadelphia: Lea and Febiger, 1984:526–537.
17. Todd R, Lippmann S, Manshadi M, Chang A. Recognition and treatment of rabbit syndrome, an uncommon complication of neuroleptic therapies. Am J Psychiatry 1983;140:1519–1520.
18. Caligiuri MP, Bracha S, Lohr JB. Asymmetry of neuroleptic-induced rigidity: development of quantitating measures and clinical correlates. Psychiatry Res 1989;30:275–284.
19. Caligiuri MP, Lohr JB, Bracha S, Jeste DV. Clinical and instrumental assessment of neuroleptic-induced parkinsonism in patients with tardive dyskinesia. Biol Psychiatry 1991;29:139–148.
20. Cummings JL. Neuropsychiatric aspects of movement disorders. In: Cummings JL. Clinical neuropsychiatry. New York: Grune and Stratton, 1985:140–162.
21. Duvoisin RC. Benign essential tremor. In: Rowland LP, ed. Merritt's textbook of neurology. Philadelphia: Lea and Febiger, 1984:525–526.
22. Shopsin B, Gershon S. Cogwheel rigidity related to lithium maintenance. Am J Psychiatry 1975;132:536–540.
23. Van Putten T, Marder SR. Behavioral toxicity of antipsychotic drugs. J Clin Psychiatry 1987;48(suppl 9):13–19.
24. Rifkin A, Quitkin F, Klein DF. Akinesia. Arch Gen Psychiatry 1975;32:672–674.
25. Marsden CD, Tarsy D, Baldessarini RJ. Spontaneous and drug-induced movement disorders in psychotic patients. In: Benson DF, Blumer D, eds. Psychiatric aspects of neurologic disease. New York: Grune and Stratton, 1975:219–266.
26. Fricchione GL. Neuroleptic catatonia and its relationship to psychogenic catatonia. Biol Psychiatry 1985;20:304–313.

27. Taylor MA, Abrams R. Catatonia. Arch Gen Psychiatry 1977;34:1223–1225.
28. Van Putten T, May PRA, Marder S, Wittmann LA. Subjective response to antipsychotic drugs. Arch Gen Psychiatry 1981;38:187–190.
29. Van Putten T. Adverse psychological (or behavioral) responses to antipsychotic drug treatment of schizophrenia. In: Rifkin A, ed. Schizophrenia and affective disorders: biology and drug treatment. Boston: John Wright, 1983.
30. Crow TJ, Johnstone EC, McClelland HA. The coincidence of schizophrenia and parkinsonism: some neurochemical implications. Psychol Med 1976;6:227–233.
31. Pearce JMS. Aetiology and natural history of Parkinson's disease. Br Med J 1978;2:1664–1670.
32. Jankovic J. Tardive syndromes and other drug-induced movement disorders. Clin Neuropharmacol 1995;18:197–214.
33. Nelli AC, Yarden PE, Guazzelli M, Feinberg I. Parkinsonism following neuroleptic withdrawal. Arch Gen Psychiatry 1989;46:383–384.
34. Hardie RJ, Lees AJ. Neuroleptic-induced Parkinson's syndrome: clinical features and results of treatment with levodopa. J Neurol Neurosurg Psychiatry 1988;51:850–854.
35. Caligiuri MP, Lohr JB, Jeste DV. Parkinsonism in neuroleptic-naive schizophrenic patients. Am J Psychiatry 1993;150:1343–1348.
36. McCreadie RG, Thara R, Kamath S, Padmavathy R, Latha S, Mathrubootham N, Menon MS. Abnormal movements in never-medicated Indian patients with schizophrenia. Br J Psychiatry 1996;168:221–226.
37. Chatterjee A, Chakos M, Koreen A, et al. Prevalence and clinical correlates of extrapyramidal signs and spontaneous dyskinesia in never-medicated schizophrenic patients. Am J Psychiatry 1995;152:1724–1729.
38. Kane JM. Commentary on the clozapine conflict. Am J Psychiatry 1996;153:1507–1508.
39. Jefferson JW, Greist JH, Ackerman DL, Carroll JA. Lithium encyclopedia for clinical practice. 2nd ed. Washington: American Psychiatric, 1987:460–461.
40. Ghadirian A-M, Annable L, Belanger M-C, Chouinard G. A cross-sectional study of parkinsonism and tardive dyskinesia in lithium-treated affective disordered patients. J Clin Psychiatry 1996;57:22–28.
41. Pies RW. Must we now consider SRIs neuroleptics? J Clin Psychopharmacol 1997;17:443–445.
42. Baldessarini RJ, Marsh ER, Kula NS. Interactions of fluoxetine with metabolism of dopamine and serotonin in rat brain regions. Brain Res 1992;579:152–156.
43. Montastruc J-L. Does fluoxetine aggravate Parkinson's disease? A pilot prospective study (letter). Mov Disord 1995;10:355–357.
44. Miller LC, Jancovic J. Metaclopramide-induced movement disorders: clinical findings and a review of the literature. Arch Intern Med 1989;149:2486–2492.
45. Kane JM. Antipsychotic drug side effects: their relationship to dose. J Clin Psychiatry 1985;46(5, Sec. 2):16–21.
46. Kane JM, Rifkin A, Woerner M, et al. Low dose neuroleptic treatment of outpatient schizophrenics. Arch Gen Psychiatry 1983;40:893–896.
47. Faraone SV, Green AI, Brown W, Yin P, Tsuang MT. Neuroleptic dose reduction in persistently psychotic patients. Hosp Comm Psychiatry 1989;40:1193–1195.
48. Chouinard G, Steinberg S. New clinical concepts on neuroleptic-induced supersensitivity disorders: tardive dyskinesia and supersensitivity psychosis. In: Stancer HC, Garfinkel PE, Rakoff VM, eds. Guidelines for the use of psychotropic drugs. New York: Spectrum, 1984:205–228.
49. Wolf ME, DeWolfe AS, Ryan JJ, et al. Vulnerability to tardive dyskinesia. J Clin Psychiatry 1985;46:367–368.
50. Mukherjee S, Rosen AM, Caracci G, Shukla S. Persistent tardive dyskinesia in bipolar patients. Arch Gen Psychiatry 1986;43:342–346.
51. Osser DN. Treatment resistant problems. In: Tupin J, Shader RI, Harnett DS, eds. Clinical handbook of psychopharmacology. 2nd ed. New York: Jason Aronson, 1988:269–328.
52. Chouinard G, Sultan S. Treatment of supersensitivity psychosis with antiepileptic drugs: report of a series of 43 cases. Psychopharmacol Bull 1990;26:337–341.
53. Clow A, Theodorou A, Jenner P, Marsden CD. Changes in rat striatal dopamine turnover and receptor activity during one year's neuroleptic administration. Eur J Pharmacol 1980;63:135–144.
54. Jellinek T, Gardos G, Cole JO. Adverse effects of antiparkinson drug withdrawal. Am J Psychiatry 1981;138:1567–1571.
55. Burke RE, Fahn S. Pharmacokinetics of trihexyphenidyl after short-term and long-term administration to dystonic patients. Ann Neurol 1985;18:35–40.
56. McEvoy JP. A double-blind crossover comparison of antiparkinson drug therapy: amantadine versus anticholinergics in 90 normal volunteers, with an emphasis on differential effects on memory function. J Clin Psychiatry 1987;48(suppl 9):20–23.
57. Hitri A, Craft RB, Fallon J, et al. Serum neuroleptic and anticholinergic activity in relationship to cognitive toxicity of antiparkinsonian agents in schizophrenic patients. Psychopharmacol Bull 1987;23(1):33–37.
58. McEvoy JP, McCue M, Freter S. Replacement of chronically administered anticholinergic drugs by amantadine in out-patient management of chronic schizophrenia. Clin Ther 1987;9:429–433.
59. Nestelbaum S, Siris SG, Rifkin A, et al. Exacerbation of schizophrenia associated with amantadine. Am J Psychiatry 1986;143:1170–1171.
60. Simpson DM, Ramos F, Ramirez LF. Death of a psychiatric patient from amantadine poisoning. Am J Psychiatry 1988;145:267–268.
61. Silver H, Geraisy N, Schwartz M. No difference in the effect of biperiden and amantadine on parkinsonian- and tardive dyskinesia-type involuntary movements: a double-blind crossover, placebo-controlled study in medicated chronic schizophrenic patients. J Clin Psychiatry 1995;56:167–170.
62. Klett CJ, Caffer E Jr. Evaluating long-term need for antiparkinson drugs by chronic schizophrenics. Arch Gen Psychiatry 1972;26:374–379.
63. Burt DR, Creese I, Snyder SH. Antischizophrenic drugs: chronic treatment elevates dopamine receptor binding in brain. Science 1977;196:326–328.
64. Gelenberg AJ. Treating extrapyramidal reactions: some current issues. J Clin Psychiatry 1987;48(suppl 9):24–27.
65. Kinon G, Sakalis G, Traficante LJ, et al. Mesoridazine in treatment-refractory schizophrenics. Curr Ther Res 1979;25:534–539.
66. Vital-Herne J, Gerbino L, Kay SR, et al. Mesoridazine and thioridazine: clinical effects and blood levels in refractory schizophrenics. J Clin Psychiatry 1986;47:375–379.
67. Osser DN, Albert LG, Figueiredo S, et al. Mesoridazine in neuroleptic-resistant psychoses. J Clin Psychopharmacol 1991;11:328–330.
68. Peuskins J & the Risperidone Study Group. Risperidone in the treatment of patients with chronic schizophrenia: a multi-national, multi-centre, double-blind, parallel-group study versus haloperidol. Br J Psychiatry 1995;166:712–726.
69. Tollefson GD, Beasley CM Jr, Tran PV, et al. Olanzapine versus haloperidol in the treatment of schizophrenia and schizoaffective and schizophreniform disorders: results of an international collaborative trial. Am J Psychiatry 1997;154:457–465.
70. Arvanitis LA, Miller BG, and the Seroquel Trial 13 Study Group. Multiple fixed doses of "Seroquel" (quetiapine) in patients with acute exacerbation of schizophrenia: a comparison with haloperidol and placebo. Biol Psychiatry 1997;42:233–246.
71. Kane J, Honigfeld G, Singer J, Meltzer H & the Clozaril Collaborative Study Group. Clozapine for the treatment-resistant schizophrenic; a double-blind comparison with chlorpromazine. Arch Gen Psychiatry 1988;45:789–796.
72. Snyder SH. Dopamine receptors, neuroleptics, and schizophrenia. Am J Psychiatry 1981;138:460–464.
73. Creese I, Burt DR, Snyder SH. Dopamine receptor binding predicts clinical and pharmacological potencies of antischizophrenic drugs. Science 1976;192:481–483.
74. Seeman P. Atypical neuroleptics: role of multiple receptors, endogenous dopamine, and receptor linkage. Acta Psychiatr Scand 1990;82:14–20.
75. Wolf ME, Deutch AY, Roth RH. Pharmacology of central dopaminergic neurons. In: Nasrallah HA, ed. Handbook of schizophrenia. Vol. 2. Neurochemistry and neuropharmacology of schizophrenia. New York: Elsevier, 1987:101–147.
76. Chiado IA, Bunney BI. Typical and atypical neuroleptics: differential effects of chronic administration on the activity of A9 and A10 nudbrain dopaminergic neurons. J Neurosci 1983;3:1607–1610.
77. Pickar D. Perspectives on a time-dependent model of neuroleptic action. Schizophrenia Bull 1988;14:256–268.
78. Farde L, Nordstrom AL, Wiesel FA, et al. Positron emission tomographic analysis of central D1 and D2 dopamine receptor occupancy in patients treated with classical neuroleptics and clozapine: relation to extrapyramidal side effects. Arch Gen Psychiatry 1992;49:538–544.
79. Kapur S, Remington G, Jones C, et al. High levels of dopamine D2 receptor occupancy with low-dose haloperidol treatment: A PET study. Am J Psychiatry 1996;153:948–950.
80. Hirschowitz J, Hitzemann R, Davidson M. A neuroendocrine predictor of optimum dosing in schizophrenia. Neuropsychopharmacol 1994;19(3S/Part 1):840S.
81. Hirschowitz J, Hitzemann R, Burr G, Schwartz A. A new approach to dose reduction in chronic schizophrenia. Neuropsychopharmacol 1991;5:103–113.
82. Baldessarini RJ, Cohen BM, Teicher MH. Significance of neuroleptic dose and plasma level in the pharmacological treatment of psychoses. Arch Gen Psychiatry 1988;45:79–91.

83. Kane JM. Neuroleptic treatment of schizophrenia. In: Nasrallah HA, ed. Handbook of schizophrenia. Vol 2. Neurochemistry and neuropharmacology of schizophrenia. New York: Elsevier, 1987:179–201.

84. Haase H-J, Janssen PAJ. The action of neuroleptic drugs. 2nd ed. New York: Elsevier, 1985.

85. McEvoy JP, Stiller RL, Everett GR. Differential therapeutic response by history during treatment with neuroleptic threshold haloperidol doses. J Clin Psychopharmacol 1987;7:368–369.

86. McEvoy JP, Hogarty GE, Steingard S. Optimal dose of neuroleptic in acute schizophrenia: a controlled study of the neuroleptic threshold and higher haloperidol dose. Arch Gen Psychiatry 1991;48:739–745.

87. McEvoy JP, Nelson L, Kamaraju LS. Neuroleptic threshold doses for schizophrenia. Symposium 87D. Scientific proceedings of the annual meeting of the American Psychiatric Association (San Francisco, CA). Washington: American Psychiatric, 1993.

88. Bolvig-Hansen L, Larsen NE. Therapeutic advantages of monitoring plasma concentrations of perphenazine in clinical practice. Psychopharmacology 1985;87:16–19.

89. Steingard S, Allen M, Schooler NR. A study of the pharmacologic treatment of medication-compliant schizophrenics who relapse. J Clin Psychiatry 1994;55:570–572.

90. Osser DN. A systematic approach to pharmacotherapy in patients with neuroleptic-resistant psychoses. Hosp Comm Psychiatry 1989;40(9):921–927.

91. Osser DN, Patterson RD. Pharmacotherapy of schizophrenia I: acute treatment. In: Soreff S, ed. Handbook for the treatment of the seriously mentally ill. Toronto: Hogrefe and Huber, 1996:91–119.

92. Osser DN, Patterson RD. Pharmacotherapy of schizophrenia II: an algorithm for neuroleptic-resistant patients. In: Soreff S, ed. Handbook for the treatment of the seriously mentally ill. Toronto: Hogrefe and Huber, 1996:121–155.

Withdrawal Dyskinesia

Anita L. Gerhard   Anthony B. Joseph

INTRODUCTION

Early observers of movement disorders associated with neuroleptics noted that reduction or discontinuation of the drug could produce new movements or exacerbate preexisting ones (1). These disorders became known as "withdrawal dyskinesias" or "withdrawal emergent dyskinesias."

As research and interest in the tardive syndromes increased, different descriptions of subtypes appeared. In some classifications "reversible" and "transient" dyskinesias overlap with what other investigators would call "withdrawal" dyskinesias.

Gardos et al distinguished among "tardive," "covert," and "withdrawal emergent" dyskinesias (2). According to their definitions, tardive dyskinesia first appears during neuroleptic administration, worsens with drug withdrawal, and may be irreversible. Covert dyskinesia does not occur during drug administration, first appears when the drug is withdrawn, and may be persistent. Withdrawal emergent dyskinesia first appears during neuroleptic withdrawal and is temporary. This classification suggests that an apparent withdrawal emergent dyskinesia that shows no sign of amelioration after 6 to 12 weeks is actually a covert dyskinesia.

For purposes of research, Schooler and Kane divide the dyskinesias into six types: "probable," "masked probable," "transient," "withdrawal," "persistent," and "masked persistent" (3).

In Jeste and Wyatt's thorough review, "acute" dyskinesia is distinguished from "withdrawal emergent" and "tardive" dyskinesias (the latter subdivided into "reversible," "intermittent," and "persistent" types) (4). The major difference between the definition of withdrawal dyskinesia proposed by Schooler and Kane and that proposed by Jeste is time course. Schooler and Kane classify as withdrawal tardive dyskinesia abnormal movements that persist for up to three months after neuroleptic withdrawal. Jeste and Wyatt draw the line at several weeks and would call a dyskinesia that disappeared spontaneously two months after neuroleptic discontinuation "reversible tardive dyskinesia" (4).

It is intuitively appealing to think of all these syndromes as representing a continuum from mild reversible dyskinesias to those that are severe and persistent. However, there is insufficient evidence to support or refute this idea (4–6).

In any case, at the current level of knowledge, it is probably academic and arbitrary where the lines between subtypes are drawn. What is important, however, is consistency in usage. Many reviewers have noted that the lack of consistent categorization makes comparisons between different investigations difficult. For the purpose of this review, Schooler and Kane's definition of withdrawal dyskinesia will be used.

DIAGNOSIS

Clinical Description and Epidemiologic Data

On appearance, withdrawal dyskinesias are the same as other varieties of tardive dyskinesia. The full range of involuntary choreiform and athetoid movements may be seen, including tongue protrusion; chewing movements; facial grimacing; eyelid fluttering; finger, hand, toe, ankle, and leg movements; ballistic movements; grunting vocalizations; and spasmodic torticollis. In children with withdrawal or persistent dyskinesia, orofacial symptoms are usually accompanied by more prominent limb and/or trunk movements (4). As with tardive dyskinesia in general, the severity of the movements that characterize withdrawal dyskinesia varies with activity and level of arousal and is made worse by anxiety.

A clinical examination alone cannot distinguish between withdrawal dyskinesias and other, less common causes of involuntary movements. Rating scales, such as the Abnormal Involuntary Movement Scale (AIMS) document only the severity of the abnormal movements, not the cause. The only definitive diagnosis that can be made on examination is what Dr Alberto O. Mascio has called the "Wrigley's syndrome," after a patient whose "tardive dyskinesia" disappeared when he removed the chewing gum from his mouth (7).

The minimum length of time or dosage of neuroleptic required to produce a withdrawal dyskinesia is not known. The typical case will begin within a few days after an abrupt dosage decrease (or discontinuance) and becomes worse as the neuroleptic is withdrawn. This initial period is followed by rapid improvement over several weeks or, more rarely, months. Withdrawal dyskinesias from depot preparations, such as fluphenazine decanoate, may take up to five weeks to appear (3). Anecdotal evidence suggests that withdrawal dyskinesia is commonly encountered after switching patients from older to atypical neuroleptics.

Withdrawal dyskinesias have been reported in association with older classes of neuroleptic. There is no evidence that different classes are more or less likely to cause a withdrawal dyskinesia, although it is hoped that atypical neuroleptics are less likely to do so (8). Withdrawal syndromes (with nausea, insomnia, etc.), however, may be more likely with drugs that have stronger anticholinergic properties (2,9). Withdrawal dyskinesias are also beginning to be reported in patients exposed to newer atypical neuroleptics (10–12).

In clinical practice it may be impossible to distinguish withdrawal dyskinesias from other tardive dyskinesias, because neuroleptics are often reinstituted after withdrawal to control the re-emergence of psychotic symptoms. In these situations care must be taken to distinguish withdrawal dyskinesias from signs of psychotic relapse (13).

The need to reinstitute neuroleptics for psychosis also complicates efforts to determine the frequency of withdrawal dyskinesias. Crane reported that 5% to 40% of previously asymptomatic patients developed dyskinesia when neuroleptics were discontinued, but in this report it is impossible to distinguish pure "withdrawal dyskinesia" from more persistent varieties (i.e., those lasting more than three months) (14). The other problem that leads to a paucity of data on withdrawal dyskinesias *per se* is that most tardive dyskinesia studies are cross-sectional (15). Those that are longitudinal usually have the point of entry into the study after a movement disorder is present on neuroleptics. Longitudinal studies that taper and discontinue neuroleptics prior to the discovery of a movement disorder are rare.

Kane et al (16) report on a sample of 70 individuals with no evidence of tardive dyskinesia whose neuroleptic was discontinued. Twenty-four (34%) showed emergent dyskinesias. Extended follow-up revealed seven as persistent, 16 as probable, and one as transient according to the research diagnostic criteria (3).

They reported the rate of emergent dyskinesia higher at the state hospital (67%) than at the voluntary (18%) or the Veterans Administration hospital (17%). In confirmation of a previous report by Levine et al, patients withdrawn from depot neuroleptic were less likely to show emergent dyskinesias than those withdrawn from oral medication (17). Age and total months of neuroleptic treatment correlated positively with emergent dyskinesias (17).

In less precise studies, Hoff and Hoffman found a 10% prevalence of withdrawal dyskinesia in 190 patients (18) and Degtwitz et al reported a prevalence of 17% in 53 patients (19).

In children the prevalence of withdrawal dyskinesia may be as high as 45% to 50%. The reported prevalence of persistent tardive dyskinesia in children ranges from 8% to 20% (4,20,21). However, in general it is believed that younger patients are more likely to improve (22). It has also been reported that stimulant medication in children can worsen withdrawal dyskinesia (23).

Differentiation from Other Syndromes

Unfortunately, neuroleptic administration or dosage increases can mask many movement disorders, regardless of etiology, and neuroleptic discontinuation or dose reductions can also unmask movements, regardless of etiology. A history of neuroleptic exposure and remission of symptoms within three months are suggestive of withdrawal dyskinesia but are not sufficient to make the diagnosis.

Even though the most common cause of withdrawal dyskinesia is a dose reduction or discontinuation of a neuroleptic drug, the clinician should not be complacent about the differential diagnosis. In these cases, the differential diagnosis is enormous and essentially the same as that of tardive dyskinesia in general (Table 10.1). A complete discussion is beyond the scope of this chapter, but a few points will be highlighted. More extensive reviews are provided in other chapters of this volume and elsewhere (4,5,24).

Other Drug Syndromes

Withdrawal dyskinesias have been reported with amoxapine, presumably due to its dopamine receptor blocking activity (25–27).

Abnormal movements in association with most other drugs occur during administration at normal or toxic levels, not during withdrawal. As Dilantin and lithium (28) are two drugs commonly prescribed along with neuroleptics, toxicity may initially be confused with withdrawal dyskinesia, if the neuroleptic dose has been decreased (29). Oral contraceptives rarely cause chorea (30). Nevertheless, when taking a medication history, the clinician should inquire specifically about the use of birth control pills, as many women do not think of them as "medication" and will not mention them spontaneously.

Pregnancy may be another complicating factor. Chorea that appears when neuroleptics are stopped in a pregnant

Table 10.1 Differential Diagnosis of Withdrawal Dyskinesia

Spontaneous oral dyskinesias (e.g., Miege's syndrome)

The tardive dyskinesias
Probable
Masked probable
Transient
Withdrawal
Persistent
Masked persistent

Other neurologic side effects of neuroleptic drugs
Acute dystonia
Drug-induced parkinsonism
Akathisia
Rabbit syndrome

Other drug and toxic syndromes that may mimic tardive dyskinesias
Drug-induced movement disorders
   Methylphenidate and other amphetamines
   Oral contraceptives
   Antidepressants
   Antimalarials
   Bromocriptine
Drug intoxications
   L-dopa
   Dilantin
   Lithium
Heavy metal intoxication (manganese, selenium)

Medical and neurologic syndromes
Acquired immunodeficiency syndrome
Postanoxic, postencephalitic, encephalitic syndromes
Wilson's disease
Huntington's disease
Rheumatic disorders (Syndenham's chorea, "St Vitus' Dance," vasculitides of lupus, etc.)
Brain neoplasm (thalamic, basal ganglia) or vascular insult
Calcification of the basal ganglia (Fahr's syndrome)
Systemic metabolic conditions affecting the brain
   Hepatic or renal failure
   Hyperthyroidism
   Hypoparathyroidism
   Hypoglycemia
Dystonias
   Dystonia musculorum deformans
   Torticollis
   Blepharospasm
   Oromandibular dystonia
Tics
   Gilles de la Tourette's syndrome
   Simple tics of childhood
   Multiple tic
Parkinsonism
   Adult and juvenile idiopathic
   Shy-Drager syndrome
   Carbon disulfide induced

Miscellaneous
Stereotyped movements of schizophrenia
Chorea gravidarum
Oral dyskinesias related to dental conditions, chewing gum, or prostheses

woman with psychosis could be due to chorea gravidarum rather than withdrawal dyskinesia (31).

Child psychiatrists are familiar with tics induced by methylphenidate, but all psychiatrists should be alert to the possibility that a patient may be abusing amphetamines and reluctant to share this information.

Lastly, L-dopa is probably the drug most likely to mimic tardive dyskinesia. Dyskinesias usually disappear when the dose is reduced, but in some cases movements reappear at the lower dose (24).

Other Medical and Neurologic Syndromes

Again, the reader is referred to Table 10.1 and the references previously mentioned. Certain medical disorders, such as Wilson's disease and Huntington's disease, can produce psychotic symptoms. As patients who have these symptoms are frequently treated with neuroleptics early in the course of the disease, both neuroleptic-induced and withdrawal dyskinesia may be present along with the underlying disorder (32).

Movement disorders have also been reported with acquired immunodeficiency syndrome, in some cases preceding other symptoms (33). It is well known that psychiatric patients have enormously high rates of concomitant medical illness (34). A patient who may have a medical or neurologic syndrome producing abnormal movements may also have a medical condition requiring treatment with a drug that produces abnormal movements and may have a withdrawal dyskinesia. Although these problems can be hard to sort out, it is important to do so. A withdrawal dyskinesia that is overlooked may mean a missed opportunity to prevent subsequent dyskinesia by considering alternatives to future neuroleptic treatment.

Finally, childhood degenerative diseases with movement disorders are rare but complicated. More extensive references are included elsewhere in this volume.

Evaluation

When a patient presents with what appears to be a withdrawal dyskinesia, a thorough medical history should be taken, detailed physical and neurologic examinations performed, and diagnostic tests ordered as indicated.

The American Psychiatric Association Task Force Report suggests the following steps in evaluating a presumed case of tardive dyskinesia: neurologic consultation, chemistry profile, thyroid function studies, liver function tests, sedimentation rate, serum ceruloplasmin, urinary copper, electroencephalogram, and in selected cases, computerized tomography scan (5). Today, many would also recommend magnetic resonance imaging.

Should every patient with a brief episode of apparent withdrawal dyskinesia receive the entire evaluation? Probably not, although some clinicians would recommend it. What is most important is a high index of suspicion and the attitude that the differential diagnosis is an ongoing process, not an "organic evaluation" to be completed and never reconsidered. Certainly, the differential diagnosis should be considered and discussed with the patient and/or family, consultation should be obtained, and the ongoing decision-making process documented in the chart.

In today's economic climate, clinicians are under pressure to order fewer diagnostic tests and special procedures. However, undiagnosed neurologic and other disorders represent additional economic costs to the health care system, not to mention the cost of human suffering and disability from potentially treatable disorders.

PROGNOSIS

What is the prognosis for withdrawal dyskinesia? By definition, the disorder is self-limited. What percentage of dyskinesias labeled "withdrawal" are just that and not misdiagnosed cases of other forms of tardive dyskinesia? As discussed in the section on epidemiologic data, there is little research to answer this question. For prognostic purposes, the clinician should be aware that even the more persistent varieties of tardive dyskinesia have remission rates as high as 30% to 35% at three months and continued improvement after three months (4,35). Some reviews are optimistic about the natural history and prognosis of tardive dyskinesia. However, methodology differs and improvement rates vary from 0% up to 92% (35,37).

Is a patient who has had a withdrawal dyskinesia more likely to have a more serious dyskinesia if neuroleptic drugs are readministered? Common sense would say yes, but there is no evidence to support or refute the hypothesis. This caution must also apply to the replacement of older neuroleptics with atypical ones, although, in general, these have lower rates of extrapyramidal side effects (38,39).

Is there any way to tell, three weeks after discontinuation of a neuroleptic, whether a movement disorder will remain a withdrawal dyskinesia or become a more persistent variety? At the present level of knowledge it is only possible to say that if there was truly no evidence, even minor, of abnormal movements during neuroleptic administration, the withdrawal syndrome is more likely to be a withdrawal dyskinesia than a covert dyskinesia. In practice, however, clinical recognition of all main extrapyramidal syndromes, especially tardive dyskinesia, is poor (40).

MANAGEMENT

Overall, the most important factors in the management of withdrawal dyskinesia are communication with the patient and time. Clinicians dread talking with patients about tardive dyskinesia before it happens, let alone after the fact. The first reaction to withdrawal dyskinesia in a patient for whom the clinician has both initiated and maintained neuroleptic treatment is often guilt-ridden: "What have I done?" The next reaction is often paralysis, as the physician agonizes over whether to say anything to the patient, hoping the problem will go away quickly before the patient or family notices.

In fact, patients often do not seem to notice or care (41), yet ignoring the problem in the expectation that it will go away is ill-advised. Both liability prevention and the therapeutic alliance are better served by addressing the problem openly and directly with the patient.

Prior to Initial Neuroleptic Treatment

The proper management of a neuroleptic-induced withdrawal dyskinesia, like the management of other tardive syndromes, begins long before the neuroleptic is given to the patient. Careful attention to diagnosis, a thorough examination to identify preexisting movements, and consideration of alternatives to neuroleptics all go a long way toward prevention.

Ideally, the process of informed consent about possible tardive dyskinesia and documentation, as detailed elsewhere (42,43) and in this volume, also begins at this point, although it may be delayed briefly due to acute psychosis.

Clinicians can also legitimately consider atypical neuroleptics as first line treatments, but it is probably premature to say definitively that they should do so (38,39,44).

During Neuroleptic Administration

Again, as described elsewhere, the clinician should use the lowest neuroleptic dosage and the shortest period of administration possible for effective treatment. Frequent assessment and documentation of any abnormal movements throughout treatment make the differential diagnosis of any future problems easier and will help distinguish true withdrawal dyskinesia from a mild but preexisting tardive syndrome that has been exacerbated by drug withdrawal.

Prior to Neuroleptic Withdrawal

When the neuroleptic is reduced or discontinued, the patient should be told that withdrawal dyskinesia is common but usually disappears within a few weeks. As discussed earlier, even patients with probable tardive dyskinesia before neuroleptic withdrawal have a better prognosis than previously believed. So that they will not be taken by surprise, such patients should be advised that the movements may be exacerbated temporarily during drug withdrawal.

Withdrawal

Just as there is no specific treatment for tardive dyskinesia, there is no specific treatment for withdrawal. If a patient has the general symptoms of a withdrawal syndrome, such as nausea, restlessness, and insomnia (2) or if the movements become so severe that they impair day-to-day activity, the clinician may want to reinstitute the neuroleptic at a lower dose and taper it more slowly. Another option, in a patient whose withdrawal dyskinesia is greatly exacerbated by anxiety, is to prescribe a benzodiazepine temporarily. A variety of other drugs (clonidine, etc.) are under investigation for more persistent varieties of tardive dyskinesia, but there is not yet enough evidence to make more specific recommendations for withdrawal dyskinesias. During the withdrawal period, careful monitoring and reconsideration of the differential diagnosis are important.

Future Treatment

A patient who has a serious relapse may require reinstitution of the neuroleptic. Alternative drugs, such as lithium, carbamazepine, valproic acid, and clozapine, should be discussed with the patient and family, and medication trials undertaken if indicated. For many patients, however, there is no viable alternative to neuroleptic treatment, and the harm of continued psychosis outweighs the risk of tardive dyskinesia. The clinician should also take note of a case report on treatment of withdrawal respiratory dyskinesia with an external magnetic field (45). Finally, even in the absence of solid evidence that withdrawal dyskinesia represents an early and perhaps more benign variant of tardive dyskinesia, it makes good clinical sense to treat it as such. Until research shows otherwise, withdrawal dyskinesia can be viewed as an opportunity for prevention of later, more persistent movement disorders.

BASIC SCIENCE

The pathophysiology of withdrawal dyskinesia and of tardive dyskinesia is unknown. It is also not known whether transient syndromes are pathophysiologically identical to or different from the late persistent dyskinesias (4,5). The most widely accepted theory to explain tardive dyskinesia has been that of dopamine receptor hypersensitivity (46).

Evidence from animal studies suggests that long-term neuroleptic treatment produces postsynaptic dopamine receptor supersensitivity in the basal ganglia, with a time course similar to that of withdrawal dyskinesias (4). Evidence in humans, however, is indirect and inconclusive.

More recently, discussion has focused on the pharmacologic and neuroendocrine heterogeneity of the tardive syndromes (47,48), and there is greater consensus that tardive dyskinesia is not a unitary disease with a single mechanism (49); a full discussion of this is beyond the scope of this chapter. Interested readers are referred to other chapters in this volume and to the previously cited references (4,5,21,50–54). It can be considered at this time, however, that experience with atypical neuroleptics raises the question of the role of the serotonergic system in extrapyramidal syndromes in general, and withdrawal dyskinesia in particular.

SUMMARY

Although definitions of withdrawal dyskinesia vary, it is clear that reduction or discontinuation of neuroleptics can lead to new or previously masked involuntary movements. The differential diagnosis remains important because neuroleptics may mask early manifestations of other movement disorders. The most important principles of management for withdrawal dyskinesia are communication with the patient, gradual discontinuation of the neuroleptic, and close monitoring. Despite several theories about mechanisms of action, the pathophysiology of withdrawal dyskinesia remains unclear.

REFERENCES

1. Uhrbrand L, Faurbye A. Reversible and irreversible dyskinesia after treatment with perphenazine, chlorpromazine, reserpine and electroconvulsive therapy. Psychopharmacologia 1960;1:408–418.
2. Gardos G, Cole JO, Tarsy D. Withdrawal syndromes associated with antipsychotic drugs. Am J Psychiatry 1978;135:1321–1324.
3. Schooler NR, Kane JM. Research diagnoses for tardive dyskinesia. Arch Gen Psychiatry 1982;39:486–487.
4. Jeste DV, Wyatt RJ. Understanding and treating tardive dyskinesia. New York: Guilford, 1982.
5. Baldessarini RJ, Cole JO, Davis JM, et al. Tardive dyskinesia: a task force report of the American Psychiatric Association. Washington: American Psychiatric Association, 1980.
6. Lohr JB, Wisniewski AA. Movement disorders: a neuropsychiatric approach. New York: Guilford, 1987.
7. Tardive dyskinesia: incidence and risk factors. Biol Ther Psychiatr 1986;9: 2–5.
8. Borison RL. Changing antipsychotic medication: guidelines on the transition to treatment with risperidone. The Consensus Study Group on resperidone dosing. Clin Ther 1996;18:592–607.
9. Chouinard G, Bradwejh J, et al. Withdrawal symptoms after long-term treatment with low-potency neuroleptics. J Clin Psychiatry 1984;45:500–502.
10. Songer DA, Schutte HM. Withdrawal dyskinesia after abrupt cessation of clozapine and benztropine. J Clin Psychiatry 1996;57:40.
11. Arnaud VS, Dewan MJ. Withdrawal—emergent dyskinesia in a patient on risperidone undergoing dosage reduction. Ann Clin Psychiatry 1996;8:179–182.
12. Perry R, Pataki C, Munoz-Silva DM, et al. Risperidone in children and adolescents with pervasive developmental disorder: pilot trial and follow-up. J Child Adolesc Psychopharmacol 1997;7:167–179.
13. Gardos G, Cole JO. Maintenance antipsychotic therapy: is the cure worse than the disease? Am J Psychiatry 1976;133:32–36.
14. Crane GE. Persistent dyskinesia. Br J Psychiatry 1973;122:395–405.
15. Glazer W, Morgenstern H. Predictors of occurrence, severity and course of tardive dyskinesia in an outpatient population. J Clin Psychopharmacol 1988;8:10–16S.
16. Kane J, Woerner M, Lieberman J. Tardive dyskinesia: prevalence, incidence and risk factors. J Clin Psychopharmacol 1988;87:52–56S.
17. Levine J, Schooler NR, Severe J, et al. Discontinuation of oral and depot fluphenazine in schizophrenic patients after one year of continuous medication: a controlled study. In: Cattabeni F, Racagni G, et al, eds. Long-term effects of neuroleptics. New York: Raven, 1980:483–493.
18. Hoff H, Hoffman G. Der persistierende extrapyramidale syndrom bei neuroleptikatherapie. Wien Med Wochenschr 1967;117:14–17.
19. Degtwitz R, Bauer MP, Gruber M, et al. Der zeitliche zusammenhang zwischen dem auftreten persistierender extrapyramidaler hyperkinesen und psychose recidiven nach abrupter unterbrechung langfristiger neuroleptischer behandlung chronisch schizophrener kranken. Arzneim Forsch 1970;20:890–893.
20. Engelhart DM, Polizos P, Waizer J. CNS consequences of psychotropic drug withdrawal in autistic children: a follow-up report. Psychopharmacol Bull 1975;11:6–7.
21. Winsberg BG, Hurwic MJ, Perel J. Neurochemistry of withdrawal emergent symptoms in children. Psychopharmacol Bull 1977;13:38–40.
22. Casey DE. In: Casey DE, Chase TN, Christensen AV, Gerlach J, eds. Dyskinesia: Research and Treatment. Berlin: Springer-Verlag, 1985:88–96.
23. Connor DF, Benjamin S, Ozbayrak KR. Case study: neuroleptic withdrawal dyskinesia exacerbated by ongoing stimulant treatment. J Am Acad Child Adolesc Psychiatry 1995;34:1490–1494.

24. Granacher RP. Differential diagnosis of tardive dyskinesia: overview. Am J Psychiatry 1981;138:1288–1297.
25. Lesser I. Case report of withdrawal dyskinesia associated with amoxapine. Am J Psychiatry 1983;140:1358–1359.
26. Weller RA, McKnelly WV. Case report of withdrawal dyskinesia associated with amoxapine. Am J Psychiatry 1983;140:1515–1516.
27. Price WA, Giannini AJ. Withdrawal dyskinesia following amoxapine therapy. J Clin Psychiatry 1986;47:329–330.
28. Reed S, Wise MG, Timmerman. Choreoathetosis: a sign of lithium toxicity. J Neuropsychiatry Clin Neurosci 1989;1:57–60.
29. Shuttleworth E, Wise G, Paulson GW. Choreoathetosis and diphenylhydantoin intoxication. JAMA 1974;230:1170–1171.
30. Nausieda PA, Koller WC, Weiner WJ, et al. Chorea induced by oral contraceptives. Neurology 1979;29:1605–1609.
31. Beresford OD, Graham AM. Chorea gravidarum. J Obstet Gynaecol Br Commonw 1950;57:616–625.
32. Tarsy D. Letter to the Editor. Am J Psychiatry 1978;135:386.
33. Nath A, Jankovic J, Pettigrew LC. Movement disorders and AIDS. Neurology 1987;37:37–41.
34. Hall RC. Unrecognized physical illness prompting psychiatric admission: a prospective study. Am J Psychiatry 1981;138:629–635.
35. Kane JM, Woerner M, Borenden M, Wegner J, Lieberman J. Integrating incidence and prevalence of tardive dyskinesia. Psychopharmacol Bull 1986;22:254–258.
36. Gardos G, Cole J, Haskell D, et al. The natural history of tardive dyskinesia. J Clin Psychopharmacol 1988;8:31–37S.
37. Casey DE, Gardos G, eds. Tardive dyskinesia and neuroleptics: from dogma to reason. Washington: American Psychiatric Association, 1986; and other chapters in this volume.
38. Masi G. Atypical neuroleptics in the treatment of early onset schizophrenia. Panminerva Med 1997;39:215–221.
39. Gutierrez-Esteinov R, Grebb JA. Risperidone: an analysis of the first three years in general use. Int Clin Psychopharmacol 1997;12(Supp. 4):3–10.
40. Weiden PG, Mann JJ, Haas G, Mattson M, Frances A. Clinical nonrecognition of neuroleptic induced movement disorders: a cautionary study. Am J Psychiatry 1987;144:1148–1153.
41. Alexopoulos GS. Lack of complaints in schizophrenics with tardive dyskinesia. J Nerv Ment Dis 1979;167:125–127.
42. Wettstein RM. Informed consent and tardive dyskinesia. J Clin Psychopharmacol 1988;8:65–70S.
43. Amabile PE, Cavanaugh JL. Legal liability for tardive dyskinesia: guidelines for practice. In: Wolf ME, Mosnaim AD, eds. Tardive dyskinesia: biological mechanisms and clinical aspects. Washington: American Psychiatric Association, 1988.
44. Casey DE. Will the new antipsychotics bring hope of reducing the risk of developing extrapyramidal syndromes and tardive dyskinesia? Int Clin Psychopharmacol 1997;12(Suppl. 1):19–27.
45. Sandyk R, Derpapas K. Successful treatment of respiratory dyskinesia with pico Tesla range magnetic fields. Int J Neurosci 1994;75:91–102.
46. Casey DE. Tardive dyskinesia. In: Meltzer HY, ed. Psychopharmacology: the third generation of progress. New York: Raven, 1987:1411–1419.
47. Lieberman J, Lesser M, Celeste J, Pollack S, Saltz B, Kane J. Pharmacologic studies of tardive dyskinesia. J Clin Psychopharmacol 1988;8:57–63S.
48. Wolf ME, Mosnaim AD, eds. Tardive dyskinesia: biological mechanisms and clinical aspects. Washington: American Psychiatric Association, 1988.
49. Yassa R, Jeste D. Tardive dyskinesia 1988: 31 years later. J Clin Psychopharmacol 1988;8:1S.
50. Deveaugh-Geiss J. Tardive dyskinesia and related involuntary movement disorders: the long-term effects of antipsychotic drugs. Boston: John Wright PSG, 1982.
51. Fann WE, Smith RC, Davis JM, Domino EF. Tardive dyskinesia: research and treatment. New York: SP Medical and Scientific Books, 1980.
52. Gardos G, Cole JO, Rapkin RM, et al. Anticholinergic challenge and neuroleptic withdrawal. Arch Gen Psychiatry 1984;41:1030–1035.
53. Perenyi A, Frecska E, Bagdy G, Revai K. Changes in mental condition, hyperkinesias and biochemical parameters after withdrawal of chronic neuroleptic treatment. Acta Psychiatr Scand 1985;72:430–435.
54. Winsberg BG, Hurwic MJ, Sverd J, Klutch A. Neurochemistry of withdrawal emergent symptoms in children. Psychopharmacology 1978;56:157–161.

Akathisia

Daniel Tarsy

HISTORICAL INTRODUCTION

The term *akathisia* (not sitting) was first introduced by Haskovec in 1901 to describe individuals unable to remain in a seated position (1). He described two cases, one of which was attributed to "hysteria" and the other to "neurasthenia." In one patient, akathisia was associated with clonic movements of the diaphragm and spasms of the larynx. Haskovec felt the movements were functional in origin and differentiated them from chorea due to neurologic disease and restlessness associated with anxiety states, depression, or psychosis.

Sicard (2) described a patient unable to remain seated, which he attributed to upper body pain and which he distinguished from Haskovec's akathisia. In reviewing Haskovec's cases, Sicard came to the conclusion that one was an example of epidemic encephalitis of the myoclonic type while the second represented tic or myoclonus. He further described three patients with a combination of forced walking (tasikinesia), diplopia, and somnolence, which he attributed to epidemic encephalitis lethargica. He noted the similarity of akathisia to similar symptoms occurring in manic excitement, certain epileptic states, phobias, dementia praecox, and depression.

Bing (3) described akathisia as part of a psychosis characterized by fear of sitting and an irresistible compulsion to stand that he distinguished from similar symptoms in Parkinson's disease in which patients could not remain in a fixed position due to discomfort of muscular rigidity. Wilson (4) described akathisia in postencephalitic parkinsonism and idiopathic Parkinson's disease, stating that although Haskovec's akathisia was originally used for cases of a "hysterical or psychopathic nature," it could be adopted for use in parkinsonism. He described immobilized patients who paradoxically complained of inability to sit who would get up and walk about "no doubt because they feel the cramping effect of fixed posture and have to move and stretch their limbs at intervals" (4). He also described a minor form of akathisia in which small changes in the positions of the feet and legs occurred together with absent motion in other body parts (4).

With the introduction of antipsychotic neuroleptic drugs in the 1950s, akathisia reappeared in large numbers of patients for the first time since the epidemic of encephalitis lethargica. Vivid descriptions of patients with inability to sit and marching like soldiers were described by several authors (5–7). The combination of akathisia with extrapyramidal signs of parkinsonism, dystonia, and choreoathetosis led to the conclusion that akathisia was also an extrapyramidal phenomenon. Historical descriptions of akathisia in postencephalitic parkinsonism and the improvement of neuroleptic akathisia with anticholinergic drugs appeared to support this assumption.

Although early descriptions (8,9) described motor restlessness and apparently involuntary movements of the feet, later accounts emphasized strong subjective feelings of internal discomfort and restlessness with a secondary need to move in order to relieve the uncomfortable sensation (10,11). Recently, this distinction has been expressed in the form of a dilemma concerning whether neuroleptic akathisia is a movement disorder, a mental disorder, or both (12). That is, are the movements secondary motor responses to extreme internal discomfort or do they represent "involuntary" dyskinesias occurring together with but independent of subjective symptoms?

ACUTE AKATHISIA

Early descriptions of neuroleptic-induced extrapyramidal reactions included graphic descriptions of patients with inability to remain seated or lying who also exhibited forced marching. Since this often occurred simultaneously with akinesia and rigidity, it was referred to by Deniker as the "hyperkinetic-hypertonic syndrome" (5). Although early European authors felt that akathisia was an extrapyramidal phenomenon, some writers were initially inclined to attribute akathisia to psychodynamic causes (13,14). Sarwer-Foner described several phenothiazine effects that he felt were psychological responses to physiologic effects of the drugs (13). By "holding down" patients physiologically, phenothiazines were thought to create feelings of increased passivity, fears of impaired body function, changes in body image, increased depression, or perceptions of sexual assault or seduction. Subsequent views allowed for both psychological and physiological interpretations. Winkelman (14), noting that akathisia had been described in psychosis, neurosis, and parkinsonism, emphasized that similar symptoms could result from anatomic abnormalities in Parkinson's disease, chemical abnormalities caused by neuroleptic drugs, or as part of a psychoneurotic process. Rather than emphasizing differences between these entities, Winkelman chose to emphasize their similarities, pointing out that drug-induced akathisia results directly from drug effects on the limbic system and indirectly from psychological reactions to extrapyramidal symptoms. Sarwer-Foner (15) later agreed, dividing "paradoxical behavioral reactions" due to phenothiazines into those that are psychodynamically and those that are neurologically determined. He described a spectrum of symptoms from mild tension and a feeling of being driven associated with drawing or pulling sensations in the legs to a more fully elaborated syndrome in which patients pace, are unable to otherwise occupy themselves, and in severe cases appear agitated. These phenomena were felt to be symptoms of neurologic dysfunction caused by direct effects of phenothiazines on the basal ganglia and their connections. Further confirmation that akathisia was a neurologic side effect without psychodynamic explanation came from descriptions of nervousness, apprehension, and agitation in psychiatrically normal patients in whom chlorpromazine was used for nonpsychiatric indications (16), descriptions in which it occurred in the absence of recognizable anxiety (17), and cases in which the subjective discomfort was markedly different from pretreatment feelings of anxiety (18). Freedman identified patients who developed akathisia following relatively low doses of phenothiazines who could not be distinguished from those without akathisia by pre-existing psychiatric or personality factors (19).

In a series of very influential articles, Van Putten (11,20,21) emphasized that subtle forms of akathisia were often overlooked by treating clinicians and might even account for descriptions of "acute toxic psychosis" (22,23) in response to phenothiazines. He emphasized that the mental component of akathisia could exist in the absence of overt physical manifestations. Although previous authors (18,24) had recognized an akathisic spectrum from subjective symptoms to overt signs, more graphic descriptions of

patients with incessant motor restlessness may have led to missing milder manifestations of the syndrome. Van Putten stated that akathisia is primarily a subjective state characterized by a strong need to move without reference to a specific type or pattern of involuntary movement (11). Similar to previous authors (25), he maintained that severely psychotic and disorganized patients were often unable to adequately describe their subjective feelings of restlessness and need to move. Discerning whether patients are upset by internal feelings of discomfort or the motor manifestations themselves may therefore be difficult in disturbed patients. Van Putten stated that akathisia may take many forms of psychiatric decompensation including anxiety, psychosis with somatic delusions, fear and paranoia, anger and rage reactions, and reexacerbations of the original psychosis (11,20). Association of these reactions with akathisic motor manifestations and prompt reversal of both psychiatric decompensation and akathisia with intramuscular administration of an anticholinergic drug was considered evidence that psychiatric decompensation was on the basis of akathisia (20). Van Putten further emphasized that subtle akathisia was an under-recognized reason for noncompliance in schizophrenic patients on neuroleptic drugs (21). In conclusion, akathisia should probably be regarded as both a mental and motor disorder (12,26). In some patients subjective symptoms predominate without externally visible signs of motor restlessness, while in others the reverse is true (26). A definite diagnosis is possible when both elements are present, while clinical judgment is required when only one or the other is present.

TARDIVE AKATHISIA

In recent years, the term *tardive akathisia* has been used to describe a subset of symptoms among patients with tardive dyskinesia. This comes from observations that many patients with chronic akathisia exhibit clinical features distinctive from acute akathisia. Their motor restlessness is associated with dyskinetic movements that are poorly responsive to anticholinergic drugs, appear to persist or exacerbate after discontinuation of neuroleptic drugs, and in many cases seem unaccompanied by subjective discomfort.

Historically, late-appearing chronic akathisia was well described in early descriptions of tardive dyskinesia. In their classical description of tardive dyskinesia, Uhrbrand and Faurbye (27) described "rocking and torsionary body movements and incessant tripping and shuffling movements so that the patient cannot stand still" in patients with irreversible orolingual dyskinesia. Although in most patients who discontinued neuroleptic treatment dyskinesia was irreversible, it was not specifically stated whether persistent akathisia was part of the "irreversible" syndrome. Kruse (9) described three patients with severe motor restlessness manifest by inability to sit or keep their legs still and distressing feelings of motor restlessness that persisted 3 to 18 months after neuroleptic withdrawal and that he referred to as "persistent muscular restlessness." Hunter et al (28) described 13 patients with persistent involuntary movements appearing after 18 months to 5 years of neuroleptic treatment. In addition to widespread choreoathetosis, "akathisia was present in all in varying degree; when severe patients could not remain seated for longer than a few minutes at a time." They emphasized that the restlessness, agitation, and distress of these patients could be mistaken for manifestations of the original psychiatric illness leading to further use of neuroleptic medications. Pryce and Edwards (29) described distress, agitation, and general restlessness occurring in combination with orofacial dyskinesia in a group of patients in whom phenothiazines had been discontinued. Kennedy et al (30) described five types of motor abnormality appearing in patients on chronic neuroleptic drugs. "Restlessness" of the trunk and limbs constituted one variety of movement disorder and was noted to have a high association with choreiform movements of the oral region. A subsequent study by this group (31) found that motor restlessness of the limbs and trunk increased significantly in patients in whom neuroleptic drugs were discontinued. Schmidt and Jarcho's description of persistent phenothiazine dyskinesias (32) included a description of "restless activity of the extremities and face and inability to sit or lie still" combined with a variety of choreoathetotic involuntary movements of the face and tongue that persisted for months to years in all five patients. Simpson (33) stated that akathisia usually appeared within a few days of initiating medication but also described "late onset akathisia, which may begin weeks, months, or years after the onset of treatment, is much more difficult to treat; in fact, it is virtually untreatable. . . . [T]he very late onset variety is frequently associated with tardive dyskinesia." Ayd (8) described akathisia as a compulsion to walk or pace together with constant shifting of the legs, tapping of the feet, and complaints of feeling jittery or anxious. Rocking movements and shifting of weight while standing were included in this description. Although acute akathisia was not distinguished from late onset akathisia, 90% of cases were said to appear within the first 73 days of initiating neuroleptic treatment suggesting a significant incidence of later-onset akathisia. Crane (34) included "shifting of weight from foot to foot" in his description of tardive dyskinesia.

The concept of tardive akathisia was addressed more specifically in the late 1970s. Forrest and Fahn (35) used the term *tardive dysphrenia and subjective akathisia* to describe persistent dyskinesia in patients no longer receiving neuroleptic drugs who exhibited combinations of akathisia and dyskinesia. They described akathisia as a syndrome of restlessness with the involuntary urge to get up and move around which is more distressing than dyskinesia. It is a "screaming inside, an unbearable feeling one is about to burst or explode with a need to move, or one is going to jump out of one's skin and it leads . . . to clinging behavior and anguished imploring of the physician to help." The observation that distressful akathisia can be a major component of tardive dyskinesia

has been reemphasized by Fahn in subsequent reports (36). In one study, 13 of 14 patients with tardive dyskinesia, most of whom were no longer receiving neuroleptic drugs, exhibited akathisia manifest as "a feeling of restlessness characterized as if the patient were going to jump out of his/her skin" (36).

Kidger et al (37) described three separate clusters or "components" of involuntary movements in patients with tardive dyskinesia. Their second "component," referred to as "peripheral tardive dyskinesia," includes involuntary movements of the trunk, arms, hands, and legs. They point out that some of these movements are ordinarily not recognized as part of tardive dyskinesia but rather as restless, fidgety movements of akathisia. Since their patients lacked subjective complaints of restlessness and inability to sit, however, it was felt they did not have akathisia. This "component" corresponds to the category of "restlessness" described by Kennedy et al (30), which also did not describe subjective distress.

A subsequent publication by this group (38) emphasized that, because phenomenologic descriptions of akathisia have varied widely, prevalence rates and results of treatment trials have been inconsistent. These authors utilized two criteria for the diagnosis of acute akathisia (38). The first criterion is subjective restlessness usually located in the lower extremities. This was previously found in 26 of 27 patients with acute akathisia (39). More general complaints of "inner restlessness" reported by many patients with acute akathisia were felt to be less specific than this condition. The second criterion was the observation of characteristic patterns of restless movements including rocking from foot to foot and walking in place. Additional characteristic movements included shuffling or tramping-like movements while seated, inability to stand without walking or pacing, and fidgety leg movements while lying down.

Studies of 82 schizophrenic patients led to the identification of three akathisia groups: acute akathisia, pseudoakathisia, and chronic akathisia (38). "Acute akathisia" refers to dose-related subjective and objective manifestations with onset of symptoms coincident with an increase in neuroleptic dose. Patients with acute akathisia were relatively young, had been receiving neuroleptic drugs for a short period of time, and had no manifestations of tardive dyskinesia. "Pseudoakathisia" refers to motor manifestations of akathisia without subjective experiences of restlessness. These patients were older, had a longer duration of neuroleptic drug treatment, and had a high incidence of orofacial and limb dyskinesia. "Chronic akathisia" refers to a group of patients fulfilling criteria for akathisia but in whom symptoms and signs did not appear coincident with an increase in drug dose and sometimes appeared with drug withdrawal. These patients resembled those with pseudoakathisia in having a high incidence of orofacial and limb dyskinesia and resembled the acute akathisia group in having a high prevalence of subjective restlessness. A particularly important observation was that 12 patients with chronic akathisia appeared to represent persistence of acute akathisia. These patients could date the onset of their symptoms months to years earlier coinciding with an increase in drug dosage. An additional report of two patients with persistent acute akathisia from the onset of neuroleptic treatment who later developed orofacial dyskinesia also suggests that persistent acute akathisia may be an antecedent of early tardive dyskinesia (40). These akathisia subdivisions suggest that acute akathisia, chronic akathisia, and pseudoakathisia may be stages in a clinical progression in which chronic akathisia represents a transitional stage of subjective symptoms and objective signs that is followed by persistent motor signs without subjective restlessness (37).

The concept of progression from acute akathisia to tardive akathisia and dyskinesia has been discussed by other investigators. Munetz and Cornes (41–43) emphasized that the clinical distinction between akathisia and tardive dyskinesia is often difficult and fraught with misdiagnoses. They described patients with "restless appearing" involuntary movements of the legs without subjective restlessness that they also referred to as pseudoakathisia and believed represents tardive dyskinesia of the lower extremities. Similar to Barnes and Braude (40), they also described patients with acute akathisia early in treatment who subsequently developed either pseudoakathisia or tardive dyskinesia (41).

Whether late-appearing tardive akathisia represents the end stage in a progression from acute akathisia remains unproven. Both studies (38,41) in which akathisia subtypes have been delineated along a spectrum from acute to chronic have been cross-sectional rather than longitudinal and do not establish this progression. An ongoing prospective study of cumulative incidence of tardive dyskinesia in patients newly placed on neuroleptic drugs indicates a correlation between early extrapyramidal side effects and subsequent appearance of tardive dyskinesia but makes no specific reference to akathisia (44,45).

Inherent in the concept of progression is the notion that the movements of acute akathisia are identical to those of late appearing chronic akathisia, but this may not be the case. Much of the motor activity in akathisia is described by patients as a voluntary effort to relieve intensely uncomfortable sensations that usually takes the form of changes in body position, standing, or pacing. In mild akathisia this can be voluntarily suppressed but in more severe states the need for persistent motor activity is sufficiently compelling to be virtually involuntary. Although in this setting it may be impossible to make a definite distinction between voluntary and involuntary motor activity, it is likely that many lower extremity and trunk movements attributable to chronic akathisia should more properly be classified as choreoathetotic dyskinesias. In one study (46), 159 psychiatric inpatients with hyperkinetic movements were divided into three subgroups with motor restlessness: there were 27 patients with motor restlesssness and a subjective need to move who lacked orofacial dyskinesia and were felt to have "definite akathisia," 79 patients who exhibited orofacial dyskinesia and

motor restlessness without a subjective need to move who were felt to have tardive dyskinesia, and an indeterminate group of 53 patients with motor restlessness without either subjective need to move or orofacial dyskinesia. Swinging of a crossed leg while seated and rapid walking were more common in the akathisia group while rubbing movements of the arms and squirming, jerky movements of the feet were more common in the tardive dyskinesia group. The authors concluded that buccolinguomasticatory movements or orofacial dyskinesia constitute a core feature of tardive dyskinesia and that such movements serve the purpose of providing an instantly recognizable sign of tardive dyskinesia. Although involuntary movements of the extremities and trunk may coexist, these are less diagnostic especially when present in the absence of orofacial dyskinesia. Whether or not "peripheral" involuntary movements of the extremities and trunk constitute an important subtype of dyskinesia, it is clear that they overlap with akathisia and by themselves are a less distinctive clinical sign.

DIAGNOSIS

The diagnosis of acute akathisia is based on the combination of subjective distress and motor restlessness following administration of an antipsychotic drug. As discussed above, patients with acute akathisia usually report subjective anxiety, inner tension, being driven to move, pulling or drawing sensations in their legs, and inability to tolerate inactivity in a seated or lying position. Subjective complaints include intense feelings of internal discomfort, tension, turmoil, irritability, impatience, or unease. Strong affective components of fright, terror, anger, rage, and anxiety may be included (11), but it is not clear if these are primary or secondary features. Such subjective sensations may be associated with a need to escape the immediate environment and in some cases have resulted in suicidal (47) or violent (48) behavior. The compelling need to move usually serves to distinguish akathisia from the anxiety, dysphoria, or psychosis that may have preceded treatment. Patients with psychotic agitation may exhibit excessive movements but usually in the form of semipurposeful movements of the upper extremities, such as hand-wringing and other repetitive activities (49). Psychotic patients with akathisia may have difficulty describing their symptoms but will usually indicate they are experiencing internal restlessness when that possibility is suggested to them (50). Objective motor manifestations of akathisia include a variety of patterns of restless motor activity. By definition, it consists of inability to remain seated but is commonly associated with repetitive shifting of weight, pacing or marching, and rocking of the trunk while standing. Continuous shuffling or tapping movements of the feet while sitting may also be present, but these are less specific and may represent choreoathetotic dyskinesia. Although in some cases the distinction will be arbitrary, an attempt should be made to decide whether the movements are variants of normal behavior, psychotic behaviors, restless movements, or choreoathetotic dyskinesias (12). Inquiries of the patients as to whether or not they are experiencing subjective distress causing a need to move are critical in making this decision (43).

Differential Diagnosis

Acute akathisia has been reported following treatments with a large variety of neuroleptic drugs as well as nonneuroleptic medications such as clozapine, serotonin reuptake inhibitor antidepressants, heterocyclic antidepressants, buspirone, and levodopa (51). In practice, neuroleptic drugs are by far the most common cause of akathisia and should be the prime consideration in cases of persistent akathisia off medication. Historically, akathisia was attributed to psychoneurosis or neurasthenia (1), but in current clinical practice this has to be considered an obscure and obsolete cause. Akathisia has also been described as one of the early manifestations of encephalitis lethargica in which it constitutes one portion of the "excitomotor syndrome" (52). Since encephalitis lethargica no longer occurs, however, this is not a practical consideration. Akathisia has also been described as a manifestation of Parkinson's disease (4,53). Although akathisia more commonly occurred in postencephalitic parkinsonism than idiopathic paralysis agitans (3,4), a recent study in which patients with Parkinson's disease were carefully questioned about symptoms of akathisia indicates a surprisingly high incidence of this symptom, although much less prominent than following neuroleptic treatment (53). Although in most cases the diagnosis of idiopathic Parkinson's disease will be apparent, the frequent combination of parkinsonism and akathisia in patients on neuroleptic drugs may create a problem in differential diagnosis. Patients with Parkinson's disease who are on L-dopa may also exhibit recurrent withdrawal akathisia at night several hours after last receiving L-dopa. Withdrawal from benzodiazepines may also produce subjective symptoms difficult to distinguish from akathisia (54).

Akathisia must also be distinguished from choreoathetotic movement disorders. Mild chorea may be limited to fidgety, restless movements of the extremities and apparent inability to keep still. Sydenham's chorea, for example, is characterized by this form of motor restlessness. Restless legs syndrome has strong clinical similarities to akathisia but can usually be distinguished by prominent subjective discomfort confined to the legs, the absence of internal feelings of anxiety or restlessness, the restriction of symptoms to when the patient is reclining, the prompt relief of symptoms by walking, and the absence of the other motor manifestations of akathisia described above.

Akathisia should be suspected in any patient who exhibits motor restlessness or psychiatric agitation shortly following initiation of neuroleptic treatment, a change to a more potent neuroleptic drug, or an increase in dose. Cyclically appearing restlessness in patients on parenteral fluphenazine esters should also suggest the diagnosis. Akathisia should be

distinguished from akathisia-like movements seen in tardive dyskinesia by the presence of subjective internal and lower extremity discomfort and relief produced by movement and changes of body position (42). The presence or absence of associated extrapyramidal signs such as cogwheel rigidity (54) does not provide a reliable basis for a diagnosis of akathisia.

Response to anticholinergic treatment has been emphasized as a reliable method of differential diagnosis. Van Putten et al (20) reported that an anticholinergic drug will reverse the symptoms and signs of akathisia and associated behavioral excitement while having no effect on agitation due to psychiatric causes. Although this may be true in some cases, the variable response of akathisia (especially late-appearing forms) to treatment (49) indicates that this may not be a reliable diagnostic tool. The use of extrapyramidal rating scales is not useful for diagnosis but should be reserved for attempts to objectively document and quantify extrapyramidal signs. Many extrapyramidal rating scales do not adequately distinguish between involuntary movements of the trunk and extremities on the basis of choreoathetotic dyskinesia or akathisia and place greater emphasis on observable motor manifestations than subjective symptoms.

Ultimately, differentiation of akathisia from tardive dyskinesia constitutes the most difficult clinical problem and, in some cases, they may remain indistinguishable. Munetz and Cornes (42) have proposed clinical criteria to help make this differentiation. It should be emphasized that akathisia should be subjectively distressing. Although tardive dyskinesia may also cause distress, this is secondary to the involuntary movements rather than the cause. The patient's appearance alone should not be the basis for concluding that subjective distress is present since dyskinetic patients often appear distressed without experiencing this subjectively. The movements of akathisia are often voluntary attempts to relieve distressing internal stimuli while those of tardive dyskinesia are involuntary movements that may cause distress. In severe akathisia, movements may be extremely compelling but nonetheless should be identifiable as voluntary. As already discussed, time of onset relative to drug exposure, location of movements in trunk or lower extremities, coexistence of other extrapyramidal signs, and response to anticholinergic drugs are not reliable for distinguishing akathisia from tardive dyskinesia.

MANAGEMENT AND TREATMENT

For many years anticholinergic drugs were purported to be an effective treatment but in clinical practice have been of limited benefit. Van Putten et al reported that biperiden given parentally was universally effective in abolishing symptoms and signs of akathisia (20). In their experience the effect was sufficiently dramatic to suggest its use as a diagnostic test for differentiation of akathisia from manic excitement or other forms of psychotic agitation (20). In a more recent study, however, Van Putten et al (50) found a high proportion of nonresponders to anticholinergic treatment in patients experiencing akathisia after a single dose of haloperidol. In an open study of diphenhydramine (an anticholinergic antihistamine) compared with diazepam, it was found that diphenhydramine in a dose of 25 mg three times daily produced no subjective or objective clinical improvement (55). DiMascio and colleagues compared the effect of benztropine to amantadine in a double-blind study and found them to be equally effective in reversal of akathisia as well as other extrapyramidal manifestations (56). Adler et al (57) compared benztropine with propranolol and placebo and found significant improvement within several days of treatment with both active drugs.

Two studies have reported that diazepam is effective in treatment of akathisia (55,58). Donlon found that diazepam 15 mg daily reduced or alleviated akathisia in 10 of 13 patients in an open-label study. Symptoms subsided within three days with subjective and objective evidence for moderate to marked relief. Gagrat and colleagues (58) studied the effect of intravenous diazepam on acute akathisia and dystonia following haloperidol. Intravenous diazepam produced significant improvement in akathisia for 120 minutes following administration, which was equal to the effect of intravenous diphenhydramine. Notwithstanding these two studies, general clinical experience with diazepam in akathisia has not been encouraging (49). In an open trial (59), lorazepam produced improvement in akathisia while clonazepam produced a similar result in a double-blind, placebo-controlled trial (60). Sodium valproate failed to improve akathisia when compared with an anticholinergic drug in one randomized study (61).

Donlon (55) commented that anticholinergic drugs "occasionally produce a favorable response in early akathisia; however, in long-term patients such as ours, these medications are generally ineffective." Thus, one problem in the evaluation of treatment studies may be that a distinction between acute and chronic akathisia is often not made (49). Lack of efficacy of anticholinergic drugs may also be due to subtherapeutic dosage. The scanty literature on anticholinergic treatment does not include a wide range of doses. In one case report, efficacy of anticholinergic treatment of akathisia was improved by monitoring of serum anticholinergic levels (62).

Influenced by reports of its efficacy in treatment of restless legs syndrome (63), Lipinski and colleagues described striking improvement in all 12 patients with akathisia treated with propranolol in an open-label study (64). Nine of these patients were said to experience complete remission of akathisia. The mean dose required to achieve greatest improvement was 30 mg daily. Onset of effect occurred within one hour of the first dose and maximum clinical response was achieved in 24 to 48 hours.

A follow-up study by the same authors (65) reported the effect of propranolol in an open-label study of 14 psychiatric hospital inpatients. These patients were a relatively spe-cialized group in that 11 were acutely manic, were being treated with lithium, and exhibited lithium tremor. Ten of these patients also displayed parkinsonism while two had mild symptoms of tardive dyskinesia. All 14 patients showed substantial improvement in akathisia with 9 of the 14 showing complete remission. Doses of propranolol ranged between 30 and 80 mg daily. Lithium tremor was controlled in most patients but little or no improvement was seen in either parkinsonism or tardive dyskinesia. There were no significant propranolol-related side effects and no patients became depressed during the first month of treatment. It should be noted that 10 patients in this study were receiving benztropine as treatment for akathisia and parkinsonism and had shown no change in akathisia on this drug. The beneficial effect of propranolol in akathisia has been confirmed in three subsequent studies by Adler and colleagues (57,66,67). In one study, propranolol was compared with placebo in a randomized, double-blind, crossover study (66). Twelve psychiatric inpatients and outpatients were studied, 11 of whom were schizophrenic. Patients were selected for study according to the presence of "akathisia-like movements" as documented by an extrapyramidal rating scale. Treatment with propranolol occurred for 6 to 10 days in a dose range of 20–60 mg. Propranolol caused a significant improvement in both subjective and objective ratings of akathisia compared with baseline and placebo ratings. Other extrapyramidal measures were unaffected. Levels of anxiety as measured by the Hamilton Anxiety Scale showed no significant change. In a separate study (67), a population of psychiatric inpatients with akathisia manifested by subjective and objective manifestations were treated with propranolol, 20–30 mg daily, and lorazepam 2 mg daily or placebo in a closed label randomized study. Subjective and objective improvement occurred with both drugs although improvement was greater with propranolol. Similar to previous studies, no improvement occurred in other extrapyramidal manifestations. A further controlled comparison of propranolol and benztropine showed them to be equally effective and both more effective than placebo (57).

Subsequent studies of beta blockers in akathisia have been carried out to determine whether effects are due to beta-1 or beta-2 receptor blockade and whether the mechanism of action is peripheral or central. Propranolol was compared with metoprolol in five psychiatric inpatients all of whom were actively psychotic at the time of the study (68). Four patients were being treated with lithium for bipolar or schizoaffective disorder. All patients demonstrated substantial improvement with propranolol and consistent but less dramatic improvement following treatment with metoprolol. By contrast, very high doses of metoprolol (200–400 mg daily) were required to produce improvement in akathisia. At these doses, metoprolol produces significant beta-2 blockade and is also less useful because of bradycardia and hypotension. Betaxolol is a relative beta-1 antagonist that was effective in reducing akathisia in low doses in four patients in an open-label study (66). These conflicting results in small open-label studies leave the issue of beta specificity unresolved for the time being.

Studies designed to determine whether peripheral or central effects of beta blockers are responsible for efficacy suggest that beta blockers with lipophilic properties that cross the blood-brain barrier are effective while beta blockers such as atenolol (69) and sotalol (70) are ineffective in treating akathisia. Although the efficacy of nadolol (71) has been interpreted to suggest a peripheral site of action, the delayed onset in effect of this mixed hydrophilic and lipophilic compound does not exclude a central mechanism of action.

Two studies concerning the effect of clonidine in akathisia have recently appeared (72,73). Zubenko and colleagues (72) treated six psychiatric inpatients in an open-label study, three of whom were manic and all six of whom were actively psychotic. All six patients showed substantial improvement in akathisia with four of the six patients showing complete remission. The dose of clonidine ranged between 0.2 and 0.8 mg. Adler and colleagues (73) confirmed these findings in six psychiatric inpatients most of whom were schizophrenics. Ratings of subjective akathisia, objective akathisia, and anxiety declined in all six patients. The latter finding may have been due to side effects of sedation and differs from the absence of any effect on anxiety scores produced by propranolol (66). Prominent sedation and hypotension in both studies will probably limit the usefulness of clonidine in treatment of akathisia.

Because of reported efficacy of opioids in treatment of restless legs syndrome (74), they have recently been studied in akathisia. Walters and colleagues compared the effect of propoxyphene, codeine, and placebo in five patients with either acute or tardive akathisia in a double-blind study (75). All patients showed a substantial to complete improvement of akathisia to opioids as determined by rating of videotapes for motor restlessness.

MECHANISMS

Early discussions of neuroleptic akathisia suggested that, similar to akathisia in postencephalitic parkinsonism and Parkinson's disease, akathisia is a subjective response to the presence of rigidity and akinesia (3,4). Some recent authors have also suggested that akathisia is primarily a sensory disturbance to which motor phenomena occur as a secondary response (10,76). If motor manifestations of akathisia are secondary to internal sensory stimuli, pathophysiologic explanations of akathisia would have to account for these abnormal sensations. However, if akathisia is primarily a form of locomotor hyperactivity associated with but not occurring in response to internal discomfort, then pathophysiologic mechanisms within the motor system would be more relevant. The assumption that akathisia is a manifestation of abnormality in the extrapyramidal system is based

entirely on its frequent coincidence with other extrapyramidal manifestations in encephalitis lethargica, postencephalitic parkinsonism, and idiopathic Parkinson's disease as well as the temporal association of akathisia with extrapyramidal effects of neuroleptic drugs. Early observations that acute dystonic reactions, parkinsonism, and akathisia could all be reversed by anticholinergic drugs, reinforced the notion that akathisia must be an extrapyramidal phenomenon.

The absence of suitable animal models for akathisia has been a limiting factor in the understanding of this disorder. Gore and Hadley (77) observed a phase of excitation or restlessness in Rhesus monkeys who were given piperazine phenothiazines. An initial sedative phase characterized by akinesia was followed by a phase of restlessness with bursts of motor activity including rolling on their backs, crawling on their bellies, leaping, attempting to escape from the observation table, assuming odd or bizarre positions, and retropulsion. This phase of restlessness was short and followed by catalepsy. The authors suggested that this phenomenon may be related to akathisia. However, subsequent studies of the acute effects of phenothiazines in other nonhuman primates described a variety of acute dyskinesias and dystonic reactions without similar descriptions of motor restlessness (78–80).

Marsden and Jenner (81) have suggested that akathisia may be a result of postsynaptic dopamine receptor blockade in cerebral dopamine-containing regions of the brain other than the corpus striatum. Thus, while blockade of dopamine receptors in the striatum and mesolimbic regions such as the nucleus accumbens inhibits locomotor activity and produces a state of akinesia or catalepsy, locomotor hyperactivity occurs following blockade of mesocortical dopamine systems. Iverson (82) showed that bilateral lesions of frontal cortex in rats caused enhancement of amphetamine-induced behavioral hyperactivity in contrast to bilateral lesions of the substantia nigra that impaired the locomotor response to amphetamine. Carter and Pycock (83,84) showed that bilateral electrolytic or 6-hydroxydopamine lesions in medial prefrontal cortex of rats enhanced the stereotypic effects of amphetamine. By contrast, intracortical injection of dopamine into the same region of frontal cortex produced a dose-dependent state of catalepsy (83). Although these results have been interpreted to indicate that catecholamines may play an inhibitory role in frontal cortex, the failure of intracortical injections of fluphenazine to enhance stereotypic or locomotor responses induced by amphetamine (83) fails to support the concept that dopamine receptor blockade in mesocortical systems enhances behavioral hyperactivity. Le Moal et al (85) described a behavioral syndrome in rats produced by high-frequency lesions of the ventral tegmental area characterized by locomotor hyperactivity, hyperreactivity, and other disturbances of complex behaviors. The ventral tegmental area contains the dopaminergic cells of origin for the mesolimbic and mesocortical neurons that innervate the frontal and cingulate cerebral cortex. Tassin and his colleagues (86) found that the locomotor hyperactivity produced by bilateral ventral tegmental area lesions in rats was dependent on ascending dopaminergic projections but not on those mediated by serotonin or nor-adrenaline. Although other investigators (87) have suggested that an increase in dopaminergic transmission in nucleus accumbens may cause locomotor hyperactivity, Tassin et al (86) found that the correlation between increased locomotor activity and decreased frontal cortex dopamine levels was much better than that observed for dopamine in nucleus accumbens, suggesting that destruction of mesocortical dopamine neurons is critical for the development of loco-motor activity.

In view of a series of recent studies demonstrating therapeutic efficacy of beta blockers in akathisia, the possibility that akathisia is due to excessive noradrenergic activity also deserves consideration. It should be noted, however, that many of these treatment studies have not adequately distinguished between acute akathisia and late-appearing akathisia. Since the pathophysiology of these two forms of akathisia may differ, the interpretation of treatment effects must be made with caution. A large number of studies have demonstrated that adrenergic drugs can produce locomotor hyperactivity in rodents. Norepinephrine nuclei located in the midbrain, some of which may project to the spinal cord, are believed to be important in some forms of locomotor activity. Bartels and colleagues (88) found that urinary excretion of norepinephrine metabolites was reduced in patients with akathisia compared to a control population. They suggested that this reflects a reduction in norepi-nephrine turnover best explained by chronic neuroleptic-induced blockade of postsynaptic alpha-receptors resulting in receptor supersensitivity. As indicated above in the section on treatment, it is not yet well established whether beta-adrenergic antagonists are acting centrally or peripherally or at beta-1 or beta-2 receptors. The reported therapeutic effect of clonidine in akathisia (72,73) may provide further evidence for a possible role of alpha-adrenergic receptors. Finally, the recent reported therapeutic effect of opioid drugs in akathisia (75) should stimulate investigations into the role of opioid mechanisms in the pathophysiology of akathisia.

A possible role of iron deficiency in akathisia has been considered in view of the putative benefit of iron treatment in restless legs syndrome and the role of iron in dopamine receptor function in experimental animals (89,90). Recent studies, however, have failed to support an association between neuroleptic-induced akathisia and iron deficiency (89,90).

REFERENCES

1. Haskovec L. L'Akathisie. Rev Neurol 1901;9:1107–1109.
2. Sicard JP. Akathisie et tasikinesie. La Press Medicale 1923;31:265–266.
3. Bing R. Textbook of nervous diseases. St. Louis: C.V. Mosby, 1939:169.
4. Wilson SAK. In: Bruce AN, ed. Neurology. Baltimore: Williams and Wilkins, 1940:118, 793.
5. Deniker P. Experimental neurological syndromes and the new drug therapies in psychiatry. Compr Psychiatry 1960;1:92–102.
6. Denham J, Carrick DJEL. Therapeutic value of thioproperazine and the importance of the associated neurological disturbances. J Mental Sci 1961;107:326–345.
7. Sirnes TB. Drug-induced extrapyramidal reactions. Acta Neurol Scand 1963;39(suppl 4):209–217.
8. Ayd FJ Jr. A survey of drug-induced extrapyramidal reactions. JAMA 1961;175:1054–1060.
9. Kruse W. Persistent muscular restlessness after phenothiazine treatment: report of three cases. Am J Psychiatry 1960;117:152–153.
10. Chien CP, DiMascio DI, DiMascio A. Drug-induced extrapyramidal symptoms and their relations to clinical efficacy. Am J Psychiatry 1967;123:1490–1498.
11. Van Putten T. The many faces of akathisia. Compr Psychiatry 1975;16:43–47.
12. Stahl S. Akathisia and tardive dyskinesia. Arch Gen Psychiatry 1985;42:915–917.
13. Sarwer-Foner GJ, Ogle W. Psychosis and enhanced anxiety produced by reserpine and chlorpromazine. Can Med Assoc J 1956;74:526–532.
14. Winkelman NW. The inter-relationship between the physiological and psychological etiologies of akathisia. In: Bordeleau JM, ed. Extrapyramidal systems and neuroleptics. Montreal: Editions Psychiatriques, 1961:563–568.
15. Sarwer-Foner GJ. Recognition and management of drug-induced extrapyramidal reactions and "paradoxical" behavioral reactions in psychiatry. Can Med Assoc J 1960;83:312–318.
16. Hollister LE, Eikenberry DT, Raffel S. Chlorpromazine in nonpsychotic patients with pulmonary tuberculosis. Am Rev Resp Dis 1960;81:562–566.
17. Hodge JR. Akathisia: the syndrome of motor restlessness. Am J Psychiatry 1959;116:337–338.
18. Freedman DX, De Jong J. Factors that determine drug-induced akathisia. Dis Nerv Sys 1961;22(suppl 2):69–76.
19. Freedman DX, De Jong J. Thresholds for drug-induced akathisia. Amer J Psychiatry 1961;117:930–931.
20. Van Putten T, Mutalpassi LR, Malkin MD. Phenothiazine induced decompensation. Arch Gen Psychiatry 1974;30:102–105.
21. Van Putten T. Why do schizophrenic patients refuse to take their drugs? Arch Gen Psychiatry 1974;31:67–72.
22. Lang AW, Moore RA. Acute toxic psychosis concurrent with phenothiazine therapy. Am J Psychiatry 1961;117:939–940.
23. Chaffin DS. Phenothiazine-induced acute psychotic reaction: the "psychotoxicity" of a drug. Amer J Psychiatry 1964;121:26–32.
24. Freyhan FA. Therapeutic implications of differential effects with new phenothiazine compounds. Amer J Psychiatry 1959;115:577–585.
25. Raskin DE. Akathisia: a side effect to be remembered. Am J Psychiatry 1972;129:121–123.
26. Sachdev P, Kruk J. Clinical characteristics and predisposing factors in acute drug-induced akathisia. Arch Gen Psychiatry 1994;51:963–974.
27. Uhrbrand L, Faurbye A. Reversible and irreversible dyskinesia after treatment with perphenazine, chlorpromazine, reserpine, and electroconvulsive therapy. Psychopharmacologia 1960;1:408–418.
28. Hunter R, Earl CJ, Thornicroft S. An apparently irreversible syndrome of abnormal movements following phenothiazine medication. Proc R Soc Med 1964;57:758–762.
29. Pryce IG, Edwards H. Persistent oral dyskinesia in female mental hospital patients. Brit J Psychiatry 1966;112:983–987.
30. Kennedy PF, Hershon HI, McGuire RJ. Extrapyramidal disorders after prolonged phenothiazine therapy. Brit J Psychiatry 1971;118:509–518.
31. Hershon HI, Kennedy PF, McGuire RJ. Persistence of extrapyramidal disorders and psychiatric relapse after withdrawal of long-term phenothiazine therapy. Brit J Psychiatry 1972;120:41–50.
32. Schmidt WR, Jarcho LW. Persistent dyskinesias following phenothiazine therapy. Arch Neurol 1966;14:369–377.
33. Simpson GM. Neurotoxicity of major tranquilizers. In: Roizin L, Shiraki H, Grcevic N, eds. Neurotoxicology. New York: Raven, 1977.
34. Crane GE. Clinical psychopharmacology in its 20th year. Science 1973;181:124–128.
35. Forrest DV, Fahn S. Tardive dysphrenia and subjective akathisia. J Clin Psychiatry 1979;40:206.
36. Fahn S. Long-term treatment of tardive dyskinesia with presynaptically acting dopamine-depleting agents. In: Fahn S, Calne DB, Shoulson I, eds. Advances in neurology. Vol. 37. Experimental therapeutics of movement disorders. New York: Raven, 1983:267–276.
37. Kidger T, Barnes TRE, Trauer T, Taylor PJ. Sub-syndromes of tardive dyskinesia. Psychol Med 1980;10:513–520.

38. Barnes TRE, Braude WM. Akathisia variants and tardive dyskinesia. Arch Gen Psychiatry 1985;42:874–878.

39. Braude WM, Barnes TRE, Gore SM. Clinical characteristics of akathisia: a systematic investigation of acute psychiatric inpatient admissions. Br J Psychiatry 1983;143:139–150.

40. Barnes TRE, Braude WM. Persistent akathisia associated with early tardive dyskinesia. Post Grad Med J 1984;60:359–361.

41. Munetz MR, Cornes CL. Akathisia, pseudoakathisia and tardive dyskinesia: clinical examples. Compr Psychiatry 1982;23:345–352.

42. Munetz MR, Cornes CL. Distinguishing akathisia and tardive dyskinesia: a review of the literature. J Clin Psychopharmacol 1983;3:343–349.

43. Munetz MR. Akathisia variants and tardive dyskinesia. Arch Gen Psychiatry 1986;143:1015.

44. Kane JM, Woerner M, Weinhold P, et al. A prospective study of tardive dyskinesia development: preliminary results. J Clin Psychopharmacol 1982;2:345–349.

45. Kane JM, Woerner M, Borenstein M, et al. Integrating incidence and prevalence of tardive dyskinesia. Psychopharmacol Bull 1986;22:254–258.

46. Lees AJ, Gibb WRG. The clinical phenomenon of akathisia. J Neurol Neurosurg Psychiatry 1986;49:861–866.

47. Drake RE, Ehrlich J. Suicide attempts associated with akathisia. Am J Psychiatry 1985;142:499–501.

48. Keckich WA. Neuroleptics. Violence as a manifestation of akathisia. JAMA 1978;240:21–85.

49. Braude WM, Barnes TRE, Gore SM. Clinical characteristics of akathisia. A systematic investigation of acute psychiatric inpatient admissions. Brit J Psychiatry 1983;143:139–150.

50. Van Putten T, May PRA, Marder SR. Akathisia with haloperidol and thiothixene. Arch Gen Psychiatry 1984;41:1036–1039.

51. Sachdev P. The identification and management of drug-induced akathisia. CNS Drugs 1995;4:28–46.

52. Marie P, Levy G. Le syndrome excito-moteur de l'encephalite epidemique. Rev Neurol 1920;36:513–537.

53. Lang AE, Johnson K. Akathisia in idiopathic parkinson's disease. Neurology 1987;37:477–481.

54. Maltbie AA, Cavenar JR, Cole JO. Akathisia diagnosis: an objective test. Psychosomatics 1977;18:36–39.

55. Donlon PT. The therapeutic use of diazepam for akathisia. Psychosomatics 1973;14:222–225.

56. DiMascio A, Bernardo DL, Greenblatt DJ, Marder JE. A controlled trial of amantadine in drug-induced extrapyramidal disorders. Arch Gen Psychiatry 1976;33:599–602.

57. Adler LA, Peselow E, Rosenthal M, Angrist A. A controlled comparison of the effects of propranolol, benztropine, and placebo on akathisia: an interim analysis. Psychopharmacol Bull 1993;29:283–286.

58. Gagrat D, Hamilton J, Belmaker RH. Intravenous diazepam and the treatment of neuroleptic-induced acute dystonia and akathisia. Am J Psychiatry 1978;135:1232–1233.

59. Bartels M, Heide K, Mann K, Schied HW. Treatment of akathisia with lorazepam: an open clinical trial. Pharmacopsychiatry 1987;20:51–53.

60. Kutcher SP, Williamson P, MacKenzie S, et al. Successful clonazepam treatment of neuroleptic-induced akathisia in older adolescents and young adults. J Clin Psychopharmacol 1989;9:403–406.

61. Friis T, Christensen TR, Gerlach J. Sodium valproate and biperiden in neuroleptic-induced akathisia, parkinsonism, and hyperkinesia. Acta Psychiatr Scand 1983;67:178–187.

62. Harris JC, Tune LE, Allen M, Coyle JT. Management of akathisia in a severely retarded adolescent male with help of an anticholinergic drug assay. Lancet 1981;2:414.

63. Ekbom KA. Restless legs and akathisia. J Swed Med Assoc 1965;62:2539–2582.

64. Lipinski JF, Zubenko GS, Barriera P, Cohen BM. Propranolol in the treatment of neuroleptic-induced akathisia. Lancet 1983;2:685–686.

65. Lipinski JF, Zubenko GS, Cohen BM, Barriera PJ. Propranolol in the treatment of neuroleptic-induced akathisia. Am J Psychiatry 1984;141:412–415.

66. Adler L, Angrist B, Peselow E, et al. Controlled assessment of propranolol in the treatment of neuroleptic-induced akathisia. Br J Psychiatry 1986;149:42–45.

67. Adler L, Angrist B, Peselow E, et al. Efficacy of propranolol in neuroleptic-induced akathisia. J Clin Psychopharmacol 1985;5:164–166.

68. Zubenko GS, Lipinski JF, Cohen BM, Barriera PJ. Comparison of metoprolol and propranolol in the treatment of akathisia. Psychiatry Res 1984;11:143–149.

69. Reiter S, Adler L, Angrist B, et al. Atenolol and propranolol and neuroleptic-induced akathisia. J Clin Psychopharmacol 1987;7:279–280.

70. Dupuis B, Catteau J, Dumon JP, et al. Comparison of propranolol, sotalol, and betaxolol in the treatment of neuroleptic-induced akathisia. Am J Psychiatry 1987;144:802–805.

71. Ratey JJ, Sorgi P, Polakoff P. Nadolol as a treatment for akathisia. Am J Psychiatry 1985;142:640–642.

72. Zubenko GS, Cohen BM, Lipinski JF, Jonas JM. Use of clonidine in treatment of neuroleptic-induced akathisia. Psychiatry Res 1984;13:253–259.

73. Adler LA, Angrist B, Peselow E, et al. Clonidine in neuroleptic-induced akathisia. Am J Psychiatry 1987;144:235–236.

74. Hening WA, Walters A, Kavey N, et al. Dyskinesias while awake and periodic movements of sleep in restless leg syndrome: treatment with opioids. Neurology 1986;36:1363–1366.

75. Walters A, Henning W, Chokroverty S, Fahn S. Opioid responsiveness in patients with neuroleptic-induced akathisia. Mov Disord 1986;1:119–127.

76. Sovner R, DiMascio A. Extrapyramidal syndromes and other neurological side effects of psychotropic drugs. In: Lipton MA, DiMascio A, Killam KF, eds. New York: Raven, 1978:1021–1032.

77. Gore EM, Hadley FV. Precataleptic restlessness induced in rhesus monkeys with phenothiazines. Fed Proc 1959;18:397.

78. Liebman J, Neale R. Neuroleptic-induced acute dyskinesias in squirrel monkeys: correlation with propensity to cause extrapyramidal side effects. Psychopharmacology 1980;68:25–29.

79. McKinney WT, Moran EC, Kraemer GW, Prange AJ Jr. Long-term chlorpromazine in rhesus monkeys: production of dyskinesias and changes in social behavior. Psychopharmacology 1980;72:35–39.

80. Meldrum BS, Anlazark GM, Marsden CD. Acute dystonia as an idiosyncratic response to neuroleptic drugs in baboons. Brain 1977;100:313–326.

81. Marsden CD, Jenner P. The pathophysiology of extrapyramidal side-effects of neuroleptic drugs. Psychol Med 1980;10:55–72.

82. Iversen S. The effect of surgical lesions to frontal cortex and substantia nigra on amphetamine responses in rats. Brain Res 1971;31:295–311.

83. Carter CJ, Pycock CJ. Studies in the role of catecholamines in frontal cortex. Br J Pharmacol 1978;62:402.

84. Carter CJ, Pycock CJ. Behavioral and biochemical effects of dopamine and noradrenaline depletion with the medial prefrontal cortex of the rat. Brain Res 1980;192:163–176.

85. Le Moal M, Cardo B, Stinus L. Influence of ventral mesencephalic lesions on various spontaneous and conditional behaviors in the rat. Physiol Behav 1969;4:567–574.

86. Tassin JP, Stinus L, Simon H, et al. Relationship between the locomotor hyperactivity induced by A 10 and the destruction of the frontocortical dopaminergic innervation in the rat. Brain Res 1978;141:267–281.

87. Pijnenburg AJJ, Honig WMM, Van der Hayden JAM, et al. Effects of chemical stimulation of the mesolimbic dopamine system upon locomotor activity. Europ J Pharmacol 1976;35:49–58.

88. Bartels M, Gaertner HJ, Golfinopoulos G. Akathisia-syndrome: involvement of noradrenergic mechanisms. J Neurol Transmission 1981;52:33–39.

89. Soni SM, Tench D, Routledge RC. Serum iron abnormalities in neuroleptic-induced akathisia in schizophrenic patients. Br J Psychiatry 1993;163:669–672.

90. Gold R, Lenox RH. Is there a rationale for iron supplementation in the treatment of akathisia? A review of the evidence. J Clin Psychiatry 1995;56:476–483.

Cognitive Akathisia: Clinical and Theoretical Aspects

ROBERT N. RUBEY   GEORGE W. ARANA

INTRODUCTION

Akathisia, which literally translated means "not to sit," has been called the "stepchild of movement disorders and an orphan of psychiatry" (1). Haskovec in 1902 first used the term to describe patients with a compulsion to move and an inability to remain seated, postulated by him to be secondary to anxiety and hysteria (2). In the 1920s, Sicard (3) and Bing (4) applied the term to patients with postencephalitic Parkinson's syndrome and Parkinson's disease who demonstrated similar symptoms, including restlessness and an inability to sit still. Ekbom described a "restless legs syndrome" in unmedicated patients with no clinical apparent psychiatric or neurologic disease who reported a constellation of symptoms including aching and restless legs with a strong desire to move (5,6).

In 1947, Sigwald et al reported the first case of drug-induced akathisia in a patient with Parkinson's disease treated with the phenothiazine promethazine (7). With the introduction of other phenothiazine antipsychotic medications in the early 1950s, reports of cognitive and motor restlessness following the use of these agents became known as neuroleptic-induced akathisia. It has been subsequently recognized that drugs other than neuroleptics may cause akathisia, including the serotonin reuptake inhibitors (SRIs) (8), so that it may be more accurate to refer to drug-induced akathisia (DIA) rather than neuroleptic-induced akathisia when drawing a distinction between the drug-induced and non-drug-induced forms of akathisia.

Although the motor and cognitive aspects of akathisia were recognized and debated, a consensus was never reached as to the importance of each. In the 1970s, reports in the literature indicated that clinicians were becoming increasingly aware of the clinical importance of cognitive akathisia, an unpleasant subjective urge to move, in patients treated with neuroleptics (9,10). The subjective restlessness of cognitive akathisia is now recognized as one of the most common neuroleptic side effects, often sufficiently distressing to the patient to induce medication noncompliance (11). It is essential that our understanding and delineation of the cognitive aspect of akathisia continue to expand.

This presentation will propose a typology for akathisia, which we believe will aid in better delineating the pathophysiology of this syndrome and, with properly designed pharmacologic studies, may help develop improved treatments for this disorder. We will describe the cognitive aspect of akathisia symptoms, briefly reviewing the literature on the distinction between the various descriptions of the syndrome, which has both cognitive and motor components. We will argue that separation of akathisia into pure cognitive akathisia, pure motor akathisia, and mixed akathisia will improve both our understanding of this entity and the therapeutics of this entity.

GENERAL REVIEW OF AKATHISIA

Neuroleptic-induced akathisia was described in the 1950s primarily as an extrapyramidal movement disorder (12). Certain investigators have defined akathisia as the subjective distress that patients experience secondary to neuroleptic therapy, whether it be a "feeling of needing to move" or nonspecific anxiety that was not apparent prior to drug treatment (13,14). In this context, the motor component may or may not be present depending on the patient's degree of inner restlessness (14,15). Certain investigators view both the subjective distress and the behavioral manifestations as essential for the diagnosis of akathisia, but differ on the relative importance of the individual factors (16,17). Moreover, several subtypes of akathisia have been proposed in an attempt to better define the presence or absence of cognitive or motor restlessness and its relationship to antipsychotic drug use (15). The array of symptoms described as components of akathisia, in conjunction with the lack of consensus on diagnostic criteria for akathisia, may have contributed to the wide range in prevalence rates reported, as well as in the efficacy data for medications used to treat the syndrome. Although the prevalence of neuroleptic-induced akathisia is generally considered to be approximately 20%, it has been reported to be from 12.5% to 75% (18,19). In proposing a typology for akathisia, we postulate that restlessness and anxiety-like symptoms induced by the use of antipsychotic medications usually, but not necessarily, consist of both cognitive and motor aspects that manifest variably in specific patients.

The onset and duration of akathisia relative to the initiation or discontinuation of antipsychotic medications varies greatly. This variability in presentation of symptoms (cognitive versus motor), in time on onset of symptoms, and in persistence of symptoms has led researchers in the field to attempt to better define and classify akathisia. Sachdev has proposed a system that describes drug-induced akathisia in terms of onset and chronicity of symptoms (20). For example, symptoms beginning within 6 weeks of initiation of drug therapy and persisting for over 3 months would be classified as chronic DIA, with acute onset. Sachdev acknowledges the lack of agreement over whether *both* cognitive and motor features must be present to make a definitive diagnosis of DIA, and also makes the telling point that the cognitive features of akathisia are often difficult to distinguish from anxiety or agitation. Lang (21) makes note of the difficulty sometimes encountered in distinguishing the mode of onset of akathisia and proposes instead a classification scheme that relies more on "prospective assessment of the patient from the time of first assessment" and that is "largely based on the classification of tardive dyskinesia . . . proposed by Schooler and Kane." Lang concurs with Sachdev that it is often difficult to separate symptoms of drug-induced akathisia from those of the underlying condition being treated.

Acute akathisia has been reported to occur within minutes of initiating or increasing dopamine antagonist compounds (22,23). Akathisia may persist despite reduction or discontinuation of the drug, resulting in chronic or persistent akathisia. Tardive akathisia is a term proposed for patients developing the motor and cognitive aspects of akathisia after chronic antipsychotic drug treatment. As in tardive dyskinesia, tardive akathisia may develop or be exacerbated by reduction or withdrawal of antipsychotic drugs and temporarily improved with increased antipsychotic dosage (24).

Some patients experience motor restlessness without any distressful subjective urge to move. Munetz and Cornes described these patients as having involuntary restlessness of tardive dyskinesia, not akathisia, and used the term pseudoakathisia to describe them (25). Other investigators,

however, defined pseudoakathisia as a variant of akathisia in which there is only motor restlessness without any cognitive restlessness (15).

It is apparent that it is often difficult to distinguish between various forms of akathisia and tardive dyskinesia. It has been proposed that these subtypes of akathisia are associated with or are a variant of tardive dyskinesia (15,16,17,25,26). In addition, there is preliminary evidence that patients with neuroleptic-induced akathisia are at increased risk for developing tardive dyskinesia (27). The lack of consensus regarding the diagnostic criteria for akathisia and the variants described briefly above, as well as the clinical phenomenologic overlap with tardive dyskinesia, serves to make specific pathophysiologically distinct subgroups difficult to understand and even more difficult to investigate systematically. However, the distinction between akathisia and tardive dyskinesia is essential to understanding the natural course of these drug-induced side effects. Further prospective studies of akathisia and its association with or possible emergence into tardive dyskinesia need to be undertaken.

The pharmacologic treatment of akathisia includes anticholinergic and dopaminergic agents, benzodiazepines, α adrenergic agonists, and β blockers, with the β blockers appearing the most promising (28–31). A recent open-label study of 17 patients with akathisia found cyproheptadine to be effective in treating symptoms in 15 of the patients (32). The majority of these reports have focused on the overall effect on akathisia without examining the cognitive and motor aspects separately. Moreover, investigators have used various akathisia rating scales, which vary in how much the cognitive and motor symptoms are weighted. In evaluating cognitive akathisia one needs to examine how the various drug treatments affect cognitive and motor akathisia differentially. Thus, the time course and specificity of therapeutics for those two forms of akathisia will also need to be studied.

COGNITIVE AKATHISIA

Cognitive akathisia has a varied clinical presentation. Patients often describe feelings of inner restlessness and anxiety, have vague somatic complaints, demonstrate strong affects of rage and terror, or even have a worsening of their psychosis without developing restless movements (10,14,33). Akathisia has been associated with dysphoric responses to neuroleptics, resulting in significant noncompliance by patients taking them (14). There have been cases reported of suicidal and homicidal behavior postulated to be secondary to the neuroleptic drugs, although clearly the etiology of this syndrome may be too complicated to determine given the illnesses being treated (34–36).

In discussing cognitive akathisia, there are some specific factors that need to be considered. As noted earlier, the degree of subjective distress may vary from very mild to very severe. Some patients experience inner restlessness and anxiety without any motor manifestations of these feelings and without feeling the desire or need to move. Consequently, the inner restlessness and anxiety would only be appreciated clinically by specifically asking the patients if they feel restless and anxious. On observation, these patients are not moving in a repetitive fashion and would deny that they feel like moving. Another possible presentation of cognitive akathisia is the lack of observable movements accompanied by the desire to move. Patients may also express inner restlessness and feel compelled to move, but may not move because of a concomitant neuroleptic-induced akinesia (i.e., parkinsonism). Furthermore, patients with cognitive restlessness may manifest their motor restlessness in subtle ways, which may not always be clinically apparent. Thus, some patients may express a desire to walk more than usual, may appear more active or involved, or might seem more anxious rather than akathetic. It is obvious that these particular types of cognitive akathisia would be very difficult to separate from anxiety and restlessness due to the psychiatric illnesses for which the patients are being treated.

Sachdev proposes that a "feeling of restlessness or inner tension or discomfort with special reference to the lower limbs" is especially characteristic of akathisia (20). Some investigators feel that cognitive symptoms alone are too nonspecific to make a reliable diagnosis of akathisia (14,15). Patients and clinicians are often unable to distinguish between drug-related inner restlessness and the underlying psychiatric illness being treated, especially if the psychiatric illness has an anxiety-related component. In an attempt to differentiate cognitive akathisia from illness-related symptoms, some investigators have proposed that the cognitive symptoms of akathisia must be relieved, to at least some degree, by antiparkinsonian medication (14). Response to antiparkinsonian medication may prove useful in making the diagnosis of cognitive akathisia, although a misdiagnosis may occur in the patient who has treatment-resistant cognitive akathisia. Rifkin suggested that the best clue to diagnosing cognitive akathisia is the presence of other related extrapyramidal symptoms (37). The presence of extrapyramidal symptoms in addition to restlessness may help the clinician consider cognitive akathisia as a diagnosis. However, not all patients with extrapyramidal symptoms who are restless have cognitive akathisia. In addition, if one suspects a patient may have neuroleptic-induced cognitive akathisia, withdrawal of the drug may help clarify the diagnosis. Although the diagnosis of neuroleptic-induced cognitive akathisia versus illness-related restlessness is difficult, it is critical in determining the appropriate treatment for the patient.

In considering cognitive akathisia (i.e., a feeling of needing to move without evidence of the motor behavior), it is essential that a thorough assessment of inner restlessness, anxiety, and a compulsion to move be completed before initiating any neuroleptic treatment. In any patient manifesting these symptoms as a component of the psychotic illness it would be impossible to delineate drug-induced symptoms from illness-related symptoms and

equally difficult to follow the time course and response to treatment. Therefore, any study of cognitive akathisia needs to be limited to patients who have not been on neuroleptics and are not experiencing symptoms of akathisia as part of their psychotic illness.

One would need to see the emergence of inner restlessness, anxiety, and the compulsion to move before any observable motor behaviorial aspect during the course of neuroleptic treatment in order to argue that the cognitive aspects are a consequence of the drug, separate from the motor component of having to move. This conclusion may also be unwarranted in patients with any mood disorder, particularly rapid-cycling bipolar patients, who may develop anxiety and restlessness as an aspect of their affective disorder. Conversely, in a situation in which a patient clearly has a motor akathisia, it is very difficult to argue about a cognitive akathisia separate from a motor akathisia given that the very experience of having to move by the patient will contaminate the cognitive aspect.

It is conceivable that the emergence of cognitive akathisia over the first week of neuroleptic treatment may actually be the result of a differential response of various psychotic symptoms, such that the anxiety and restlessness continue unabated whereas other psychotic symptoms improve. In other words, the inner restlessness, anxiety, and compulsion to move may have been present throughout the preneuroleptic treatment phase, but were shrouded by other psychotic symptoms. These psychotic symptoms may respond differentially, with the nonakathisia-like symptoms resolving sooner than the akathisia-like symptoms, resulting in the unmasking of the underlying psychotic restlessness. In any event, any study of this cognitive akathisia aspect of neuroleptic treatment needs to be done with careful pretreatment screening.

PROPOSED TYPOLOGY FOR AKATHISIA

It is generally accepted that akathisia usually occurs within the first week of initiation or increase in neuroleptic therapy; however, the range of akathisia onset has been reported to be hours to months (12,16,17,38–41). In addition, it is generally accepted that the cognitive aspects of akathisia precede and later coexist with the motor aspect (16). To date, there has been no study of the time course of cognitive versus motor akathisia in patients who are treated with neuroleptics. Our proposed typology for akathisia includes a cognitive aspect, a motor aspect, and then a mixed akathisia in which both components are clinically apparent. As shown in Figure 12.1, cognitive akathisia may precede or follow motor akathisia, which is consistent with the clinical subtypes previously discussed. Thus, if one assumes a constant neuroleptic level for a fixed period of time to be a point *A* in Figure 12.1, a given patient may manifest symptoms as shown in Figure 12.1a, and another patient may present as in Figure 12.1b. To complicate the issue further, to our knowledge there are no reported data on

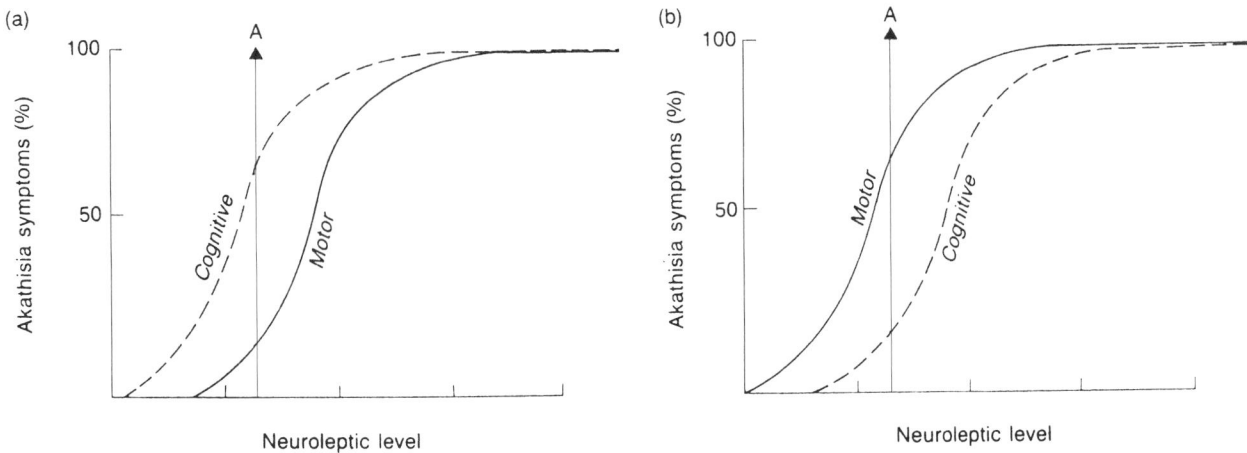

FIGURE 12.1   *A model for differential cognitive and motor symptoms of neuroleptic-induced akathisia. Point A represents constant neuroleptic concentration for a fixed period of time.*

whether different neuroleptics, that is, butyrophenones versus phenothiazines, affect the time course of cognitive and motor akathisia differentially.

Careful studies need to be done in psychotic patients who, prior to study, do not have restlessness, anxiety, or compulsion to move their extremities. These patients, after initiation of neuroleptics, need to be followed closely in order to detect the emergence of cognitive versus motor akathisia. The cognitive akathisia would essentially be the development of anxiety, restlessness, and a compulsion to move without clinically apparent manifestations of movement (Fig. 12.1a). A possible confounding factor in such a study would be the development of neuroleptic-induced parkinsonism, especially akinesia, which may mask motor akathisia. Accordingly, if a patient develops akathisia and parkinsonism concomitantly, it confounds the picture with regard to whether the patient has only cognitive akathisia or mixed akathisia with the motor akathisia symptoms overridden by the parkinsonism (Fig. 12.1b). Therefore, in evaluating these patients longitudinally, parkinsonism symptoms need to be monitored continually. Thus, the ideal cognitive akathisia patient would be the individual who is not manifesting any motor hyperkinesis or parkinsonian symptoms but is complaining of anxiety and restlessness that were not apparent at the onset of the treatment (Fig. 12.1a). The assessment of the differential development of motor versus cognitive akathisia will also be contaminated with the emergence of parkinsonian symptoms.

Once a time course has been established for the onset of cognitive versus motor akathisia, one can begin to look at the differential manifestations of these two forms of akathisia depending on the neuroleptic used. Freedman and DeJong reported that the risk of developing akathisia depended on the individual's sensitivity and the neuroleptic used (41). Other investigators have indicated that the more potent neuroleptics (e.g., haloperidol, trifluoperazine) are associated with a higher frequency of akathisia than less potent neu-

roleptics (e.g., chlorpromazine, thioridazine) (19,42,43). However, we are unaware of any reported data comparing the different effects of the various classes of neuroleptics on cognitive and motor akathisia. This could be accomplished using the same paradigm outlined earlier for studying the time course of cognitive and motor akathisia.

In addition to the time course of the development of motor and cognitive akathisia and the variable development of motor and cognitive akathisia with different neuroleptic agents, illness variables need to be evaluated. Thus, the question arises whether patients with schizophrenia versus psychotic mood illnesses are more or less likely to develop either of these forms of akathisia and whether akathisia medications are likely to treat these various forms of akathisia successfully.

THEORETICAL IMPLICATIONS

The implications of a "pure cognitive akathisia" in which there is clearly no motor restlessness and no extrapyramidal symptoms but clearly a cognitive/affective change with neuroleptics raise the theoretic possibility that the cognitive aspects induced by neuroleptics may be either anatomically or physiologically subserved differently than the motor aspects. If cognitive akathisia is distinct from motor akathisia, it also may prove to be a useful model for evaluating and understanding drug-free, illness-related psychomotor agitation. Marsden and Jenner have suggested that the mesocortical dopaminergic system was involved in the development of akathisia (44). In an attempt to differentiate the pathophysiology of cognitive and motor akathisia, Munetz and Cornes hypothesized that prolonged neuroleptic use may lead to a denervation-like supersensitivity in the mesolimbic system, resulting in cognitive akathisia, and in the nigrostriatal system, resulting in pseudoakathisia (25). However, recent studies demonstrating the effective treatment of patients with both cognitive and motor akathisia with β antagonists (e.g., propranolol) and α agonists (e.g., clonidine) suggest that the etiology of akathisia may result from noradrenergic interaction with the dopaminergic system (30,31,45,46).

FUTURE DIRECTIONS OF RESEARCH ON COGNITIVE AKATHISIA

To our knowledge there are no studies of patients with pure cognitive akathisia without motor akathisia. Although there are many inherent difficulties in clinically assessing pure cognitive akathisia, carefully designed studies of cognitive akathisia would help in elucidating the pathophysiology of cognitive akathisia and thus possibly the pathophysiology of illness-related psychomotor agitation in non-neuroleptic-induced cases. A particularly useful paradigm would be a double-blind placebo-controlled study of patients with pure cognitive akathisia comparing the β antagonist propranolol and the anticholinergic agent benztropine. The data from such a study would help elucidate which neuronal systems were more involved with cognitive akathisia. If the majority of patients responded to the β antagonist, that would be additional evidence of noradrenergic involvement; conversely, a majority response to the benztropine would imply involvement of the cholinergic and dopaminergic system. To further investigate the pathophysiology of cognitive akathisia, one would substitute various drugs in the above paradigm to evaluate other receptor systems, such as benzodiazepines to investigate the benzodiazepine/γ-aminobutyric acid complex and its effect on cognitive akathisia. Such studies would help determine if cognitive akathisia is a separate definable pathophysiologic entity from motor and mixed akathisia, and, if it is, may have implications for our understanding of the mechanism of psychiatric illness-related psychomotor agitation.

REFERENCES

1. Stahl SM. Akathisia variants and tardive dyskinesia [letter]. Arch Gen Psychiatry 1986;43:915–917.
2. Haskovec L. Akathisia. Arch Bohemes Med Clin 1902;3:193–200.
3. Sicard JA. Akathisia and tasikinesia. Presse Med 1923;31:265–266.
4. Bing R. Ueber einige Bemerkenswerte Beleiterscheinungen der "Extrepyramidalen Rigiditat" (Akathisia—Mikrographie—Kinesia Paradox). Schweiz Med Wochenschr 1923;4:167–171.
5. Ekbom KA. Asthenia crurum parathestica (irritable legs). Acta Med Scand 1944;118:197.
6. Ekbom KA. Restless legs syndrome. Neurology 1960;10:868–873.
7. Sigwald J, Grossiord A, Duriel P, Dumont G. Le traitement de la maladie de Parkinson et des manifestations extrepyramidales par le diethylaminoethyl n-thiophyenylamine (2987 RP): resultats d'une anee d'application. Rev Neurol 1947;79:683–687.
8. Lipinski JR Jr, Mallya A, Zimmerman P, et al. Fluoxetine-induced akathisia: clinical and theoretical implications. J Clin Psychiatry 1989;50:339–342.
9. Raskin D. Akathisia: a side effect to be remembered. Am J Psychiatry 1972;129:345–347.
10. Van Putten T. The many faces of akathisia. Compr Psychiatry 1975;16:43–47.
11. Van Putten T. Why do schizophrenic patients refuse to take their drugs? Arch Gen Psychiatry 1974;31:67–72.
12. Ayd FJ. A survey of drug-induced extrapyramidal reactions. JAMA 1961;175:1054–1060.
13. Crane GE, Naranjo ER. Motor disorders induced by neuroleptics. Arch Gen Psychiatry 1971;24:179–184.
14. Van Putten T, Marder SR. Behavioral toxicity of antipsychotic drugs. J Clin Psychiatry 1987;48(suppl 9):13–19.
15. Barnes TRE, Braude WM. Akathisia variants and tardive dyskinesia. Arch Gen Psychiatry 1985;42:874–878.
16. Stahl SM. Akathisia and tardive dyskinesia. Arch Gen Psychiatry 1985;42:915–917.
17. Gibb WRG, Lees AJ. The clinical phenomenon of akathisia. J Neurol Neurosurg Psychiatry 1986;49:881–886.
18. Freyhan FA. Extrapyramidal symptoms and other side effects in trifluoperazine—clinical and pharmacological aspects. Philadelphia: Lea & Febiger, 1958.
19. Van Putten T, May PRA, Marder SR. Akathisia with haloperidol and thiothixene. Arch Gen Psychiatry 1984;41:1036–1039.
20. Sachdev P, Loneragan C. Research diagnostic criteria for drug-induced akathisia: conceptualization, rationale, and proposal. Psychopharmacology 1994;114:181–186.
21. Lang A. Withdrawal akathisia: case reports and a proposed classification of chronic akathisia. Mov Disord 1994;9:188–192.
22. Barnes TRE, Braude WM, Hill DJ. Acute akathisia after oral droperidol and metaclopramide preoperative medication. Lancet 1982;ii:48–49.
23. Jungman E, Schoffling K. Akathisia and metaclopramide. Lancet 1982;ii:221.
24. Braude WM, Barnes TRE. Late-onset akathisia: an indicant of covert dyskinesia: two case reports. Am J Psychiatry 1983;140:611–612.
25. Munetz MR, Cornes CL. Akathisia, pseudoakathisia and tardive dyskinesia: clinical examples. Compr Psychiatry 1982;23:345–352.
26. Munetz MR, Cornes CL. Distinguishing akathisia and tardive dyskinesia: a review of the literature. J Clin Psychopharmacol 1983;3:343–350.
27. Barnes TRE, Braude WM. Persistent akathisia associated with early tardive dyskinesia. Postgrad Med J 1984;60:51–53.
28. Gelenberg AJ. General principles of treatment of extrapyramidal syndromes. Clin Neuropharmacol 1983;6(suppl 1):S52–S56.
29. DiMascio A, Bernardo DL, Greenblatt DJ, Marder JE. A controlled trial of amantadine in drug-induced extrapyramidal disorders. Arch Gen Psychiatry 1976;33:599–602.
30. Lipinski JF, Zubenko GS, Cohen BM, Barreira PJ. Propranolol in the treatment of neuroleptic-induced akathisia. Am J Psychiatry 1984;141:412–415.
31. Adler LA, Angrist B, Peselow E, Corwin J, Malansky R, Rotrosen J. A controlled assessment of propranolol in the treatment of neuroleptic-induced akathisia. Br J Psychiatry 1986;149:42–45.
32. Weiss D, Aizenberg D, Hermesh H, et al. Cyproheptadine treatment in neuroleptic induced akathisia. Br J Psychiatry 1995;167:483–486.
33. Van Putten T, Mutalipassi LR, Malkin MD. Phenothiazine induced decompensation. Arch Gen Psychiatry 1974;30:102–105.
34. Drake RE, Ehrlich J. Suicide attempts associated with akathisia. Am J Psychiatry 1985;142:499–501.
35. Schulte JR. Homicide and suicide associated with akathisia and haloperidol. Am J Forensic Psychiatry 1985;6:3–7.
36. Shaw ED, Mann JJ, Weider PJ, et al. A case of suicidal and homicidal ideation and akathisia in a double-blind neuroleptic crossover study [letter]. J Clin Psychopharmacol 1986;6:196–197.
37. Rifkin A. Extrapyramidal side effects: a historical perspective. J Clin Psychiatry 1987;48(suppl 9):3–6.
38. Kendler KS. A medical student's experience with akathisia. Am J Psychiatry 1976;133:454–455.
39. Tarsey D. Movement disorders with neuroleptic drug treatment. Psychiatr Clin North Am 1984;7:453–471.
40. Akathisia and antipsychotic drugs [editorial]. Lancet 1986;ii:1131–1132.
41. Freedman DX, DeJong J. Factors that determine drug-induced akathisia. Dis Nerv Syst 1961;22:69–76.
42. Marsden CD, Tarsey D, Baldessarini RJ. Spontaneous and drug induced movements in psychotic patients. In: Benson DF, Blymer D, eds. Psychiatric Aspects of Neurologic Disease. New York: Grune & Stratton, 1975.
43. Szabadi E. Akathisia: a distressing complication of neuroleptic treatment. Compr Ther 1986;13:3–6.
44. Marsden C, Jenner P. The pathophysiology of extrapyramidal side effects of neurologic drugs. Psychol Med 1980;10:55–72.
45. Adler LA, Angriest B, Peselow E, Reitano J, Rotrosen J. Clonidine in neuroleptic-induced akathisia. Am J Psychiatry 1987;144:235–236.
46. Gelenberg AJ. Treating extrapyramidal reactions: some current issues. J Clin Psychiatry 1987;48(suppl 9):24–27.

Acute Neuroleptic-Induced Dystonia

Daniel E. Casey

HISTORICAL INTRODUCTION

Neuroleptic antipsychotic drugs have been associated with acute extrapyramidal motor syndromes (EPS) since these drugs were introduced into clinical practice in the 1950s. It was once thought that antipsychotic and motor side effects were inextricably linked. This perspective is now widely recognized to be incorrect because these two separate effects involve distinct brain regions. The antipsychotic effects are hypothesized to occur in the limbic or prefrontal cortex, whereas the motor side effects implicate the basal ganglia. However, the therapeutic index for neuroleptic drugs is very narrow because the doses required for antipsychotic effects very often produce motor symptoms (1).

The changing patterns of neuroleptic use over the past four decades have produced striking increases in the prevalence of acute extrapyramidal symptoms, particularly the acute dystonic syndrome. The first neuroleptics, reserpine and sparine, were low potency, slow-acting agents that only occasionally produced acute dystonia. In the early 1960s a survey of all extrapyramidal syndromes noted a 2.3% rate of acute dystonia (2). [Historical note: At that time acute dystonia was also called acute dyskinesia or dyskinesia because tardive dyskinesia was not labeled as such until 1964 (3).] The gradual increase in the use of high-potency neuroleptics, such as haloperidol, and the use of higher drug dosages have led to much higher rates of acute dystonia. In contrast to the 2.3% rate in 1961, a survey in 1980 observed a 39% prevalence rate (4). A later study of high-risk (young, male) patients treated with high-potency neuroleptics reported acute dystonia in over 90% of the patients (5).

DIAGNOSIS

Clinical Description

Acute dystonia is a syndrome of briefly sustained or fixed abnormal posture(s) caused by involuntary muscular contraction. It includes symptoms of torticollis, trismus, oculogyric crises, laryngeal-pharyngeal constriction, tongue protrusion, or bizarre positions of the limbs and trunk. Occasionally when the mouth or pharynx is involved it is difficult to observe the abnormal muscular contractions, and the diagnosis must rely on the patient's complaint of difficulty swallowing, throat tightening, or thickness in the tongue.

Risk Factors

Several different risk factors play an important role in determining vulnerability to acute dystonia. These are generally categorized as patient characteristics, drug factors, and temporal aspects.

Patient Characteristics

Age is the most important risk factor in acute neuroleptic-induced dystonia. Children and young adults are highly vulnerable to acute dystonia, whereas there is a virtual absence of this syndrome in the elderly. Gender also plays an important role, as males are nearly twice as susceptible to acute dystonia as females. This contrasts with the increased risk in females for tardive dyskinesia (6). Prior dystonic reactions to neuroleptics are potent predictors of future vulnerability to these symptoms when reexposure to the same drug dose and type occurs (7).

Drug Factors

Neuroleptic drug characteristics also strongly influence acute dystonia rates. The association with dosage is complicated. There is an inverted U-shaped curve function between the prevalence of dystonia and neuroleptic dosage. Most acute dystonia occurs with moderate to high doses of neuroleptics; there is a decrease in the prevalence when megadoses (over approximately 2000 mg/day of chlorpromazine equivalence) are used. Thus, the very low doses and the very high doses of neuroleptics produce less dystonia (4,7).

Drug potency is positively correlated with dystonia. The low-milligram, high-potency compounds (e.g., haloperidol, fluphenazine) produce high rates of dystonia, whereas the high-milligram low-potency compounds (e.g., thioridazine, chlorpromazine) produce much lower rates (4,8). The relative balance of dopamine receptor blocking and anticholinergic properties intrinsic to each neuroleptic drug also correlates with both its milligram potency and propensity to produce EPS (8).

This receptor-blocking ratio has been proposed as an explanation of why clozapine (which has a low dopamine-acetylcholine antagonism ratio) has an exceptionally low rate of acute EPS. However, other factors have been suggested as an explanation of clozapine's special acute extrapyramidal syndrome profile (9). Serotonin-dopamine antagonists also have low EPS rates, including dystonia, at doses that have antipsychotic efficacy (10–12). It has been hypothesized that blockade of serotonin type 2 receptors may be a mechanism for mitigating EPS (13). However, further research is necessary to clarify this issue because these drugs also antagonize several other neurotransmitter receptor subtypes.

Temporal Aspects

Time since last neuroleptic exposure is an essential aspect of understanding acute dystonia. The vast majority of cases (greater than 95%) occur within the first 5 days of starting or rapidly increasing neuroleptic doses (2,4). Only rarely is acute dystonia seen after this time. If such symptoms do occur, this should lead one to consider that the patient has taken a larger neuroleptic dose than prescribed, combined his or her neuroleptic with other neuroleptics or alcohol, has not been taking anti-EPS medicines, or may have a separate underlying medical disorder.

Differential Diagnosis

For a diagnosis of acute neuroleptic drug-induced dystonia to be valid, the patient must have been exposed to neuroleptic drugs within the past few days. Sometimes this is not known, so other diagnoses must be considered. Psychiatric syndromes of hysteria or malingering are part of the differential diagnosis, though they do not commonly occur. It is best to give the patient the benefit of the doubt and consider neuroleptic drug-induced acute dystonia as the cause of abnormal postures or complaints of muscular con-

tractions in the mouth or throat region if there is any reason to believe the patient has had access or exposure to neuroleptics in the prior 5 days (14).

Neurologic or endocrinologic (hyperthyroidism) diseases may also produce dystonia. Occasionally, temporal lobe seizures produce bizarre behavior as well as peculiar posture. Central nervous system viral or bacterial infections, as well as trauma or space-occupying lesions, are rare causes of acute dystonia.

Other drugs besides those typically used to treat schizophrenia can cause acute dystonia. Any compound with dopamine receptor blockade properties has the potential to cause dystonia, particularly in the high-risk patient. Some antiemetic agents, such as prochlorperazine (Compazine), are well known for their dystonia-producing ability. This is particularly common in children. Metoclopramide (Reglan), a dopamine antagonist that is widely used for diabetic gastroparesis, can cause acute dystonia as well as the other extrapyramidal syndromes of akathisia, drug-induced parkinsonism, or tardive dyskinesia (15). Drug overdoses such as those with phenytoin can also produce dystonic postures that are part of a much broader clinical picture of neurologic dysfunction.

Finally, other uncommon idiopathic neurologic syndromes may have dystonia as a component. These include focal or regional dystonias such as torticollis, oromandibular dystonia, or blepharospasm. They are usually easily distinguished from drug-induced dystonia by the absence of neuroleptics and the slow onset of weeks to months.

MANAGEMENT

Prophylaxis

Considerable controversy surrounds the issue of prophylaxis with anti-EPS medicines to prevent the onset of acute dystonia and other extrapyramidal syndromes. Proponents of prophylaxis argue that dystonic episodes can be dangerous, such as laryngeal-pharyngeal dystonia. Opponents of prophylaxis argue that the anti-EPS medicines have their own side effects as drawbacks, such as memory impairment, blurred vision, and dry mouth. As expected, both sides of the controversy contend that their approach is the best method for achieving the maximum benefit with the minimum side effects, thus fostering a therapeutic alliance with the patient that encourages treatment compliance.

Prophylaxis is highly appropriate when there is a high risk of EPS, predisposition to EPS, and detrimental sequelae, such as paranoid patients believing external forces are controlling them. A review of the studies examining the effectiveness of initial anti-EPS prophylaxis indicates that it is clearly efficacious (1). Several studies (two prospective and three retrospective) found a statistically significant benefit. On the other hand, if there is a low likelihood of EPS, treatment with only a neuroleptic drug and no anti-EPS agent until extrapyramidal syndromes develop is the pre-ferred strategy because the risk of undesirable side effects from anti-EPS agents outweighs the limited potential benefit of prophylaxis.

An informed judgment about whether to use anti-EPS prophylaxis is best made by considering patient characteris-tics (age, sex, prior EPS), drug properties (milligram potency, dosage, intrinsic anticholinergic activity), and temporal aspects when drug treatment is initiated (1,4). If initial pro-phylaxis is used for acute dystonia, it is recommended that the anti-EPS agent is slowly tapered after the first week of treatment since acute dystonia rarely occurs beyond the fifth day of neuroleptic therapy. It is important to slowly taper the anti-EPS drugs because sudden discontinuation may cause a rebound acute dystonic reaction.

Treatment

Treating acute dystonic reactions is less controversial. Parenteral or oral administration of anticholinergics (e.g., benztropine [Cogentin], biperidine [Akineton]) or an antihistaminic (e.g., diphenhydramine [Benadryl]) is so uniformly effective in reversing acute dystonia that a failure to improve after one to three doses over a few hours should stimulate the search for other uncommon causes of dysto-nia associated with underlying medical illnesses. Only in rare situations may it be necessary to try a parenteral benzodi-azepine after the anticholinergic agents have failed.

BASIC SCIENCE

Although neuroleptic drugs have been used for more than 35 years, little is known about the pathophysiology of acute dystonia. It is tempting to speculate that acute dystonia is due to the onset of dopamine receptor blockade that occurs within a few hours of starting neuroleptics. However, most dystonic reactions do not occur until several hours to a few days after initiating neuroleptic therapy, and these reactions often occur during the time of falling rather than rising neuroleptic blood levels (16).

This discrepancy between blood level and acute dysto-nia time course is central to the conflicting theories of whether acute dystonia is due to *increased* or *decreased* stri-atal dopamine neurotransmission. Increased dopamine syn-thesis and release provoked by the compensatory dopamine feedback system after acute neuroleptic administration has been proposed as the underlying pathophysiology of dysto-nia (17,18). Evidence for this increased striatal dopamine activity hypothesis includes the observation that levodopa can cause dyskinesias resembling acute dystonia in idiopathic parkinsonian patients and in lesioned monkeys receiving large parenteral doses (19,20). Direct intrastriatal application of dopamine can also cause acute dystonia in monkeys (21). These data have contributed to the "mismatch" hypothesis of neuroleptic-induced acute dystonia, which proposes that the compensatory increased dopamine release associated

with neuroleptic therapy overrides dopamine receptor blockade as neuroleptic levels in the blood and brain decline. Against this hypothesis is the observation that dopamine agonists such as amphetamine, apomorphine, and levodopa can have therapeutic benefits in neuroleptic-induced acute dystonia.

In contrast, the hypothesis of decreased striatal dopamine function as the neurochemical basis of neuroleptic drug-induced acute dystonia comes from the observation that neuroleptics block dopamine receptors in close correlation to their clinical potency in humans and pharmacologic activities in animals (22,23). Further evidence for this hypothesis comes from studies examining dopamine func-tion in nonhuman primates. Pretreatment with dopamine synthesis inhibitors or depleters exacerbated haloperidol-induced acute dystonia (24,25). The beneficial effects of dopamine agonists in the clinic also support this hypothe-sis. Further evidence is the observation that pargyline, a monoamine oxidase inhibitor, also reduced acute dystonia in monkeys (26).

Other neurotransmitters, particularly serotonin, have been proposed as playing a role in acute dystonia and EPS. Sero-tonin prevents catalepsy in rodents (27), but the effects in nonhuman primates and patients have only received minimal investigation. In one study, serotonin antagonism modestly reduced dystonia (28), but another investigation noted no effect (29), perhaps because only two minimal doses were used. Newly developed drugs with widely varying degrees of serotonin and dopamine antagonism have also been studied and found to have variable liability for dystonia in monkeys (30,31). For example, haloperidol and risperidone have very different ratios of dopamine-serotonin antagonism, but have similar EPS liability when doses of 10 mg/day or more are used (10). The advantage of risperi-done is that it has antipsychotic efficacy at doses of 6 mg/day or less, whereas the benefits of haloperidol in this dose range remain to be fully elucidated. Other compounds with relatively high ratios of serotonin-dopamine antago-nism and low EPS at effective antipsychotic doses include clozapine, olanzapine, and sertindole. Thus, these novel com-pounds with low EPS may owe their unique profile, at least in part, to the better antipsychotic efficacy as well as lower EPS liability from serotonin receptor subtype 2 antagonism (13).

In summary, acute dystonia is an increasingly prevalent side effect of antipsychotic drug therapy as more potent neuroleptics are being used at moderate to high dosages. Symptoms usually occur within the first 5 days of starting neuroleptic therapy in patients at high risk. Differential diagnoses include the psychiatric syndromes of hysteria or malingering, neurologic syndromes of seizures, central nervous system infections, trauma, idiopathic dystonic syn-dromes, and endocrinopathies. Additionally, other drug causes of acute dystonia must be considered. Managing acute dystonia includes considering the strategy of prophylaxis with anti-EPS medicines. This is best decided after a careful consideration of patient characteristics (age, sex, prior EPS), drug factors (dose, milligram potency, anticholinergic activity), and temporal aspects. Treating acute dystonia is almost always effective with parenteral anti-EPS medicines. The underlying pathophysiology of acute dystonia is unknown. Two conflicting theories of either increased or decreased striatal dopamine function have been proposed. There is a renewed interest in understanding acute dystonia, as well as the other acute extrapyramidal syndromes, because it is recognized that elucidating the pathophysiology of these disorders will lead to the possibility of developing new antipsychotic drugs that are free of acute extrapyramidal syndromes.

ACKNOWLEDGMENTS

This work was supported in part by funds from the Veterans Affairs Research Program, NIMH grant MH 36657, and core grant RP00163. The typescript was prepared by Crystal Berger.

REFERENCES

1. Casey DE, Keepers GA. Neuroleptic side effects: acute extrapyramidal syndromes and tardive dyskinesia. In: Casey DE, Vibeke Christensen A, eds. Psychopharmacology: current trends. Berlin: Springer-Verlag, 1988:74–93.
2. Ayd FJ. A survey of drug-induced extrapyramidal reactions. JAMA 1961;75:1054–1060.
3. Faurbye A, Rasch PJ, Bender Peterson P, et al. Neurologic symptoms in the pharmacotherapy of psychoses. Acta Psychiatr Scand 1964;40:10–26.
4. Keepers GA, Clappison VJ, Casey DE. Initial anticholinergic prophylaxis for neuroleptic-induced extrapyramidal syndromes. Arch Gen Psychiatry 1983;40:1113–1117.
5. Boyer WF, Bakalar NH, Lake CR. Anticholinergic prophylaxis of acute haloperidol-induced dystonic reactions. J Clin Psychopharmacol 1987;7:164–166.
6. Casey DE. Tardive dyskinesia. In: Meltzer HY, ed. Psychopharmacology: the third generation of progress. New York: Raven, 1987:1411–1419.
7. Keepers GA, Casey DE. Prediction of neuroleptic-induced dystonia. J Clin Psychopharmacol 1986;7:342–344.
8. Snyder S, Greenberg D, Yamamura H. Antischizophrenic drugs and brain cholinergic receptors. Arch Gen Psychiatry 1974;31:58–61.
9. Casey DE. Clozapine: neuroleptic-induced EPS and TD. Psychopharmacology 1989;99:S47–S53.
10. Marder SR, Meibach RC. Risperidone in the treatment of schizophrenia. Am J Psychiatry 1994;151(6):825–835.
11. Beasley CM, Sanger T, Satterlee W, et al. Olanzapine versus placebo: results of a double blind, fixed-dose olanzapine trial. Psychopharmacology 1996;124:159–167.
12. van Kammen DP, McEvoy JP, Targum SD, et al. A randomized, controlled, dose-ranging trial of sertindole in patients with schizophrenia. Psychopharmacology 1996;124:168–175.
13. Meltzer HY, Matsubara S, Lee JC. Classification of typical and atypical antipsychotic drugs on the basis of dopamine D-1, D-2 and serotonin pKi values. J Pharmacol Exp Ther 1989;251:238–246.
14. Casey DE. The differential diagnosis of tardive dyskinesia. Acta Psychiatr Scand 1981;63(suppl 291):71–87.
15. Casey DE. Metoclopramide side effects. Ann Int Med 1983;98:673–674.
16. Garver DL, Davis JM, Dekirmenjian H, et al. Dystonic reactions following neuroleptics: time course and proposed mechanisms. Psychopharmacology 1976;47:199–201.
17. Marsden CD, Jenner P. The pathophysiology of extrapyramidal side-effects of neuroleptic drugs. Psychol Med 1980;10:55–72.
18. Kolbe H, Clow A, Jenner P, Marsden CD. Neuroleptic-induced acute dystonic reactions may be due to enhanced dopamine release onto supersensitive postsynaptic receptors. Neurology 1981;31:434–439.
19. Sassin JF. Drug-induced dyskinesia in monkeys. In: Meldrum BS, Marsden CD, eds. Primate models of neurological disorders: advances in neurology, vol. 10. New York, Raven Press, pp 47–54.
20. Parkes JD, Bedard P, Marsden CD. Chorea and torsion in parkinsonism. Lancet 1976:155.
21. Cools AR, Hendricks G, Korten J. The acetylcholine-dopamine balance in the basal ganglia of rhesus monkeys and its role in dynamic, dystonic, dyskinetic, and epileptoid motor activities. J Neural Transm 1974;36:91–105.
22. Creese I, Burt DR, Snyder SH. Dopamine receptor binding predicts clinical and pharmacological potencies of antischizophrenic drugs. Science 1976;192:481–483.
23. Liebman J, Neale R. Neuroleptic-induced acute dyskinesias in squirrel monkeys: correlation with propensity to cause extrapyramidal side effects. Psychopharmacology 1980;68:25–29.
24. Casey DE, Gerlach J, Christensson E. Dopamine, acetylcholine, and GABA effects in acute dystonia in primates. Psychopharmacology 1980;70:83–87.
25. Neale R, Gerhardt S, Liebman J. Effects of dopamine agonists, catecholamine depletors, and cholinergics and GABAergic drugs on acute dyskinesias in squirrel monkeys. Psychopharmacology 1984;82:20–26.
26. Heintz R, Casey DE. Pargyline reduces/prevents neuroleptic-induced parkinsonism in older schizophrenics. Biol Psychiatry 1987;93:207–213.
27. Balsara JJ, Jadhav JH, Chandorkar AC. Effects of drugs influencing central serotonergic mechanisms on haloperidol-induced catalepsy. Psychopharmacology 1979;62:687–690.
28. Korsgaard S, Gerlach J, Christensson E. Behavioral aspects of serotonin-dopamine interaction in the monkey. Eur J Pharmacol 1985;118:245–252.
29. Povlsen UJ, Noring U, Laursen AL, Korsgaard S, Gerlach J. The effects of serotonergic and anticholinergic drugs in haloperidol-induced dystonia in cebus monkeys. Clin Neuropsychol Pharmacol 1986;9(1):84–90.
30. Casey DE. Serotonergic aspects of acute extrapyramidal syndromes in nonhuman primates. Psychopharmacology Bull 1989;25(3):457–459.
31. Casey DE. Behavioral effects of sertindole, risperidone, clozapine and haloperidol in cebus monkeys. Psychopharmacology 1996;124:134–140.

Oculogyric Crisis

Sheldon Benjamin

I lift up mine eyes unto the mountains from whence my help cometh. ★

HISTORY

Among the neuropsychiatric lessons of the encephalitis lethargica (Von Economo's encephalitis) epidemic of 1916–1927 was the concept of linkage of disorders of motion and disorders of emotion. Much of what is known about oculogyric crisis (OGC), or acute extraocular muscle spasm, stems from experience gained in the wake of that epidemic.

Encephalitis Lethargica

Encephalitis lethargica typically presented with a flu-like prodrome and signs of brainstem encephalitis, including rigidity, akinesia, hypersomnolence, and cranial nerve abnormalities, especially of the eyes. Ophthalmoplegia, ptosis, and abnormal pupillary responses were common. Von Economo enumerated many other presentations as well, including a form in which the onset included hyperkinesia and insomnia (5). Many patients presented with psychiatric symptoms or parkinsonism, having had an occult initial infection. As did most neuropsychiatric sequelae, recurrent OGC tended to emerge when the acute phase of the illness was subsiding. In the chronic phase, up to 30% of patients developed postencephalitic parkinsonism.

In 1921 Oeckinghaus (6) published the first case report this century of postencephalitic OGC, that of a 15-year-old girl who developed forced upward eye deviation and euphoria 1 month after awakening from the acute hypersomnolent phase of encephalitis lethargica. OGC was known then in the German literature as *Blickkrampf* or *Schauanfälle* (7). The first American case, that of a streetcar conductor who was fired from his job "because, while on duty, his eyes turned up, and he could not get them down," was reported by Hohman (7). Jelliffe (1–4) reviewed over 200 cases of postencephalitic OGC that had been reported in the literature in the ensuing 10 years. He regarded OGC as a compulsive tic whose origin could best be understood through psychoanalysis. Jelliffe's monograph (2) was attacked in the pages of *Psychoanalytic Quarterly* (8) for its lack of consideration of the heterogeneity of OGC and for its emphasis on symptom content rather than form. Jelliffe offered the quotation with which this chapter begins as an interpretation of the guilt/punishment theme in the analysis of a young girl with the syndrome.

At least three types of crises occurred during the chronic phase of encephalitis lethargica: oculogyric crisis, autonomic crisis (primarily sweating), and respiratory crisis (usually breath holding). There was no agreement among clinicians as to the prevalence of OGC in chronic encephalitis lethargica, though it was regarded as the most common of the three types of crises. OGC prevalence figures ranged from 1% to 30% (9,10). The attacks tended to occur almost exclusively in those postencephalitic patients who went on to develop parkinsonism (11). The coexistence of parkinsonism and oculogyric crisis was considered pathognomonic for postencephalitic parkinsonism when trying to differentiate it from the idiopathic variety.

Postencephalitic OGC tended to be recurrent. Attacks lasted from seconds to hours and occurred most often in the afternoons and evenings. In some patients, OGC occurred predictably at regular intervals. The eyes would

---

★ Quotation from Psalm 121 offered by a patient of the author's as part of an explanation for his repeated oculogyric crises. This same verse was quoted in one of Smith Ely Jelliffe's 1929 case reports as evidence of underlying guilt in a young girl with postencephalitic oculogyric crisis (1–4).

deviate upward, or upward and laterally, though they would occasionally be directed downward or in fixed convergence spasm. Vertical nystagmus often occurred during the initial upward eye movements. Once the OGC was fully developed, the eyes would remain tonically deviated at the extreme of gaze. The patient would be unable to voluntarily move the eyes to normal position, except very briefly with tremendous effort. Some patients could briefly suppress the movements by forced eye closure. The condition was usually painless, though it seldom occurred in isolation. Table 14.1 lists the associated symptoms that were often reported.

In many patients who suffered from stereotypic paroxysmal psychiatric symptoms during their oculogyric crises, the disappearance of psychiatric symptoms at the conclusion of a crisis and the absence of those symptoms between crises were striking. Schwab et al divided the associated paroxysmal psychiatric symptoms into eight subtypes: anxiety attacks; attacks of compulsive thinking, counting, and word use; paroxysmal depression; paranoid attacks; attacks of strange feeling in the limbs; schizoid reactions (depersonalization); states of severe agitation and tension (similar to akathisia); and fatigue states (12).

In patients with recurrent OGC, individual attacks could be precipitated by fatigue, emotional stress, or suggestion. McCowan and Cook reported a patient whose attacks could be precipitated by revolving while waltzing (13). Other known precipitants included prolonged voluntary visual fixation, bright light, being reminded of prior psychic trauma, or withdrawal from sedative injections. In most cases, however, no precipitants were known.

A prodrome was often described. This could be irritability, depression, suicidal thoughts, or compulsive thoughts for hours to days preceding the attack, or a feeling of anxiety, panic, or fear just before the attack. Onuaguluchi (9)

reported that all patients had a preoccupied staring expression with or without nystagmus just prior to their ocular movements. Some patients were lethargic or somnolent after their crises had concluded, whereas others found their crises could be terminated by sleep.

Treatments commonly tried for postencephalitic OGC included hyoscine (scopolamine) hydrobromide, sodium phenobarbitone (14), stramonium, atropine, and amphetamines. Amphetamines often completely abolished the oculogyric crises, but only slightly improved the parkinsonian symptoms (15,16).

In his book *Awakenings*, Oliver Sacks described the tragedy of postencephalitic parkinsonism and the great hope that accompanied the advent of L-dopa therapy (17). In addition to a dramatic increase in mobility, oculogyric crises were decreased or eliminated. However, after a brief honeymoon period, L-dopa toxicity often resulted in rebound OGC even worse than the patient had had originally. In a series of 25 postencephalitic patients treated with L-dopa, all 5 with severe OGC had remissions lasting from 2 weeks to 5 months. They then developed a toxic reaction and their OGC recurred in a crescendo fashion until it was much worse than it had been before treatment. One patient without preexisting OGC developed it during L-dopa treatment. Several patients developed OGC "status" until the dose of L-dopa was lowered (18). Many of these patients walked a tightrope between akinesia and OGC without L-dopa and dyskinesias, OGC status, and mental status deterioration with L-dopa (17).

Oculogyric Crisis in the Pre–Encephalitis Lethargica Era

Although the literature on oculogyric crisis in the preneuroleptic era derives largely from the encephalitis lethargica experience, OGC-like ocular movements had long been known to occur. In Raphael's sixteenth-century painting *Transfiguration*, a conjugate upward eye deviation was depicted in what the painter felt was an epileptic. Medical historians have documented European epidemics in previous centuries that strongly resembled the encephalitis lethargica epidemic (19). The "Schlafkrankheit" of 1580, the "febris comatosa" that swept London from 1672–1675, the Tubingen "catarrhal fever" of 1712–1713, and the "Italian Nona" of 1889–1890 are some examples (19,20).

In his 1695 pamphlet *De Febre Lethargica in Strabismus Utrisque Oculi Desinente* (Fig. 14.1), Johann Peter Albrecht of Hildesheim described a 20-year-old woman who developed a febrile illness associated with headache and hypersomnolence, followed by fixed upward eye deviation after recovery from the acute phase (2). Jelliffe (2) cited reports of OGC-like movements in syphilis, multiple sclerosis, epilepsy, Parkinson's disease, and various brain tumors before the era of Von Economo's encephalitis.

Table 14.1   Signs and Symptoms Reported During Postencephalitic Oculogyric Crisis

Synchronous turning of head and eyes in same direction	Headache
	Ocular pain
Torsion of trunk and limbs	Vertigo
Retrocollis	Helplessness
Mutism	Anxiety attacks
Palilalia	Compulsive thinking, counting, word use
Inability to close eyes	
Eye blinking	Paroxysmal depression
Jaw spasms	Recurrent fixed ideas
Conjunctival congestion	Paranoia
Lacrimation	Strange feelings in the limbs
Pupillary dilatation	Depersonalization
Sialorrhea	Fugue states
Respiratory dyskinesia	Psychomotor excitement
Increased blood pressure and heart rate	Violence
Facial flushing	Obscene language

CLINICAL FEATURES

Today, OGC usually occurs as a side effect of antipsychotic drug treatment. It is one of the acute dystonic reactions, the earliest occurring of the three major categories of acute neuroleptic side effects: acute dystonic reactions, akathisia, and neuroleptic-induced parkinsonism.

Dystonias are hyperkinetic movement disorders characterized by sustained and twisting involuntary movements. They can be classified several ways, including by etiology and by distribution (21). Primary dystonia refers to the idiopathic or hereditary torsion dystonias, whereas secondary dystonia refers to dystonias associated with other conditions. OGC is a secondary or symptomatic dystonia that can be classified as a focal dystonia when it occurs in isolation, or as a segmental dystonia when there are other associated facial and neck movements.

Although they can occur at any time in the course of neuroleptic treatment, dystonic reactions typically occur in the 72 hours following initiation of treatment, following an abrupt increment in antipsychotic dosage or potency, or following a switch to parenteral neuroleptic therapy (22). OGC is the most common of the ocular dystonic reactions, which also include blepharospasm, periocular twitches (winking), and protracted staring episodes (23).

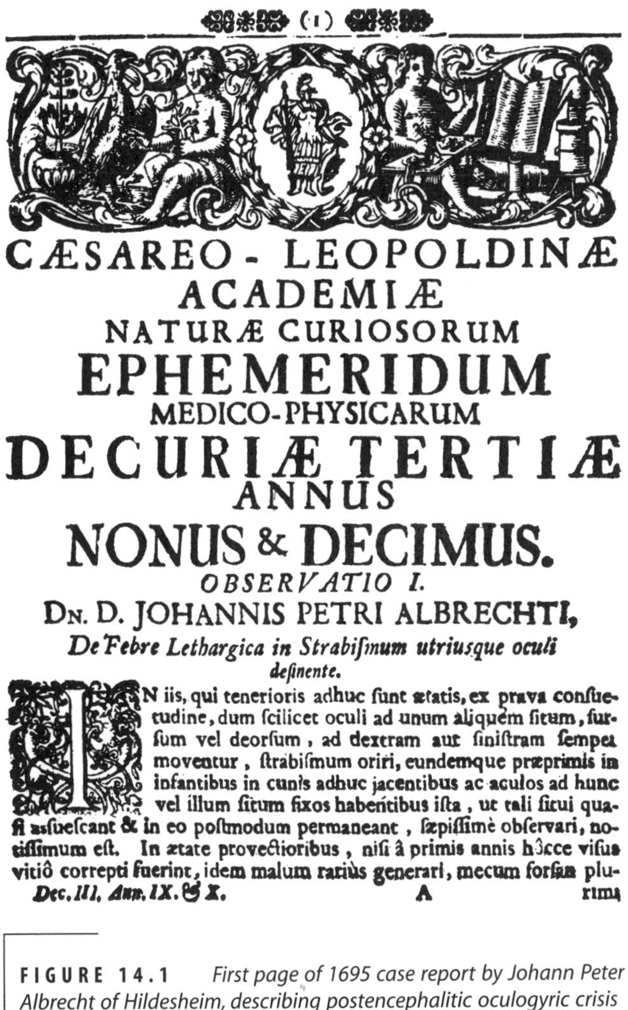
(1)

CÆSAREO - LEOPOLDINÆ
ACADEMIÆ
NATURÆ CURIOSORUM
EPHEMERIDUM
MEDICO-PHYSICARUM
DECURIÆ TERTIÆ
ANNUS
NONUS & DECIMUS.
OBSERVATIO I.
Dn. D. JOHANNIS PETRI ALBRECHTI,
De Febre Lethargica in Strabismum utriusque oculi desinente.

IN iis, qui tenerioris adhuc sunt ætatis, ex prava consuetudine, dum scilicet oculi ad unum aliquem situm, sursum vel deorsum, ad dextram aut sinistram semper moventur, strabismum oriri, eundemque præprimis in infantibus in cunis adhuc jacentibus ac oculos ad hunc vel illum situm fixos habentibus ista, ut tali situi quasi assuescant & in eo postmodum permaneant, sæpissimè observari, notissimum est. In ætate provectioribus, nisi à primis annis hocce visus vitiô correpti fuerint, idem malum rariùs generari, mecum forsan plu-

Dec. III. Ann. IX. & X. A rimi

FIGURE 14.1 *First page of 1695 case report by Johann Peter Albrecht of Hildesheim, describing postencephalitic oculogyric crisis in a young woman. Reproduced from Jelliffe S. Psychopathology of forced movements and the oculogyric crises of lethargic encephalitis. New York: Nervous and Mental Disease, 1932.*

Estimates of the frequency of neuroleptic-induced OGC are scarce in the literature. Acute dystonic reactions have been estimated to occur in from 2.3% (22) to 11.9% (24) of neuroleptic-treated individuals. One reason for the difference in these two figures is that higher-potency neuroleptics were introduced in the interim. In a multicenter collaborative study of 1152 consecutive neuroleptic-treated individuals, Swett (25) found a 10.1% incidence of acute dystonic reactions. Of those patients with dystonic reactions, the frequencies of the most common types were as follows: torticollis, 30%; glossal dystonia, 17%; trismus, 15%; OGC, 6%; and opisthotonos, 3.5%. Sachdev estimated an OGC incidence of 4% based on a population of 100 schizophrenic outpatients with greater than 6 months' neuroleptic exposure (34). Acute dystonic reactions occur twice as often in males than in females (22) and are most frequent in adolescents and young adults. Acute dystonic reactions in children younger than 15 years tend more often to look like generalized dystonia (22). Their occurrence increases with neuroleptic potency and dosage (25). The likelihood of acute dystonic reactions increases with increasing initial neuroleptic doses and decreasing interdose intervals (24).

Few other factors have been identified that clearly predispose certain neuroleptic-treated individuals to dystonic reactions. Hypoparathyroidism has been associated with a lowered threshold for dystonic reactions to prochlorperazine (26). Hypocalcemia and hypomagnesemia have been implicated as factors predisposing some patients to dystonia (27). Alcohol (28), emotional stress, fatigue (29), and suggestion (24) have all been found to precipitate OGC in vulnerable individuals. Increased susceptibility to acute dystonic reactions has been alleged in patients with family histories of dystonia musculorum deformans and neuroleptic-induced dystonic reactions (30). In fact, a prochlorperazine challenge has been advocated as a screening test for heterozygote family members of patients with torsion dystonia (31).

The onset of a crisis may be paroxysmal or stuttering over several hours. There may be a prodrome of malaise or restlessness for several hours, or of a fixed stare for several moments, followed by the characteristic sustained maximal upward deviation of the eyes, often such that only the sclerae are visible. As in postencephalitic OGC, the eyes may also converge, deviate upward and laterally, or deviate downward. Patients may be able to force their eyes to normal position for an instant with effort and discomfort, but the eyes quickly resume their deviated position. Blinking or forced eye closure may also bring down the eyes for an instant. Associated signs and symptoms occur similar to those seen in postencephalitic OGC. The most frequently reported associated findings are backward (retrocollis) and lateral (torticollis) flexion of the neck, widely opened mouth, protruded tongue, and ocular pain (22,23). The typical presentation is depicted in Figure 14.2. Blepharospasm or autonomic discharge may also occur. A wave of exhaustion follows some episodes. Compared with the postencephalitic variety, neuroleptic OGC is less often associated with parkinsonism, which tends to develop slightly later in the course of neuroleptic therapy than acute dystonic reactions. Also, OGC tended to occur without torticollis or retrocollis in postencephalitic patients.

Apart from the observation that OGC is frequently associated with anxiety, few authors in the neuroleptic era have commented on the presence or absence of stereotyped psychiatric symptoms during or preceding OGC. Transient recurrence of auditory hallucinations has been described during acute OGC (32) and what was called tardive OGC

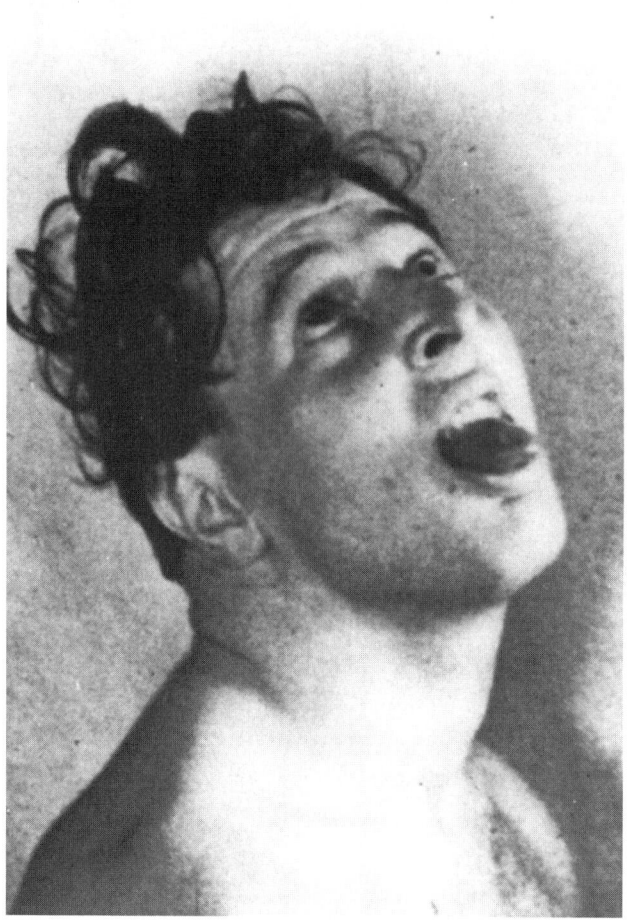

FIGURE 14.2 *Oculogyric crisis with torticollis and tongue protrusion. Reproduced by permission from Delay J, Deniker P. Drug-induced extrapyramidal syndromes. In: Vinken PJ, Bruyn GW, eds. Handbook of clinical neurology, volume 6: diseases of the basal ganglia. Amsterdam: North-Holland Publishing, 1968:248–266.*

(33). Sachdev reported co-occurrence of psychiatric symptoms in four chronic cases and one acute case of OGC (34). Leigh and colleagues described two patients with psychiatric symptoms during neuroleptic-induced OGC (35). Four schizophrenic patients whose oculogyric crises included appearance or exacerbation of psychotic symptoms have been described (36). One author observed concurrent psychiatric symptoms in a case of OGC but concluded they could be explained psychologically (29).

In my experience, the association of chronic OGC with stereotyped emotional or cognitive symptoms is frequent but often overlooked. Table 14.2 describes a series of 10 neuroleptic-treated patients I examined in public-sector mental health facilities. All had greater than 5 years' neuroleptic exposure. All were evaluated for chronic OGC episodes. All 10 had stereotyped psychiatric symptoms associated with their OGC. In no case had this association been appreciated by the attending psychiatrist. Half were not recognized to have been suffering from OGC at all, but were believed to have periodic exacerbations of their psychiatric disorders. All patients reported resolution of the psychiatric concomitants along with the ocular dystonia when episodes were treated with anticholinergic agents. The spontaneous resolution of the stereotyped psychiatric symptoms when OGC abates is most striking.

Differential Diagnosis

The presentation of oculogyric crisis is so characteristic that differential diagnosis is almost never an issue. What can be a problem, however, is failure of clinicians to recognize the disorder. It may be misdiagnosed as a psychogenic or hysterical symptom because of its tendency to recur under conditions of emotional arousal and in association with psychiatric symptoms. In the series of individuals with chronic OGC described earlier, for example, only half had been recognized as having OGC prior to consultation. Since OGC typically occurs in the setting of acute psychosis, it is not uncommon for patients to offer delusional interpretations of their oculogyric movements, such as the one suggested by the biblical quotation at the beginning of this chapter. Inexperienced clinicians may be misled into diagnosing a psychogenic disorder when the patient suffering from OGC voluntarily brings his or her eyes down for an instant or when movements can be influenced by suggestion. A lesson learned from the encephalitis lethargica experience is that motor symptoms appearing to be purely psychogenic can prove to have a neurologic basis.

Although there is seldom any question as to the differential diagnosis of neuroleptic OGC, a few neurologic conditions with eye movements resembling OGC should be mentioned. Forced conjugate gaze deviations often occur in Tourette's syndrome, though they are usually less sustained than those of either neuroleptic or postencephalitic OGC [37]. Generalized absence seizures might occasionally cause conjugate upgaze episodes, but these are easily distinguished

Table 14.2 Associated Symptoms in 10 Cases of Chronic OGC

Age, Sex	Diagnosis	Associated Symptoms	OGC Known?
31, M	Schizophrenia, substance abuse	Delusion (computer attacks), anxiety	No
31, F	Schizophrenia	Visual hallucinations, delusion (religious)	No
30, F	Psychotic depression	Increased psychosis, anxiety, agitation	Yes
31, F	Schizophrenia	Anxiety, agitation	Yes
27, M	Schizophrenia	Auditory hallucinations (repetitive), anxiety, agitation, compulsive thoughts of trauma	Yes
43, M	Schizotypal personality	Compulsive thoughts; spacey, repetitive speech	No
56, M	Schizoaffective disorder, alcohol abuse	Delusion (attracted to the lights)	Yes
36, F	Bipolar disorder, posttraumatic stress disorder, substance abuse	Disorganized, disoriented (unlike regular side effects)	Yes
34, M	Schizophrenia	Metamorphopsia, compulsive thoughts (religious)	No
38, F	Schizoaffective disorder	Anxiety, compulsive thoughts (worries)	No

Note: Based on author's study of 10 patients with chronic oculogyric crisis seen in the University of Massachusetts Medical Center neuropsychiatry clinics. The last column indicates whether the OGC had been known to the referring clinician. All patients had greater than 5 years' neuroleptic exposure.

by the shorter duration of eye movements (seconds), the absence of communication during the episode, the absence of discomfort, the patient's lack of recall for the episode, the presence of characteristic electroencephalographic abnormalities, and the failure to respond to agents used in treating dystonia.

Table 14.3 lists the reported causes of OGC, including encephalitis, medications, neurodegenerative diseases, benign syndromes, and focal lesions. A benign self-limited childhood syndrome of oculogyric crisis, ataxia, and clumsiness has been described (38). The childhood degenerative disorder of neuronal intranuclear hyaline inclusion disease includes OGC (39,40).

Those conditions associated with focal pathology tend to include either basal ganglionic or midbrain lesions. OGC has been described in basal ganglia stroke syndromes (41,42). Apart from encephalitis lethargica, other conditions involving the midbrain have also been linked to OGC (43,44). The syndrome of dopa–responsive dystonia (DRD), which has both familial and sporadic forms, occasionally includes OGC (45–49). Lamberti et al (49), reporting a patient who had been symptomatic with dystonia for 19 years and with OGC for 13 years prior to treatment, suggested that the frequency of OGC in DRD would be greater except that low-dose L-dopa effectively treats both dystonia and OGC. Interestingly, their patient had "emotional stress" during each OGC attack.

Antipsychotic drug therapy is certainly the most common etiology of modern-day OGC. Although the newer atypical antipsychotic agents tend to cause extrapyramidal side effects (EPS) less frequently than do traditional neuroleptics, atypical neuroleptics can give rise to the entire range of acute EPS, including dystonic reactions and OGC (50,51). When it appears that there is no history of recent antipsychotic exposure, a history of recent antiemetic treatment with prochlorperazine or metaclopramide may sometimes be discovered. Phenothiazine antiemetic treatment is

Table 14.3 Reported Causes of Oculogyric Crisis

Drugs	Conditions
Antipsychotics (including phenothiazine antiemetics)	Postencephalitic parkinsonism
Amantadine (54)	Tourette's syndrome (37)
Benzodiazepines (54)	Multiple sclerosis (64, 65)
Carbamazepine (55–57)	Neurosyphilis (66)
Chloroquine (54)	Head trauma (66)
Droperidol (58)	Bilateral paramedian thalamic infarction (41)
Isotretinoin (59)	Juvenile Parkinson's disease (67)
L-Dopa[a] (18)	Lesions of fourth ventricle and cerebellum (64)
Lithium[b] (60)	
Metoclopramide (61)	Cystic glioma of third ventricle with positional OGC (43)
Nifedipine[b] (62)	Familial juvenile amaurotic idiocy (Spielmeyer-Vogt disease)[b] (68)
Reserpine (54)	
Tricyclic antidepressants (54)	Neuronal intranuclear inclusion disease (40)
Gabapentin (63)	Herpes encephalitis (44)
	Benign OGC, clumsiness, ataxia syndrome of childhood (38)
	Familial Parkinson-dementia syndrome (69)
	Dopa-responsive dystonia (45–49)
	Bilateral putaminal hemorrhages (42)

[a] OGC resulted from interaction of L-dopa and postencephalitic parkinsonism.
[b] Patients described were also on a neuroleptic. The reported drug may have served to lower the threshold for neuroleptic OGC.

frequently repeated every 4 hours, resulting in an increased risk of dystonic reaction, especially in children and young adults. L-Dopa–related OGC tends to occur in the setting of L-dopa toxicity, when other dyskinesias occur. Some of the case reports listed in Table 14.3 (e.g., lithium and nifedipine) may actually represent lowering of the neuroleptic OGC threshold by another agent rather than direct causation of OGC. Finally, there are still occasional case reports of encephalitis followed by parkinsonism and OGC that strongly resemble encephalitis lethargica (52,53).

A chronic form of OGC has also been described in neuroleptic-treated individuals (34,35,70–73). Cases with onset years after beginning neuroleptic treatment and associated with other signs of tardive dyskinesia have been described as tardive OGC by some authors (34,71–74). One author (51) has labeled a case of clozapine-induced recurrent OGC without any other signs of dyskinesia as tardive OGC due to late onset only. FitzGerald and Jankovic (73) treated four patients in whom OGC developed in the setting of established tardive dyskinesia or tardive dystonia. They used dopamine-depleting agents rather than standard anticholinergic regimens due to the concurrent dyskinesia and made a compelling argument that their cases represented tardive OGC.

Most case reports of chronic OGC are inconsistent with respect to reporting neuroleptic dosage, potency, or changes in prn medication preceding OGC onset. In most cases, there are several differences between chronic OGC syndromes and tardive dyskinesia. Chronic OGC typically responds readily to anticholinergic therapy, neuroleptic discontinuation, or to decrease in neuroleptic dosage or potency. Choreoathetoid tardive dyskinesia is typically exacerbated by all these factors. Tardive dystonia is exacerbated by all these factors except anticholinergic therapy. Although there are exceptions, most patients with tardive dyskinesia are unaware of their movements, whereas most patients with chronic OGC are aware of the attacks and find them unpleasant. OGC has even been held by one author (75) to be a key feature differentiating acute from tardive dystonia. Apart from late onset, there is little similarity in most cases between chronic OGC and other tardive disorders.

MANAGEMENT

Since OGC can be extremely frightening and since it responds readily to treatment, the patient should be examined and treated immediately, while at the same time offered reassurance. Once the patient is able to be interviewed comfortably, a more thorough history should be sought. Table 14.4 lists several points to cover in eliciting the patient's history and investigating an episode of OGC. Important variables include recent changes in neuroleptic regimen, recent addition of an agent known to activate neuroleptic OGC, or presence of any of the reported predisposing or precipitating factors. Attention should be paid to associated psychiatric symptoms. One would not want to increase the dosage of the offending agent for psychotic features that are actually part of the oculogyric crisis.

The diagnosis of neuroleptic OGC can be established quickly with a brief examination and a glance at the patient's record. For severe crises or crises associated with pain, acute treatment should be administered parenterally to

Table 14.4   Evaluation of the Patient with Oculogyric Crises

Drug Exposure	**Known Precipitants**
Length of neuroleptic treatment	Recent alcohol ingestion
Neuroleptic dosage	Exhaustion
Interdose interval	Emotional trauma
Recent change to depot neuroleptics	Recent addition of drug reported to release OGC (see Table 14.2)
Description of Attack	
Eye position	**Predisposing Factors**
Ability to briefly bring eyes down voluntarily	History of dystonia sensitivity
	Family history of primary torsion dystonia
Diplopia or visual blurring	Family history of neuroleptic
Frequency of Attacks	dystonia sensitivity
Time of day	Hypocalcemia
Regularity or periodicity	Hypoparathyroidism
	Brain damage
Associated Features	Basal ganglia
Pain	Midbrain
Torticollis/Retrocollis	
Oromandibular dystonia	**Differential Diagnosis**
Glossal dystonia	History of seizures
Psychiatric symptoms	History of Tourette's syndrome or tic disorder
Severe anxiety	
Hallucinations	History of encephalitis
Delusions	History of postencephalitic parkinsonism
Compulsive thoughts	
Psychomotor agitation	
Prodrome	
Anxiety	
Precipitous depression	
Compulsive thinking	
Staring	

avoid any delay in relieving the patient's symptoms. Benztropine (Cogentin) 2 mg or diphenhydramine (Benadryl) 50 mg intramuscularly (IM) or intravenously (IV) will usually abort an OGC attack. If not, the dose should be repeated in 30 minutes. If there is no response, diazepam 5–10 mg IV or lorazepam 1 mg IM or IV (76) should be administered slowly to avoid respiratory depression. Korczyn and Goldberg (77) advocate parenteral benzodiazepines as a first-line therapy of dystonic reactions because of the more widespread familiarity with their parenteral administration, and their beneficial associated anxiolytic effects.

Once the acute attack has subsided, the patient should be given an oral antiparkinsonian agent such as benztropine or trihexyphenidyl in divided doses for 2 weeks. These agents are preferred over diphenhydramine treatment, which is also effective in OGC, in order to avoid unnecessary sedation. If the patient is on depot neuroleptics, the clinician can expect the crises to recur, so oral therapy may have to be continued for a longer time. Table 14.5 lists the treatment alternatives for oculogyric crisis. In the past, some clinicians have recommended a single dose of 10–30 mg oral diazepam as a first-line treatment in mild to moderate crises because of its rapid bioavailability and relatively long duration of

Table 14.5   Agents Used in the Treatment of Oculogyric Crises

Acute Attack[a]
Benztropine (Cogentin) 2 mg IV/IM
Diphenhydramine (Benadryl) 25–50 mg IV/IM
Diazepam (Valium) 5–10 mg IV
Lorazepam (Ativan) 1 mg IV/IM

Follow-up Treatment[b]
Benztropine (Cogentin) 2–6 mg/day
Trihexyphenidyl (Artane) 4–15 mg/day
Diphenhydramine (Benadryl) 25–100 mg/day
Diazepam 10–30 mg/day
Amantadine (Symmetrel) 100–300 mg/day

[a] Repeat in 30 minutes if no response.
[b] All follow-up treatment should be given in divided doses due to longer half-life of neuroleptics compared with antiparkinson agents.

Table 14.6   Disorders of Motion and Emotion

Extrapyramidal Disorders with Cognitive or Psychiatric Symptoms	Psychiatric Disorders with Motor Symptoms
Encephalitis lethargica	Schizophrenia
Oculogyric crisis	Depression
Parkinson's disease	Mania
Huntington's disease	Anxiety
Wilson's disease	Obsessive–compulsive disorder
Idiopathic basal ganglia calcification (Fahr's disease)	Attention deficit disorder with hyperactivity
Tourette's syndrome	
Progressive supranuclear palsy	
Meige's syndrome	
Akathisia*	
Tardive dyskinesia*	

* Cognitive correlates of these disorders have been reported in the literature, but the issue of causation remains unclear.

action. Symptom resolution follows in 30 to 60 minutes. Some patients initially treated with only 10 mg require repeat 10-mg doses at 8 and 12 hours (24). Treatment with a benzodiazepine may be helpful if significant anxiety develops secondary to OGC. However, when anxiety occurs as a psychiatric symptom of the OGC itself, it usually resolves with anticholinergic treatment as well. Left untreated, an acute dystonic reaction subsides within 24 hours. If no pharmacologic agents of any kind are available, the crisis may resolve within a few hours if the patient is placed in a quiet, darkened room (24).

If recurrent OGC becomes a problem, the patient can be given a low-potency or atypical neuroleptic, neuroleptic dosage can be lowered, or the interdose interval can be increased. Serum calcium should be checked in the event of recurrent crises.

When a patient is begun on neuroleptics, the risk of dystonic reaction should be discussed if the patient's mental status allows. In the setting of acute psychosis, when the development of a dystonic reaction might be most detrimental to a fragile doctor-patient alliance, prophylactic administration of anticholinergic agents may afford some protection against dystonia. A 7-day course of benztropine 2 mg twice a day was shown to prevent acute dystonic reactions without any drug-related morbidity in one placebo-controlled study of patients 18 to 40 years old (78).

BASIC SCIENCE

Basal Ganglia as Limbic-Motor Crossroads

The mechanism of oculogyric crisis is not yet understood. Schwab and colleagues (12) were especially interested in OGC because they felt that the study of the neural correlates of the associated paroxysmal psychiatric symptoms could shed light on the etiology of the primary psychiatric symptoms they so strongly resembled. A number of condi-

tions exist that, like oculogyric crisis, involve a combination of involuntary movement and psychiatric symptoms. Table 14.6 lists some of these, including primarily extrapyramidal disorders associated with psychotic, affective, obsessive–compulsive, and dementia symptoms and attention deficits, and primarily psychiatric disorders associated with disorders of movement.

Anxiety, emotional distress, suggestion, and environmental variables have been shown to precipitate oculogyric crises in vulnerable individuals. Similar emotional exacerbation of movement disorders occurs in tremor, tic, and tardive dyskinesia, the latter increasing in depression and decreasing in mania (79–81). Many abnormal involuntary movements, including OGC and tics, can be voluntarily suppressed briefly. At first OGC was held to be a hysterical symptom due to these observations. McCowan and Cook (13) argued against any supposition that hysteria should be so pervasive in postencephalitics when it was comparatively rare in the general population. They postulated that the same lesions that caused postencephalitic motor manifestations also resulted in abnormal motor responses to psychic stimuli, thus foreshadowing what we are now beginning to learn about the neuroanatomy and neurochemistry of limbic-basal ganglionic connections. The basal ganglia have been widely investigated as a crossroads of limbic and motor function. In recent years the basal ganglia's striatal "input zone," composed of the caudate and putamen, has been expanded to include the ventral striatum (nucleus accumbens septi and some of the olfactory tubercles). Similarly, the pallidal "output zone" of the basal ganglia has been expanded to include the nondopaminergic part of the substantia nigra and the ventral pallidum (80). Projections to the striatum have been demonstrated from the midbrain ventral tegmental area, hippocampus, amygdala, and cingulum.

Extrapyramidal striatal, septal, and nigral nuclei all receive limbic input, creating an anatomic substrate for the interplay of emotion and motion (78).

Psychodynamic Theory

Although now of historical significance only, Jelliffe's theory that OGC was a symptom of obsessive-compulsive neurosis was widely accepted for many years. He was able to discover emotional trauma predating the initial attack in his patients and postulated that the ocular deviations and psychomotor excitement were rituals secondary to repressed guilt and the need for punishment. He saw the problem as related to loss of ego repression due to cortical destruction (1–3).

Midbrain Pathology

A number of theories on the pathophysiology of OGC come from the encephalitis lethargica experience. Von Economo showed that cerebral cortical lesions in encephalitis lethargica were nonspecific and inconsistent, but the areas of greatest damage were the substantia nigra, cerebral peduncles, midbrain tegmentum, and the deep gray matter surrounding the third ventricle and aqueduct (5). Since encephalitis lethargica principally involved the midbrain, it was suggested that OGC was the result of mesencephalic inflammation (7). Note that both the nigrostriatal and the mesolimbic ascending dopamine pathways mentioned previously originate in the midbrain. There have been no reported evoked potential studies investigating midbrain function in OGC-prone individuals. Nor have there been any reports of searches for midbrain pathology on postmortem examination of patients suffering from recurrent neuroleptic OGC. However, invoking a focal degenerative process would be difficult given the increased incidence of OGC and dystonia in young individuals (82).

Epileptiform abnormalities in OGC patients have been sought without success (35), though "tonic eye fits" were held as a possible epileptic manifestation by investigators early in the century. Upward gaze deviation has been evoked in monkeys by bilateral or midline mesencephalic stimulation (35). Two midbrain structures, the rostral interstitial nucleus of the medial longitudinal fasciculus and the interstitial nucleus of Cajal, appear to be important in control of vertical gaze. Impairment of normal activity in these centers can contribute to vertical gaze deficits (83). Devinsky (84) reviewed two efferent pathways from the midbrain in which a lesion could lead to OGC. The first arises from the substantia nigra pars reticularis and projects to the superior colliculus. The second projects from the pars reticularis and pars compacta of the substantia nigra, as well as from the ventral tegmental area to the midbrain tegmentum.

Against the existence of a specific anatomic lesion as a cause of OGC is the observation that ocular movements during a crisis are occasionally lateral, downward, or convergent, and that during some crises, the direction of ocular deviation has been observed to change. Further evidence against such a lesion is that full extraocular movements within the confines of the upper extent of the visual field have been demonstrated during OGC (35). Leigh and colleagues (35) have proposed a hypothesis for the origin of OGC based on the "corollary discharge" model of how the brain monitors eye movements. According to their model, OGC occurs when the brain's saccade generator receives erroneous information causing it to generate excessive upward saccades. This generator is driven by the difference (the motor error) between desired eye position and the brain's estimate of current eye position.

Vestibular Theory

Onuaguluchi advocated the vestibular theory of OGC (9). It is well known that bilateral caloric stimulation produces tonic upward deviation of the eyes. Bilateral caloric stimulation would precipitate an attack in patients with postencephalitic OGC. Up to 40% of patients had true vertigo during their OGC attacks, and most had some degree of vertical nystagmus. Onuaguluchi believed two criteria were necessary for the development of OGC: an irritative brainstem lesion in the vestibular pathway and a source of vestibular stimulation. Wax obstruction of an auditory canal and revolving during dancing were cited as two examples of the sort of stimulation necessary. He felt that the initial OGC attack came on suddenly without emotional symptoms and that conditioning was responsible for the coincidence of psychiatric symptoms during further attacks.

Sleep Theory

Hall (11) believed that OGC represented a sleep disorder. He pointed out the centrality of sleep disorders, either hypersomnolent or insomniac, in the acute encephalitic phase, the observation that OGC happened more often in the latter half of the day when fatigue was a factor, and that OGC attacks were usually followed by sleep. His argument was that the gaze deviations of OGC were not active muscle spasms but were identical to the position that eyes normally assume in sleep. As evidence he cited Bell's observation that, in sleep, when the eyelids are closed, the eyes wander upward. Since OGC included eye positions other than just upward deviation, Hall observed the eye positions in sleep of 206 individuals and found that 54% moved upward, 38% remained forward, 5% moved downward, and 3% moved laterally. Further, eye position in some subjects was identical on consecutive nights, but in others it differed. Finally, he noted the absence of forehead wrinkling during the fully developed oculogyric attack, just as during eye movement in sleep, in contrast with the prominent forehead wrinkling during volitional extreme upgaze. Thus, he felt that OGC represented inhibition of normal extraocular muscle tone. It is still arguable whether OGC represents a positive or negative symptom.

Dopamine and "Psychomotility" Disorders

Several neurotransmitters, including dopamine, serotonin, norepinephrine, GABA (γ-aminobutyric acid), and somatostatin, are involved in both psychiatric and movement disorders (78,80). As the site of action of the most commonly implicated agent in OGC, the dopamine system may be a way of explaining why oculogyric crisis is so intimately bound up with psychiatric symptoms. The three principal dopaminergic pathways of the brain are the nigrostriatal, projecting from dopaminergic nigral neurons to striatal receptors; the mesolimbic, projecting from the midbrain ventral tegmental area to the nucleus accumbens, amygdala, limbic striatum, and parts of the frontal cortex; and the tuberoinfundibular, within the hypothalamic-pituitary axis (78). The first two pathways may explain the coincidence of involuntary movements and psychiatric symptoms in many extrapyramidal diseases. Cummings feels that the two components, psychiatric and motor, of many of the syndromes in Table 14.6 are so universal that these conditions should be classified as "psychomotility disorders" (78).

Although neuroleptics affect neurotransmitters other than dopamine, dopamine is implicated in acute dystonias since relatively selective dopamine antagonists such as pimozide also cause them. Both dopamine hypofunction and paradoxical dopamine hyperfunction have been postulated to cause OGC and other acute dystonias (82). The former model is explained by the acute effects of dopamine receptor blockade and is supported by the ability of dopamine agonists to suppress neuroleptic-induced dystonia in primates. This would explain L-dopa's initial ability to suppress OGC in postencephalitic parkinsonism; however, the existence of L-dopa–induced dystonia and crises during toxicity favors a dopamine hyperfunction model. The dopamine hyperfunction model, suggested by Marsden and Jenner (82), could be explained by increased dopamine release due to failure of feedback inhibition caused by neuroleptic blockade of presynaptic dopamine receptors. The released dopamine is then postulated to act at an unblocked subpopulation of supersensitive postsynaptic receptors. Increased dopamine turnover is found only on acute administration of dopamine-blocking agents and is diminished by anticholinergic agents, an obvious parallel with acute dystonic reactions (82). Presynaptic dopamine mechanisms have been implicated in neuroleptic-induced dystonia in animals. Acute neuroleptic-induced dystonia can be prevented in primates by blocking presynaptic catecholamine synthesis combined with depletion of presynaptic dopamine stores (85). It should be noted that the baboons used in the above experiments did not manifest OGC during their dystonic reactions, so it remains possible that OGC has a different mechanism than other forms of acute dystonic reaction.

If the dopamine hyperfunction model is accurate, a further explanation is needed as to why so few individuals actually develop acute dystonic reactions to neuroleptics. One possibility, suggested by Garver and colleagues (86), is that the intracellular neuroleptic level is more critical than the plasma level in the generation of dystonic reactions. In comparing individuals with and without dystonic reactions, they found that despite equal plasma levels, the red blood cell levels of neuroleptics in the symptomatic group were six times higher at the onset of the dystonic reaction than the levels in the asymptomatic group.

The above arguments bear some similarity to the dopamine receptor hypersensitivity hypothesis of tardive dyskinesia. Nasrallah has suggested that dystonia might be considered a manifestation of acute dopamine hyperactivity (with rebound increased dopamine release), and tardive dyskinesia a manifestation of chronic dopamine hyperactivity (with postsynaptic receptor supersensitivity) (71). Munetz (72) reported a case of a patient with OGC who went on to develop tardive dyskinesia, but cautioned against interpreting this as an increased tendency toward tardive dyskinesia in patients with acute dystonic reactions.

SUMMARY

The syndrome of neuroleptic-induced oculogyric crisis bears a striking resemblance to postencephalitic oculogyric crisis, with the exception that the latter was usually associated with parkinsonism. Apart from anxiety secondary to the ocular dystonia, the association of psychiatric symptoms with oculogyric crisis, well known in the postencephalitic era, has not often been commented on in the neuroleptic OGC literature. The associated psychiatric symptoms may be important to the understanding of the etiology of OGC and should be inquired about when examining patients. Acute OGC is easily recognized and usually responds rapidly to treatment. Chronic OGC, too, can be easily recognized and treated when clinicians are aware of the frequently co-occurring cognitive and psychiatric symptoms of the attack. The mechanism of OGC remains unknown, but a number of theories have been advanced over the years. Among the most promising avenues for exploration in the understanding of OGC and other "psychomotility disorders" are dysfunction of ascending dopaminergic pathways originating in the midbrain and dysfunction of limbic-basal ganglionic connection circuits.

REFERENCES

1. Jelliffe S. Psychological components in postencephalitic oculogyric crises: contribution to a genetic interpretation of compulsion phenomena. Arch Neurol Psychiatry 1929;21:491–532.
2. Jelliffe S. Psychopathology of forced movements and the oculogyric crises of lethargic encephalitis. New York: Nervous and Mental Disease, 1932.
3. Jelliffe S. Oculogyric crises: psychopathologic considerations of the affective states. Arch Neurol Psychiatry 1930;23:1227–1247.
4. Jelliffe S. Oculogyric crises as compulsion phenomena in postencephalitis: their occurrence, phenomenology, and meaning. J Nerv Ment Dis 1929;69:59–68, 165–184, 278–297, 415–426, 531–551, 666–679.

5. Von Economo C. Encephalitis lethargica: its sequelae and treatment. London: Oxford University, 1931.

6. Oeckinghaus W. Encephalitis epidemica und Wilsonsches Krankheitsbild. Dtsch Z Nervenkr 1921;72:294–309.

7. Hohman L. Forced conjugate upward movements of the eyes in post-encephalitic parkinson's syndrome. JAMA 1925;84:1489–1490.

8. Kubie L. Psychopathology of forced movements in oculogyric crises. Psychoanal Q 1933;2:622–626.

9. Onuaguluchi G. Crises in post-encephalitic parkinsonism. Brain 1961;84:395–415.

10. Wimmer A. Tonic eye fits in chronic epidemic encephalitis. Acta Psychiatr Neurol 1926;1:173–187.

11. Hall A. Chronic epidemic encephalitis with special reference to the ocular attacks. Br Med J 1931;2:833–837.

12. Schwab R, Fabing H, Prichard J. Psychiatric symptoms and syndromes in parkinson's disease. Am J Psychiatry 1951;107:901–907.

13. McCowan P, Cook L. Oculogyric crises in chronic epidemic encephalitis. Brain 1928;51:285–309.

14. Onuaguluchi G. Drug treatment of parkinsonism and its assessment. In: Vinken P, Bruyn G, eds. Handbook of clinical neurology. Amsterdam: North-Holland, 1968:218–226.

15. Davis P, Stewart W. The use of benzedrine sulfate in post encephalitic parkinsonism. JAMA 1938;110:1890–1892.

16. Matthews R. Symptomatic treatment of chronic encephalitis with benzedrine sulfate. Am J Med Sci 1938;195:448–452.

17. Sacks O. Awakenings. New York: E. P. Dutton, 1973.

18. Sacks O, Kohl M. L-dopa and oculogyric crises. Lancet 1970;2:215–216.

19. Crookshank F. Influenza: essays by several authors. London: William Heinemann, 1922.

20. Sacks O. Parkinsonism—a so-called new disease. Br Med J 1971;4:111.

21. Jankovic J, Fahn S. Dystonic syndromes. In: Jankovic J, Tolosa E, eds. Parkinson's disease and movement disorders. Baltimore: Urban and Schwarzenberg, 1988.

22. Ayd F Jr. A survey of drug-induced extrapyramidal reactions. JAMA 1961;125:1054–1060.

23. Lees A. Tics and related disorders. New York: Churchill Livingstone, 1985.

24. Ayd F Jr. Early onset neuroleptic-induced extrapyramidal reactions: a second survey. In: Coyle J, Enna S, eds. Neuroleptics: neurochemical, behavioral, and clinical perspectives. New York: Raven, 1983.

25. Swett C Jr. Drug-induced dystonia. Am J Psychiatry 1975;132:532–555.

26. Schaaf M, Payne C. Dystonic reactions to prochlorperazine in hypoparathyroidism. N Engl J Med 1966;275:991–995.

27. Alexander P, van Kammen D, Bunney W. Serum calcium and magnesium levels in schizophrenia: possible relationship to extrapyramidal symptoms. Arch Gen Psychiatry 1979;36:1372–1377.

28. Lutz E. Neuroleptic-induced akathisia and dystonia triggered by alcohol. JAMA 1976;236:2422–2423.

29. Bumpass E, Knoll J III. Emotional factors in oculogyric crisis. J Nerv Ment Dis 1982;170:366–370.

30. Rupniak N, Jenner P, Marsden C. Acute dystonia induced by neuroleptic drugs. Psychopharmacology 1986;88:403–419.

31. Marsden C, Harrison M, Bundey S. Natural history of idiopathic torsion dystonia [comment following paper by Eldridge R]. In: Eldridge R, Fahn S, eds. Advances in neurology. New York: Raven, 1976.

32. Chiu L. Transient recurrence of auditory hallucinations during acute dystonia. Br J Psychiatry 1989;115:110–113.

33. Sachdev P, Tang W. Psychotic symptoms preceding ocular deviation in a patient with tardive oculogyric crises. Aust N Z J Psychiatry 1992;26:666–670.

34. Sachdev P. Tardive and chronically recurrent oculogyric crises. Mov Disord 1993;8:93–97.

35. Leigh R, Foley J, Remler B, Civil R. Oculogyric crisis: a syndrome of thought disorder and ocular deviation. Ann Neurol 1987;22:13–17.

36. Thornton A, McKenna P. Acute dystonic reactions complicated by psychotic phenomena. Br J Psychiatry 1994;164:115–118.

37. Frankel F, Cummings J. Neuro-ophthalmic abnormalities in Tourette's syndrome: functional and anatomic implications. Neurology 1984;34:359–361.

38. Campistol J, Prats J, Garaizar C. Benign paroxysmal tonic upgaze of childhood with ataxia. A neuro-ophthalmological syndrome of familial origin? Dev Med Child Neurol 1993;35:431–434.

39. Parker J J Jr. Neuronal intranuclear hyaline inclusion disease associated with premature coronary atherosclerosis. J Clin Neurol Ophthalmol 1987;7:244–249.

40. Haltia M, Somer H, Palo J, Johnson W. Neuronal intranuclear inclusion disease in identical twins. Ann Neurol 1984;15:316–321.

41. Kakigi R, Shibasaki H, Katafuchi Y, et al. The syndrome of bilateral paramedian thalamic infarction associated with oculogyric crisis. Rinsho Shinkeigaku 1986;26:1100–1105.

42. Shimpo T, Fuse S, Yoshizawa A. Retrocollis and oculogyric crisis in association with bilateral putaminal hemorrhages. Rinsho Shinkeigaku 1993;33:40–44.

43. Heimburger R. Positional oculogyric crises. Case report. J Neurosurg 1988;69:951–953.

44. Matsumura K, Sakuta M. Oculogyric crisis in acute herpetic brainstem encephalitis. J Neurol Neurosurg Psychiatry 1987;50:365–366.

45. Deonna T. Dopa-sensitive progressive dystonia of childhood with fluctuations of symptoms—Segawa syndrome and possible variants. Neuropediatrics 1986;17:81–85.

46. Nygaard T, Duvoisin R. Hereditary dystonia-parkinsonism syndrome of juvenile onset. Neurology 1986;36:1424–1428.

47. Rajput A. Levodopa in dystonia musculorum deformans. *Lancet* 1973;1:432.

48. Rondot P, Ziegler M. Dystonia—L-dopa responsive or juvenile parkinsonism? J Neural Transm Suppl 1983;19:273–281.

49. Lamberti P, de Mari M, Iliceto G, et al. Effect of L-dopa on oculogyric crises in a case of dopa-responsive dystonia. Mov Disord 1993;8:236–237.

50. Faulk R, Gilmore J, Jensen E, Perkins D. Risperidone-induced dystonic reaction. Am J Psychiatry 1996;153:577.

51. Dave M. Tardive oculogyric crises with clozapine. J Clin Psychiatry 1994;55:264–265.

52. Espir M, Spalding J. Three recent cases of encephalitis lethargica. Br Med J 1956;1:1141–1144.

53. Rail D, Scholtz C, Swash M. Post-encephalitic parkinsonism: current experience. J Neurol Neurosurg Psychiatry 1981;44:670–676.

54. Fraunfelder F. Drug induced ocular side effects and drug interactions. 3rd ed. Philadelphia: Lea and Febiger, 1989.

55. Berchou R, Rodin E. Carbamazepine-induced oculogyric crisis. Arch Neurol 1979;36:522–523.

56. Henry E. Oculogyric crisis and carbamazepine. Arch Neurol 1980;37:326.

57. Arnstein E. Oculogyric crisis: a distinct toxic effect of carbamazepine. J Child Neurol 1986;1:289–290.

58. Dingwall A. Oculogyric crisis after day case anaesthesia. Anaesthesia 1987;42:565.

59. Bigby M, Stern R. Adverse reactions to isotretinoin. A report from the adverse drug reaction reporting system. J Am Acad Dermatol 1988;18:543–552.

60. Sandyk R. Oculogyric crisis induced by lithium carbonate. Eur Neurol 1984;23:92–94.

61. Berkman N, Frossard C, Moury F. Oculogyric crisis and metaclopramide. Bull Soc Ophthalmol Fr 1981;81:153–155.

62. Singh I. Prolonged oculogyric crisis on addition of nifedipine to neuroleptic medication regime. Br J Psychiatry 1987;150:127–128.

63. Reeves A, So E, Sharbrough F, Krahn L. Movement disorders associated with the use of gabapentin. Epilepsia 1996;37:988–990.

64. Roy F. Ocular differential diagnosis. Philadelphia: Lea and Febiger, 1975.

65. Barton J, Cox T, Calne D. Involuntary ocular deviations and generalized dystonia in multiple sclerosis: a case report. J Neuroophthalmol 1994;14:160–162.

66. Cogan D. Neurology of the ocular muscles. Springfield: Charles Thomas, 1956.

67. Shimizu N, Mizuno M. Oculomotor characteristics of parkinsonism in comparison with those of cerebellar ataxia. J Neural Transm Suppl 1983;19:233–242.

68. Sorenson J, Parnas J. A clinical study of 44 patients with juvenile amaurotic family idiocy. Acta Psychiatr Scand 1979;59:449–461.

69. Mata M, Dorovini-Zis K, Wilson M, Young A. New form of familial parkinson-dementia syndrome: clinical and pathologic findings. Neurology 1983;33:1439–1443.

70. Benjamin S, Coldwell C. Co-occurrence of psychiatric symptoms in acute and chronic oculogyric crisis. Abstract. New Orleans: American Neuropsychiatric Association Annual Meeting, 1999.

71. Nasrallah H, Pappas N, Crowe R. Oculogyric dystonia in tardive dyskinesia. Am J Psychiatry 1980;137:850–851.

72. Munetz M. Oculogyric crises and tardive dyskinesia. Am J Psychiatry 1980;137:1628.

73. FitzGerald P, Jankovic J. Tardive oculogyric crises. Neurology 1989;39:1434–1437.

74. Sachdev P. The association of tardive oculogyric crises with obsessional thoughts. Br J Psychiatry 1991;158:720–721.

75. Burke R, Kang U. Tardive dystonia: clinical aspects and treatment. In: Jankovic J, Tolosa E, eds. Facial dyskinesias. New York: Raven, 1988.

76. Hyman S, Arana G, Rosenbaum J. Handbook of psychiatric drug therapy. Boston: Little, Brown, 1995.

77. Korczyn AD, Goldberg GJ. Intravenous diazepam in drug-induced dystonic reactions. Br J Psychiatry 1972;121:75–77.

78. Cummings J. Psychosomatic aspects of movement disorders. Adv Psychosom Med 1985;13:111–132.

79. DePotter R, Linkowski P, Mendlewicz J. State-dependent tardive dyskinesia in manic-depressive illness. J Neurol Neurosurg Psychiatry 1983;46:666–668.

80. Cutler N, Post R. State-related dyskinesias in manic-depressive illness. J Clin Psychopharmacol 1982;2:350–354.

81. Weiner W, Werner T. Mania-induced remission of tardive dyskinesia in manic-depressive illness. Ann Neurol 1982;12:229–230.

82. Marsden C, Jenner P. The pathophysiology of extrapyramidal side-effects of neuroleptic drugs. Psychol Med 1980;10:55–72.

83. King W, Leigh R. Rhysiology of vertical gaze. In: Lennerstrand G, Zee D, Zeller E, eds. Functional basis of ocular motility disorders. Oxford: Pergamon Press, 1982.

84. Devinsky O. Neuroanatomy of Gilles de la Tourette's syndrome: possible midbrain involvement. Arch Neurol 1983;40:508–514.

85. Meldrum B, Anlezark G, Marsden C. Acute dystonia as an idiosyncratic response to neuroleptics in baboons. Brain 1977;100:313–326.

86. Garver D, Davis J, Dekirmenjian H, et al. Pharmacokinetics of red blood cell phenothiazine and clinical effects: acute dystonic reactions. Arch Gen Psychiatry 1976;33:862–866.

Tardive Dystonia

STANLEY FAHN

INTRODUCTION

The spectrum of the tardive dyskinesia syndromes consists of classic tardive dyskinesia (manifested as rhythmic movements), tardive dystonia, tardive akathisia, and more infrequent disorders of tardive tics and tardive myoclonus (Table 15.1) (1). Distinctions among them not only depend on the clinical phenomena making each one unique, but also on their natural history, their characteristic susceptibility related to age and gender, and their clinical pharmacology. Why there should be separate tardive entities when all have the same etiology, namely, exposure to dopamine receptor blocking agents (DRBA), is unknown. The scope of this chapter will be solely on tardive dystonia.

CLINICAL FEATURES

The seminal paper making tardive dystonia a distinct entity was that of Burke et al in 1982 (2). Although persistent dystonic movements as a complication of DRBA had been noted previously (3), the feature of dystonia was not recognized as representing a distinct form of the tardive dyskinesia spectrum. Studies have now elucidated that it has a different epidemiology, pharmacology, and natural history (4). It is important to distinguish between acute dystonic reactions and tardive dystonia, both of which occur as a complication of DRBA (Table 15.1). Acute dystonic reactions were well characterized shortly after the introduction of DRBA into clinical psychiatry. Acute dystonic reactions occur in the first few days after administration of these drugs, affecting predominantly children and young adults, and males more often than females (5). Acute dystonic reactions fade within a couple of days if left untreated (responding dramatically to parenteral anticholinergics, antihistaminics, or benzodiazepines). Tardive dystonia tends to

occur after chronic use of DRBA, even though it has been reported to occur in one patient after only 3 weeks (2), and it persists. It is also difficult to treat, and does not respond acutely to parenteral anticholinergics, antihistaminics, or benzodiazepines.

In the chapter on idiopathic torsion dystonia (Fahn, Chapter 77), it is noted that idiopathic dystonia affects all ages, tending to progress with childhood onset to involve many body parts (generalized dystonia) and to remain local or segmental with adult onset. The clinical appearance of tardive dystonia is very similar. However, opisthotonic posturing and retrocollis tend to be more common in tardive than in idiopathic dystonia (4). Another clinical feature separating the two is that some patients with generalized tardive dystonia obtain some relief by walking, whereas generalized idiopathic dystonia is usually exacerbated by walking. The most common site for tardive dystonia is the cranial and neck region, both in children and in adults. For idiopathic dystonia, the most common site in adults is also the cranial and cervical region, but in children involvement is mainly in the legs, trunk, and arms.

In contrast to the predilection for adult onset of classic tardive dyskinesia, which appears as rhythmic movements, tardive dystonia affects all ages, with a mean of about 40 years (4). There is no apparent age preference, in contrast to the bimodal distribution of idiopathic torsion dystonia with one early peak in childhood and another later peak in adulthood (6). Like idiopathic dystonia, both genders are equally affected, but men have a slightly younger age of onset than women (4). Children may have leg involvement and a generalized form of dystonia, whereas adults tend to have focal and segmental dystonia (4), thereby resembling symptoms of idiopathic dystonia. Tardive dystonia appears to be less common than classic tardive dyskinesia. The prevalence of tardive dystonia in chronic psychiatric inpatients has been

Table 15.1 Neurologic Complications of Dopamine Receptor Blocking Agents

Acute syndromes
   Acute dystonic reaction
   Acute akathisia
Drug-induced parkinsonism
Neuroleptic malignant syndrome
Tardive dyskinesia syndromes
   Classic chorea (withdrawal emergent syndrome)
   Rhythmic movements (classic tardive dyskinesia)
   Persistent dystonia (tardive dystonia)
   Persistent akathisia (tardive akathisia)
   Persistent myoclonus (tardive myoclonus)

reported to be between 1.5% and 2% (7,8). In the series reported by Kang et al (4), the duration of exposure to DRBA ranged from 3 weeks to 40 years, with a mean of 7 years. Twenty percent of patients with tardive dystonia had developed this disorder within 1 year of exposure.

Often patients with tardive dystonia have features of other tardive syndromes, particularly classic tardive dyskinesia (rhythmic movements) and tardive akathisia. The presence of these other clinical phenomena aids in the differential diagnosis of tardive dystonia versus idiopathic dystonia. Tardive akathisia and tardive dystonia are usually the most disabling of the tardive syndromes.

TREATMENT

The treatment strategies for tardive dystonia are derived from the treatment approaches for idiopathic dystonia on the one hand and for classic tardive dyskinesia on the other. As with tardive dyskinesia, it is important to discontinue the offending DRBA if clinically possible. If it is not possible, then this drug should be continued at the lowest affective dosage, and a dopamine depleter, such as reserpine or tetrabenazine, added. If the DRBA can be discontinued, one can either treat with reserpine (or tetrabenazine) or with high-dosage anticholinergics. Approximately 50% of patients respond to dopamine depleters, and slightly less to anticholinergics (4).

If a patient requires continuing use of an antipsychotic drug, it seems prudent to reduce the dosage to as low a level as clinically feasible, then add a dopamine depleter to control the tardive dystonia.

REFERENCES

1. Fahn S. The tardive dyskinesias. In: Mathews WB, Glaser GH, eds. Recent advances in clinical neurology, vol. 4. Edinburgh: Churchill Livingstone, 1984:229–260.
2. Burke RE, Fahn S, Jankovic J, et al. Tardive dystonia: late-onset and persistent dystonia caused by antipsychotic drugs. Neurology 1982;32:1335–1346.
3. Druckman R, Seelinger D, Thulin B. Chronic involuntary movements induced by phenothiazines. J Nerv Ment Dis 1962;135:69–76.
4. Kang UJ, Burke RE, Fahn S. Natural history and treatment of tardive dystonia. Mov Disord 1986;1:193–208.
5. Ayd FJ Jr. A survey of drug-induced extrapyramidal reactions. JAMA 1961;175:1054–1060.
6. Fahn S. Concept and classification of dystonia. In: Fahn S, Marsden CD, Calne DB, eds. Advances in neurology, vol. 50, Dystonia 2. New York: Raven, 1988:1–8.
7. Yassa R, Nair V, Dimitry R. Prevalence of tardive dystonia. Acta Psychiatr Scand 1986;73:629–633.
8. Friedman JH, Kucharski LT, Wagner RL. Tardive dystonia in a psychiatric hospital. J Neurol Neurosurg Psychiatry 1986;50:801–803.

Neuroleptic Malignant Syndrome

ANTHONY L. PELONERO   JAMES L. LEVENSON   ANANDA K. PANDURANGI

HISTORY

Neuroleptic malignant syndrome (NMS) is an uncommon adverse side effect of antipsychotic drugs. The syndrome is characterized by severe rigidity, tremor, fever, altered mental status, autonomic dysfunction, and elevated serum creatine phosphokinase (CPK) and white blood cell count (WBC). Neuroleptics, introduced for clinical use in 1952, were first reported to have caused such a syndrome by Delay et al (1). The syndrome's name derives from the French *syndrome malin des neuroleptiques*, which translates into English as neuroleptic malignant syndrome (2).

Many case reports of NMS, from many countries, have been published since the 1960s, and similar syndromes that were described early in the neuroleptic era may in retrospect have been cases of NMS that were not termed as such (2). A number of excellent reviews on NMS have been published, including those by Kurlan (3), Levenson (4), Pearlman (5), Addonizio et al (6), Lazarus et al (2), and Shalev et al (7). NMS is a severe, life-threatening condition, and the patient will often appear acutely ill; it can be difficult to diagnose and treat, and complicates further psychiatric treatment.

INCIDENCE AND DEMOGRAPHICS

Although NMS was originally thought to be rare, a number of case reports and other studies has created a different impression. Systematic retrospective estimates of incidence vary from 0.02% to 3.23% of psychiatric inpatients receiving neuroleptics (2). This wide variation results from differences in diagnostic criteria for NMS, patient populations sampled (e.g., acute versus chronic mentally ill), hospital type (e.g., state hospital versus university), and treatment style (e.g., high- versus low-dose neuroleptics), as well as the lim-

itations of retrospective study designs. Prospective studies in two different Boston psychiatric hospitals found NMS incidence rates of 0.07% and 0.9% (8,9). A prospective study of inpatients treated with neuroleptics at a large psychiatric hospital in China determined an NMS rate of 0.12% (12 of 9,792 patients), or 1.23 cases per 1,000 inpatients exposed to neuroleptics (10). A survey comparing consecutive 31-month and 47-month intervals during 1984–1990 found a "nearly tenfold decrease" in estimated frequency, from 1.10% ± 0.40% to 0.15% ± 0.05%. The decrease was attributed to greater awareness, early detection and treatment of medication side effects, and decreased risk factors (11). In any case, the incidence will always vary in a given patient population depending on the frequency of risk factors.

NMS has been reported in patients of all ages, and about twice as often in men than in women. Most cases have occurred in patients between the ages of 20 and 50 years, likely paralleling peak neuroleptic use. There is usually a history of neuroleptic therapy in patients with suspected NMS, but not always. Virtually all neuroleptics are capable of inducing NMS, including the atypical antipsychotic clozapine (12,13). Risperidone, an antipsychotic with serotonin and dopamine D_2 blocking activity, has also been the focus of a number of case reports associating the drug with NMS (14–16). The antiemetic metoclopramide (17–19) and amoxapine, a tricyclic antidepressant, have also been reported to cause NMS (20,21), presumably because of their dopamine-blocking properties.

Underlying diagnoses most commonly are schizophrenia or affective disorders, but NMS also occurs in other conditions where neuroleptics have been used, including dementia, delirium, other psychoses, mental retardation, and anxiety disorders. NMS (or very similar syndromes) has also been reported in patients with extrapyramidal disorders, including Parkinson's disease, Wilson's disease, Huntington's chorea, and striatonigral degeneration, who have received neuroleptics or dopamine depleting agents or have had dopamine agonists abruptly withdrawn (22–25).

CLINICAL EVALUATION

Both physiologic and environmental factors have been suggested to predispose for the development of NMS. High on the list of conditions suspected to promote NMS is dehydration (26,27). Patients with prior episodes of NMS are at higher risk. Receiving high doses of neuroleptics, especially by intramuscular injection, may also be a risk factor for NMS (28). However, Lazarus et al (2) concluded that NMS appeared not to be dose related, often occurring at therapeutic levels. Other suggested risk factors include a rapid rate of neuroleptic loading, depot neuroleptics, prolonged use of restraints, receiving other medications with neuroleptics (especially lithium), poorly controlled neuroleptic-induced extrapyramidal symptoms (EPS), treatment-resistant EPS, withdrawal of antiparkinsonian medications, an affective disorder diagnosis, alcoholism, phase of menstrual cycle (29), organic brain syndrome or previous brain injury, primary extrapyramidal disorder (e.g., Parkinson's disease, Huntington's disease), iron deficiency, and catatonia. Although there have been reports of familial clustering (30), genetically transmitted risk for NMS has not been considered clinically significant.

On physical examination, patients with NMS will typically have fever (>37°C), muscle rigidity, altered consciousness, and autonomic dysfunction. Muscle rigidity that is unresponsive to anticholinergic treatment may be the first sign of NMS or may be simultaneously identified with increased temperature. Rigidity may range from muscle hypertonicity to severe, lead pipe rigidity. Parkinsonian findings are common in NMS, but other movement disorders may be present at the same time (3). Neurologic dysfunction may include tremors, abnormal reflexes, bradykinesia, chorea, dystonias (including opisthotonos, trismus, blepharospasm, and oculogyric crisis), nystagmus and opsoclonus, dysphagia, dysarthria, aphonia, and seizures.

Altered consciousness may range from a decreased awareness of one's surroundings or confusion to obtundation or total unresponsiveness. Other mental status abnormalities may occur, such as agitation or delirium, and the distinction between what mental abnormalities are from the original psychiatric illness and what are due to NMS can be difficult.

Autonomic dysfunction in NMS is manifested in a number of findings. Hypertension, postural hypotension, and labile blood pressure are often identified along with tachycardia and tachypnea when measuring vital signs. Other autonomic disturbances may consist of sialorrhea, diaphoresis, skin pallor, and urinary incontinence. Physical signs of dehydration, such as dry mucous membranes, sunken eyes,

and increased skin turgor, are important to note. Myoglobinuria may be revealed by dark urine that does not contain red blood cells.

In the diagnostic evaluation of suspected NMS, in addition to a careful history and physical examination, physicians will usually find it helpful to obtain a number of laboratory examinations. CPK levels are often elevated in NMS secondary to skeletal muscle damage, and can reach very high levels (>100,000). CPK may also be elevated by the use of intramuscular injections or restraints in the psychiatric patient, but usually at lower levels (<600) than in NMS. Serial CPK measurements obtained during treatment of a patient with NMS will typically show falling levels with resolution of the syndrome. Falling CPK levels concurrent with fever spikes correctly led to a search for infection in a patient with NMS and acquired immune deficiency syndrome (31). WBC is often elevated, with a range between 10,000 and 40,000/mm^3 commonly reported; a WBC shift to the left may or may not be found.

In addition to CPK level and WBC, other important tests to rule out other etiologies of the symptoms include urinalysis; electrolytes, including calcium and magnesium; kidney, liver, and thyroid function tests; lumbar puncture; electroencephalogram (EEG); and computed tomography (CT) or magnetic resonance imaging (MRI) scan of the head. Other studies such as blood gases, coagulation studies, blood cultures, toxicology screen, and determination of serum lithium level should be done if appropriate. Electromyography and muscle biopsy are not useful, often showing only nonspecific changes, if any.

DIAGNOSIS

Diagnostic criteria have been proposed for NMS; however, this is somewhat of a controversial area among investigators. A number of systems have been suggested for diagnosing NMS (4,32–34). Diagnostic criteria evolved in the literature as case reporting grew and series of cases were reviewed. Lazarus et al (2) concluded that "hyperthermia and muscle rigidity are cardinal features of NMS" (p. 23) and proposed their own set of criteria, consisting of treatment with neuroleptics within 7 days prior to onset of the syndrome, hyperthermia, muscle rigidity, the exclusion of systemic or neuropsychiatric illness that could account for the syndrome, and three of the following: change in mental status, tachycardia, change in blood pressure, tachypnea, CPK elevation or myoglobinuria, leukocytosis, and metabolic acidosis.

Patients believed to be in the early stages of NMS have been described, as have patients with mild forms of NMS that did not progress to the full-blown syndrome, some despite continued neuroleptic therapy (35–37). With the current diagnostic criteria for NMS, some of these cases would not qualify for the diagnosis, although withdrawing the offending neuroleptic is still advisable if early NMS is suspected. We are not at the point of being able to say who will develop full-blown NMS, and the risk of morbidity and even mortality deserves serious consideration.

Differential Diagnosis

The majority of patients receiving neuroleptics who develop fever and rigidity will have conditions other than NMS, making the differential diagnosis of prime importance. Although active steps must be taken to rule out other conditions, NMS should not be regarded entirely as a diagnosis of exclusion because of the importance of promptly withholding neuroleptics in cases where NMS is suspected. At the same time, physicians must be careful not to conclude prematurely that the diagnosis is NMS in patients who may have a medical cause for a fever (e.g., aspiration pneumonia) superimposed on neuroleptic-induced EPS (38).

A very large number of conditions could be considered in the differential diagnosis of NMS if each sign, particularly fever or catatonia, were examined individually. Here we will focus on those conditions that may present with several or even all the signs of NMS (Table 16.1). Malignant hyperthermia (MH) is a hypermetabolic state of skeletal muscle most frequently associated with the administration of halogenated inhalation anesthetic agents and succinylcholine. Originally thought to be an autosomal dominant trait, MH is now viewed as having a multifactorial pattern of inheritance. The clinical presentation is identical to NMS, and rhabdomyolysis and death are common outcomes. Intravenous dantrolene sodium is specifically therapeutic in MH, and oral dantrolene is effective as preoperative prophylaxis. The diagnosis of MH (or of the trait) is reliably established by exposing biopsied muscle tissue to caffeine or halothane in vitro, which results in a hypercontractile response when compared with normal muscle. Muscle tissue from NMS patients does not demonstrate the same effect. In most cases NMS and MH can be distinguished clinically by the different settings and drug exposures. In addition, no family histories of hyperthermia have been documented in patients with NMS. Cross-reactivity between triggering agents has not been found (39).

Table 16.1   Differential Diagnosis of NMS

Malignant hyperthermia
Lethal catatonia
Heatstroke
Severe extrapyramidal reactions
CNS infections
CNS mass lesions
Allergic drug reactions
Toxic encephalopathies
Hyperthyroidism
Tetany
Parkinson's disease and other neurologic disorders

Lethal catatonia is a syndrome in which mutism, extreme motor excitement, clouding of consciousness, and fever may progress to severe autonomic disturbances, stupor and coma, and death. Mann et al (40) have suggested that lethal catatonia should be regarded as a final common pathway for a variety of psychiatric and medical illnesses. They conceptualize NMS as one (iatrogenic) cause of lethal catatonia. Others regard functional lethal catatonia and NMS as separate entities that can be clinically differentiated, pointing out, among other differences, that lethal catatonia begins with extreme psychotic excitement, whereas NMS begins with severe muscle rigidity (41). Whatever the relationship is between NMS and lethal catatonia, in practice the distinction may be very difficult if not impossible (42). In any case, neuroleptics should be discontinued since they are usually ineffective in lethal (or severe) catatonia (2,40).

Neuroleptics may cause other adverse effects that may be confused with NMS. Heatstroke is a risk because neuroleptics suppress central heat loss mechanisms, resulting in increased vulnerability to hot environments and marked exertion. Although hot environmental conditions may increase the risk for NMS (43), most cases of NMS have occurred under normal temperature conditions. Heatstroke is also distinguished by hot, dry skin, rather than the diaphoresis seen in NMS, and by the absence of rigidity.

Neuroleptics can cause severe EPS, even resulting in rhabdomyolysis (4) or catatonia (44), but such patients do not manifest marked fever, leukocytosis, or autonomic disturbances unless a secondary complication has developed such as infection or pulmonary embolus. Causes of rhabdomyolysis other than NMS or severe dystonia that are frequent in severely ill psychiatric patients include immobilization, restraints, dehydration, malnutrition, multiple intramuscular injections, alcoholism, and trauma.

Central nervous system (CNS) infections, including meningitis, encephalitis, or neurosyphilis, may mimic NMS. Lumbar puncture and EEG should lead to the distinction. Except for a few cases of slightly elevated cerebrospinal fluid (CSF) protein, the CSF in NMS does not demonstrate the changes in glucose, white cells, or protein expected in CNS infections. A CT or MRI scan is useful in ruling out brain abscesses and other structural lesions.

Allergic drug reactions may produce fever and autonomic instability but not rigidity. Signs of allergy should be looked for, including rash, wheezing, urticaria, and eosinophilia. Various toxic encephalopathies may resemble NMS, including those due to strychnine, tetanus, botulism, anticholinergic delirium, lithium toxicity, and hyperthermia induced by other psychotropic drugs (tricyclic antidepressants, monoamine oxidase inhibitors, stimulants, and hallucinogens) (2). NMS itself may be viewed as a toxic encephalopathy. Hyperthyroidism and hypocalcemic or hypomagnesemic tetany must also be considered and are easily tested for. Parkinson's disease and other neurologic disorders may include rigidity, trauma, and autonomic neuropathy but not leukocytosis, fever, or elevated CPK.

A diagnosis of NMS must first be considered before specific treatments of the syndrome can be implemented. A thorough evaluation as suggested should enable the clinician to rule out the many neurologic, toxic, infectious, or metabolic causes with similar clinical pictures. Work-up also serves to identify possible concurrent medical illnesses and complications of NMS.

COMPLICATIONS

As implied by the use of the word *malignant* in NMS, death as a result of NMS or its life-threatening complications may occur. Levinson and Simpson (38) reported that 79% of NMS patients make a full recovery; the mortality in their series was 8%. Temporally reviewing 202 case reports, Shalev et al (7) noted a decreasing mortality of 11.6%, probably attributable to better recognition of the syndrome and earlier intervention. In their review, NMS patients with organic mental disorders had significantly higher mortality than patients with functional psychoses, as did patients who developed myoglobinuria and renal failure.

Complications of NMS are often physiologic consequences of severe rigidity and the immobilization that comes with it. Poor oral intake leads to dehydration, increasing the risk of rhabdomyolysis, which in turn may lead to acute renal failure. Deep venous thrombosis and pulmonary embolism may occur as other consequences of rigidity, immobilization, and dehydration, and account for about one-fourth of fatalities in NMS (45). Difficulty swallowing combined with altered mental status may lead to aspiration and pneumonia, and patients may need to be intubated and receive ventilatory support. Other causes of pulmonary failure include adult respiratory distress syndrome (especially with rhabdomyolysis) (46) and shock lung.

Many other serious complications of NMS or its treatment have been reported; myocardial infarction, disseminated intravascular coagulation, and sepsis are examples (4). Cerebellar neuronal degeneration has been attributed to hyperpyrexia from NMS (47). Persons with lithium in their system during NMS, even at nontoxic levels, may be particularly at risk for cerebellar damage and ataxia from hyperthermia (2). Indeed, a range of persistent neurologic abnormalities after resolution of NMS is possible, including neuropsychological (cognitive) impairments (48). Most patients recover from NMS without any cognitive impairment, and new dysfunction usually is attributable to very high fever, hypoxia, or other complications, rather than to NMS per se.

TREATMENT

Stopping neuroleptic treatment is of primary importance. After recognition and discontinuation of neuroleptics, the usual clinical course of NMS runs 2 to 14 days (2,6).

Prolonged cases have occurred in patients who received long-acting preparations (49). Discontinuation of anticholinergics and lithium is also recommended. Dopamine agonist medications such as amantadine, however, should be continued if already in use; their withdrawal may worsen the NMS.

Many patients require a high level of supportive care in an intensive care unit, including antipyretics, cooling blanket, oxygen, intravenous fluids to correct dehydration and electrolyte abnormalities, and antihypertensive treatment. Some patients require intubation and ventilator support. Subcutaneous heparin is recommended to guard against deep venous thrombosis and pulmonary embolism. Dialysis may be needed if renal failure develops, but is ineffective for removing neuroleptics because they are strongly protein bound.

Attention to nutritional support is important because most patients cannot eat due to altered mental status or rigidity with esophageal spasm, and may have already been malnourished before developing NMS. NMS is a very stressful syndrome, particularly because of increased body temperature and the energy expenditure of prolonged rigidity, and good nutrition helps minimize rhabdomyolysis and other tissue damage.

It is important to make an analysis of the risks versus the benefits of drug treatment before initiating pharmacotherapy for NMS. We recommend starting supportive care first and observing for 1 to 3 days; if the patient's condition does not improve or worsens, then consider pharmacologic interventions. A patient may benefit from supportive treatment alone without risking further morbidity. In other words, the temptation to rush into drug treatment should be regarded with some skepticism.

A number of somatic treatments have been tried for NMS, with mixed results. The dopamine agonists bromocriptine, amantadine, apomorphine, lisuride, and carbidopa-levodopa have a theoretical and clinical rationale in the treatment of NMS, and there are many case reports supporting their use. Bromocriptine may be the preferred choice of these dopamine agonists (2).

Dantrolene, a muscle relaxant, has been used in NMS based on its efficacy in malignant hyperthermia. Dantrolene is specifically recommended for severe hyperthermia, and may relieve this by relaxing skeletal muscle. Dantrolene can cause a drug-induced hepatitis; therefore, liver function tests should be checked during its use. The simultaneous use of bromocriptine and dantrolene for an individual with NMS may be warranted. Bromocriptine is usually given in divided doses of 7.5–45.0 mg per day. Dantrolene can be given by intravenous bolus, 1–10 mg per kilogram, or orally in divided doses of 50–600 mg per day (2).

Due to the absence of controlled studies of drug therapy for NMS, the reported effectiveness of specific drug treatments may be illusory. Rosenberg and Green (50) found that the "addition of dantrolene or bromocriptine significantly shortened the time to clinical response," whereas a prospective series of 24 cases did not find bromocriptine or dantrolene markedly important in bringing about improvement (51). A case-control analysis of 734 cases by Sakkas et al (52) concluded that dantrolene, bromocriptine, and amantidine seemed to be most effective in treating NMS.

Other somatic treatments tried with mixed results include benzodiazepines, barbiturates, verapamil, and curare. Electroconvulsive therapy (ECT) has received much attention as a treatment for NMS, with mixed results, and for the underlying psychiatric condition, with good results (53). The length of treatment is often about 10 days; medications and other therapies are gradually withdrawn while recovery is monitored via vital signs, CPK levels, and other features that were abnormal for that particular individual.

Re-treatment of the Primary Illness

Psychosis itself carries severe morbidity and significant risk of mortality, and restarting neuroleptics in a patient who has experienced NMS may be necessary due to continued psychiatric illness (54). Before resuming antipsychotic therapy, however, first consider non-neuroleptic therapies, such as lithium, carbamazepine, or ECT. Note that there have been a few cases of NMS attributed to the atypical antipsychotic drug clozapine (12,13). Should restarting a neuroleptic be deemed necessary, switch to a neuroleptic in a different chemical class and with a lower D_2 affinity than the one that produced the NMS. The availability of the serotonin-dopamine antagonist antipsychotics (SDA) clearly has increased the number of treatment options. It should be noted, though, that both risperidone and clozapine have been associated with cases of NMS (14,55). Based on case report literature, clozapine may be the preferred antipsychotic for patients in whose treatment a neuroleptic is essential. However, this entails exposing the patient to the serious risks associated with clozapine, such as seizure and agranulocytosis.

Monitoring vital signs and CPK level is advisable to identify NMS relapse early in order to stop the neuroleptic as soon as possible. In any case, re-treatment with neuroleptics should be reserved for those patients with a clear-cut psychosis. A discussion of the risks and benefits of re-treatment with the patient and his or her family is advisable, and obtaining informed consent may be prudent.

A review of 41 cases of neuroleptic therapy following resolution of NMS reported that the risk of relapse was less if at least 5 days passed from recovery to rechallenge (56). There was no relation with patient age, sex, or the drug used. Susman and Addonizio (57) suggested that the use of high-potency neuroleptics is possibly a risk factor for recurrence and also stressed the need for complete recovery from NMS before reintroducing a neuroleptic. Rosebush et al (58) recommend a minimum of 2 weeks after recovery of NMS before reintroducing neuroleptics and found potency and dosage less important than time factor. Lazarus et al (2)

concluded in their review that "recurrences appear to correlate more closely with the dopamine antagonist potency of the drug involved."

Although fatal recurrences have been reported (27), patients can have neuroleptics reintroduced safely with monitoring. After discharge from a hospital, long-term outcome after NMS can be good, even with continued neuroleptic therapy for primary psychiatric illness (59).

PREVENTION

Decreasing the putative risk factors for NMS includes early detection and treatment of neuroleptic-induced side effects. Avoidance of dehydration, of physical restraints for long durations, and of numerous intramuscular injections also decreases risk. Fostering nutrition along with hydration is recommended.

Early recognition of the syndrome can limit morbidity, but the clinician must have an index of suspicion for early recognition. Gelenberg et al (60) stressed the importance of screening for a history of NMS in patients being readmitted to a hospital for psychiatric treatment. Additionally, there has been the suggestion that vunerability to NMS may be familial (30); a family history of NMS should be heeded.

Some psychiatrists and anesthesiologists remain fearful about anesthetizing patients who have a history of NMS; however, it has now been well documented that patients who have had NMS are at no extra risk from anesthesia (59,61).

THE BIOLOGY OF NMS

The pathophysiology of NMS remains to be fully understood. Reduced dopaminergic activity secondary to neuroleptic-induced dopamine blockade has been considered as mediating the symptoms of NMS since the early recognition of this syndrome, and remains the most viable and accepted theoretical explanation. However, this theory is limited in that it does not explain why NMS occurs in a very small number within the large population of patients who receive neuroleptics and other dopamine-blocking drugs. Thus, other factors critical to initiating the syndrome or facilitating the progression of isolated symptoms have to be invoked to explain its idiosyncratic occurrence. These might include genetic, constitutional, environmental, and iatrogenic pharmacologic factors. Few studies have been designed to address or define the role of such factors.

Genetic, constitutional, or immunological mechanisms are suggested by case reports of previously physically healthy persons developing NMS after a single dose of neuroleptic (5,30,62). Whereas Iwahashi et al (63) found evidence in a single case to suggest polymorphism of the gene for CYP450 2D6 in a patient with NMS, Ueno et al (64) could not replicate this in a series of nine patients. Horn et al (65) reported necrosis in the anterior and lateral hypothalamic nuclei of a patient with NMS, and Gertz et al (66) found low melanin content in the substantia nigra of a young patient with schizophrenia who succumbed to NMS. In a case-control study, Keck et al (28) confirmed that psychomotor agitation, dosage of neuroleptic administered, number of intramuscular injections, and rate of neuroleptic dosage increase were all significant factors associated with NMS. The exact manner in which these factors operate or whether they are even necessary for NMS remains to be established.

Another question in understanding the pathophysiology of NMS is the sequence in which the various components of the syndrome develop. For example, if muscular rigidity were the first sign, extrapyramidally mediated CNS dopaminergic dysfunction can account for it. Subsequent hyperthermia could be secondary to muscle-related peripheral mechanisms of heat generation. On the other hand, if the rise in temperature were the first manifestation, both endogenous central thermodysregulation and exogenous factors such as dehydration and excessive motor activity (often seen in patients prior to developing NMS) might cause the hyperthermia. Hyperthermia in turn might, by inactivating the regulatory protein GTP (guanosine 5′-triphosphate), enhance neuroleptic binding to the dopamine receptors (67), leading to excessive rigidity. Addonizio et al (6) concluded from their retrospective review of NMS cases that in most patients EPS occurs before temperature rise, suggesting that muscle contraction was a factor in the hyperthermia. Mental changes and EPS were also found to be the initial manifestations in another review of 153 cases of NMS (68). Further prospective study is needed and should include the course and outcome of patients who develop incomplete forms of NMS. A better understanding of the pathophysiologic sequence of NMS could enlighten pharmacotherapy.

Previous reviews of NMS (2,3) have discussed in detail human temperature-regulating mechanisms. It has been recognized that dopamine plays a major role in the hypothalamic regulation of temperature. If these mechanisms are interfered with by the administration of neuroleptics or withdrawal of dopaminergic agents, hyperthermia can result. Weinberg and Twersky (69) have suggested that heat-dissipating systems such as vasodilation may be impaired in NMS. Dopamine receptors may be instrumental in mediating some responses involved in thermoregulation, and blockade of these receptors by neuroleptics may alter this regulation, resulting in hyperthermia as seen in NMS patients (3). To date there are no direct studies of temperature regulation in NMS patients.

The extrapyramidal effects of neuroleptic drugs mediated by their ability to block the D_2 receptor in the striatum are well recognized, but why does the rigidity in NMS not respond to the usual anticholinergic drugs? Several possible explanations can be considered: the rigidity of NMS is so severe that it does not respond to the usual doses of anticholinergics, or the presence of hyperthermia perpetuates

rigidity and renders these drugs ineffective, or the rigidity seen in NMS is qualitatively different from that seen commonly in the neuroleptic-induced acute parkinsonian syndrome.

Striatal and hypothalamic dopamine receptor blockade may both be involved in NMS (44). In addition to the case report–based epidemiological data, several other lines of evidence support the involvement of dopaminergic blockade in NMS, and there is not much controversy regarding this. Toru et al (70) reported NMS-like states following withdrawal of antiparkinsonian drugs. Verhoeven et al (71) reported decreased CSF homovanillic acid (HVA) in a patient with NMS, whereas Tollefson and Garvey (72) reported a case where there was decreased HVA but increased 3,4,dihydroxyphenyl acetic acid. Nisijima and colleagues (73,74) reported that HVA levels in the CSF of patients during the active phase of NMS and after recovery were significantly decreased compared with those of the controls. This contrasts with our knowledge that HVA rises in CSF following acute neuroleptic treatment in non-NMS patients (75) and might return to normal or decrease when treatment is continued over a long period of time. Nisijima et al (73,74) emphasize the reduction in HVA levels in these patients within a short period of 3 weeks and suggest that this unusual finding may be a characteristic finding in active NMS. These authors also studied other monoamine metabolites and report that whereas levels of 5-hydroxyindoleacetic acid (a serotonin metabolite) were insignificantly decreased during the active phase of NMS and remained decreased after improvement compared with controls, noradrenaline levels were slightly higher during active phase and returned to normal after recovery from NMS. Levels of γ-aminobutyric acid (GABA) were significantly lower. It is well known that prolactin is under the direct inhibitory control of hypothalamic dopamine; studies on prolactin would provide a test of these dopamine tracts and complement metabolic studies. We are aware of a single case report where serum prolactin was followed (76). Finally, the therapeutic benefit reportedly obtained in patients with NMS from bromocriptine, a direct dopamine agonist, would also support the dopamine theory of NMS, although there are no controlled studies of this treatment.

Other neurotransmitter abnormalities in NMS in addition to dopaminergic dysfunction have been considered. Feibel and Schiffer (77) and Gurrera and Romero (78) have reported elevated plasma and urinary catecholamines in a patient with NMS. A hypernoradrenergic state might be a factor in NMS and may explain the cardiovascular instability. Lew and Tollefson (79) have suggested mechanisms involving GABA because of the effectiveness of benzodiazepines in some cases of NMS. They suggest that benzodiazepines may have an indirect dopaminergic effect mediated by GABA. Increased cholinergic activity and relative imbalance in the norepinephrine-dopamine ratio have also been suggested in NMS. The data to support these theories are so far weak.

In view of the clinical similarities between MH and NMS, the presence of a primary skeletal muscle pathologic condition in NMS has been investigated. There are conflicting results in this regard. Some investigators (80,81) have found abnormal contractile response of muscle tissue from NMS subjects to halothane and fluphenazine, whereas others have not (82–84). It is unlikely that NMS is a variant of MH, given the safety with which NMS patients have received anesthesia and the safety with which MH patients have received neuroleptics. Kurlan et al (3) noted that research has demonstrated that "phenothiazines produce complex effects on muscle, including displacement of membrane-bound calcium ions, antagonism of calmodulin, uncoupling of mitochondrial oxidation, and perturbation of glucose and cholesterol metabolism" (p. 117). They wonder whether any of these mechanisms are linked to the pathogenesis of NMS. We are currently unable to answer these questions.

LEGAL ISSUES

Although the legal issues surroundings NMS are not unique, they are worthy of careful consideration. Malpractice litigation regarding NMS is quite common, though little attention has been paid to this in the literature (85,86). The dramatic symptom picture, the associated morbidity and mortality, and the name of the syndrome itself all seem to draw the interest of plaintiffs' attorneys. As one would expect, NMS lawsuits range from those that appear justified to the spurious and frivolous. An example of the former would be the continued administration of neuroleptics, especially by IM injection, despite the development of full-blown symptoms of NMS and even after a consultant's suggestion that NMS be considered. At the other end of the spectrum, some attorneys and their expert witnesses will see NMS lurking behind any catastrophic outcome in a psychotic patient receiving neuroleptics, particularly if fever or rigidity has occurred. Physicians have been sued for not using dantrolene or bromocriptine to treat NMS, or for not using them "quickly enough" or in "sufficiently high doses" (in the opinion of the plaintiff's expert witness). Other litigation has questioned the use of neuroleptics in patients who had a prior history of NMS or NMS-like symptoms.

For clinical as well as risk management reasons, we would advise the following steps whenever NMS is considered a possibility. Seek early consultation from psychiatric and medical or neurological colleagues. Document a broad differential diagnosis and rationally narrow it down. Whenever NMS is seriously under consideration it is best to consider withholding neuroleptics, keeping in mind that the risks of continuing neuroleptics must be weighed against the risks of withholding them (i.e., the patient's danger to self and others). Given the circumstances under which NMS develops, the clinician may feel too busy to worry about the paperwork, but documentation of one's thinking will reduce

liability risk and need not be tediously detailed. Although patients with mild symptoms suggestive of possible NMS may be appropriately managed in psychiatric settings, more seriously ill patients should be transferred out of freestanding psychiatric hospitals to general hospitals where expertise in psychiatry, neurology, and critical care is available (87). Informing families during or after an episode of NMS (and patients who have sufficiently recovered) is also an important step in eliminating the misunderstandings that are the breeding ground for future lawsuits. Are physicians who prescribe neuroleptics obligated to inform patients about the risk of NMS? Acutely psychotic patients are often incapable of sufficient understanding. Since NMS is rare and its onset unpredictable, the value of warning patients about NMS is questionable. It would be more sensible to inform patients about the importance of reporting high fever, rigidity, or abnormal movements.

Physicians who serve as expert witnesses in cases where mismanagement is alleged should retain objectivity and humility, eschewing 20/20 hindsight. There is no test that can definitively rule NMS in or out. In our opinion, there is no proven specific treatment for NMS, despite statements in the literature to the contrary. There is no unanimity among experts regarding the value of dantrolene, bromocriptine, and other "specific" treatments. There is no way to validly predict which patients will develop a first or recurrent episode of NMS. On the other hand, known risk factors should have been heeded and NMS recognized if the symptoms were sufficiently severe. The standard of care for the recognition of NMS has shifted considerably over the past 15 years, with literally hundreds of case reports and reviews throughout the medical literature. NMS belongs in the differential diagnosis of any patient receiving a neuroleptic who develops a high fever or severe rigidity. Finally, although specific treatment remains controversial, supportive treatment is critical and widely supported by consensus (e.g., rapid cooling for extremely high fever, hydration, and apparent anticoagulation).

REFERENCES

1. Delay J, Pichot P, Lemperiere T, et al. Un neuroleptique majeur non phenothiazine et non reserpine, l'haloperidol, dans le traitement des psychoses. Ann Med Psychol 1960;118(1):145–152.
2. Lazarus A, Mann SC, Caroff SN. The neuroleptic malignant syndrome and related conditions. Washington, DC: American Psychiatric, 1989.
3. Kurlan R, Hamill R, Shoullson I. Neuroleptic malignant syndrome. Clin Neuropharmacol 1984;7(2):109–120.
4. Levenson JL. Neuroleptic malignant syndrome. Am J Psychiatry 1985;142(10):1137–1145.
5. Pearlman CA. Neuroleptic malignant syndrome: a review of the literature. J Clin Psychopharmacol 1986;6(5):257–273.
6. Addonizio G, Susman VL, Roth SD. Neuroleptic malignant syndrome: review and analysis of 115 cases. Biol Psychiatry 1987;22(8):1004–1020.
7. Shalev A, Hermesh H, Munitz H. Mortality from neuroleptic malignant syndrome. J Clin Psychiatry 1989;50(1):18–25.
8. Gelenberg AJ, Bellinghausen B, Wojcik JD, et al. A prospective survey of neuroleptic malignant syndrome in a short-term psychiatric hospital. Am J Psychiatry 1988;145(4):517–518.

9. Keck PE, Sebastianelli J, Pope HG, McElroy SL. Frequency and presentation of neuroleptic malignant syndrome in a state psychiatric hospital. J Clin Psychiatry 1989;50(9):352–355.

10. Deng MZ, Chen GQ, Phillips MR. Neuroleptic malignant syndrome in 12 of 9,792 Chinese inpatients exposed to neuroleptics: a prospective study. Am J Psychiatry 1990;147(9):1149–1155.

11. Keck PE, Pope HG, McElroy SL. Declining frequency of neuroleptic malignant syndrome in a hospital population. Am J Psychiatry 1991;148(7):880–882.

12. Pope HG, Cole JO, Choras PT, Fulwiler CE. Apparent neuroleptic malignant syndrome with clozapine and lithium. J Nerv Ment Dis 1986;174(8):493–495.

13. Muller T, Becker T, Fritze J. Neuroleptic malignant syndrome after clozapine plus carbamazepine [letter]. Lancet 1988;2:1500.

14. Dave M. Two cases of risperidone-induced neuroleptic malignant syndrome. Am J Psychiatry 1995;152(8):1233–1234.

15. Singer S, Richards C, Boland RJ. Two cases of risperidone-induced neuroleptic malignant syndrome. Am J Psychiatry 1995;152(8):1234.

16. Najara JE, Enikeev ID. Risperidone and neuroleptic malignant syndrome: a case report [letter]. J Clin Psychiatry 1995;56(11):534–535.

17. Friedman LS, Weinrauch LA, D'Elia JA. Metoclopramide-induced neuroleptic malignant syndrome. Arch Intern Med 1987;147(8):1495–1497.

18. Patterson JF. Neuroleptic malignant syndrome associated with metoclopramide. South Med J 1988;81(5):674–675.

19. Brower RD, Dreyer CF. Neuroleptic malignant syndrome in a child treated with metoclopramide for chemotherapy-related nausea [letter]. J Child Neurol 1989;4(3):230–232.

20. Madakasira S. Amoxapine-induced neuroleptic malignant syndrome. Drug Intell Clin Pharm 1989;23(1):50–55.

21. Taylor NE, Schwartz HI. Neuroleptic malignant syndrome following amoxapine overdose. J Nerv Ment Dis 1988;176(4):249–251.

22. Friedman JH, Feinberg SS, Feldman RG. A neuroleptic malignant-like syndrome due to levodopa therapy withdrawal. JAMA 1985;254(19):2792–2795.

23. Gibb WRG. Neuroleptic malignant syndrome in striatonigral degeneration. Br J Psychiatry 1988;153:254–255.

24. Kontaxakis V, Stefanis C, Markidis M, Tserpe V. Neuroleptic malignant syndrome in a patient with Wilson's disease [letter]. J Neurol Neurosurg Psychiatry 1988;51(7):1001–1002.

25. Bower DJ, Chalasani P, Ammons JC. Withdrawal-induced neuroleptic malignant syndrome [letter]. Am J Psychiatry 1994;151(3):451–452.

26. Itoh H, Ohtsuka N, Ogita K, et al. Malignant neuroleptic syndrome—its present status in Japan and clinical problems. Folia Psychiatrica Neurologica Japonica 1977;31(4):565–576.

27. Harsch HH. Neuroleptic malignant syndrome: physiological and laboratory findings in a series of nine cases. J Clin Psychiatry 1987;48(8):328–333.

28. Keck PE, Pope HG, Cohen BM, et al. Risk factors for neuroleptic malignant syndrome. Arch Gen Psychiatry 1989;46(10):914–918.

29. Mizuta E, Kuno S. Hormones and Parkinson's disease. Reply. Neurology 1995;45(5):1028–1029.

30. Otani K, Horiuchi M, Kondo T, et al. Is the predisposition to neuroleptic malignant syndrome genetically transmitted? Br J Psychiatry 1991;158(6):850–853.

31. Burch EA, Montoya J. Neuroleptic malignant syndrome in an AIDS patient [letter]. J Clin Psychopharmacol 1989;9(3):228–229.

32. Addonizio G, Susman VL, Roth SD. Symptoms of neuroleptic malignant syndrome in 82 consecutive inpatients. Am J Psychiatry 1986;143(12):1587–1590.

33. Roth SD, Addonizio G, Susman VL. Diagnosing and treating neuroleptic malignant syndrome [letter]. Am J Psychiatry 1986;143(5):673.

34. Pope HG, Keck PE Jr, McElroy SL. Frequency and presentation of neuroleptic malignant syndrome in a large psychiatric hospital. Am J Psychiatry 1986;143(10):1227–1233.

35. VanPutten T, Beckson M, Marder SR. The neuroleptic malignant syndrome manifested as a prolonged confusional state [letter]. J Clin Psychopharmacol 1988;8(3):229–230.

36. Clarke CE, Shand D, Yuill GM, Green MHP. Clinical spectrum of neuroleptic malignant syndrome [letter]. Lancet 1988;2:969–970.

37. McCarthy A, Bourke S, Fahy J, et al. Fatal recurrence of neuroleptic malignant syndrome. Br J Psychiatry 1988;152:558–559.

38. Levinson DF, Simpson GM. Neuroleptic-induced extrapyramidal symptoms with fever: heterogeneity of the 'neuroleptic malignant syndrome.' Arch Gen Psychiatry 1986;43(9):839–848.

39. Keck PE, Caroff SN, McElroy SL. Neuroleptic malignant syndrome and malignant hyperthermia: end of a controversy? J Clin Neuropsychiatry Clin Neurosci 1995;7(2):135–144.

40. Mann SC, Caroff SN, Bleier HR, et al. Lethal catatonia. Am J Psychiatry 1986;143(11):1374–1381.

41. Castillo E, Rubin RT, Holsboer-Trachsler E. Clinical differentiation between lethal catatonia and neuroleptic malignant syndrome. Am J Psychiatry 1989;146(3):324–328.

42. Levenson JL. Clinical differentiation between lethal catatonia and neuroleptic malignant syndrome [letter]. Am J Psychiatry 1989;146(9):1241.

43. Shalev A, Hermesh H, Munitz H. The role of external heat load in triggering the neuroleptic malignant syndrome. Am J Psychiatry 1988;145(1):110–111.

44. Stoudemire A, Luther JS. Neuroleptic malignant syndrome and neuroleptic-induced catatonia: differential diagnosis and treatment. Int J Psychiatry Med 1984;14(1):57–63.

45. van Agtamael MA, van Harten PN. Malignant neuroleptic syndrome: complete anticoagulant treatment or not? Ned Tijdschr Geneeskd 1992;136(38):1870–1872.

46. Johnson SB, Alvarez WA, Freinhar JP. Rhabdomyolysis in retrospect: psychiatric patients predisposed to this little-known syndrome. Int J Psychiatry Med 1987;17(2):163–171.

47. Lee S, Merriam A, Kim TS, et al. Cerebellar degeneration in neuroleptic malignant syndrome: neuropathologic findings and review of the literature concerning heat-related nervous system injury. J Neurol Neurosurg Psychiatry 1989;52(3):387–391.

48. Rothke S, Bush D. Neuropsychological sequelae of neuroleptic malignant syndrome. Biol Psychiatry 1986;21(8–9):838–841.

49. Legras A, Hurel D, Dabrowski G, et al. Protracted neuroleptic malignant syndrome complicating long-acting neuroleptic administration. Am J Med 1988;85(6):875–878.

50. Rosenberg MR, Green M. Neuroleptic malignant syndrome. Review of response to therapy. Arch Intern Med 1989;149(9):1927–1931.

51. Rosebush P, Stewart T. A prospective analysis of 24 episodes of neuroleptic malignant syndrome. Am J Psychiatry 1989;146(6):717–725.

52. Sakkas P, Davis JM, Hua J, Wang Z. Pharmacotherapy of neuroleptic malignant syndrome. Psychiatry Ann 1991;21(3):157–164.

53. Scheftner WA, Shulman RB. Treatment choice in neuroleptic malignant syndrome. Convuls Ther 1992;8(4):267–279.

54. Pelonero AL, Levenson JL, Silverman JL. Neuroleptic therapy following neuroleptic malignant syndrome. Psychosomatics 1985;26(12):946–948.

55. Sachdev P, Kruk J, Kneebone M, Kissane D. Clozapine-induced neuroleptic malignant syndrome: review and report of new cases. J Clin Psychopharmacol 1995;15(5):365–371.

56. Wells AJ, Sommi RW, Crismon ML. Neuroleptic rechallenge after neuroleptic malignant syndrome: case report and literature review. Drug Intell Clin Pharm 1988;22(6):475–480.

57. Susman VL, Addonizio G. Recurrence of neuroleptic malignant syndrome. J Nerv Ment Dis 1988;176(4):234–241.

58. Rosebush PI, Stewart TD, Gelenberg AJ. Twenty neuroleptic rechallenges after neuroleptic malignant syndrome in 15 patients. J Clin Psychiatry 1989;50(8):295–298.

59. Levenson JL, Fisher JG. Long-term outcome after neuroleptic malignant syndrome. J Clin Psychiatry 1988;49(4):154–156.

60. Gelenberg AJ, Bellinghausen B, Wojcik JD, et al. Patients with neuroleptic malignant syndrome histories: what happens when they are rehospitalized? J Clin Psychiatry 1989;50(5):178–180.

61. Addonizio G, Susman VL. ECT as a treatment alternative for patients with symptoms of neuroleptic malignant syndrome. J Clin Psychiatry 1987;48(3):102–105.

62. Konikoff F, Kuritzky A, Jerushalmi Y, Theodor E. Neuroleptic malignant syndrome induced by a single injection of haloperidol [letter]. Br Med J 1984;289:1228–1229.

63. Iwahashi K. CYP2D6 genotype and possible susceptibility to the neuroleptic malignant syndrome. Biol Psychiatry 1994;36(11):781–782.

64. Ueno S, Otani K, Kaneko S, et al. Cytochrome P-450 2D6 gene polymorphism is not associated with neuroleptic malignant syndrome. Biol Psychiatry 1996;40:72–74.

65. Horn E, Lach B, Lapierre Y, Hrdina P. Hypothalamic pathology in the neuroleptic malignant syndrome. Am J Psychiatry 1988;145(5):617–620.

66. Gertz H-J, Schmidt LG. Low melanin content of substantia nigra in a case of neuroleptic malignant syndrome. Pharmacopsychiatry 1991;24(3):93–95.

67. Creese I, Hamblin MW, Leff SE, Sibley DR. CNS dopamine receptors. In: Iversen LL, Iversen SD, Snyder SH, eds. Handbook of psychopharmacology, vol. 17. New York: Plenum, 1983:81–138.

68. Velamoor VR, Norman RM, Caroff SN, Mann SC. Progression of symptoms in neuroleptic malignant syndrome. J Nerv Ment Dis 1994;182(3):168–173.

69. Weinberg S, Twersky RS. Neuroleptic malignant syndrome. Anesth Analg 1983;62(9):848–850.
70. Toru M, Matsuda O, Makiguchi K, Sugano K. Neuroleptic malignant syndrome-like state following withdrawal of antiparkinsonian drugs. J Nerv Ment Dis 1981;169(5):324–327.
71. Verhoeven WMA, Elderson A, Westenberg HGM. Neuroleptic malignant syndrome: successful treatment with bromocriptine. Biol Psychiatry 1985;20(6):680–684.
72. Tollefson GD, Garvey MJ. The neuroleptic syndrome and central dopamine metabolites. J Clin Psychopharmacol 1984;4(3):150–153.
73. Nisijima K, Ishiguro T. Neuroleptic malignant syndrome: a study of CSF monoamine metabolism. Biol Psychiatry 1990;27(3):280–288.
74. Nisijima K, Ishiguro T. Cerebrospinal fluid levels of monoamine metabolites and gamma-aminobutyric acid in neuroleptic malignant syndrome. J Psychiatry Res 1995;29(3):233–244.
75. Bowers MB, Heninger GR. Cerebrospinal fluid homovanillic acid patterns during neuroleptic treatment. Psychiatry Res 1981;4(3):285–290.
76. Hashimoto F, Sherman CB, Jeffery WH. Neuroleptic malignant syndrome and dopaminergic blockade. Arch Intern Med 1984;144(3):629–630.
77. Feibel JH, Schiffer RB. Sympathoadrenomedullary hyperactivity in the neuroleptic malignant syndrome: a case report. Am J Psychiatry 1981;138(8):1115–1116.
78. Gurrera RJ, Romero JA. Sympathoadrenomedullary activity in the neuroleptic malignant syndrome. Biol Psychiatry 1992;32(4):334–343.
79. Lew T, Tollefson GD. Chlorpromazine-induced neuroleptic malignant syndrome and its response to diazepam. Biol Psychiatry 1983;18(12):1439–1444.
80. Caroff S, Rosenberg H, Gerber JC. Neuroleptic malignant syndrome and malignant hyperthermia [letter]. Lancet 1983;1:244.
81. Downey GP, Caroff S, Beck S, et al. Neuroleptic malignant syndrome patient with unique clinical and physiologic features. Am J Med 1984;77(2):338–340.
82. Tollefson G. A case of neuroleptic malignant syndrome: in vitro muscle comparison with malignant hyperthermia. J Clin Psychopharmacol 1982;2(4):266–270.
83. Scarlett JD, Zimmerman R, Berkovic SF. Neuroleptic malignant syndrome. Aust N Z J Med 1983;13(1):70–73.
84. Bond WS. Detection and management of the neuroleptic malignant syndrome. Clin Pharm 1984;3(3):302–307.
85. Blair DT, Dauner A. Neuroleptic malignant syndrome: liability in nursing practice. J Psychosoc Nurs Ment Health Serv 1993;31(2):5–12.
86. Lannas PA, Packar JV. A fatal case of neuroleptic malignant syndrome. Med Sci Law 1993;33(1):86–88.
87. Lazarus A. Should meuroleptic malignant syndrome be treated in a private psychiatric hospital or a general hospital? Gen Hosp Psychiatry 1990;12(4):245–247.

Tardive Tourette's: Tardive Dyskinesia Form Fruste or a Distinct Clinical Syndrome?

Jeffrey A. Lieberman   Bruce L. Saltz

Various tardive syndromes have been reported to occur as a consequence of chronic neuroleptic treatment (1). The best known and most prevalent of these is tardive dyskinesia (TD) (2). TD is an abnormal, involuntary, hyperkinetic movement disorder, usually choreoathetoid in nature, which is believed to arise from the sustained chemical denervation of dopamine (DA) neuronal systems in the basal ganglia produced by neuroleptic treatment (1). Depending on how broadly or narrowly TD is defined, other tardive syndromes also have been included in this diagnostic category, among them tardive dystonia (3,4), tardive akathisia (5–8), tardive myoclonus (9), and tardive parkinsonism (10). There is some debate as to whether these are valid clinical entities, although they have, to varying degrees, come to be accepted. Other tardive syndromes have also been described in the literature that are somewhat more controversial, such as tardive psychosis (11) and tardive dysmentia (12). This latter category of controversial syndromes also includes the so-called tardive Tourette's syndrome (TTS) (13,14), where motor and phonic tics characteristic of idiopathic Gilles de la Tourette's syndrome (TS) have arisen following chronic neuroleptic exposure. However, questions have been raised concerning the validity of this allegedly drug-induced phenomenon, including whether patients may have exhibited symptoms of TS prior to neuroleptic treatment that had gone undetected, whether the TTS symptoms that occur are qualitatively similar to those of TS, and whether TTS is caused by drug treatment or simply is TS that spontaneously occurs coincident with neuroleptic exposure.

There have been 10 reports of TTS in the world English-language literature. Fog et al (15) reported three patients with chronic schizophrenia who developed Tourette-like symptoms. The first was a 22-year-old man with "simple schizophrenia." After 2 years of neuroleptic treatment, he developed head and body tics as well as grunting when

withdrawn from haloperidol. The duration of symptoms while off drugs was not reported. Symptoms diminished "somewhat" upon reinstitution of haloperidol (dosage not specified). Subsequent treatment with pimozide and tetrabenazine, separately and together, was ineffective. Their dosage and temporal relationship to haloperidol were not specified. Follow-up treatment with biperiden at unspecified doses yielded a "fairly good response." Results of computed tomography (CT) scanning of the head and neurologic examination were negative. There was no information about family history provided.

The second patient was a 58-year-old man with an 18-year history of schizophrenia, treated with various phenothiazines and haloperidol. He presented with brief episodes of arm movements, echolalia (involuntary repetition of another person's words or sentences), door slamming, and shouting that were sudden in onset. Information was not provided about the clinical context of these symptoms, such as whether the patient was concurrently psychotic or whether symptoms were temporally associated with dosage changes. Separate treatment trials with pimozide and tetrabenazine "somewhat" diminished symptoms. Improvement increased when these drugs were combined. Thioridazine was the most efficacious treatment, but the dosage and duration of treatment were not reported. No information about family history was provided, but results of a standard neurologic examination were said to be normal. A head CT scan showed cortical atrophy.

The third individual was seen at age 55 with a 14-year history of paranoid schizophrenia and treatment with various neuroleptics, mostly phenothiazines. There had been a history of echopraxia since childhood, but no other cognitive dysfunction or abnormal motor activity. At age 50, he developed echopraxia, echolalia, howling, and a slight unspecified dyskinesia without evidence of motor tics. There was no information about psychopathology. The temporal relationship of symptoms to drug or dosage changes was not provided. Symptoms "nearly disappeared" with pimozide treatment as well as with perphenazine. Family history was not stated. Results of neurologic examination were otherwise normal. Head CT scan showed atrophy with sclerotic plaques in the left caudate nucleus.

Klawans et al (16) reported the development of a Tourette-like syndrome in three individuals after chronic neuroleptic exposure. The first was a 28-year-old woman with a 10-year history of paranoid schizophrenia and idiopathic seizure disorder since age 2, treated with chlorpromazine, phenobarbital, and dilantin. Upon discontinuation of the neuroleptic after 6 years, she exhibited facial twitching, followed by shoulder and arm twitching. A few months later she developed spontaneous barking and clicking vocalizations and bruxism. Haloperidol 30 mg/day incompletely controlled the tics. Neologisms and bizarre thoughts characterized her behavior at this time. Her family history was unremarkable, but no report was made about investigation of other neurologic disorders.

The second patient was a 35-year-old woman with a 12-year history of paranoid schizophrenia treated alternately with haloperidol, chlorpromazine, and fluphenazine. At age 20, she began to exhibit spontaneous bruxism, barking, grunting, and coprolalia. Later she exhibited palilalia (involuntary repetition of words or sentences), echolalia, facial tics, and blepharospasm at a time when no psychotic signs were present. No information on the family history or neurologic examination was provided.

The third patient was a 71-year-old woman with a 20-year history of trifluoperazine 4–6 mg/day for nonpsychotic anxiety. At age 70, the trifluoperazine was discontinued for surgery and there developed persistent bruxism, facial tics, buccofaciolingual dyskinesia, spontaneous grunting, and stereotyped low-pitched counting, as well as occasional echolalia. Results of neurologic examination were otherwise unremarkable. No information about treatment outcome or family history was provided.

De Veaugh-Geiss (17) described the case of a 65-year-old man with an 8-year history of neuroleptic treatment (thioridazine 100 mg/day for 4 years and perphenazine 4–12 mg/day for 2 years). Treatment was complicated by persistent tremor and rigidity even while off neuroleptics. After 4 years of treatment, he developed involuntary movements of his head, neck, and mouth, and chorea in all extremities. Rapid neuroleptic discontinuation led to mental status deterioration, urinary incontinence, and motor restlessness. The slower reduction of neuroleptic dose caused no initial change in motor activity but prevented deterioration in mental status. After 2 months, his previous motor symptoms were reduced, but were replaced by orofacial tics and spontaneous grunting and barking. These symptoms disappeared 6 months after medication withdrawal. There was no family history and no other known personal neurologic illness.

Mueller and Aminoff (18) described the case of a 27-year-old man with early-onset autism characterized by failure to speak or socialize, head banging, self-biting, rocking, and preoccupation with certain household objects. He was treated for more than 12 years with thioridazine 800–2,000 mg/day, supplemented for 1 to 2 years with fluphenazine, and later switched to chlorpromazine 200 mg/day for 3 years, followed by lithium carbonate 3,000 mg/day for 1 to 2 years. Three weeks after all medication was stopped, he developed head nodding and torticollis, repetitive tongue clucking, clicking guttural noises, truncal rocking, choreoathetoid finger movements, lip smacking, and licking. He also exhibited right-hand flapping. All adventitious movements and vocalizations other than rocking disappeared with the institution of haloperidol 6 mg/day. Results of neurologic examination and laboratory studies were otherwise unremarkable.

Seeman et al (19) reported the case of a 26-year-old woman with a 4-year history of schizophrenia treated with electroconvulsive therapy, chlorpromazine, haloperidol, perphenazine, and trifluoperazine. After 3 years, she developed grimacing and spontaneous giggling while receiving fluphenazine. She subsequently developed eye blinking, bruxism, and finger rolling. She made lewd remarks to male colleagues, grunted frequently, and talked aloud to herself. These behaviors were uncharacteristic for her and in marked contrast to her usual introverted personality. A few months after the fluphenazine was stopped, the motor symptoms began to improve, with total resolution by the fourth month. No information was provided on family history or other neurologic assessment.

Stahl (20) reported the case of an autistic 28-year-old man with a 2-year history of sniffing, grunting, coprolalia, tics of the face, neck, torso and diaphragm, and involuntary limb movements. Early childhood behavior had included bizarre sounds, poor understanding of spoken language, flapping, and rocking activity. After age 13, neuroleptics were prescribed continuously at doses of 200 mg of chlorpromazine or thioridazine because of "bizarre behavior." Diazepam and phenobarbital were also occasionally prescribed. All symptoms were completely suppressed by a brief trial of haloperidol (dose unspecified).

Pary (21) described a 19-year-old woman with a 7-year history of schizophrenia treated continuously with one or more neuroleptics (in daily doses exceeding 2,000 mg in chlorpromazine equivalents). At age 19, she developed paroxysmal eye blinking, episodic cursing and hissing, as well as facial grimacing, without other abnormal involuntary motor activity. Treatment with haloperidol up to 100 mg/day initially reduced the cursing and later diminished her hissing, eye blinking, delusions, and hallucinations. Family history was unremarkable, and results of neurologic and laboratory studies were not suggestive of other neuromedical disorders.

Lal and AlAnsari (22) reported the case of an 18-year-old man with childhood-onset schizophrenia who developed transient involuntary movements (nature unknown) at age 10 after a few months of treatment with thioridazine (25–50 mg/day). Upon reexposure to this medication at age 13, he developed burping and whistling noises. When medication was withdrawn, he became paranoid and exhibited choreiform and ballistic movements of his upper extremities and shoulders, with bruxism, blepharospasm, torticollis, lip pursing, and tongue movements. He also exhibited spontaneous vocalizations such as grunting, barking, sniffing, coughing, whistling, throat clearing and spitting, echolalia, palilalia, and coprolalia. Movements could be voluntarily suppressed for brief periods. Speech was incoherent, but other aspects of his mental status were not reported. Results of neurologic examination and laboratory studies were otherwise normal. Family history was noncontributory. All involuntary activity remitted after 5 months of medication washout.

DISCUSSION

In light of the fact that there is a substantial prevalence of tardive dyskinesia (23) in neuroleptic-treated patients and an estimated incidence of 4% per year of continuous neuroleptic exposure (24), the occurrence of TTS (at least in so far as it has been reported) is quite rare. Assuming that this is not the result of underdetection and reporting, the infrequency of the condition would suggest that it is a rare variant of more typical TD in the same way that tardive dystonia is an infrequent and more severe variant of TD (4), or that it can only occur in vulnerable individuals, that is, those with a genetic diathesis to tic disorders or TS. The cases described in the articles reviewed show phenomenologic overlap with the symptoms of idiopathic TS. At the same time, they include many other neurobehavioral symptoms that are qualitatively different from those traditionally seen in TS (25,26). These patients appear to exhibit admixtures of Tourette-like symptoms along with involuntary movements that commonly occur in TD, as well as the behavioral pathology associated with their primary psychiatric disorder. Clearly, however, the occurrence of Tourette-like symptoms can be more problematic for patients because their effects are often disruptive to those around them rather than simply quietly disfiguring to patients, as is usually the case with classic forms of TD. In addition, the natural history of the Tourette-like symptoms in the cases described is markedly different from that seen in idiopathic TS, which has its onset in childhood.

There is a theoretical rationale to support both pathologic models of this putative side-effect syndrome. TD is believed to result from a disturbance of DA neuronal systems of the substantia nigra and corpus striatum that is produced by chronic neuroleptic treatment (27). In rodents, sustained antagonism of DA neurotransmission produces an upregulation of postsynaptic DA type 2 receptors in the caudate nucleus and behavioral hyperactivity and enhanced stereotypic behaviors in response to DA agonist stimulation (27).

Similarly, the pathophysiologic basis of TS is hypothesized to involve increased DA neural tone in the basal ganglia nuclei (28,29). Thus, both conditions are believed to arise from hyperactive DA neural systems in basal ganglia structures. In view of this, it is plausible to suggest that sustained neuroleptic exposure could produce DA supersensitivity in the striatal regions that are involved in TS and thus mimic a lesion that occurs idiopathically in TS patients. It is also possible that the pharmacologic effects of neuroleptic treatment could provoke the pathophysiologic process in the striatum of TS in patients who are genetically vulnerable but previously were asymptomatic, and thereby precipitate the onset of symptoms.

There is insufficient data in the literature with which to validate the existence of TTS as a variant of TD or as the pharmacologic induction of idiopathic TS in patients predisposed to the disorder. Evidence that would be useful in this regard would come from family history; studies; treatment trials using agents that are effective in idiopathic TS, such as clonidine (30), although clonidine may also have some efficacy in TD (31); and biologic investigations, for example, positron emission tomography and neurochemical measures of central nervous system DA.

In summary, it appears from review of the literature that TTS occurs in neuroleptic-treated patients at a low frequency. The course and treatment response of TTS are comparable with classic TD. Risk factors for the development of TTS have not been identified. Whether this condition arises solely as a consequence of neuroleptic exposure or occurs in patients physiologically predisposed to TS or other idiopathic tic disorders cannot yet be determined. It is our speculative conclusion that TTS does occur, albeit rarely, and is an infrequent variant of chronic drug-induced extrapyramidal side-effect syndrome.

ACKNOWLEDGMENTS

This study was supported by a Research Scientist Development Award (MH-00537) and grant (MH-41646) to Dr Lieberman and the Mental Health Clinical Research Center (MH-41960) of LIJMC-Hillside Hospital from the National Institute of Mental Health.

REFERENCES

1. Jeste DV, Wisniewski AA, Wyatt RJ. Neuroleptic-associated tardive syndromes. Pychiatr Clin N Am 1986;9:183–192.
2. Baldessarini RJ, Cole JO, Davis M, et al. Tardive dyskinesia: task force report. Washington, DC: American Psychiatric Association, 1980.
3. Davis RJ, Cummings JL. Clinical variants of tardive dyskinesia. Neuropsychiatry Neuropsychol Behav Neurol 1988;1:31–38.
4. Burke RE, Fahn S, Jankovic J, et al. Tardive dystonia: late onset and persistent dystonia caused by antipsychotic drugs. Neurology 1982;32:1335–1346.
5. Gardos G, Cole JO, Tarsy D. Withdrawal syndromes associated with antipsychotic drugs. Am J Psychiatry 1978;135:1321–1324.
6. Munetz MR, Cornes CL. Akathisia, pseudoakathisia, and tardive dyskinesia: clinical examples. Compr Psychiatry 1981;23:345–352.
7. Munetz MR, Cornes CL. Distinguishing akathisia and tardive dyskinesia: a review of the literature. J Clin Psychopharmacol 1983;3:343–350.

8. Braude WM, Barnes TRE, Gore SM. Clinical characteristics of akathisia: a systematic investigation of acute psychiatric inpatient admissions. Br J Psychiatry 1983;143:137–150.

9. Lohr JB, Jeste DV. Neuroleptic induced movement disorders: acute and subacute disorders. In: Cavenar JO Jr, ed. Psychiatry. Philadelphia: JB Lippincott (in press).

10. Tarsy D. Movement disorders with neuroleptic drug treatment. Psychiatr Clin North Am 1984;7:458.

11. Chouinard G, Jones B. Neuroleptic induced supersensitivity psychosis. Am J Psychiatry 1980;137:16–21.

12. Wilson IC, Garbutt JC, Lanier CF, Moylan J, Nelson W, Prange AJ Jr. Is there a tardive dysmentia? Schizophr Bull 1983;9:187–192.

13. Klawans HL, Falk DR, Nausieda PA. Gille de la Tourette's syndrome after long term chlorpromazine therapy. Neurology 1978;28:1064–1066.

14. Stahl SA. Tardive Tourette's syndrome in an autistic patient after long-term neuroleptic administration. Am J Psychiatry 1980;137:1267–1269.

15. Fog R, Pakkenberg H, Regeur L, Pakkenberg B. "Tardive" Tourette's syndrome in relation to long-term neuroleptic treatment of multiple tics. In: Friedhoff AJ, Chase TN, eds. Gilles de la Tourette's syndrome. New York: Raven, 1982:419–421.

16. Klawans HL, Nausieda PA, Goetz CC, Tanner CM, Weiner WJ. Tourette-like symptoms following chronic neuroleptic therapy. In: Friedhoff AJ, Chase TN, eds. Gilles de la Tourette's syndrome. New York: Raven, 1982:415–418.

17. De Veaugh-Geiss J. Tardive Tourette's syndrome. Neurology 1980;30:562–563.

18. Mueller J, Aminoff MJ. Tourette-like syndrome after long term neuroleptic drug treatment. Br J Psychiatry 1982;141:191–193.

19. Seeman MV, Patel J, Pyke J. Tardive dyskinesia with Tourette-like syndrome. J Clin Psychiatry 1981;42:357–358.

20. Stahl SA. Tardive syndrome in an autistic patient after long-term neuroleptic administration. Am J Psychiatry 1980;137:1267–1269.

21. Pary RJ. The "psychotic" curse. Am J Psychiatry 1979;136:715–716.

22. Lal S, AlAnsari E. Tourette-like syndrome following low dose short-term neuroleptic treatment. Can J Sci Neurol 1986;13:125–128.

23. Woerner MG, Kane JM, Lieberman JA, et al. The prevalence of tardive dyskinesia. J Clin Psychopharmacol 1991;11:34–42.

24. Kane JM, Woerner M, Weinhold P, et al. A prospective study of tardus dyskinesia development: preliminary results. J Clin Psychopharmacol 1982;2:345–349.

25. Golden GS. Movement disorders in children: Tourette's syndrome. J Dev Behav Pediatr 1982;3:209–216.

26. Shapiro AK, Shapiro ES, Bruun RD, Sweet RD. Gille de la Tourette's syndrome. New York: Raven, 1978.

27. Lieberman JA. Dopamine pathophysiology in tardive dyskinesia. Psychiatr Ann 1989;19:289–296.

28. Feinberg M, Carroll BJ. Effects of dopamine agonists and antagonists in Tourette's disease. Arch Gen Psychiatry 1979;36:979–985.

29. Messiha FS, Knopp W. A study of endogenous dopamine metabolism in Tourette's disease. Dis Nerv Syst 1976;37:470–473.

30. Ferre RC. Tourette's disorder and the use of clonidine. A. Am Acad Child Psychiatry 1982;21:294–297.

31. Nishikawa T, Tanaka M, Tsuda A, Koga I, Uchida Y. Clonidine therapy for tardive dyskinesia and related syndromes. Clin Neuropharmacol 1984;7:239–244.

Rabbit Syndrome

Daniel E. Casey

HISTORY

Neuroleptic (antipsychotic) drugs have been associated with involuntary movement disorders since these drugs were originally introduced for the treatment of schizophrenia and other psychoses. Although it was originally hypothesized that patients must necessarily experience motor side effects as part of achieving antipsychotic benefits, this has been widely shown not to be the case. However, neuroleptic-induced motor side effects do commonly occur, affecting 50% to 75% of patients receiving these drugs (1).

These motor side effects are classified into two broad categories. Symptoms that occur at the initiation of neuroleptic treatment and that may continue during treatment are grouped as acute extrapyramidal syndromes (EPS). The most common syndromes are dystonia, parkinsonism, and akathisia. These symptoms typically resolve when neuroleptics are discontinued. The second type of abnormal movement disorder is the late-onset tardive dyskinesia (TD) syndrome, which occurs after extended neuroleptic treatment and may or may not resolve (2).

The rabbit syndrome is another neuroleptic drug-induced disorder. Although there are only a few reports about this syndrome, it is probably best conceptualized as an acute EPS phenomenon. It was first described in 1972 (3) as "perioral muscular movements strikingly imitating the rapid, chewing-like movements of a rabbit's mouth." These movements did not involve the tongue and were limited exclusively to the territory of the oral and masticatory muscles. This clinical picture was immediately labeled "the rabbit syndrome" (3).

DIAGNOSIS

Clinical Description

As noted in the initial description, the primary signs of rabbit syndrome involve rapid perioral movements. These are principally in the vertical plane and do not involve horizontal, or rotatory jaw motions. Although the tongue was not affected in the initial report, subsequent descriptions have noted occasional tongue tremors associated with these perioral movements. Polygraphic assessments show a frequency range of 2.5 to 5.5 cycles/second (4–6), which is typical of both idiopathic and neuroleptic drug-induced parkinsonism. Most of the case reports and small group studies also note that the large majority of patients with rabbit syndrome also have other signs of drug-induced parkinsonian tremor, rigidity, and bradykinesia involving the face, limbs, or trunk. Only rarely does the perioral tremor occur in isolation during neuroleptic treatment.

Prevalence

The true rate of occurrence of the rabbit syndrome is difficult to estimate because there are so few studies in this area. Approximately only 30 patients have been included in case reports and small investigations. However, the actual number of patients with perioral tremor alone or in combination with other signs of drug-induced parkinsonism is likely to be considerably higher. The low rate of reporting for rabbit syndrome is probably due to the lack of awareness that this symptom is characterized as a separate syndrome, as well as the prompt and effective therapy available for treating this symptom. One study of rabbit syndrome prevalence found that it occurred at a rate of 2.3% to 4.4%, depending on which patient population was studied (7). If neuroleptic-treated patients only were considered, 6 (4.4%) of 137 patients demonstrated the rabbit syndrome. However, none of the 129 patients receiving concomitant neuroleptics plus anticholinergics exhibited this syndrome. If both groups are combined, as is usually seen in a broad representative group of patients receiving neuroleptic therapy with or without anticholinergics, the expected prevalence will be approximately 3% (7). Other reports find prevalence rates of 2.3% and 1.5% (8,9).

Risk Factors

Several specific variables related to patient demographics, drug treatment characteristics, and temporal aspects can influence the expression of rabbit syndrome.

Patient Demographics

Age   The majority of patients described with rabbit syndrome are over 45 years old, but these symptoms can be seen in younger patients as well. The age distribution may be related to the observation that drug-induced parkinsonism is more common in older patients (10), though this is not uniformly true (11). Additionally, it may reflect the lore that tremor is more common in older patients whereas bradykinesia is more likely to be observed in younger patients.

Sex   The female-to-male ratio of rabbit syndrome appears to be approximately 2:1. However, this ratio is subject to wide variation because only a few patients have been reported in the literature.

Psychiatric Diagnosis   Rabbit syndrome is most commonly described in schizophrenic patients, since schizophrenics are the most likely to receive neuroleptics. However, rabbit syndrome has been described in other psychotic patients (bipolar affective disorders, schizoaffective schizophrenia, and the demented elderly) and nonpsychotic patients receiving neuroleptics (3–6,12,13,14). Preexisting central nervous system injury has also been speculated as a risk factor, but there is insufficient information to address this issue conclusively.

Drug Treatment Variables

Drug Dose   No studies have specifically addressed the relationship between drug dose and rabbit syndrome. However, it appears that this syndrome is associated with low to intermediate neuroleptic doses. Higher doses produce more generalized signs of parkinsonism, which would take clinical precedence over isolated perioral tremor. Additionally, rabbit syndrome symptoms usually decrease or disappear when the neuroleptic dose is lowered and can

increase or recur when neuroleptic therapy is increased or reinstituted.

Drug Type   High-potency, low-milligram neuroleptics (e.g., haloperidol, fluphenazine) are most commonly associated with the rabbit syndrome. However, the symptoms have also been reported with many other neuroleptics, including the low-potency, high-milligram types (e.g., chlorpromazine, thioridazine). This difference in liability of EPS is also seen in the traditional signs of drug-induced parkinsonism. One case has been reported with the antidepressant imipramine (15). The rabbit syndrome has not been reported with antianxiety agents or sedative hypnotics.

Temporal Aspects

The exact onset of rabbit syndrome is difficult to pinpoint because most cases were not followed prospectively to identify the time course for developing perioral tremor. This symptom is usually described as occurring with chronic neuroleptic therapy (3,5), but it has been reported to occur as soon as the second week of neuroleptic treatment (12). Clinical experience indicates that it can occur at any time during neuroleptic treatment, which includes the first few weeks, several months, many years, and decades of neuroleptic therapy. This time course is also consistent with the time course for the onset of drug-induced parkinsonism and again supports the concept that the rabbit syndrome is another acute EPS.

Differential Diagnosis

Other movement disorders that may either be drug-related or spontaneously occurring phenomena need to be distinguished from the rabbit syndrome (16). TD is the most important differential diagnosis to make because the implications for treatment and prognosis are very different (see Treatment, below). TD is characterized by choreic and athetotic symptoms in the tongue, mouth, and other facial parts. These symptoms usually occur irregularly and are less frequent than the rapid rhythmical perioral tremor of rabbit syndrome. Also, one often sees limb (hands or feet) choreoathetosis or truncal dyskinesias associated with TD. Pharmacologic differences between these two syndromes are also useful. TD increases or is unchanged by anticholinergic agents, whereas the rabbit syndrome generally improves with these compounds. Polygraphic recordings also show important differences between TD and rabbit syndrome. TD may increase, remain unchanged, or decrease with concentration tests and motor performance tasks, whereas rabbit syndrome uniformly increases under these conditions (5).

Distinguishing the rabbit syndrome from drug-induced parkinsonism is principally an academic exercise since the two disorders are at least closely related and probably represent slightly different points along the pathophysiologic continuum of the same disorder. The distinguishing feature is whether the primary symptom is isolated perioral tremor (with or without secondary tremor or bradykinesia in other parts of the body) or a predominance of typical parkinsonian symptoms without perioral tremor.

It is important to recognize that both TD and the acute EPS of rabbit syndrome, drug-induced parkinsonism, or other acute extrapyramidal syndromes can coexist. In these patients the clinical picture can change from TD to acute EPS and back to TD again in a matter of seconds (5).

Finally, it is necessary to separate the rabbit syndrome from spontaneously occurring abnormal movements. These can occur in untreated schizophrenics (stereotypies, which are usually bizarre movements and not as rhythmical as rabbit syndrome), focal dystonias of oromandibular dystonia (forced mouth gaping or grimacing), and mild idiopathic parkinsonism. The clinical features specific to each of these syndromes and the absence of neuroleptic drugs are used to make this last group of differential diagnoses (16).

TREATMENT

Dopaminergic Influences

The first approach in treating a patient with the rabbit syndrome is to reduce the neuroleptic dose. It may take a few to several days before a decrease in the symptoms is seen due to the long half-lives of neuroleptic drugs, especially in those patients who have received drugs for a long time and may have large tissue stores of neuroleptics.

Very little information is available about adding dopaminergic agonists to treat rabbit syndrome. One case report of successful therapy with amantadine (13) conflicts with other case reports of unsuccessful amantadine treatment (10,14). The efficacy of amantadine may depend on the neuroleptic dosage and the severity of perioral tremor, as amantadine may be too weak an agonist in some cases to offset the neuroleptic-induced effects. This weak dopamine agonist effect is one of the limitations of amantadine in treating either drug-induced or idiopathic parkinsonism. Other strategies to consider for enhancing dopamine transmission include the indirect dopamine agonist levodopa plus carbidopa or a direct agonist like bromocriptine. However, caution is warranted because of the concern that extended dopamine agonists may aggravate the underlying psychosis.

Cholinergic Influences

Standard anticholinergic therapy is almost uniformly effective in reducing or eliminating the rabbit syndrome. Typical drugs tried are benztropine, trihexyphenidil, and procyclidine, but there is no reason why other anticholinergic or antihistaminic agents would not also be beneficial. As expected, the rabbit syndrome may recur in some cases if these drugs are decreased or discontinued. Occasionally, intravenous or intramuscular anticholinergic administration was ineffective, whereas oral treatment for several days

with the same compounds in the same patients was beneficial.

Parenteral physostigmine has been used to temporarily aggravate the rabbit syndrome as a diagnostic challenge test (13). This response of increasing symptoms is also similar to drug-induced and idiopathic parkinsonism, which further supports the classification of rabbit syndrome as an acute EPS. However, parenteral physostigmine can have serious side effects, including respiratory distress, tachycardia, or seizures. Thus, it should not be used routinely for evaluating the rabbit syndrome.

Other

Benzodiazepines, such as diazepam or chlorazepate, may be partially effective, but have not been widely studied. They are not recommended as the first line of treatment intervention since they do not clearly have efficacy and do have the problem of potential dependence liability with chronic treatment, which is often needed to treat the rabbit syndrome if neuroleptic dosage cannot be decreased. A few other agents, such as phenytoin and L-tryptophan, were ineffective in this syndrome (6,12–14).

BASIC SCIENCE

The clinical phenomenology and pharmacologic profile of the rabbit syndrome strongly support the proposal that it is best characterized as an acute EPS. These symptoms are hypothesized to occur from an imbalance between the inversely related dopaminergic and cholinergic influences in the basal ganglia. Neuroleptics decrease dopaminergic influences by blocking dopamine receptors, thus producing a relative cholinergic excess. Effective interventions then include decreasing the neuroleptic blockade by reducing the neuroleptic dose or augmenting dopaminergic mechanisms with dopamine agonists. Conversely, reducing the relative cholinergic excess by adding anticholinergics is also effective. One case report with single photon emission computed tomography (SPECT) noted decreased cerebral perfusion in the basal ganglia while the movement disorder was present and a return to normal perfusion when symptoms resolved (15).

Data from polygraphic studies show that the rabbit syndrome is a distinctly different phenomenon than the abnormal movements seen in TD. These differences can be seen in patients at rest and during mental concentration tasks, as well as in motor performance tests and in the sleep electroencephalogram in non-REM phases.

In summary, the rabbit syndrome is an uncommonly reported neuroleptic drug-induced side effect characterized by perioral movements. This syndrome is best understood as a subtle sign or form fruste of drug-induced parkinsonism and commonly occurs with other subtle parkinsonian signs of tremor, rigidity, or bradykinesia. The pharmacologic profile of rabbit syndrome is identical to treatment strategies for drug-induced parkinsonism. Although this disorder is not frequently recorded, it probably occurs quite commonly and is effectively managed by reducing neuroleptic dosage or adding antiparkinson agents.

ACKNOWLEDGMENTS

This work was supported in part by funds from the Veterans Affairs Research Program, NIMH grant MH 36657, and core grant RP00163. The typescript was prepared by Crystal Berger.

REFERENCES

1. Casey DE, Keepers GA. Neuroleptic side effects: acute extrapyramidal syndromes and tardive dyskinesia. In: Casey DE, Vibeke Christensen A, eds. Psychopharmacology: current trends. Berlin: Springer-Verlag, 1988:74–93.
2. Casey DE. Tardive dyskinesia. In: Meltzer HY, ed. Psychopharmacology: the third generation of progress. New York: Raven Press, 1987:1411–1419.
3. Villeneuve A. The rabbit syndrome—a peculiar extrapyramidal reaction. Can Psych Assoc J 1972;17(2):69–72.
4. Jus K, Jus A, Villeneuve A. Polygraphic profile of oral tardive dyskinesia and of rabbit syndrome: for quantitative and qualitative evaluation. Dis Nerv Syst 1973;34(1):27–32.
5. Jus K, Jus A, Villeneuve A, Villeneuve R. Influence of concentration and motor performance on tardive dyskinesia and rabbit syndrome. Can Psych Assoc J 1973;18(4):327–330.
6. Jus K, Jus A, Gautier J, et al. Studies on the action of certain pharmacological agents on tardive dyskinesia and on the rabbit syndrome. Int J Clin Pharmacol 1974;9(2):138–145.
7. Yassa R, Samarthji L. Prevalence of the rabbit syndrome. Am J Psychiatry 1986;143(5):656–657.
8. Inada T, Yagi G, Kaijima K, et al. Clinical variants of tardive dyskinesia in Japan. Jpn J Psychiatry Neurol 1991;45(1):67–71.
9. Chiu HFK, Lam LCW, Chung DWS, et al. Prevalence of the rabbit syndrome in Hong Kong. J Nerv Ment Dis 1993;181(4):264–265.
10. Ayd FJ. A survey of drug-induced extrapyramidal reactions. JAMA 1961;175:1054–1060.
11. Keepers GA, Clappison VJ, Casey DE. Initial anticholinergic prophylaxis for neuroleptic-induced extrapyramidal syndromes. Arch Gen Psychiatry 1983;40:1113–1117.
12. Todd R, Lippmann S, Manshadi M. Recognition and treatment of rabbit syndrome, an uncommon complication of neuroleptic therapies. Am J Psychiatry 1983;140(11):1519–1520.
13. Weiss KJ, Ciraulo DA, Shader RI. Physostigmine test in the rabbit syndrome and tardive dyskinesia. Am J Psychiatry 1980;137(5):627–628.
14. Sovner R, Dimascio A. The effect of benztropine mesylate in the rabbit syndrome and tardive dyskinesia. Am J Psychiatry 1977;134(11):1301–1302.
15. Fornazzari L, Ichise M, Remington G, Smith I. Rabbit syndrome, antidepressant use, and cerebral perfusion SPECT scan findings. J Psychiatry Neurol 1991;16(4):227–229.
16. Casey DE. The differential diagnosis of tardive dyskinesia. Acta Psychiatr Scand 1981;63(suppl 291):71–87.

Special Lithium-Induced Movement Disorders

Jonathan M. Himmelhoch

Je trouve très raisonnable la croyance celtique que les âmes de ceux que nous avons perdus sont captives dans . . . une chose inanimée . . . il en est ainsi de notre passé. Il est caché hors de son domaine . . . en quelque objet materiel . . . il depend du hasard que nous le rencontrions avant de mourir.

—*Proust*, A la Recherche du Temps Perdu

For Proust it was the magical powers of a tea-soaked *petite madeleine* that revived a forgotten past. A critical lesson of the psychopharmacologic era is that neurons also have forgotten pasts and hidden patterns that can be reactivated by chance exposure to inciting pharmacologic stimuli: sometimes by reexposure to agents used before, sometimes by the precipitous discontinuation of agents to which the neuron has been chronically exposed, sometimes by encounters with new agents that unveil previously altered cellular mechanisms, and sometimes even by environmental perturbations that imitate the situation in which an agent had previously been used. It is in this Proustian light that we can best understand such phenomena as the resistance of a naive user to psychedelic agents, tolerance and withdrawal from opiates and sedatives, neurologic kindling, flashbacks, and especially the tardive effects of neuropharmacologic agents.

The exposure of neural tissue, even briefly then, to psychoactive agents is not necessarily an innocent event; chronic exposure is surely not. The organism may seem to forget, it may even die without giving up the slightest behavioral clue to its exposure, but on occasion there is a *petite madeleine neurochimique* that either evokes neural memory of old exposures or makes the hidden consequences of ongoing treatments manifest.

Beitman (1) has described a case that suggests lithium may reinvoke a long-past neuroleptic-induced dyskinesia. In this chapter we will describe four cases in which lithium seems to be the provocative agent in awakening quiescent motor disorders. In the latter two cases, the original neural insult was probably the effect of exposure to neuroleptics. In the other two, although neuroleptics played a role, the original insult was probably long-quiescent, post-streptococcal illness.

CLINICAL CASES

Lithium-Associated Chorea

A 45-year-old black woman was admitted to Western Psychiatric Institute and Clinic (WPIC) during her first psychotic manic episode, which was readily controlled on thioridazine 600 mg/day. At age 14 she had well-documented rheumatic fever. She had not experienced Sydenham's chorea, but had been known as "nervous" since that time. She was discharged after 3 weeks on 100 mg thioridazine. She was placed on 900 mg lithium carbonate in the outpatient clinic, but at a lithium level of 0.9 mmol/l she developed classic chorea: bilateral quasipurposive movements of fingers, wrists, elbows, and shoulders. The chorea dissipated after 2 weeks and she thereafter responded well to lithium.

A 59-year-old white woman was admitted to WPIC in the midst of a psychotic manic episode of the type she had repeatedly experienced since 1946. She had been treated with many kinds of neuroleptics. She once developed a tardive dyskinesia on haloperidol, which had abated. At age 16 she had glomerular nephritis. On admission she had been off drugs for 2 months. Attempts to treat her with lithium resulted first in a mild recurrence of her dyskinesia and then in the development of florid bilateral chorea of her arms. Both movement disorders disappeared after 10 to 14 days of lithium treatment.

In both these cases the unmasking of neuroleptic-related motor symptoms by lithium salts is less important than the advent of chorea, because the possibility exists that lithium salts uncovered the neuronal vestiges of ancient poststreptococcal syndromes. Nausieda et al (2) have pointed out phenytoin's similar ability to uncover quiescent choreiform disorders. In the following cases neuroleptic-induced akathisia is greatly magnified by lithium treatment.

Akathetic Somnambulism

A 53-year-old woman was treated for 15 years with neuroleptics for manic-depressive psychosis. Lithium therapy had allowed discharge from residential care in a veteran's hospital, but after 3 years she became manic again. Haloperidol was reluctantly added. She became severely akathetic. Even asleep her akathisia was observable. She would arise like la somnambula *and pace the floor. Her akathetic somnambulism recurred in subsequent manic episodes managed without neuroleptics.*

A 35-year-old man had a 12-year history of manic-depressive psychosis. Early manic episodes were treated with neuroleptics. Later he achieved better mood control on lithium carbonate, but experienced a manic breakthrough that forced the adjunctive use of haloperidol. He developed akathisia, and then akathetic somnambulism. Akathisia became the driving force behind all waking and sleeping behavior. His motor syndrome recurred in future manic episodes, some treated with lithium alone.

Although this virulent form of akathisia occurred only during psychotic manic episodes, in both cases it looked more like a toxic drug effect than a mood-dependent state. It also resembled the "organic driveness" of patients with brainstem lesions (3). Neuroleptics have been reported to produce a most severe form of somnambulism (4). In our patients, however, somnambulism occurred in subsequent episodes in the absence of neuroleptics and in the presence of lithium salts.

DISCUSSION

Since the original publication of this chapter there have been a fairly large number of clinical reports about lithium effects on the neostriatum. In many cases, lithium is used as a co-drug for control of mood swings, most often with neuroleptics, but verapamil, divalproex sodium, and clonazepam have also been part of the induction of neostriatal pathophysiology. Reed et al (5) report cases of choreoathetosis in two patients, the first additionally treated with clonazepam, the second with butyrophenone. From these two cases and from a review of the literature, the authors rather strongly opine that choreoathetosis is almost always a sign of lithium toxicity, accompanied by signs of neurotoxicity such as delir-

ium and cerebellar dysfunction. In their review 44% of patients with choreoathetosis went on to develop permanent movement disorders (not always the original choreiform disorders). Moreover, 63% of the patients who developed permanent involuntary motor deficits were taking both lithium and a neuroleptic. In those cases that proved reversible, the chorea took an average of 7 days to disappear.

Helmuth et al (6) in a letter to the *Journal of Clinical Psychopharmacology* describes a similar case after the addition of verapamil to the regimen of a patient on full therapeutic doses and serum levels of lithium salts. The interactions of lithium and calcium channel blockers have not been completely described, but it is entirely within reason that verapamil might drive lithium from the extracellular to the intracellular department even if it does not act through changes in renal function. Once again, either excess lithium dosing or blood levels is promulgated as the cause of a neostriatal movement disorder, rather than some special genetic or acquired vulnerability of the basal ganglia to lithium.

Finally, Matsis et al (7) report lithium-associated chorea that is accompanied by hypercalcemia (see the above case on verapamil) and hyperamylasemia. They describe a 71-year-old woman who had had over the years previous good responses to lithium carbonate in both her depressive and hypomanic/manic phase. When she began to appear depressed and withdrawn on this occasion, her baseline lithium dosage was increased, as it had been in past depressions. She rapidly became confused and manifested choreiform movements. These symptoms of acute toxicity evanesced when lithium was stopped. When lithium was reinstituted, her chorea recurred. Moreover, she also experienced an increase in serum calcium, parathormone and amylase—all without any modicum of pancreatitis. The authors offer the case as another example of obvious lithium toxicity, although they never explain her elevation of calcium, parathormone, and amylase—indeed, they never explain her chorea.

A similar experience has come about regarding lithium-associated parkinsonism. Holroyd and Smith (8) report three cases of disabling parkinsonism after institution of lithium treatment. Although one of these cases showed obvious and severe lithium toxicity, the other two showed, in the authors' words, no other sign of lithium toxicity (implying, of course, that these two patients were experiencing toxic reactions, with disabling parkinsonism as their sole indication of neurotoxicity). Their motor disorder disappeared upon discontinuation of lithium and, upon reinstitution of this salt, showed no recurrences unless their serum level rose to 0.7 mEq/l or above. Lecamwasam et al (9) reported chronic lithium toxicity presenting as Parkinson's disease. A 71-year-old man, long stable on the same dose of maintenance lithium, became encephalopathic after 9 years. His encephalopathy was almost certainly due to lithium intoxication. Lithium was stopped, mania ensued, and lithium was recommenced at lower doses than his previous maintenance regimen. He was stable again for 8 more years, but then presented with a parkinsonian syndrome. He was taking no other medications. He died in the hospital when he had an acute myocardial infarction while his physicians were investigating the parameters of his motor disorder. Microscopic examination of his brain revealed neurologic cellular damage entirely typical of chronic lithium intoxication and no evidence of pathology of cells in his striatum or substantia nigra, nor was their evidence of any other neurodegenerative condition. The authors conclude that his parkinsonism was an atypical manifestation of chronic lithium intoxication.

The majority of clinicians and investigators seem to agree, therefore, that the motor disorders associated with lithium pharmacology are manifestations of lithium toxicity. In general they agree with Axelsson and Nilsson (10), who investigated 37 lithium-treated patients on two occasions 7 years apart. The average lithium exposure in the group was 8.2 years, and every subject had been exposed to neuroleptics. Psychiatric status and side effects were evaluated; the Abnormal Involuntary Movement Scale (AIMS) was used to assess motor pathology. Eight percent of the patients showed involuntary movement disorders on first measure; 16% showed them 7 years later. Women were more vulnerable than men and hence were selected for further analysis, which showed that severe involuntary movements were associated with female gender, early onset of affective illness, low body weight, the occurrence of dementia in first-degree relatives, and, finally, with higher 12-hour serum lithium levels. The upshot of the report is that neostriatal pathology occurs almost exclusively because of exposure to toxic intracellular concentrations of lithium over time.

However, our experience is quite different, at least in one significant respect: patients with abnormal movements often had experienced preexisting insults to their basal ganglia. These patients were young, showed their disorders upon first exposure to unremarkable serum concentrations of lithium, and each and every one either lost his or her disorder (especially chorea) over time or could be treated quite effectively by lowering lithium doses and adding other mood stabilizers. If lithium toxicity is the culprit, therefore, the concept of toxicity must be expanded considerably. First, as others have noted, the toxic level of lithium decreases with age (11). Second, earlier conceptualizations of therapeutic lithium dosage and serum levels have to be down-tuned to exclude that degree of lithium exposure that can produce elevated thyroid-stimulating hormone, increases in polydypsia or polyurea, subtle problems in motor coordination and effectiveness, or, finally, blocked creativity with or without decreased libido. In summary, any previous central neuronal exposure—be it to streptococcal antibodies or substances such as neuroleptics and other psychoactive drugs—that produces even temporary changes in receptor

patterns and receptor affinities in the neostriatum must be considered.

There is, in fact, no reason to reject such an expanded definition of lithium excess and toxicity. The former case argued so well by Axelsson and Nilsson reflects situations in which there is decreased neuronal mass and, by inference, decreases in the number and changes in the sensitivity of both postbasal ganglia and prebasal ganglia receptors. The latter case simply pushes the beginning backward in time to include any exposure of said receptors that leads to upward or downward changes in sensitivity or to very early changes in receptor number, before actual neuronal loss has occurred. Recent changes in NIMH guidelines lowering maintenance lithium doses and maintenance serum levels reflect the same extended definition of lithium toxicity (12). Indeed, our group considers any patient who complains that their lithium maintenance regimen has produced chronic anergia, impaired imagination, decreased sexual function, or loss of his or her accustomed level of motor coordination to be experiencing lithium toxicity. If protection against relapse requires higher lithium regimens, we recommend that lithium doses be cut and maintenance of mood augmented with carbamazepine, divalproex sodium, lamotrigine, clonazepam, neurontin, clozapine, or, in very special situations, minimal doses of neuroleptics.

So far we have dealt with motor disorders that could reflect preexisting neurotransmitter receptor changes, actual loss of neuronal mass, or both. In the following discussion we will deal with those disorders that invariably are accompanied by mass effects:

1. Myoclonus and serotonin syndrome.
2. Creutzfeldt-Jakob–like syndromes that represent an intensification of myoclonic disorders associated with lithium administration, often when lithium is accompanied by serotonergic antidepressants.
3. Cerebellar disorders that result from acute central nervous system and cerebellar exposure to high concentrations of lithium, either from acute overdoses, from chronic long-term mismanagement with excessive lithium dosages, or from acute lithium intoxication that results from hemoconcentration—especially from that provoked by lithium-induced nephrogenic diabetes (NDI).

If one were to trace the development of loss of neuronal mass from lithium toxicity, the pathway would begin with the induction of myoclonus, then move into the realms of neuroleptic malignant syndromes, which in turn might lead to dementiform states—some representing generalized cortical and subcortical injury, some showing more specific features divided between those clinical symptoms reflecting Creutzfeldt-Jakob–type (spongiform encephalopathic) presentations and those symptoms reflective of pure cerebellar degeneration without dementia. The trigger for such devastation ranges from a single episode of severe, acute lithium toxicity to long-term, heavy-handed use of lithium producing chronic low-grade toxic lithium exposure and, perhaps most important, episodes of severe toxicity tantamount to dehydration with prerenal azotemia—most specifically that in the wake of lithium-induced NDI.

In the last type of case, there seems to be too casual an acceptance of polydypsia and polyurea by clinicians (13). They look at such symptoms as merely an annoyance to lithium maintenance regimens. Conversely, there seems to be no clinical recognition that even mild polydypsia and polyurea represent the beginnings of dehydration and prerenal failure. The lithium patient with NDI lives constantly on the precipice of dehydration and resultant acute lithium toxicity. In the University of Pittsburgh Research Affective Disorders Clinic, the advent of even early signs of NDI is an indicator to lower lithium dosage and fill in any gaps in mood stabilization with an antikindling anticonvulsant, particularly carbamazepine when NDI crops up (13).

From a study of 748 patients in a lithium clinic, Merikangas and Himmelhoch (14) have shown that the appearance of clinically significant myoclonus almost always occurs in the context of combined lithium regimens. Moreover, they have been able to show that in lithium-antidepressant combinations the more serotonergic antidepressants are the culprits in the manifestation of increasingly frequent and serious myocionic jerks. Of particular note are lithium and monoamine oxidase inhibitor (MAOI) and lithium and selective serotonin reuptake inhibitor (SSRI) combinations. Lithium by itself seems to have little connection with the induction of myoclonus. These observations have been supported by recent literature that also targets lithium in combination with serotonin-active antidepressants. Of particular interest in Muly and associate's (15) report of serotonin syndrome produced by a combination of fluoxetine and lithium. Serotonin syndrome, which is manifested by myoclonic jerks, fever and decreased core body temperature control, perceptual distortions, and severe gastrointestinal symptoms, can lead to dementia or death. It is most often seen when serotonergic substances are used in the presence of irreversible MAOIs, leading to high central concentrations of serotonin (16).

Sometimes myoclonic syndromes related to various lithium regimens progress to Creutzfeldt-Jakob–like spongioform encephalopathic deterioration (17,18,19). Lithium regimens associated with this outcome include lithium and levodopa (18) and lithium and nortriptyline (19), but the condition has been seen associated with pure, acute lithium toxicity. Finelli (20) describes a case caused by lithium and nortriptyline: a patient on lithium and nortriptyline developed progressive neurological deterioration consisting of worsening cognitive impairment, myoclonus, parkinsonism, an abnormal electroencephalogram (EEG), and fasciculations. The patient was considered for brain biopsy to diagnose Creutzfeldt-Jakob disease, but complete clinical recovery followed on withdrawal from lithium and nortriptyline. Indeed, reversibility is the distinguishing feature of this pharmacologic imitation of a disease that is fundamentally irreversible. This universal effect of lithium and central nervous system drug combinations and of lithium toxicity must be kept in mind, lest such patients be exposed to costly, invasive, and unnecessary neuroinvestigative procedures.

The most important myoclonic syndrome associated with lithium treatment is neuroleptic malignant syndrome (NMS) either with or without catatonia. Although previous lithium toxicity can increase a patient's vulnerability to this potentially lethal drug-treatment complication (21), NMS essentially never occurs without parallel use of neuroleptics. Even lithium-clozapine combinations (22) can produce severe myoclonus, which remits if lithium is stopped. Nevertheless, it is lithium-neuroleptic combinations that are almost always involved in the induction of rigidity, fever, an increased muscle isoenzyme of creatinine phosphokinase, autonomic dysfunction, delirium, and prerenal azotermia—the cardinal features of increasingly severe neuroleptic malignant syndrome.

Hermesh et al (23) investigated the occurrence of neuroleptic malignant syndrome in two prospectively followed series of psychiatric inpatients (120 in the first group, 103 in the second). Bipolar disorder and patients treated with depot injections of neuroleptics were significantly overrepresented. Lithium-haloperidol combinations have become symbolic of this problem, but there is nothing special about butyrophenones, since any neuroleptic, especially one given intramuscularly, can interact with lithium in the induction of NMS.

Keck et al (24) have used porcine stress syndrome, a genetic disorder in swine that spontaneously leads to a syndrome similar enough to NMS to be used as a possible animal model for NMS. They administered either haloperidol, lithium, or the two drugs combined to both susceptible and resistant pigs. Porcine stress syndrome was produced in two out of three susceptible animals and one out of three normally resistant ones with lithium and haloperidol combined, but it was not triggered in either susceptible or resistant pigs by lithium alone or by haloperidol alone.

Thus, evidence continues to accumulate that although lithium itself at therapeutic doses cannot produce NMS (or pseudoparkinsonism), it facilitates these most dangerous side effects of the neuroleptics. There is no systematic evidence to tease out how much it is the lithium molecule per se that facilitates NMS versus how necessary the particular vulnerability of bipolar patients to NMS is for lithium facilitation of motor anomalies that progress to catatonia. At present it seems that both the illness and its primary treatment interact in increasing the frequency and intensity of these neuroleptic side effects. Bipolar illness is consistently observed as a factor associated with an increased incidence of NMS.

The occurrence of NMS is particularly predicted by agitation and motor excitement, but not by psychosis (25). Bipolar I mood elevation can present a panoply of excited and agitated states. Kraepelin (26) described manic excitement ranging from grandiose manic psychosis to melancholia agitata (mixed mania) through manic stupor, which is indistinguishable from catatonic stupor. Taylor and Abrams (27) have identified catatonic stupor as a switch state belonging to severe bipolar I disorder, an opinion supported at least in part by Bunney et al (28) and Himmelhoch et al (29). Therefore, it can be seen that the mechanism for catatonia is already in place as part of the pathophysiology of manic psychosis. The increase in NMS seen in bipolar illness treated with neuroleptics and lithium may simply follow the same pathophysiologic pathway as manic stupor. No comparison of the incidence of NMS in bipolar I disorder (with manic psychosis) with that in bipolar II disorder (which never manifests mood elevation more than hypomania) has been made, but there is every indication that NMS should occur far more frequently in bipolar I patients, perhaps exclusively when bipolar I patients are experiencing severe or mixed mania.

Although NMS may simply occur as a pharmacologic intensification of the pathophysiology of severe bipolar disorder, cerebellar degeneration, the last of the lithium-related motor disorders to be discussed, seems to occur purely as a result of lithium poisoning. Neuroleptic malignant syndrome occurs stepwise, and it is not until full-blown NMS is manifest that cellular death occurs from high concentrations of intracellular lithium. Saran et al (30) performed a prospective electroencephalographic study on 21 patients treated with lithium–neuroleptic combinations. Fourteen of the patients were bipolar, seven schizophrenic. They were each administered a baseline EEG, and then a repeat study 10 to 14 days after combination therapy began. Five of 11 patients receiving lithium-haloperidol showed EEG abnormalities, whereas none of the 10 on other neuroleptics did. But the special toxicity of haloperidol and lithium was not the major finding (nor has it panned out to the degree that other neuroleptics should not be given very carefully in the presence of lithium salts). The authors concluded that the EEG was measuring evidence of neurotoxicity (in all likelihood lithium neurotoxicity) and of potential mass effect from cellular loss. Li et al (31) have shown how lithium-haloperidol combination reduces inosital phosphate, a critical substance in the cycle of second messenger function, hence reducing neurotransmitter information transfer in the frontal cortex and striatum. These reductions lead to intracellular accumulation of inosital and linked lipid fragments that is premonitory of cell death.

Cerebellar degeneration only occurs if there is cellular destruction, and cellular loss is caused only by lithium intoxication. To emphasize this point, Naramoto et al (32) report the autopsy results from a patient with cerebellar degeneration in immediately preceding NMS. This case might be considered that rare report of a pure lithium-induced NMS, but autopsy revealed complete loss of Purkinje cerebellar cells and mild destruction of other cerebellar cell types that had to have preceded NMS and are more typical sequelae of severe lithium toxicity. In this case, loss of central tem-

perature control and death followed, evidence of NMS, but proceeding from the most severe lithium exposure. The most important cause of cerebellar degeneration comes from the volume contraction that ensues in patients with severe lithium-induced NDI, which in turn leads to neurotoxic lithium concentration (11,33). Patients in this situation develop dysarthria, nystagmus, and gait disturbances. The highest serum lithium levels seen at the author's clinic have occurred in the context of NDI (34). As stated before, these cases have provoked us to substitute antikindling, anticonvulsant mood stabilizers for any lithium increment that produces polydypsia and polyurea. We have not experienced a single case of NDI or of significant lithium toxicity since this decision was made—all while preserving our previous efficacy in mood stabilization.

In general, lithium salts cause a range of motor disorders, from those that involve subtle, state-related, reversible effects all the way to those that produce neuronal death, hypersensitization of receptors, and loss of function and are sometimes lethal. It is the subtle effects and interactions that probably tell us most about the sites and mechanisms of lithium efficacy, for they occur by keeping said mechanisms in operation and either exaggerating or diminishing receptor-related and ionophoric activity. They also often depend on previous neurologic exposures experienced by the patient.

In these patients lithium seems to have an almost archaeologic quality that uncovers ancient, quiescent insults to one specialized group of neurons or another. In general, these findings support the observations of numerous investigators that lithium facilitates dyskinetic symptoms (35) and that dyskinetic symptoms augur poor lithium response (36). But others have reported that lithium can be used to treat tardive dyskinesia (37). Pert et al (38) have demonstrated that in animals lithium pretreatment blocks the development of neuroleptic-induced receptor supersensitivity. This conundrum is partially answered by the observation that a critical factor in determining the effects of lithium salts is the state of the organism when it is treated. In this sense, the only difference between Pert's observations and ours is the timing of the administration of lithium. Recent observations on membrane function by Mallinger et al (39,40) may help explain this state-dependent quality of lithium treatment. In carefully done experiments on lithium transport systems, these investigators have stoichiometrically demonstrated that during lithium treatment at a clinically significant concentration, excess cellular sodium may be extruded from erythrocytes (the model used) by increased activity of the membrane sodium-potassium pump, which has electrogenic properties and thereby could augment the cell's membrane potential. In potential counterweight, however, the phloretin-sensitive lithium countertransport system becomes increasingly less effective because of decreasing substrate affinity for lithium, thereby increasing intracellular lithium concentrations that are more and more difficult to extrude. Moreover, membrane detritus, such as phosphatidyl inosital and choline, contribute to the state-dependent effects of lithium. This web of membrane effects is the most probable pathway for lithium's efficacy and its oscillating collection of contradictory motor effects.

REFERENCES

1. Beitman BD. Tardive dyskinesia reinduced by lithium carbonate. Am J Psychiatry 1978;135:229–1230.
2. Nausieda PA, Koller WC, Klawans HL, Weiner WJ. Phenytoin and choreic movements. N Engl J Med 1978;298:1093–1094.
3. Luchins DJ, Sherwood PM, Gillin C, et al. Filicide during psychotropic-induced somnambulism: a case report. Am J Psychiatry 1978;135:1404–1405.
4. Kahn E. Organic driveness: a brainstem syndrome and an experience with case reports. N Engl J Med 1934;210:748–756.
5. Reed SM, Wise MG, Timmerman I. Choreoathetosis: a sign of lithium toxicity. J Neuropsychiatry Clin Neurosci 1989;1:57–60.
6. Helmuth D, Ljaljevic Z, Ramirez L, Meltzer HY. Choreoathetosis induced by verapamil and lithium treatment. J Clin Psychopharmacol 1989;9:454–455.
7. Matsis PP, Fisher RA, Tasman-Jones C. Acute lithium toxicity—chorea, hypercalcemia and hyperamylasemia. Aust N Z J Med 1989;19:718–720.
8. Holroyd S, Smith D. Disabling parkinsonism due to lithium: a case report. J Geriatr Psychiatry Neurol 1995;8:118–119.
9. Lecamwasam D, Synek B, Moyles K, Ghose K. Chronic lithium neurotoxicity presenting as Parkinson's disease. Int Clin Psychopharmacol 1994;9:127–129.
10. Axelsson R, Nilsson A. On the pathogenesis of abnormal involuntary movements in lithium-treated patients with major affective disorder. Eur Arch Psychiatry Clin Neurosci 1991;241:1–7.
11. Van der Velde CD. Toxicity of lithium carbonate in elderly patients. Am J Psychiatry 1971;127:115–117.
12. Consensus Development Panel. NIMH/NIH Consensus Development Conference Statement. Mood disorders: pharmacologic prevention of recurrences. Am J Psychiatry 1985;142:469–476.
13. Himmelhoch JM. On the failure to recognize lithium failure. Psychiatr Ann 1994;24:241–250.
14. Merikangas JR, Merikangas KR, Himmelhoch JM. Serotonergic activity and drug-induced myoclonus. Proc Am Psychiatric Assoc New Res 1986;139:95.
15. Muly EC, McDonald W, Steffens D, Book S. Serotonin syndrome produced by a combination of fluoxetine and lithium. Am J Psychiatry 1993;150:1565.
16. Sternbach H. The serotonin syndrome. Am J Psychiatry 1991;148:705–713.
17. Kemperman CJ, Notermans SL. Creutzfeldt-Jakob like syndrome due to lithium toxicity. J Neurol Neurosurg Psychiatry 1989;52:291.
18. Primavera A, Brusa G, Poeta MG. A Creutzfeldt-Jakob like syndrome due to lithium toxicity. J Neurol Neurosurg Psychiatry 1989;52:423.
19. Broussolle E, Setiey A, Moene Y, et al. Reversible Creutzfeldt-Jakob like syndrome induced by lithium plus levodopa treatment. J Neurol Neurosurg Psychiatry 1989;52:686–687.
20. Finelli PF. Drug-induced Creutzfeldt-Jakob like syndrome. J Psychiatry Neurosci 1992;17:103–105.
21. Joseph JK, Thomas K. Lithium toxicity—a risk factor for neuroleptic malignant syndrome. J Assoc Physicians India 1991;39:572–573.
22. Lemus CZ, Lieberman JA, Johns CA. Myoclonus during treatment with clozapine and lithium: the role of serotonin. Hillside J Clin Psychiatry 1989;11:127–130.
23. Hermesh H, Aizenberg D, Weizman A, et al. Risk for definite neuroleptic malignant syndrome. A prospective study in 223 consecutive inpatients. Br J Psychiatry 1992;161:254–257.
24. Keck PE Jr, Seeler DC, Pope HG Jr, McElroy SL. Porcine stress syndrome: an animal model for the neuroleptic malignant syndrome? Biol Psychiatry 1990;28:58–62.
25. Velamoor VR, Norman RM, Caroff SN, et al. Progression of symptoms in neuroleptic malignant syndrome. J Nerv Ment Dis 1994;182:168.
26. Kraepelin E. Manic-depressive insanity and paranoia (1921). Edinburgh: E&S Livingstone, 1987:106–107.
27. Taylor MA, Abrams R. Catatonia: prevalence and importance in the manic phase of manic depressive illness. Arch Gen Psychiatry 1977;34:1223–1225.
28. Bunney W, Murphy D, Goodwin F, et al. The "switch process" in manic-depressive illness. I. A systematic study of sequential behavior change. Arch Gen Psychiatry 1972;27:295–302.
29. Himmelhoch JM, Coble P, Kupfer DJ, Ingenito J. Agitated psychotic depression associated with severe hypomanic episodes: a rare syndrome. Am J Psychiatry 1976;133:765–771.
30. Saran A, Addy O, Foliart RH, et al. Electroencephalographic changes and other indices of neurotoxicity with haloperidol-lithium therapy. Neuropsychobiology 1989;20:152–157.
31. Li R, Wing LL, Wyatt RJ, Kirch DG. Effects of haloperidol, lithium, and valproate on phosphoinositide turnover in rat brain. Pharmacol Biochem Behav 1993;46:323–329.
32. Naramoto A, Koizumi N, Itoh N, Shigematsu H. An autopsy case of cerebellar degeneration following lithium intoxication with neuroleptic malignant syndrome. Acta Pathologica Japonica 1993;43:55–58.
33. Lee R, Jampol L, Brown W. Nephrogenic diabetes insipidus and lithium intoxication: complications of lithium carbonate therapy. N Engl J Med 1971;284:93–94.
34. Forrest J, Cohen A, Toretti J, et al. On the mechanism of lithium-induced diabetes insipidus in man and the rat. J Clin Invest 1974;53:1115–1123.
35. Branchey MH, Charles J, Simpson GM. Extrapyramidal side effects in lithium maintenance therapy. Am J Psychiatry 1976;133:444–445.
36. Himmelhoch JM, Neil JF, May SJ, et al. Age, dementia, dyskinesias and lithium response. Am J Psychiatry 1980;137:941–945.
37. Reda FA, Escobar JI, Scanlan JM. Lithium carbonate in the treatment of tardive dyskinesia. Am J Psychiatry 1975;132:560–562.
38. Pert A, Rosenblatt JE, Sivit C, et al. Long-term treatment with lithium prevents the development of dopamine receptor supersensitivity. Science 1978;201:171–173.
39. Mallinger AG, Hanin I, Himmelhoch JM, et al. Stimulation of cell membrane sodium transport activity by lithium: possible relationship to therapeutic action. Psychiatry Res 1987;22:49–59.
40. Mallinger AG, Himmelhoch JM, Thase ME, et al. Reduced cell membrane affinity for lithium ion during maintenance treatment of bipolar affective disorder. Biol Psychiatry 1990;27:795–798.

Antidepressant-Induced Myoclonus

Carmen Z. Lemus   Jeffrey A. Lieberman

INTRODUCTION

Myoclonus is defined as the rapid, involuntary contraction of a single muscle or group of muscles. There are two major types of myoclonus: arrhythmic myoclonus and segmental or rhythmic myoclonus. Arrhythmic myoclonus is characterized by irregular jerking movements that may be precipitated by sensory stimulation or by purposeful activity. It is associated with numerous disorders of the central nervous system (CNS), in cases of brain damage due to anoxia, infection, or trauma, and as a reaction to certain drugs and toxic agents. Typically, the movements disappear during sleep.

Segmental myoclonus presents with rhythmic muscle jerks that are not stimulus sensitive and may persist during sleep. It is usually due to lesions of the brainstem or spinal cord.

Of all pharmacologic compounds used in medical therapeutics, antidepressant drugs, including lithium, are among those that most frequently cause myoclonus. Antidepressant drugs are widely used compounds with proven efficacy in the treatment of affective disorders. More recently, indications for their use have expanded to include certain anxiety disorders, phobic states, chronic pain, and eating disorders. They are divided into two main categories: heterocyclic antidepressants (HCAs) and monoamine oxidase inhibitors (MAOIs).

MONOAMINE OXIDASE INHIBITORS

MAOIs bind irreversibly to monoamine oxidase (MAO), the degradation enzyme of monoamines. This produces an increase in the concentration and availability of serotonin (5-HT), dopamine (DA), norepinephrine (NE), and phenylethylamine, which is believed to be the mechanism by which MAOIs exert their antidepressant effect (1). Two types of MAO have been identified. MAO type A (MAO-A) primarily degrades 5-HT and NE and accounts for approximately 20% of the CNS MAO. MAO type B (MAO-B) degrades mostly DA and phenylethylamine and constitutes 80% of the MAO in the human brain (2).

The MAOIs that are currently available commercially (phenelzine, isocarboxazid, tranylcypromine) inhibit both types of MAO. Experimental agents that function as selective MAOIs have also been developed. Clorgyline and myclobemide inhibit MAO-A, whereas L-deprenyl and pargyline inhibit MAO-B. MAO-A inhibitors are considered more effective antidepressants than MAO-B inhibitors (3).

Neuromuscular effects of MAOIs have been extensively reported in the literature. Dally and Rhode (4) reported the occurrence of muscle twitching in treatment trials with various MAOIs, and suggested that it was particularly common with phenelzine. Several years later Goldberg (5) described episodes of increased neuromuscular activity with muscle twitching and involuntary movements of the extremities emerging at high doses of any MAOI. In another study, 14 depressed patients were treated with either 45 or 60 mg/day of phenelzine for 6 months. Two patients (14%) experienced muscle twitches that emerged after 2 to 3 months of treatment (6). A case of myoclonus and episodic delirium associated with therapeutic doses of phenelzine has been described by White (7). The patient was a 55-year-old woman who developed involuntary jerking movements of her legs, and cramps. These symptoms emerged after 44 days of treatment with 45 mg/day of phenelzine, prescribed for agoraphobia and generalized anxiety. A week later the patient showed behavioral signs of toxicity consisting of disorientation, depersonalization, hallucinations, and delusions. Phenelzine was discontinued and lorazepam 3 mg/day was started. The myoclonus and delirium disappeared by the seventh day.

Myoclonic activity has also been reported with selective MAOIs. Cohen et al (8) reported a case of myoclonus and hypomania that developed after 10 days of treatment with clorgyline. The patient was a 51-year-old man who experienced severe jerking movements in different body parts, which were precipitated by loud noises and exacerbated by anxiety. As the drug dose was decreased, the movements and hypomania abated.

The addition of another drug to an MAOI is also known to cause myoclonus. Several cases of myoclonus have developed after the 5-HT precursor L-tryptophan (20–50 mg/kg) was introduced. These symptoms included ataxia, hyperreflexia, spontaneous jerking movements of the legs, ankle clonus, and dysarthria, and disappeared within 24 hours after stopping the tryptophan (9). Glassman and Platman (10) described one patient who abruptly experienced muscle twitching, myoclonus, and hyperreflexia after ingesting 18 g of tryptophan while taking phenelzine. In this case the symptoms also subsided 24 hours after stopping the tryptophan. Another case involved a 26-year-old woman who was treated with 20 mg of tranylcypromine for 4 days. One hour after taking 2 g of L-tryptophan, she developed muscle jerks of the mouth, trunk, and extremities, and ocular movements (11). Similar cases have been reported by others (Table 20.1) (12,13).

HETEROCYCLIC ANTIDEPRESSANTS

HCAs block the reuptake of neurotransmitters released into the synapse, thereby increasing the availability of these neurotransmitters (14). In addition, they produce "downregulation" of postsynaptic receptors (15).

HCAs, although not entirely selective, act preferentially on either NE or 5-HT. The tertiary amine HCAs (imipramine, amitriptyline, trimipramine, clomipramine) are more potent inhibitors of 5-HT uptake, whereas the secondary amine HCAs (nortriptyline, desipramine) are more potent NE reuptake inhibitors (16).

Myoclonic activity has been frequently reported in HCA overdoses (17). A review of 100 cases of HCA overdose reported myoclonic movements in 43% of the subjects (18). These movements were characterized by twitching or jerkiness of the distal extremities and were precipitated by tactile or auditory stimuli.

Myoclonus had been considered an unusual complication of HCA treatment at therapeutic dosages (19). However, there have been several reports in the literature of myoclonic movements appearing during routine HCA treatment in patients with no prior history of neurologic disease.

In 1970, three cases of intention myoclonus were reported during treatment with imipramine and amitriptyline, which disappeared upon drug discontinuation (20). Another report involved a 25-year-old woman who experienced intermittent twitching and myoclonic movements of one hand on 150 mg/day of amitriptyline. Reducing the dose to 100 mg/day was effective in abolishing the movements. A subsequent increase to 125 mg/day produced a reemergence of violent, jerking movements (21). A similar report by the same group described myoclonic jerking of the limbs in a patient after the fifth day of treatment with 125 mg/day of amitriptyline (22). Other cases of HCA-induced myoclonus have been reported with clomipramine (23).

The only prospective study of myoclonus secondary to HCA therapy was conducted by Garvey and Tollefson (24). Of 98 patients who were starting treatment with HCAs, 39 (40%) experienced myoclonic movements. Most of these patients developed myoclonus within 1 month of initiating therapy. No group differences were found between patients with myoclonus and unaffected patients with respect to age, gender, and mean dose of antidepressants. This study suggests that the sensitivity of detection methods has a significant effect on the reported rates of drug-induced myoclonus.

Table 20.1   Reports of MAOI-Induced Myoclonus

Drug	No. of Patients	Comments	Reference
Phenelzine	2 of 14	Muscle twitching	Evans et al (6)
Phenelzine	1	Myoclonus of legs, delirium	White (7)
Clorgyline	1	Myoclonus of different body parts and hypomania; movements precipitated by loud noises	Cohen et al (8)
Pheniprazine + L-tryptophan	7	Myoclonus of the legs, ataxia, hyperreflexia, ankle clonus, dysarthria	Oates and Sjoerdsma (9)
Phenelzine + L-tryptophan	1	Muscle twitching, myoclonus, hyperreflexia	Glassman and Platman (10)
Tranylcypromine + L-tryptophan	1	Myoclonus of mouth, trunk, and extremities; ocular movements	Baloh et al (11)
Phenelzine + L-tryptophan	3	Myoclonus of legs, hyperreflexia, diaphoresis	Levy et al (13)
Phenelzine + L-tryptophan	1	Myoclonus of jaw, trunk, and limbs; hyperreflexia; ocular movements	Thomas and Rubin (12)
Phenelzine + imipramine	1	Muscle tension, twitching, myoclonus	Howarth (25)
Clorgyline + clomipramine	2	Myoclonus, hyperreflexia, cardiac irritability, "serotonin syndrome"	Insel et al (26)

Several authors have reported the emergence of myoclonus following a switch from an MAOI to an HCA. Howarth (25) described muscle tension, twitching, and clonus in an elderly patient switched from phenelzine to imipramine. A more unusual presentation is reported by Insel et al (26), who described two cases treated unsuccessfully with clorgyline. After the clorgyline trial both patients were medication free for 4 weeks. In spite of this washout period they developed myoclonic movements, hyperreflexia, and cardiac irritability after their first dose of clomipramine 100 mg administered orally. The reintroduction of clomipramine 6 weeks later did not produce any adverse effects. The authors noted the similarity between this presentation and the "serotonin syndrome" described in the animal pharmacology literature (27).

Two cases of myoclonus that developed after the addition of lithium to an HCA were reported (28). In one case the myoclonus improved but did not disappear after nortriptyline was maintained at 75 mg/day and lithium was discontinued. Once nortriptyline was stopped and treatment with desipramine was begun, the myoclonus disappeared within 1 week. The second patient developed myoclonic jerks of the upper and lower extremities on a combination of nortriptyline 125 mg/day, lithium 900 mg/day (lithium level 0.93 mmol/l), and propranolol 40 mg/day given for lithium-induced tremor. When lithium was decreased to 600 mg/day the movements disppeared.

NEW ANTIDEPRESSANTS

A series of new antidepressants have been marketed with chemical structures and pharmacology different from the classic HCAs and MAOIs. We will briefly discuss two of these new compounds that have been reported to cause myoclonus.

Maprotiline has been available in the United States since 1981. It is a tetracyclic compound derived by the addition of an ethylene bridge to the basic tricyclic structure (29). It is considered a relatively selective noradrenergic reuptake blocker with no inhibitory effect on 5-HT reuptake in vivo (30). Kettl and DePaulo (31) reported the occurrence of myoclonic jerks of the face in a 60-year-old woman within 1 week of starting treatment with maprotiline 50 mg/day. Despite this, the dose was raised to 75 mg/day and lithium was added. At this point the myoclonus worsened, with severe jerks of both arms and myoclonic jerks of her face that prevented her from speaking normally. Maprotiline and lithium were discontinued, and the movements disappeared within 3 days. Of interest is the fact that the patient had experienced the same symptoms previously while being treated with an unnamed HCA.

Another case report involved a 54-year-old woman who developed involuntary contractions of her extremities 4 days after her dose of maprotiline was increased from 150 to 200 mg/day (32). The movements were severe enough to cause the patient to lose grasp of objects, spill beverages, and fall several times. She also had contractions of pharyngeal muscles with resultant dysphonia. Maprotiline was stopped for 24 hours and reinstituted at 150 mg/day for 5 months without reemergence of myoclonus. Reexposure to a higher dose reproduced the myoclonus.

Trazodone is another new antidepressant commercially available in the United States since 1982. It is a phenylpiperazine derivative of triazolopyridine that causes selective but weak inhibition of 5-HT reuptake (33). One report in the literature describes a 38-year-old woman who developed myoclonus while receiving therapeutic doses of trazodone (34). The myoclonus gradually disappeared within 1 week of trazodone discontinuation (Table 20.2).

Table 20.2 Reports of Tricyclic and Other Antidepressant-Induced Myoclonus

Drug	No. of Patients	Comments	Reference
Tricyclic Antidepressants			
Amitriptyline	2	Twitching and jerking movements of upper extremities; intention myoclonus; abnormal EEG	Lippman et al (21,22)
Imipramine, amitriptyline	3	Intention myoclonus	Darcourt et al (20)
Clomipramine	15	Myoclonus of lower limbs appearing during sleep	Casas et al (23)
Imipramine, desipramine, amitriptyline, doxepin, trazodone, maprotiline, nortriptyline	30 of 98	Myoclonus of jaw, upper and lower extremities	Garvey and Tollefson (24)
Nortriptyline + lithium	2	Myoclonus of upper and lower extremities. Improvement with lithium discontinuation and switch from nortriptyline to desipramine.	Devanand et al (28)
Nontricyclic Antidepressants			
Maprotiline	1	Involuntary contractions of limb and pharyngeal musculature	DeCastro (32)
Trazodone	1	Myoclonic jerks of upper extremities	Patel et al (34)
Maprotiline + lithium	1	Myoclonus of arms and face, worsened when lithium was added	Kettl and DePaulo (31)

CLINICAL FEATURES

The phenomenology of antidepressant-induced myoclonus includes muscle twitching and jerking movements. Twitching movements can develop in isolated muscle groups or become generalized and experienced by the patient as a shivering sensation. Muscle jerks typically involve, in decreasing order of frequency, the lower extremities, upper extremities, trunk, neck, and face. The muscle jerks have been described during rest, as well as during the first stages of sleep. They may worsen with volitional activity, interfere with ambulation, and cause the patient to fall or lose grasp of objects. Contractions of the face and pharyngeal musculature may cause dysphonia. Findings on neurologic examination include diffuse hyperreflexia, unsustained ankle clonus, nystagmus, and tremor. The Babinski reflex is absent. There is no evidence of cerebellar dysfunction or cranial nerve involvement.

Electroencephalogram (EEG) recordings show paroxysmal abnormalities with bursts of sharp waves, spikes, and spike and slow wave activity of 2–4.5 Hz lasting 1 to 3 seconds. One study reported simultaneous sleep EEG, electro-oculogram, and electromyogram recordings in several patients being treated with phenelzine (35). They observed multiple rhythmic and arrhythmic single motor unit discharges in non–rapid eye movement (non-REM) periods, and sustained bursts in single and multiple muscle groups during REM periods. Muscle activity was present over 75% of the total sleep time.

Some investigators have postulated that the appearance and severity of myoclonus is dose related. The multiple reports showing an improvement in symptoms with a decrease in dosage would tend to support this claim. However, a study conducted by Casas et al (23) on a sample of 30 outpatients found no significant differences in the plasma levels of clomipramine or its metabolite desmethylclomipramine among subjects who developed myoclonus and a comparison group. The authors concluded that the development of myoclonic movements is related to individual idiosyncratic factors.

Antidepressant-induced myoclonus appears to be a totally reversible phenomenon that in most cases can be treated successfully by simply removing the responsible agent. The movements tend to improve within 24 hours of drug discontinuation, and full recovery usually occurs by the seventh day. In some cases stopping the antidepressant for 24 hours and then reintroducing it at a lower dose is sufficient to manage the adverse effects (21,22,32). When the myoclonus appears after the addition of a second medication (e.g., lithium, L-tryptophan) to an ongoing antidepressant trial, removal of the second agent may be enough, and treatment can continue with the original antidepressant.

It is important to note that serotonergic drugs that are used in the treatment of posthypoxic action myoclonus (5-hydroxytryptophan [5-HTP], MAOI plus L-tryptophan) can produce or exacerbate antidepressant-induced myoclonus, suggesting basic differences in the underlying pathophysiology.

NEUROCHEMICAL MECHANISMS

Antidepressant-induced myoclonus has been related to increased serotonergic neurotransmission. We will discuss the relevant preclinical and clinical evidence.

Preclinical Studies

Administration of the 5-HT precursor 5-HTP to guinea pigs has been shown to produce myoclonic movements (36,37). These movements are dose dependent and correlate with increases in brain 5-HT content (36). They are abolished by the 5-HT antagonists methysergide, methergoline, and cyproheptadine, but not by DA or NE receptor blockers (36–39). The myoclonic response to 5-HTP is also significantly decreased by blocking the conversion of 5-HTP to 5-HT (40) and can be enhanced by pretreatment with 5-HT reuptake inhibitors, peripheral aromatic amino acid decarboxylase inhibitors, and MAOIs (41,42).

Luscombe et al (43) conducted the most comprehensive study to date of guinea pig myoclonus, using a variety of compounds that act on the serotonergic system. The 5-HT agonists 5-methoxy-*N*, *N*-dimethyltryptamine, *N,N*-dimethyltryptamine, and LSD, and the 5-HT precursors tryptophan and tryptamine in conjunction with pargyline pretreatment all produced dose-dependent myoclonus. In contrast, the piperazine-containing agonist MK-212, quipazine, and 1-(*m*-trifluoromethylphenyl)-piperazine, even at very high doses, elicited only weak and intermittent myoclonus. Myoclonus was potently inhibited by pretreatment with the 5-HT antagonists methergoline and cyproheptadine, whereas methysergide, mianserin, and BW501C67 had little or no effect. 5-HT reuptake blockers varied in their ability to produce myoclonus. Pretreatment with clomipramine, paroxetine, and ORG6582 strongly potentiated myoclonus, whereas femoxetine, desipramine, and fluoxetine did not (Table 20.3). In the same study, DA and NE antagonists failed to inhibit the behavioral response.

Changes in postsynaptic receptors may also contribute to the development of myoclonus in laboratory animals. After induction of 5-HT receptor supersensitivity with chronic methysergide pretreatment, Klawans et al (44) were able to increase the myoclonic response to 5-HTP. Using a different paradigm, Stewart et al (38) produced postsynaptic supersensitivity by presynaptic denervation with the neurotoxin 5,7-dihydroxytryptamine. Following 5-HTP injection, lesioned rats developed myoclonus, whereas control rats showed increased locomotor activity but no myoclonus.

The activity of the enzyme MAO is believed to be important in the production of myoclonus. Neurologically intact rats developed a strong myoclonic response following

Table 20.3 Summary of the Ability of Serotonin Agonists or Precursors to Induce Myoclonus, Serotonin Antagonists to Antagonize 5-HTP-Induced Myoclonus, and Serotonin Reuptake Blockers to Potentiate 5-HTP-Induced Myoclonus in the Guinea Pig

Serotonin Agonists or Precursors	
Did produce myoclonus	**Did not produce myoclonus**
5-methoxy-*N,N*-dimethyltryptamine	Quipazine
	MK-212
N,N-dimethyltryptamine	1-(*m*-trifluoromethylphenyl)-piperazine
d-LSD	
5-HTP (+ carbidopa)	Tryptophan
Tryptophan (+ pargyline)	Tryptamine
Tryptamine (+ pargyline)	
Serotonin Antagonists	
Potently antagonized myoclonus	**Weak or no effect on myoclonus**
Methergoline	Mianserin
Cyproheptadine	Methylsergide
	BW 501C67
Serotonin Reuptake Blockers	
Strongly potentiated myoclonus	**Little or no potentiation of myoclonus**
Chlorimipramine	Femoxetine
Paroxetine	Fluoxetine
ORG6582	Desmethylimipramine

Modified, with permission of Pergamon Press, from Luscombe G, Jenner P, Marsden CD. Pharmacological analysis of the myoclonus induced by 5-hydroxytryptophan in the guinea pig suggests the presence of multiple 5-hydroxytryptamine receptors in the brain. Neuropharmacology 1981;20:819.

pretreatment with pargyline (38). Likewise, in unlesioned rats pretreated with a nonselective MAOI, 5-HTP and L-tryptophan produced myoclonus (45).

Luscombe et al have also examined the 5-HT receptor subtypes mediating the myoclonic response (46). Focusing on the brainstem, the area of the brain believed to initiate myoclonus in the guinea pig (37), they demonstrated specific binding sites for the 5-HT1 receptor, but weak and inconsistent binding for the 5-HT2 receptor. In addition, the 5-HT1 ligand was displaced by indole-containing 5-HT agonists but not by piperazine-containing agonists. They concluded that the myoclonus is mediated by 5-HT1 receptors.

The above findings suggest that increases in 5-HT availability, decreases in 5-HT catabolism, loss of presynaptic inactivation, and postsynaptic supersensitivity may all play a role in the induction of myoclonic activity. The relative importance of these mechanisms continues to be investigated.

Clinical Studies

Clinical evidence seems to support the role of 5-HT in the induction of antidepressant-induced myoclonus. The HCAs most commonly implicated (clomipramine, amitriptyline, and imipramine) are all 5-HT reuptake inhibitors. L-Tryptophan and lithium in combination with antidepres-

sants may also precipitate myoclonic episodes. Both these agents increase serotonergic activity. Tryptophan administration increases brain tryptophan and 5-HT levels, as well as the concentration of its major metabolite, 5-hydroxyindoleacetic acid (47). Lithium enhances serotonergic transmission in the rat forebrain, which is believed to underlie its ability to augment antidepressant response (48).

Using the same strategy described in the preclinical literature, Lieberman et al (35) gave 3–9 g/day of L-tryptophan to patients pretreated with phenelzine. L-Tryptophan aggravated the neuromuscular effects. These symptoms were reversed by methysergide and cyproheptadine. Administration of these antagonists to patients receiving phenelzine diminished the neuromuscular side effects.

Another method of assessing 5-HT involvement in myoclonus is to study the selective MAOIs. Because MAO-A degrades primarily 5-HT, a selective MAO-A inhibitor such as clorgyline would be expected to cause more myoclonus than a selective MAO-B inhibitor. In effect, there are several reports of myoclonus secondary to clorgyline, whereas L-deprenyl seems to cause these side effects much less frequently, even when given in combination with L-tryptophan (49). In our review of the literature we have come across only one case of myoclonus during treatment with L-deprenyl (50).

Although the evidence suggests that increased serotonergic activity may be responsible for the appearance of myoclonus in patients treated with antidepressants, the involvement of other neurotransmitters needs to be considered. All the antidepressants reviewed act on other neurotransmitter systems besides 5-HT to a greater or lesser extent. Even the selective MAOIs lose their selectivity at high doses, and crossover inhibition can occur. Moreover, the 5-HT model cannot explain the reports of myoclonus during maprotiline treatment (31,32). Maprotiline has no inhibitory effect on 5-HT reuptake in vivo (30) and is considered a relatively selective NE reuptake inhibitor (30,51).

DA activity may also be an important factor in relation to 5-HT-mediated myoclonus. Myoclonus activity induced in guinea pigs by tranylcypromine and 5-HTP was suppressed by the DA agonists apomorphine and 3,4-dihydroxyphenylethylamine (39). This suppression of 5-HTP-induced myoclonus by a DA agonist could in turn be reversed by the DA antagonists haloperidol and pimozide.

More studies are needed to pharmacologically characterize the mechanisms involved in antidepressant-induced myoclonus in human subjects. The preclinical literature supports the use of selective agonists and antagonists as a useful strategy. Measurement of monoamine metabolites in cerebrospinal fluid, although of limited value by itself, may provide further insights when done in conjunction with pharmacologic probes. The expanded clinical use of selective 5-HT reuptake inhibitors (e.g., fluoxetine, fluvoxamine) may also shed light on the role of serotonergic overactivity in the causation of antidepressant-induced myoclonus.

REFERENCES

1. Robinson DS, Nies A, Ravaris L, Ives JO, Bartlett D. Clinical pharmacology of phenelzine. Arch Gen Psychiatry 1978;35:629–635.
2. Yang HYT, Neff NH. The monoamine oxidases of brain: selective inhibition with drugs and consequences for the metabolism of the biogenic amines. J Pharmacol Exp Ther 1974;189:733–740.
3. Murphy DL, Aulakh CS, Garrick NA, Sunderland T. Monoamine oxidase inhibitors as antidepressants: implications for the mechanism of action of antidepressants and the psychobiology of the affective disorders and some related disorders. In: Meltzer HY, ed. Psychopharmacology: the third generation of progress. New York: Raven, 1987:545–552.
4. Dally PJ, Rhode P. Comparison of antidepressant drugs in depressive illnesses. Lancet 1961;i:18–20.
5. Goldberg LI. Monoamine oxidase inhibitors. Adverse reactions and possible mechanisms. JAMA 1964;190:456.
6. Evans DL, Davidson J, Raft D. Early and late side effects of phenelzine. J Clin Psychopharmacol 1982;2:208–210.
7. White PD. Myoclonus and episodic delirium associated with phenelzine: a case report. J Clin Psychiatry 1987;48:340–341.
8. Cohen RM, Pickar D, Murphy DL. Myoclonus-associated hypomania during MAO-inhibitor treatment. Am J Psychiatry 1980;137:105–106.
9. Oates JA, Sjoerdsma A. Neurologic effects of tryptophan in patients receiving a monoamine oxidase inhibitor. Neurology 1960;10:1076–1078.
10. Glassman AH, Platman SR. Potentiation of a monoamine oxidase inhibitor by tryptophan. J Psychiatr Res 1969;7:83–88.
11. Baloh RW, Dietz J, Spooner JW. Myoclonus and ocular oscillations induced by L-tryptophan. Ann Neurol 1982;11:95–97.
12. Thomas JM, Rubin EH. Case report of a toxic reaction from a combination of tryptophan and phenelzine. Am J Psychiatry 1984;141:281–283.
13. Levy AB, Bucher P, Votolato N. Myoclonus, hyperreflexia and diaphoresis in patients on phenelzine–tryptophan combination treatment. Can J Psychiatry 1985;30:434–436.
14. Baldessarini RJ. The basis for amine hypothesis in affective disorders. A critical evaluation. Arch Gen Psychiatry 1975;32:1087–1093.
15. Sulser F. New perspectives on the mode of action of antidepressant drugs. Trends Pharmacol Sci 1979;1:92–94.
16. Rudorfer MV, Potter WZ. Pharmacokinetics of antidepressants. In: Meltzer HY, ed. Psychopharmacology: the third generation of progress. New York: Raven, 1987.
17. Starkey IR, Lawson AAH. Poisoning with tricyclic and related antidepressants—a ten year review. Q J Med 1980;193:33–49.
18. Noble J, Matthew H. Acute poisoning by tricyclic antidepressants: clinical features and management of 100 patients. Clin Toxicol 1969;2:403–421.
19. Sovner R, DiMascio A. Extrapyramidal syndromes and other neurological side effects of psychotropic drugs. In: Lipton MA, DiMascio A, Killan K, eds. Psychopharmacology: a generation of progress. New York: Raven, 1978.
20. Darcourt G, Fadeuilhe A, Lavagna J, et al. Trois cas de myoclonies d'action au cors de traitements par l'imipramine et l'amitriptyline. Rev Neurol 1970;122:141–142.
21. Lippman S, Moskovitz R, O'Tuama L. Tricyclic-induced myoclonus. Am J Psychiatry 1977;134:90–91.
22. Lippman S, Tucker D, Wagemaker H, Schulte T. A second report of tricyclic-induced myoclonus. Am J Psychiatry 1977;134:585–586.
23. Casas M, Garcia-Ribera C, Alvarez E, Udina C, Queralto JM, Grau JM. Myoclonic movements as a side-effect of treatment with therapeutic doses of clomipramine. Int J Psychopharmacol 1987;2:333–336.
24. Garvey MJ, Tollefson GD. Occurrence of myoclonus in patients treated with cyclic antidepressants. Arch Gen Psychiatry 1987;44:269–272.
25. Howarth E. Possible synergistic effects of the new thymoleptics. J Ment Sci 1961;107:100–108.
26. Insel TR, Roy BF, Cohen RM, Murphy DL. Possible development of the serotonin syndrome in man. Am J Psychiatry 1982;139:954–955.
27. Squires RF. Monoamine oxidase inhibitors: animal pharmacology. In: Iversen L, Iversen S, Snyder S, eds. Handbook of psychopharmacology. vol. 14. New York: Plenum, 1978.
28. Devanand DP, Sackeim HA, Brown RP. Myoclonus during combined tricyclic antidepressant and lithium treatment. J Clin Psychopharmacol 1988;8:446–447.
29. Blackwell B. Newer antidepressant drugs. In: Meltzer HY, ed. Psychopharmacology: the third generation of progress. New York: Raven, 1987:1041–1049.
30. Baumann PA, Maitre L. Neurobiochemical aspects of maprotiline (Ludiomil) action. J Int Med Res 1979;7:391–400.
31. Kettl P, DePaulo JR. Maprotiline-induced myoclonus. J Clin Psychopharmacol 1983;3:264–265.
32. DeCastro RM. Antidepressants and myoclonus: case report. J Clin Psychiatry 1985;46:284–287.
33. Riblet LA, Taylor DP. Pharmacology and neurochemistry of trazodone. J Clin Psychopharmacol 1981;1(suppl 1):17–22.
34. Patel HC, Bruza D, Yeragoni V. Myoclonus with trazodone. J Clin Psychopharmacol 1988;8:152.
35. Lieberman JA, Kane JM, Reife R. Neuromuscular effects of monoamine oxidase inhibitors. J Clin Psychopharmacol 1985;5:221–228.
36. Klawans HL, Goetz C, Weiner WJ. 5-Hydroxytryptophan-induced myoclonus in guinea pigs and the possible role of serotonin in infantile myoclonus. Neurology 1973;23:1234–1240.
37. Chadwick D, Hallett M, Jenner P, Marsden CD. 5-Hydroxytryptophan-induced myoclonus in guinea pigs. J Neurol Sci 1978;35:157–165.
38. Stewart RM, Campbell A, Sperk G, Baldessarini RJ. Receptor mechanisms in increased sensitivity to serotonin agonists after dihydroxytryptamine shown by electronic monitoring of muscle twitches in the rat. Psychopharmacology 1979;60:281–289.
39. Volkman PH, Lorens SA, Kindel GH, Ginos JZ. L-5-Hydroxytryptophan-induced myoclonus in guinea pigs: a model for the study of central serotonin–dopamine interactions. Neuropharmacology 1978;17:947–955.
40. Stewart RM, Growdon JH, Cancian D, Baldessarini RJ. 5-Hydroxytryptophan induced myoclonus: increased sensitivity to serotonin after intracranial 5,7-dihydroxytryptamine in the adult rat. Neuropharmacology 1976;15:449–455.
41. Nakumura M, Fukushima H, Kitagawa S. Effects of amitriptyline and isocarboxazid on 5-hydroxytryptophan-induced head twitches in mice. Psychopharmacology 1976;48:101.
42. Klawans HL, Carvey PM, Tanner CM, Goetz CG. Drug-induced myoclonus. In: Fahn S, Marsden CD, VanWoert M, eds. Advances in neurology. vol. 43. New York: Raven, 1986:251–264.
43. Luscombe G, Jenner P, Marsden CD. Pharmacological analysis of the myoclonus induced by 5-hydroxytryptophan in the guinea pig suggests the presence of multiple 5-hydroxytryptamine receptors in the brain. Neuropharmacology 1981;20:819.
44. Klawans HL, D'Amico DJ, Nausieda PA, Weiner WJ. The specificity of neuroleptic- and methysergide-induced behavioral supersensitivity. Psychopharmacology 1977;55:49–52.
45. Grahame-Smith DG. Studies in vivo on the relationship between brain tryptophan, brain 5-HT synthesis and hyperactivity in rats treated with a monoamine oxidase inhibitor and L-tryptophan. J Neurochem 1971;18:1053.
46. Luscombe G, Jenner P, Marsden CD. Correlation of [³H] 5-hydroxytryptamine (5-HT) binding to rat brainstem preparations and the production and prevention of myoclonus in guinea pig by 5-HT agonists and antagonists. Eur J Pharmacol 1984;104:235.
47. Fernstrom JD, Wurtman RJ. Brain serotonin content: physiological dependence on plasma tryptophan levels. Science 1971;173:149–152.
48. DeMontigny C, Cournoyer G, Mousette R, Langlois R, Caille G. Lithium carbonate addition in tricyclic resistant unipolar depression. Arch Gen Psychiatry 1983;40:1327–1334.
49. Mendlewicz J, Youdim MBH. Antidepressant potentiation of 5-hydroxytryptophan by L-deprenyl, an MAO "type B" inhibitor. J Neural Transm 1978;43:279–286.
50. Mann JJ, Aarons SF, Wilner PJ, et al. A controlled study of the antidepressant efficacy and side effects of (−)-Deprenyl. A selective monoamine oxidase inhibitor. Arch Gen Psychiatry 1989;46:45–50.
51. Maitre L, Waldmeier PC, Greengrass PM, Jackel J, Sedlacek S, Delini-Stula A. Maprotiline—its position as an antidepressant in the light of recent neuropharmacological and neurobiochemical findings. J Int Med Res 1975;3(suppl 2):2–15.

Spontaneous and Drug-Induced Disorders of Movement in the Elderly

Bruce L. Saltz   Jeffrey A. Lieberman

Since the advent of antipsychotic medications in the 1950s, innumerable reports have appeared in the medical literature about the neuroleptic-induced neuromuscular disorder tardive dyskinesia. Research into the prevalence of this disorder has been complicated by multiple methodologic issues, including the variability in diagnostic criteria and the potential for false positive cases. The diagnostic differentiation of "spontaneous" from drug-induced neuromuscular disorders has been particularly troublesome because of the lack of knowledge about pathophysiologic mechanisms.

The classification of movement disorders is replete with problems of specificity. For example, even the expression "movement disorder" may be a misnomer because abnormalities of static posture are often a feature (sometimes exclusively) of these very conditions. Many of the terms used to represent signs and symptoms are applied differently by different examiners and may overlap in meaning (e.g., dystonia, dyskinesia, tics, athetosis, chorea, myoclonus). Table 21.1 (1) contains a list of definitions and descriptions that may be used to identify these phenomena accurately and reliably.

Recognition of nonmotor signs and symptoms that may coexist with such disorders of movement is important for proper diagnostic formulation. For example, the association of pregnancy and chorea may suggest gravidarum chorea, whereas the association of intellectual dysfunction with chorea may be more suggestive of Huntington's disease. Table 21.2 (2–4) contains a list of medical conditions in which abnormal movements are found. Motor phenomena may be a principal feature of a primary movement disorder (e.g., Sydenham's chorea, senile chorea, Huntington's disease), or they may occur as a common association (e.g., in Alzheimer's disease) or uncommon association (e.g., in polycythemia vera).

The scientific literature indicates that elderly individuals are more likely than younger people to be afflicted by certain kinds of adventitious neuromuscular conditions (e.g., Huntington's disease, Parkinson's disease, myoclonus in Creutzfeldt-Jakob disease) (5–9). The clinicopathologic characteristics of these disorders have been well described (10–12). Thus, a number of neurobehavioral disorders must be considered in the differential diagnosis of tardive dyskinesia, which also occurs with greater frequency in the elderly (13–29).

Kane and Smith (30) reviewed 56 prevalence surveys of tardive dyskinesia in psychiatric populations. They compared the results with the prevalence rates of "spontaneous dyskinesias" in 19 samples of untreated individuals, and found average prevalence rates of 20% in neuroleptic-treated individuals and 5% in untreated individuals. However, direct comparison of rates must be made with caution because of possible differences in many other important variables, such as age, gender, cumulative drug exposure, diagnosis, and history of other extrapyramidal phenomena.

Kane et al (31) studied 151 individuals (38% male) attending two senior citizen community centers: 6 with a history of psychiatric illness, 17 with a history of neurologic illness, 1 after partial mandibulectomy, and 127 healthy elderly (mean age: 72.3 years). Using criteria applied to tardive dyskinesia rating scores derived from the Simpson dyskinesia scale (SDS) (1) modified by the addition of a global severity item, 4% (5 of 127) were found to have abnormal involuntary movement scores (AIMS) of mild severity or greater (all were women). The researchers pointed out that if individuals with "questionably positive" ratings were included, the prevalence rate increased to 8%.

In a study that has been widely quoted, Owens et al (32) surveyed 1,227 inpatients' case notes and identified 635 with a diagnosis of schizophrenia who had been hospitalized for more than a year, 524 of whom met Feighner's criteria on present state examination, without evidence of a discrete neurologic condition. Five hundred and ten remained in the

Table 21.1 Types of Adventitious Movements

Dyskinesia	Generic term that refers to excessive or abnormal involuntary movement that can be subcharacterized depending on rhythmicity, speed, repetition, and other characteristics
Tremor	Rhythmic oscillatory movements that may occur at different frequencies and that may be present at rest or during action
Tic	Transient complex coordinated movements that appear suddenly, such as eye blinking and head turning; vocal activity may be involved
Chorea	Brief, irregular, nonrhythmic contractions, usually purposeless, often coarse or quick
Athetosis	Continuous, slow, writhing movements
Hemiballismus	Wild uncontrollable flinging movements of the extremities
Dystonia	Involuntary motor activity that is terminated with sustained contractions at the end of the movement; frequently twisting in character; sometimes the sustained contraction is present only while the affected body part is active
Myoclonus	Lightning-like movements secondary to contractions or inhibition of contraction of single muscles or groups of muscles
Akathisia	Restlessness characterized by inability to sit or stand still

Table 21.2 Conditions in which Adventitious Movements Can Be Identified

Congenital or Hereditary
Acanthocytosis, acute intermittent porphyria, ataxia telangiectasia, atrophy, benign familiar chorea, cerebral palsy, dystonia musculorum deformans, glutaric acidemia, Hallervorden-Spatz, hereditary lipidoses, Huntington's disease, Lesch-Nyhan syndrome, olivopontocerebellar degeneration, perinatal injury (e.g., anoxia, kernicterus), Wilson's disease

Inflammatory or Infectious
Brain tumors, diphtheria, Henoch-Schönlein purpura, Creutzfeldt-Jakob disease, Lyme disease, multiple sclerosis, periarteritis nodosa, pertussis, rheumatoid arthritis, serum sickness, subacute sclerosing panencephalitis, Sydenham's chorea, syphilis, systemic lupus erythematosus, varicella, other encephalitides

Toxic/Metabolic
Amphetamines, carbon monoxide, dilantin, hypernatremia, hepatic encephalopathy, hypocalcemia, hypoglycemia, hypokalemia, L-dopa, lithium, manganese, mercury, methyl bromide, methylphenidate, neuroleptics, oral contraceptives, parathyroid disease, strychnine, thyroid disease

Psychogenic
Mannerisms associated with illnesses such as schizophrenia

Posttraumatic Syndromes
Subdural hematoma

Miscellaneous
Alzheimer's disease, Brueghel's syndrome, cerebrovascular accidents, edentulous dyskinesia, epilepsy, idiopathic torsion dystonia, Meige's syndrome, Parkinson's disease, Pick's disease, polycythemia, progressive supranuclear palsy, senile chorea, Tourette's syndrome, transient facial myokymia

hospital during the study, and 65 had never been treated. At initial examination, 50% had some kind of abnormal movement, and 411 were reexamined 12 to 18 months later. Ages of the neuroleptic-treated individuals ranged from 21 to 91 years (mean: 56.9 years). Ages of the untreated individuals ranged from 29 to 90 years (mean: 66.7 years). The prevalence rates of AIMS at different severity levels were compared for those with and those without a history of neuroleptic exposure. No statistical differences were found at any severity level in any body region using either AIMS or SDS for abnormal involuntary movements. The prevalence of abnormal movements using an AIMS threshold of 2 or greater (33) in those free from neuroleptic exposure was 53.2% (76.6% using SDS). The difference in rates between scales was mostly due to the inclusion of tremor in SDS. Facial movements were predominant. Using a criterion value of greater than or equal to 3 reduced the prevalence rate to 36.2%. The authors concluded that spontaneous involuntary movement disorders can be a feature of severe chronic schizophrenia unmodified by neuroleptic drugs.

One additional factor noted by the authors was that 8.5% of the total population studied may have had cerebral lesions undetected by routine clinical examination, with 5% to 6% having suffered infarctions. Because patients in the neuroleptic-free group were older (average age: 66.7 ± 11.7 years), the authors concluded that the abnormal movements may represent some age-related neurologic condition, such as senile chorea or mouthing.

Villeneuve et al (34) examined four samples of elderly individuals for the purpose of assessing the frequency of some release phenomena and iterative activities and their association with psychiatric illness and psychotropic medications, principally neuroleptics. They looked for four different types of abnormal movements:

1. Hypertonia: increased rigidity in motor and psychological fields, typically *gegenhalten* (a particular form of motor rigidity also called "negativism" or "opposition hypertonia.") Operationally, they counted any resistance of the forearm to passive movement and did not separately distinguish parkinsonism.
2. Tonic transmission: in contrast to opposition hypertonia, once the initial resistance to movement has been overcome, this movement is pursued automatically by the patient as long as a contact (even a light one) is maintained by the examiner's hand.
3. Spontaneous oral movements: protrusion of tongue, suction of tongue, chewing movements.
4. Other stereotyped activities: kneading, folding, smoothing, thumbing, polymorphic movements of the hands, legs, or whole body.

The total number of patients was 155 (55 men, 100 women): 56 with organic brain syndromes (group I), 30 of whom had senile dementia; 51 with functional psychoses (group II), mostly schizophrenic, average age 70.9 years; and 16 with chronic schizophrenia (group III) untreated by neuroleptics (all women). Also examined were 32 "normal, healthy elderly" (group IV) from a private nursing home, average age 76.3 years, of whom 34% were men. The groups were not perfectly matched by age or total amount of neuroleptic exposure. Most of the individuals in the first two groups were still receiving neuroleptics.

Hypertonia was seen in 50%, 37%, 19%, and 0%, in groups I, II, III, and IV, respectively. Tonic transmission was seen in 16%, 12%, 19%, and 0%, respectively. Oral movements were seen in 30%, 32%, 31%, and 0% respectively, often associated with oral release phenomena like pouting, sucking, and the palmomental reflex. Stereotyped activities were seen only in groups I and II, at 16% and 4% respectively, primarily in senile dementia. The authors concluded that release phenomena and iterative activities were seen significantly more frequently in patients with "organic brain syndromes" than in controls, and that individuals older than 50 may be more susceptible to neuroleptic-induced dyskinesias or reversible neurologic complications.

In 1972, Altrocchi (35) described the case of a 64-year-old woman with no prior neuroleptic exposure who developed spontaneous jaw opening and "restlessness of her tongue." She had worn dentures for 17 years prior to that point, but they fit her well until several months prior to the onset of her dyskinesia. She later developed constant involuntary jaw opening with dystonia and difficulty in chewing, but no dysphagia. New dentures did not help. Symptoms worsened with stress and fatigue, but disappeared with sleep. Past medical history was positive for progressive bilateral exophthalmos, which had occurred 22 years earlier and was treated by orbital decompression surgery followed years later by pituitary radiation because of disease progression. At that point, thyroid supplementation (1.5 grains/day) was initiated, along with prednisone 5 mg/day. The oral dyskinesia was much improved on first exposure to chlorpromazine 100 mg and trihexyphenidyl 6 mg, but when movements reappeared upon drug withdrawal, they could not be suppressed by reinstitution of the drug.

Later, Marsden et al (36–38) reported on the dystonic variant of dyskinesia in their description of 39 cases of blepharospasm–oromandibular dystonia syndrome (Brueghel's syndrome). These individuals exhibited prolonged spasms of contraction of mouth and jaw muscles, distinct from the chewing, lip smacking, or tongue rolling choreiform movements of oral dyskinesia. These individuals had no personal or family history of this or other neurologic or mental deficit or use of known offending drugs at the onset of illness. Among the 39 cases (36% male), 13 had isolated blepharospasm, 17 had blepharospasm and oromandibular involvement, and 9 had oromandibular involvement only. The average duration of symptoms was 5 years, and the peak age at onset was in the sixth decade. The author likened these diseases to focal manifestations of the syndrome of

adult-onset torsion dystonia. No consistent abnormalities were seen on skull radiographs, brain scans, electroencephalograms (EEG), cerebrospinal fluid, or plasma calcium and copper studies when done.

Lieberman et al (39) have suggested that tardive dystonia is a valid subtype of tardive dyskinesia with different pathophysiologic and pharmacologic characteristics. Differences in mechanisms may also exist between dystonic and nondystonic "spontaneous" dyskinesias.

Another report of dystonia, this time in a nonelderly patient without restriction to the orofacial region, was made by Altrocchi and Forno (40). They reported neuropathologic findings of a 44-year-old man with "spontaneous oral facial dyskinesia." He developed involuntary contraction of the frontalis muscle, followed 2 months later by prominent involuntary jaw opening. For 6 years, his mouth remained open much of the time, associated with facial grimacing and difficulty speaking, chewing, and swallowing. Later he developed an intermittently dystonic right leg and retrocollis, associated with mild cogwheel rigidity of the arms and akathisia in all limbs. His symptoms progressively worsened, with severe dysphagia leading to cachexia and death from aspiration pneumonia. He had no known family history of movement disorders, and no prior personal exposure to neuroleptics, amphetamines, L-dopa, tricyclic antidepressants, antihistamines, phenytoin, lithium, anticholinergics, or benzodiazepines. Laboratory studies were unrevealing, including chemistry screen, ceruloplasmin, serum antinuclear antibody (ANA), skull films, electromyography (EMG), slit lamp, bilateral carotid angiography, spinal tap, and pneumoencephalography. Pathologic examination revealed no gross atrophy of cortical or subcortical structures, except for slight flattening of the caudate nuclei. Microscopic abnormalities were present only in the dorsal halves of the caudate and putamen, consisting of uneven cell loss with gliosis, giving a mosaic appearance. The authors concluded that this pattern may have been caused by a selective vulnerability of functionally or metabolically different cell populations within the caudate and putamen to an unidentified insult.

Dystonia has also been associated with a basal ganglia disorder that shares some features with Parkinson's disease. Rafal and Friedman (41) reviewed the charts of 30 patients with limb dystonia in progressive supranuclear palsy (PSP; diagnostic criteria not specified). The dystonia was rated on the scale of Burke et al (42). A positive rating required the continuous presence of dystonia in more than one limb, and a score of 3 or greater (1 = mild dystonia without limitation of limb function; 2 = moderate dystonia with some preservation of function; 3 = severe dystonia preventing useful function; 4 = extreme dystonia with pain, deformity, or soft tissue damage). Patients who developed dystonia late in the course of PSP or secondary to L-dopa or other medications were excluded. Eight individuals met these criteria. Their charts were further reviewed for evidence of degree of ophthalmoparesis and neck dystonia. Limb dystonia did not correlate with the presence or severity of neck dystonia or degree of ophthalmoparesis. No patient had a history of cerebrovascular disease. All had normal head computed tomography (CT) scans. One patient, who died with severe hemiplegic dystonia and severe right upper extremity intention tremor, had severe neuronal loss, gliosis, and neurofibrillary changes in the substantia nigra, colliculi, peritectal and periaqueductal regions, subthalamic nucleus, and globus pallidus. Atrophy and neurofibrillary changes were seen in the cerebral cortex and hippocampus. Severe neuronal loss was seen in the dentate region of the cerebellum bilaterally. The authors concluded that limb dystonia may be a common early feature of PSP.

Several reports describe nondystonic orofacial dyskinesias, which suggests that both local (e.g., dental) and central nervous system processes must be considered when evaluating such motor differences. Koller (43,44) studied 75 (49% male) consecutive elderly demented and nondemented individuals (mean age: 68.6 years) without tooth extractions, who were seen as part of a study of aging. Also studied were 75 (99% male) patients (mean age: 62 years) with total or partial tooth removal in a Veteran's Administration dental clinic. Patients with exposure to medications known to cause abnormal movements or with recognizable neurologic disorders were excluded. AIMS was used to characterize movements. Also tested were the ability to keep the tongue protruded for 30 seconds, and double simultaneous stimulation and two-point discrimination on tongue and gingiva. Twelve (16%) of 75 edentulous patients and none of 75 nonedentulous patients had orofacial dyskinesia. In the dyskinesia patients, 8 had had total tooth extractions, and 4 had had partial. These had been performed an average of 17.8 years before. Five of 12 wore dentures, 1 of 12 wore partial dentures, and 6 of 12 wore no dentures. The abnormal movements consisted mostly of lip smacking, lip pursing, lateral deviation, and protrusion of the tongue and jaw. Six reported the average time of onset as 1.9 years prior to evaluation. Sixty-three of 75 edentulous patients (53 with total tooth removal, 10 with at least all teeth missing from one jaw) did not have facial dyskinesia. All were male (mean age: 59.4 years, range: 29–84 years). Tooth removal averaged 12.3 years prior to evaluation, and all but 6 patients wore dentures. The authors concluded that not all orofacial movements in the elderly are due to neuroleptic-induced tardive dyskinesia. Many orofacial dyskinesias are related to dental problems such as absence of needed dentures or presence of ill-fitting dentures.

Woerner et al (45) examined 2,250 individuals at three psychiatric and two geriatric sites, including 400 healthy elderly volunteers in an NIMH-sponsored prevalence survey of tardive dyskinesia. The healthy elderly sample, age range 60 to 79 years (mean ± SD = 73 ± 7 years) was 29.2% male and mostly Caucasian. Five of 400 (40% male) exhibited abnormal movements that would have met criteria for "case" designation but had no prior neuroleptic exposure. Thus, the prevalence rate was 1.25%. Among the 293

untreated patients in a medical geriatric hospital constituting another subsample in this prevalence survey, the rate of "spontaneous dyskinesia" was 4.8%. The role of denture use was examined in the total sample. Users were subdivided into two groups: those who did and those who did not wear dentures at the time of examination. Users not wearing dentures at the time of examination were found to be at increased risk of being rated "positive" as a "case" of tardive dyskinesia, especially between the ages of 35 and 55. Younger patients (less than 55 years) wearing dentures were also more prone to be classified as positive for tardive dyskinesia, but the increased risk was less than that seen in users not wearing dentures. Regression analysis was performed to adjust for effects of age, gender, site, and duration of neuroleptic use. Individuals who had dentures but did not wear them were 3.5 times more likely to be rated as having tardive dyskinesia than those without dentures. Users who wore dentures were at slightly elevated risk to be rated tardive dyskinesia positive when compared with nonusers. The authors did not speculate about alternative pathophysiologic mechanisms.

Sutcher et al (46) described four patients who had been seen in a university neuropsychiatric unit for orofacial dyskinesias that had not responded to treatment with trihexyphenidyl and benadryl. The subjects (one man, three women) ranged in age from 45 to 72 years. Three had complete upper and lower dentures, one had complete upper dentures and a removable partial lower denture, and all had grossly incorrect occlusions. They had various combinations of oral, facial, and cervical dyskinesias, and some had attendant problems with speech or muscle pain. All had moderate improvement in many symptoms with progressive alterations in new dental prosthetics. The author pointed out that most people with ill-fitting dentures do not develop these problems, but suggested that the cause of neuromuscular problems in some may be related to periodontal proprioception abnormalities.

Some cases of antihistamine- and benzodiazepine-associated dyskinesias and dystonias have been reported (47,48), but comprehensive evaluations of local oral pathology, non-CNS, toxic, metabolic, infectious, or other neuromedical disorders that could have caused these apart from medication were not always done.

A variety of different lesions in the basal ganglia, cerebellum, and cerebral cortex have been associated with spontaneous movement disorders. Although there have been a number of case reports about clinical and pathologic correlates of spontaneous movement disorders, no large controlled studies have been done in this area.

Alcock (49) described the neuropathology in two men (aged 56 and 62) who exhibited dyskinesias (of ungraded severity) and who had no known family history of movement disorders. The older patient showed a marked decrease of total cell counts in the caudate and putamen, with an apparent increase in number in the globus pallidus, which was otherwise normal in appearance and accounted for by the shrinkage in the structure's total size. No changes in the cerebral cortex or blood vessels were seen. The younger patient showed a small reduction in cell count in the caudate and a marked reduction in the putamen. Likewise, no cerebral cortex or blood vessel changes were seen.

Cerebrovascular disease may be a risk factor for the development of abnormal involuntary motor activity. Certain cerebrovascular diseases are more prevalent in the elderly (e.g., stroke). Appenzeller and Biehl (50) reported 11 cases of elderly edentulous individuals (aged 55 to 95, nine men, two women) with "mouthing" and a variety of neuromedical and psychiatric presentations. Two of the men (aged 72 and 74 years), who had no prior history of "phenothiazine" exposure, exhibited significant microscopic cell loss in the cerebellum. The first patient had a prior history of tuberculosis, subtotal gastrectomy for adenocarcinoma, and a subdural hematoma. The second had a history of recurrent seizures and multiple pathologic neurologic signs consistent with one or more strokes.

Abbruzzese et al (51) reported EMG features of four elderly hypertensive patients with a history of sudden-onset vascular hemichorea. All had generalized cardiovascular disease but none had a family history of movement disorder or signs of "mental deterioration." Only one had an otherwise abnormal neurologic examination with signs of a previous contralateral hemiparesis. All but one had abnormal CT scans with small multiple ischemic lesions always involving inter alia and contralateral basal ganglia. EMG showed gross irregularity and random variability of burst duration and of muscle activation order.

Modern imaging techniques have been used to detect structural brain changes that are associated with disorders of movement. Berkovic et al (52) found bilateral striatal hypodensities on CT scans of three men (aged 4, 18, and 47 years) with generalized dystonia. Pettigrew and Jankovic (53) reported on a series of 22 patients with hemidystonia from cerebrovascular disease, perinatal or childhood trauma, neural storage disease, neurodegenerative disease, lesions after thalamotomy, or encephalitis. Sixteen (73%) had CT evidence of contralateral basal ganglia disease, history of hemiparesis, or both. In older patients, onset of hemidystonia appeared up to 6 months after injury. Marsden (38) studied 28 patients with focal or hemidystonia due to tumor, arteriovenous malformation, hemorrhage, infarction, or hemiatrophy. All had CT evidence of lesions in either the caudate nuclei, the lentiform nucleus, or the thalamus. Kartin et al (54) described a case of a 74-year-old man with multiple pyramidal and extrapyramidal signs in the setting of hypoparathyroidism many years after a thyroidectomy. CT showed evidence of basal ganglia calcification. Kase et al (55) have reported on another uncommon type of dyskinesia known as hemiballismus. It is frequently self-limited but often responsive to antidopaminergic therapy. Many cases have been associated with CT evidence of basal ganglia hemorrhage or infarction.

There is evidence that magnetic resonance imaging (MRI) may be superior to CT scanning in the identification of such lesions, whether or not there exist other manifestations of brain disease. Biller et al (56), for example, described two patients with hemiballismus that exhibited MRI evidence of lacunar infarctions in the subthalamic nucleus not seen on cranial CT scans. Tabaton et al (57) reported a case of generalized chorea due to MRI-documented bilateral lacunar infarcts of the caudate nucleus, putamen, and deep frontal white matter.

Research into the incidence and prevalence of tardive dyskinesia has been complicated by the difficulty of differentiating this entity from idiopathic causes of dyskinesia. Indeed, these other conditions may even serve as vulnerability factors for the development of drug-induced dyskinesia, further confounding the problem. Current evidence indicates that although idiopathic dyskinesia is considerably less common than neuroleptic-associated (tardive) dyskinesia, such adventitious movements can develop in association with a wide variety of neuromedical conditions, several of which are more prevalent in the elderly. Therefore, for both clinical and research purposes, it is important to be able to recognize the signs and symptoms of these other conditions and, in so far as possible, to establish their etiology and diagnosis. For the most part, this can be accomplished by thorough history taking, including family history, combined with relevant physical and laboratory examinations in the evaluation of these disorders. For example, if the medical history suggests the coexistence of any cognitive dysfunction, then conditions as disparate as Alzheimer's disease, stroke, and neurosyphilis must be high in the differential diagnosis. Likewise, if the family history is positive for Huntington's disease, this entity must be seriously considered.

The conditions listed in Table 21.2 highlight several main categories of illness that may exhibit dyskinesia. The temporal relationship between dyskinesia onset and other elements of the medical history is extremely important and has implications for diagnosis and improved understanding of pathophysiology and treatment as well. For example, onset of choreoathetoid finger movements 3 months after initiation of oral prednisone therapy for chronic obstructive pulmonary disease may be an important observation. It may point to the need to switch to inhalant forms of therapy if tolerated. If movements developed in the context of recently initiated neuroleptic therapy for behavioral agitation, then these medications may be individually or synergistically responsible for the new symptom. If a thorough history and physical examination do not reveal the etiology, then screening laboratory tests such as complete blood count, chemistry and toxicology profiles, fluorescent titer antibody studies, EEG, and CT or MRI scans may be useful.

There are no known unifying theories or pathophysiologic mechanisms of movement disorders. It would be difficult to hypothesize similar mechanisms for chorea associated with proprioceptive abnormalities (such as might occur with stroke) and chorea associated with neurodegenerative processes (such as might occur with Alzheimer's disease). However, it is possible that many etiologies of dyskinesia have a final common pathophysiologic pathway, such as the release of pallidal and thalamic activity that occurs secondary to striatal neuron loss, which normally has a modulating effect on the pallidum (in the setting of intact upper motor neuronal pathways) (12). Whether the disruption of basal ganglia dysfunction develops secondary to cerebrovascular disease (e.g., stroke) or chemical denervation (e.g., neuroleptic blockade of dopamine receptors), the end result is similar. Obviously, the ability to treat acutely or prevent development of these adventitious movements depends on the specificity of the diagnosis achieved and its proximity to the hypothetical "final common pathway." For example, the treatment of choice for drug-induced dyskinesia would be drug discontinuation in individuals who do not require continuous exposure because of relapse of the underlying condition. This approach would not be relevant in the treatment of disabling dyskinesia associated with Alzheimer's disease or Huntington's disease or subthalamic nucleus stroke. The former conditions may be symptomatically responsive to chemical manipulations of striatal dopamine receptors, as might be accomplished with neuroleptic agents, although the benefits obtained would have to be measured against other less desirable effects of these medications. Some investigators have utilized surgical techniques to lesion the cortical spinal tract or the medial segment of the globus pallidus or ventrolateral nucleus of the thalamus (12). Clearly, further research is needed into the pathophysiologic mechanisms of these motor phenomena in order to more clearly identify and distinguish them for clinical and research purposes.

ACKNOWLEDGMENTS

This study was supported by a Research Scientist Development Award (MH-00537) and grant (MH-41646) to Dr Lieberman and the Mental Health Clinical Research Center (MH-41960) of LIJMC-Hillside Hospital from the National Institute of Mental Health.

REFERENCES

1. Simpson GM, Lee JH, Zoubok B, Gardos G. A rating scale for tardive dyskinesia. Psychopharmacology 1979;64:171–179.
2. Duvoisin RC. Chorea. In: Duvoisin RC, ed. Seminars in neurology, vol. 2. Thieme Stratton, 1982:351–358.
3. Fahn S. The extrapyramidal disorders. In: Wyngaarden JB, Smith LH Jr, eds. Cecil textbook of medicine. 17th ed. Philadelphia: WB Saunders, 1985:2069–2078.
4. Kaufman DM. Involuntary movement disorders. In: Clinical neurology for psychiatrists. 2nd ed. New York: Harcourt Brace Jovanovich, 1985:333–338.
5. Margolin DI, Marsden CD. Episodic dyskinesias and transient cerebral ischemia. Neurology 1982;32:1379–1380.
6. Hurwitz LJ, Montgomery DAD. Persistent choreoathetotic movements in liver disease. Arch Neurol 1965;13:421.
7. Saris S. Chorea caused by caudate infarction. Arch Neurol 1983;40:590–591.
8. Oppenheimer DR. Diseases of the basal ganglia, cerebellum, and motor neurons. In: Adams JH, Corsellis JAN, Duchen W, eds. Greenfield's neuropathology. 4th ed. New York: John Wiley, 1984:699–747.

9. Pakkenberg H, Fog R. Spontaneous oral dyskinesia—results of treatment with tetrabenazine, pimozide, or both. Arch Neurol 1974;31:352–353.
10. Dunlap CB. Pathological changes in Huntington's chorea, with special reference to corpus striatum. Arch Neurol Psychiatry 1927;18:867.
11. Vonsattel JP, Ferrante RJ, Richardson EP. Neuropathologic classification of Huntington's disease. J Neuropathol Exp Neurol 1983;42:345.
12. Adams RD, Victor M, eds. Degenerative diseases of the nervous system. In: Principles of neurology, 4th ed. New York: McGraw Hill, 1989:921–967.
13. Mehta D, Mehta S, Mathew P. TD in psychogeriatric patients: a five year follow-up. J Am Geriatr Soc 1977;25:545–547.
14. Weiner WJ, Klawans HL. Lingual–facial–buccal movements in the elderly. I. Pathophysiology and treatment. J Am Geriatr Soc 1973;21:314–317.
15. Weiner WJ, Klawans HL. Lingual–facial–buccal movements in the elderly. II. Pathogenesis and relationship to senile chorea. J Am Geriatr Soc 1973;21:318–320.
16. McGeer PL, McGeer EG, Suzuki JS. Aging and extrapyramidal function. Arch Neurol 1977;34:33–35.
17. Casey DE. Spontaneous and tardive dyskinesia: clinical and laboratory studies. J Clin Psychiatry 1985;46:42–47.
18. Bourgeois M, Bouilh P, Tignol J, Yesavage J. Spontaneous dyskinesias vs. neuroleptic-induced dyskinesias in 270 elderly subjects. J Nerv Ment Dis 1980;168:177–178.
19. Varga E, Sugarman AA, Varga V, Zomorodi A, Zomorodi W, Menken M. Prevalence of spontaneous oral dyskinesia in the elderly. Am J Psychiatry 1982;139:329–331.
20. Chacko RC, Root L, Marmion J, Molinari V, Adams GL. The prevalence of tardive dyskinesia in geropsychiatric outpatients. J Clin Psychiatry 1985;46:55–57.
21. Crane GE, Smeets RA. Tardive dyskinesia and drug therapy in geriatric patients. Arch Gen Psychiatry 1974;30:341–343.
22. Delwaide PJ, Desseilles M. Spontaneous buccolingual–facial dyskinesia in the elderly. Acta Neurol Scand 1977;56:256–262.
23. Smith JM, Baldessarini RJ. Changes in prevalence, severity, and recovery in tardive dyskinesia with age. Arch Gen Psychiatry 1980;37:1368–1373.
24. Toennissen IM, Casey DE, McFarland BH. Tardive dyskinesia in the aged—duration of treatment relationships. Arch Gen Psychiatry 1985;42:278–284.
25. Klawans HL, Barr A. Prevalence of spontaneous lingual–facial–buccal dyskinesias in the elderly. Neurology 1982;32:558–559.
26. Blowers AJ, Borison RL. Dyskinesias in the geriatric population. Brain Res Bull 1983;11:175–178.
27. Blowers AJ, Borison RL, Blowers CM, Bicknell DJ. Abnormal involuntary movements in the elderly [letter]. Br J Psychiatry 1981;139:363–364.
28. Brandon S, McClelland HA, Protheroe C. A study of facial dyskinesia in a mental hospital population. Br J Psychiatry 1971;118:171–184.
29. Edwards H. The significance of brain damage in persistent oral dyskinesia. Br J Psychiatry 1970;116:271–275.
30. Kane JM, Smith JM. Tardive dyskinesia, prevalence and risk factors. Arch Gen Psychiatry 1982;39:473–481.
31. Kane JM, Weinhold P, Kinon B, Wegner J, Leader M. Prevalence of abnormal involuntary movements ("spontaneous dyskinesias") in the normal elderly. Psychopharmacology 1982;77:105–108.
32. Owens DGC, Johnstone EC, Frith CD. Spontaneous involuntary disorders of movement. Arch Gen Psychiatry 1982;39:452–461.
33. Guy W. ECDEU Assessment manual for psychopharmacology. Department of Health, Education, and Welfare. Washington, DC: Government Printing Office, 1976:534–537.
34. Villeneuve A, Turcotte J, Bouchard M, Cote JM, Jus A. Release phenomena and iterative activities in psychiatric geriatric patients. Can Med Assoc J 1974;110:147–153.
35. Altrocchi PH. Spontaneous oral–facial dyskinesia. Arch Neurol 1972;26:506–512.
36. Marsden CD. Motor disorders in basal ganglia disease. Hum Neurobiol 1984;2:245–250.
37. Marsden CD, Obesso JA, Zarranz JJ, Lang AE. The anatomical basis of symptomatic hemidystonia. Brain 1985;108:463–483.
38. Marsden CD. Blepharospasm–oromandibular dystonia syndrome (Brueghel's syndrome), a variant of adult-onset torsion dystonia? J Neurol Neurosurg Psychiatry 1976;39:1204–1209.
39. Lieberman JA, Alvir J, Mukherjee S, Kane JM. Treatment of tardive dyskinesia with bromocriptine. A test of the receptor modification strategy. Arch Gen Psychiatry 1989;46:908–913.
40. Altrocchi PH, Forno LS. Spontaneous oral facial dyskinesia: neuropathology of a case. Neurology 1983;33:802–805.

41. Rafal RD, Friedman JH. Limb dystonia in progressive supranuclear palsy. Neurology 1987;37:1546–1549.

42. Burke RE, Fahn S, Marsden CD, Bressman SB, Moskowitz C, Friedman J. Validity and reliability of a rating scale for the primary torsion dystonias. Neurology 1985;35:73–77.

43. Koller WC. Edentulous orodyskinesia. Ann Neurology 1983;13:97–99.

44. Koller WC. Prevalence of spontaneous lingual–facial–buccal dyskinesias [letter]. Neurology 1983;33:669–670.

45. Woerner MG, Kane JM, Lieberman JA, et al. The prevalence of tardive dyskinesia. J Clin Psychopharmacol 1991;11:34–42.

46. Sutcher HD, Underwood RB, Beatty RA, Sugar O. Orofacial dyskinesia, a dental dimension. JAMA 1971;216:1459–1463.

47. Thach BT, Chase TN, Bosma JF. Oral–facial dyskinesia associated with prolonged use of antihistaminic decongestants. N Engl J Med 1976;293:486–487.

48. Kaplan SR, Murkofsky C. Oral–buccal dyskinesia symptoms associated with low dose benzodiazepine treatment. Am J Psychiatry 1978;135:1558–1559.

49. Alcock NS. A note on the pathology of senile chorea (nonhereditary). Brain 1936;59:376–387.

50. Appenzeller O, Biehl JP. Mouthing in the elderly: a cerebellar sign. J Neurol Sci 1968;6:249–260.

51. Abbruzzese G, Brusa G, Dall'Agata D, Morena M, Spadavecchia L, Favale E. Electrophysiological analysis of motor control in patients with vascular hemichorea. Ital J Neurol Sci 1987;8:357–362.

52. Berkovic SF, Karpati G, Carpenter S, Lang AE. Progressive dystonia with bilateral putaminal hypodensities. Arch Neurol 1987;44:1184–1187.

53. Pettigrew LC, Jankovic J. Hemidystonia: a review of 22 patients and a review of the literature. J Neurol Neurosurg Psychiatry 1985;48:650–657.

54. Kartin P, Zupevc M, Pogacnik T, Cerk M. Calcification of basal ganglia, postoperative hypoparathyroidism, and extrapyramidal, cerebellar, pyramidal motor manifestations. J Neurol 1982;227:171–176.

55. Kase CS, White JL, Joslyn JN, Williams JP, Mohr JP. Cerebellar infarction in the superior cerebellar artery distribution. Neurology 1985;35:705–711.

56. Biller J, Graff-Radford NR, Smoker WR, Adams HP Jr, Johnston P. MR imaging in "lacunar" hemiballismus. J Comput Assist Tomogr 1986;10:793–797.

57. Tabaton M, Mancardi G, Loeb C. Neurology 1985;35:588–589.

Crack Dancing and Other Movement Disorders Related to Cocaine Use

Barbara S. Koppel   Michael Daras

Increased motor activity with stereotyped behavioral patterns has been noted in experimental animals (1,2) as well as in humans (3) after use of cocaine or other stimulants. Stereotyped cocaine-related obsessive-compulsive behavior in humans, including repetitive sorting of objects, nail polishing, furniture rearranging, washing of dishes, and fastidious bathing, has been described (3). A clear association between cocaine use and abnormal movements was first made by Kumor et al (4), who reported an increased incidence of dystonic movements in seven volunteer regular cocaine users injected with haloperidol. A similar observation was made by Hegarty et al (5): 19 (42%) of 45 hospitalized psychiatric patients who had regularly used cocaine before admission developed dystonic reactions to neuroleptics, as compared with 10 (14%) of 71 nonusers. Choy-Kwong and Lipton (6,7) reported a threefold increase of dystonic reactions to neuroleptics in patients with a history of cocaine use. Dystonic reactions in the absence of neuroleptics have been observed during both intoxication (8,9) and withdrawal from cocaine (6,10). In extreme cases, dystonia may evolve into a neuroleptic malignant–like syndrome that has been fatal (11,12).

Cocaine use may exacerbate other movement disorders, such as tics in Tourette's syndrome patients who may have been in remission or adequately controlled on treatment (13–16). De novo appearance of tics has also been described, which has been speculated to be due to uncovering an undiagnosed case of this common disorder (16). One case of opsoclonus-myoclonus lasting 4 weeks after cocaine use has been reported (17).

Choreoathetoid movements resembling tardive dyskinesia or Huntington's disease have been reported in seven patients (18,19). These were self-limited, with a maximum duration of 6 days. One patient developed transient parkinsonian features (19). Akathisia after cocaine use was noted in patients treated with flupentixol for depression; its severity caused an aversion to cocaine (20). Spanish-speaking cocaine users refer to the buccolingual dyskinesias as *boca torcida*, or twisted mouth, while the generalized dyskinesias have been labeled "crack dancing" by cocaine users.

CLINICAL FEATURES

Dystonia in cocaine users is similar to idiopathic and drug-induced dystonia, consisting of torticollis (3,5,15), masseter spasm (9), and facial spasm (7). Less common symptoms include tremor of the head and hand or postural tremor (16), and akinesia or akathisia (4). Akathisia occurred in five patients 3 to 9 days from the first dose of flupentixol and in one after the second dose, immediately following a crack binge (20). It was associated with severe restlessness and other extrapyramidal symptoms, and subsided spontaneously.

Tics include barking, coprolalia or other obscene vocalizations, eye blinking, hand shaking, facial or extremity jerking, shoulder shrugging, and stereotyped facial gesturing. Obsessive-compulsive behavior including copropraxia has been described (16). The tics observed in cocaine users are usually induced by snorting cocaine, suggesting that lower doses are adequate to block dopamine reuptake and exacerbate Tourette's syndrome. In the two women without a personal or family history of tics, larger doses of cocaine, either by intranasal bingeing for 24 hours or intravenous injection for 3 days, were required to produce motor and vocal tics.

Opsoclonus-myoclonus presented in a 26-year-old woman who was a regular weekend snorter of cocaine, with vertigo, nausea, vomiting, ataxia and "dancing eyes." Limb myoclonus and trunk movements increased with action;

nystagmus was continuously present and increased on any direction of gaze. Results of all studies were negative, and symptoms subsided over 4 weeks (17).

Choreoathetosis (18,19) can involve the distal extremities, face, tongue, eyes, or rarely the trunk. It is more common in women, and in our series half the patients had prior neuroleptic or methylphenidate exposure. Although akathisia was noticeable to family or friends, the patients themselves often denied any unpleasant sensations accompanying their abnormal movements. One patient whose abnormal movements had persisted for 9 months complained of muscle soreness, but most patients complained only of agitation or confusion, or were brought to the hospital involuntarily (19). In one patient with AIDS who presented with inability to walk, parkinsonian-like bradykinesia and rigidity persisted for 1 week (19).

MANAGEMENT

Most cocaine-induced movement disorders resolved spontaneously, and in fact may be useful in alerting family members of a patient's relapse into drug abuse. In patients with psychosis, agitation, or confusion ("crack attack"), neuroleptics should be used with care due to the risk of precipitating dystonia or even neuroleptic malignant syndrome. Trihexyphenidyl has been somewhat helpful in managing dystonia (16). Tics lasted from 90 minutes to 4 months (15), but required no treatment. The patient with opsoclonus-myoclonus (17) received valproic acid, clonazepam, and lorazepam, but with only moderate response. Choreoathetosis has been treated with low doses of haloperidol (18,19) and diphenhydramine but showed no response to diazepam (19). Most symptoms resolved within a week; patient reassurance may be all that is required. Four of the patients with flupentixol-cocaine–related akathisia responded to benztropine, diphenhydramine, or diazepam (20). The other two had spontaneous remission of their symptoms at the end-of-dose crash.

PATHOGENETIC MECHANISMS

By blocking the reuptake of dopamine, cocaine potentiates dopaminergic neurotransmission in various sites. In the basal ganglia, this leads to abnormal involuntary movements such as chorea and dystonia. In the mesolimbic system, cocaine's effects are euphoria and sexual excitation, and in the hypothalamus it may cause elevated temperature and depressed appetite. This effect is probably mediated by a dopamine transporter (21,22), a 619–amino acid protein that has been isolated in the ventral tegmental and substantia nigral regions of the rat brain (23,24). Estrogen receptors may predispose women to abnormal movements, as women outnumber men in most series. Female rats can also be sensitized by a single injection of cocaine, whereas males cannot (25).

The initial observation that chronic cocaine use leads to striatal dopamine depletion (26) was considered essential in explaining cocaine reinforcement. Subsequent reports of decreased tyrosine hydroxylase activity (27) leading to lower dopamine production, and of a decreased number of post-synaptic dopamine receptor sites (28), suggest that dopamine depletion may be a compensatory mechanism against dopaminergic overstimulation. Failure to downregulate dopamine concentration in the basal ganglia may be responsible for the recurrence of the abnormal movements with repeated cocaine use in some patients. Just as drug craving is primed in opposite ways by D_1 and D_2 receptor activation, as shown in the rat model (29), effects on D_1 and D_2 receptors in motor regions may cause dyskinesias or lack of movement, as described in our series. The involvement of other catecholamines by cocaine may contribute to the pathophysiology of movement disorders, but further research is required to clarify any potential effect.

The epidemiology of movement disorders in cocaine users has not been studied because of its inherent difficulties. However, the number of published reports on cocaine-related abnormal movements and the presence of street names to describe them (crack dancing and *boca turcida*) suggest that they may be more common than physicians recognize.

REFERENCES

1. Johanson C-E, Fischman MW. The pharmacology of cocaine related to its abuse. Pharmacol Rev 1989;41:3–52.
2. McDougle CJ, Goodman WK, Delgado PL, et al. Pathophysiology of obsessive-compulsive disorder. Am J Psychiatry 1989;146:1350–1351.
3. Weiner WJ, Sanchez-Ramos JR. Movement disorders and dopaminergic stimulant drugs. In: Lang AE, Weiner WJ, eds. Drug-induced movement disorders. Mount Kisco, NY: Futura Publishing, 1992:315.
4. Kumor K, Sherer M, Jaffe J. Haloperidol-induced dystonia in cocaine addicts. Lancet 1986;2:1341–1342.
5. Hegarty AM, Lipton RB, Merriam AE, Freeman K. Cocaine as a risk factor for acute dystonic reactions. Neurology 1991;41:1670–1672.
6. Choy-Kwong M, Lipton RB. Dystonia related to cocaine withdrawal: a case report and pathogenic hypothesis. Neurology 1989;39:996–997.
7. Choy-Kwong M, Lipton RB. Cocaine withdrawal dystonia. Neurology 1990;40:863–864.
8. Merab J. Acute dystonic reaction to cocaine. Am J Med 1988;84:564.
9. Farrell PE, Diehl AK. Acute dystonic reaction to crack cocaine. Ann Emerg Med 1991;20:322.
10. Rebischung D, Daras M, Tuchman AJ. Dystonic movements associated with cocaine use. Ann Neurol 1990;28:267.
11. Daras M, Kakkouras L, Tuchman AJ, Koppel BS. Rhabdomyolysis and hyperthermia after cocaine abuse: a variant of the neuroleptic malignant syndrome? Acta Neurol Scand 1995;92:161–165.
12. Kosten TR, Kleber HD. Rapid death during cocaine abuse: a variant of the neuroleptic malignant syndrome? Am J Drug Alcohol Abuse 1988;14:335–346.
13. Mesulam M-M. Cocaine and Tourette's syndrome. N Engl J Med 1986;315:398.
14. Factor SA, Sanchez-Ramos JR, Weiner J. Cocaine and Tourette's syndrome. Ann Neurol 1988;23:423–424.
15. Pascual-Leone A, Dhuna A. Cocaine-associated multifocal tics. Neurology 1990;40:999–1000.
16. Cardoso FEC, Jankovic J. Cocaine-related movement disorders. Mov Disord 1993;8:175–178.
17. Scharf D. Opsoclonus-myoclonus following the intranasal usage of cocaine. J Neurol Neurosurg Psychiatry 1989;52:1447–1448.
18. Habal R, Sauter D, Olowe O, Daras M. Cocaine and chorea. Am J Emerg Med 1991;9:618–620.

19. Daras M, Koppel BS, Atos-Radzion E. Cocaine-induced choreoathetoid movements ("crack dancing"). Neurology 1994;44:751–752.

20. Gawin FH, Khalsa-Denison ME, Jatlow P. Flupentixol-induced aversion to crack cocaine. N Engl J Med 1996;334:1340–1341.

21. Kuhar MJ, Ritz MC, Boja JW. The dopamine hypothesis of the reinforcing properties of cocaine. Trends Neurosci 1991;14:299–302.

22. Woolverton WL, Johnson KM. Neurobiology of cocaine abuse. Trends Pharmacol Sci 1992;13:193–200.

23. Shimada S, Kitayama S, Lin CL, et al. Cloning and expression of a cocaine-sensitive rat dopamine transporter complementary DNA. Science 1991;254:576–579.

24. Kilty JE, Lorang D, Amara SG. Cloning and expression of a cocaine-sensitive rat dopamine transporter. Science 1991;254:578–579.

25. Glick SD, Hinds PA. Sex differences in sensitization to cocaine-induced rotation. Eur J Pharmacol 1984;99:119–120.

26. Dackis CA, Gold MS. New concepts in cocaine addiction: the dopamine depletion hypothesis. Neurosci Biobehav Rev 1985;9:469–477.

27. Trulson ME, Babb S, Joe JC, Raese JD. Chronic cocaine administration depletes tyrosine hydroxylase immunoreactivity in the rat brain nigral striatal system: quantitative light microscopic studies. Exp Neurol 1986;94:744–756.

28. Volkow ND, Fowler JS, Wolf AP, et al. Effects of chronic cocaine abuse on postsynaptic dopamine receptors. Am J Psychiatry 1990;147:719–724.

29. Self DW, Barnhart WJ, Lehman DA, Nestler EJ. Opposite modulation of cocaine-seeking behavior by D1- and D2-like dopamine receptor agonists. Science 1996;271:1586–1589.

Dementias and Neurodegenerative Disorders

The Neurology of Huntington's Disease

Merit E. Cudkowicz   Joseph B. Martin   Walter J. Koroshetz

INTRODUCTION

Huntington's disease (HD) is an autosomal dominant, uniformly progressive neurodegenerative disorder of midlife onset characterized clinically by movement disorder (chorea), personality changes, and dementia (1). The pathogenesis is unknown and there are currently no effective therapies; there has, however, been considerable recent progress in HD research. Experimental and genetic findings provide new understanding of the pathophysiology of the delayed striatal in HD. The gene abnormality responsible for HD has been located near the tip of the short arm of chromosome four (2). The mutation is an unstable expansion of a trinucleotide repeat (CAG) located in the presumed coding region of a novel gene called "huntington" (3). The neuropathologic pattern of cell death and neurochemical changes in HD can be mimicked in animals by intrastriatal injection of certain excitotoxins that activate the N-methyl-D-aspartate (NMDA) glutamate receptor and by intrastriatal or systemic injection of toxins that block mitochondrial oxidative phosphorylation (4,5). These findings have led to an excitotoxic theory and an energy metabolism theory of Huntington's pathophysiology. A transgenic animal mouse model of HD was recently generated (6). This animal model and others could potentially lead to the development of effective therapies to prevent the genetically programmed neuronal death that inevitably occurs in HD.

EPIDEMIOLOGY

The prevalence of affected persons with HD in the United States is approximately 5 to 10 persons per 100,000 (7,8). There are two to four times as many asymptomatic gene carriers. There are no gender or definite racial predispositions and the disease is found throughout the world.

Prevalence rates are particularly high in selected genetically segregated areas, such as the Lake Maracaibo region of Venezuela (9). Genetic studies in families with apparent new mutations show that rarely an expansion of the triplet repeat occurs resulting in new occurrences of the phenotype.

Because symptoms of HD are typically not manifest until individuals are in midlife, inheritance does not influence reproduction and the gene continues to be transmitted in an autosomal dominant fashion. Genetic studies in families with apparent new mutations show that rarely an expansion of the triplet repeat occurs resulting in new occurrence of the phenotype.

In the New England population, the mean age of onset of motor symptoms in HD is approximately 37 years (10). The severity of the neuropathologic involvement at autopsy varies inversely with age of onset and directly with disease duration (10). In patients with juvenile or adolescent onset, the mean duration of illness is 12 years and the neuronal loss at autopsy is more widespread. In those with onset closer to the mean, the average duration of illness is 15 to 20 years and the degree of neuronal loss is less severe (10). Elderly HD patients often die of other causes and show the least atrophy despite relatively long duration of illness.

MOLECULAR GENETICS

HD is an autosomal dominant disease. Each child of a person with the HD gene has a 50% chance of inheriting the disease gene. Using DNA restriction fragment length polymorphisms, it was determined that the gene abnormality responsible for HD is located near the tip of the short arm of chromosome four (2). The actual mutation is an unstable expansion of a trinucleotide repeat (CAG) located in the presumed coding region of the novel gene, hunting-ton. Unstable expansions of CAG and other trinucleotide repeats have recently been identified in other neurologic disorders including myotonic dystrophy, fragile X, dentato-rubro-pallidal-luysian atrophy, Machado-Joseph disease, a form of autosomal dominant spinocerebellar atrophy, and spinomuscular atrophy type 1 (Kennedy's syndrome). The repeat length in normal individuals ranges between 12 and 34 with a peak in the distribution curve at 19. The repeat length in affected individuals with HD ranges between 37 and 86 with a peak in the distribution curve at 45. Age of onset in juvenile HD patients is predicted in part by the extent of the CAG expansion; this does not hold true in adult onset cases. The repeat length is fairly constant throughout most tissues with the exception of the male germ cells. Expansion of repeat length occurs in sperm from affected individuals and is believed responsible for the vari-ation of repeat length and onset age between affected fathers and their affected children.

The gene involved in HD encodes a protein called "huntingtin." The expanded CAG repeat causes an abnor-mally elongated polyglutamine tracts near the amino termi-nus. The function of the normal huntingtin protein is currently unknown. Homozygote knockout mice for the huntington gene show gross abnormalities in embryonic development and die before reaching fetal maturity. Heterozygote knockout mice for the huntington gene are normal. Both the normal and expanded huntingtin protein and its mRNA are located in all cells of the body and in all brain regions. The protein is found in the cytoplasm of neurons and along the axon and may be concentrated in synaptic regions (11). Intraneuronal nuclear inclusions reac-tive to huntingtin have been found in the brain of HD transgenic mice and patients with HD (12,13).

Genetic testing, with polymerase chain reaction (PCR), is now widely available to confirm the clinical diagnosis of HD and can aid individuals at risk for HD to plan their future. Only a small proportion of at-risk individuals are currently tested, and it is unlikely that genetic testing will substantially reduce the incidence of the disease. This new technology carries with it new challenges. Throughout the world, a significant proportion of those who approach testing centers eventually change their minds and decide against going through with testing. It is critical that patients are provided adequate genetic counseling prior to genetic testing.

PATHOLOGY OF HUNTINGTON'S DISEASE

The clinical symptoms of HD arise from impairment of motor, emotional, and cognitive processes. The major neu-rologic abnormalities are thought to result from the degen-eration and nerve cell loss in the striatum, which is the site of the earliest and most profound cell loss. Extrastriatal atrophy also occurs in HD, and there is frequently a 30% reduction in overall brain weight and 20% to 30% reduc-tion in cortical area (14). Degeneration of pyramidal pro-jection neurons in cortex has also been demonstrated (15). Neuronal loss has been reported to occur in various other areas of the brain (16) including the globus pallidum, sub-thalamic nucleus (17), substantia nigra (pars reticulata), and hypothalamus (18).

Studies of the striatal degeneration in HD have revealed specific features that provide clues to its pathogenesis. The atrophy is most severe dorsally and medially in the caudate and dorsally in the putamen. Changes in these areas, espe-cially in the tail of the caudate, are already seen in the least affected brains, Vonsattel grades 1 and 2 (19). In more advanced cases, there is atrophy also in the ventral-lateral striatum. Even in advanced cases, the most ventral part of the striatum—the nucleus accumbens—remains relatively spared. The striatum is organized into "patches," which stain for opiate receptors, substance P, and met-enkephalin, and "matrix," which stains for acetylcholinesterase, somatostatin, and neuropeptide Y (20). The matrix area has been found to differentially degenerate in patients with HD (21). The cause of these topographical gradients of degeneration has not been elucidated.

There is also a characteristic pattern of cell loss in the striatum of patients with HD (1). The medium spiny neurons are preferentially destroyed in HD. Eighty to ninety percent of striatal neurons are medium spiny cells. They contain GABA, with substance P or enkephalin, and receive the majority of glutamatergic afferents from the cortex and dopaminergic afferents from the nigra. Reports that in early stage HD there is preferential loss of enkephalin staining in globus pallidus (and substance P in the substantia reticulata), as opposed to normal substance P staining in the internal globus pallidus, suggests that there may be another level of vulnerability within the class of spiny neurons. Those neurons projecting to lateral globus pallidus may be more susceptible than those projecting to medial globus pallidus (22). In contrast to the loss of spiny projection neurons, the aspiny interneurons, which stain for NADPH diaphorase and contain nitric oxide synthase (NOS) are preferentially spared (1). Nitric oxide has been implicated in neuronal death in a variety of experimental studies (23). To under-stand how the (CAG)n expansion in the huntington gene, present in all cells from birth, leads to the very specific cell type and regional neuronal vulnerability remains the intri-guing challenge of HD neurobiology.

PATHOGENESIS OF HD

The pathology in HD can be mimicked to some extent by striatal injections of NMDA receptor agonists. The injection of NMDA agonists (quinolinic acid) produces caudate lesions and causes death of intrinsic neurons but not of affer-ent processes and relative sparing of NADPH (NOS posi-tive) cells (24,25). There is early and preferential loss of NMDA receptors in HD postmortem tissue, consistent with a role of NMDA activation in HD cell death (26). However, no direct evidence has been extracted to indicate that there is excess excitatory stress in HD. Excitatory synaptic function is the driving force behind many neuronal processes and it is possible that a variety of cellular defects could ultimately lead to cell death by an excitotoxic pattern. Excitotoxic death has been associated with brain ischemia, growth factor withdrawal, damage by free radicals, disordered energy metabolism, and disordered intracellular calcium homeostasis.

Another major hypothesis of the pathogenesis of HD suggests that there is an underlying defect in cellular metabolism in HD. The two hypotheses may be tightly linked. Neuronal excitation is closely linked to neuronal metabolic energy requirements and excitatory mechanisms contribute to cell death in metabolically compromised cells, that is, in brain ischemia. A recent study of platelets from patients with HD demonstrated a specific defect in mitochondrial function (27). The striatum may be especially sensitive to metabolic compromise (28). Patients with mitochondrial cytopathies frequently have lesions in the basal ganglia (29). Indeed, Leber's disease has occurred coincident with striatal degeneration (30).

Agents that compromise neuronal metabolic function simulate an excitotoxic pattern of cell death that can be blocked by antagonists of specific glutamate receptors (31). In addition the systemic administration of the mitochondrial toxin, 3-nitroprorionic acid, causes selective destruction of the striatum in animals and humans. Prefeeding rats with agents that may improve mitochondrial function—such as coenzyme Q10 and nicotinamide—markedly reduced the striatal toxicity of 3-NP and malonate. The lesions appear to be caused by a secondary excitotoxic mechanism since 3-NP and malonate have no direct depolarizing effects on neurons (32). The lesions induced by these agents are blocked by removal in vivo of excitatory cortical inputs (25) or by excitatory amino acid antagonists in vitro (33). These studies suggest that an interaction between compromised mitochondrial function and NMDA receptor activation can lead to the selective neuronal vulnerability typical of HD.

Using ^{1}H-NMR spectroscopy, we and others have found that patients with clinical HD have elevated brain lactate levels. Lactate is produced in brain during physiologic stimulation. Large lactate production has been seen during seizure, acute stroke, and acute excitotoxin lesions, conditions in which the demand of robust excitatory transmission may exceed the neuronal supply of ATP. Elevated brain lactate is also found in the brains of patients with mitochondrial disorders, conditions in which glycolysis is enhanced due to impaired oxidative metabolism. This technique has been used to screen for drugs that decrease the brain lactate in HD. The therapeutic potential of this strategy is yet to be tested. However, the power of advanced MR technology to provide morphologic and physiologic measures of central nervous system disease and disease progression seems certain.

DIAGNOSIS OF EARLY HD

Most neurologists require chorea to make the diagnosis of HD. "At risk" individuals, however, do not have chorea or noticeable disability but may have so-called soft neurologic signs. Such persons have been systematically followed by the clinical team evaluating the large Venezuelan kindred and the presence of soft signs seems to portend future onset of chorea (34). In diagnosed patients, an inability to perform rapid, tapping movements with the tongue is almost a universal finding. Other signs (35) present in early HD include an inability to rapidly tap fingers in sequence, dysdiadochokinesia, abnormalities of voluntary gaze, and inability to maintain tongue protrusion. There is also a prechoreic movement disorder in some patients. Not uncommonly the spouse of a patient with newly diagnosed HD will report that the patient developed restless movements during sleep several years before the onset of chorea. Many newly diagnosed patients are described as becoming "fidgety" several years prior to coming to medical attention. These individuals have an increased frequency of stereotyped movements that are qualitatively identical to "restless" or "fidgety" movements seen in normal individuals. Though signs of abnormal motor control are usually present when chorea manifests, it is yet unclear which "soft signs" are specific enough to justify a diagnosis of HD in the absence of chorea.

A subset of patients develop disabling psychiatric syndromes before the onset of chorea. Depression is common in patients with diagnosed HD and often precedes onset of symptoms. Individuals at risk for HD have an increased propensity for suicide around the age when first symptoms are expected. A small subset of Huntington's patients develop psychosis and their thought disorder can precede the onset of chorea.

The diagnosis of HD is psychologically devastating to individuals who have seen their parent, sibling, or other close relative become progressively disabled. It is therefore important that it not be issued without clinical certainty. It is compelling to conclude that the development of psychologic and motor system abnormalities in an "at risk" individual marks the onset of HD. Many of the "soft" signs discussed above, however, are not specific for HD and may result from other pathologic processes.

CLINICAL HD

The clinical manifestations of HD have a range of presentations that depend on the age of onset. Patients with a family history of HD usually first come to medical attention with the onset of chorea. Patients themselves may notice incoordination when attempting tasks that require exactly timed and executed limb or finger movements. It is not unusual that patients report unexplained falls, slight unsteadiness walking, a tendency to drop objects, or a change in handwriting. In the majority, a major change in the character of an individual's emotional life occurs prior to the time of diagnosis. An increased tendency for anxiety, anger, or frustration is common along with withdrawal from social interactions and interests. A subset of patients exhibit a hypersomatization disorder, alcohol abuse, antisocial behavior, aimless wandering, or occasionally a hypomanic state.

Cognitive Abnormalities

Signs of cognitive impairment are frequently evident at the time of onset of chorea. A history is commonly obtained that an individual who was functioning at a high level in the workplace had increasing difficulty performing his job in the past few years. The difficulties usually encountered involve substantial impairments in the construction and execution of mental plans rather than the loss of a specific skill, for example, memory, communicative, or arithmetic ability. Patients commonly have deficits in concentration, attention, and planning. In many cases, the newly diagnosed patient seemingly applies himself to a mental task with full attention but is grossly incorrect and slow. Simple tasks require greater than normal effort. A major feature of HD is a tendency for the patient to attempt fewer activities and to require more time to complete those that are attempted.

Memory function is also impaired in HD, visual memory more so than verbal memory. Patients perform poorly on tests of short-term memory but never demonstrate the complete amnestic deficit that is seen in Korsakoff's or Alzheimer's disease (24). Even patients with the most severe disease may still recognize relatives or retain some primitive interest. Patients usually recall a subset of recent personal events, but their reports are sparse and sometimes incorrect due to forgetting or disordered recall of sequence. Patient comprehension of detailed instructions may require multiple repetitions, but long-term registration may still be possible. Learning new skills is rare after the diagnosis of HD. Tongue and finger movements often appear apraxia. There is often a mimical apraxia for facial movements.

Psychiatric Syndromes

Some disorder of emotion, personality, or affect invariably occurs in patients with HD. The psychiatric disorders in HD may be extreme, and in most areas of this country psychiatric hospitals provide the best available setting to manage a subset of patients with HD safely.

A chronic atypical depressive state is common. This may manifest as sadness, with feelings of hopelessness, guilt, anhedonia, hypersomatization, and irritability. Sleep disorders and social withdrawal occur commonly in HD; appetite is usually increased. As expected, depressive mood disturbances are cloaked in concern for the future of the individual and the family. Suicide and suicidal thoughts are a major problem in this patient population. It reflects in part a desire

not to prolong one's life through the end stages of the illness, but in some patients it is clearly mixed with impulsivity and/or an endogenous mood disorder. Fluctuations in severity of the atypical mood disorder also attest to its endogenous nature. Antidepressant therapy in patients with HD often causes some partial benefit in their dysthymic disorder but only rarely renders the patient euthymic. Electroconvulsive therapy has been used with mixed, but some definite, benefit in severely involuted patients. Sociopathic behavior is also not uncommon in HD; in some it occurs in the context of a paranoid or idiosyncratic thought disorder and remits when the thought disorder is controlled. In others, sociopathic behavior stems from chronic problems with lack of emotional control.

Disordered emotional control is perhaps the most common, difficult management issue in caring for a large number of patients with HD. Patients with physical and cognitive disability who become intermittently very irritable, demanding, or verbally or physically abusive strain their supports in the home, community, or institution. Sudden displays of anger of less-defined emotional upset may be triggered by apparently trivial events and are occasionally dangerous. They occur in those with minimal cognitive changes as well as in those with more advanced disease. Clonazepam, fluoxetine, valproate, neuroleptics, betaadrenergic antagonists, or carbamazepine can be of limited benefit in controlling this behavior. Some professionals have developed individual interactive techniques that effectively calm patients with HD.

There is an abnormality in changing sets and a severe limitation of the range of thought in many patients. Obsessional thought and behavior are also seen in a significant proportion of patients with HD. The occurrence of these symptoms may have as its basis the caudate hypometabolism that has been reported both in patients with HD and in patients with obsessive-compulsive disease. HD patients with obsessional concerns may respond to treatment with fluoxetine or clomipramine.

Chorea

Chorea is an involuntary set of flowing or jerky movements about multiple joints (30,31). Some choreic movements, especially those seen distally in the extremities, are rapid though slower than myoclonus. More commonly choreic movements resemble abnormally quick voluntary movements such as the rapid raising of the eyebrows or shrugging of the shoulder. Slower movements, lasting a second or longer, are called "choreoathetotic movements" and are more writhing or flowing and resemble the jerking of a string puppet. In the late stages of the illness, movements may slow down and become athetotic or simply reflect the change of one dystonic posture to another. Choreatic movements increase in frequency with stress and disappear during sleep. Chorea is commonly exacerbated by walking. It can be voluntarily suppressed for brief periods. Patients are sometimes unaware of their involuntary movements or do not appreciate the extent of their movements.

Chorea contributes to the patient's disability first because it is unsightly and an embarrassment for the patient. Chorea of the trunk and legs in combination with poor postural control may cause gait instability and falling. Large amplitude chorea in the upper extremities can interfere with all voluntary movements. The degree of chorea varies; some patients have continuous choreic movements in all extremities while awake, whereas others may never develop more than a few choreic jerks each minute.

Experimental studies have tried to address the basis of choreas. Dopamine agonists commonly cause chorea in patients with Parkinson disease and worsen chorea in patients with HD, whereas dopamine antagonists lessen chorea in patients with HD. This has led to the hypothesis that chorea is due to a relative hyperactivity of dopaminergic neurotransmission in HD. Definitive evidence of hyperactivity of the dopaminergic system in HD has been difficult to confirm. Experimentally, lesion studies have shown that various means of decreasing the output of the subthalamic nucleus in monkeys cause ballism (34), an involuntary movement disorder bearing resemblance to some of the choreic movements in HD patients. Chorea and ballism are thought perhaps to have a common pathophysiologic basis. In addition, putamenal injections of gamma-aminobutyric acid (GABA), which causes functional inhibition of the subthalamic nucleus, also cause chorea in the monkey. Our knowledge of the basal ganglia circuit predicts that striatal degeneration, as in HD, would also lead to decreased output from the subthalamic nucleus (less inhibition of the inhibitory lateral globus pallidal neurons projecting to the subthalamic nucleus = increased subthalamic inhibition). This functional abnormality may lie at the basis of chorea in early HD if, as described, the projections (enkephalinergic) to lateral globus pallidus are disproportionately degenerated (35,36). As the projections to medial globus pallidus (substance P containing) degenerate in the later stages of HD, the model also predicts the clinical finding that rigidity replaces chorea. Further support for these ideas comes from a neuropathologic comparison of nonchoreic, rigid, juvenile cases with choreic juvenile cases. As predicted by the model, the rigid cases showed degeneration of terminals in both the medial and the lateral globus pallidus, the choreic case only in the lateral globus (39).

Abnormalities of Voluntary Movements

Most patients with HD have abnormalities in voluntary motor control, which more than chorea is the source of their greatest motoric disability. Huntington in his original report noted that patients had great difficulty with tongue movements (40). Fast repetitive tongue movements, such as tapping the tongue against the upper lip, are uniformly slow, dysrhythmic, or even impossible to perform. Repetitive

sequential movements with the fingers are usually slow or dysrhythmic. The breakdown of motor performance when patients are asked to perform patterns of movements has been reported in controlled studies (41). Although it is more difficult to observe in the choreic patient, most choreic HD patients show significant bradykinesia in their performance of trajectory as well as patterned movements (41,42). This is more apparent in patients with the bradykinetic variety of HD. Clinically apparent disorders of gaze (43,44) include 1) slow saccadic velocity, 2) difficulty suppressing head movement or blink on shifting gaze, and 3) increased latency between the command to refixate and the saccadic response. Smooth pursuit movements are broken by inappropriate fixation and followed by a corrective saccade.

Motor incoordination contributes to the severe disability in HD. Patients lose the ability to perform accurate motor patterns. Feeding, dressing, and washing eventually become impossible. Later in the illness, patients may retain only grasping ability with their hands, and all trajectory movements become slow and are inaccurately timed and placed. Some dysarthria in speech probably occurs in very early stage HD and progresses until speech is practically unintelligible. The dysarthria is caused by a combination of uncoordinated control of respiratory, tongue, facial, and pharyngeal musculature. There is a tendency in some patients to speak explosively and enunciate poorly. Most patients develop a dysphonia characterized by a tight spastic sound with poor volume control and consisting almost entirely of vowel sounds. Swallowing becomes hazardous in the later stages of the illness. Some patients have a tendency to overfill the mouth with food and have frequent choking. Most have discoordinated swallowing movements that affect swallowing liquids and solids. The use of a straw to deliver liquid to the back of the mouth and dietary changes may be necessary. In the final stages of the illness, aspiration of oral secretions leads to pneumonia, which is often the cause of death.

Posture and Gait

Posture frequently is abnormal. Even early on, the head may be held slightly flexed forward or to one side while the resting position of the hand often demonstrates abnormal extension at the metacarpalphalangeal joints of the index and middle fingers with dorsiflexion at the wrist. There may be an increased lordotic or scoliotic posture when standing. Many but not all patients with HD have a gait abnormality that is separate from chorea. Unexplained falling is common even early in the illness. Sometimes falls are due to problems with visual–spatial processing, which results in tripping over or bumping into objects. Falls while walking down stairs are especially common. The maintenance of accurate balance is also affected in most patients. Only rarely can patients walk tandem or stand on one foot for longer than 20 seconds. Patients lose the normal rhythm of walking. Their steps vary in length, often misstepping to the side. The base of their gait sometimes widens to accommodate the inaccuracy in balance. Feet are often placed too far laterally and there is an abnormal variation in the length of each step. This causes patients to walk in a jerky side-to-side path. The gait disorder most resembles a cerebellar ataxia and patients are often considered to be intoxicated. It is further aggravated by choreic movements that often are more prominent while walking. In some patients walking appears to be composed entirely of a series of choreic trunk and leg movements. In the late stages of HD, patients cannot walk or stand due to their imbalance.

Clinical Variants of Huntington's Disease

There is wide variability in some of the manifestations of HD. This is expressed by the range of onset age between childhood and senescence. It is also seen in the expression of various clinical phenotypes. All have striatal degeneration, although some have additional sites of neuropathologic change that may account for the varied clinical characteristics. Since the atypical forms occur in families with patients who demonstrate more typical manifestations, variability is probably caused by modifier genes rather than different forms of the HD gene defect.

Patients who do not develop chorea until they are past 60 years old often are affected less severely by Huntington's (45). The diagnosis in certain families in which the history suggests exclusively late-onset chorea has been confirmed by genetic analysis of the mutation (46). Although triplet repeat numbers correlate with age of onset in a population of subjects with HD, it is not very helpful in predicting age of onset in a given patient. Some patients are misdiagnosed as having senile chorea. Patients in their 80s with only minimal disability are evidence that the HD mutation can be attenuated, but the mechanism by which this occurs is unknown.

Juvenile Huntington's Disease

Children or young adults affected with HD usually become the most severely disabled. They more frequently inherit the gene from an affected father. The diagnosis of juvenile HD is often missed. It often presents with progressive rigidity without chorea (47,48). Bradykinesia without true rigidity occurs in some patients. Juvenile patients may also develop a seizure disorder. Disabling cognitive abnormalities occur early. When bradykinesia is pronounced, saccadic eye movements are always slow, as are other voluntary movements. The pathology in the juvenile cases is usually more widespread. The magnetic resonance imaging (MRI) scan shows a markedly increased T2 signal in the caudate, putamen, and periventricular white matter and a decreased signal in the globus pallidus (49). Not infrequently, patients with early adult onset also present with a bradykinetic form of HD with slow saccadic eye movements. Patients with the bradykinetic form of HD may have prominent myoclonus (50).

TREATMENT

There is no effective treatment for the neuronal degeneration in HD. The physician faces the challenging task of assisting patients to live as fully as possible with their neurologic limitations and their anxiety about the future.

Early in the illness, disability is caused primarily by the patient's reaction to the diagnosis combined with a dysphoric mood disorder and cognitive deficits. Depression and anxiety states are common and can be helped with psychologic counseling and either tricyclic antidepressants or benzodiazepines. A sleep disorder with frequent restless movements may cause sleep deprivation (51). Clonazepam at bedtime is often beneficial. If chorea is disabling, tetrabenazine, haloperidol, or clonazepam may improve function (52). Most patients are less impaired if medicated at low doses rather than medicated to suppress chorea. Clonazepam is occasionally of benefit in the management of chorea. The motor dysfunction in HD is exacerbated by weight loss, and occasionally dramatic improvement occurs if patients are placed on very high caloric diets that enable weight gain.

Patients and family members must be warned about the loss of driving skills, which is an inevitable consequence of HD. A myriad of social, interpersonal, financial, and medical problems plague those with disabling HD, so a team consisting of a social worker, psychological counselor, and neurologist is most effective. The lack of appropriate long-term care facilities for patients with late-stage illness or HD patients with psychiatric manifestations is a source of much anxiety on the part of patients, family, and medical staff. Patients with serious emotional dyscontrol present difficult management problems. Phenothiazines have some limited effectiveness in controlling destructive behavior. Relaxation therapy and trials of lithium, tegretol, fluoxetine, valproate, benzodiazepines, or high dose beta-adrenergic blockers may be helpful.

The finding that excitotoxins and mitochondrial inhibitors produce striatal lesions that resemble HD pathology offers hope that a strategy may emerge. A surge of interest in the clinical manifestation of HD has fueled and been fueled by the above-mentioned basic science successes. Small clinical pilot trials aimed at slowing the progression of HD are underway or have been performed with vitamin E, idebenone, baclofen, coenzyme Q10, and lamotrigine. A European group has begun a program of fetal cell transplant. An American group has begun a program of fetal pig striatal transplantation. A large multicenter group, the Hungtington's Study Group, has been formed to collect clinical data in a uniform fashion among centers. The aim of the group is to be poised to conduct large clinical trials of promising medications when the nature of the Huntington gene is identified.

FUTURE EFFORTS

The goals of future research in HD have been crystallized by the discovery of the HD mutation. Work is underway to learn 1) the biologic function of the normal huntingtin protein, 2) the biologic function of the huntingtin protein containing an expanded (CAG)n trinucleotide repeat, 3) the effect of the HD mutation in a transgenic mouse, and 4) the rules that underly the instability of the mutation during transmission from parent to child. Most believe that the autosomal dominant HD mutation causes the huntingtin protein with its expanded stretch of polyglutamines to take on a new, destructive function. Characterization of the cell biologic effect of the mutation may lead to ideas for therapy. The generations of a transgenic mouse model of HD will critically advance the effort to understand the illness and to test potential therapeutic strategies. Understanding how the expanded trinucleotide repeat might be influenced to contract during transmission from parent to child could obliterate the illness within a generation.

REFERENCES

1. Kowall NW, Ferrante RJ, Martin JB. Patterns of cell loss in Huntington's disease. Trends Neurosci 1987;10:24–29.
2. Gusella JF, Wexler NS, Conneally PM, et al. A polymorphic DNA marker genetically linked to HD. Nature 1983;306:234–238.
3. Huntington's Disease Collaborative Research Group. A novel gene containing a trinucleotide repeat that is expanded and unstable on Huntington's disease chromosomes. Cell 1993;72:971–983.
4. Beal MF, Kowall NW, Ellison DW, et al. Replication of the neurochemical characteristics of HD by quinolinic acid. Nature 1986;321:168–171.
5. Ferrante RJ, Kowall NW, Beal MF, et al. Morphologic and histochemical characteristics of a spared subset of striatal neurons in HD. J Neuropathol Exp Neurol 1987;46:12–27.
6. Mangiarini L, Sathasivam K, Seller M, et al. Exon 1 of the HD gene with an expanded CAG repeat is sufficient to cause a progressive neurological phenotype in transgenic mice. Cell 1996;87:493–506.
7. Hayden MR. Huntington's chorea. New York: Springer-Verlag, 1981.
8. Harper PS, ed. Huntington's disease. London: WB Saunders, 1991.
9. Shoulson I, Penney JB, et al. HD in Venezuela: neurologic features and functional decline. Neurology 1986;36:244–249.
10. Myers RH, Vonsattel JP, Stevens T, et al. Clinical and neuropathologic assessment of severity in HD. Neurology 1988;38:341–347.
11. Strong TV, Tagle DA, Valdes JM, et al. Widespread expression of the human and rat Huntington's disease gene in brain and nonneural tissues. Nat Genet 1993;5:259–265.
12. Davies SW, Turmaine M, Cozens B, et al. Formation of neuronal intranuclear inclusions underlies the neurological dysfunction in mice transgenic for the HD mutation. Cell 1997;90:537–548.
13. DiFiglia M, Sapp E, Chase KO, et al. Aggregation of Huntingtin in neuronal intranuclear inclusions and dystrophic neurites in brain. Science 1997;277:1990–1993.
14. de la Monte SM, Vonsattel JP, Richardson EP. Morphometric demonstration of atrophic change in the cerebral cortex. J Neuropathol Exp Neurol 1988;47:516–525.
15. Cudkowicz M, Kowall NW. Degeneration of pyramidal projection neurons in Huntington's disease cortex. Ann Neurol 1990;27:200–204.
16. Bruyn GW. Neuropathological changes in Huntington's chorea. In: Barbeau A, Chase TN, Paulson GW, eds. Huntington's Chorea, 1872–1972. Advances of Neurology. Vol 1. New York: Raven, 1973:399–403.
17. Lange N, Thorner G, Hopf A, Schroder HF. Morphometric studies of the neuropathological changes in choreatic disease. J Neurol Sci 1976;28:401–425.
18. Kremer HPH, Roos RAC, Dingjan G, et al. Atrophy of the hypothalamic lateral tuberalnucleus in Huntington's disease. J Neuropathol Exp Neurol 1990;49:371–382.
19. Vonsattel JP, Myers RH, Stevens TJ, et al. Neuropathological classification of Huntington's disease. J Neuropathol Exp Neurol 1985;44:559–577.
20. Graybiel AM. Neurotransmitters and neuromodulators in the basal ganglia. Trends Neurosci 1990;13:244–254.
21. Ferrante RI, Kowall NW, Richardson EP. Patch-matrix distribution of cholecystokinin and cytochrome oxidase activity in normal and Huntington's disease striatum. Soc Neurosci 1988;14:1046. Abstract.
22. Reiner A, Albin RL, Anderson HD, et al. Differential loss of striatal projection neurons in Huntington disease. Proc Natl Acad Sci USA 1988;85:5733–5737.
23. Dawson TM, Dawson VL, Snyder SH. A novel neuronal messenger molecule in brain—the free radical, nitric oxide. Ann Neurol 1992;32:297–311.
24. Beal MF, Kowall NW, Ellison DW, et al. Replication of the neurochemical characteristics of HD by quinolinic acid. Nature 1986;321:168–171.
25. Beal MF, Hyman BT, Koroshetz WJ. Do defects in mitochondrial energy metabolism underlie the pathology of neurodegenerative diseases? Trends Neurosci 1992;16:125–131.
26. Young AB, Greenamyre JT, Hollingsworth Z, et al. NMDA receptor losses in putamen from patients with Huntington's disease. Science 1988;241:981–983.
27. Parker WD Jr, Boyson SJ, Lauder AS, Parks JK. Evidence for a defect in NADH: ubiquinone oxidoreductase (complex I) in Huntington's disease. Neurology 1990;40:1231–1234.
28. Miyoshi K. Experimental striatal necrosis induced by sodium azide. Acta Neuropathol 1967;9:199–216.
29. Montpetit V, Andermann F, Carpenter S, et al. Subacute necrotizing encephalomyelopathy. Brain 1971;94:1–30.
30. Novotny EJ, Singh G, Wallace DC, et al. Leber's disease and dystonia: a mitochondrial disease. Neurology 1986;36:1053–1060.
31. Ferrante RJ, Kowall NW, Cippolloni PB, et al. Excitotoxin lesions in primates as a model for Huntington's disease: Histopathologic and neurochemical characterization. Exp Neurol 1993;119:46–71.
32. Riepe M, Hori N, Ludolph AC, et al. Inhibition of energy metabolism by 3-nitropropionic acid activates ATP-sensitive potassium channels. Brain Res 1992;586:61–62.
33. Ludolph AC, Seelig MO, Ludolph A, et al. 3-Nitropropionic acid decreases cellular energy levels and causes neuronal degeneration in cortical explants. Neurodegeneration 1992;1:21–28.
34. Penney JB, Young AB, Shoulson I, et al. Huntington's disease in Venezuela: 7 years of follow up of at risk and symptomatic individuals. Neurology 1988;38(suppl 1):358.
35. Folstein SE, Leigh RJ, Parhad IM, Folstein MF. The diagnosis of HD. Neurology 1986;36:1279–1283.
36. Bergman N, Wichman T, DeLong MR. Reversal of experimental parkinsonism by lesions of the subthalamic nucleus. Science 1990;249:1436–1438.
37. Albin R, Young AB, Penny J. Functional anatomy of movement disorders. Trends Neurosci 1989;12:366–375.
38. Sapp E, Ge P, Aizawa H, et al. Evidence for a preferential loss of enkephalin immunoreactivity in the external globus pallidus in low grade Huntington's disease using high resolution image analysis. Neuroscience 1995;64:397–404.
39. Albin RL, Reiner A, Anderson HD, et al. Striatal and nigral neuron subpopulations in rigid Huntington's disease: implication for the functional anatomy of chorea and rigidity-akinesia. Ann Neurol 1990;27:357–365.
40. Huntington G. On chorea. Med Surg Rep 1872;26:317–321.
41. Thompson PD, Berardelli A, Rothwell JC, et al. The coexistence of bradykinesia and chorea in Huntington's disease and its implications for theories of basal ganglia control of movement. Brain 1988;111:223–244.
42. Hefter N, Homerg N, Lange NW, et al. Impairment of rapid movement in HD. Brain 1987;110:585–612.
43. Leigh RJ, Newman SA, Folstein SE, et al. Abnormal ocular motor control in HD. Neurology 1983;33:1268–1275.
44. Lasker AG, See DS, Hain TC, et al. Saccades in HD: initiation defects and distractibility. Neurology 1987;37:364–370.
45. Myers RN, Sax DS, Schoenfeld M, et al. Late onset of HD. J Neurol Neurosurg Psychiatry 1985;48:530–534.
46. Koroshetz WJ, Myers RH, Mastromauro C, et al. Late life Huntington's disease: Its implications for the diagnosis of "new" families and spontaneous mutations. Neurology 1989;39(suppl 1):128.

47. Jervis GA, Thiells NY. Huntington's chorea in childhood. Arch Neurol 1963;9:244–257.

48. Bittenbender JB, Quadvasel FA. Rigid and akinetic forms of Huntington's chorea. Arch Neurol 1962;7:275–288.

49. Sax DS, Buonnano FS. Putamenal changes in spin-echo MRI signal in bradykinetic/rigid forms of Huntington's disease. Neurology 1986;36(suppl 1):314.

50. Vogel CM, Drury I, Terry LC, Young AB. Myoclonus in adult Huntington's disease. Ann Neurology 1991;29:213–215.

51. Huggins M, Block M, Karani S, et al. Ethical and legal dilemmas arising during predictive testing for adult onset disease: the experience of Huntington's disease. Am J Hum Genet 1990;47:4–12.

52. Hansotia P, Wall R, Berendes R. Sleep disturbances and severity of HD. Neurology 1985;35:1672–1674.

Behavioral Aspects of Huntington's Disease

Jonathan H. Woodcock

INTRODUCTION

Huntington's disease (HD) is a familial, progressive, degenerative illness producing both mental and motor symptoms. Since the description by George Huntington in 1872, cognitive, behavioral, and psychologic aspects of the mental deterioration have been noted (1). The cognitive symptoms involve a progressive, inexorable dementia. Throughout the course, but often more notably early on, behavioral and psychologic changes may predominate.

DIFFICULTIES IN BEHAVIORAL EVALUATION

A number of factors complicate the evaluation of mental symptoms in HD. Although the inheritance is dominant and the penetrance complete, the time of onset is variable and the development of symptoms is insidious. Often the first symptoms are of a psychologic or behavioral nature, and thus fall into categories of human experience that may not clearly be considered pathologic. This is especially true in families that have been stressed by the occurrence of the disease in parents and possibly siblings, with attendant emotional, social, and financial disruption. Often symptoms develop during times of parental responsibilities, leading to emotional developmental disruption and stress for the children at risk (2–5). The responsibilities of caring for a progressively impaired parent and concerns regarding the development of early symptoms as harbingers of the illness in oneself bring stress responses that may not be easily distinguished from early symptoms (6,7).

The availability of presymptomatic polymorphic DNA marker screening techniques can add another form of stress. While many of those at risk indicated a desire to take advantage of low morbidity, high-accuracy screening tests before they were actually available, now that such tests have been developed, a significant proportion of those at risk are not interested in taking advantage of them (8). The presumed advantages of knowledge of more refined estimates of genetic risk may be over-shadowed by the burden of that same knowledge. In a genetically dominant condition, for each person who does participate and learns of lower than 50/50 risk, another will learn of higher risk. Those persons must find ways of coping with that knowledge. Their families and those providing the screening information must provide needed support.

CATEGORIES OF BEHAVIORAL DESCRIPTION

The behavioral sciences provide a number of paradigms for the description and understanding of neuropsychiatric impairments. It is essential that the full range of these tools be considered in the evaluation of any neuropsychiatric illness, particularly one with the multidimensional manifestations of HD. The careful evaluation of behavioral, affective, cognitive, psychologic, and functional–adaptive dimensions is important, not principally for heuristic goals, but because it can lead to treatments, interventions, and supports for the patient, family, and social systems that will enhance quality of life.

CATEGORIES OF IMPAIRMENT

Studies of impairments in HD have utilized the major disciplines and approaches of the clinical behavioral sciences. Behavioral syndromes have been described using the phenomenologic tools of recent descriptive psychiatric nosology. Cognitive function has been studied using neuropsychologic testing protocols. Emotional and psychologic studies have focused on characterologic and coping functions accompanying the stresses faced by patients and their families. Adaptive and functional living skills have been investigated using standardized rating instruments.

Neuropsychiatric Behavioral Syndromes

The major studies that have catalogued the neuropsychiatric behavioral syndromes in HD are summarized in Table 24.1. These studies differ both in the referral population being described and in the diagnostic criteria used. The studies that were based on a behaviorally impaired referral group are indicated, as are those based on an unselected population. Several conclusions can be drawn from these studies in spite of their differences in design (16). There is a very high prevalence of major psychiatric disorders in HD, ranging from 68% to 95%. Major affective disorders contribute substantially to this pathology, particularly major depression. Thought disorders and personality disorders are also prominently represented.

Folstein et al have reported a very high prevalence of affective disease in HD (15). In a series of 88 consecutive patients with HD, 41% met DSM-III (17) criteria for major affective disorder. Major depressive disorder was identified in 32% of this group and bipolar disorder in 9%. (Depres-

sive episodes required a one-month duration rather than two weeks as in DSM-III.) By comparison, the lifetime prevalence in 128 spouses and in-laws of the probands was 2%. These rates in HD are considerably higher than that found in catchment area studies. Life-time prevalence in the range of 3% to 7% for major depressive episode and 0.6% to 1.1% for manic episode is found in the general population (18). The onset of affective disorder preceded that of HD in 23 of 34 patients with available data. In those patients, affective disorder preceded HD from 2 to 20 years, with a mean of 5.1 years. Six of the 34 patients had concurrent onset, and in five the HD preceded the affective disorder. Antidepressant and electroconvulsive treatment was found to be effective in the depressed group. The presence of affective disorder predicted affective disorder in other patients with HD within the same family. This association of affective disorder and HD was limited to certain families. It was suggested that this association of manic–depressive illness and HD represented either a genetic heterogeneity in HD or a genetic linkage between the two disorders.

Mindham et al (19) compared psychiatric syndromes occurring before the onset of dementia in Alzheimer's

Table 24.1 Neuropsychiatric Syndromes in HD [Prevalence (%)]

Reference	9[a]	10	11	12[b]	13[b]	14[a]	15[b]
Year	1964	1967	1970	1979	1979	1983	1983
n	155	82	334	45	11	30	88
Affective (total)	11			42	63	37	46
Major depression	9	12	25		27[c]	17	32
Dysthymic					18[d]	20	5
Manic	2	5			18		9
Thought disorder							
Total	13	11	33	20		20	
Paranoid						3	
Schizophrenic	13	11	33	20		10	3
Other					18	7	
Anxiety						7	
Intermittent explosive						7	
Personality disorder							
Total	0	4	8	18		34	
Paranoid						7	
Somatization						13	
Antisocial						7	2
Unlabeled						7	
Alcohol/drug abuse							10
Irritable/withdrawn					18		
Other diagnoses	10	11					32
None		5		20			32

[a] Referred with behavioral problems.
[b] Unselected.
[c] Bipolar, depressed.
[d] "Demoralization."

disease (AD) and HD. The frequency of affective disorders in the HD group was twice that in AD, indicating again an increased occurrence of affective illness in HD, independent of the dementing process itself.

Suicide

Death by suicide has been associated with HD since George Huntington's original report (1). Wexler (6) found that half of 35 people at risk thought they would commit suicide if they became ill. Suicide ranks as the tenth leading cause of death in the United States, but is the third or fourth cause of death in patients with HD. Farrer (20) found suicide to be the cause of death in 5.7% of 440 deceased patients with HD, about four times that in the general population. Farrer reported that 27.6% of 831 patients attempted suicide at least once.

Schoenfeld et al (21) found that in a group of 157 deceased patients with HD in whom the cause of death was established, 12.7% had committed suicide. Those in the 10 to 49 year age group were three times as likely to commit suicide as the general population. Those in the 50 to 69 year age group were 23 times more likely. That study also reported a rate of suicide in males four times higher than in females, corresponding to the gender difference in the general population. The prevalence of suicide was four times higher in those suspected of having HD compared with those already diagnosed. The mean age of death of 342 deceased patients was 54.8 years, compared with a mean of 47.7 years among those who committed suicide.

In a survey of 831 patients with HD, Farrer found that lethal attempts occurred more often among the first attempts made (20). There were 5.9 attempted suicides per suicide, comparable with the ratio for the general population. Completed suicide was twice as common in men (7.7%) as compared with women (3.2%), but women were more likely to attempt suicide and made more repeated attempts. No established relationship between suicide and age at onset or any clinical presentation of HD was found.

By comparison, about one-third of the 440 HD deaths of known cause studied by Farrer were due to pneumonia or other infectious disease. Another quarter resulted from illnesses related to senescence including cardiovascular disease, stroke, and cancer. Other disability related causes of death included choking (5.7%) and accidents (3.2%). Death was attributed merely to HD in 20.9%.

Cognitive Function

Cognitive decline, although progressive, does appear to be quite variable (22). There is less global impairment than in AD, especially early on when deficits have focal characteristics and certain intellectual functions are spared. Relative strengths include orientation to time and place, recognition of family and friends, insight into the disease process, sense of humor, and social intelligence. Distinct apraxias, agnosias, and aphasias are absent. Speech comprehension is maintained very late, well after intelligible speech production is lost (17).

There is considerable evidence that subtle but measureable evidence of cognitive decline is present for many years before clinical diagnosis is certain (23–25). Early signs include problems with verbal memory and visuospatial function (26). Patients often first complain of difficulty with organization, planning, and sequential arrangement of information. They may feel easily overwhelmed by too much information (27). Other difficulties include calculations and verbal fluency, in spite of retained capacity for naming until later in the course (28).

The memory impairment may be related more to retrieval than to encoding processes as verbal recognition is relatively spared (29,30). This suggests that there may be an impairment in the ability to systematically search stored information in an organized fashion (31). Attentional phases of information processing and cognitive processes that are part of appreciation of the meaning of stimuli remain relatively intact (32). Butters et al have suggested that patients with HD were unable to store new information efficiently (33). On tests of learning new material, logical memory, and associative learning, impairment is evident in recently diagnosed HD (34).

Several differences are found in comparison of HD with other dementing illnesses. The memory deficit for remote events tends to span past periods of life equally, in comparison with the memory deficit in Korsakoff's amnesia (KA), which may show sparing of very remote events and periods (29).

Patients with KA also may have relative sparing of skill or procedure learning that is not content specific. Patients with HD, on the other hand, have particular difficulty in this area (29,35–37). On comparison, patients with KA have decreased verbal recognition compared with patients with HD, but relatively spared procedural learning.

Differences in perceptuospatial capacities between HD and AD have been described (38–40). Tests of egocentric spatial judgment or directional sense tend to be impaired in HD in comparison with AD. In contrast, visuoconstructive ability and route learning are impaired in AD and relatively spared in HD. Brouwers et al offers a neuropathologic explanation (39). In the early stages of HD there is neuronal loss in the caudate and putamen. Later this extends to the frontal and occipital cortices. In AD the characteristic findings are most prominent in the hippocampus and temporo-parietal cortex. Lesions in the left frontal cortex have been reported to affect directional sense (40). This contrasts to deficits in manipulation of extrapersonal space, as affected by lesions in the right parietal cortex. The neuropathologically based predictions would therefore be for difficulties with egocentric space or directional sense in HD, and with extrapersonal space in AD.

Apathy may be marked fairly early in the course, but does not correlate with the degree of dementia (14). With affective arousal and encouragement, patients are able to demonstrate significant cognitive abilities that appear impaired when they are left to function without encouragement. They may explain this apathy by complaining of feeling fatigued, uninterested, or anxious when more active.

Emotional Reactions

A variety of pathologic emotional reactions and their correlates have been described in HD, including family stress and disruption, child abuse, and personality disorders (3–5,41–43).

Caine and Shoulson (14) found that irritability, labile affect, and suspiciousness were very common, although not clearly differentiated from premorbid characteristics. Irritability may be marked and at times associated with unpredictable, aggressive responses. Patients reported feeling that their responses were out of their control, and later regretted them. Among 30 patients with HD who were referred with behavioral problems, they described 10 with significant personality disorders: antisocial (two); paranoid (two); somatization (four); and unlabelled (two).

Fedio et al (44) found high overt anxiety, concern about suicidal ideation, and a wide range of personal and social difficulties. Personality assessment often showed dependence, introversion, and concern about anger.

Conduct disorder was found in 28 (25%) of 112 offspring of HD probands by Folstein et al (2). This was more common with earlier onset of illness in the HD parent and when the non-HD parent had a psychiatric illness. Both of these factors would be expected to contribute to disorganization in the household of origin for these offspring. Affective disorder occurred in 20 (18%) of these offspring and occurred more often if similar symptoms occurred in the parent with HD. Affective disorder, but not conduct disorder, was considered a possible early manifestation of HD.

Functional Disability

Shoulson and Fahn (45) have described a scale of functional disabilities in HD that rates activities of daily living, dressing, eating, and handling finances. This instrument has been used to correlate functional decline with treatment (46), progression of radiologic features (47), and progression in impairments of cognition, affect, and motor control (48).

Mayeux et al (48) retrospectively reviewed the progression of HD in 48 patients, comparing intellectual impairment, depression, motor impairment, and functional disability. Intellectual capacity, as measured by a brief mental status instrument, correlated significantly with functional capacity. There was also a significant correlation between depression scores based on the Brief Psychiatric Rating Scale (BPRS) (49) and functional capacity. In a calculation of partial correlations, intellectual capacity and depression contributed significantly to functional disability, but motor disability did not. They did question whether somatic features of depression could be reliably differentiated from physical symptoms inherent to HD. This distinction is especially intriguing in view of the finding that although antidepressants benefit the somatic features of depression in HD, they do not alter the depressed mood or ideational elements of the depressive syndrome (14).

A lack of self-initiated activities contributes to the functional incapacity in HD. This situational apathy could be overcome with encouragement and structure. It did not prevent eager, sustained participation in planned, structured events (14). Caine and Shoulson also found that in four of five severely incapacitated patients, major psychiatric disorders were the principle source of disability, whereas in the fifth patient, a combination of dementia and psychopathology was the source of disability. They found that functional disability correlated significantly with both dementia and with psychopathology, although the latter two did not correlate with each other (14).

The parental line of transmission has been found to have an impact on the progression of impairments in HD (50,51). Patients with early onset are more likely to have inherited the HD gene from their father. They are prone to a more rapid course and to have the rigid–akinetic form of the illness rather than the choreic–hyperkinetic form. Conversely, late-onset patients are more likely to have a slower course, maternal transmission, and less severe neuropathologic features (52).

In a study of eye movements in a group of mildly affected patients with HD, those with onset of symptoms before age 30 were compared with those with later onset (53). The patients with onset before age 30 were more likely to have inherited the illness from their father (70%). Among the patients with onset after age 30, 70% inherited HD from their mother. In the patients with earlier onset, saccade speed was reduced. This reduction correlated with age of onset, but not to duration, indicating a greater severity of eye movement abnormalities in the group with earlier onset.

Neuropathologic involvement has been correlated with progression of physical disability (54). Physical disability at death was determined retrospectively for 163 patients with HD whose postmortem brain specimens were studied neuropathologically. In 23 of these cases, cell counts were completed in the head of the caudate. The number of neurons correlated significantly with physical disability rating, onset age (positively), and duration (negatively). Offspring of affected fathers had an average age of onset $5\frac{1}{2}$ years earlier than those with affected mothers. All seven patients with onset before age 20 had affected fathers.

TREATMENT OF BEHAVIORAL PROBLEMS

The most important treatment for patients with HD consists of general supportive care, including reduction of stress and of performance demands. Even so, specific behavioral symptoms that might respond to pharmacologic intervention should be considered. The most important of these is depression, followed by anxiety and thought disorder.

The treatment of mental symptoms may be overlooked in patients with HD as treating professionals and family alike may assume that despondency, hopelessness, helplessness, inertia, anxiety, and even anhedonia are normal and understandable reactions to the stress and horror of progressive disability. Thought disorder, as well, might be considered inherent to the dementing process. These presumptions have some basis. But the depressive syndrome, particularly its endogenous or somatic components, often does respond to antidepressant treatment or to electroconvulsive therapy (13–15,55). While the ideational component of depression may persist, improvement in endogenous symptoms may lead to improvement in functional capacity.

Antipsychotic treatment of thought disorder may also be effective, although probably less often than antidepressant treatment. Anxiety symptoms may respond to anxiolytics and antidepressants (14). In some instances, combination of antidepressants and antipsychotics may be necessary to achieve a response (13), just as in the treatment of delusional depression.

Chorea may respond to treatment with dopamine blockers or depleters of presynaptic dopamine (56,57). Gait disorder, however, has not responded similarly (58).

The importance of general care is emphasized in a report by Leopold and Kagel (59) demonstrating the efficacy of a behavioral program for the management of dysphagia. Improvement lasted up to 3 years.

Careful assessment of emotional and behavioral symptoms is as much the basis of rational and potentially helpful therapy in HD as in any neuropsychiatric disorder. Identification of treatable target symptoms is to be preferred to less specific, broad syndromic approaches.

CONCLUSION

Caine and Shoulson have noted that HD presents an instructive paradigm of pathogenesis in neuropsychiatric disorders (14). Although HD is syndromically recognizable with high accuracy, genetically dominant (presumably on the basis of a point mutation), and fully penetrant, its unitary genetic pathogenesis results in a broad variety of neuropsychiatric syndromes. This dissociation challenges the assumption of modern psychiatric nosology that typologically unified neuropsychiatric syndromes are based on unitary pathologies. The common genetic pathology in HD apparently affects a number of disparate final common pathways underlying behavior.

This distinction is supported by the finding of Kurlan et al (60) of a pattern of CSF metabolites [corticotropin-releasing factor (CRF) and 5-hydroxyindoleacetic acid (5-HIAA)] in depressed patients with HD different from that reported in depressed patients without HD. Although CRF concentration did correlate with the severity of depression in HD, neither it nor 5-HIAA differed in the depressed patients in comparison with the nondepressed patients, suggesting that depression in HD may have a biochemical basis distinct from that of other forms of depression.

In spite of these considerations, a symptomatic and functional approach to treatment interventions yields encouraging results. Depression and anxiety respond to standard treatments. Thought disorder may also respond to antipsychotic medication, even if with lesser frequency. Multidimensional handicaps respond to multidisciplinary support. While progression cannot be ultimately stayed, function can be supported, symptoms can be treated, relationships can be strengthened, and self-esteem can be sustained.

REFERENCES

1. Huntington G. On chorea. Med Surg Rep 1872;26:317–321.
2. Folstein SE, Franz L, Jensen BA, et al. Conduct disorder and affective disorder among the offspring of patients with Huntington's disease. Psychol Med 1983;13:45–52.
3. Pearlstein LS, Brill CB, Mancall EL. Child abuse in Huntington's disease. Pediatrics 1982;70:630–632.
4. Haus MB, Koeppen AH. Huntington's chorea: its impact on the spouse. J Nerv Ment Dis 1980;168:209–214.
5. Tyler A, Harper PS, Davies K, Newcome RG. Family breakdown and stress in Huntington's chorea. J Biosoc Sci 1983;15:127–138.
6. Wexler NS. Genetics "Russian roulette": the experience of being at risk for Huntington's disease. In: Kessler S, ed. Genetic counseling: psychological dimensions. New York: Academic, 1979:190–220.
7. Wexler N. Huntington's disease. In: Jeste D, Wyatt RJ, eds. Neuropsychiatric movement disorders. Washington: American Psychiatric, 1984:53–65.
8. Quaid KA, Brandt J, Folstein SE. The decision to be tested for Huntington's disease (letter). J Am Med Assoc 1987;257:3362.
9. Brothers C. Huntington's chorea in Victoria and Tasmania. J Neurol Sci 1964;1:405–420.
10. Healthfield KWG. Huntington's chorea. Brain 1967;90:203–232.
11. Bolt JMW. Huntington's chorea in the west of Scotland. Br J Psychiatry 1970;116:259–270.
12. Lieberman A, Dziatolowski M, Neophytides A, et al. Dementias of Huntington's and Parkinson's disease. In: Chase TN, Wexler NS, Barbeau A, eds. Advances in neurology. Vol. 23. Huntington's disease. New York: Raven, 1979:273–280.
13. Folstein SE, Folstein MF, McHugh PR. Psychiatric syndromes in Huntington's disease. In: Chase TN, Wexler NS, Barbeau A, eds. Advances in neurology. Vol. 23. Huntington's disease. New York: Raven, 1979:281–289.
14. Caine ED, Shoulson I. Psychiatric syndromes in Huntington's disease. Am J Psychiatry 1983;140:728–733.
15. Folstein SE, Abbott MH, Chase GA, et al. The association of affective disorder with Huntington's disease in a case series and in families. Psychol Med 1983;13:537–542.
16. Jeste DV, Karson CN, Wyatt RJ. Movement disorders and psychopathology. In: Jeste D, Wyatt RJ, eds. Neuropsychiatric movement disorders. Washington: American Psychiatric, 1984:119–150.
17. American Psychiatric Association. Diagnostic and statistical manual of mental disorders. 3rd ed. Washington: APA, 1980.
18. Robins LN, Helzer JE, Weissman MM, et al. Lifetime prevalence of specific psychiatric disorders in three sites. Arch Gen Psychiatry 1984;41:959–967.
19. Mindham RHS, Steele C, Folstein MF, Lucas J. A comparison of the frequency of major affective disorder in Huntington's disease and Alzheimer's disease. J Neurol Neurosurg Psychiatry 1985;48:1172–1174.

20. Farrer LA. Suicide and attempted suicide in Huntington's disease: implications for preclinical testing of persons at risk. Am J Med Genet 1986;24:305–311.
21. Schoenfeld M, Myers RH, Cupples LA, et al. Increased rate of suicide among patients with Huntington's disease. J Neurol Neurosurg Psychiatry 1984;47:1283–1287.
22. Folstein SE, Folstein MF. Psychiatric features of Huntington's disease. Psychol Dev 1983;2:193–206.
23. Lyle OE, Gottesman II. Premorbid psychometric indicators of the gene for Huntington's disease. J Consult Clin Psychol 1977;45:1011–1022.
24. Lyle OE, Gottesman II. Subtle cognitive deficits as 15 to 20 year precursors of Huntington's disease. In: Chase TN, Wexler NS, Barbeau A, eds. Advances in neurology. Vol. 23. Huntington's disease. New York: Raven, 1979:227–238.
25. Jason GW, Pajurkova EM, Suchowersky O, et al. Presymptomatic neuropsychological impairment in Huntington's disease. Arch Neurol 1988;45:769–773.
26. Josiassen RC, Curry LM, Mancall EL. Development of neuropsychological deficits in Huntington's disease. Arch Neurol 1983;40:791–796.
27. Caine ED, Fisher JM. Dementia in Huntington's disease. In: Frederiks JAM, ed. Handbook of clinical neurology. Vol. 2. Neurobehavioral disorders. Amsterdam: Elsevier, 1985:302–310.
28. Butters N, Grady M. Effect of predistractor delays on the short-term memory performance of patients with Korsakoff's and Huntington's disease. Neuropsychologia 1977;13:701–705.
29. Butters N, Wolfe J, Martone M, et al. Memory disorders associated with Huntington's disease: verbal recall, verbal recognition and procedural memory. Neuropsychologia 1985;23:729–743.
30. Moss MB, Albert MS, Butters N, Payne M. Differential patterns of memory loss among patients with Alzheimer's disease, Huntington's disease, and alcoholic Korsakoff's syndrome. Arch Neurol 1986;43:239–246.
31. Butters N, Wolfe J, Granholm E, Martone M. An assessment of verbal recall, recognition and fluency abilities in patients with Huntington's disease. Cortex 1986;22:11–32.
32. Weingartner H, Caine ED, Ebert MH. Encoding processes, learning, and recall in Huntington's disease. In: Chase TN, Wexler NS, Barbeau A, eds. Advances in neurology. Vol. 23. Huntington's disease. New York: Raven, 1979:215–226.
33. Butters N, Tarlow S, Cermak LS, et al. A comparison of the information processing deficits of patients with Huntington's chorea and Korsakoff's syndrome. Cortex 1976;12:134–144.
34. Butters N, Sax D, Montgomery K, Tarlow S. Comparison of the neuropsychological deficits associated with early and advanced Huntington's disease. Arch Neurol 1978;35:585–589.
35. Butters N. The clinical aspects of memory disorders: contributions from experimental studies of amnesia and dementia. J Clin Neuropsychol 1984;6:17–36.
36. Cohen N, Squire LR. Preserved learning and retention of pattern analyzing skills in amnesia: dissociation of knowing how and knowing that. Science 1980;210:207–210.
37. Martone M, Butters N, Payne M, et al. Dissociations between skill learning and verbal recognition in amnesia and dementia. Arch Neurol 1984;41:965–970.
38. Potegal M. A note on spatial-motor deficits in patients with Huntington's disease: a test of a hypothesis. Neuropsychologia 1971;9:233–235.
39. Brouwers P, Cox C, Martin A, et al. Differential perceptual–spatial impairment in Huntington's and Alzheimer's dementias. Arch Neurol 1984;41:1073–1076.
40. Butters N, Soeldner C, Fedio P. Comparison of parietal and frontal lobe spatial deficits in man: extrapersonal vs personal (egocentric) space. Percept Mot Skills 1972;34:27–34.
41. Dewhurst K, Oliver JE, McKnight AL. Socio-psychiatric consequences of Huntington's disease. Br J Psychiatry 1970;116:255.
42. Oliver JE, Dewhurst KE. Six generations of ill-used children in a Huntington's pedigree. Postgrad Med J 1969;45:757.
43. Dewhurst K. Personality disorder in Huntington's disease. Psychiatr Clin 1970;3:221.
44. Fedio P, Cox CS, Neophytides A, et al. Neuropsychological profile of Huntington's disease: patients and those at risk. In: Chase TN, Wexler NS, Barbeau A, eds. Advances in Neurology. Vol. 23. Huntington's disease. New York: Raven, 1979:239–255.
45. Shoulson I, Fahn S. Huntington's disease: clinical care and evaluation. Neurology 1979;29:1–3.
46. Shoulson I. Huntington's disease: a prospective evaluation of functional capacities in patients treated with neuroleptics and antidepressants. Neurology 1981;31:1333–1335.
47. Shoulson I, Plassche W, Odoroff C. Huntington's disease: caudate atrophy parallels functional impairment. Neurology 1982;32:143.
48. Mayeux R, Stern Y, Herman A, et al. Correlates of early disability in Huntington's disease. Ann Neurol 1986;20:727–731.
49. Overall JE, Gorham DR. Brief psychiatric rating scale. Psychol Rep 1962;10:799–812.
50. Myers RH, Goldman D, Bird ED, et al. Maternal transmission in Huntington's disease. Lancet 1983;i:29:208–210.
51. Farrer LA, Conneally PM. Predictability of phenotype in Huntington's disease. Arch Neurol 1987;44:109–113.
52. Myers RH, Sax DS, Schoenfeld M, et al. Late onset of Huntington's disease. J Neurol Neurosurg Psychiatry 1985;48:530–534.
53. Lasker AF, Zee DS, Hain TC, et al. Saccades in Huntington's disease: slowing and dysmetria. Neurology 1988;38:427–431.
54. Myers RH, Vonsattel JP, Stevens TJ, et al. Clinical and neuropathologic assessment of severity in Huntington's disease. Neurology 1988;38:341–347.
55. Whittier JR, Haydn G, Crawford J. Effect of imipramine on depression and hyperkinesis in Huntington's disease. Am J Psychiatry 1962;118:79.
56. Shoulson I, Goldblatt D. Huntington disease: effect of tetrabenazine and antipsychotic drugs on motoric features. Neurology 1981;31(suppl):79.
57. Girotti F, Carella F, Scighano G, et al. Effect of neuroleptic treatment on involuntary movements and motor performances in Huntington's disease. J Neurol Neurosurg Psychiatry 1984;47:848–852.
58. Koller WC, Trimble J. The gait abnormality of Huntington's disease. Neurology 1985;35:1450–1454.
59. Leopold NA, Kagel MC. Dysphagia in Huntington's disease. Arch Neurol 1985;42:57–60.
60. Kurlan R, Caine E, Rubin A, et al. Cerebrospinal fluid correlates of depression in Huntington's disease. Arch Neurol 1988;45:881–883.

Huntington's Disease Neuropathology

Jean Paul G. Vonsattel

INTRODUCTION

Huntington disease (HD) is an autosomal dominant neurodegenerative disease with mid-life onset characterized by involuntary movements and psychiatric and cognitive alterations (1). The course of the disease is relatively slow; death occurs 12 to 15 years from the time of symptomatic onset (2). The gene abnormality is located on chromosome 4 (3,4); it consists of an expanded and unstable trinucleotide (CAG) repeat (5). The number of CAG repeats in the normal population varies between 6 and 34; in contrast, the number of CAG repeats in HD varies between 37 and more than 100. The number of these repeats is unstable through meiotic transmission (6,7). Up to 95% of patients with the clinical and pathologic hallmarks of HD have an expanded CAG allele; a few individuals with the phenotype of HD have been reported to have CAG repeat lengths in the normal range (5,7,8).

Atrophy of the striatum (caudate nucleus (CN), putamen, and globus pallidus (GP)) (9) is the neuropathologic hallmark of HD (10,11). Neostriatal neuronal loss first involves the medial CN adjacent to the lateral ventricle, the dorsal putamen, and the tail of the caudate nucleus (TCN); the nucleus accumbens is spared until late in the course of the disease (12). The rate of degeneration of neostriatal neurons varies according to their class. The aspiny neurons are less prone to degeneration than are the spiny ones (13–16). Biochemical data corroborate these observations (17–21). To some extent, the neurochemical and neuropathologic changes seen in HD striatum can be obtained in animal models following overstimulation of striatal glutamate receptors, supporting an excitotoxic theory of the pathophysiology of HD (22–25). Efforts are currently devoted to identifying the primary cause of the genetically programmed, premature neuronal death that occurs in HD.

NEUROPATHOLOGIC HISTORY

Anton (26) and Lannois and Paviot (27) were the first to identify striatal abnormalities associated with movement disorders. Jelgersma later correlated the atrophy of the CN with chorea in HD (28). Alzheimer attributed chorea of HD mainly to atrophy of the striatum (29). Much less consistent neuropathologic changes in HD were described in the claustrum (30–32), hypothalamus (33), hypothalamic lateral tuberal nucleus (34,35), amygdala (36,37), hippocampal formation (38), subthalamic region (29,39,40), thalamus (41, 42), nucleus coeruleus (43,44), red nucleus (45), substantia nigra (39,46), superior olivary nucleus, pons and medulla oblongata (1,29,31,32,43,47,48), cerebellum (32,36,48–55), and spinal cord (29,49,50,52).

Although most observers have suggested the opposite, Pfeiffer (41) and Dunlap (10) found the putamen to be more involved than the CN in HD. Kiesselbach (49) and Dunlap (10) noted atrophy of the white matter. The neuropathologic features characteristic of HD may be summarized as the gradual atrophy (loss of neurons with gliosis) of the neostriatum (30). The severity of the neuropathologic changes in the neostriatum increases along the antero-posterior, latero-medial, and ventro-dorsal axes (12). The GP is also affected, but to a lesser extent (30,49,56). In the cerebral cortex subtle changes, especially neuronal loss, occur (30,31,57–60). Volumetric loss of the cerebral white matter is gradual with the progression of the disease and may be striking (10,49).

ANATOMY AND NOMENCLATURE OF THE BASAL GANGLIA

The basal ganglia consists of the corpus striatum and the amygdaloid nucleus or archistriatum, which is part of the limbic system (9). Because of their functions, it would be reasonable to include the subthalamic nucleus and substantia nigra in the basal ganglia.

The corpus striatum consists of the neostriatum (CN and putamen) and paleostriatum (globus pallidus). The GP is divided into external (GPe) and internal (GPi) segments. The neostriatum is commonly referred to as the "striatum" (9). The "lenticular nucleus" is a descriptive definition of both the putamen and the GP. The substantia nigra has two main zones: the pars reticulata (SNr) and the pars compacta (SNc). The pars reticulata contains neurons morphologically similar to those in the GPi; the pars compacta contains neurons that are pigmented in the adult. The nucleus accumbens is the ventral anterior part of the neostriatum, where the CN and putamen fuse.

With cresyl violet as least two groups of neurons can be distinguished in the neostriatum (61). One group consists of small- or medium-sized type and a second of large neurons (40 μm in diameter and larger). The ratio of small-medium to large neostriatal neurons averages 175:1 (range 130:1 to 258:1) (62). Golgi and ultrastructural studies identify at least five general categories of neurons. The two main categories consist of neurons with spiny dendrites (spiny neurons) and neurons with smooth dendrites (aspiny neurons) (63,64). Both the spiny (which are the most numerous) and aspiny neurons are represented by large- and small-medium-sized neurons (63). Spiny neurons have distant connections and often are referred to as projection neurons; they contain gamma-aminobutyric acid, enkephalin, dynorphin, substance P, or calbindin (65–68). Aspiny neurons or interneurons have local connections and contain nicotinamide adenine dinucleotide phosphate diaphorase, somatostatin, neuropeptide Y, cholecystokinin, or acetylcholine (67–72).

The primate neostriatum can be divided into two compartments: the striosomes and the matrix (73,74). However, recent data suggest that this compartmentalization might be more complex (75). The intensity of histochemical staining for acetylcholinesterase is weak in the 300 to 600 μm-wide discrete zones referred to as "striosomes". The staining is intense in the matrix, which surrounds the striosomes (66,74). Calbindin, a neuronal cytoplasmic calcium-binding protein, is abundant in the matrix and rare in the striosomes (76). Afferents to the striosomes originate in the SNc, prefrontal cortex, and limbic system. Efferents from the striosomes terminate in the SNc. Afferents to the matrix originate in the motor and somatosensory cortices, and in the parietal, occipital, and frontal cortices. Efferents from the matrix terminate in the SNr, GPi, and GPe (76–78).

PHYSIOLOGIC CONSIDERATIONS

The basal ganglia concerned with motor functions can be conceptualized physiologically as two compartments: one for input (CN and putamen) and one for output (GP, subthalamic nucleus, and substantia nigra).

The entire cerebral cortex projects onto the striatum (79–81). Specific cortical areas send projections to selected portions of the CN and putamen, or input compartment. The output nuclei are the GPi, SNr, and ventral pallidum; their target nuclei are located in the thalamus, which has an excitatory action upon the cortex.

Two major pathways (a direct and an indirect) connect the input compartment to the output nuclei. The direct pathway arises from inhibitory neostriatal (CN and putamen) efferents to the GPi. The indirect pathway also arises from the neostriatum but passes first to the GPe, subthalamic nucleus, and SNr, and then to the GPi, which sends projections to the thalamus. The two efferent systems of the basal ganglia have apparently opposing effects upon the output nuclei and thalamic target nuclei. It seems likely that decreases in GPi-SNr discharges facilitate movements initiated in the cortex and that increases in GPi-SNr discharges inhibit cortically initiated movements (82).

There is evidence that early in the course of HD there is a selective loss of striatal neurons that give rise to the indirect pathway (83–86). This neuronal loss reduces the inhibitory action of the GPe upon the subthalamic nucleus, which becomes hypofunctional and causes reduction of the inhibitory action of the GPi upon the thalamus. This subsequent disinhibition of the thalamus leads to choreiform movements. Albin et al (85) have shown pathologic evidence supporting the hypothesis that chorea might result from preferential loss of striatal neurons projecting to the GPe, and that rigid-akinetic HD might be due to the additional loss of striatal neurons projecting to the GPi.

NEUROPATHOLOGY

Atrophy of the striatum is the neuropathologic hallmark of HD. Five grades (0 to 4) of neuropathologic severity of striatal involvement can be distinguished (12). Grade 0 defines cases of clinically diagnosed HD without discernible abnormality of the striatum as judged by conventional neuropathologic (macroscopic and microscopic) standards. In grade 1, neuropathologic changes of the striatum can only be recognized microscopically. In grades 2 and 3, gross striatal atrophy is mild to severe, respectively. In grade 4, the brain is diffusely smaller than normal with the brunt of the atrophy involving the striatum, where 95% or more of neurons are lost. There is good correlation between the overall atrophy of the brain and that of the striatum, although there are exceptions. The neuropathologic definition of clinically well-established HD can be summarized as a diffuse atrophy of the brain with the brunt of the degenerative changes involving the striatum (12,29).

External Examination of the Brain

Eighty percent of brains from patients who have died with HD show atrophy on external examination of the brains as evidenced by widened sulci and shrunken gyri, particularly in the frontal lobes. The remaining 20% do not show gross abnormality.

The mean weight of 138 brains was 1067 g (normal about 1350 g). The mean weights of 163 brains that were classified according to grade were as follows: 1240 g for grades 0 and 1, 1140 g for grade 2, 1120 g for grade 3, and 995 g for grade 4 (12).

The ventricular system is widened in HD. Measurement of 162 left or right lateral ventricles of HD brains gave a mean volume of 16.3 cc (range: 8 to 46 cc; normal about 7 cc). The mean left or right ventricular volume in the series of 138 brains classified according to grade was as follows: 11.7 cc for grade 1, 15.5 cc for grade 2, 16.8 cc for grade 3, and 20.2 cc for grade 4. The frontal horns and atria are more widened than the temporal and occipital horns.

Coronal Sections

Coronal sections are apparently normal in 5% of the HD brains. Usually, the cerebral cortex is thinner than normal. There is volumetric reduction of the white matter, striatum, and thalamus (Fig 25.1). De La Monte et al (87) morphometrically evaluated five standardized coronal brain slices in 30 patients with HD. There was a 21% to 29% loss in the cerebral cortex, a 29% to 34% loss in the white matter, a 28% loss in the thalamus, a 57% loss in the CN, and a 64% loss in the putamen.

Striatum

The most striking changes in HD are exhibited in the striatum, where there is volumetric reduction, neuronal loss, and reactive astrogliosis (Figs 25.1–25.3). The extent and distribution of these changes depend on the degree of illness at the time of death. The striatal pattern of neuronal loss and gliosis is distinctive and probably pathognomonic for HD as judged by our observations of more than 1000 HD brains that we have evaluated systematically during the past 12 years. These pathologic striatal characteristics are the quin-

tessence of the grading system applied to HD brains and are invaluable for the differential diagnosis.

As previously stated, five grades of striatal neuropathologic severity can be distinguished, each grade reflecting the extent and distribution of neuronal loss and gliosis (Fig 25.4). The assignment of a grade is based on striatal findings on both gross and microscopic examinations of three standardized coronal sections. One coronal section includes the head of the caudate nucleus (HCN), putamen, and nucleus accumbens; this level is referred to as "CAP" (caudate, accumbens, putamen) (see Fig 25.1). The next coronal section includes the CN, putamen, and both the external and internal segments of the globus pallidus (level

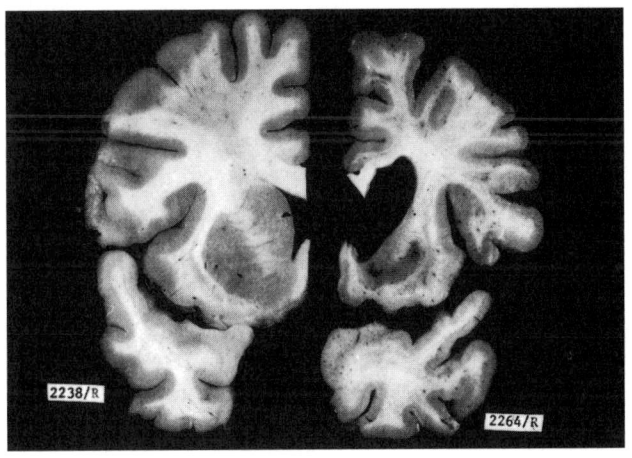

FIGURE 25.1 *Coronal sections through the head of caudate nucleus (HCN), nucleus accumbens, and putamen (level CAP). The section on the left is that of a 34-year-old man (suicide, brain weight 1,680 g); the section on the right is that of a 48-year-old man with HD (brain weight 1,100 g, grade 3/4), the atrophy strikingly involves the neostriatum and white matter; cortical thinning is not obvious.*

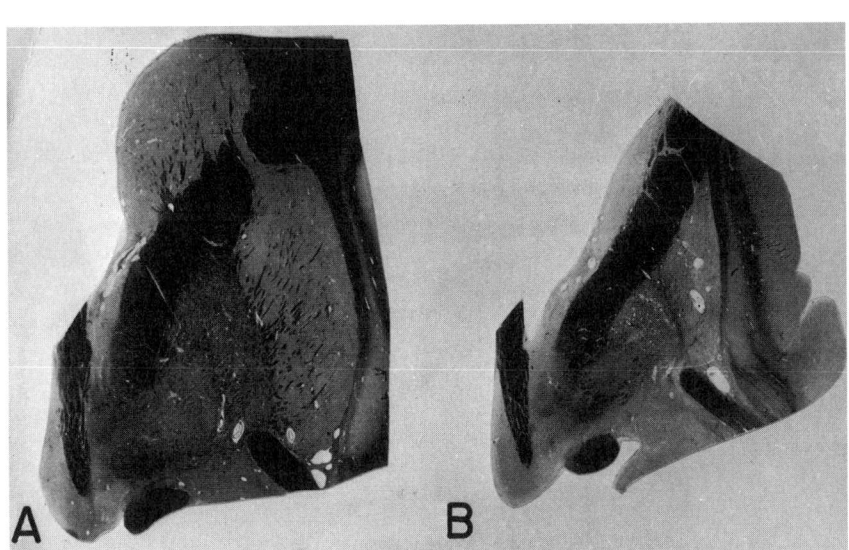

FIGURE 25.2 *Microphotographs showing coronal sections through the HCN, putamen, external and internal segments of the globus pallidus (level GP) of a 41-year-old man without neurological abnormality (A) and of a 43-year-old man with HD (B). The HD sample shows severe atrophy of the striatum; the dorso-medial border of the lenticular nucleus is concave medially; and the external segment of the globus pallidus is relatively more atrophic than the internal segment. (Luxol fast blue, counterstained with hematoxylin and eosin [LHE], original magnification ×2.5.)*

GP) (see Fig 25.2). The third coronal section contains the TCN at the level of the lateral geniculate body (LGB); it may provide the only visible change on gross examination early in the course of the disease. In addition, this section contains the body of the caudate nucleus (BCN) and the thalamus (including the centrum medianum) at the midpoint of the sagittal axis between the frontal and occipital poles.

Grade 0. Grade 0 is assigned to brains from patients with definite genetic or clinical evidence for the diagnosis of HD, yet without any gross or microscopic abnormality sugges-

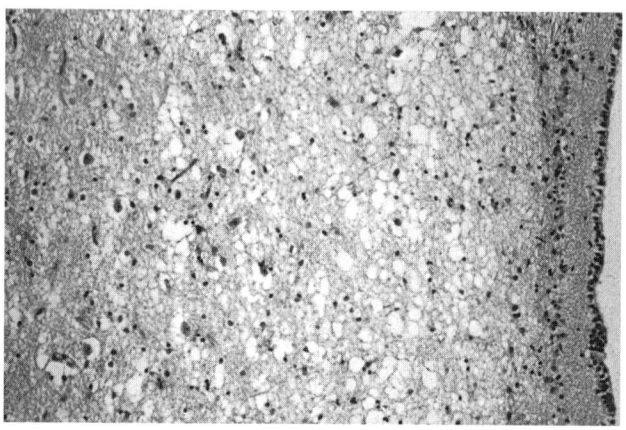

FIGURE 25.3   *Huntington's disease grade 3/4. Microphotograph of the HCN at midpoint between the dorsal and ventral limits of the neostriatum at level CAP. It shows the ependymal lining, subependymal glial layer, and, in continuity, the loosely textured caudate parenchyma, which gradually becomes denser in the opposite direction of the ependymal surface. Neuronal loss is very severe in the loose textured zone, whereas there are scattered neurons in the denser area. (LHE, original magnification ×100.)*

tive of HD on examination of the brain. The grade 0 brains are grossly indistinguishable from normal brains despite a cell count indicating a 30% to 40% neuronal loss and no significant increase in the number of astrocytes or reactive astrocytosis. These subtle changes might not be appreciated without quantitative study.

No neuropathologic change could be identified by conventional examination of 15 brains from patients at risk for HD; three of them turned out to have inherited the HD gene, indicating that the striatum of a pre-symptomatic carrier of the HD mutation appears normal (7).

Grade 1. Macroscopically, the striatum is apparently normal with the exception of the TCN, which is much smaller than normal; atrophy of the BCN may already be obvious. Neuronal loss and astrogliosis are evident in the TCN and less so in the BCN. A moderate fibrillary astrocytosis is present especially in the medial HCN and in the dorsal half of the putamen (see Fig 25.4); neuronal loss is mild and may be barely perceptible on general survey of the slides. Cell count, however, shows that more than 50% of neurons are lost in the HCN (12). The GP is apparently normal on gross and microscopical examination.

Grade 2. Macroscopically, the atrophy of the TCN is severe. The BCN is about half its normal size. At level CAP, atrophy of the HCN and of the putamen might be subtle or is evident; the medial outline of the HCN is only slightly convex but still bulges into the lateral ventricle. At level GP, striatal atrophy ranges from subtle to obvious.

Neuronal loss and gliosis are severe in the BCN and in the TCN, conspicuous in the medial HCN and in the dorsal half of the putamen; they are less pronounced in the paracapsular portion of the HCN and in the ventral portion of the putamen (see Fig 25.4). The nucleus accumbens and GP are apparently normal.

Grade 3. Macroscopically, the neostriatum is severely reduced in size; however, the atrophy of the nucleus accum-

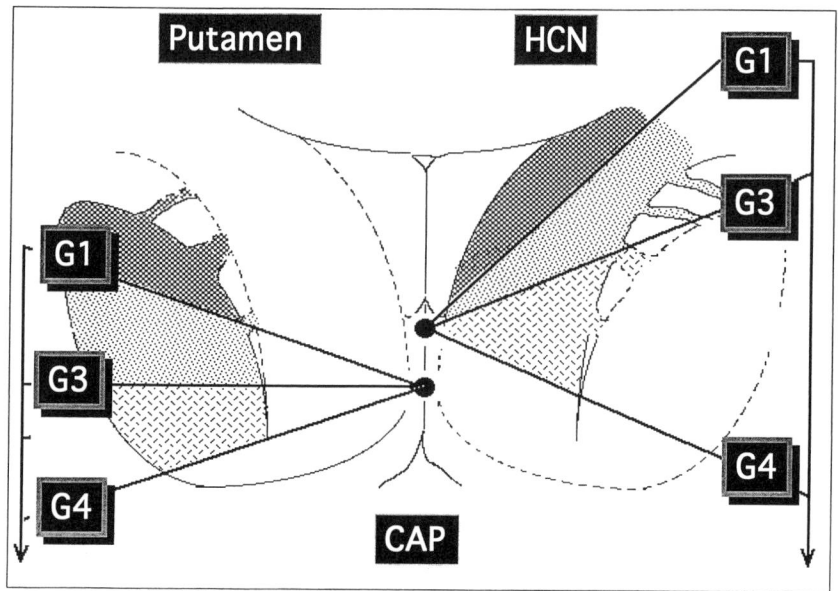

FIGURE 25.4   *Schematic coronal section at level CAP (caudate, accumbens, putamen) illustrating the topographical progression of the neuropathologic changes in the putamen (left) and in the HCN (right) during the course of the disease (the volumetric changes are not represented). Neuronal loss and gliosis are first seen in the dorsomedial portion of the HCN, dorsal third of the putamen, and dorsal caudoputaminal bridges (grade 1 [G1]). Later in the course of the disease, the changes reach the ventral third of the anterior neostriatum with relative preservation of the nucleus accumbens (grade 2 [not shown] and grade 3 [G3]). Most of the ventral third of the anterior neostriatum is involved in the end stage of the disease (grade 4 [G4]), however, to a lesser extent than it is dorsally.*

bens is less striking. The medial outline of the HCN forms a straight line or is slightly concave medially (see Fig 25.1, right). The BCN is reduced by about 75%; the TCN consists of a barely visible stripe. The dorso-medial outline of the lenticular nucleus is straight or slightly concave medially (see Fig 25.2). The GP is smaller than normal, especially the GPe. The white matter bundles of the lentiform nuclei are thinner than normal or blurred (see Fig 25.2). There is atrophy of the ansa lenticularis and thinning of the anterior limb of the internal capsule.

Neuronal loss and fibrillary astrocytosis are especially conspicuous in the TCN, BCN, paraventricular portion of the HCN, and dorsal half of the putamen (see Fig 25.3). There is relative preservation of the paracapsular portion of the HCN. The nucleus accumbens is usually normal; however, occasional reactive astrocytes might be present dorsally (Fig 25.5). Slight fibrillar astrocytosis is present especially in the lateral third of the GPe; the GPi is microscopically within normal limits.

Grade 4. Grade 4 is characterized by extreme atrophy of the neostriatum. At level CAP, the HCN is shrunken and yellow-brown. Its medial contour is concave, as is the anterior limb of the internal capsule. The putamen is atrophic with a concave dorso-medial outline. The nucleus accumbens is smaller than normally expected but is relatively prominent in comparison with the adjacent HCN or putamen. At the level of GP, the HCN consists of a thin strip. The putamen is much smaller than normal, often with widened perivascular spaces in its ventral third. The medullary laminae of the GP are thinner than normal and blurred as are the lenticular white matter bundles. There is about a 50% reduction of the GP, the external segment being more involved than the internal segment.

Neuronal loss and gliosis are extremely severe and diffuse throughout the neostriatum; the neuropil is often loosely

textured, especially in the paraventricular regions. The bridges between the HCN and the putamen show neuronal loss and gliosis, but less severely than in the main part of the CN or putamen; and the dorsal bridges are more involved than the ventral ones (Figs 25.6 and 25.7). Neuronal depletion and gliosis are less severe in the nucleus accumbens than in the adjacent HCN or putamen. The GP is remarkable for the presence of fibrillary astrocytosis, especially in the GPe; neurons are smaller than usual and are more closely packed together than in age-matched controls.

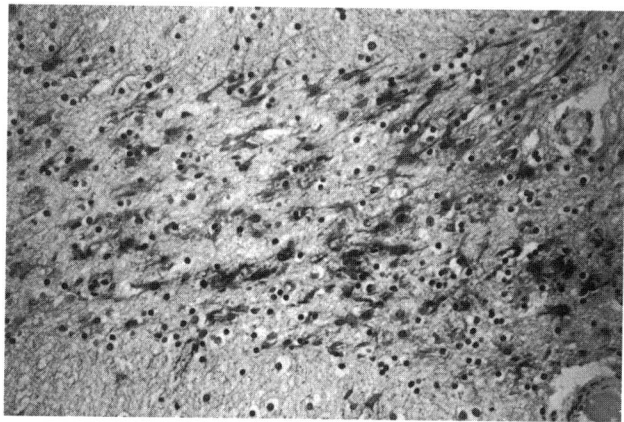

FIGURE 25.6 *Huntington's disease grade 4/4 (same case as Fig 25.7). Microphotograph of the dorsal, caudo-putaminal gray matter bridge at level CAP showing severe reactive astrocytosis confined to the gray matter bordered dorsally and ventrally by white matter. (Glial fibrillary acidic protein [GFAP], original magnification ×160.)*

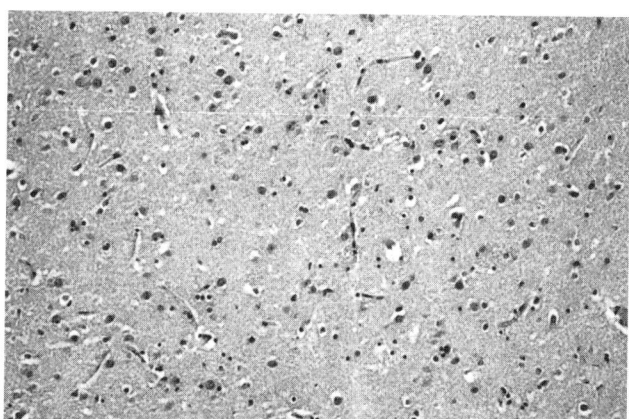

FIGURE 25.5 *Huntington's disease grade 3/4. Microphotograph of the nucleus accumbens, which is relatively preserved when compared with a more dorsal area of the HCN (see Fig 25.3). Neuronal density and neuropil texture are apparently normal; reactive gliosis is mild. (LHE, original magnification ×100.)*

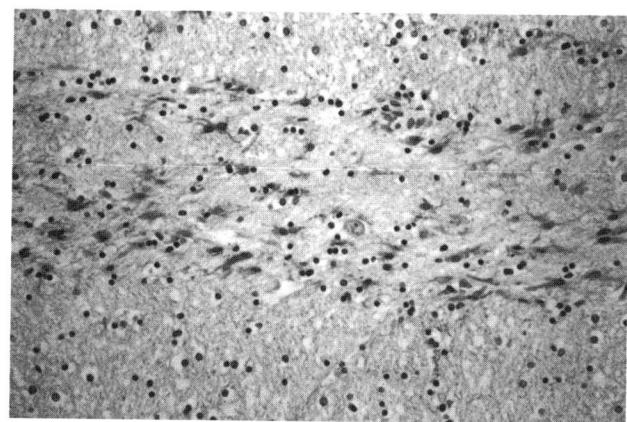

FIGURE 25.7 *Huntington's disease grade 4/4 (same case as Fig 25.6). Microphotograph of the ventral, caudo-putamenal gray matter bridge at level CAP showing reactive astrocytosis that is less severe than in the dorsal bridge (see Fig 25.6) illustrating the dorsoventral gradient of decreasing neurophatological severity so characteristically present in HD. (GFAP, original magnification ×160.)*

The distribution of 214 HD brains categorized according to grade between July 1993 and July 1996 is shown in Table 25.1 indicating that grade 3 HD brains are those encountered most frequently (see Figs 25.1 and 25.2B).

In grade 2, the neostriatal gradients of increased severity of neuronal loss and gliosis along the antero-posterior, ventro-dorsal, and latero-medial axes are discrete and probably pathognomonic for HD (see Fig 25.4). The identification of these gradients is crucial in making the diagnosis of HD, especially in the early stages of the disease when there are few if any striatal changes visible on gross examination, with the exception of the TCN. Indeed, the TCN is atrophic early in the course of the disease.

Caution should be exercised in making the diagnosis of HD grade 1, especially when the tissue is not optimally prepared or when changes due to an acute or remote hypoxic-ischemic event are present. In these instances, it is advisable to evaluate the length of the CAG repeat for a final diagnostic statement. Careful examination of the TCN is essential in these cases since atrophy is always present early in the course of the disease. One should be aware, however, that segments of the TCN might be absent in brains from patients without any neurologic or psychiatric disorder. Therefore, prior to concluding that the TCN is atrophic, one must scrutinize it in its entirety. In early stages of HD the atrophy of the TCN is always associated with some involvement of the medial half of the BCN, and must be confirmed microscopically.

Grade 0 brains are rare. The frequency of grade 0 might depend to some extent on the experience of the neuropathologist: the more experienced the neuropathologist, the higher the probability of identifying subtle striatal changes in a very early stage of the disease.

Hedreen and Folstein (88) have shown that scattered islands of astrocytosis and neuronal loss involve the neostriatum before the ventrally progressive wave of generalized neuronal loss, and that they correspond to striosomes. These islands may be specific for HD; their histologic demonstration is important for the pathologic differential diagnosis of this disease especially in its early stage.

Unusual Neostriatal Findings

Less than 5% of the HD brains show unusual neostriatal microscopic changes. They consist of the presence of one to five (rarely more) discrete round or oval islets with ill-defined borders of relatively intact parenchyma present in the anterior neostriatum. The cross-sections of the islets measure about 100 mm. The number of neurons in these islets is the same as or slightly lower than in the normal neostriatum, but the number of astrocytes is increased (89). These islets are larger than striosomes, but their nature is poorly understood. They are more frequently seen in patients whose symptoms appear earlier and develop faster than in HD patients with the usual neostriatal lesions. Local variation in neuronal loss and gliosis is occasionally noticed in the anterior neostriatum (56). In these instances, however, the atrophic and relatively spared zones are ill-defined. Occasionally there are thin, gliotic bands projecting from the most severely involved areas (dorsal HCN or putamen) into the ventral, relatively preserved parts. These cases might represent intermediary forms between those with the usual neostriatal lesions and those with discrete islets.

Selective or Variable Rates of Degeneration of Neostriatal Neurons

Spiny or projection neurons bear the brunt of the degenerative process in HD (15). Aspiny or interneurons tend to be more resistant or to degenerate later in the course of the disease (14,16,90,91). However, the extreme atrophy of the neostriatum and the loss of 95% of the neostriatal neurons in grade 4 suggest that both the spiny and aspiny neurons are vulnerable.

Reiner et al (83) evaluated whether there was a differential loss among neostriatal projection neurons in 17 HD brains. They found that enkephalin-containing neurons projecting to the GPe were much more affected than substance P-containing neurons projecting to the GPi. This observation was confirmed by Sapp et al (92) and Richfield et al (93). Each of these three studies found a grade-related decline in the striatal enkephalin immunoreactivity or in the number of preproenkephalin-labeled neurons.

Matrix–Striosomes

The compartmentalization (matrix–striosomes) is preserved in the HD neostriatum, where the decrease in the surface of the matrix is striking while that of the striosomes is relatively unchanged (16). However, neuronal loss and gliosis involve both compartments (94). As mentioned previously, gliosis and neuronal loss were found to first occur in the striosomes, as evidenced by the evaluation of brains of patients who died at an early stage of the disease (88).

Cerebral Cortex and White Matter

The cerebral cortex and white matter do not show any specific macroscopic or microscopic changes as judged by conventional neuropathologic examination; the exception is a volumetric reduction that is more pronounced in the white matter than in the cortex. It was noted that the loss of white matter was more striking than that of gray matter with the exception of the striatum as early as 1914 (10,49). As stated

Table 25.1   Distribution of 214 Graded HD Brains Categorized Between July 1993 and July 1996

Grade	1	2	3	4
Total (*n*)	8	35	111	60
Percentage	3.7	16.4	51.9	28.0

previously, de la Monte et al (87) found a 21% to 29% volumetric cortical loss and a 29% to 34% loss of white matter in HD. The extent of these losses correlates with the grade of neuropathological severity. However, within the same grade of neuropathologic severity, for example grade 3, the cortical and white matter loss may vary. At time, the atrophy of both cortex and white matter is somewhat proportional to that of the striatum; there are cases with striatal changes of grade 3 but with only slight volumetric reduction of cortex and white matter.

Dunlap (10) found the HD cortex (*n* = 30) to be "slightly thinner than in the controls (*n* = 30), but the difference was very little." Terplan's illustration in 1924 (56) (reproduced by Hallervorden in his often quoted review published in 1957 (52)) compares a normal cerebral cortex with that of a HD patient with severe neuronal loss. The control brain was from a 20-year-old executed convict, the other was from a 38-year-old woman with a 10-year history of chorea and with gangrene of the lungs found at autopsy (these details are to be found in Terplan's publication but not in Hallervorden's review). Zalneraitis et al (95) found little or no appreciable neuronal loss, normal astrocytes, and a relatively normal content of glial fibrillary protein in the cortex of 14 HD brains.

Morphometric studies of the prefrontal cortex in 81 HD brains (grades 2 to 4) and 23 normal age-matched controls showed a loss of large pyramidal neurons in layers III, V, and VI in HD; neuronal loss was striking in grade 4; there was no increase in glial cells in the HD cortex (60). Cudkowicz and Kowall performed cell counts in the cortex including Brodmann areas 8, 9, and 24 of eleven patients with HD (three grade 2; seven grade 3; and one grade 4) and of six age-matched controls (58). They found a depletion of long projecting neurons but a normal number of local circuit neurons in HD brains when compared to the controls. Contrary to Sotrel et al (60), Cudkowicz and Kowall did not find a correlation between the grades and the severity of cortical neuronal loss. Hedreen et al compared Brodmann area 10 of five HD brains (grade 4) with five age-matched controls (59). They found cortical thinning, a 57% neuronal loss in layer VI, and a 71% loss in layer V in the HD samples.

According to our experience, the extent of cortical atrophy depends on the stage of the disease: it is most pronounced in grades 3 and 4, while the cortex is apparently normal in grades 1 and 2. There is no reactive gliosis across the grades. It can be extremely difficult to identify cortical abnormalities in HD (96). The volumetric loss of white matter is severe in grades 3 and 4 without any apparent microscopic abnormality.

Thalamus, Hypothalamus, and Substantia Nigra

The thalamus is normal on gross and microscopic examination in grades 1 and 2. It is smaller than normal in grade 3 and even more so in grade 4. Astrocytosis and neuronal loss in the centrum medianum are the only microscopic abnormalities regularly observed in grade 4 and, to a lesser extent, grade 3 brains.

Another pathologic feature of HD is the neuronal loss that correlates with the grade in both the lateral nucleus of the hypothalamus (34,35) and SNr (96). The SNr is markedly atrophic and the neuronal density is decreased, especially in grades 3 and 4; the SNc is thinner than normal yet its number of neurons remains normal in all grades (39,96). The loss of neuropil results in a relative increased density of pigmented neurons, especially in grades 3 and 4.

Subthalamic Nucleus and Red Nucleus

Personal experience indicates that the subthalamic nucleus and red nucleus show mild to moderate volumetric reduction in grades 3 and 4 without any recognizable microscopic alteration except for the presence of occasional reactive astrocytosis in some end-stage cases. These nuclei are apparently normal in grades 1 and 2. They were atrophic and gliotic with scattered argyrophilic neurons in a single brain that, in addition to the characteristic features of HD, displayed those of progressive supranuclear palsy.

Cerebellum

There are no specific cerebellar HD changes recognizable by conventional neuropathologic examination. The cerebellum is normal on gross and microscopic examination in grades 1 and 2; there is gross atrophy without microscopic abnormality in grades 3 and 4. Cortical neuronal loss, when present, is often associated with hypoxic-ischemic events.

We were unable to reliably differentiate 25 HD cases from 25 non-HD cases in a blind evaluation of 50 slides from systematically selected blocks of the dentate nucleus with the cortical ribbon dorsal to it. Dunlap (10) found the cerebellum to be morphologically normal in 29 of 30 HD cases; one was atrophic.

Juvenile HD patients usually have severe cerebral and cerebellar atrophy with striatal features of grade 4 at the time of autopsy. Byers et al reported the neuropathologic data of four juvenile HD patients all with severe cerebellar atrophy (48). The hippocampal formation was available in three of the four patients; of these three hippocampi, two were abnormal. Forty percent of juvenile HD patients have seizures, which may be accountable for cerebellar or hippocampal neuronal loss (53).

The brainstem and spinal cord show volumetric reduction in grades 3 and 4, without any significant microscopical abnormality.

CAG REPEATS: NEUROPATHOLOGY AND GENE EXPRESSION

As stated previously, HD appears to be caused by an expansion of an unstable CAG repeat on chromosome 4p16.3

within a coding region of a gene referred to as "IT15" (for "Interesting Transcript") (5,97). Juvenile onset patients typically have repeat lengths of more than 60 units, while most mid-life onset patients have repeat lengths in the 40 to 50 unit range, and those with late onset usually have 37 to 40 units. These numbers of repeats correlate inversely with age of onset or with age at death (7,8,98–100).

Correlation of CAG repeat lengths and grades using 310 brains from clinically diagnosed HD patients showed that repeat stretches of 37 to 40 units occurred in all grades and that the largest alleles (>50 units) occurred only in grades 3 and 4. These observations indicate that there is no larger threshold repeat size associated with grade 4, and that the largest alleles influence the rate of striatal atrophy (7). There is a definite correlation between the CAG lengths and grades of neuropathologic severity, or the neostriatal extent of neuronal loss and gliosis (101,102).

The gene involved in HD may be translated as a variable polyglutamine segment in the cytosolic protein product huntingtin. The HD mutation does not eliminate the expression of huntingtin, as evidenced by its presence in cells from HD homozygotes. The HD huntingtin is larger than the normal huntingtin (100,103); and it can be distinguished from the normal huntingtin with specific antibodies (104).

Investigations using in situ hybridization (with RNA probes constructed from cDNA subclones making up the composite sequences of IT15) and immunochemistry (with antisera directed at peptides predicted by the DNA sequence upstream and downstream of the CAG repeats) revealed widespread expression of IT15. Indeed, it is expressed in all brain regions and in other organs of both HD and control samples (99,100,105–109). Regional cerebral expression of IT15 is apparently proportional to neuronal density. The highest levels are seen in the cerebellum, hippocampus, cerebral cortex, SNc, and pontine nuclei, with intermediate levels in the neostriatum and with low levels in the GP (109). IT15 expression predominates in neurons and is weak in glial cells. The mechanism by which CAG repeats are expanded and translated into a polyglutamine segment in huntingtin leading to neuronal death (especially in the striatum) is unknown. The function of the normal huntingtin is not known although it might play a role in microtubule-mediated transport or vesicle function (110). The HD expansion of the polyglutamine repeat perhaps induces a toxic gain of function possibly through interactions with other proteins. Li et al recently identified a protein (huntingtin-associated protein or HAP-1) that binds to huntingtin and whose normal function is unknown; the binding of HAP to huntingtin is enhanced by an expanded polyglutamine repeat (111).

Exceptionally, HD-like neuropathology can occur in the absence of expanded CAG repeats (7). The identification of such brains by careful neuropathologic evaluation, by saving fresh frozen samples for nucleic acid studies, and by genotyping family members could unveil an as yet unknown sub-category of striatal degeneration. Clarification of this putative subcategory of brains would be invaluable in the process of understanding the mechanism whereby an expanded CAG allele becomes deleterious to certain classes of neurons in specific areas.

ACKNOWLEDGMENTS

I thank Dr. E. D. Bird, director of the Brain Tissue Resource Center, McLean Hospital, Belmont, MA, for his support. I am truly grateful to Timothy Wheelock, Lisa Kanaley-Andrews, Wendy Hobbs, Stephanie Lenzi, and Lynne M. Kelley for their excellent technical assistance. I gratefully acknowledge Larry Cherkas for his photography and advice. I also express my appreciation to the numerous pathologists who referred case material to the Brain Tissue Resource Center. I am especially grateful to the families of the patients for providing brain tissue for research.

This work was supported in part by NIH grants NINCDS 31862 (Brain Tissue Resource Center) and NS 16367 (Huntington's Disease Center Without Walls); and by grants from the Vaughn Foundation and Hereditary Disease Foundation.

REFERENCES

1. Martin JB, Gusella JF. Huntington's disease. Pathogenesis and management. Seminars in medicine of the Beth Israel Hospital, Boston. N Engl J Med 1986;315:1267–1276.
2. Myers RH, Vonsattel JP, Stevens TJ, et al. Clinical and neuropathologic assessment of severity in Huntington's disease. Neurology 1988;38:341–347.
3. Gusella JF, Wexler NS, Conneally PM, et al. A polymorphic DNA marker genetically linked to Huntington's disease. Nature 1983;306:234–238.
4. Gusella JF. Huntington's disease. In: Harris H, Hirschhorn K, eds. Advances in human genetics. Vol. 20. New York: Plenum, 1991:125–151.
5. The Huntington's Disease Collaborative Research Group. A novel gene containing a trinucleotide repeat that is expanded and unstable on Huntington's disease chromosomes. Cell 1993;72:971–983.
6. Read AP. Huntington's disease: testing the test. Nat Genet 1993;4:329–330.
7. Persichetti F, Srinidhi J, Kanaley L, et al. Huntington's disease CAG trinucleotide repeats in pathologically confirmed post-mortem brains. Neurobiol Dis 1994;1:159–166.
8. Andrew SE, Goldberg YP, Kremer B, et al. The relationship between trinucleotide (CAG) repeat length and clinical features of Huntington's disease. Nat Genet 1993;4:398–403.
9. Carpenter MB, Sutin J. Human neuroanatomy. 8th ed. Baltimore/London: Williams & Wilkins, 1983:579–586.
10. Dunlap CB. Pathologic changes in Huntington's chorea. Arch Neurol Psychiatry (Chicago) 1927;18:867–943.
11. Stone TT, Falstein EI. Pathology of Huntington's chorea. J Nerv Ment Dis 1938;88:773–797.
12. Vonsattel J-P, Myers RH, Stevens TJ, et al. Neuropathological classification of Huntington's disease. J Neuropathol Exp Neurol 1985;44:559–577.
13. Dawbarn D, De Quidt ME, Emson PC. Survival of basal ganglia neuropeptide Y-somatostatin neurones in Huntington's disease. Brain Res 1985;340:251–260.
14. Ferrante RJ, Kowall NW, Beal MF, et al. Selective sparing of a class of striatal neurons in Huntington's disease. Science 1985;230:561–563.
15. Graveland GA, Williams RS, DiFiglia M. Evidence for degenerative and regenerative changes in neostriatal spiny neurons in Huntington's disease. Science 1985;227:770–773.
16. Ferrante RJ, Kowall NW, Beal MF, et al. Morphologic and histochemical characteristics of a spared subset of striatal neurons in Huntington's disease. J Neuropathol Exp Neurol 1987;46:12–27.

17. Bird ED, Iversen LL. Huntington's chorea. Post-mortem measurement of glutamic acid decarboxylase, choline acetyltransferase and dopamine in basal ganglia. Brain 1974;97:457–472.

18. Aronin N, Cooper PE, Lorenz LJ, et al. Somatostatin is increased in the basal ganglia in Huntington's disease. Ann Neurol 1983;13:519–526.

19. Beal MF, Bird ED, Langlais PJ, Martin JB. Somatostatin is increased in the nucleus accumbens in Huntington's disease. Neurology 1984;34:663–666.

20. Beal MF, Ellison DW, Mazurek MF, et al. A detailed examination of substance P in pathologically graded cases of Huntington's disease. J Neurol Sci 1988;84:51–61.

21. Beal MF, Mazurek MF, Ellison DW, et al. Somatostatin and neuropeptide Y concentrations in pathologically graded cases of Huntington's disease. Ann Neurol 1988;23:562–569.

22. Beal MF, Kowall NW, Ellison DW, et al. Replication of the neurochemical characteristics of Huntington's disease by quinolinic acid. Nature 1986;321:168–171.

23. Ellison DW, Beal MF, Mazurek MF, et al. Amino acid neurotransmitter abnormalities in Huntington's disease and the quinolinic acid animal model of Huntington's disease. Brain 1987;110:1657–1673.

24. DiFiglia M. Excitotoxic injury of the neostriatum: a model for Huntington's disease. Trends Neurosci 1990;13:286–289.

25. Roberts RC, Ahn A, Swartz KJ, et al. Intrastriatal injections of quinolinic acid or kainic acid: differential patterns of cell survival and the effects of data analysis on outcome. Exp Neurol 1993;124:274–282.

26. Anton G. Über die Beteiligung der grossen basalen Gehirnganglien bei Bewegungstörungen und insbesondere bei Chorea. Jahrbücher Psychiatr Neurol (Lpz) 1896;14:141–181.

27. Lannois M, Paviot J. Deux cas de la chorée héréditaire avec autopsies. Arch Neurol (Paris) 1897;4:333–334.

28. Jelgersma G. Neue anatomische Befunde bei Paralysis agitans und bei chronischer Chorea. Neurol Centralblatt 1908;27:995–996.

29. Alzheimer A. Über die anatomische Grundlage der Huntingtonschen Chorea und der choreatischen Bewegungen überhaupt. Neurol Centralblatt 1911;30:891–892.

30. Bruyn GW. Huntington's chorea; historical, clinical and laboratory synopsis. In: Vinken PJ, Bruyn GW, eds. Handbook of clinical neurology. Vol. 6. Amsterdam: Elsevier, 1968:298–378.

31. Forno LS, Jose C. Huntington's chorea: a pathological study. In: Barbeau A, Chase TN, Paulson GW, eds. Advances in neurology. Vol. 1. Huntington's chorea. New York: Raven, 1973:453–470.

32. Rodda RA. Cerebellar atrophy in Huntington's disease. J Neurol Sci 1981;50:147–157.

33. Bruyn GW. Neuropathological changes in Huntington's chorea. In: Barbeau A, Chase TN, Paulson GW, eds. Advances in neurology. Vol. 1. Huntington's chorea. New York: Raven, 1973:399–403.

34. Kremer HPH, Roos RAC, Dingjan G, et al. Atrophy of the hypothalamic lateral tuberal nucleus in Huntington's disease. J Neuropathol Exp Neurol 1990;49:371–382.

35. Kremer HPH, Roos RAC, Dingjan GM, et al. The hypothalamic lateral tuberal nucleus and the characteristics of neuronal loss in Huntington's disease. Neurosci Lett 1991;132:101–104.

36. Davison C, Goodhart SP, Shlionsky H. Chronic progressive chorea. The pathogenesis and mechanism; a histopathologic study. Arch Neurol Psychiatry (Chicago) 1932;27:906–928.

37. Bruyn GW, Bots G, Dom R. Huntington's chorea: Current neuropathological status. In: Chase TN, Wexler NS, Barbeau A, eds. Advances in neurology. Vol. 23. Huntington's disease. New York: Raven, 1979:83–93.

38. Spargo E, Everall IP, Lantos PL. Neuronal loss in the hippocampus in Huntington's disease: a comparison with HIV infection. J Neurol Neurosurg Psychiatry 1993;56:487–491.

39. Schroeder K. Zur Klinik und Pathologie der Huntingtonschen Krankheit. J Psychologie Neurol 1931;43:183–201.

40. Lange H, Thörner G, Hopf A, Schröder KF. Morphometric studies of the neuropathological changes in choreatic diseases. J Neurol Sci 1976; 28:401–425.

41. Pfeiffer JAF. A contribution to the pathology of chronic progressive chorea. Brain 1913;35:276–292.

42. Dom R, Malfroid M, Baro F. Neuropathology of Huntington's chorea. Neurology 1976;26:64–68.

43. Zweig RM, Koven SJ, Hedreen JC, et al. Linkage to the Huntington's disease locus in a family with unusual clinical and pathological features. Ann Neurol 1989;26:78–84.

44. Zweig RM, Ross CA, Hedreen JC, et al. Locus coeruleus involvement in Huntington's disease. Arch Neurol 1992;49:152–156.

45. Lange HW. Quantitative changes of telencephalon, diencephalon, and mesencephalon in Huntington's chorea, postencephalitic, and idiopathic parkinsonism. Verh Anat Ges 1981;75:923–925.

46. Oyanagi K, Takeda S, Takahashi H, et al. A quantitative investigation of the substantia nigra in Huntington's disease. Ann Neurol 1989;26:13–19.

47. Bonduelle M, Gruner J, Bouygues P. Chorée de Huntington avec paraplégie spasmodique. Deux cas familiaux. Étude anatomique. Remarque sur les relations de la surdité et des lésions de l'olive supérieure. Rev Neurol (Paris) 1953;88:126–131.

48. Byers RK, Gilles FH, Fung C. Huntington's disease in children. Neurology 1973;23:561–569.

49. Kiesselbach G. Anatomischer Befund eines Falles von Huntingtonscher Chorea. Monatsschr Psychiatrie Neurol (Berl) 1914;35:525–543.

50. Spielmeyer W. Die anatomische Krankheitsforschung am Beispiel einer Huntingtonschen Chorea mit Wilsonschem Symptombild. Z Neurol Psychiatrie 1926;101:701–728.

51. Birnbaum G. Chronisch-progressive Chorea mit Kleinhirnatrophie. Archiv Psychiatrie 1941;114:160–182.

52. Hallervorden J. Huntingtonsche Chorea (Chorea chronica progressiva hereditaria). In: Lubarsch O, Henke F, Rössle R, eds. Handbuch der speziellen pathologischen Anatomie und Histologie (XIII/1 Bandteil A). Berlin: Springer Verlag, 1957:793–822.

53. Fau R, Chateau R, Tommasi M, et al. Étude anatomo-clinique d'une forme rigide et myoclonique de maladie de Huntington infantile. Rev Neurol 1971;124:353–366.

54. Castaigne P, Escourolle R, Gray F. Chorée de Huntington et atrophie cérébelleuse. A propos d'une observation anatomo-clinique. Rev Neurol 1976;132:233–240.

55. Jeste DV, Barban L, Parisi J. Reduced Purkinje cell density in Huntington's disease. Exp Neurol 1984;85:78–86.

56. Terplan K. Zur pathologischen anatomie der chronischen progressiven chorea. Virchows Arch 1924;252:146–176.

57. Roizin L, Stellar S, Liu JC. Neuronal nuclear-cytoplasmic changes in Huntington's chorea: electron microscope investigations. In: Chase TN, Wexler NS, Barbeau A, eds. Advances in neurology. Vol. 23. Huntington's disease. New York: Raven, 1979:95–122.

58. Cudkowicz M, Kowall NW. Degeneration of pyramidal projection neurons in Huntington's disease cortex. Ann Neurol 1990;27:200–204.

59. Hedreen JC, Peyser CE, Folstein SE, Ross CA. Neuronal loss in layers V and VI of cerebral cortex in Huntington's disease. Neurosci Lett 1991;133: 257–261.

60. Sotrel A, Paskevich PA, Kiely DK, et al. Morphometric analysis of the prefrontal cortex in Huntington's disease. Neurology 1991;41:1117–1123.

61. Bielschowsky M. Einige Bemerkungen zur normalen und pathologischen Histologie des Schweif- und Linsenkerns. J Psychologie Neurol 1919;25:1–11.

62. Schröder KF, Hopf A, Lange H, Thörner G. Morphometrisch-statistische Strukturanalysen des Striatum, Pallidum und Nucleus subthalamicus beim Menschen. I. Striatum. J Hirnforsch 1975;16:333–350.

63. Graveland GA, Williams RS, DiFiglia M. A Golgi study of the human neostriatum: neurons and afferent fibers. J Comp Neurol 1985;234:317–333.

64. DiFiglia M, Carey J. Large neurons in the primate neostriatum examined with the combined Golgi-electron microscopic method. J Comp Neurol 1986;244:36–52.

65. Steiner H, Gerfen CR. Cocaine-induced c-fos messenger RNA is inversely related to dynorphin expression in striatum. J Neurosci 1993;13:5066–5081.

66. Graybiel AM, Ragsdale CW Jr. Biochemical anatomy of the striatum. In: Emson PC, ed. Chemical neuroanatomy. New York: Raven, 1983:427–504.

67. Nieuwenhuys R. Chemoarchitecture of the brain. Berlin: Springer Verlag, 1985.

68. Selden N, Geula C, Hersh L, Mesulam M-M. Human striatum: chemoarchitecture of the caudate nucleus, putamen and ventral striatum in health and Alzheimer's disease. Neuroscience 1994;60:621–636.

69. Cooper PE, Fernstrom MH, Rorstad OP, et al. The regional distribution of somatostatin, substance P and neurotensin in human brain. Brain Res 1981;218:219–232.

70. Sagar SM, Beal MF, Marshall PE, et al. Implications of neuropeptides in neurological diseases. Peptides 1984;5:255–262.

71. Morton AJ, Nicholson LFB, Faull RLM. Compartmental loss of NADPH diaphorase in the neuropil of the human striatum in Huntington's disease. Neuroscience 1993;53:159–168.

72. Colmers WF, Bleakman D. Effects of neuropeptide Y on the electrical properties of neurons. Trends Neurosci 1994;17:373–379.

73. Graybiel AM, Ragsdale CW Jr. Fiber connections of the basal ganglia. In: Cuénod M, Kreutzberg GW, Bloom FE, eds. Development and chemical specificity of neurons. Amsterdam: Elsevier, 1979:239–283.

74. Goldman-Rakic PS. Cytoarchitectonic heterogeneity of the primate neostriatum: subdivision into island and matrix cellular compartments. J Comp Neurol 1982;205:398–413.

75. Selemon LD, Gottlieb JP, Goldman-Rakic PS. Islands and striosomes in the neostriatum of the rhesus monkey: non-equivalent compartments. Neuroscience 1994;58:183–192.

76. Gerfen CR, Herkenham M, Thibault J. The neostriatal mosaic: II. Patch- and matrix-directed mesostriatal dopaminergic and non-dopaminergic systems. J Neurosci 1987;7:3915–3934.

77. Ragsdale CW Jr, Graybiel AM. The fronto-striatal projection in the cat and monkey and its relationship to inhomogeneities established by acetylcholinesterase histochemistry. Brain Res 1981;208:259–266.

78. Gerfen CR, Baimbridge KG, Thibault J. The neostriatal mosaic: III. biochemical and developmental dissociation of patch-matrix mesostriatal systems. J Neurosci 1987;7:3935–3944.

79. Selemon LD, Goldman-Rakic PS. Longitudinal topography and interdigitation of corticostriatal projections in the rhesus monkey. J Neurosci 1985; 5:776–794.

80. Whitworth RH Jr, LeDoux MS, Gould HJ III. Topographic distribution of connections from the primary motor cortex to the corpus striatum in *Aotus trivirgatus*. J Comp Neurol 1991;307:177–188.

81. Graybiel AM, Aosaki T, Flaherty AW, Kimura M. The basal ganglia and adaptive motor control. Science 1994;265:1826–1831.

82. Alexander GE, Crutcher MD. Functional architecture of basal ganglia circuits: neural substrates of parallel processing. Trends Neurosci 1990;13:266–271.

83. Reiner A, Albin RL, Anderson KD, et al. Differential loss of striatal projection neurons in Huntington disease. Proc Natl Acad Sci USA 1988;85:5733–5737.

84. Albin RL, Young AB, Penney JB. The functional anatomy of basal ganglia disorders. Trends Neurosci 1989;12:366–375.

85. Albin RL, Reiner A, Anderson KD, et al. Striatal and nigral neuron subpopulations in rigid Huntington's disease: implications for the functional anatomy of chorea and rigidity-akinesia. Ann Neurol 1990;27:357–365.

86. Albin RL, Young AB, Penney JB, et al. Abnormalities of striatal projection neurons and N-methyl-d-aspartate receptors in presymptomatic Huntington's disease. N Engl J Med 1990;322:1293–1298.

87. de la Monte SM, Vonsattel JP, Richardson EP Jr. Morphometric demonstration of atrophic changes in the cerebral cortex, white matter, and neostriatum in Huntington's disease. J Neuropathol Exp Neurol 1988;47:516–525.

88. Hedreen JC, Folstein SE. Early loss of neostriatal striosome neurons in Huntington's disease. J Neuropathol Exp Neurol 1995;54:105–120.

89. Vonsattel J-P, Myers RH, Bird ED, et al. Maladie de Huntington: sept cas avec îlots néostriataux relativement préservés. Rev Neurol 1992;148:107–116.

90. Ferrante RJ, Beal MF, Kowall NW, et al. Sparing of acetylcholinesterase-containing striatal neurons in Huntington's disease. Brain Res 1987;411:162–166.

91. Kowall NW, Ferrante RJ, Martin JB. Patterns of cell loss in Huntington's disease. Trends Neurosci 1987;10:24–29.

92. Sapp E, Ge P, Aizawa H, et al. Evidence for a preferential loss of enkephalin immunoreactivity in the external globus pallidus in low grade Huntington's disease using high resolution image analysis. Neuroscience 1995;64:397–404.

93. Richfield EK, Maguire-Zeiss KA, Cox C, et al. Reduced expression of preproenkephalin in striatal neurons from Huntington's disease patients. Ann Neurol 1995;37:335–343.

94. Ferrante RJ, Kowall NW, Richardson EP Jr. Cellular composition of striatal patch and matrix compartments in Huntington's disease. Soc Neurosci 1989;15:935. Abstract.

95. Zalneraitis EL, Landis DMD, Richardson EP Jr, Selkoe DJ. A comparison of astrocytic structure in cerebral cortex and striatum in Huntington's disease. Neurology 1981;31:151.

96. Richardson EP Jr. Huntington's disease: some recent neuropathological studies. Neuropathol Appl Neurobiol 1990;16:451–460.

97. Gusella JF, MacDonald ME, Ambrose CM, Duyao MP. Molecular genetics of Huntington's disease. Arch Neurol 1993;50:1157–1163.

98. Snell RG, MacMillan JC, Cheadle JP, et al. Relationship between trinucleotide repeat expansion and phenotypic variation in Huntington's disease. Nat Genet 1993;4:393–397.

99. Duyao M, Ambrose C, Myers R, et al. Trinucleotide repeat length instability and age of onset in Huntington's disease. Nat Genet 1993;4:387–392.

100. Persichetti F, Ambrose CM, Ge P, et al. Normal and expanded Huntington's disease gene alleles produce distinguishable proteins due to translation across the CAG repeat. Mol Med 1995;1:374–383.

101. Furtado S, Suchowersky O, Rewcastle B, et al. Relationship between trinucleotide repeats and neuropathological changes in Huntington's disease. Ann Neurol 1996;39:132–136.

102. Penney JB, Vonsattel J-P, MacDonald ME, et al. CAG repeat number governs development rate of pathology in Huntington's disease. Ann Neurol 1997;41:689–692.

103. Gusella JF, MacDonald ME. Huntington's disease and repeating trinucleotides. N Engl J Med 1994;330:1450–1451.

104. Trottier Y, Devys D, Imbert G, et al. Cellular localization of the Huntington's disease protein and discrimination of the normal and mutated form. Nat Genet 1995;10:104–110.

105. Hoogeveen AT, Willemsen R, Meyer N, et al. Characterization and localization of the Huntington disease gene product. Hum Mol Genet 1993;2:2069–2073.

106. Li S-H, Schilling G, Young WS III, et al. Huntington's disease gene (IT15) is widely expressed in human and rat tissues. Neuron 1993;11:985–993.

107. Dure LS IV, Landwehrmeyer GBL, Golden J, et al. IT15 gene expression in fetal human brain. Brain Res 1994;659:33–41.

108. Strong TV, Tagle DA, Valdes JM, et al. Widespread expression of the human and rat Huntington's disease gene in brain and nonneural tissues. Nat Genet 1994;5:259–263.

109. Landwehrmeyer GB, McNeil SM, Dure LS IV, et al. Huntington's disease gene: regional and cellular expression in brain of normal and affected individuals. Ann Neurol 1995;37:218–230.

110. DiFiglia M, Sapp E, Chase K, et al. Huntingtin is a cytoplasmic protein associated with vesicles in human and rat brain neurons. Neuron 1995;14:1075–1081.

111. Li X-J, Li S-H, Sharp AH, et al. A huntingtin-associated protein enriched in brain with implications for pathology. Nature 1995;378:398–402.

Parkinson's Disease and Parkinsonism

Morgan L. Levy   Jeffrey L. Cummings

HISTORICAL INTRODUCTION

James Parkinson described the syndrome that came to bear his name in 1817. He noted the occurrence of tremor, alterations of gait and posture, hypophonia, dysgraphia, and sialorrhea. He believed the senses and intellectual function to be spared but observed that many of the patients were unhappy. Since Parkinson's original description, understanding of Parkinson's disease (PD) and the parkinsonian syndrome has expanded dramatically (1).

There are several major milestones in the evolution of understanding PD. In 1959, Oleh Hornykiewicz discovered low levels of dopamine in the brains of PD patients, demonstrating for the first time that levels of a specific neurotransmitter correlated with a disease of the brain. The observation led to dramatically successful therapy with dopamine replacement strategies. The dopamine hypothesis of schizophrenia gained prominence when dopamine therapy produced psychosis and dopamine blocking therapy produced parkinsonism. These findings propelled the study of other catecholamines such as serotonin and norepinephrine, which soon were found to be correlated with mood and anxiety disorders.

In this chapter, "PD" will refer to the classic idiopathic syndrome, whereas "parkinsonism" or "parkinsonian syndrome" will be used in reference to all other akinetic syndromes that resemble PD. Among the causes of parkinsonism included in this chapter are degenerative, vascular, metabolic, toxic, infectious, traumatic, and neoplastic disorders (Table 26.1).

DIAGNOSIS

Parkinson's Disease

The prevalence of PD reported in different studies varies between 84 and 187 per 100,000; the mean age of onset is 58 to 62 years (range; 40 to 70 years); and men are somewhat more likely to develop the disorder (2). Untreated PD progresses from onset to death in 8 to 10 years (range; 1 to 30 years). Contemporary therapeutic interventions have extended the life expectancy of patients so that the terminal phases are usually postponed for 13 to 14 years after appearance of the first symptoms. Most cases are sporadic and twins generally lack concordance. In some cases, however, it is inherited in an autosomal dominant pattern and a family history of either PD or essential tremor are risk factors for the disease. Other risk factors include advancing age, exposure to pesticides or heavy metals (Fe, Mn, Al), drinking well water in certain areas, and living in rural communities. Cigarette smoking has been associated with reduced risk of PD (3,4).

Motor disturbances in PD include tremor, rigidity, bradykinesia, and loss of righting reflexes. Autonomic abnormalities and oculomotor dysfunction are found in most patients. The typical PD *tremor* is a low-frequency (four to six cycles per second) large-amplitude rest tremor that is present when the patient is awake but in repose and disappears when the affected limb is called into action and when the patient sleeps. The tremor typically involves the hands and may sometimes affect the head, lips, tongue, trunk, or legs. Many PD patients have a higher-frequency lower-amplitude action tremor in addition to their rest tremor. *Cogwheel rigidity* is present in the upper limbs and occasionally in the neck, whereas *plastic rigidity* is more common in the lower extremities. The cogwheel phenomenon results from the co-occurrence of tremor and rigidity. *Bradykinesia* is one of the most pervasive elements of PD and contributes to the slowness of movement, start hesitation, impaired repetitive movements, freezing episodes, en block movements, diminished arm swing, micrographia, facial masking, and sialorrhea. The typical posture of PD includes flexion of trunk, knees, elbows, and neck, and the gait is

Table 26.1   Differential Diagnosis of Parkinsonism

Degenerative Disorders	Drug-Induced and Toxic Parkinsonism
Idiopathic Parkinson's disease	Neuroleptic agents
Progressive supranuclear palsy	Phenothiazines
Huntington's disease (rigid variant)	Butyrophenones
Striatonigral degeneration	Thioxanthenes
Shy-Drager syndrome	Benzamides
Idiopathic basal ganglia calcification	Reserpine
Guamanian Parkinsonism-dementia complex	Alphamethyldopa
Machado-Joseph disease	Lithium
Neuroacanthocytosis	Diazepam (high doses)
Lewy body dementia	Monoamine oxidase inhibitors
Hallervorden-Spatz disease	Calcium channel blocking agents
Olivopontocerebellar atrophy	Cytosine arabinoside
Spinocerebellar degenerations	Cyanide
Pallidal degeneration syndromes	Selective serotonin reuptake inhibitors
Ceroid lipofuscinosis	Organophosphates
Mitochondrial encephalopathy	Manganese
Type 3 (adult) GM1 gangliosidosis	Carbon monoxide
	MPTP
Vascular Parkinsonism	
Lacunar state	**Miscellaneous Disorders**
Binswanger's disease	Hydrocephalus
	Brain tumors
Infection-Related Parkinsonism	Subdural hematomas
Postencephalitic parkinsonism after epidemic encephalitis	Syringomesencephalia
Transient parkinsonism after acute viral encephalitis	Trauma
Jakob-Creutzfeldt disease	
AIDS	
Neurosyphilis	
Metabolic Causes of Parkinsonism	
Hypothyroidism	
Hypoparathyroidism	
Non-Wilsonian hepatocerebral degeneration	
Wilson's disease	

characterized by short steps, diminished step height, and festination. Balance is impaired and the patient has difficulty with retropulsion or propulsion or both and fails to make the appropriate postural adjustments. Seborrhea, impotence, constipation, and postural hypotension are among the signs of autonomic dysfunction in PD; impaired convergence, limited up-gaze, and lid retraction are the most common neuro-ophthalmologic abnormalities (5).

Cognitive dysfunction exists in a majority of PD patients and approximately 40% have overt dementia (6). Bradyphrenia (slow thinking) and executive function impairment are the most striking aspects of cognitive dysfunction in nondemented PD patients. Memory, visual–spatial ability, verbal fluency, and naming may be mildly impaired, and the pattern of deficits in these domains also suggests abnormalities of frontal-subcortical systems or executive dysfunction. Cortical features of dementia such as aphasia, amnesia, agnosia, and apraxia can occur and likely signify the presence of cortical Lewy bodies, Alzheimer's-type pathology, or both.

Behavioral alterations are common in both treated and untreated PD. A premorbid parkinsonian personality described as stoic, introverted, and inflexible may exist in some patients but is not uniformly present and may change considerably with disease onset (7). Clinically significant depression occurs in 40% of PD patients and anxiety disorders are common. Depression is frequently not severe; self-punitive ideation is not frequent and suicide is rare. Severity of depression does not correlate with disability and preliminary evidence suggests there is greater depression with right hemiparkinsonism than left (8). Anxiety disorders are present in approximately one-third of PD patients and the most frequent diagnoses are generalized anxiety disorder, social phobia, and panic disorder (9). Finally, therapy with dopaminergic agents may produce formed visual hallucinations, persecutory delusions, anxiety, depression, mania, hypersexuality, and sleep disturbance; anticholinergic therapy may produce delirium with or without psychotic features (10).

The principal neuropathologic changes in PD are depigmentation and loss of cells in the substantia nigra with Lewy body formation in many of the remaining neurons. Similar changes also occur in the locus ceruleus, dorsal motor nucleus of the vagus nerve, nucleus basalis of Meynert, and the ventral tegmental area of the midbrain as well as other subcortical nuclei. Deficiency of dopamine is the main neurotransmitter alteration; there are less marked deficits of norepinephrine, acetylcholine, serotonin, and several neuromodulators. Some patients have Alzheimer type neuropathologic changes or Lewy bodies in the cerebral cortex (11).

Structural imaging has limited utility in PD and most parkinsonian syndromes but functional imaging, such as positron emission tomography (PET), can directly assess neurotransmitter activity in the nigrostriatal dopaminergic system using [^{18}F] fluorodopa (FD) as a tracer. Most causes of parkinsonism, including PD, are associated with reduced striatal FD compared with normal aging or other causes of dementia. PD can be further differentiated from other causes of parkinsonism because it is associated with particularly low levels of FD in the putamen. Fluorodopa PET is also useful for detecting preclinical PD and for following the disease progression over time (12). [^{18}F]fluorodeoxyglucose PET may be normal or may demonstrate global reduction in cerebral metabolism, especially severe in the frontal lobes (13). Patients with PD-related dementia syndromes may have a temporal-parietal pattern of hypometabolism indistinguishable from the pattern seen in AD patients (14). Treatment of PD is described below.

Other Degenerative Parkinsonian Syndromes

Table 26.1 lists the parkinsonian syndromes to be considered in the differential diagnosis of PD. Several of these disorders are described in more detail in other chapters of this volume but will be mentioned briefly here to contrast them with classical PD.

Progressive supranuclear palsy (PSP) is identified in 5% of patients referred for a parkinsonian disorder. It typically begins in the sixth decade of life and is characterized by a progressive course lasting 4 to 12 years. Clinical findings include supranuclear ophthalmoplegia, axial rigidity, pseudobulbar palsy, and dementia (15). The eye movement disorder may progress from an initial paralysis of volitional vertical gaze to a complete nuclear ophthalmoplegia. Rigidity involves the trunk and neck with less affect on the limbs. Pseudobulbar palsy is manifested by severe dysarthria, dysphagia, expressionless facies, sialorrhea, and exaggerated facial, masseter, and pharyngeal reflexes. A subcortical dementia is present with bradyphrenia, memory impairment, loss of ability to manipulate information, and mood and personality changes (16). Apathy is often severe. Pathological changes include cell loss, neurofibrillary tangles and granulovacuolar degeneration concentrated in the globus pallidus, subthalamic nucleus, red nucleus, substantia nigra, superior colliculus, periaqueductal gray matter, pontine tegmentum, and the dentate nucleus of the cerebellum. Dopamine is the only neurotransmitter that is consistently deficient in PSP (17); dopamine receptors are also decreased and the disorder is usually refractory to L-dopa therapy.

Huntington's disease is a neurodegenerative disorder caused by an expanded CAG trinucleotide repeat on the IT15 gene on chromosome 4. It is inherited in an autosomal dominant pattern, begins in midlife, and manifests a progressive dementia with motor system abnormalities. The most common motor disturbance is chorea but a minority of patients exhibit an akinetic–rigid parkinsonian syndrome. Six percent of adults and as many as one-third of juveniles with Huntington's disease begin with a predominance of parkinsonian symptoms; a portion of these will later develop chorea and conversely a number of patients who initially manifest the typical choreic syndrome will manifest parkinsonism late in the course of their disease (18). Atrophy of the caudate nuclei with enlargement of the frontal horns of the lateral ventricles is evident on x-ray computed tomography or magnetic resonance images of the brain. Pathologically, the patients are found to have a marked depopulation of the small ganglion cells of the putamen and caudate nuclei. The principal neurotransmitter of these neurons is gamma-aminobutyric acid (GABA) and this agent is preferentially depleted. The parkinsonian symptoms of Huntington's disease may improve following L-dopa therapy, but the course of the illness and the intellectual decline is unaltered by treatment.

Lewy body dementia (LBD) frequently presents with psychiatric symptoms such as depression, agitation, delusions, and hallucinations early in the course. Cognitive symptoms can progress rapidly and relentlessly but often fluctuate and relatively lucid intervals may occur. Patients may have mild extrapyramidal symptoms, gait disturbance, orthostatic hypotension, unexplained falls, and transient clouding and/or loss of consciousness. Almost all PD patients have cortical Lewy bodies and almost all LBD patients have brainstem and diencephalic Lewy bodies in the same distribution as previously described for PD. Behavioral symptoms can be difficult to treat due to increased neuroleptic sensitivity, but the novel antipsychotic agents such as olonzapine or clozapine appear to be safe and effective (19,20).

Multiple system atrophy (MSA) (comprising striatonigral degeneration, Shy-Drager syndrome, and sporadic olivopontocerebellar atrophy) is a degenerative disease found in 8% to 10% of brains from parkinsonian brain banks. Mean age at onset is 53 years (range; 33 to 76 years) and average survival is 10 years (range; 33 to 76 years). Parkinsonism, autonomic dysfunction, and cerebellar signs are the cardinal features and all three occur in the vast majority of cases but with considerable variability in specific manifestations. Any one of the cardinal features may predominate. Cognitive dysfunction may appear to be minimal but most patients have frontal system impairment and a number develop overt dementia late in the course. Oligodendroglial cytoplasmic inclusions characterize MSA and are found, along with cell loss and gliosis, in the striatum, substantia nigra, inferior olives, pons, cerebellum, and spinal cord (21).

Idiopathic basal ganglia calcification (Fahr's disease) produces mental status alterations, motor system disturbances, and dense calcification of the basal ganglia, thalamic nuclei, and subcortical white matter. Behavioral changes include ubiquitous mood disturbances and dementia; psychosis occurs in approximately 50% of reported cases (8). Choreoathetotic or parkinsonian syndromes may be present. Perivascular calcific deposits are evident in the involved nuclei, and in most cases the calcification is readily visualized by x-ray computed tomography. The mood disorder and psychotic symptoms may improve with antidepressant or antipsychotic therapy.

Guamanian parkinsonism-dementia complex is a syndrome occurring primarily in the Chamorro people of Guam and consisting of a unique combination of dementia and parkinsonism. One-third of the patients have evidence of upper and lower motor neuron dysfunction. Autopsy studies demonstrate neuronal loss and abundant neurofibrillary tangles in the cerebral cortex, basal ganglia, cerebellum, and brainstem (22).

Machado-Joseph disease (also known as Azorean disease) is an autosomal dominant neurodegenerative disorder caused by an unstable CAG trinucleotide repeat on chromosome 14q32.1 and is associated with a diverse array of neurologic signs (23). The typical clinical picture includes parkinsonism, ophthalmoplegia, fasciculations, ataxia, and extensor plantar responses (24). Pathological investigations reveal neuronal loss and gliosis in the substantia nigra, pontine nuclei, putamen, spinal cord, and cranial nerve nuclei.

Corticobasal degeneration may be misdiagnosed as PD. Cortical and subcortical symptoms can occur: most patients develop akinesia, rigidity, and apraxia in one arm or leg that progresses ipsilaterally then contralaterally, and a striking asymmetry persists late in the course. Cortical signs include marked limb apraxia and visuospatial disorders. Pathology reveals frontoparietal and substantia nigra degeneration with characteristic swollen achromatic neurons (25).

Neuroacanthocytosis is a rare, recently recognized syndrome. A variety of behaviors have been observed in the disease including parkinsonism, chorea, tics, and fasciculations (26). Most patients exhibit a peripheral neuropathy. Laboratory examination reveals an elevated number of acanthocytes when red blood cell morphology is studied.

Hallervorden-Spatz disease is an autosomal recessive disorder that typically begins in childhood and produces progressive dementia, bradykinesia, rigidity, spasticity, and dystonia. Rarely, the disease onset is delayed until middle or late life and parkinsonism is the predominant clinical manifestation (27). Histologic studies of the brain reveal axonal spheroids and deposits of iron pigments in the globus pal-

lidus, caudate nucleus, and substantia nigra. There is marked loss of dopamine in the nigrostriatal system. No effective therapy has been described.

Additional neurodegenerative disorders that commonly include parkinsonian symptoms include autosomal dominant cerebellar atrophy, primary pallidal atrophies, spinodentatonigral degeneration, and corticodentatonigral degeneration (28–34).

Rare inborn errors of neuronal metabolism that may present with a parkinsonian syndrome include ceroid lipofuscinosis, mitochondrial encephalopathy, and type 3 (adult) GM1 gangliosidosis (35–37).

Vascular Parkinsonism

Multiple subcortical infarctions produce a syndrome with parkinsonian features. The syndrome is usually complicated by pyramidal signs resulting from injury to descending white matter tracts (corticobulbar and corticospinal). Tremor is infrequent, but akinesia, rigidity, flexed posture, shuffling gait, and dysarthria form a clinical syndrome resembling PD. Dementia, depression, and psychosis are common behavioral manifestations. The disorder can usually be distinguished from PD by the absence of tremor, presence of brisk muscle stretch reflexes and extensor plantar responses, history of hypertension and of stroke, and stepwise progression (38,39). Computerized tomography or magnetic resonance imaging reveal lacunar infarctions and ischemic injury of subcortical white matter (Fig 26.1).

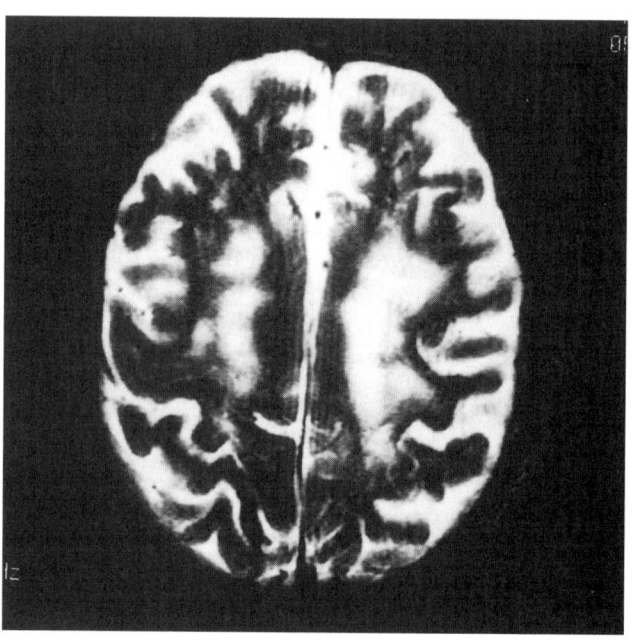

FIGURE 26.1   *An example of subcortical vascular disease producing parkinsonism.*

Infection-Related Parkinsonism

The epidemic of encephalitis lethargica that spread throughout the world from 1919 to 1926 left in its wake a large number of patients with postencephalitic parkinsonism. The extrapyramidal syndrome developed immediately in some patients and was delayed for months or years after the acute episode in others. Akinesia and rigidity were the most common extrapyramidal symptoms of the syndrome, but some patients exhibited tremor, myoclonus, chorea, or tics in addition to the parkinsonism. Oculogyric crises with episodes of forced gaze deviation, often in association with stereotyped thinking, were nearly unique to this parkinsonian syndrome (40). Behavioral disorders also were common in postencephalitic parkinsonism: children developed hyperactivity and conduct disorders and adults frequently suffered from personality changes, mood disorders, or obsessions and compulsions. The principal pathological changes involved the substantia nigra, but there were often widespread lesions involving the basal ganglia, thalamus, hypothalamus, and, to a lesser extent, the cerebral cortex. New cases of encephalitis lethargica and postencephalitic parkinsonism are rare and the disorder is now rarely seen.

Acute transient parkinsonism has been observed in the course of several types of viral encephalitis including Eastern equine encephalitis, Western equine encephalitis, Coxsackie B encephalitis, measles encephalitis, Murray Valley encephalitis, chicken pox encephalitis, and Japanese B encephalitis (40,41).

Jakob-Creutzfeldt disease is characterized by a rapidly progressive dementia syndrome with prominent myoclonus and combined pyramidal and extrapyramidal disturbances (11). The disease is due to a prion infection of the central nervous system, and autopsy studies reveal spongiform changes and gliosis in cortical and subcortical structures.

Infection with the human immunodeficiency virus (HIV) produces the acquired immunodeficiency syndrome (AIDS) and frequently leads to brain dysfunction with dementia. The intellectual deterioration may be accompanied by a variety of neurologic symptoms including parkinsonism (42).

A parkinsonian syndrome occasionally occurred in the course of syphilis. Spirochetal invasion of the brain in general paresis involves predominantly the frontal lobe, but other structures can be affected and basal ganglionic changes produce akinesia and rigidity (31).

Metabolic Causes of Parkinsonism

A parkinsonian appearance does not necessarily indicate the occurrence of irreversible structural damage to the basal ganglia; parkinsonism also can be a product of metabolic abnormalities. Hypothyroid patients exhibit psychomotor retardation and superficially resemble PD. Abnormalities of tone and tremor are typically absent. In hypoparathyroidism, calcium deposits accumulate in the basal ganglia and the patients develop parkinsonism with gait and posture changes, hypertonia, bradykinesia, and loss of righting reflexes (43). Non-Wilsonian hepatocerebral degeneration is a chronic metabolic encephalopathy produced by hepatic dysfunction and shunting of blood flow around the liver into the general circulation. The syndrome is dominated by dementia and chorea but parkinsonism may also occur (31).

Wilson's disease is an autosomal recessive disorder of copper metabolism in which the liver is unable to metabolize copper normally. Serum ceruloplasmin levels are low and urinary copper levels are typically elevated. Dystonia and cerebellar signs are the most common motor manifestations of Wilson's disease, but rigidity, bradykinesia, micrographia, and gait and postural abnormalities of a parkinsonian type are not unusual (44). Behavioral changes are frequent in Wilson's disease and include depression, delusions, mania, emotional lability, and personality changes. Bilateral putamenal lesions may be evident on computerized tomograms or magnetic resonance imaging.

Drug-Induced and Toxic Parkinsonism

A wide array of drugs, metals, and toxins are capable of inducing parkinsonism. The agents most likely to produce a parkinsonian syndrome are the dopamine receptor-blocking neuroleptic agents including phenothiazines, butyrophenones, thioxanthenes, and benzamides (31). Most of these drugs are used in the treatment of major psychiatric illnesses, but some phenothiazines (e.g., compazine) and benzamides (e.g., reglan) are used in the management of gastrointestinal illnesses and may easily be overlooked as potential causes of brain dysfunction. Parkinsonism occurs in 10% to 50% of patients treated with therapeutic doses of neuroleptic agents, and the syndrome appears to be more likely to occur in older patients. Bradykinesia and rigidity are the parkinsonian features most likely to be produced by neuroleptic drugs; tremor is less frequently observed. The parkinsonism usually reverses within 10 days of stopping the neuroleptic agent or initiating treatment with an anticholinergic drug or amantadine hydrochloride, but symptoms occasionally persist for many months (45).

Reserpine and alphamethyldopa, antihypertensive agents that act by interfering with catecholamine function at the synapse, produce parkinsonism in 5% to 30% of treated patients (46). Other agents capable of inducing reversible parkinsonian signs include lithium, high doses of diazepam, monoamine oxidase inhibitors, calcium channel blocking agents, and cytosine arabinoside (47–51).

Permanent parkinsonism has been reported following exposure to cyanide, organophosphates, manganese, carbon monoxide, and 1-methyl-4-phenyl-1,2,3,6-tetrahydropyridine (MPTP), a by-product of meperidine synthesis (52–56).

Miscellaneous Parkinsonian States

In addition to the disorders described above, parkinsonism also has been observed with obstructive hydrocephalus, brain tumors compressing or invading the midbrain or basal ganglia, subdural hematomas, syringomesencephalia, trauma, and dementia pugilistica, the syndrome emerging after repeated head injuries in boxers (31,32–35).

MANAGEMENT

Management of Parkinsonism

The treatment of parkinsonism is partially determined by the etiology of the symptom complex. Metabolic, toxic, and structural causes of parkinsonism all require slightly different therapeutic approaches. When the disorder is metabolic in nature—hypothyroidism, hypoparathyroidism, non-Wilsonian hepatolenticular degeneration—the primary treatment efforts are directed at the underlying disorder. Wilson's disease is treated with a low copper diet and penicillamine. Early introduction of therapy may prevent the emergence of neurologic symptoms, and established symptoms may be reversed if tissue destruction has not occurred. Residual symptoms that present after the causative condition has been corrected are treated in the same way as idiopathic PD discussed below.

Neuroleptic agents are the most common cause of drug-induced parkinsonism. The first step in management of this syndrome is to re-evaluate the need for neuroleptic treatment and reduce the drug dosage to the minimum necessary level. Many patients, however, require ongoing antipsychotic therapy and discontinuation of the agent will be impossible. In such cases, parkinsonian symptoms may be ameliorated by anticholinergic drugs or amantadine hydrochloride. The latter enhances dopaminergic function. The two classes of agents are equally efficacious but amantadine may produce fewer side-effects (61,62).

Management of Parkinson's Disease

Motor Symptoms

The principal therapeutic modalities useful in the treatment of idiopathic PD and other parkinsonian syndromes caused by structural brain changes are dopamine precursor therapy and administration of dopamine receptor agonists and use of agents with putative neuroprotective effects. Dopamine does not cross the blood-brain barrier, but L-dopa, the biochemical precursor of dopamine, readily enters the brain through active transport mechanisms. L-dopa is administered orally and is commonly given in conjunction with a peripheral dopa-decarboxylase inhibitor such as carbidopa to prevent the conversion of L-dopa to dopamine peripherally. Coadministration of carbidopa results in higher brain levels of dopamine and limits the side-effects produced by peripheral L-dopa catabolism. Potential side-effects of L-dopa therapy include chorea, tics, vivid dreams and

nightmares, hallucinations, delusions, and confusional states. Nausea and orthostatic hypotension are encountered occasionally.

Early responses to therapy are often dramatic with patients having nearly complete resolution of symptoms. With prolonged therapy, however, response failure and motor fluctuations may become apparent. The patients experience on-off effects in which there are abrupt transitions from an akinetic and rigid state to normal motor function or even to hyperkinetic states with levodopa-induced dyskinesias (63). For this reason, L-dopa therapy should be delayed until the disability begins to interfere with daily function. Anticholinergic agents and amantadine hydrochloride may be useful as initial adjunctive agents in the treatment of PD, but they are rarely sufficiently efficacious to be used alone for extended periods.

Precursor therapy depends on the integrity of at least a portion of the normal neuronal population of the substantia nigra to metabolize L-dopa to dopamine and transport the product to the synaptic terminals in the striatum. When the functioning cell population is too small, precursor therapy is ineffective and other means of stimulating striatal receptors must be found. Bromocriptine, an ergot derivative, is a direct dopamine receptor agonist that is used in conjunction with L-dopa and may continue to provide antiparkinsonian relief after the beneficial effects of L-dopa have been exhausted. Its longer serum half-life (approximately eight hours, as opposed to four hours for L-dopa) results in a smoother response pattern and the early introduction of bromocriptine may prevent the emergence of response fluctuations seen with chronic L-dopa therapy (64). Pergolide, a semisynthetic ergoline dopamine agonist, is 10 times more potent than bromocriptine and has a half-life of 12 to 24 hours.

Two non-ergot selective dopaminergic receptor agonists, pramipexole and ropinerole, may be used as monotherapy prior to the initiation of treatment with L-dopa or in conjunction with the latter to extend its longevity in the course of the illness. These two agents have a high affinity for the D_2 dopamine receptor family and pramipexole has its highest affinity for the D_3 receptor among the D_2-type receptors (65,66). Pramipexole and ropinerole have a beneficial effect on motor performance and have been reported to induce fewer dyskinesias than conventional dopamine agonists that have effects on multiple receptor types. They also may have beneficial neuropsychiatric effects; patients on these agents appear to be less likely to manifest depression syndromes than patients undergoing other types of therapy.

Tolcapone, a catechol-o-methyl transferase (COMT) inhibitor with effects on peripheral and central COMT, may enhance the effectiveness of L-dopa by reducing its metabolism. Tolcapone is used as an adjunctive agent.

Selegiline, a selective MAO-B inhibitor at low doses, may reduce the dose of L-dopa required for symptomatic relief, slow deterioration, and delay the need for L-dopa by six to nine months (67,68). Selegiline's effect may be due to catecholamine-mediated symptomatic relief or it could confer neuroprotection through its antioxidant effect.

Surgical treatment of PD has received renewed interest in recent years. Stereotactic ventromedial pallidotomy reduces dyskinesias but should be reserved for PD patients with disabling hyperkinesias. Ventrolateral thalamotomy is useful in patients with asymmetric tremors as the predominant manifestation. Two treatments currently in experimental stages of development are high-frequency electrical stimulation of the ventral intermediate thalamic nucleus and striatal implantation of a dopamine-rich neural graft. Considerable technical difficulties currently limit the utility of these procedures (69).

Psychiatric Symptoms

Depression in PD can be treated with an antidepressant agent or electroconvulsive therapy (8). L-dopa may occasionally induce depression and mixed dopamine agonists, anticholinergics, amantadine, and selegiline have little antidepressant potential. Selective dopamine agonists have antidepressant effects. Nortriptyline and desipramine are relatively safe and effective provided they are initiated at low dose to avoid potentiating the hypotensive effect of L-dopa. They can also be effective for comorbid anxiety disorders, especially panic disorder. Other antidepressants have not been well studied in PD patients. Serotonin reuptake inhibitors are free of hypotensive and anticholinergic effects. While they have been reported to produce extrapyramidal symptoms in some patients, they are the agents most commonly used to treat depression in PD. Selegiline and antidepressants cannot be administered simultaneously because of the danger of precipitating the serotonin syndrome. Buproprion and lithium can potentiate the effects of L-dopa, but lithium alone has been reported to occasionally produce extrapyramidal symptoms.

Electroconvulsive therapy is the safest and most effective treatment for depression, and about half of PD patients will experience significant but usually temporary reduction in their motor symptoms independently of the effect on their psychiatric symptoms (70). Psychotherapy should be made available to every PD patient early in their course to hasten acceptance of their new condition and to help mobilize their resources for a struggle against a relentless illness.

Psychotic symptoms such as visual hallucinations and persecutory delusions are rare in untreated PD but commonly occur in the course of treatment with anti-PD drugs. When they occur prior to initiation of treatment they may suggest the existence of LBD. Delirium should be suspected in delusional patients and may be caused by anticholinergic agents or underlying systemic disease such as urinary tract or respiratory system infection. Dopa-agonists and L-dopa commonly produce psychotic symptoms in a clear sensorium. Traditional neuroleptics frequently fail to ameliorate these psychotic symptoms without producing significant extrapyramidal symptoms. The atypical antipsychotic clozapine has relatively little effect on the nigrostriatal portion of the dopaminergic system and has been shown to be both safe and effective in PD at low doses (25–50 mg), but the risk of agranulocytosis increases with age (20). Olanzapine and quetiapine may be safer alternatives. Selective 5-HT$_3$ antagonists such as odansetron have the potential to reduce psychotic symptoms but have received limited study.

BASIC SCIENCE

Akinesia and rigidity are the core symptoms of parkinsonism and executive dysfunction is a frequent finding. Tremor commonly accompanies these abnormalities in PD but is an inconstant and nonessential element of other parkinsonian syndromes. Recent approaches to understanding the pathophysiology of these symptoms have focused on the five frontal-subcortical circuits that run parallel from the frontal lobe through the striatum, pallidum, and thalamus (71). Involvement of the circuit organization in the medial frontal area and projecting through the putamen produces akinesia, whereas involvement of the dorsolateral prefrontal-subcortical circuit and medial frontal-subcortical circuit produce executive dysfunction and apathy, respectively. Oculomotor abnormalities are mediated by dysfunction of the circuit beginning in the frontal eye fields.

Increased muscle tone appears to result from an imbalance between competing inhibitory and disinhibitory neural pathways within the subcortical motor circuit, which runs from the sensorimotor cortex through the putamen, pallidum, thalamus and back to the cortex. Between the striatum and thalamus there are two pathways: the direct pathway decreases thalamic inhibition and the indirect pathway through the subthalamic nucleus increases thalamic inhibition. Dopaminergic projections from the substantia nigra to the striatum appear to regulate or stabilize this inhibitory/disinhibitory balance (72), and loss of dopamine results in unopposed thalamic inhibition and parkinsonism.

Akinesia is not a product of rigidity but is an independent component of the parkinsonian syndrome. The symptom encompasses impaired movement initiation, slowed execution of motor acts, prolonged central processing time involving the planning of intended movements, and loss of associated movements. Akinesia is manifested clinically by diminished spontaneity, paucity of gestures, prolonged response delays, and decreased verbal output. Fatigue, apathy, and loss of motivation are common subjective accompaniments of the akinetic syndrome (73,74). Executive dysfunction includes perseveration, difficulty shifting set, impaired higher-order attention, and poor abstraction and concept formation. These behavioral and neuropsychological symptoms are mediated by fronto-subcortical circuits that run parallel to but separate from the motor circuit. Sometimes called the "complex loop," these projections originate in frontal association cortex and enter the striatum at the caudate whereas the "motor loop" enters the putamen. Dopamine-mediated stabilization of the inhibitory/disinhibitory balance between direct and indirect pathways probably occurs in this circuit in the same fashion as described for the motor circuit (72).

ACKNOWLEDGMENTS

This project was supported by the Department of Veterans Affairs, an NIA Alzheimer's Disease Center grant (AG10123), an Alzheimer's Disease Research Center of California grant, and the Sidell-Kagan Foundation.

REFERENCES

1. Jankovic J. International classification of diseases, tenth revision: neurologic adaptation (ICD-10NA): extrapyramidal and movement disorders. Mov Disord 1995;10:533–540.
2. Martilla RJ. Epidemiology. In: Koller WC, ed. Handbook of Parkinson's disease. New York: Marcel Dekker, 1987:35–50.
3. Morens DM, Grandinetti A, Reed D, et al. Cigarette smoking and protection from Parkinson's disease: false association or etiologic clue? Neurology 1995;45:1041–1051.
4. Grandinetti A, Morens DM, Reed D, MacEachern D. Prospective study of cigarette smoking and the risk of developing idiopathic Parkinson's disease. Am J Epidemiol 1994;139:1129–1138.
5. Barbeau A. Parkinson's disease: clinical features and etiopathology. In: Vinken PJ, Bruyn GW, Klawans HL, eds. Handbook of clinical neurology. Vol 5 (49). Extrapyramidal disorders. New York: Elsevier Science, 1986:87–152.
6. Cummings JL. The dementias of Parkinson's disease. Eur Neurol 1988;28(suppl 1):15–23.
7. Hubble JP, Koller WC. The parkinsonian personality. Adv Neurol 1995;65:43–48.
8. Cummings JL. Depression and Parkinson's disease: a review. Am J Psychiatry 1992;149:443–453.
9. Menza MA, Robertson-Hoffman DE, Bonapace AS. Parkinson's disease and anxiety: comorbidity with depression. Biol Psychiatry 1993;34:465–470.
10. Factor SA, Molho ES, Podskalny GD, Brown D. Parkinson's disease: drug-induced psychiatric states. Adv Neurol 1995;65:115–138.
11. Cummings JL, Benson DF. Dementia; a clinical approach. 2nd ed. Boston: Butterworths, 1992.
12. Snow BJ. Fluorodopa PET scanning in Parkinson's disease. Adv Neurol 1996;69:449–457.
13. Brooks DJ. PET studies on the early and differential diagnosis of Parkinson's disease. Neurology 1993;43(suppl 6):S6–S16.
14. Read SL, Miller BL, Mena I, et al. SPECT in dementia: clinical and pathological correlation. J Am Geriatr Soc 1995;43:243–247.
15. Steele JC, Richardson JC, Olszewski J. Progressive supranuclear palsy. Arch Neurol 1964;10:333–359.
16. Albert ML, Feldman RG, Willis AL. The "subcortical dementia" of progressive supranuclear palsy. J Neurol Neurosurg Psychiatry 1974;37:121–130.
17. Kish SJ, Chang LJ, Mirchandani L, et al. Progressive supranuclear palsy: relationship between extrapyramidal disturbances, dementia, and brain neurotransmitter markers. Ann Neurol 1985;18:530–536.
18. Bruyn GW. Huntington's chorea. Historical, clinical and laboratory synopsis. In: Vinken PJ, Bruyn GW, eds. Handbook of clinical neurology. Vol. 6. Diseases of the basal ganglia. New York: American Elsevier, 1968:298–378.
19. Beck BJ. Neuropsychiatric manifestations of diffuse Lewy body disease. J Geriatr Psychiatry Neurol 1995;8:189–196.
20. Musser WS, Akil M. Clozapine as a treatment for psychosis in Parkinson's disease: a review. J Neuropsychiatry Clin Neurosci 1996;8:1–9.
21. Quinn NP, Wenning GK. Multiple system atrophy. Adv Neurol 1996;69:413–419.
22. Rodgers-Johnson P, Garruto RM, Yanagihara R, et al. Amyotrophic lateral sclerosis and parkinsonism-dementia on Guam: a 30-year evaluation of clinical and neuropathologic trends. Neurology 1986;36:7–13.
23. Sudarsky L, Coutinho P. Machado-Joseph disease. Clin Neurosci 1995;3:17–22.
24. Romanul FCA, Fowler HL, Radvany J, et al. Azorean disease of the nervous system. N Engl J Med 1977;296:1505–1508.
25. Rinne JO, Lee MS, Thompson PD, Marsden CD. Corticobasal degeneration. A clinical study of 36 cases. Brain 1994;117:1183–1196.
26. Spitz MC, Jankovic J, Killian JM. Familial tic disorder, parkinsonism, motor neuron disease, and acanthocytosis: a new syndrome. Neurology 1985;35:366–370.
27. Jankovic J, Kirkpatrick JB, Blomquist KA, et al. Late-onset Hallervorden-Spatz disease presenting as familial parkinsonism. Neurology 1985;35:227–234.
28. Duvoisin RC, Chokroverty S, Lepore F, Nicklas W. Glutamate dehydrogenase deficiency in patients with olivopontocerebellar atrophy. Neurology 1983;33:1322–1326.
29. Harding AE. The hereditary ataxias and related disorders. New York: Churchill Livingstone, 1984.
30. Jellinger K. Pallidal, pallidonigral, and pallidoluysionigral degenerations including association with thalamic and dentate degenerations. In: Vinken PJ, Bruyn GW, Klawans HL, eds. Handbook of clinical neurology. Vol 5 (49). Extrapyramidal disorders. New York: Elsevier Science, 1986:445–463.
31. Koller WC. Classification of parkinsonism. In: Koller WC, ed. Handbook of Parkinson's disease. New York: Marcel Dekker, 1987:51–80.
32. Narabayashi H. Cerebellodiencephalic interactions in olivopontocerebellar atrophy. In: Duvoisin RC, Plaitakis A, eds. The olivopontocerebellar atrophies. New York: Raven, 1984:87–95.
33. Serratrice GT, Toga M, Pellissier JF. Chronic spinal muscular atrophy and pallidonigral degeneration: report of a case. Neurology 1983;33:306–310.
34. Weir RL, Fan KJ. Spinocerebellar degeneration with parkinsonian features: a clinical and pathological report. Ann Neurol 1981;9:87–89.
35. Ohta K, Tsuji S, Mizuno Y, et al. Type 3 (adult) GM1 gangliosidosis: case report. Neurology 1985;35:1490–1494.
36. van Erven PMM, Gabreels FJM, Ruitenbeek W, Reiner WO, Fischer JC. Mitochondrial encephalopathy. Association with an NADH dehydrogenase deficiency. Arch Neurol 1987;44:775–778.
37. Vercruyssen A, Martin JJ, Ceuterick C, et al. Adult ceroid-lipofuscinosis: diagnostic value of biopsies and of neurophysiological investigations. J Neurol Neurosurg Psychiatry 1982;45:1056–1059.
38. Critchley M. Arteriosclerotic parkinsonism. Brain 1929;52:23–83.
39. Ishii N, Nishihara Y, Imamura T. Why do frontal lobe symptoms predominate in vascular dementia with lacunes? Neurology 1986;36:340–345.
40. Duvoisin RC, Yahr MD. Encephalitis and parkinsonism. Arch Neurol 1965;12:227–239.
41. Howard RS, Lees AJ. Encephalitis lethargica. A report of four recent cases. Brain 1987;110:19–33.
42. Nath A, Jankovic J, Pettigrew LC. Movement disorders in AIDS. Neurology 1987;37:37–41.
43. Friedman JH, Chiucchini I, Tucci JR. Idiopathic hypoparathyroidism with extensive brain calcification and persistent neurologic dysfunction. Neurology 1987;37:307–309.
44. Starosta-Rubinstein S, Young AB, Kluin K, et al. Clinical assessment of 31 patients with Wilson's disease. Correlations with structural changes on magnetic resonance imaging. Arch Neurol 1987;44:365–370.
45. Marsden CD, Jenner P. The pathophysiology of extrapyramidal side-effects of neuroleptic drugs. Psychol Med 1980;10:55–72.
46. Tarsy D. Neuroleptic-induced extrapyramidal reactions: classification, description, and diagnosis. Clin Neuropharm 1983;6(suppl 1):S9–S26.
47. Luque FA, Selhorst JB, Petruska P. Parkinsonism induced by high-dose cytosine arabinoside. Mov Disord 1987;2:219–222.
48. Micheli F, Pardal MF, Gatto M, et al. Flunarizine- and cinnarizine-induced extrapyramidal reactions. Neurology 1987;37:881–884.
49. Suranyi-Cadotte BE, Nestoros JN, Nair NPV, et al. Parkinsonism induced by high doses of diazepam. Biol Psychiatry 1985;20:451–460.
50. Teusink JP, Alexopoulos GS, Shamoian CA. Parkinsonian side effects induced by a monoamine oxidase inhibitor. Am J Psychiatry 1984;141:118–119.
51. Tyrer P, Alexander MS, Regan A, Lee I. An extrapyramidal syndrome after lithium therapy. Brit J Psychiatry 1980;36:191–194.
52. Ballard PA, Tetrud JW, Langston JW. Permanent human parkinsonism due to 1-methyl-4-phenyl-1,2,3,6-tetrahydropyridine (MPTP): seven cases. Neurology 1985;35:949–956.
53. Davis KL, Yesavage JA, Berger PA. Possible organophosphate-induced parkinsonism. J Nerv Ment Dis 1978;166:222–225.
54. Klawans HL, Stein RW, Tanner CM, Goetz CG. A pure parkinsonian syndrome following acute carbon monoxide intoxication. Arch Neurol 1982;39:302–304.
55. Mena I, Court J, Fuenzalida S, et al. Modification of chronic manganese poisoning. New Engl J Med 1970;282:5–10.
56. Uitti RJ, Rajput AH, Ashenhurst EM, Rozdilsky B. Cyanide-induced parkinsonism: a clinicopathologic report. Neurology 1985;35:921–925.

57. Corsellis JAN, Bruton CJ, Freeman-Browne D. The aftermath of boxing. Psychol Med 1973;3:270–303.

58. Hardy RC, Stevenson LD. Syringomesencephalia. J Neuropath Exp Neurol 1957;16:365–370.

59. Miodrag A, Das TK, Shepherd RJ. Normal pressure hydrocephalus presenting as Parkinson's syndrome. Postgrad Med J 1987;63:113–115.

60. Roth RL, Bebin J. Cerebral hemispheric tumors and extrapyramidal signs and symptoms. Neurology 1958;8:277–284.

61. DiMascio A, Bernardo DL, Greenblatt DJ, Marder JE. A controlled trial of amantadine in drug-induced extrapyramidal disorders. Arch Gen Psychiatry 1976;33:599–602.

62. Fann WE, Lake R. Amantadine versus trihexyphenidyl in the treatment of neuroleptic-induced parkinsonism. Am J Psychiatry 1976;133:940–943.

63. Quinn NP. Levodopa. In: Koller WC, ed. Handbook of Parkinson's disease. New York: Marcel Dekker, 1987:317–337.

64. Le Witt PA. Therapy with dopaminergic drugs in Parkinson's disease. In: Koller WC, ed. Handbook of Parkinson's disease. New York: Marcel Dekker, 1987:381–402.

65. Piercey MF. Pharmacology of pramipexole, a dopamine D3-preferring agonist useful in treating Parkinson's disease. Clin Neuropharm 1998;21:141–151.

66. Schrag AE, Brooks DJ, Brunt E, et al. The safety of ropinerole, a selective nonergoline dopamine agonist, in patients with Parkinson's disease. Clin Neuropharm 1998;21:169–175.

67. Olanow CW, Hauser RA, Gauger L, et al. The effect of deprenyl and levodopa on the progression of Parkinson's disease. Ann Neurol 1995;38:771–777.

68. Parkinson's Study Group. Effects of tocopherol and deprenyl on the progression of disability in early Parkinson's disease. N Engl J Med 1993;328:176–183.

69. Olanow CW, Marsden CD, Lang AE, Goetz CG. The role of surgery in Parkinson's disease management. Neurology 1994;44(suppl 1):S17–S20.

70. Faber R, Trimble MR. Electroconvulsive therapy in Parkinson's disease and other movement disorders. Mov Disord 1991;6:293–303.

71. Cummings JL. The frontal-subcortical circuits and human behavior. Arch Neurol 1993;50:873–880.

72. Saint-Cyr JA, Taylor AE, Nicholson K. Behavior and the basal ganglia. Adv Neurol 1995;65:1–28.

73. Lance JW, McLeod JG. A physiological approach to clinical neurology. Boston: Butterworths, 1981.

74. Mandell AJ, Markham CH, Tallman FF, Mandell MP. Motivation and ability to move. Am J Psychiatry 1962;119:544–549.

The "On–Off" Phenomenon in Parkinson's Disease

Marie-Helene Saint-Hilaire   Robert G. Feldman

INTRODUCTION

The "on–off" phenomenon in Parkinson's disease consists of abrupt variations in mobility in patients on chronic L-dopa therapy. The patients alternate between periods when parkinsonian signs are relatively severe (the "off" state) and intervals when parkinsonism is replaced by increased mobility accompanied by involuntary movements (the "on" state). This clinical picture was first described soon after the advent of L-dopa therapy (1) and is now a familiar problem in the long-term treatment of Parkinson's disease with L-dopa. About 50% of patients will experience motor fluctuations in response after five years of treatment (2). First, there appears a gradual shortening of the duration of action of single doses of L-dopa with a "wearing-off" effect, which progresses to rapid dose-related changes (predictable "on–off") and finally to abrupt random swings, seemingly unrelated to the timing of medication doses. This unpredictable "on–off" effect is also called "yo-yoing" (3,4). This chapter will focus on the description and pathogenesis of these random oscillations in functional status.

CLINICAL DESCRIPTION

The switching between "on" and "off" periods occurs many times during the day and is unrelated to the timing of L-dopa doses. The transition from one state to another is usually completed within five minutes. Improvements in mobility are commonly preceded by a flurry of stereotyped dyskinesias, often presenting as flexion-extension movements of both legs or resembling more complex mannerisms such as performing aerobic exercises, stamping a foot, rotating the head, or handwringing (3). Patients are aware that they are going to switch to the "on" state and feel that these rituals will hasten the transformation. Akinesia seems

to disappear instantaneously and the patients attain maximal mobility with obvious dyskinesias for a variable period of 15 minutes to 2 hours (4). The return to the "off" state may be heralded by the reappearance of the tremor in the presence of dyskinesias before the rapid return of the akinetic state over one to two minutes. This is often associated with autonomic manifestations including pallor, profuse sweating, palpitations, and extreme lassitude (3). In some patients, return to the "off" state is associated with a significantly depressed mood that disappears when they turn back "on."

PATHOPHYSIOLOGY OF THE "ON–OFF" PHENOMENON

The pathophysiology of the "on–off" phenomenon is still not completely understood but several excellent studies have increased our understanding of the problem. The factors involved can be divided as central and peripheral. The central mechanisms consist of presynaptic and postsynaptic changes caused by progression of the disease and the effects of chronic L-dopa therapy on dopaminergic receptors. Peripheral mechanisms involve the pharmacokinetics of L-dopa and its dose–response relationship (5).

Central Mechanisms

Presynaptic Mechanisms

The degeneration of presynaptic dopamine terminals plays an important role in the development of motor fluctuations. Clinically, it has been observed that patients with the "on–off" phenomenon usually have fairly severe baseline parkinsonian signs and many are wheelchair-bound or bedridden if L-dopa is stopped (4). This has also been observed in patients with 1-methyl-4-phenyl-1,2,3,6-

tetrahydropyridine (MPTP) induced parkinsonism who have severe disability at the onset (stages 4 and 5 of Hoehn and Yahr) and develop fluctuations within one year of starting L-dopa treatment (6,7). A study of motor score deterioration after cessation of L-dopa infusions (8) showed that the efficacy half-time of L-dopa decreased with increasing severity of the fluctuations. The initial decay slope in motor scores and the severity of motor fluctuations were best predicted by the severity of parkinsonian symptoms.

The clinical response to L-dopa depends largely on the ability of the brain to decarboxylate it to dopamine. A study of central and peripheral measurements of L-dopa and the dopamine metabolite homovanillic acid (HVA) levels in patients on chronic L-dopa therapy (9) showed that clinical improvement after one dose of carbidopa/L-dopa correlated very highly with cerebrospinal fluid HVA levels, but not with cerebrospinal fluid and serum concentrations of L-dopa.

Assessments of central pharmacokinetics of L-dopa support that fluctuations are at least partly a consequence of a reduction in the rate of conversion of L-dopa to dopamine and perhaps diminished capacity for the storage of dopamine. In rats with nigral lesions and dopamine depletion, the elevation of striatal dopamine after a dose of L-dopa is shorter than in control animals (10). In monkeys treated with MPTP, there is marked decrease in striatal aromatic amino acid decarboxylase, which appears to decrease the rate of L-dopa metabolism in that region (11). In humans, positron emission tomography (PET) imaging using 6-[^{18}F]-fluorodopa shows reduced radioisotope accumulation in the striatum, particularly the putamen, in patients with Parkinson's disease (12). In addition, the decrease of the striatal activity is more marked in patients with the "on–off" phenomenon than in patients without fluctuations (13). Sequential plasma and cerebrospinal fluid (CSF) levodopa and CSF dopamine sulfate levels were measured in patients with advanced Parkinson's disease after a dose of L-dopa (14). The clinical response to L-dopa correlated precisely with L-dopa and dopamine sulfate levels in the CSF, indicating that in patients with advanced Parkinson's disease, there is a diminished capacity to store dopamine synthesized from exogenous L-dopa. Thus motor fluctuations reflect in part the decreased capacity to buffer oscillations in L-dopa levels that occur with periodic oral administration.

Postsynaptic Mechanisms

Alterations in the pharmacodynamics of postsynaptic dopamine receptors play a major role in the pathogenesis of the "on–off" phenomenon.

In patients with "on–off," the antiparkinsonian response to an infusion of L-dopa is shorter than the half-life of L-dopa itself after the infusion is stopped (8). This cannot be explained by the presynaptic loss of buffering capacity and implies the contribution of postsynaptic factors. This is supported by studies of apomorphine infusions that have shown

that the duration of the antiparkinsonian effect of apomorphine declines with progression of the disease (15,16). The response to apomorphine was shortest in patients with "on–off" but was also shortened in patients with "wearing-off" compared to stable responders and patients who were never treated (15). Because the effect of apomorphine does not depend on presynaptic mechanisms, the diminished duration of response is most likely caused by alterations of the postsynaptic function. These alterations are thought to result from chronic oral L-dopa therapy, with pulsatile stimulation of dopamine receptors. Patients with "on–off" show a steeper dose–response slope to an intravenous injection of L-dopa compared to patients with a stable response or patients who were never treated (17). Although the threshold to observe an antiparkinsonian effect is the same in all patients, the threshold to induce dyskinesias decreases as fluctuations worsen. This results in the narrowing of the therapeutic window that is observed clinically in patients with fluctuations. The threshold dose for the antiparkinsonian effect correlates with the severity of the symptoms, while the threshold for dyskinesias and the dose–response slope correlate with the duration of L-dopa therapy. The dose–response slope and the threshold for antiparkinsonian effect and dyskinesias can be modified by long-term L-dopa infusions (18). After 7 to 12 days of continuous infusion, motor fluctuations significantly decrease, the dose–response curve shifts to the right, and the threshold for dyskinesias increases with widening of the therapeutic window. After cessation of the infusion, the clinical benefits last for about six days on oral L-dopa therapy. Thus the pharmacodynamic changes contributing to severe motor fluctuations can be modified by continuous dopamine replacement. These results also underline the role of chronic intermittent L-dopa therapy in the development of these pharmacodynamic alterations.

The exact nature of these postsynaptic changes remains unclear. Studies on the effect of chronic L-dopa therapy in animals have led to contradictory results, reporting increase, decrease, or no change in striatal dopamine receptor function (19). In classic pharmacologic terms, receptors become supersensitive following denervation, and the continuous application of an agonist is expected to lead to desensitization. However, supersensitivity of the receptors is exaggerated if the agonist is given at intervals longer than its pharmacological half-life (20). Similarly, the dopaminergic system manifests behavioral supersensitivity after chronic L-dopa therapy but not after continuous treatment (21,22). In addition, the normal interactions between D_1 and D_2 dopamine receptors might be affected by chronic L-dopa administration, which appears to sensitize D_2 receptors and downregulate D_1 receptors (23). Autoradiography studies in rats have shown that this is associated with increased metabolism in the D_2-mediated striatopallidal-subthalamic (indirect) pathway and decreased activity in the D_1 receptor-mediated striatonigral (direct) pathway (24). The balance of activity in the two parallel pathways of the basal ganglia is affected. The increased sensitivity to L-dopa manifested by the increased dose–response slope is consistent with increased D_2 receptor sensitivity. On the other hand, excessive D_1 stimulation might result in abnormal involuntary movements (25).

Peripheral Mechanisms

Role of Peripheral L-dopa Pharmacokinetics

The improvement of "off" periods with intravenous infusions of L-dopa in patients with Parkinson's disease stresses the dependence of motor function on the delivery of L-dopa to the striatum. This delivery itself is dependent on the absorption of L-dopa, its plasma half-life, and its transport across the blood-brain barrier.

L-dopa is absorbed in the proximal small intestine by a saturable large neutral amino acid transport system (26). Slowing of gastric emptying by meals (27) or by medications such as anticholinergics will delay the absorption of L-dopa and increase its decarboxylation by the gastric mucosa (28). Direct duodenal delivery of the drug will increase its absorption (29).

Factors influencing the absorption of L-dopa are important because its plasma half-life is very short. The elimination half-life generally fits a two-compartment model, with a rapid distribution phase (42 ± 8 minutes), representing the distribution of L-dopa into various tissues, followed by a slower elimination phase (92 ± 3 minutes) representing the metabolism of L-dopa (30). These values do not differ between patients who had a stable response to L-dopa, patients with "wearing off," and patients with "on-off" (30), showing that fluctuations are not caused by differences in the peripheral metabolism of the drug between these three groups (31).

The last factor influencing the bioavailability of L-dopa to the brain involves its transport through the blood-brain barrier by a saturable carrier system that also transports large neutral amino acids (32). This transport of L-dopa into the brain is dependent on its plasma concentration and on the concentration of the other large neutral amino acids competing for the same carrier system. An elevation of these large neutral amino acids can reduce the effect of L-dopa (27) whereas a diet low in protein decreases the "on–off" phenomenon (33). In addition, 3-O-methyldopa, a major metabolite of L-dopa, is also transported into the brain by the same carrier system and may compete with L-dopa (34). The relative importance of 3-O-methyldopa is debatable. Although its concentration in the plasma seems to represent a small portion of the total large neutral amino acids (35), it has been observed that the "on–off" phenomenon was more frequent in patients with high 3-O-methyldopa-dopa ratios (36). This ratio has clinical relevance only in patients who have had the disease for more than five years, suggesting that patients with a shorter duration of illness can compensate for pharmacokinetic factors. The fact that more advanced patients are sensitive to these factors is supported by the observation that the protein redistribution diet is effective in severe fluctuators but is not useful in stable responders (37).

Dose–Response Relationship

During intravenous L-dopa infusions, it has been observed that the plasma L-dopa level has to reach a certain threshold to produce a clinical response and that this response is "all or nothing" (38). Above this threshold, increasing the rate of infusion of L-dopa will not improve the motor function but will increase the duration of the response (5). Low infusion rates, resulting in plasma L-dopa levels nearer to "threshold," may be associated with occasional spontaneous "off" periods (38). These observations suggest that the current therapeutic approach to motor fluctuations, decreasing each dose of medication and increasing the frequency, may itself be a factor in the development of the "on–off" phenomenon (5). The peak plasma concentration achieved with each dose of L-dopa will be nearer to threshold, and even a small decrease in absorption or transport of the drug may result in plasma L-dopa concentrations that do not reach the minimum effective concentration to produce a clinical response. Thus the response to each dose will be more variable (5), and it has been clinically observed that unpredictable fluctuators tend to take more frequent doses at shorter intervals. In addition, there can be overlapping of individual doses, and in patients with long response latency to L-dopa, the "off" period following one dose can occur after the next dose is taken and becomes effective (38). In fact, returning to a three-times-a-day regimen of a standard dosage may restore a predictable response at the expense of increase of "off" time (39).

CONCLUSION AND IMPLICATION FOR TREATMENT

The main factors implicated in the development of the "on–off" phenomenon are delayed alterations in the pharmacodynamics of postsynaptic dopamine receptors—a consequence of the periodic oral administration of L-dopa—and the progressive loss of dopaminergic neurons. Another factor is the pharmacokinetics of L-dopa itself. The availability of L-dopa depends on its absorption, peak plasma level, and transport across the blood-brain barrier. Modification of any of these factors in advanced Parkinson's disease may lead to a subthreshold dopamine level with no subsequent clinical response. Patients in the early phase of the disease appear able to buffer these variations in the availability of L-dopa.

Although the treatment of the "on–off" phenomenon remains difficult, it is likely from these observations that maintaining above-threshold, constant levels of L-dopa or the development of long-acting dopaminergic drugs may be beneficial. Adjunctive treatment with dopamine agonists is the approach most frequently used but has been so far ineffective in eliminating fluctuations in severely affected patients. New agonists such as cabergoline or Pramipexole might prove more effective, as well as subcutaneous infusions of Lisuride or apomorphine (40,41,42). Constant duodenal delivery of L-dopa (43) or hourly intake of a liquid form of L-dopa (44) can be helpful to maintain more stable blood levels. A protein redistribution diet (37) or proportioned 7:1 carbohydrate-protein diet (45) can improve the transport of L-dopa across the blood-brain barrier by decreasing competition with large neutral amino acids. Catechol-O-methyl transferase (COMT) inhibitors, Entacapone and Tolcapone, have been shown to improve fluctuations by increasing the peripheral half-life of L-dopa and reducing the formation of 3-O-methyldopa that may decrease competition for transport across the blood-brain barrier (46,47). Tolcapone also has a central effect to decrease dopamine metabolism. Restorative surgery such as the implantation of human or porcine fetal cells in the striatum is still considered experimental, but could result in long-term improvements.

REFERENCES

1. Cotzias GC, Papavasiliou PS, Gelline R. Modification of parkinsonism: chronic treatment with L-dopa. N Engl J Med 1969;280:337.
2. Sweet RD, McDowell FH. Plasma dopa concentrations and the "on-off" effect after chronic treatment of Parkinson's disease. Neurology 1974;24:953–956.
3. Barbeau A. The clinical physiology of side effects in long-term L-dopa therapy. In: McDowell FH, Barbeau A, eds. Advances in neurology. Vol. 5. New York: Raven, 1974.
4. Marsden CD, Parkes JD. On-off effects in patients with Parkinson's disease on chronic levodopa therapy. Lancet 1976;i:292–296.
5. Hardie RJ, Lees AJ, Stern GM. On-off fluctuations Parkinson's disease: a clinical and neuropharmacological study. Brain 1984;107:487–506.
6. Langston JW. MPTP-induced parkinsonism: "How good a model is it?" In: Fahn S, Marsden D, Jenner P, Teychenne P, eds. Recent developments in Parkinson's disease. New York: Raven, 1986.
7. Langston JW, Ballard P. Parkinsonism induced by 1-methyl-4-phenyl-1,2,3,6-tetrahydropyridine: implications for treatment and the pathogenesis of Parkinson's disease. Can J Neurol Sci 1984;11:160–165.
8. Fabbrini G, Mouradian MM, Juncos JL, et al. Motor fluctuations in Parkinson's disease: central pathophysiological mechanisms, part I. Ann Neurol 1988;24:366–371.
9. Durso R, Szabo G, Davoudi H, Feldman RG. Central levodopa metabolism may limit drug efficacy in chronically treated Parkinson disease. Neurology 1988;38(suppl 1):257.
10. Spencer SE, Wooten GF. Altered pharmacokinetics of L-dopa metabolism in rat striatum deprived of dopaminergic innervation. Neurology 1984;34:1105–1108.
11. Burns RS, Kopin I, Weiss V, et al. Decreased LAAAD in striatum influences brain L-dopa metabolism in MPTP-treated rhesus monkey with severe parkinsonism. Neurology 1991;41(suppl 1):378.
12. Martin WRW, Stoessl AJ, Adam MJ, et al. Positron emission tomography in Parkinson's disease: glucose and dopa metabolism. In: Yahr M, Bergman K, eds. Advances in neurology. Vol. 45. Parkinson's disease. New York: Raven, 1986.
13. Leenders KL, Palmer AJ, Quinn N, et al. Brain dopamine metabolism in patients with Parkinson's disease measured with positron emission tomography. J Neurol Neurosurg Psychiatry 1986;49:853–860.
14. Cedarbaum JM, Olanow CW. Dopamine sulfate in ventricular cerebrospinal fluid and motor function in Parkinson's disease. Neurology 1991;41(suppl 1):379.
15. Bravi D, Mouradian MM, Roberts JW, et al. Wearing-off fluctuations in Parkinson's disease: contribution of postsynaptic mechanisms. Ann Neurol 1994;36:27–31.
16. Grandas F, Gancher ST, Rodriguez M, et al. Differences in the motor response to apomorphine between untreated and fluctuating patients with Parkinson's disease. Clin Neuropharmacol 1992;15:13–18.
17. Mouradian MM, Juncos JL, Fabbrini G, et al. Motor fluctuations in Parkinson's disease: central pathophysiological mechanisms, part II. Ann Neurol 1988;24:372–378.
18. Mouradian MM, Heuser IJE, Baronti F, Chase TN. Modification of central dopaminergic mechanisms by continuous levodopa therapy for advanced Parkinson's disease. Ann Neurol 1990;27:18–23.
19. Jenner P, Boyce S, Marsden CD. Effect of repeated L-dopa administration on striatal dopamine receptor function in the rat. In: Fahn S, Marsden D, Jenner P, Teychenne P, eds. Recent developments in Parkinson's disease. New York: Raven, 1986.
20. Post RM. Intermittent versus continuous stimulation: effect of time on the development of sensitization or tolerance. Life Sci 1980;26:1275–1282.
21. Juncos JL, Engber TM, Raisman R, et al. Continuous and intermittent levodopa differentially affect basal ganglia function. Ann Neurol 1989;25:473–478.
22. Weick BG, Engber TM, Susel Z, et al. Responses of substantia nigra pars reticulata neurons to GABA and SKF 38393 in 6-hydroxydopamine–lesioned rats are differentially affected by continuous and intermittent levodopa administration. Brain Res 1990;523:16–23.
23. Engber TM, Susel Z, Juncos JL, Chase TN. Continuous and intermittent levodopa differentially affect rotation induced by D1 and D2 dopamine agonists. Eur J Pharmacol 1989;168:291–298.
24. Engber TM, Susel Z, Kuo S, Chase TN. Chronic levodopa treatment alters basal and dopamine agonist-stimulated cerebral glucose utilization. J Neurosci 1990;10:3889–3895.
25. Blanchet PJ, Grondin R, Bedard PJ. Dyskinesia and wearing-off following dopamine D1 agonist treatment in drug-naive 1-Methyl-4-Phenyl-1,2,3,6-tetrahydropiridine-lesioned primates. Mov Disord 1996;11:91–94.
26. Wade DN, Merrick PT, Morris JL. Active transport of L-dopa in the intestine. Nature 1973;242:463–465.
27. Nutt JG, Woodward WR, Hammerstad JP, et al. The on-off phenomenon in Parkinson's disease: relation to levodopa absorption and transport. N Engl J Med 1984;310:483–488.
28. Rivera-Calimlin L, Dujovne CA, Morgan JP, et al. Absorption and metabolism of L-dopa by the human stomach. Eur J Clin Invest 1971;1:313–320.
29. Shuh L, Sage JI, Heikkila RE, Duvoisin RC. Continuous intradermal infusion of levodopa (LD) produce steady plasma LD levels which correlate with improvement of motor fluctuations in parkinsonian patients. Neurology 1987;37(suppl 1):277.
30. Fabbrini G, Juncos J, Mouradian MM, et al. Levodopa pharmacokinetic mechanisms and motor fluctuations in Parkinson's disease. Ann Neurol 1987;37(suppl 1):277.
31. Gancher ST, Nutt JG, Woodward WR. Peripheral pharmacokinetics of levodopa in untreated, stable and fluctuating parkinsonian patients. Neurology 1987;37:940–944.
32. Pardridge WM. Kinetics of competitive inhibition of neutral amino acid transport across the blood brain barrier. J Neurochem 1977;28:103–108.
33. Pincus JH, Barry K. Control of the on-off phenomenon with dietary manipulation. Ann Neurol 1986;20:149.
34. Wade LA, Katzman R. 3-O-methyldopa uptake and inhibition of L-dopa at the blood brain barrier. Life Sci 1975;17:131–136.
35. Nutt JG, Woodward WR, Gancher ST, Merrick D. 3-O-methyldopa and the response to levodopa in Parkinson's disease. Ann Neurol 1987;21:584.
36. Muradas V, Abravia V, Mena MA, Yebenes J. The significance of biologic and pharmacokinetic factors in the pathophysiology of abnormal responses to levodopa therapy in Parkinson's disease. Neurology 1987;37(suppl 1):261.
37. Karstaldt P, Pincus JH. Protein redistribution diet remains effective in patients with fluctuating parkinsonism. Arch Neurol 1992;49:149–151.
38. Nutt JG. On-off phenomenon, relation to levodopa pharmacokinetics and pharmacodynamics. Ann Neurol 1987;22:535–540.
39. Quinn N, Marion MH, Stocchi F, et al. Intravenous dopamine agonist studies in Parkinson's disease. In: Fahn S, Marsden D, Jenner P, Teychenne P, eds. Recent developments in Parkinson's disease. New York: Raven, 1986.
40. Hughes AJ, Bishop S, Kleedorfer B, et al. Subcutaneous apomorphine in Parkinson's disease: response to chronic administration for up to five years. Mov Disord 1993;8(2):165–170.
41. Baronti F, Mouradian MM, Davis TL. Continuous Lisuride effects on central dopaminergic mechanisms in Parkinson's disease. Ann Neurol 1992;32:776–781.
42. Geminiani G, Fetoni V, Genitrini S, et al. Cabergoline in Parkinson's disease complicated by motor fluctuations. Mov Disord 1996;11:495–500.
43. Cedarbaum JM, Silvestri M, Kutt H. Sustained enteral administration of levodopa increases and interrupted infusion decreases levodopa dose requirements. Neurology 1990;40:995–997.

44. Kurth MC, Tetrud JW, Irwin I. Oral levodopa/carbidopa solution versus tablets in Parkinson patients with severe fluctuations: a pilot study. Neurology 1993;43:1036–1039.

45. Saint-Hilaire M, Feldman RG, Thomas CA, et al. Proportioned carbohydrate: protein diet in the management of Parkinson's disease. Neurology 1996;44(suppl 2):246.

46. Mannisto P, Kaakkola S, Nissinen E, et al. Properties of novel effective and highly selective inhibitors of catechol-o-methyltransferase. Life Sci 1988;43:1465–1471.

47. Davis TL, Roznoski M, Burns RS. Effects of tolcapone in Parkinson's patients taking L-dihydroxyphenylalanine/carbidopa and selegiline. Mov Disord 1995;10:349–351.

Akinesia in Parkinsonism

Hirotaro Narabayashi

INTRODUCTION

Akinesia is a commonly and sometimes vaguely used term in clinical neurology to describe a group of difficulties in motor activity in patients with Parkinson's disease (PD). It is not as clearly defined as rigidity and tremor are; it includes a wide variety of motor difficulties, such as slowness of movement, disturbances of skill in performing delicate coordinated movements (i.e., complex finger and arm movements), and poverty or lack of movements (e.g., such as loss of arm swinging while walking). Difficulty in performing two different movements simultaneously, as pointed out by Marsden, may describe another aspect of akinesia (1). Loss or poverty of facial expression, masking of the face, and soft voice or unclearness of speech also constitute a part of so-called akinesia. In walking, slowness and unsteadiness of gait, including difficulty of postural control or even lessening of walking drive, are also often included in the term *akinesia*. These are the symptoms that constitute the difficulty with and lowering of motor activities. This chapter deals with an analysis classifying several types of motor difficulties within akinesia and attempts to interpret the complex mechanisms underlying it (2–4).

SECONDARY AKINESIA DUE TO RIGIDITY

Muscle rigidity, which is one of the essential symptoms of parkinsonism, results in difficulties with motor performance. Rigidity produces cocontraction of antagonistic muscles, thus producing disturbances of reciprocal innervation and of smooth performance of voluntary movement. In such instances, elimination of rigidity by stereotaxic thalamotomy using a microelectrode in the ventrolateral (VL; also known as VIM) nucleus of the thalamus produces immediate abolition of akinetic symptoms, such as slowness and lack of skill in coordinating movements (5). Difficulties of separate and individual movement and counting of fingers, supination–pronation of the hand, shoulder rotation, and joint movements at hip, knee, and ankle are usually immediately improved and almost normalized. Such immediate changes are easily and routinely observable on the operating table within a few seconds after making a small confined electrocoagulation lesion of about 4 mm diameter within the VL nucleus. The VL nucleus is understood to receive the afferent projection from the pallidum internum (GPi), where rigidity is generated by striatal dopamine (DA) deficiency in parkinsonism (6).

Such akinesia, which can be completely relieved by the thalamic lesion, is therefore interpreted as an akinesia secondary to rigidity. Clear recognition of secondary akinesia is important, as it provides further understanding of the mechanisms of akinesia. Figure 28.1 illustrates an example of improvement of reciprocal innervation and simple movements when moderate rigidity is totally abolished by surgery.

PRIMARY AKINESIA

Barbeau (7) stressed the importance of akinesia that still remains after alleviation of rigidity by surgical treatment. Observations on unilaterally operated patients with bilateral parkinsonism often indicate that some difficulty of movement or akinesia remains even after successful surgery that completely eliminated rigidity and tremor on the contralateral side of the body. This is one of the reasons why surgical treatment has a limited effect. Nevertheless, L-dopa improves the remaining akinesia as well as rigidity itself; this has made L-dopa treatment preferable to surgical treatment. Using a neurochemical interpretation, nigrostriatal DA deficiency thus produces both rigidity and akinesia (7,8).

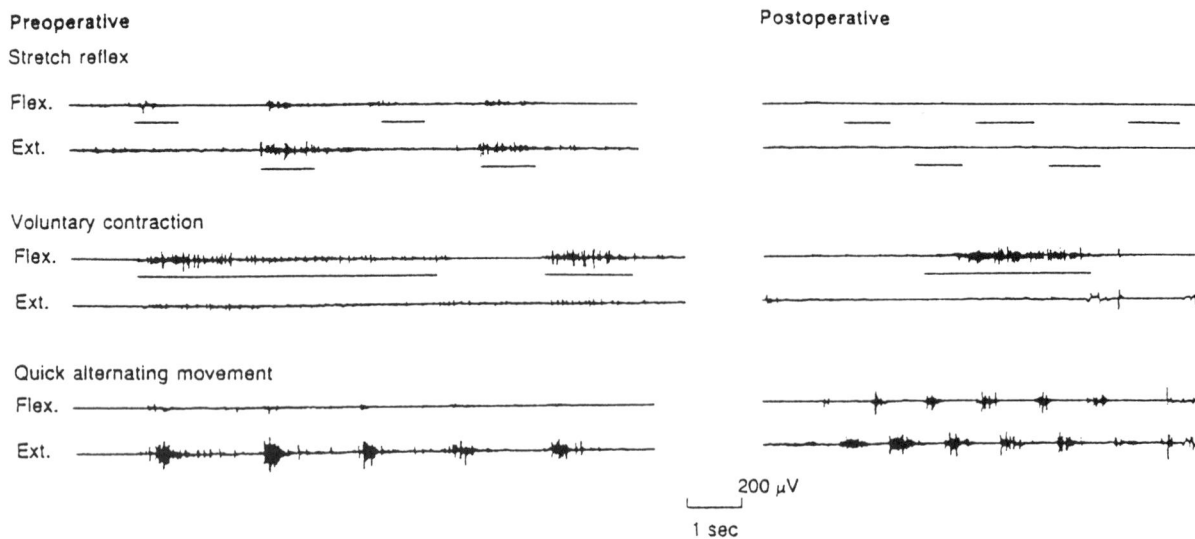

FIGURE 28.1   *Disturbance of reciprocal muscle contraction in the rigid state.* Upper two recordings: *increase of tonic stretch reflex discharges indicating rigidity. Underline indicates the period of passive stretch of muscle. Postoperatively there is no rigidity.* Middle two recordings: *voluntary contraction, indicated by underline, causes codischarge in antagonist muscle preoperatively, which disappeared after surgery.* Lower two recordings: *Quick repetitive flexion–extension movement is slow and causes cocontraction of antagonist muscles preoperatively; with alleviation of rigidity, the movement becomes smoother and faster postoperatively. Flex., forearm flexor muscle. Ext., forearm extensor muscle.*

Such akinesia, independent from and not secondary to rigidity, may be designated as "primary akinesia". Primary akinesia produces only lack or poverty of movements. The most elegant description was that made by Martin (9) about the lack of facial expression and blinking, and a decrease of arm swing and of other movements that one habitually sees in normal people, such as slight fidgeting with the hands, folding and unfolding the arms, and crossing the legs. Primary akinesia remaining after thalamic surgery responds well to L-dopa, which Hughes et al (10) have described as producing the same effect as on the unoperated side.

Since primary akinesia becomes neither better nor worse following lesions of the pallidothalamic projection either at the VL thalamus or at the pallidum, neural structures responsible for primary akinesia might be different from those for rigidity. Mechanisms of primary akinesia are still unknown. One of the relevant factors seems to be a lowering of the drive for movements possibly related to pathophysiology of the caudate nucleus and/or of the limbic system.

On the other hand, a possible role of truncal rigidity in producing primary akinesia should be considered. Bilaterally affected cases have more severe primary akinesia than do cases of hemiparkinsonism. The latter usually show almost complete normalization after alleviation of rigidity and tremor by surgery on the contralateral thalamus. They present minimal or no akinesia postoperatively. But bilaterally affected cases have akinesia that remains after successful surgery on one side. This raises the question as to whether primary akinesia in the bilateral cases is due to rigidity of truncal muscles, which cannot completely be abolished by the unilateral procedure. Because bilateral surgery is better avoided when one performs a classic thalamotomy, it is not known whether primary akinesia can be eliminated after bilateral improvement of rigidity or whether the truncal rigidity is a cause of primary akinesia.

With the introduction of microelectrode techniques in stereotaxic surgery, for the highly accurate identification of target structures, localization of target neurons of micrometer size became possible (6). As a result, the size of lesions is now much smaller, and they are confined only within the subnuclei to be lesioned. At present, by using this new, advanced, and sophisticated technique, bilateral procedures with intervals of more than one year between the two sides can be performed safely without adverse effects on speech or in the psychologic sphere, particularly in patients below the age of 60. From our previous observations (11,12), two bilaterally operated younger patients in whom tremor and rigidity were satisfactorily removed by surgery remained almost normal in their daily life and jobs without medication. They presented with no primary akinesia postoperatively. The other nine cases live almost normally by taking a lower dose of L-dopa than preoperatively [e.g., 2–3 Sinemet (10/100) daily]. These observations may indicate that primary akinesia is also highly improved when rigidity is alleviated satisfactorily and bilaterally.

This question has not been fully elucidated, but the existence of rigidity on both sides of the body must be more important in producing primary akinesia than is usually believed. If bilateral rigidity is a main cause of primary akinesia, the term *primary* must be reconsidered.

PSYCHOMOTOR AKINESIA

Psychomotor akinesia manifests itself in postural difficulty, gait-freezing, and psychological changes such as depressive mood or bradyphrenia. Frozen gait has long been described in the symptomatology of parkinsonism. It is often observed in bilaterally affected rigid cases, and is therefore considered to be due, at least partly, to rigidity of the legs and trunk. However, in well-treated cases of PD under long-term L-dopa medication, it was gradually recognized that marked freezing of gait is observed without rigidity as a cause of a severe inability to walk in the chronic stage. Increased doses of L-dopa in these cases often makes freezing worse. Furthermore, Narabayashi et al (13) reported cases of "pure akinesia," which presented only gait-freezing from the beginning of the disease without any sign of rigidity or tremor. In these cases muscles are often even hypotonic. L-dopa administration produces no improvement, and can even make the symptom worse. Freezing was analyzed to be difficulty of rhythm formation in performing repetitive movements (14,15).

In parkinsonism, reduction in the activity of tyrosine hydroxylase (TH) is well-established. According to Nagatsu et al (16), dopamine β hydroxylase (DβH), the synthesizing enzyme for norepinephrine (NE), is also decreased. Further reduction of DβH activity is found when the disease becomes long-standing (17). This finding suggests a possible role of NE deficiency in producing freezing symptoms, which tend to appear in the later stage of the disease during long-term treatment with L-dopa.

In order to compensate for the deficiency of NE (17), the author began a trial of L-threo-3,4-dihydroxyphenylserine (L-threo-DOPS), the synthesized precursor of NE. A double-blind study of the usefulness of the substance proved its mild effect on freezing symptoms in chronic PD cases during long-term L-dopa treatment and in the pure akinesia cases (18,19). Although the neural mechanisms underlying this effect or even those responsible for freezing in gait itself are not fully explained, it is highly probable that NE deficiency has some important role in the generation of specific motor symptoms such as freezing.

Another important observation during L-threo-DOPS administration is the activating effect the drug has on emotion. Lowered emotional levels, which lead to an akinetic state, are elevated, as demonstrated by analysis using psychometric tests and clinical observation.

Figure 28.2 demonstrates one case with marked improvement of frozen gait and of depressive traits when L-threo-DOPS 600 mg was administered. In a few cases, diffuse slowing in electroencephalograms became slightly improved and frequency of the waves increased about 0.5 Hz together with relative activation of the hypokinetic state. Influences

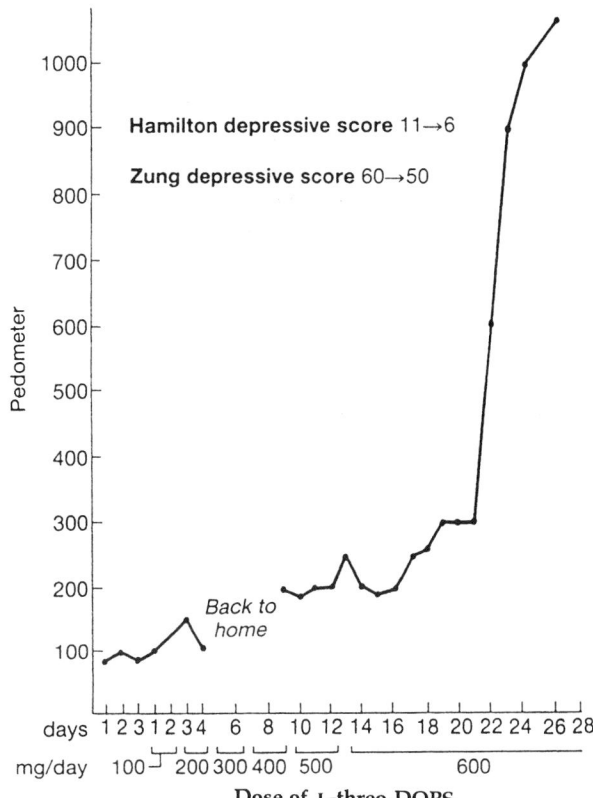

FIGURE 28.2 *A case of idiopathic parkinsonism in a 74-year-old with a three-year disease history and a Hoehn-Yahr stage of IV. Improvement of gait is shown by a pedometer, and changes in depression by the Hamilton test.*

on the latency and the size of the somatosensory evoked potentials are being investigated.

SUMMARY

Akinesia in parkinsonism is one of the most common terms used in the daily clinical practice of neurology; however, it is a term that has not been precisely defined. Rigidity is one of the most important causes of akinesia. This is secondary akinesia as defined by the author. Primary akinesia can be defined as unrelated to rigidity, but its generating mechanisms are still not fully explained. There is some possibility that truncal rigidity causes this type of akinesia.

On the other hand, deficiency of NE may play an important role in the genesis of freezing gait and emotional hypoactivity. Lowering of emotional activity may also possibly be related to akinesia in a wider sense. Akinesia is not a simple symptom, but it may involve disorders of muscle tone as well as emotional tone.

The importance of recognizing the three types of akinesia analyzed in this chapter is that they never appear together at the beginning of the disease. Secondary akinesia due to rigidity of muscles appears first and primary akinesia usually appears several years later. Psychomotor akinesia manifests in the chronic stage of the disease, usually several years later. The gradual addition of these different types of akinesia results in the progressive worsening of the clinical picture. In the late stage of the disease, the presence of all three types of akinesia severely incapacitates the patient. Details of these analyses based on neuropathology and clinical studies are described in other papers by the author (20,21).

REFERENCES

1. Marsden CD. The mysterious motor function of the basal ganglia: The Robert Wartenberg lecture. Neurology 1982;32:514–539.
2. Narabayashi H. Clinical analysis of akinesia. J Neural Transm 1980;(suppl 16):129–136.
3. Narabayashi H. Pharmacological basis of akinesia in Parkinson's disease. J Neural Transm 1983;(suppl 19):143–151.
4. Narabayashi H. Akinesia in parkinsonism: pharmacological and physiological analysis. In: Struppler A, Weindl A, eds. Electromyography and evoked potentials. Berlin: Springer Verlag, 1985.
5. Ohye C, Tsukahara N, Narabayashi H. Rigidity and disturbance of reciprocal innervation. Confin Neurol 1964;26:24–40.
6. Narabayashi H. Lessons from stereotaxic surgery using microelectrode techniques in understanding parkinsonism. Mt Sinai J Med 1988;55:50–57.
7. Barbeau A. Contributions of levodopa therapy to the neuropharmacology of akinesia. In: Siegfried J, ed. Parkinson's disease. Vol. 1. Bern: Hans Huber Publishers, 1972:151–174.
8. Hornykiewicz O. Biochemical and pharmacological aspects of akinesia. In: Siegfried J, ed. Parkinson's disease. Vol. 1. Bern: Hans Huber Publishers, 1972:127–149.
9. Martin JP. The basal ganglia and posture. London: Pitman Medical Publishing, 1967.
10. Hughes RC, Polgar JG, Weighman D, Walton JN. L–dopa in parkinsonism and the influence of previous thalamotomy. Br Med J 1974;I:7–13.
11. Narabayashi H. Surgical treatment in the era of levodopa and other pharmacological treatment. In: Stern G, ed. Parkinson's disease. London: Chapman and Hall, 1990:597–646.
12. Narabayashi H, Maeda T, Yokochi F. Long-term follow-up study of nucleus ventralis intermedius and ventrolateralis thalamotomy using a microelectrode technique in parkinsonism. Appl Neurophysiol 1987;50:330–337.
13. Narabayashi H, Imai H, Yokochi M, et al. Cases of pure akinesia without rigidity and tremor and with no effect by L–dopa therapy. In: Birkmayer W, Hornykiewicz O, eds. Advances in parkinsonism. Basle: Roche, 1976:335–342.
14. Nakamura R, Nagasaki H, Narabayashi H. Arrhythmokinesia in parkinsonism. In: Birkmayer W, Hornykiewicz O, eds. Advances in parkinsonism. Basle: Roche, 1976:258–268.
15. Narabayashi H, Nakamura R. Clinical neurophysiology of freezing in parkinsonism. In: Delwaide PJ, Agnoli A, eds. Clinical neurophysiology in parkinsonism. Amsterdam: Elsevier, 1985:49–57.
16. Nagatsu T, Wakui Y, Kato T, et al. Dopamine beta-hydroxylase activity in cerebrospinal fluid of parkinsonian patients. Biomed Res 1982;3:95–98.
17. Narabayashi H, Kondo T, Hayashi A, et al. L–threo-3,4-dihydroxyphenylserine treatment for akinesia and freezing of parkinsonism. Proc Jpn Acad 1981;57(Ser. B):351–354.
18. Narabayashi H, Kondo T, Yokochi F, Nagatsu T. Clinical effects of L–threo-3,4-dihydroxyphenylserine in cases of parkinsonism and pure akinesia. In: Yahr MD, Bergmann KJ, eds. Advances in neurology. Vol. 45. New York: Raven, 1986:593–602.
19. Narabayashi H, Kondo T. Results of a double-blind study of L–threo-DOPS in parkinsonism. In: Fahn S, Marsden CD, Calne D, Goldstein M, eds. Recent developments in Parkinson's disease. Vol. 2. New Jersey: Macmillan Healthcare Information, 1987:279–291.
20. Narabayashi H. Three types of akinesia in the progressive course of Parkinson's disease. In: Narabayashi H, Nagatsu T, Yanagisawa N, Mizuno Y, eds. Advances in neurology. Vol. 60. New York: Raven, 1993:18–24.
21. Narabayashi H. The neural mechanisms and progressive nature of symptoms of Parkinson's disease—based on clinical, neurophysiological and morphological studies. J Neural Transm 1995;10:63–75.

Parkinsonism–Dementia Complex of Guam

Michael A. Schwarzschild   J. Stephen Fink

INTRODUCTION

Parkinsonism and dementia together are found in hyperendemic proportion among the Chamorro people of Guam. This disorder is probably a clinical variant of a form of amyotrophic lateral sclerosis (ALS) present in high incidence on islands of the Western Pacific. Parkinsonism-dementia complex (PDC) is a late-onset, chronic degenerative condition manifested by parkinsonism, cognitive dysfunction, and, in approximately half of cases, features of ALS. It is a uniformly fatal condition resulting in death usually within four to six years. Since its discovery following World War II, PDC has been the focus of extensive epidemiologic and biochemical investigations. Additional geographic clusters of similar disorders have been identified among the Chamorro people of other Mariana Islands, in the Kii peninsula of Japan, and among the Auyu and Jakai people of West New Guinea (1). The etiology of these conditions has not been determined. However, animal models, new neuropathologic techniques applied to PDC, and continued epidemiologic investigations have provided evidence for novel pathogenetic mechanisms for this unique disease complex and suggest that PDC is a neurodegenerative disease resulting from "environmental" insults.

HISTORY AND EPIDEMIOLOGY

Although ALS had been described more than 100 years ago in the Western Pacific and referred to as "lytico," the first clinical description of Parkinson's disease on Guam was in 1936 (2). "Hereditary paralysis" had been reported on Guam as early as 1900 (3). In 1953, parkinsonism, sleep disorder, and cognitive impairment were described in a number of individuals (who were thought to have had viral encephalitis) during a survey of ALS in the Mariana Islands (4). Later,

in 1961, the pathology of neurofibrillary tangles described in 22 patients with parkinsonism, cognitive impairments, and ALS suggested a unique disorder distinct from classical ALS (5).

On the islands of Guam and Rota in the Mariana Islands, the incidence of PDC is limited to the indigenous Chamorros and to Filipino laborers who emigrated to Guam after World War II and maintained residence for 15 to 26 years before the onset of symptoms (6). The risk of PDC or ALS in U.S. construction workers between 1945 and 1954 and Armed Forces veterans during World War II was not increased (7,8). Together with the observations that Chamorros born on Guam and migrating to the U.S. mainland or elsewhere after age 18 are at increased risk for PDC or ALS (9,10), these data suggest a minimum of 15 years' exposure to the environment of Guam may be required to be at risk to develop PDC. The observation that up to 70% of the normal Chamorro population have neurofibrillary tangles, and in 15% the appearance of these tangles is indistinguishable from PDC, is consistent with a necessary period of environmental exposure to be at risk for PDC (11,12). The declining incidence of PDC and ALS in Guam since 1955 and a shift toward older age of onset (13–15) suggest that the etiology of PDC may be environmental factor(s) that are now less prevalent.

Recently, a high prevalence of isolated dementia (i.e., without parkinsonism) has been appreciated in this region and has accordingly been named "Marianas dementia" (16). Preliminary neuropathologic findings in this condition are typical of Guamanian PDC (17). A less rapid decline in the incidence for PDC compared with ALS on Guam (18) together with the emergence of Marianas dementia may represent a shift in the clinical manifestations of a single disease. Such clinical evolution over just a few decades would argue against prominent genetic factors. It may be most consistent with an environmental etiology in which the changing neurologic pattern reflects the increasing time between the putative period of maximal exposure and the clinical presentation.

CLINICAL CHARACTERISTICS

Like Guamanian ALS, PDC is more frequent in males with onset in mid-life, although its average onset is 10 years later than that of ALS (19–21). Parkinsonism, dementia, or both may be the initial clinical presentation. The extrapyramidal features are prominent akinesia with flexed posture. Rigidity usually affects the axial and proximal musculature. Abnormal postural reflexes may be present. Unlike idiopathic Parkinson's disease, rest tremor is infrequent and, when present, tremor is usually a rapid, action type. Pyramidal tact signs are often present. Other signs include dysarthria, dysphagia, oculomotor abnormalities, frontal release signs, and prominent autonomic dysfunction (21a). In later stages, a generalized flexed posture is characteristic and accompanied by deformities of the extremities. The prominence of axial rigidity, the infrequency of rest tremor, and the presence of supranuclear gaze weakness in most patients (22) suggest that the parkinsonism in PDC may be clinically more closely related to progressive supranuclear palsy than to idiopathic Parkinson's disease.

Progressive cognitive abnormalities are characteristic of PDC and, in approximately 30% of cases, may be the presenting sign. The dementia of PDC is global, involving memory, reasoning, orientation, and personality change. Aphasia and apraxia are not common. In PDC upper motor neuron signs are present in 50% to 94% of patients; lower motor neuron signs are present in 17% to 46% (3,23–25). Hypertension, diabetes, obesity, bony fractures, or hyperuricemia are common. Parkinsonism and dementia with ALS may present simultaneously, as parkinsonism-dementia followed by ALS or as amyotrophy/spasticity followed by parkinsonism-dementia. Although at least 50% of PDC patients develop ALS, only 5% of patients with Guamanian ALS develop parkinsonism-dementia (21). The existence of a combined PDC/ALS clinical presentation, together with the neuropathologic similarities of combined PDC/ALS and PDC or ALS alone, support the notion that Guamanian ALS, PDC, and combined PDC/ALS represent a clinical continuum of a single disease.

Progressive parkinsonism and dementia, perhaps with motor neuron signs, with onset in mid-late life in a population in certain islands in the Western Pacific secures the diagnosis of PDC. Clinical course is progressive with death typically occurring within six years, even with symptomatic therapy using dopaminergic agonists. Laboratory findings, which are not specific for PDC, are not particularly useful in establishing the diagnosis. There is progressive slowing of the electroencephalogram (EEG) alpha rhythm and computerized tomography (CT) scans reveal cortical atrophy. Similar to idiopathic Parkinson's disease, homovanillic acid

and 5-hydroxyindolacetic acid, metabolites of dopamine and serotonin, respectively, are reduced (26). However, routine cerebrospinal fluid (CSF) analysis is unremarkable or may show slightly increased protein. Other laboratory abnormalities include increases in IgA and reductions in IgM, resulting in a reversed serum albumin/globulin ratio (21).

Other conditions that may present as parkinsonism and dementia, such as idiopathic Parkinson's disease and Alzheimer's disease, are uncommon on Guam. A variant of ALS presenting with parkinsonism, dementia, and ALS features may occur in "corticostriatospinal degeneration" (27). Other conditions may present with prominant parkinsonism and motor neuron disease including Azorean disease, pallidopyramidal and pallidonigral degeneration, multiple system atrophies, neuroacanthocytosis, and parkinsonism with Friedreich's tabes or Charcot-Marie-Tooth disease (24). The geographical focus of PDC in the Western Pacific, however, usually need not make these other clinical presentations a problem in the differential diagnosis of PDC.

Neuropathologic findings have been extensively described and include cortical atrophy, ventricular dilatation, and depigmentation of the substantia nigra and locus coeruleus (7,28–30). There is widespread neuronal degeneration most prominent in cortex, amygdala, temporal cortex and frontal cortex, Ammon's horn, nucleus basalis of Meynert, globus pallidus, thalamus, periaqueductal grey, substantia nigra, hypothalamus, and brainstem motor nuclei. Neurofibrillary tangles are frequent in the residual neurons and are similar to those of Alzheimer's disease, but are infrequent in the spinal cord and peripheral nervous system. Using conventional methods, occasional neurofibrillary tangles have been found in the spinal cords of 22% to 37% of patients with Guamanian ALS and 30% to 63% of patients with PDC (29,31). Hippocampal neurofibrillary tangles in Guam ALS and PDC are similar in composition to those found in Alzheimer's disease, containing hyperphosphorylated tau protein, paired helical filaments, ubiquitin, phosphorylated neurofilament, and Alz-50 (32–36). Using antibodies to tau protein and ubiquitin, it has been demonstrated that neurofibrillary tangles are more numerous in the spinal cords of Guam ALS and PDC than previously found with conventional methods (37).

The specific antigenic composition of neurofibrillary tangles and other neuropathologic features seen in both Alzheimer's disease and PDC (38) suggest a common pathogenetic mechanism. However, senile plaques, a common feature of Alzheimer's Disease, are rarely found in PDC, nor are amyloid plaques seen using a sensitive antibody to the beta(A4)-amyloid protein (39). The presence of pure neurofibrillary tangles formation without beta(A4) suggests that the pathogenetic mechanism of PDC may be different from that of Alzheimer's disease or other disorders in which beta(A4) plaques are seen, such as dementia pugilistica. In Chamorros with no known neurological disease, neurofibrillary tangles are present in over 70% of autopsied specimens, and in 15% of these the density and pattern was indistinguishable from PDC (11,12). Although the significance of this finding is not understood, the presence of neurofibrillary tangles in the neurologically normal Guamanian population in frequency exceeding age-matched, non-Guamanians is consistent with widespread environmental factors contributing to PDC pathogenesis.

Unlike idiopathic Parkinson's disease, Lewy bodies are uncommonly seen in Guam ALS or PDC. Of note, the neuropathology of progressive supranuclear palsy (which displays clinical features closely resembling the parkinsonism in PDC) also includes neurofibrillary tangles. However, the biochemical features of the tau protein component of neurofibrillary tangles in PDC are distinct from those in progressive supranuclear palsy (and are, in fact, similar to those in Alzheimer's disease) (36). Using antisera to basal ganglia neuropeptides it has been demonstrated that the striatal efferent system appears to be preserved in both idiopathic Parkinson's disease, Alzheimer's disease, and in PDC (40).

There is, however, more severe loss of substantia nigra dopaminergic cell bodies in PDC than in Parkinson's disease, suggesting a difference in midbrain neuropathology. Guamanian PDC patients, like idiopathic Parkinson's disease, have decreased striatal ^{18}F-6-fluorodopa uptake as measured using positron emission tomography (PET) (41). This confirms a presynaptic dopaminergic lesion in PDC and, together with the preservation of striatal output pathways, is consistent with the dopa-responsiveness of PDC patients (42). Guamanian ALS patients and two normal Guamanian subjects who did not have evidence of extrapyramidal disease also had reduced ^{18}F-6-fluorodopa uptake. The presence of subclinical nigrostriatal damage in Guam ALS and in normal Guamanian subjects is consistent with the notion that Guam ALS and PDC are a single disease with a spectrum of clinical presentation resulting from a widespread environmental factor on Guam.

ETIOLOGY: A NEUROTOXIC DISORDER?

Perhaps the most interesting aspect of PDC has been the intensive investigation of its etiology. Failure to find linkage to gene markers (such as HLA antigens, red blood cell enzymes, blood groups, and immunoglobulin allotypes) and the results of pedigree analysis of high incidence villages and prospective case control registries provide additional evidence that genetic factors do not play a major role in PDC (43,44). Epidemiologic findings also fail to support a genetic hypothesis. Offspring of affected PDC persons do not have an increased risk of PDC. Zhang and colleagues found that of 140 affected PDC persons, 121 had siblings with PDC, but only eight had offspring with PDC (13). Additionally, none of nine doubly affected couples had offspring who developed PDC.

The well-documented high level of familial aggregation of PDC (20,44a) is likely to have been the result of common

environmental exposures. It is probable, however, that genetic susceptibility plays a role in the eitology of PDC (44a,45), together with an environmental risk factor that may have a latency period before demonstrating clinical effect. Three specific genetic hypotheses based on the linkage of ALS, Alzheimer's disease, and Parkinson's disease to identified genes were recently dismissed after no correlation was found between Guamanian neurodegenerative disease and Cu/Zn superoxide dismutase gene mutations, apolipoprotein E alleles, or CYP2D6 alleles, respectively (46,47,47a).

Several lines of epidemiological evidence argue strongly for an environmental cause of PDC. Chamorros on the islands of Guam and Rota have a greater incidence and mortality from PDC and Guam ALS that Chamorros on Saipan, Tinian, and more northerly Mariana Islands (48). Chamorros who migrated from Guam to other environments have a decreased risk of PDC (14). These findings implicate environmental factors on Guam and Rota, rather than genetics, as important factors in the pathogenesis of PDC. The downward trend in age-adjusted incidence rates of PDC on Guam and the entire Mariana archipelago is in favor of a change in an important environmental factor, perhaps as the result of recent socioeconomic changes on Guam (13–15,49).

The decline in incidence rates has not been accompanied by a change in the pathologic features of PDC (31). There is also an upward trend in age of onset of PDC among Chamorros on Guam (14). A fivefold to tenfold increased risk of developing ALS and PDC is maintained for up to three decades when Chamorros (who have had at least 18 years' exposure to the Guam environment) move to the U.S. mainland or when Filipinos migrate to Guam and remain there for at least 13 years (6). These lines of evidence suggest that infectious, toxic, dietary, or other environmental factors are important to the pathogenesis of PDC (50).

Although the clinical presentation and neuropathology are not inconsistent with a viral etiology (51), no direct proof of an infectious agent has been found. Virus has not been isolated from brain tissue cultures, viral nucleic acids have not been identified, and PDC or ALS has not been successfully transmitted to other laboratory animals (52–54).

It has been hypothesized that the critical environmental factor in the pathogenesis of PDC is chronic nutritional deficiency of calcium and magnesium (55–58). The resulting secondary hypoparathyroidism that results from impaired dietary intake of calcium and magnesium may lead to increased intestinal absorption of potentially toxic metals such as aluminum and manganese and neuronal deposition in patients with PDC and Guam ALS. The intraneuronal accumulation of metals may interfere with axonal transport and produce abnormal neurofilament synthesis and the accumulation of neurofibrillary tangles (59). In favor of this hypothesis is the finding of mild abnormalities of calcium metabolism in some Guam ALS and PDC patients (57) and deposition of aluminum, calcium and silicon in neurofibrillary tangle-containing neurons in Guam ALS and PDC patients (49,58,60,61).

However, there are opponents of the hypothesis that calcium and magnesium deficiency leads to heavy metal accumulation and consequently PDC (13,18,62). No correlation has been found between the concentrations of various elements from soil and water sources, including calcium and magnesium, and district-specific incidence rates of PDC (13). Moreover, low levels of calcium in certain rivers of Guam have not been confirmed (63). Recent attempts to correlate Guamanian neurodegenerative disease with calcium metabolism and body stores of heavy metals (e.g., aluminum) have shown no clear differences between patients and island control subjects (64). Nevertheless, in the absence of biologic (and environmental) samples obtained at the time of a putative peak in toxin exposure, the calcium metabolism/heavy metal hypothesis remains a possibility.

It was proposed more than three decades ago that Guam ALS and PDC were linked to a toxin contained in cycad seed (65). Six international conferences held between 1962 and 1972 sought to investigate the relationship between the use of the toxic seed of the false sago palm *Cycas circinalis* for food and medicine among the Chamorro and the high incidence of ALS and PDC on Guam. A cycad toxin, beta-N-methylamino-L-alanine (BMAA) was identified, but because of the low concentrations of this convulsant amino acid in cycad seeds and its failure to induce in rats neurologic damage similar to ALS/PDC, BMAA was not felt to be the toxic factor in PDC (66,67). The cycad hypothesis was revived in 1986 when Spencer and colleagues (68,69) demonstrated the induction of a motor disorder in 13 cynomolgus monkeys within 2 to 12 weeks of ingesting large amounts of BMAA. In these monkeys, more prolonged treatment was required to produce extrapyramidal signs (which were responsive to L-dopa). Neuropathologic examination showed signs of neuronal damage in the motor cortex and less damage to anterior horn cells. The basal ganglia, hippocampus, and cerebellum were similar to controls except for one monkey treated for 13 weeks that showed neuritic swellings in the pars compacta of the substantia nigra. The cellular mechanism of action of BMAA may be similar to that of a structurally related, plant-derived neurotoxic amino acid, beta-N-oxalylamino-L-alanine (BOAA), which induces corticospinal (but not extrapyramidal) deficiency in primates and is implicated in human lathyrism, an upper motor neuron disease resulting from excess intake of the chickling pea *Lathyrus sativus* (70,71). L-BOAA and L-BMAA act directly or indirectly at glutamate receptors (69,72).

While the revived interest in the cycad hypothesis has persisted and been supported by some epidemiologic data (13,18), a role for BMAA in PDC has increasingly been questioned. The syndrome in BMAA-fed monkeys resembles ALS more than PDC, was nonprogressive after dosing was stopped, and displays neuropathology without characteristic neurofibrillary tangles (69,73). It has been argued that the doses of BMAA in cycad flour are too low to produce a neurotoxic syndrome in humans (74). Garruto et al (75) have also demonstrated that cycad does not potentiate the pyramidal and extrapyramidal neuropathology produced by low calcium plus a toxic metal diet.

Another cycad toxin, cycasin, was identified several decades ago but was initially discounted as a candidate for ALS/PDC of Guam. Although it is present in cycad seed at a high concentration and acts as a strong alkylating agent and potent carcinogen, neurotoxicity was not appreciated in early animal studies (76,77). More recent investigations, however, have demonstrated cycasin neurotoxicity in cortical neurons in vitro (78) as well as in spinal cords of animals fed cycasin (79). In addition, cycasin concentrations in regional flour samples is tightly correlated with ALS/PDC incidence on Guam (73,80). Whether exposure to cycasin or an as yet unidentified cycad (or other dietary/environmental) toxin causes PDC remains an open question.

The most serious problem with the environmental toxin hypothesis of PDC is that latency for a clinical effect must occur to explain the increased risk for PDC/ALS of emigrated Chamorros that is maintained for decades. Some PDC-ALS patients have had a single cycad exposure or cycad use several decades before the onset of symptoms (81). Latency for clinical effect could occur following a toxic neuronal insult without symptoms, which only becomes symptomatic with age-related central nervous system changes. This has been suggested to occur in Parkinson's and Alzheimer's diseases (82). Although provocative, this explanation for several late-life neurodegenerative diseases, including PDC, remain to be proven. However, the geographic focus of PDC in the Chamorro population may continue to provide a unique opportunity to identify new biological mechanisms that may be important to the pathogenesis of more common neurodegenerative diseases.

ACKNOWLEDGMENTS

We thank Drs. L.T. Kurland, D.P. Perl, and P.S. Spencer for their thoughtful comments.

REFERENCES

1. Garruto RM, Yase Y. Neurodegenerative disorders of the western Pacific: the search for mechanisms of pathogenesis. Trends Neurosci 1986;9:368–374.
2. Yase Y, Chen KM, Brody JA, Toyokura Y. A historical note on parkinsonism-dementia complex of Guam. Neuro Med (Tokyo) 1978;8:583–589.
3. Elizan TS, Hirano A, Abrams BM, et al. Amyotrophic lateral sclerosis and the parkinsonism-dementia complex of Guam: neurologic reevaluation. Arch Neurol 1966;14:356–368.
4. Mulder DW, Kurland LT, Iriarte LLG. Neurological disease on the island of Guam. US Armed Forces Med J 1954;5:1724–1739.
5. Malamud N, Hirano A, Kurland LT. Pathoanatomic changes in amyotrophic lateral sclerosis on Guam: special reference to the occurrence of neurofibrillary changes. Arch Neurol 1961;5:401–415.

6. Garruto RM, Gajdusek DC, Chen KM. Amyotrophic lateral sclerosis and parkinsonism-dementia among Filipino migrants to Guam. Ann Neurol 1981;10:341–350.

7. Brody JA, Hirano A, Scott RM. Recent neuropathologic observations in amyotrophic lateral sclerosis and the parkinsonism-dementia complex of Guam. Neurology 1971;21:528–536.

8. Brody JA, Edgar AH, Gillespie MM. Amyotrophic lateral sclerosis: no increase among US construction workers in Guam. JAMA 1979;240:551–552.

9. Eldridge R, Ryan R, Rosario J, Brody JA. Amyotrophic lateral sclerosis and the parkinsonism-dementia complex in a migrant population from Guam. Neurology 1969;19:1029–1037.

10. Garruto RM, Gajdusek DC, Chen KM. Amyotrophic lateral sclerosis among Chamorro migrants from Guam. Ann Neurol 180;8:612–619.

11. Anderson FH, Richardson EP, Okazaki H, Brody J. Neurofibrillary degeneration on Guam: frequency in Chamorros and non-Chamorros with no known neurologic disease. Brain 1979;102:65–77.

12. Chen L. Neurofibrillary changes on Guam. Arch Neurol 1981;38:16–18.

13. Zhang Z-X, Anderson DW, Mantel N. Geographic patterns of Parkinson-dementia complex on Guam: 1956 through 1985. Arch Neurol 1990;47:1069–1074.

14. Zhang Z-X, Anderson DW, Lavine L, Mantel N. Patterns of acquiring parkinsonism-dementia complex on Guam: 1944 through 1985. Arch Neurol 1990;47:1019–1024.

15. Garruto RM, Yanagihara R, Gadjusek DC. Disappearance of high incidence amyotrophic lateral sclerosis and parkinsonism-dementia on Guam. Neurology 1985;35:193–198.

16. Lavine L, Steele JC, Wolfe N, et al. Amyotrophic lateral sclerosis/parkinsonism-dementia complex in southern Guam: is it disappearing? Adv Neurol 1991;56:271–285.

17. Perl DP, Hof PR, Steele JC, et al. Neuropathologic studies of a pure dementing syndrome (Marianas dementia) among the inhabitants of Guam, a form of amyotrophic lateral sclerosis/parkinsonism-dementia complex. Brain Path 1994;4:529. Abstract.

18. Reed D, Labarthe D, Chen KM, Stallones R. A cohort study of amyotrophic lateral sclerosis and parkinsonism-dementia on Guam and Rota. Am J Epidemiol 1987;125:92–100.

19. Kurland LT, Mulder DW. Epidemiological investigations of amyotrophic lateral sclerosis. I: preliminary report on geographic distribution, with special reference to the Mariana Islands, including clinical and pathologic observations. Neurology 1954;4:438–448.

20. Kurland LT, Mulder DW. Epidemiological investigations of amyotrophic lateral sclerosis. II: familial aggregations indicative of dominant inheritance. Neurology 1955;5:182–196.

21. Chen K-M, Chase TN. Parkinsonism-dementia. In: Vinken PJ, Bruyn GW, Klawans HL, eds. Handbook of clinical neurology. Vol. 49. Amsterdam: Elsevier, 1986:167–183.

21a. Low PA, Ahlskog JE, Petersen RC, et al. Autonomic failure in Guamanian neurodegenerative disease. Neurology 1997;49:1031–1034.

22. Lepore FE, Steele JC, Cox TA, et al. Supranuclear disturbances of ocular motility in lytico-bodig. Neurology 1988;38:1849–1853.

23. Hirano A, Kurland LT, Krooth RS, Lessell S. Parkinsonism-dementia complex, an endemic disease on the island of Guam. I: clinical features. Brain 1961;84:642–661.

24. Lessell S, Hirano A, Torres JM, Kurland LT. Parkinsonism-dementia complex: epidemiological considerations in the Chamorros of the Mariana Islands and California. Arch Neurol 1962;7:377–385.

25. Chen KM, Tsuji S, Gajdusek DC, Gibbs CJ. Studies on the natural history of amyotrophic lateral sclerosis and parkinsonism-dementia of Guam: II. motor neuron involvement and postural deformities in advanced stage. Neurology 1979;29:578.

26. Brody JA, Chase TN, Gordon EK. Depressed monoamine catabolite levels in cerebrospinal fluid of patients with parkinsonism-dementia of Guam. N Engl J Med 1970;282:947–950.

27. Weiner WJ, Lang AE. Movement disorders: a compehensive survey. Mt. Kisco, NY: Futura, 1989:181–184.

28. Hirano A, Malamud N, Kurland LT. Parkinsonism-dementia complex, an endemic disease on the island of Guam. II: pathological features. Brain 1961;84:662–679.

29. Hirano A, Malamud N, Elizan TS, Kurland LT. Amyotrophic lateral sclerosis and the parkinsonism-dementia complex of Guam: further pathologic studies. Arch Neurol 1966;15:35–51.

30. Hirano A, Zimmerman HM. Alzheimer's neurofibrillary changes: a topographic study. Arch Neurol 1962;7:227–242.

31. Rodgers-Johnson P, Garruto RM, Yanagihara R, et al. Amyotrophic lateral sclerosis and parkinsonism-dementia on Guam: A 30-year evaluation of clinical and neuropathological trends. Neurology 1986;36:7–13.

32. Kosik KS, Joachim CJ, Selkoe DJ. Microtubule-associated protein tau (T) is a major antigenic component of paired helical filaments in Alzheimer disease. Proc Natl Acad Sci 1986;83:4044–4043.

33. Shankar SK, Yanagihara R, Garruto RM, et al. Immunocytochemical characterization of neurofibrillary tangles in amyotrophic lateral sclerosis and the parkinsonism-dementia complex of Guam. Ann Neurol 1989;25:146–151.

34. Love S, Saitoh T, Quijada S, et al. Alz-50, ubiquitin and tau immunoreactivity of neurofibrillary tangles, Pick bodies and Lewy bodies. J Neuropathol Exp Neurol 1988;47:393–405.

35. Joachim CL, Morris JH, Kosik KS, Selkoe DJ. Tau antisera recognize neurofibrillary tangles in a range of neurodegenerative disorders. Ann Neurol 1987;22:514–520.

36. Buée-Scherrer V, Buée L, Hof PR, et al. Neurofibrillary degeneration in amyotrophic lateral sclerosis/parkinsonism-dementia complex of Guam: Immunochemical characterization of tau proteins. Am J Path 1995;68:924–932.

37. Matsumoto S, Hirano A, Goto S. Spinal cord neurofibrillary tangles of Guamanian amyotrophic lateral sclerosis and the parkinsonism-dementia complex: an immunohistochemical study. Neurology 1990;40:975–979.

38. Perl DP, Steele JC, Loerzel A, et al. Amyotrophic lateral sclerosis/parkinsonism-dementia complex of Guam as a model of Alzheimer's disease. In: Iqbal K, McLachlan DRC, Winblad B, et al., eds. Alzheimer's disease: Basic mechanisms, diagnostic and therapeutic strategies. New York: John Wiley, 1991:375–381.

39. Gentleman SM, Perl D, Allsop D, et al. Beta(A4)-amyloid protein and parkinsonism-dementia complex of Guam. Lancet 1991;337:55–56.

40. Goto S, Hirano A, Matsumoto S. Immunohistochemical study of the striatal efferents and nigral dopaminergic neurons in parkinsonism-dementia complex on Guam in comparison with those in Parkinson's and Alzheimer's diseases. Ann Neurol 1990;27:520–527.

41. Snow BJ, Peppard RF, Guttman M, et al. Positron emission tomographic scanning demonstrates a presynaptic dopaminergic lesion in lytico-bodig: the amyotrophic lateral sclerosis and parkinsonism-dementia complex of Guam. Arch Neurol 1990;47:870–874.

42. Holden EM, Brody JA, Chase TN. Parkinsonism-dementia of Guam: treatment with levodopa and L-alpha-dopahydrazine. Neurology 1974;24:263–265.

43. Brody JA, Kirk RL, Wilson RM, et al. Search for a red cell enzyme or serum protein marker in amyotrophic lateral sclerosis and the parkinsonism-dementia complex of Guam. Am J Med Genet 1983;14:299–305.

44. Garruto RM, Plato CC, Schanfield MS, et al. Blood groups, immunoglobulin allotypes and dermatographic frequencies in patients with amyotrophic lateral sclerosis and parkinsonism-dementia of Guam. Am J Med Genet 1983;14:289–298.

44a. McGeer PL, Schwab C, McGeer EG, et al. Familial nature and continuing morbidity of the amyotrophic lateral sclerosis–parkinsonism dementia complex of Guam. Neurology 1997;49:400–409.

45. Bailey-Wilson JE, Plato CC, Elston RC, et al. Potential role of an additive genetic component in the cause of amyotrophic lateral sclerosis and parkinsonism-dementia in the Western Pacific. Am J Med Genet 1993;45:68–76.

46. Figlewicz DA, Garruto RM, Krizus A, et al. The Cu/Zn superoxide dismutase gene in ALS and parkinsonism-dementia of Guam. Neuroreport 1994;5:557–560.

47. Waring SC, O'Brien PC, Kurland LT, et al. Apolipoprotein E allele in Chamorros with amyotrophic lateral sclerosis/parkinsonism-dementia complex. Lancet 1994;343:611.

47a. Chen X, Xia Y, Gresham LS, et al. ApoE and CYP2D6 polymorphism with and without parkinsonism–dementia complex in the people of Chamorro, Guam. Neurology 1996;47:779–784.

48. Yanagihara RT, Garruto RM, Gajdusek DC. Epidemiological surveillance of amyotrophic lateral sclerosis and parkinsonism-dementia in the Commonwealth of the northern Mariana Islands. Ann Neurol 1983;13:79–86.

49. Kurland LT. Amyotrophic lateral sclerosis and the Parkinson's disease complex on Guam linked to an environmental neurotoxin. Trends Neurosci 1988;11:51–54.

50. Reed DM, Brody JA. Amyotrophic lateral sclerosis and parkinsonism-dementia on Guam, 1945–1972: I. descriptive epidemiology. Am J Epidemiol 1975;101:287–301.

51. Hudson AJ, Rice GPA. Similarities of Guamanian ALS/PD to post-encephalitic parkinsonism/ALS: possible viral cause. Can J Neurol Sci 1990;17:427–433.

52. Gibbs CJ, Gajdusek DC. An update on long-term in vivo and in vitro studies designed to identify a virus as the cause of amyotrophic lateral sclerosis, parkinsonism-dementia and Parkinson's Disease. In: Rowland LP, ed. Human motor neuron diseases. New York: Raven, 1982.

53. Kohne DE, Gibbs CJ, White L, et al. Virus detection by nucleic acid hybridization: examination of normal and ALS tissue for the presence of polio virus. J Gen Virol 1982;56:223–233.

54. Viola MV, Myers JC, Gann KL, et al. Failure to detect poliovirus genetic information in amyotrophic lateral sclerosis. Ann Neurol 1979;5:402–403.

55. Garruto RM, Fukatsu R, Yanagihara R, et al. Imaging of calcium and aluminum in neurofibrillary tangle-bearing neurons in parkinsonism-dementia of Guam. Proc Natl Acad Sci USA 1984;81:1875–1879.

56. Yase Y. Pathogenesis of amyotrophic lateral sclerosis. Lancet 1972;2:292–296.

57. Yanagihara RY, Garruto RM, Gajdusek DC, et al. Calcium and vitamin D metabolism in Guamanian Chamorros with amyotrophic lateral sclerosis and parkinsonism-dementia. Ann Neurol 1984;15:42–48.

58. Garruto R, Swyt C, Yanagihara R, et al. Intraneuronal co-localization of silicon with calcium and aluminum in amyotrophic lateral sclerosis and parkinsonism with dementia of Guam. N Engl J Med 1986;11:711–712.

59. Gajdusek DC. Hypothesis: interference with axonal transport of neurofilament as a common pathogenetic mechanism in certain diseases of the central nervous system. N Engl J Med 1985;312:714–719.

60. Perl DP, Gajdusek DC, Garruto RM, et al. Intraneuronal aluminum accumulation in amyotrophic lateral sclerosis and Parkinsonism-dementia of Guam. Science 1982;217:1053–1055.

61. Good PF, Perl DP. Aluminum in Alzheimer's. Nature 1993;362:418.

62. Heitz L, Zolan W, Ellis-Neill L, et al. Guam's Piga Spring: a source of confusion: the ALS/parkinsonism-dementia complex. Neurology 1988;38 (suppl 1):310.

63. Spencer PS. Guam ALS/parkinsonism-dementia: a long-latency neurotoxic disorder caused by "slow toxin(s)" in food? Can J Neurol Sci 1987;14 (suppl 3):347–357.

64. Ahlskog JE, Waring SC, Kurland LT, et al. Guamanian neurodegenerative disease: investigation of the calcium metabolism/heavy metal hypothesis. Neurology 1995;45:1340–1344.

65. Whiting MG. Toxicity of cycads. Econ Bot 1963;17:271–302.

66. Polsky FI, Nunn PB, Bell EA. Distribution and toxicity of alpha-amino-beta-methylaminopropionic acid. Fed Proc 1972;31:1473–1475.

67. Vega A, Bell EA. Alpha-amino-beta-methylpropionic acids: a new amino acid from seeds of Cycas circinalis. Phytochemistry 1967;6:759–762.

68. Spencer PS, Nunn PB, Hugon J, et al. Motor neurone disease on Guam: possible role of a food neurotoxin. Lancet 1986;1:965.

69. Spencer PS, Nunn PB, Hugon J, et al. Guam amyotrophic lateral sclerosis-parkinsonism-dementia linked to a plant excitant neurotoxin. Science 1987;237:517–522.

70. Spencer PS, Ludolph A, Dwivedi MP, et al. Lathyrism: evidence for the role of the neuroexcitatory amino acid BOAA. Lancet 1980;2:1066–1067.

71. Spencer PS, Schaumberg HH. Lathyrism: a neurotoxic disease. Neurobeh Toxicol 1983;5:625–629.

72. Nunn PB, Seelig M, Zagoren JC, Spencer PS. Stereospecific acute neuronotoxicity of "uncommon" plant amino acids linked to human motor-system disease. Brain Res 1987;410:375–379.

73. Kisby GE, Ellison M, Spencer P. Content of the neurotoxins cycasin (methylazoxymethanol β-D-glucoside) and BMAA (β-N-methylamino-L-alanine) in cycad flour prepared by Guam Chamorros. Neurology 1992;42:1336–1340.

74. Duncan MW, Steele JC, Kopin IJ, Markey SP. 2-Amino-3-(methylamino)-propanoic acid (BMAA) in cycad flour: an unlikely cause of amyotrophic lateral sclerosis and the parkinsonism-dementia of Guam. Neurology 1990;40:767–772.

75. Garruto RM, Yanagihara R, Gajdusek DC. Cycads and amyotrophic lateral sclerosis/parkinsonism dementia. Lancet 1988;2:1079.

76. Laquer GL, Mickelson O, Whiting MG, Kurland LT. Carcinogenic properties of nuts from cycas circinalis L. indigenous to Guam. J Natl Cancer Inst 1963;31:919–951.

77. Yang MG, Mickelson O, Campbell ME, et al. Cycad flour used by Guamanians: effects produced in rats by long-term feeding. J Nutr 1966;90:153–156.

78. Kisby GE, Ross SM, Spencer P, et al. Cycasin and BMAA: candidate neurotoxins for Western Pacific amyotrophic lateral sclerosis/parkinsonism-dementia complex. Neurodegeneration 1992;1:73–82.

79. Shimizu T, Yasuda N, Kono I, et al. Hepatic and spinal lesions in goats chronically intoxicated with cycasin. Jpn J Vet Sci 1986;8:1291–1295.

80. Zhang ZX, Anderson DW, Mantel N, et al. Motor neuron disease on Guam: geographic and familial occurrence, 1956–85. Acta Neurol Scand 1996;94:51–59.

81. Steele JC, Guzman T. Obsservations about amyotrophic lateral sclerosis and the parkinsonism-dementia complex of Guam with regard to epidemiology and etiology. Can J Neurol Sci 1987;14(suppl 3):358–362.

82. Calne DB, Eisen A, McGeer E, Spencer PS. Alzheimer's disease, Parkinson's disease, and motorneuron disease: abiotrop(h)ic interaction between aging and environment. Lancet 1986;2:1067–1069.

Depression, Dementia, and Parkinson's Disease

GRAEME D. HAMMOND-TOOKE   MARTIN POLLOCK

HISTORICAL INTRODUCTION

In addition to the classic features of tremor, bradykinesia, rigidity, and postural disturbance, patients with idiopathic Parkinson's disease (PD) may be depressed, demented, or have cognitive disturbances without overt dementia. The frequency with which these features occur and their relationship to the underlying disease has become clearer in recent years.

In Parkinson's original description, published in 1817, patients with PD were stated to be intellectually unimpaired (1). Later, Charcot and Vulpian (2) considered that psychic impairment was generally present, and Parant (3) described mental abnormalities in parkinsonian patients that he divided into "personality change," "weakening of the intellectual faculties," and "symptoms of insanity proper" (4).

Descriptions of depression as a feature of PD include those of Patrick and Levy (5), Mjönes (6), and Celesia and Wanamaker (7), who described three categories of psychiatric disturbance in PD: dementia, depression, and acute psychotic disorder. While the exact frequency of depression in PD is uncertain, the major controversy is whether the depression is "reactive" or "endogenous," occurring as an integral feature of the disease or resulting from an independent constitutional or genetic predisposition to mood disorder that is aggravated by PD (4).

With regard to dementia in PD, there is disagreement between those who consider it to be due to coincidental Alzheimer's disease (AD) (8) and those who believe it is due to PD itself. Both AD and PD are associated with cell loss from the nucleus basalis of Meynert, suggesting both diseases are extremes of a spectrum, so that simultaneous occurrence of the two diseases may be more than fortuitous (9). Of relevance to these issues are the concepts of "subcortical dementia" and "bradyphrenia."

The term *subcortical dementia* was introduced by Albert et al (10) to describe the intellectual impairment seen in progressive supranuclear palsy. The concept is an anatomical one, implying a dementia due to dysfunction in subcortical structures. It has been used to describe cognitive disturbances in Huntington's disease (HD), Wilson's disease, and PD. It is characterized by forgetfulness, slowing of thought processes, alteration in mood and personality, and decreased ability to manipulate acquired knowledge. It contrasts with "cortical dementia" typified by AD and characterized by amnesia, aphasia, apraxia, and agnosia (11). Whether neuropathologic and neuropsychologic evidence support the separation of "cortical" and "subcortical" dementias is controversial (12,13).

The term *bradyphrenia* was introduced by Naville (14) to describe a syndrome seen commonly in PD and parkinsonism due to encephalitis lethargica. While sometimes used synonymously with "subcortical dementia," the term implies that thinking is slow but intelligence is normal. It is characterized by "decreased voluntary attention, spontaneous interest, initiative, and capacity for effort and work, with objective and subjective fatigability and slight diminution of memory" (15,16). In a sense, this is the cognitive equivalent of bradykinesia and its presence in PD favors a common pathogenesis for the motor and cognitive disturbances.

DEPRESSION IN PD

Prevalence

The reported prevalence of depression in PD varies markedly (from 4% to 70%, with a mean of 40%) (17) due to differences in criteria, methodology, and the characteristics of the population studied (18). Most studies have shown that approximately 35% to 40% of parkinsonian patients have significant depression (19). Most have found no relationship between depression and the patients' current age, age of onset, or length of illness (17). Some have found depression in PD more common in women (17,20) or in younger, less disabled patients (21,22) but most investigators report no consistent relationship with age or gender (18). Depression is more common in PD than other equally severe chronic diseases (23), but *major* depression may be no more frequent than in age- and sex-matched physically disabled controls (24).

Clinical Features

Depression in PD is usually of mild to moderate intensity and characterized by dysphoria, pessimism, somatic symptoms, and, in some cases, mild intellectual impairment (18). Patients do not tend to hold a negative view of themselves, lack guilt or self-blame, and seldom commit suicide (25). As a similar pattern is found in arthritis sufferers, it has been suggested that the depression of PD is merely the result of a chronic, disabling illness. Mayeux (18) suggests that most patients have an organic affective disorder when depression occurs during or prior to the development of PD, but reactive depression is more likely in those who become depressed in the first year of their PD. Santamaria et al (26) claimed that the depression is mainly of the dysthymic or major depression type, but, according to Cummings, slightly more than half of depressed patients with PD meet criteria for a major depressive episode and slightly less than half have dysthymia or minor depression (17). The presence of "vegetative signs" in PD, of course, complicates the distinction between reactive and endogenous depression.

Another feature of depression in PD is the frequent association with anxiety, and this may represent a specific subtype of depression in PD (27,28). There is a relative lack of delusions and hallucinations (29) and a low suicide rate despite a high frequency of suicidal ideation (17).

Relationship of Depression to Parkinsonism

The temporal relationship between depression and parkinsonism varies, but in up to 40% of cases the depression precedes the neurological symptoms (26,30). Such patients tend to have a younger age of onset and less severe disease (21,31). There is some evidence that PD patients have a personality profile characterized by introversion that increases with the onset of disease and is closely correlated with depression (32).

The relationship between depression and the duration or severity of PD remains uncertain (5,30). Most authors have found no relationship between mood and motor manifestations, but there is a limited relationship between the severity of disability and the presence of mood changes (17). Brown and MacCarthy (29) found an association between depression and disability both initially and at one-year

follow-up. Severely disabled patients tended to be more depressed, but depression was not related to fluctuation in level of disability or rate of progression. Patients who became more disabled with time became more depressed, with increased dysphoria and pessimism, although self-blame, guilt, and somatic symptoms were not significantly worsened. Perhaps progress of disability is a better predictor of depression than the absolute level of disability. Santamaria et al (26) found no difference in frequency or severity of depression in mild than in advanced PD. It is unclear whether the side of onset of parkinsonism is related to depression; some studies suggest greater depression with right hemiparkinsonism (33,34).

There may be a subtype of PD with more frequent depression, characterized by increased rigidity and bradykinesia and lower age of onset and positive family history (35). Families have been described with autosomal dominant parkinsonism, depression, and alveolar hypoventilation (36).

Apathy may be present with or without depression, and is associated with deficits in tests of verbal memory and time-dependent tasks (34).

Neurochemical Aspects

Mayeux et al (30) reported an association between depression in PD and decreased cerebrospinal fluid 5-hydroxyindoleacetic acid (CSF 5-HIAA). There was little correlation between severity of depression and the level of 5-HIAA, but the greatest reduction was in patients with major depression. Lower CSF 5-HIAA was associated with psychomotor retardation and loss of self-esteem in both parkinsonian and nonparkinsonian depression. No correlation between depression and CSF 4-methoxy-3-hydroxyphenylglycol (MHPG), a dopamine metabolite, was demonstrated. Nevertheless, other authors suggest that dopaminergic mechanisms may play a role (37,38).

Studies disagree as to the value of the dexamethasone suppression test in PD with depression (19,20). The test is often abnormal in PD but is not sensitive or specific enough to serve as a marker for depression.

Single photon emission computerized tomography (SPECT) studies have shown correlations between depression and impaired dorsolateral frontal lobe perfusion (39), as has also been reported in idiopathic depression (17). Impaired perfusion has also been found in anteromedial regions of medial frontal cortex, cingulate cortex (40), caudate nuclei, and orbitofrontal cortex (41).

Pharmacological Aspects and Treatment

Some reports suggest that L-dopa has a mood elevating effect, but this could be due to an improvement in motor symptoms (18). Some studies showed no effect (42) and others have reported re-emergence of affective symptoms (43). In one case, L-dopa may have resulted in suicide (44).

Cantello et al (45) assessed fluctuations in mood in relation to "mobile" and "immobile" periods in L-dopa–treated PD with end-of-dose deterioration, using subjects with active rheumatoid arthritis as controls. Worsening mood during temporary immobility was more marked in patients with PD, suggesting a correlation with fluctuating central dopaminergic function.

Unfortunately, very few controlled studies of pharmacologic treatment of depression in PD have been performed and further research is required (46). Many depressed parkinsonians respond to treatment with tricyclic antidepressants (47) or electroconvulsive therapy (48). Improvement in bradykinesia and rigidity has been observed with both forms of treatment (18). Trials of 5-hydroxytryptophan have resulted in varying responses, including increased bradykinesia and rigidity, decreased tremor, and improved or worsened depression (30).

Brown and MacCarthy (29) suggest that mildly disabled patients with depression are best treated by better control of parkinsonian symptoms. In more severely disabled patients, this is likely to be ineffective and direct treatment of the depression may be indicated. The same applies in cases where guilt and self-blame are present—features not "typical" of parkinsonian depression.

DEMENTIA IN PD

Prevalence

Estimates of the prevalence of dementia in PD vary enormously (49), largely due to differences in defining dementia, assessing it, and patient selection. The DSM-IV criteria for dementia require memory impairment and disturbance of at least one other cognitive function sufficient to interfere with social or occupational activities (50). Few studies have used these criteria, and their use in parkinsonism is complicated by motor dysfunction.

Brown and Marsden (51) consider that the true frequency of dementia in PD lies between 15% and 20%. Since most parkinsonians are elderly, there is the possibility of coincidental AD, but the frequency of dementia is probably 10% to 15% greater than expected.

Stern et al (52) reported the following risk factors for dementia: age greater than 70, a PD rating scale score greater than 25, depression, confusion, or psychosis on L-dopa, and facial masking as a presenting sign. Age is a critical determining factor in the rate and type of cognitive decline in PD and late onset cases have a much higher rate of dementia.

Clinical Features

The cognitive disturbance in PD ranges from specific cognitive deficits, demonstrated by detailed neuropsychologic examination, to overt dementia, and there is a continuous spectrum between these two extremes (53). It does not necessarily follow that isolated cognitive defects are the precursor of parkinsonian dementia, but there is evidence that cognitive defects do progress (54,55). There is evidence of a preclinical phase of dementia and tests of verbal fluency may be a good predictor of later dementia (56).

Dementia in PD is in many ways similar to that of AD but is milder and less rapidly progressive (49). PD is characterized, moreover, by a paucity of dysphasia, apraxia, and agnosia, prominent features of AD and other "cortical" dementias. Brown and Marsden (57) highlighted evidence for fundamental differences between the two diseases. These include impaired visuoperceptual matching in PD, a task performed normally by AD patients (58). There may be selective impairment in the dating of historical photographs in PD, while AD caused difficulties in recognition of the scenes as well (59). Freedman and Oscar-Berman (60) found impairment in both AD and PD in frontal lobe tasks, including tests of tactile original and tactile reversal learning. Patients with AD were impaired on tactile original learning, and both groups were impaired on tactile reversal learning, with the AD group making more perseverative errors. Such differences suggest separate mechanisms for dementia in the two diseases.

Cummings suggested that there are three types of dementia in PD: a relatively mild subcortical dementia, a more severe form with a wider range of cognitive impairment but neuropathologically distinct from AD, and a third severe dementia with subcortical and cortical involvement that may reflect basal ganglia and Alzheimer-type pathology (61).

Specific Cognitive Impairment in PD

Neuropsychologic testing reveals specific impairments in most parkinsonian patients, even in the absence of overt dementia (49), and in early onset PD (62). The pattern of impairment suggests frontostriatal dysfunction (63,64). Patients have disorders mainly of problem solving, memory, and attention (65). They are less capable of changing strategies for solution of cognitive problems and have impaired performance if they have to solve a problem by means of internally generated strategies.

Visuospatial impairment has been frequently reported, but it is possible that primary disturbances of executive functions may be responsible for these findings. Impaired tasks include route finding, pursuit tracking, and judgment of the visual and postural vertical (49). Such tasks are performed poorly even when they include no motor component (66). In some studies, however, no abnormality of visuospatial function has been observed (67,68), especially when tasks requiring speed of motor performance are omitted (69). Wilson et al (70) showed that, when age and verbal intelligence are controlled, PD patients show no deficit on purely spatial tasks.

Disturbances of attentional control may be present in PD. There is no deficit of focused attention, but patients cannot divide their attention between two different tasks and they cannot shift attention from an externally cued task to an internally controlled one (65,71). Downes et al (72) postulated a deficit in inhibitory attentional processes and an impairment in the maintenance of internal representations that control action.

Memory deficits include impairment of both immediate and long-term memory, verbal and nonverbal memory, and in tasks using visual, auditory, and somatosensory stimuli. Tests have included digit span, immediate recall of drawings, and delayed recall of prose (11). Usually they are impaired on free recall paradigms but not in cued recall and recognition (73). On recognition tasks, patients tend to fare better than those with AD (74). Parkinsonians are disproportionately impaired in their ability to temporally order or sequence new information (75). Patients with PD are able to use semantic encoding, but usually do not do so spontaneously. Evidence suggests that the impairment in memory may involve the retrieval stage, as retrieval cues improve performance, and recall of past events is impaired with no temporal gradient (11). PD patients have disturbances of explicit memory rather than of automatic (modality monitoring and word frequency estimation) or implicit (word and picture fragment identification) memory tasks (76). Taylor suggested apparent memory impairment was due to lack of spontaneous organization of material to be memorized (77). These findings demonstrate a distinction between the true amnestic syndrome of AD and basal ganglia disorders.

Language impairment has generally been reported to be absent (18), but a few reports have shown deficits in naming and verbal fluency in PD (78–80). The "tip of the tongue" phenomenon, described by Matison et al (79) may be a manifestation of bradyphrenia or bradykinesia rather than a language dysfunction. Cummings et al (81) have demonstrated language disturbance to be more severe in AD than in PD with dementia of comparable severity. Nevertheless, impaired verbal fluency may be a good predictor of future dementia in PD.

Sequencing may be disturbed in PD as demonstrated by the picture arrangement subtest of the Wechsler adult intelligence scale (WAIS), in which cartoons must be placed in a logical order to tell a story (59). Patients are impaired in concept shifting and planning as demonstrated by the "Tower of London" test and card sorting tests, respectively (65). A set-shifting deficit, with inability to change cognitive attitude in response to environmental requirements, has been demonstrated using the Wisconsin card sort (82) and the Stroop word-color test (83). The set-shifting deficit appears to be a primary cognitive impairment in PD and presumably arises from dysfunction of the nigrostriatal–dorsolateral prefrontal cortex complex loop (84). Reitan and Boll (85) have demonstrated difficulty in logical analysis and in abstract reasoning.

Many of the above functions may be the result of a disturbance of "executive functions." Baddeley's tripartite model includes a central executive responsible for controlling nonroutine current mental activities by coordinating and supervising subordinate short-term memory processes and retrieval of information from long-term memory (86). The two subordinate systems are the phonological loop system, responsible for speech-based information, and the visuospatial sketchpad. A disturbance in the central executive may explain some of the disparate results in the literature concerning set shifting and visuospatial tasks and explain the attentional, memory, and planning deficits of PD.

Bradyphrenia in PD

Bradyphrenia may be a feature of PD (87,88). This implies slowing of cognitive processes, usually associated with impaired concentration and apathy (16). It is demonstrated by applying tests of different cognitive complexity that require the same motor responses and comparing the patient's reaction times, or by demonstrating accurate performance of cognitive tests given sufficient time. Sager and Sullivan (75) showed on a stimulus-recognition test that PD patients were selectively impaired at shorter stimulus intervals, unlike patients with AD.

Not all agree that there is bradyphrenia in PD. Rogers et al (88) reported that cognitive slowing was only significant in patients who had structural lesions outside the corpus striatum on computerized tomography or who had depression. Medicated PD patients were able to mentally rotate alphanumeric or figural stimuli as rapidly as normal healthy controls (89). In another study, no slowing was demonstrated on a memory scanning task (90).

The Relationship Between Dementia and Parkinsonism

Intellectual impairment in PD is related to the severity of motor dysfunction, especially bradykinesia, but not to duration of disease (91). There may also be a correlation between dementia and age of onset of PD to the extent that there may be two types of disease: an early onset form causing motor disturbance only and responding well to therapy, and a late-onset form with intellectual disturbance, fulminant course, and poor response to therapy (18).

One of the authors (M.P.) has described the findings in 39 patients with idiopathic PD (92). Visuospatial and perceptuomotor dysfunction and Mini-Mental Status Examination scores paralleled the extrapyramidal deficit. Patient age closely correlated with motor and cognitive function but age of onset did not appear to be a predictive variable.

Portin and Rinne (93) found that the course of parkinsonian disability and cognitive deterioration is similar but with some discrepancies. Visuomotor deterioration and impaired daily activities were more related to cognitive change than to parkinsonian disability. Old age, pretreatment cognitive decline, deteriorating response to L-dopa (but not pretreatment parkinsonian disability and disease duration) were of predictive value.

Hietanen and Teravainen (94) have compared early- and late-onset cases of PD. While they found that later age of onset (greater than 60 years) is associated with a higher incidence of dementia but with marked variability, they also showed cognitive disturbances in early-onset cases. They concluded there may be chance occurrence of AD in the older age group.

It is unclear whether the side of onset affects dementia in PD. Increased cognitive decline has been reported both with left-sided onset (95) and bilateral onset (96), while Finali et al found no relation to side of onset (97).

The Relationship Between Dementia and Depression in PD

Depressed parkinsonians may also be demented. Mayeux (18) demonstrated a correlation between severity of depression and deficits in attention, calculation, and recall. The relationship was thought to be independent because of the weak correlation found between depression and disease severity. Depression exacerbates some memory and language impairment associated with PD, influencing the quantity rather than quality of cognitive impairment (98). Patients with PD and depression tend to have more marked frontal lobe dysfunction that those without mood alterations (17). On tests of bradyphrenia, patients with primary depressive illness have shown psychomotor slowing comparable in degree with patients with PD (83). Mortimer et al (91), however, found poor correlation between depression and dementia and concluded that depression alone could not account for the incidence of cognitive impairment in PD.

Electrophysiologic Correlates

Electroencephalography (EEG) reveals a higher incidence of abnormalities in PD than in the normal population, although in the majority the EEG is normal (99). Previous studies failed to distinguish between demented and non-demented parkinsonians on EEG, but Korczyn et al (99) showed a correlation between slowing of the dominant EEG frequency and degree of dementia, although EEG abnormalities were more strongly related to motor disability. Increased amplitudes in the theta and delta ranges, with relatively decreased alpha amplitude, have been found in demented PD patients (100).

Goodin and Aminoff (101) studied long-latency auditory evoked potentials in PD and were able to distinguish AD, PD, and Huntington's disease (HD). N1, N2, and P3 peak latencies were prolonged in demented PD compared with the nondemented group and normal controls. Prolongation of the N1 latency distinguished demented parkinsonian group from patients with AD.

Okuda et al studied pattern reversal visual evoked potentials in PD using large checks and found a significant negative correlation between the P100 latency and the Mini-Mental Status Examination score (102).

An impairment in "processing negativity," an event-related potential that reflects neuronal activity during selective attention, has been correlated with poor performance on "frontal" neuropsychological tests in parkinsonian patients (103).

Radiological Correlates

Pneumoencephalography and computerized tomography (CT) have shown an increased incidence of cortical atrophy and ventricular enlargement in PD, with mental impairment related to ventricular dilatation but not to cerebral atrophy (18). Lichter et al (92) demonstrated no difference between parkinsonians and controls. There was, however, a correlation between the block design subtest of the WAIS and the bicaudate diameter and width of the anterior interhemispheric fissure. This test also correlated with certain indices of cortical and subcortical volume atrophy. Korczyn et al (99) found only intercaudate distance and width of the third ventricle correlated with dementia, and pointed out that the latter parameter correlates with cognitive decline in AD. In a more recent study, there was a significant correlation between neuropsychologic deficits and atrophy in specific brain areas (104).

A SPECT study showed cognitive function closely related to temporal lobe perfusion, while frontal lobe abilities were more linked to frontal perfusion and the presence of depression (105). In another study, 12 of 13 demented PD patients had significantly less blood flow in frontal lobes, although some had hypoperfusion in a other areas as well, probably reflecting Alzheimer's or other pathology (106). In a further study, cortical perfusion defects were highly correlated with cognitive impairment. The pattern of SPECT abnormality in most demented patients with PD was similar to that seen in AD (107).

In a study using positron emission tomography (PET), diffuse glucose hypometabolism in the cerebral cortex was seen in PD with dementia (108). In the study of Peppard et al (109), the pattern of glucose hypometabolism seen in the demented patients with PD resembled that described in patients with AD, with a global decrease in glucose metabolism, and more severe abnormalities observed in the temporo-parietal regions.

Neuropathologic Correlates

The pathology in parkinsonian dementia involves both cerebral cortex and subcortical structures. The two main types of change are those associated with AD (neurofibrillary tangles and plaques) and Lewy bodies (110). These may be associated with damage to the nucleus basalis of Meynert and with depleted cholinergic input to the cortex.

Senile plaques, neurofibrillary tangles, and granulovacuolar degeneration, hallmarks of AD, are common in brains of patients with PD (111) but it is not clear how this relates to the cognitive disturbances. Although Boller et al (66) showed a significant correlation between intellectual impairment and Alzheimer change, this has not been a consistent finding. Conversely, Lewy bodies may be seen in Alzheimer brains (112). Degeneration of the nucleus basalis of Meynert, the locus coeruleus, and dorsal raphe nucleus are commonly seen in both PD and AD, and cell loss from the nucleus basalis of Meynert may be more frequent in demented than nondemented PD (112).

In a recent study, Alzheimer-type pathology was thought to be the major pathological determinant of cognitive change in PD (113). In another study, a neuropathologic staging based on the distribution of neurofibrillary tangles correlated with psychological status in both AD and PD (114).

Lewy bodies may be seen in the cerebral cortex as well as in the basal ganglia. They are widely scattered in moderate numbers in diffuse Lewy body disease (115). A moderate scattering of Lewy bodies in limbic regions is seen in 5% to 10% of parkinsonians, and these patients often have dementia (116).

Zweig and colleagues found that the presence of dementia was associated 1) with significantly lower locus coeruleus neuronal count and greater neuronal loss within the ventral tegmental area, nucleus basalis of Meynert, and possibly the medial (but not the lateral) substantia nigra pars compacta, and 2) with more Lewy bodies in the anterior cingulate gyrus (117).

The neuropathologic substrate for dementia in PD is by no means clear. It seems likely, however, that dementia in PD is not always associated with Alzheimer changes (118), and it is uncertain whether Alzheimer changes are more frequent than expected by chance (112).

Neurochemical Correlates

Cortical choline acetyltransferase deficiency has been found in PD with and without Alzheimer changes (119). This is the neurochemical marker best correlated with severity of dementia in both PD and AD, but deficiency has also been seen in PD in the absence of dementia (120). Javoy-Agid and Agid (121) found decreased dopamine in cortical projection areas receiving fibers from the dopamine-containing neurons of the mesencephalon and they suggested that this may play a role in cognitive impairment. Reduced cortical noradrenaline and serotonin levels are found in both AD and PD, but no correlation with dementia has been shown in the latter (112).

Cash et al (122) showed decreased norepinephrine, 3-methoxy-4-hydroxyphenylglycol (MHPG), and homovanillic acid (HVA) levels in demented parkinsonians, but not in parkinsonians without intellectual impairment. Mayeux et al (123) found a correlation between CSF MHPG and a continuous performance task and reaction times in parkinsonians; patients with bradyphrenia had the highest levels. Reduced cortical serotonin has been demonstrated in AD and PD, and reduced somatostatin-like immunoreactivity has been found in the frontal cortex of demented parkinsonians (112).

Tau proteins are a biochemical marker for AD and have been demonstrated to be more pronounced in demented PD patients compared to nondemented PD patients in the prefrontal area, temporal cortex, and entorhinal cortex but not in the occipital or cingulate cortices. This suggests that lesions of the prefrontal cortex may significantly contribute to the occurrence of cognitive changes, at least in some patients with PD (124).

Pharmacologic Aspects

A number of investigators have suggested an association between dementia and poor response to treatment in PD (18). One study divided patients into four groups: untreated, good response to treatment, fluctuation, and poor response to treatment (125). All groups displayed deficits in psychomotor tests and in several tests of frontal lobe dysfunction, but only the poor response group was impaired on all tests. Ability to respond to dopamine replacement appeared to be more important than disease duration, length of treatment, or severity of motor impairment.

All anti-parkinsonian drugs may produce mental side effects, including behavioral changes, confusional states, or psychosis (91). Anticholinergics may lead to a confusional state and decreased memory function; monoamine oxidase inhibitors may potentiate certain side effects when used in combination with other compounds; and ergot alkaloids often induce severe psychiatric complications (126). L-dopa treatment may produce little effect on cognition, apart from nonspecific arousal and alleviation of concomitant depression (126).

A few reports have implicated both anticholinergics (127) and L-dopa as causing a permanent dementia (128). However, a high incidence of parkinsonian dementia was established by epidemiologic studies in the pre-L-dopa era (129), and it seems unlikely that the dementia of PD is drug-induced. Lieberman et al reported no differences in frequency of dementia between treated and untreated patients (130).

In contrast, several studies have suggested beneficial effects of L-dopa on cognition, and dementia may improve in the short term after starting L-dopa therapy (131). Cooper et al showed that while anticholinergic drugs produced impairment in processes underlying the immediate registration of information, dopaminergic therapy produced improvement on a task dependent on working memory and cognitive sequencing (132). Mohr et al (133) studied changes in cognitive function during fluctuations in L-dopa-treated parkinsonism. Changes in motor status were accompanied by selective improvement in delayed verbal memory, although this did not reach control levels during mobile periods. Rafal et al (134) showed no response of bradyphrenia to L-dopa treatment. Another study demonstrated that L-dopa improved verbal fluency but impaired performance on certain other tests of frontal lobe function (135). Malapani et al (136) found abnormalities in concurrent auditory and visual choice reaction tasks during "off" periods but not at times of maximal clinical benefit.

Other Parkinsonian Syndromes

Dementia is a prominent feature of parkinsonian syndromes other than idiopathic PD. Mindham (137) reported that the prevalence of dementia was similar irrespective of the type of parkinsonism, but a number of studies have suggested that arteriosclerotic parkinsonism is associated with a higher rate of dementia (129). Postencephalitic parkinsonism appears to cause dementia at a rate comparable with idiopathic PD. Dementia is prominent in the parkinsonism-dementia complex of Guam, a rapidly progressive form of parkinsonism associated with widespread neurofibrillary change and neuronal loss (91). In progressive supranuclear palsy, depression and ultimately dementia are characteristic features. Patients differ from AD in the relative sparing of language and comprehension deficits, and resemble PD in abnormalities of frontal lobe tests, including set-shifting, sequencing, and verbal fluency (138). Dementia is almost invariable in cortico-striatonigral degeneration and is common in Fahr's disease, a familial idiopathic calcification of the basal ganglia (4). Cognitive changes have been described in parkinsonism due to l-methyl-4-phenyl-1,2,3,6-tetrahydropyridine (MPTP) (139).

Robbins et al studied patients with idiopathic PD, multiple system atrophy, and progressive supranuclear palsy and concluded that these basal ganglia disorders share a distinctive pattern of cognitive deficits on tests of frontal lobe dysfunction, but that there are differences in the exact nature of the impairments (140). Striato-nigral degeneration manifests a dysexecutive syndrome similar to that of PD and less severe than progressive supranuclear palsy (141). Diffuse Lewy body disease typically causes a progressive cortical dementia (115).

ETIOLOGY

Depression

Depression in PD may be a reaction to a chronic disabling illness, an organic depressive state that is augmented by the pathologic and neurochemical consequences of PD, an integral feature of the disease itself, or a combination of these (4).

Undoubtedly, some patients become depressed because they have a disabling disease, but there is evidence that depression is more frequent than in other equally disabling diseases and there are often features of major depression

including vegetative disturbances and psychomotor retardation (18). Patients may have a history of depression prior to the start of PD, their mood may fluctuate with their motor state, and they may respond to L-dopa, tricyclic antidepressants, and electroconvulsive therapy (48). Such features suggest the presence of organic depression, although mania and bipolar features are rare (30).

PD causes deficits not only in dopaminergic pathways but also in noradrenergic, cholinergic, serotonergic, and peptidergic systems (112). Parkinsonian mood disturbances have been attributed to impairment of the mesocortical and mesolimbic dopaminergic pathways (45). These structures degenerate in PD and have been shown to be involved in the psychophysiologic reinforcement and reward processes that may be involved in depression. The relationship between mood and "on-off" motor changes would support this view. Alternatively, there is evidence of a correlation between mood and disturbed serotonin metabolism. A relationship between low brain serotonin, decreased CSF 5-HIAA, and primary depression is well-established (30).

Thus PD is associated with abnormalities in at least two neurotransmitter systems that have been implicated in depression, which supports the view that this complication is often a feature of the disease itself.

Dementia

Dementia in PD may be due to the simultaneous occurrence of AD (coincidentally or because PD and AD are simply part of a spectrum of neuronal degeneration (9) or an integral feature of the disease on the basis of "subcortical" pathology (12). Parkinsonian syndromes other than idiopathic PD may produce dementia by other mechanisms.

Estimates of the prevalence of dementia in idiopathic PD suggest that this is more common than would be expected by chance, but Quinn et al (112) argued that clinical AD occurs in only a proportion of those with pathologic features of disease and suggested that subclinical degrees of AD may combine with PD to cause dementia. In other words, AD is more likely to become clinically evident if the patient has PD as well. This may increase the prevalence of dementia in parkinsonians as compared with age-matched populations.

Alternatively, dementia as an integral part of PD is supported by neuropsychologic studies suggesting a different pattern of dementia in PD as compared with AD and by studies linking cognitive defects to the dysfunction in dopaminergic systems. The strong correlation between extrapyramidal and cognitive functions, especially between tests of visuospatial and perceptuomotor function and bradykinesia (92), favors the view that the specific cognitive deficits of PD are predominantly related to degeneration of the nigrostriatal and mesocortical dopaminergic systems (91). Changes in cognitive function during motor fluctuations (133) and evidence of cognitive deficits in MPTP parkinsonism, which has more restricted dopaminergic system pathology (139), further support this. Specific involvement of "frontal lobe" cognitive function in PD may reflect the close associations between the striatum and frontal cortex (135).

It is therefore likely that a proportion of demented parkinsonians have cognitive decline related to Alzheimer changes. It is also likely that the "subcortical" changes of PD can cause specific cognitive impairments and possibly bradyphrenia. It is less clear whether these specific cognitive impairments can combine to cause significant dementia without the superimposition of other pathology.

In our opinion it is unreasonable to blame either depression or dementia in PD on any one cause or on degeneration in any single system. It is a complex disease with multiple sites of neuropathology and multiple neurotransmitter abnormalities. It may well coexist at times with subclinical or overt AD. The fact that it results in disturbances of brain function other than purely motor is hardly surprising.

REFERENCES

1. Parkinson J. An essay on the shaking palsy. London: Sherwood, Neely and Jones, 1817.
2. Charcot JM, Vulpian A. De la paralysie agitante. Gaz Hebdom Méd Chir 1861;8:765–767.
3. Parant V. Paralysis agitans: insanity associated with. In: Tuke DH, ed. Dictionary of psychological medicine. London: Churchill Livingstone, 1892.
4. Whitlock FA. The psychiatric complications of Parkinson's disease. Aust NZ J Psychiatry 1986;20:114–121.
5. Patrick HT, Levy DM. Parkinson's disease: a clinical study of 146 case. Arch Neurol Psychiatry 1922;7:710–720.
6. Mjönes H. Paralysis agitans: a clinical and genetic study. Acta Psychiatr Neurol 1949;24(suppl 54):1–195.
7. Celesia GL, Wanamaker WM. Psychiatric disturbance in Parkinson's disease. Dis Nerv Syst 1972;33:577–583.
8. König H. Zur psychopathologie der paralysis agitans. Arch Psychiatr Nervenkr 1912;50:285–305.
9. Rossor MN. Parkinson's' disease and Alzheimer' disease as disorders of the isodendritic core. Br Med J 1981;2:1588–1590.
10. Albert M, Feldman RG, Willis AL. The "subcortical dementia" of progressive supranuclear palsy. J Neurol Neurosurg Psychiatry 1974;37:121–130.
11. Brown RG, Marsden CD. "Subcortical dementia" the neurophysical evidence. Neuroscience 1988;2:363–387.
12. Cummings JL. Subcortical dementia: neuropsychology, neuropsychiatry and pathophysiology. Br J Psychiatry 1986;149:682–697.
13. Whitehouse PJ. The concept of subcortical dementia: another look. Ann Neurol 1986;19:1–6.
14. Naville F. Les complications et les sequelles mentales de l'encephalite epidemique. Encephale 1922;17:369–375.
15. Wilson SAK. Progressive lenticular degeneration: a familial nervous disease associated with cirrhosis of the liver. Brain 1912;34:295–509.
16. Rogers D. Bradyphrenia in Parkinson's disease. Br J Hosp Med 1988;39:128–130.
17. Cummings JL. Depression and Parkinson's disease: a review. Am J Psychiatry 1992;149:443–454.
18. Mayeux R. Depression and dementia in Parkinson's disease. In: Marsden CD, Fahn S, eds. Movement disorders. London: Butterworths, 1981:75–95.
19. Pfeiffer RF, Hsieh HH, Dierks MJ, et al. Dexamethasone suppression test in Parkinson's disease. Adv Neurol 1986;45:439–442.
20. Warburton JW. Depressive symptoms in parkinsonian patients referred for thalamotomy. J Neurol Neurosurg Psychiatry 1967;30:368–370.
21. Santamaria J, Tosala E, Valles A. Parkinson's disease with depression: a possible subgroup of patients with idiopathic parkinsonism. Neurology 1986;36:1130–1133.
22. Brown RG, MacCarthy B, Gotham A-M, et al. Depression and disability in Parkinson's disease: a follow-up of 132 cases. Psychol Med 1988;18:49–55.
23. Robins AH. Depression in patients with parkinsonism. Br J Psychiatry 1976;128:141–145.
24. Hantz P, Caradoc-Davies G, Caradoc-Davies T, et al. Depression in Parkinson's' disease. Am J Psychiatry 1994;151:1010–1014.
25. Gotham A-M, Brown RG, Marsden CD. Depression in Parkinson's disease: a quantitative analysis. J Neurol Neurosurg Psychiatry 1986;49:381–389.
26. Santamaria J, Tolosa ES, Vallés A, et al. Mental depression in untreated Parkinson's disease of recent onset. Adv Neurol 1986;45:443–446.
27. Menza MA, Robertson-Hoffman DE, Bonapace AS. Parkinson's disease and anxiety: comorbidity with depression. Biol Psychiatry 1993;34:465–470.
28. Henderson R, Kurlan R, Kersun JM, Como P. Preliminary examination of the comorbidity of anxiety and depression in Parkinson's disease. J Neuropsychiatry Clin Neurosci 1992;4:257–264.
29. Brown RG, MacCarthy B. Psychiatric morbidity in patients with Parkinson's disease. Psychol Med 1990;20:77–87.
30. Mayeux R, Stern Y, Cote L, Williams JBW. Altered serotonin metabolism in depressed patients with Parkinson's disease. Neurology 1984;34:642–646.
31. Todes CJ, Lees AJ. The pre-morbid personality of patients with Parkinson's disease. J Neurol Neurosurg Psychiatry 1985;48:97–100.
32. Hubble JP, Venkatesh R, Hassanein RE, et al. Personality and depression in Parkinson's disease. J Nerv Ment Dis 1993;181:657–662.
33. Direnfeld LK, Albert ML, Volicer L, et al. Parkinson's disease: the possible relationship of laterality to dementia and neurochemical findings. Arch Neurol 1984;41:935–941.
34. Starkstein SE, Preziosi TJ, Bolduc PL, Robinson RG. Depression in Parkinson's disease. J Nerv Ment Dis 1990;178:27–31.
35. Haltenhof H, Schroter C. Depression beim Parkinson-syndrome. Eine Literaturubersicht. Fortschritte der Neurologie-Psychiatrie 1994;62:94–101.
36. Bhatia KP, Daniel SE, Marsden CD. Familial parkinsonism with depression: a clinicopathological study. Ann Neurol 1993;34:842–847.
37. McCance-Katz EF, Marek KL, Price LH. Serotonergic dysfunction in depression associated with Parkinson's disease. Neurology 1992;42:1813–1814.
38. Brown AS, Gershon S. Dopamine and depression. J Neural Transm 1993;91:75–109.
39. Jagust WJ, Reed BR, Martin EM, et al. Cognitive function and regional cerebral blood flow in Parkinson's disease. Brain 1992;115:521–537.
40. Ring HA, Bench CJ, Trimble MR, et al. Depression in Parkinson's disease: a positron emission study. Brit J Psychiatry 1994;165:333–339.
41. Mayberg HS, Starkstein SE, Sadzot B, et al. Selective hypometabolism in the inferior frontal lobe in depressed patients with Parkinson's disease. Ann Neurol 1990;28:57–64.
42. Marsh GG, Markham CH. Does levodopa alter depression and psychopathology in parkinsonian patients? J Neurol Neurosurg Psychiatry 1973;36:925–935.
43. Mindham RHS, Marsden CD, Parkes JD. Psychiatric symptoms during L-dopa therapy for Parkinson's disease and their relationship to physical disability. Psychol Med 1976;6:23–33.
44. Raft D, Newman M, Spencer R. Suicide on L-dopa. South Med J 1972;65:312.
45. Cantello R, Gilli M, Riccio A, Bergamasco B. Mood changes associated with end of dose deterioration in Parkinson's disease: a controlled study. J Neurol Neurosurg Psychiatry 1986;49:11892–11990.
46. Klaassen T, Verhey FR, Sneijders GH, et al. Treatment of depression in Parkinson's disease: a meta-analysis. J Neuropsychiatry Clin Neurosci 1995;7:281–286.
47. Laitinen L. Desipramine in treatment of Parkinson's' disease. Acta Neurol Scand 1969;45:109–113.
48. Lebensohn Z, Jenkins RB. Improvement of parkinsonism in depressed patients treated with ECT. Am J Psychiatry 1975;132:283–285.
49. Growdon JH, Corkin S. Cognitive impairments in Parkinson's disease. Adv Neurol 1986;45:383–392.
50. American Psychiatric Association. Diagnostic and statistical manual of mental disorders. 4th ed. Washington: American Psychiatric Association, 1994.
51. Brown RG, Marsden CD. How common is dementia in Parkinson's disease? Lancet 1984;ii:1262–1265.
52. Stern Y, Marder K, Tang MX, Mayeux R. Antecedent clinical features associated with dementia in Parkinson's disease. Neurology 1993;43:1690–1692.
53. Girotti F, Marano R, Grazzi L, et al. Cognitive impairment in Parkinson's disease. J Neural Transm 1986;(suppl 22):163–170.
54. Caparros-Lefebvre D, Blond S, Pecheux N, et al. Evaluation neuropsychologique avant et apres stimulation thalamique chez 9 parkinsoniens. Rev Neurol 1992;148:117–122.

55. Piccirilli M, D'Alessandro P, Finali G, Piccinin GL. Neuropsychological follow-up of parkinsonian patients with and without cognitive impairment. Dementia 1994;5:17–22.
56. Jacobs D, Marder K, Cote LJ, et al. Neuropsychological characteristics of preclinical dementia in Parkinson's disease. Neurology 1995;45:1691–1696.
57. Brown RG, Marsden CD. "Subcortical dementia": the neuropsychological evidence. Neuroscience 1988;25:363–387.
58. Sahakian BJ, Morris RG, Evenden JL, et al. A comparative study of visuospatial memory and learning in Alzheimer-type dementia and Parkinson's disease. Brain 1988;111:695–718.
59. Sagar HJ, Cohen NJ, Sullivan EV, et al. Remote memory function in Alzheimer's disease and Parkinson's disease. Brain 1988;111:185–206.
60. Freedman M, Oscar-Berman M. Tactile discrimination learning deficits in Alzheimer's and Parkinson's disease. Arch Neurol 1987;44:394–398.
61. Levin BE, Tomer R, Rey GJ. Cognitive impairments in Parkinson's disease. Neurol Clin 1992;10:471–485.
62. Tsai CH, Lu CS, Hua MS, et al. Cognitive dysfunction in early onset parkinsonism. Acta Neurol Scand 1994;89:9–14.
63. Channon S, Jones MC, Stephenson S. Cognitive strategies and hypothesis testing during discrimination learning in Parkinson's disease. Neuropsychologia 1993;31:75–82.
64. Owen AM, James M, Leigh PN, et al. Fronto-striatal cognitive deficits at different stages of Parkinson's disease. Brain 1992;115(pt 6):1727–1751.
65. Berger HJC, van Spaendonck KPM, Horstink MWIM, Cools AR. Can cognitive assessment contribute to the diagnostics of Parkinson's disease? Focus on Parkinson's Disease 1995;7:52–57.
66. Boller F, Passafiumi D, Keefe NC, et al. Visuospatial function in Parkinson's disease. Brain 1986;109:987–1002.
67. Brown RG, Marsden CD. Visuospatial function in Parkinson's disease. Brain 1986;109:987–1002.
68. Della Sala S, Di Lorenzo G, Giodano A, Spinnier H. Is there a specific visuospatial impairment in parkinsonism? J Neurol Neurosurg Psychiatry 1986;49:1258–1265.
69. Stelmach GE, Philips JG, Chau AW. Visuospatial processing in parkinsonians. Neuropsychologia 1989;27:485–493.
70. Wilson RS, Gilley DW, Tanner CM, Goetz CG. Ideational fluency in Parkinson's disease. Brain Cognition 1992;20(2):236–244.
71. Brown RG, Marsden CD. Internal vs. external cues and the control of attention in PD. Brain 1988;111:323–345.
72. Downes JJ, Sharp HM, Costall BM, et al. Alternating fluency in Parkinson's disease. An evaluation of the attentional control theory of cognitive impairment. Brain 1993;116(pt 4):887–902.
73. Pillon B, Deweer B, Agid Y, Dubois B. Explicit memory in Alzheimer's, Huntington's, and Parkinson's diseases. Arch Neurol 1993;50(4):374–379.
74. Flowers KA, Pearce I, Pearce JMS. Recognition memory in Parkinson's disease. J Neurol Neurosurg Psychiatry 1984;47:1174–1181.
75. Sagar HJ, Sullivan EV. Patterns of cognitive impairment in dementia. In: Kennard C, ed. Recent advances in clinical neurology. No. 5. Edinburgh: Churchill Livingstone, 1988.
76. Appollonio I, Grafman J, Clark K, et al. Implicit and explicit memory in patients with Parkinson's disease with and without dementia. Arch Neurol 1994;51(4):359–367.
77. Taylor AE, Saint-Cyr JA, Lang AE. Memory and learning in early Parkinson's disease: evidence for a "frontal lobe syndrome." Brain Cogn 1990;13:211–232.
78. Lees AR, Smith E. Cognitive deficits in early stages of Parkinson's disease. Brain 1983;106:257–270.
79. Matison R, Mayeux R, Rosen J, Fahn S. "Tip of the tongue" phenomenon in Parkinson's disease. Neurology 1982;32:567–570.
80. Jacobs DM, Marder K, Cote LJ, et al. Neuropsychological characteristics of preclinical dementia in Parkinson's disease. Neurology 1995;45(9):1691–1696.
81. Cummings JL, Darkins A, Mendez M, et al. Alzheimer's disease and Parkinson's disease: comparison of speech and language alterations. Neurology 1988;38:680–684.
82. Taylor AE, Saint-Cyr JA, Lang AE, Kenny FF. Frontal lobe dysfunction in Parkinson's disease: the cortical focus of neostriatal outflow. Brain 1986;109:845–883.
83. Hietanen M, Teravainen H. Cognitive performance in early Parkinson's disease. Acta Neurol Scand 1986;73:151–159.
84. Cronin-Golomb A, Corkin S, Growdon JH. Impaired problem solving in Parkinson's disease: impact of a set-shifting deficit. Neuropsychologia 1994;32(5):579–593.
85. Reitan RM, Boll TJ. Intellectual and cognitive function in Parkinson's disease. J Consult Clin Psychol 1971;37:364–369.
86. Dalrymple-Alford JC, Kalders AS, Jones RD, Watson RW. A central executive deficit in patients with Parkinson's disease. J Neurol Neurosurg Psychiatry 1994;57(3):360–367.
87. Wilson RS, Kaszniak AW, Klawans HL, Garron DC. High speed memory scanning in parkinsonism. Cortex 1980;16:67–72.
88. Rogers D, Lees AJ, Smith E, et al. Bradyphrenia in Parkinson's disease and psychomotor retardation in depressive illness: an experimental study. Brain 1987;110:761–776.
89. Duncombe ME, Bradshaw JL, Iansek R, Phillips JG. Parkinsonian patients without dementia or depression do not suffer from bradyphrenia as indexed by performance in mental rotation tasks with and without advance information. Neuropsychologia 1994;32(11):1383–1396.
90. Howard LA, Binks MG, Moore AP, Playfer JR. How convincing is the evidence for cognitive slowing in Parkinson's disease? Cortex 1994;30(3):431–443.
91. Mortimer JA, Christensen KJ, Wekster DD. Parkinsonian dementia. In: Frederiks JAM, ed. Handbook of clinical neurology. Vol. 46 (Revised series 2). Neurobehavioural disorders. Amsterdam: Elsevier, 1985:371–384.
92. Lichter DG, Corbett AJ, Fitzgibbon GM, et al. Cognitive and motor dysfunction in Parkinson's disease. Clinical, performance, and computed tomographic correlations. Arch Neurol 1988;45:854–860.
93. Portin R, Rinne UK. Predictive factors for cognitive deterioration in dementia in Parkinson's disease. Adv Neurol 1986;45:413–416.
94. Hietanen M, Teravainen H. The effect of age of disease onset on neuropsychological performance in Parkinson's disease. J Neurol Neurosurg Psychiatry 1988;51:244–249.
95. Tomer R, Levin BE, Weiner WJ. Side of onset of motor symptoms influences cognition in Parkinson's disease. Ann Neurol 1993;34(4):579–584.
96. Viitanen M, Mortimer JA, Webster DD. Association between presenting motor symptoms and the risk of cognitive impairment in Parkinson's disease. J Neurol Neurosurg Psychiatry 1994;57(10):1203–1207.
97. Finali G, Piccirilli M, Rizzuto S. Neuropsychological characteristics of parkinsonian patients with lateralized motor impairment. J Neural Transm 1995;9(2–3):165–176.
98. Troster AI, Stalp LD, Paolo AM, et al. Neuropsychological impairment in Parkinson's disease with and without depression. Arch Neurol 1995;52(12):1164–1169.
99. Korczyn AD, Inzelberg R, Treves T, et al. Dementia of Parkinson's disease. Adv Neurol 1986;45:399–403.
100. Neufeld MY, Blumen S, Aitkin I, et al. EEG frequency analysis in demented and nondemented parkinsonian patients. Dementia 1994;5(1):23–28.
101. Goodin DS, Aminoff MJ. Electrophysiological differences between demented and nondemented patients with Parkinson's disease. Ann Neurol 1987;21:90–94.
102. Okuda B, Tachibana H, Kawabata K, et al. Correlation of visual evoked potentials with dementia in Parkinson's disease. Nippon Ronen Igakkai Zasshi 1992;29(6):475–479.
103. Stam CJ, Visser SL, Op de Coul AA, et al. Disturbed frontal regulation of attention in Parkinson's disease. Brain 1993;116(5):1139–1158.
104. Starkstein SE, Leiguarda R. Neuropsychological correlates of brain atrophy in Parkinson's disease: a CT-scan study. Mov Disord 1993;8(1):51–55.
105. Jagust WJ, Reed BR, Martin EM, et al. Cognitive function and regional cerebral blood flow in Parkinson's disease. Brain 1992;115(2):521–537.
106. Sawada H, Udaka F, Kameyama M, et al. SPECT findings in Parkinson's disease associated with dementia. J Neurol Neurosurg Psychiatry 1992;55(10):960–963.
107. Liu RS, Lin KN, Wang SJ, et al. Cognition and 99Tcm-HMPAO SPECT in Parkinson's disease. Nucl Med Commun 1992;13(10):744–748.
108. Sasaki M, Ichiya Y, Hosokawa S, et al. Regional cerebral glucose metabolism in patients with Parkinson's disease with or without dementia. Ann Nucl Med 1992;6(4):241–246.
109. Peppard RF, Martin WR, Carr GD, et al. Cerebral glucose metabolism in Parkinson's disease with and without dementia. Arch Neurol 1992;49(12):1262–1268.
110. Gibb WRG, Luthert PJ. Dementia in Parkinson's disease and Lewy body disease. In: Burns A, Levy R, eds. Dementia. London: Chapman and Hall, 1994.
111. Hakim AH, Mathieson G. Dementia in Parkinson's disease: a neuropathological study. Neurology 1979;29:1209–1214.
112. Quinn NP, Rossor MN, Marsden CD. Dementia and Parkinson's disease: pathological and neurochemical consequences. Br Med Bull 1986;42:86–90.
113. de Vos RA, Jansen EN, Stam FC, et al. "Lewy body disease": clinico-pathological correlations in 18 consecutive cases of Parkinson's disease with and without dementia. Clinical Neurol Neurosurg 1995;97(1):13–22.

114. Bancher C, Braak H, Fischer P, Jellinger KA. Neuropathological staging of Alzheimer lesions and intellectual status in Alzheimer's and Parkinson's disease patients. Neurosci Lett 1993;162(1–2):179–182.

115. Kosaka K. Dementia and neuropathology in Lewy body disease. Adv Neurol 1993;60:456–463.

116. Yoshimura M. Cortical changes in the parkinsonian brain: a contribution to the delineation of diffuse Lewy body disease. J Neurol 1983;229:17–32.

117. Zweig RM, Cardillo JE, Cohen M, et al. The locus ceruleus and dementia in Parkinson's disease. Neurology 1993;43(5):986–991.

118. Chiu HC, Mortimer JA, Slager U, et al. Pathologic correlates of dementia in Parkinson's disease. Arch Neurol 1986;43:991–995.

119. Hornykiewicz O, Kiosh SJ. Neurochemical basis of dementia in Parkinson's disease. Can J Neurol Sci 1984;11(suppl):185–190.

120. Ruberg M, Ploska A, Javoy-Agid F, Agid Y. Muscarinic binding and choline acetyl transferase activity in parkinsonian subjects with reference to dementia. Brain Res 1982;232:129–139.

121. Javoy-Agid F, Agid Y. Is the mesocortical dopaminergic system involved in Parkinson's disease? Neurology 1980;30:1326–1330.

122. Cash R, Dennis T, L'Heureux R, et al. Parkinson's disease and dementia: norepinephrine and dopamine in locus coeruleus. Neurology 1987;37:42–46.

123. Mayeux R, Stern Y, Sano M, et al. Clinical and biochemical correlates of bradyphrenia in Parkinson's disease. Neurology 1987;37:1130–1134.

124. Vermersch P, Delacourte A, Javoy-Agid F, et al. Dementia in Parkinson's disease: biochemical evidence for cortical involvement using the immunodetection of abnormal Tau proteins. Ann Neurol 1993;33(5):445–450.

125. Taylor AE, Saint Cyr JA, Lang AE. Parkinson's disease: cognitive changes in relation to treatment response. Brain 1987;110:35–51.

126. Saint-Cyr JA, Taylor AE, Lang AE. Neuropsychological and psychiatric side effects in the treatment of Parkinson's disease. Neurology 1993;43(12 suppl 6):S47–52.

127. Nishiyama K, Mizuno T, Sakuta M, Kurisaki H. Chronic dementia in Parkinson's disease treated by anticholinergic agents. Neuropsychological and neuroradiological examination. Adv Neurol 1993;60:479–483.

128. Wolf SM, Davis RL. Permanent dementia in idiopathic parkinsonism treated with levodopa. Arch Neurol 1973;29:276–278.

129. Pollock M, Hornabrook RW. The prevalence, natural history and dementia of Parkinson's disease. Brain 1966;89:429–448.

130. Lieberman A, Dziatolowski M, Kupersmith M, et al. Dementia in Parkinson's disease. Ann Neurol 1979;6:355–359.

131. Sweet RD, McDowell FH, Feigenson JS, et al. Mental symptoms in Parkinson's disease during chronic treatment with levodopa. Neurology 1976;26:305–310.

132. Cooper JA, Sagar HJ, Doherty SM, et al. Different effects of dopaminergic and anticholinergic therapies on cognitive and motor function in Parkinson's disease. A follow-up study of untreated patients. Brain 1992;115(6):1701–1725.

133. Mohr E, Fabbrini G, Ruggieri S, et al. Cognitive concomitants of dopamine system stimulation in parkinsonian patients. J Neurol Neurosurg Psychiatry 1987;50:1192–1196.

134. Rafal RD, Posner MI, Walker JA, Friedrich FJ. Cognition and the basal ganglia: separating mental and motor components of performance in Parkinson's disease. Brain 1984;107:1083–1094.

135. Gotham AM, Brown RG, Marsden CD. "Frontal" cognitive function in patients with Parkinson's disease "on" and "off" levodopa. Brain 1988;111:299–321.

136. Malapani C, Pillon B, Dubois B, Agid Y. Impaired simultaneous cognitive task performance in Parkinson's disease: a dopamine-related dysfunction. Neurology 1994;44(2):319–326.

137. Mindham RHS. Psychiatric symptoms in parkinsonism. J Neurol Neurosurg Psychiatry 1970;33:188–191.

138. Maher ER, Smith EM, Lees AJ. Cognitive defects in the Steele-Richardson-Olszewski syndrome (progressive supranuclear palsy). J Neurol Neurosurg Psychiatry 1985;48:1234–1239.

139. Stern Y, Langston JW. Intellectual changes in patients with MPTP-induced parkinsonism. Neurology 1985;35:1506–1509.

140. Robbins TW, James M, Owen AM, et al. Cognitive deficits in progressive supranuclear palsy, Parkinson's disease, and multiple system atrophy in tests sensitive to frontal lobe dysfunction. J Neurol Neurosurg Psychiatry 1994;57(1):79–88.

141. Pillon B, Gouider-Khouja N, Deweer B, et al. Neuropsychological pattern of striatonigral degeneration: comparison with Parkinson's disease and progressive supranuclear palsy. J Neurol Neurosurg Psychiatry 1995;58(2):174–179.

The Etiology of Parkinson's Disease

Barry J. Snow

INTRODUCTION

The etiology of Parkinson's disease remains unknown. This is despite continual speculation since the original description of the disease by James Parkinson in 1817 (1). Parkinson suspected that the location of the lesion was in the upper spinal cord, but he did not offer an opinion as to the cause of the disease. He did record the suggestions of his patients, however, which were quite reasonable and included "indulgence in spirituous liquors," "long lying on damp ground," and "considerable exertion of the involved limb."

The syndrome of parkinsonism is characterized by tremor, rigidity, bradykinesia (slowness of movement), and impaired postural reflexes. While this syndrome may be due to a variety of causes, the majority of patients have so-called idiopathic or primary Parkinson's disease. The remainder have secondary parkinsonism due to a variety of causes including drugs, multiple system atrophies, metabolic disturbances, and perhaps viral infections.

Before exploring the cause of Parkinson's disease, it is worthwhile to consider the pattern of progression of the disease. In particular, it is important to separate the cause from pathogenetic process as these separate components often become confused with each other. The cause of Parkinson's disease is the triggering event—this may be some external factor or an internal event, perhaps on the basis of genetic susceptibility. Once triggered, the pattern of progression suggests that the process is self-sustaining—this is the pathogenesis (2). It is possible that more than one trigger can result in the same self-sustaining pathogenic process (3). Once the process is begun, there is nerve cell dysfunction followed by cell loss. Eventually there is sufficient loss of cells so that the patient develops symptoms of Parkinson's disease. The disease then progresses through various stages of severity. Finally the patient enters a stage of L-dopa-related complications. These may occur at a stage when the disease itself is no longer progressing or is progressing much more slowly than at the early stages of clinical disease.

TRIGGERING EVENTS

Genetics

There is no obvious genetic pattern of inheritance for the majority of patients with Parkinson's disease. This does not, however, exclude the possibility of a hereditary trait with poor penetrance or a genetic susceptibility to an external trigger (4). Several families have been described with dominantly inherited parkinsonism. Most have had features that distinguish them from sporadic Parkinson's disease. A few families have had otherwise typical Parkinson's disease, however (5). This suggests that at least some Parkinson's disease has a genetic basis.

Further support for the possibility of a genetic basis for Parkinson's disease comes from careful family studies. With good case ascertainment, various studies have shown an approximately twofold increased risk of parkinsonism in the relatives of patients with Parkinson's disease (6).

An increased familial risk of Parkinson's disease does not distinguish shared environmental exposure from a genetic factor, however; this issue is best addressed in twin studies. There have been three studies comparing the frequency of parkinsonism in the co-twins of monozygotic and dizygotic patients with Parkinson's disease (7–10). No difference in the frequency of parkinsonism was demonstrated in any of these studies leading to the conclusion that there was not a primary genetic component to the disease. These studies are confounded by the difficulties with definition and diagnosis of Parkinson's disease, and when different criteria are applied to these studies, it is possible to produce a result that supports the hypothesis of a genetic basis for Parkinson's disease (11).

Taken together, it is reasonable to conclude that there is a genetic component to the etiology of Parkinson's disease but that some external factor probably influences the likelihood of developing the disease.

Environmental Toxins

The lack of a strong genetic factor for the trigger of Parkinson's disease diverts attention to the possibility of an environmental toxin. No satisfactory candidate was identified until the early 1980s when a group of drug addicts in California developed parkinsonism and were found to have injected 1-methyl-4-phenyl-1,2,3,6-tetrahydropyridine (MPTP), a synthetic heroin (12,13). MPTP-induced parkinsonism bears a remarkable similarity to Parkinson's disease. The clinical features are almost identical apart from a lower frequency of tremor. Patients are responsive to L-dopa, and they develop the typical L-dopa-related complications of motor fluctuations, dyskinesias, and hallucinations. Animals exposed to MPTP demonstrate loss of pigmented cells from the substantia nigra with an associated loss of dopamine from the striatum (14). Low-dose exposure to MPTP produces a distribution of striatal dopamine loss that is similar to the distinctive pattern seen in Parkinson's disease (15–18). Aged monkeys treated with MPTP develop intraneuronal inclusions with similarities to Lewy bodies (16).

MPTP is unlikely to be responsible for Parkinson's disease, however. Intensive searches have not revealed environmental equivalents with similar toxicity for nigral dopaminergic neurones. A number of cases have been described with toxin-induced parkinsonism. These include patients exposed to hexanes, toluene, and petroleum products (19–21). Insufficient numbers of these patients have been seen to determine how closely their condition mimics Parkinson's disease.

Infections

Encephalitis lethargica occurred in pandemics from 1919 until 1926 (22). Large numbers of survivors were left with neurologic sequelae, including a form of progressive parkinsonism. Despite important clinical differences between the two conditions, this experience led to the suggestion that Parkinson's disease was caused by a viral infection. Poskanzer and Schwab predicted that Parkinson's disease would disappear in the 1980s as the last of the postencephalitic patients died (23). The continuing occurrence of Parkinson's disease has disproved this theory, but other viral causes have been sought. Parkinsonism may occur after the acute phase of measles, Japanese B encephalitis, and Western equine encephalitis (24–26). In these conditions, the syndrome is even less like Parkinson's disease than encephalitis lethargica

in that it always occurs immediately following infection and there is subsequent improvement.

Two recent observations suggest that viral infection may produce parkinsonism. Lin et al described a patient with typical parkinsonism following an acute flu-like illness, but no virus was identified (27). The patient had prominent signal changes of the substantia nigra on magnetic resonance imaging (MRI) that improved as the parkinsonism improved. Positron emission tomography (PET) revealed a pattern of dopaminergic deficit similar to Parkinson's disease with reduced fluorodopa uptake, indicating impaired dopaminergic transmission, and increased raclopride binding, indicating upregulation of dopamine receptors. Takahashi et al infected mice with a neurovirulent strain of influenza A virus and demonstrated sensitivity for the ventral substantia nigra and hippocampus (28). These findings raise the possibility that viral infections, perhaps specifically influenza A, could induce Parkinson's disease. The problem with any theory postulating an infectious cause for Parkinson's disease is that the disease does not present in clusters or epidemics. In addition, attempts to transmit viruses or prions have been unsuccessful.

An intriguing observation by Kohbata and Beamann suggested that infection with *Nocardia asteroides* could induce damage to the substantia nigra (29). Following experimental introduction of infection, there is both clinical and pathologic evidence for substantia nigra damage. Nocardia is widespread in the soil and, if it does cause human parkinsonism, could explain the increased risk of Parkinson's disease in agricultural workers (30,31). A case-controlled study did not show an increased frequency of *Nocardia* antibodies in patients with Parkinson's disease compared with controls (32).

Recently, the twin studies mentioned under *Genetics*, above, have been further reinterpreted to support a hypothesis that prion analogues may cause Parkinson's disease (33). The authors make the point that the rate of Parkinson's disease seems to be similarly increased in both monozygotic and dizygotic twins. They suggest that this could be due to shared exposure to a prion.

PATHOGENESIS

While the triggering event remains unknown, there are a number of candidates for the ongoing pathogenetic process. Parkinson's disease is almost invariably progressive. Usually the progression is continuous without step-wise advances. This pattern of progression is not consistent with repeated exposure to an environmental toxin. Thus the triggering event, whatever that is, must set off a self-sustaining mechanism leading to ongoing loss of dopaminergic neurons. Cross-sectional studies of substantia nigra cell counts at postmortem and analysis of clinical deficits both suggest that the decline in dopaminergic function is not linear but rather decelerating in an exponential pattern (2,34). This pattern is compatible with two mechanisms: an event or a process (35).

The "event hypothesis" suggests that the external insult kills some neurons and damages others. These damaged neurons have reduced survival potential. They die off successively and produce an exponential pattern of clinical decline. The "process hypothesis" suggests that the initial event causes the development of an ongoing mechanism that engages healthy neurones.

Three main possibilities for an ongoing process have been suggested: auto-oxidation, excitotoxins, and disturbances of mitochondrial function. The main pathway for the destruction of dopamine in the synaptic cleft is by oxidation by two forms of the enzyme monoamine oxidase (36). This leads to the formation of hydrogen peroxide and free radicals of oxygen. If left uncontrolled, free radicals can damage lipid membranes and lead to the destruction of neurones (37). Multiple mechanisms exist to control free radicals. Some of these seem to be deficient in Parkinson's disease (38). The outstanding question is whether these changes are the primary cause of the ongoing degeneration or simply secondary effects of degeneration due to another cause (39). Stemming from the oxidative theory of Parkinson's disease, several trials of the monoamine oxidase inhibitor selegiline have shown an apparent slowing of the progression of Parkinson's disease (40,41). While these results were initially greeted with much enthusiasm, subsequent scrutiny has shown that all the benefit may be explained by a symptomatic effect. Monoamine oxidase inhibition by selegiline does not slow the progression of Parkinson's disease (42,43).

Excitatory neurotransmitters such as glutamate are toxic to neurons in vitro and may play a role in the pathogenesis of Parkinson's disease (44). There are large excitatory inputs from the cortex to the basal ganglia. Some of these synapse with the terminals of the nigrostriatal dopaminergic neurons and could be toxic to those neurons. If proven, the excitotoxic theory has obvious therapeutic implications. Consistent with this idea is the report that the weak *N*-methyl-D-aspartate (NMDA) antagonist amantadine may prolong the survival of patients with Parkinson's disease (45). The development of nontoxic glutamate antagonists will lead to further interest in therapeutic trials to slow the progression of Parkinson's disease.

A further possible pathogenic mechanism for Parkinson's disease is a failure of energy production by disturbances of mitochondrial function. Studies of mitochondrial Complex I activity in platelets and substantia nigral tissue suggest that there may be a failure in Parkinson's disease (46–48). Further support for the hypothesis that mitochondrial function may be disturbed in Parkinson's disease is that the mechanism of MPTP toxicity is via inhibition of Complex I activity. In a way analogous to the oxidative issue described above, however, it is difficult to determine if mitochondrial dysfunction causes or is a result of the ongoing neurodegenerative process.

The search for the cause of Parkinson's disease is hampered by several features of the condition. First, it is difficult to diagnose. While the fully developed syndrome is unmistakable, parkinsonism (as distinct from Parkinson's disease) is associated with many conditions. Two postmortem studies have shown a misdiagnosis rate on the order of 25% (49,50). The misdiagnosed patients would have an important effect on the outcome of epidemiologic and therapeutic studies of Parkinson's disease. Second, there may be a substantial preclinical period before symptoms become apparent (51). Both animal and human experiments suggest that approximately 50% of substantia nigra dopaminergic neurones must be lost before clinical parkinsonism develops. If the progression of disease is slow, then this could mean that there is a very long preclinical period, perhaps up to 40 years. If this is the case, then the search for a transient exposure to an environmental toxin will be very difficult. If the progression of the disease is exponential, however, then the preclinical period would be much shorter—on the order of five years (2,52). This does not exclude the possibility of a triggering event many years before the start of exponential neuronal loss with a subsequent short latency to the onset of symptoms.

Finally, the remarkable range in clinical presentation and progression and the already known multiple causes of parkinsonism raise the possibility that what we know as Parkinson's disease is in fact a common expression of damage to the substantia nigra by multiple causes (3). If there is a range of potential triggering factors, then it will be very difficult to identify the cause of Parkinson's disease and develop preventive strategies. On the other hand, it still may be possible to determine what produces the ongoing process. If it is due to auto-oxidation or excitotoxicity, then it seems likely that protective mechanisms could be developed that slow the progression of disease. If the ongoing degeneration is due to an event with subsequent slow death of damaged neurones, then salvage measures using growth factors, perhaps delivered by molecular medicine techniques, may prove able to slow and reverse the dopaminergic deficits of Parkinson's disease.

REFERENCES

1. Parkinson J. An essay on the shaking palsy. London: Sherwood, Neely and Jones, 1817.
2. Lee CS, Schulzer M, Mak E, et al. Clinical observations on the rate of progression of idiopathic parkinsonism and a mathematical model of pathogenesis. Brain 1994;117:501–507.
3. Calne DB. Is "Parkinson's disease" one disease? J Neurol Neurosurg Psychiatry 1989;52:18–21.
4. Duvoisin RC, Golbe LI. Kindreds of dominantly inherited Parkinson's disease: keys to the riddle. Ann Neurol 1995;38:355–356.
5. Wszolek ZK, Pfeiffer B, Fulgham JR, et al. Western Nebraska family (family D) with autosomal dominant parkinsonism. Neurology 1995;45:502–505.
6. Marder K, Tang M, Mejia H, et al. Risk of Parkinson's disease among first degree relatives. Neurology 1996;47:155–160.
7. Duvoisin RC, Eldridge R, Williams AC. Twin study of Parkinson's disease. Neurology 1981;31:77–80.
8. Vieregge P, Schiffke KA, Friedrich HJ, et al. Parkinson's disease in twins. Neurology 1992;42:1453–1461.
9. Marsden CD. Parkinson's disease in twins. J Neurol Neurosurg Psychiatry 1987;50:105–106.

10. Martilla RJ, Kaprio J, Koskenvuo MD, Rinne UK. Parkinson's disease in a nationwide twin cohort. Neurology 1988;38:1217–1219.

11. Johnson WG, Hodge SE, Duvoisin RC. Twin studies and the genetics of Parkinson's disease—a reappraisal. Mov Disord 1990;5:187–194.

12. Davis GE, Williams AC, Markey SP, et al. Chronic parkinsonism secondary to intravenous injection of meperidine analogues. Psychiatry Res 1979;1:249–254.

13. Langston JW, Ballard PA, Tetrud JW, Irwin I. Chronic parkinsonism in humans due to a product of meperidine-analog synthesis. Science 1983;219:979–980.

14. Burns RS, Chiueh CC, Markey SP, et al. A primate model of parkinsonism: selective destruction of dopaminergic neurons in the pars compacta of the substantia nigra by N-methyl-4phenyl-1,2,3,6-tetrahydropyridine. Proc Natl Acad Sci 1983;80:4546–4550.

15. Moratalla R, Quinn B, DeLanney LE, et al. Differential vulnerability of primate caudate-putamen and striosome-matrix dopamine systems to the neurotoxic effects of 1-methyl-4-phenyl-1,2,3,6-tetrahydropyridine. Proc Natl Acad Sci USA 1992;89:3859–3863.

16. Forno LS, DeLanney LE, Irwin I, Langston JW. Similarities and differences between MPTP-induced parkinsonism and Parkinson's disease. Neuropathologic considerations. Adv Neurol 1993;60:600–608.

17. Hantraye P, Varastet M, Peschanski M, et al. Stable parkinsonian syndrome and uneven loss of striatal dopamine fibres following chronic MPTP administration in baboons. Neuroscience 1993;53:169–178.

18. Perez-Otano I, Oset C, Luquin MR, et al. MPTP-induced parkinsonism in primates: pattern of striatal dopamine loss following acute and chronic administration. Neurosci Lett 1994;175:121–125.

19. Pezzoli G, Barberi S, Ferrante C, Zecchinelli A. Parkinsonism due to n-hexane exposure. Lancet 1989;2:874.

20. Uitti RJ, Snow BJ, Shinotoh H, et al. Parkinsonism induced by solvent abuse. Ann Neurology 1994;35:616–619.

21. Tetrud JW, Langston JW, Irwin I, Snow BJ. Parkinsonism caused by petroleum waste ingestion. Neurology 1994;44:1051–1054.

22. Duvoisin RC, Yahr MD. Encephalitis and parkinsonism. Arch Neurol 1965;12:227–239.

23. Poskanzer DC, Schwab RS. Cohort analysis of Parkinson's syndrome: evidence for a single etiology related to sub-clinical infection around 1920. J Chron Dis 1963;16:961–973.

24. Shoji H, Watanabe M, Itoh S, et al. Japanese encephalitis and parkinsonism. J Neurol 1993;240:59–60.

25. Sasco AJ, Paffenberger RSJ. Measles infection and Parkinson's disease. Am J Epidemiol 1985;122:1017–1031.

26. Goto A. A follow-up study of Japanese B encephalitis. Psychiat Neurol Jpn 1962;64:236–266.

27. Lin S-K, Lu C-S, Vingerhoets FJG, et al. Isolated involvement of substantia nigra in acute transient parkinsonism: MRI and PET observations. Parkinsonism Relat Disord 1995;1:67–72.

28. Takahashi M, Yamada T, Nakajima S, et al. The substantia nigra is a major target for neurovirulent influenza A virus. J Exp Med 1995;181: 2161–2169.

29. Kohbata S, Beaman BL. L-dopa-responsive movement disorder caused by Nocardia asteroides localized in the brains of mice. Infect Immun 1991;59:181–191.

30. Tanner CM. The role of environmental toxins in the etiology of Parkinson's disease. Trends Neurosci 1989;12:49–54.

31. Tanner CM. Epidemiological clues to the cause of Parkinson's disease. In: Fahn S, Marsden CD, eds. Movement disorders. 3rd ed. London: Butterworths, 1993:124–146.

32. Hubble JP, Cao T, Kjelstrom JA, Koller WC, Beaman BL. Nocardia species as an etiologic agent in Parkinson's disease: serological testing in a case-control study. J Clin Microbiol 1995;33:2768–2769.

33. Sommer SS, Rocca WA. Prion analogues and twin studies in Parkinson's disease. Neurology 1996;46:273–275.

34. Fearnley JM, Lees AJ. Ageing and Parkinson's disease: substantia nigra regional selectivity. Brain 1991;114:2283–2301.

35. Calne DB. Is idiopathic parkinsonism a consequence of an event or a process? Neurology 1994;44:5–10.

36. Oreland L. Monoamine oxidase, dopamine and Parkinson's disease. Acta Neurol Scand 1991;81(suppl):60–65.

37. Cohen G. The pathobiology of Parkinson's disease: biochemical aspects of dopamine neuron senescence. J Neural Transm 1983;19(suppl):89–103.

38. Fahn S, Cohen G. The oxidant stress hypothesis in Parkinson's disease: evidence supporting it. Ann Neurol 1992;32:804–812.

39. Calne DB. The free radical hypothesis in idiopathic parkinsonism: evidence against it. Ann Neurol 1992;32:799–803.

40. The Parkinson Study Group. Effect of deprenyl on the progression of disability in early Parkinson's disease. N Engl J Med 1989;321:1364–1371.

41. Tetrud JW, Langston JW. The effect of deprenyl (selegiline) on the natural history of Parkinson's disease. Science 1989;245:519–522.

42. Parkinson Study Group. Impact of deprenyl and tocopherol treatment on Parkinson's disease in DATATOP subjects not requiring levodopa. Ann Neurol 1996;39:29–36.

43. Parkinson Study Group. Impact of deprenyl and tocopherol treatment on Parkinson's disease in DATATOP patients requiring levodopa. Ann Neurol 1996;39:37–45.

44. Turski L. Excitatory amino acid antagonists and Parkinson's disease. In: Rinne UK, Nagatsu T, Horowski R, eds. International workshop, Berlin: Parkinson's disease. Bussum, Netherlands: Medicom, 1991:97–112.

45. Uitti RJ, Rajput AH, Ahlskog JE, et al. Amantadine treatment is an independent predictor of impaired survival in Parkinson's disease. Neurology 1996;46:1551–1556.

46. Mizuno Y, Ohta S, Tanaka M. Deficiencies in Complex I subunits of the respiratory chain in Parkinson's disease. Biochem Biophys Res Commun 1989;163:1450–1455.

47. Schapira AHV, Cooper JM, Dexter DT, et al. Mitochondrial Complex I deficiency in Parkinson's disease. J Neurochem 1990;54:823–827.

48. Parker WD, Boyson SJ, Parks JK. Abnormalities of the electron transport chain in idiopathic Parkinson's disease. Ann Neurol 1989;26:719–723.

49. Hughes AJ, Daniel SE, Kilford L, Lees AJ. Accuracy of clinical diagnosis of idiopathic Parkinson's disease: a clinico-pathological study of 100 cases. J Neurol Neurosurg Psychiatry 1992;3:181–184.

50. Rajput AH, Rozdilsky B. Accuracy of clinical diagnosis in parkinsonism—a prospective survey. Can J Neurol Sci 1991;18:275–278.

51. Shults CW. Future perfect? Presymptomatic diagnosis. neural transplantation, and trophic factors. In: Cederbaum JM, Gancher ST, eds. Neurologic clinics: Parkinson's disease. Philadelphia: Saunders, 1992;567:592.

52. Shinotoh H, Vingerhoets FJG, Schulzer M, Snow BJ. The presymptomatic period in a patient with idiopathic parkinsonism. Parkinsonism and related disorders 1996;2:127–130.

The Side Effects of Chronic Treatment in Parkinson's Disease

CYNTHIA L. COMELLA   CAROLINE M. TANNER

INTRODUCTION

The drugs that are effective in the treatment of Parkinson's disease (PD) may be categorized into two classes. Dopaminergic agents are those that activate dopamine receptors either directly or indirectly. Included in this class are the indirect agonists such as amantadine, the direct acting agonists such as bromocriptine, and precursor agents such as L-dopa. The second class of drugs are the anticholinergic compounds.

With the introduction of dopaminergic agents, specifically L-dopa, in the 1960s, it was possible to prolong the life expectancy and lessen the disability of many patients with PD (1). However, it was not long after the introduction of L-dopa into clinical use that drug-induced side effects were described (2). These adverse effects can be divided into peripheral and central effects. The latter will be the focus of this chapter.

The centrally mediated adverse effects of chronic L-dopa therapy can be categorized into cognitive and behavioral disorders and motor abnormalities. The former include sleep abnormalities, hallucinations, psychosis, and confusional states. The motor effects include chorea, dystonia, myoclonus, and asterixis (3–9). These will be discussed in this chapter. The oscillations in motor performance will be reviewed in another chapter in this volume.

COGNITIVE AND BEHAVIORAL COMPLICATIONS

Diagnosis

The cognitive and behavioral changes encountered in PD can be separated into those resulting from the chronic administration of antiparkinsonian medications and those due to progression of the underlying degenerative disease. This distinction may be difficult, as dopaminergic drugs may exacerbate underlying mental dysfunction without being the causative agent. The cognitive and behavioral abnormalities that appear to be related to dopaminergic drugs are sleep disturbances, hallucinations, psychosis, and confusional states. Those that are likely to be related to the underlying degenerative disease are depression and dementia.

Sleep

Sleep disorders are a common complaint of the parkinsonian population, affecting as many as 74% of patients (10). The sleep disruption reported in PD may be related to three factors: akinesia, drug therapy, and depression.

The most common polysomnographic sign associated with PD is sleep fragmentation. Although this disorder has been reported as a side effect of dopaminergic therapy (10), formal sleep studies demonstrated increased sleep fragmentation in patients without treatment that resolved to baseline after treatment (11), suggesting that sleep fragmentation is more likely to be related to the symptoms of PD. In support of this, in a questionnaire study, Goetz et al found that akinesia and pain occurring during maximal parkinsonian symptoms can disrupt sleep, which may improve with an increase in medication (12).

Abnormal dream phenomena are associated with chronic dopaminergic therapy (10). The dreams are vivid ones, which seem very real, featuring persons and events from the patient's remote past. Nightmares, which are frightening, very real, and often paranoid in nature, and night terrors in which the patient screams out and thrashes about in sleep, but upon awakening is amnesic for the event, also occur (13). Less frequently reported sleep events in treated patients include nocturnal vocalizations, in which the patient calls out during sleep, somnambulism, and myoclonus (10,14).

Hallucinations and Psychosis

In most cases, the hallucinations are visual and lifelike, taking the form of people, sometimes relatives and friends from the past. There may be many people in the room, some of them familiar, although commonly, their faces will appear indistinct. Others may report seeing a solitary figure who appears repeatedly but does not speak. The hallucinations may feature animals, scurrying across the floor and furniture or appearing to enter through a closed window or door. Rarely, the images have a more fantastic quality. Inanimate objects may sprout legs and amble through the room. Miniature people may appear on window sills or under the bed (15). Ceilings and floors may appear to be in motion. Doors may seem to open and close.

Although the hallucinations may have an eerie quality, they are usually nonthreatening and after the initial few occurrences, are recognized by the patient as being distinct from reality (16,17). In some cases, however, the hallucinations may be of a more threatening nature, with menacing figures and strange creatures. The patient may believe that the figures in the hallucination are real and that they are going to do harm. Sometimes, the patient may seek protection from these images through the local authorities.

Although the hallucinations are most commonly visual, occasionally they may be auditory and feature voices that talk to the patient. Although the quality of the hallucinations may differ, there are a few characteristics that these phenomena tend to have in common. In any single patient, the hallucinations tend to be stereotyped, featuring the same images repeatedly. In addition, the hallucinatory events typically occur during the evening hours (18).

Anticholinergic drug toxicity or the advanced stages of chronic dopaminergic drug toxicity may produce a toxic delirium. This is characterized by confusion, agitation, hallucinations, and, sometimes, autonomic nervous system lability with tachycardia, mydriasis, and fever. These hallucinations are usually more unformed and lack a coherent theme.

Psychiatric disturbances related to chronic dopaminergic therapy occur in 20% to 30% of chronically treated patients (19). Psychotic reactions to L-dopa may be categorized as early-onset and late-onset psychosis (20). Early-onset psychotic reactions usually occur within weeks of drug initiation in patients who have a past history of a severe psychiatric disorder or a "nervous breakdown." L-dopa appears to exacerbate an underlying psychotic tendency in these patients. Late-onset psychosis, which occurs after several years of therapy in patients with no previous psychiatric history, typically affects those who have already experienced abnormal dream phenomena or hallucinations (20).

The latter psychosis typically is a paranoid delusional state, although obsessional and depressive qualities have also been described (21). It often presents in patients with an otherwise clear sensorium (17), although a toxic confusional state can coexist (19).

Other Behavioral Manifestations

There have been reports of hypersexuality occurring with chronic dopaminergic treatment of PD (C.M. Tanner, personal communication) (22). Although infrequent, this side effect, when it occurs, may be disabling. The patient, most typically male, becomes preoccupied with sexual intercourse and makes persistent attempts to satisfy these urges. The excessive demands may embarrass and exhaust the patient's spouse, and when directed toward those outside the home, may cause social and legal problems.

Euphoria, manifested by excessive self-confidence, and anxiety with apprehension, irritability, and autonomic overactivity may rarely occur with chronic dopaminergic therapy.

Dementia

Dementia occurs in 14% to 75% of PD patients (16,23–26), occurring up to 10 times more frequently in this group than in the general population of the same age (27).

Dopaminergic agents do not cause a progressive dementia. In fact, L-dopa may actually benefit some aspects of cognitive dysfunction in PD (28,29). The major clinical importance of dementia in relationship to drug therapy is that demented patients are more likely to develop adverse psychiatric reactions to a variety of drugs used to treat their disease, including amantadine, anticholinergics, and dopaminergic agents (30,31).

Anticholinergic agents frequently affect cognitive function. They may cause confusion or memory loss, even in patients without clinically significant dementia before treatment. They are particularly difficult to use in older patients as a toxic confusional state may occur in up to 90% of these patients (32).

Basic Science

Sleep

The effect of L-dopa on sleep architecture is not clear. There are reports of changes with both acute and chronic dopaminergic treatment. An acute, parenteral infusion of L-dopa or apomorphine, a dopamine agonist, is reported to induce sleep and cause a suppression of rapid eye movement (REM) and slow wave sleep in both controls and previously untreated PD patients (33,34). This effect is blocked by pretreatment with dopamine receptor antagonists (35). Kales et al report that within the first days of beginning oral L-dopa treatment in four untreated PD patients there is a decrease of REM in three and an increase in REM in one, with no effect on sleep induction or slow wave sleep (35,36).

The reports of the effects of chronic oral L-dopa differ. Schmidt and Knopp report that sleep studies in two patients after one month of treatment demonstrated an increase in REM sleep (37). Concomitant diazepam use, however, may have confounded this result. Kales et al report that one month after the start of L-dopa therapy, the sleep changes noted on initiation of treatment had returned to baseline, pretreatment levels in their four patients (35,36), a finding similar to the report by Greenburg and Pearlman (38). Askenasy and Yahr (11) also report no significant changes in REM sleep with chronic L-dopa treatment. This group, however, finds that sleep fragmentation is significantly improved by drug-related normalization of muscle activity, as demonstrated in five patients by analysis of polysomnographic records and simultaneous electromyography. Goetz et al observe that self-reported sleep disruption tends to occur more frequently in patients with pain related to parkinsonian symptoms, suggesting that in some PD patients, sleep disturbance is the result of the disease and not the treatment (12). In one study of patients with dysphoric dreams, the only abnormality is an absence of K-complexes and sleep spindles (10).

Serotonin plays a crucial role in sleep (39,40). Some studies in animals show that the acute administration of L-dopa causes a depletion of central serotonin (41,42). The subsequent administration of L-tryptophan, a serotonin precursor, reverses this depletion (43). Hence, it has been suggested that L-dopa's effect on sleep may be mediated through alterations in serotonin activity.

Hallucinations and Cognitive and Behavioral Disorders

Drug-induced hallucinations are typically late side effects of treatment. In contrast to drug-related dyskinesias, which can occur within months of treatment onset, hallucinations usually develop after several years of therapy. Reduction or discontinuation of dopaminergic or anticholinergic agents eliminates the hallucinations in most cases, but will leave the patient functionally disabled in most cases.

The pathogenesis of hallucinations in PD is unknown. They are believed to be induced by dopaminergic agents based on empiric observations. Although hallucinations occur rarely in untreated PD or in others with midbrain pathology, the occurrence of hallucinations in 33% of chronically treated PD patients (44) suggests that either disease duration or chronic dopaminergic treatment are important to their production. It is difficult to separate these, as patients with long disease duration are more likely to be treated with dopaminergic agents and those who remain untreated may have difficulty communicating. Empiric evidence supporting the role of dopaminergic agents is obtained from experiences treating hallucinating PD patients. These patients usually improve with a decrease or discontinuation of dopaminergic drugs, and the hallucinations tend to worsen with an increase of the drugs. Direct-acting dopaminergic agonists are even more likely to cause hallucinations and other behavioral abnormalities than L-dopa.

Classically, hallucinogens have been classified as aminergic or anticholinergic. The associated clinical states are distinctive. Aminergic hallucinations usually occur with a clear sensorium and feature vivid, fantastic images (45), whereas anticholinergic hallucinations typically occur associated with a toxic delirium and feature poorly formed images.

The typical hallucination in chronic PD is most similar phenomenologically to those produced by aminergic hallucinogens such as LSD. This drug is postulated to produce hallucinations by altering central serotonergic activity (45). Goetz et al, however, observe that in PD patients, identical hallucinations could result from increasing either L-dopa or anticholinergic drugs, suggesting a common pathogenesis (46).

The paranoid delusional state that can develop with chronic dopaminergic therapy usually occurs in the same clinical context as hallucinations. The psychosis usually appears in a patient who has had hallucinatory episodes in the past. Moskovitz et al postulated that this suggests a kindling phenomenon similar to that reported in epilepsy, where continued dopaminergic stimulation results in agonist-induced hypersensitivity involving a progressively greater population of neurons (17).

Sleep abnormalities have been hypothesized to be the initial manifestation of a progressive psychiatric disorder due to chronic dopaminergic therapy (10). This hypothesis is based on the observation that, of the patients who develop hallucinations as a result of treatment, almost all report preceding sleep disturbances. Sleep fragmentation, vivid dreams, and nightmares are the most common. Nocturnal myoclonus, while less common, is reported to be always associated with other abnormalities of sleep (10) and a good predictor of daytime hallucinations. This hypothesis, however, needs further testing.

Dementia

The mechanism of the toxic confusional state in demented PD patients treated with L-dopa is unknown. Anticholinergic-related amnesia and delirium are better understood. They result from disruption of central cholinergic systems. In healthy subjects, parenteral scopolamine, an anticholinergic drug, causes deficits of information encoding and retrieval of old information, sparing attentiveness. These deficits are reversible by physostigmine, a centrally acting acetylcholinesterase inhibitor (47–49). Furthermore, scopolamine in a small dose that does not affect certain memory tasks in nonparkinsonian subjects significantly alters the performance of these tasks in nondemented PD patients (31), suggesting that even PD patients who are cognitively intact are more at risk for developing cognitive impairment with anticholinergic agents than are normals.

Treatment

Sleep

Sleep abnormalities may improve with the avoidance of late evening doses of dopaminergic agents or a reduction in the total dose. Sleep onset insomnia and sleep fragmentation may also improve with the use of amitriptyline in low doses (14). Those with abnormal dream events or myoclonus may not be helped by amitryptyline, or may even worsen with the use of this drug. L-tryptophan and 5-hydroxytryptophan may be of benefit (50,51), but the clinical efficacy has yet to be convincingly demonstrated (52). Benzodiazepines or other hypnosedatives may cause confusion and should be avoided.

Hallucinations and Psychosis

The clinical management of the mental effects of chronic PD therapy is difficult. The aim is to eliminate the hallucinations without significantly worsening motor function. Reduction of drugs, while often effective, can result in the reemergence of life-threatening motor disability.

As a general principle, the first step is to remove those drugs with the poorest therapeutic index. A decrease or discontinuation of amantadine (53–55) may be useful. As amantadine is excreted unchanged through the kidney, this is particularly important in patients with abnormal renal function. A decrease in anticholinergic drugs, if tolerated by the patient, may also result in improvement in cognition and behavior. Anticholinergic drugs must be tapered slowly, as acute anticholinergic withdrawal may significantly exacerbate the symptoms of PD (56).

Although haloperidol and other dopamine receptor antagonists may alleviate drug-induced psychosis, these agents often cause an unacceptable exacerbation of parkinsonian symptoms. Small doses of thioridazine given at bedtime may improve hallucinations without worsening PD, but these patients should be watched closely. Clozapine, a potent antipsychotic agent with special affinity for mesolimbic areas, may effectively treat psychosis with minimal extrapyramidal effects (57–59).

Drug Holiday

The temporary withdrawal of dopaminergic agents, or drug holiday (DH), may be considered in those patients who manifest both increasing symptoms of PD and adverse effects of treatment. DH has been reported to benefit this group of patients for periods of six months to two years (56,60–63). The benefit is temporary and any single patient may require more than one DH during the course of treatment. During the period of drug withdrawal, patients may become completely immobilized due to the reemergence of PD symptoms. In most cases, they need complete care. Hospitalization is required to prevent and treat the complications of DH, including deep venous thrombosis, pulmonary embolism, aspiration pneumonia, urinary tract infections, inability to swallow, and depression during the period of maximal disability (56,64,65). Some have argued that the risk of these complications may outweigh the benefit (65,66). However, in selected patients hospitalized in centers experienced with DH and with careful attention to pulmonary hygiene, nutritional needs, maintenance of joint mobility through physical therapy, and prophylaxis of venous thrombosis, DH may be an effective means of extending the period of drug efficacy (3,4,56,60,61,67).

DOPA DYSKINESIAS

Dopa dyskinesias (DD) occur in 30% to 90% of patients on chronic L-dopa therapy (unpublished observations) (9,68). In contrast to the cognitive and behavioral complications of dopaminergic therapy, which usually occur after years of treatment, DD can occur as early as four weeks after treatment is begun, with up to 50% of patients developing DD by the end of the first year of therapy (8,69).

A variety of abnormal involuntary movements may be associated with chronic treatment of PD, including chorea, dystonia, myoclonus, and asterixis.

Diagnosis

Chorea

Choreic movements may involve face, tongue, hands, limbs, and trunk. These movements are rapid and nonstereotyped (3,70–72). Ballistic movements, which are more violent, flinging movements involving proximal musculature, may also occur. Involvement of respiratory muscles, manifested by panting, inspiratory spasms, and subjective sensations of dyspnea can happen and are sometimes confused with primary lung disease (73). The movements tend to become more severe with continued treatment and may progress to involve more body regions. Not only is chorea a cosmetic problem, it may also interfere with functional activity, impairing eating, swallowing, speech, ambulation, and respiratory status.

In most cases, chorea occurs at the time of maximal drug effect ("peak dose") and coincides with the greatest degree of clinical improvement. In this pattern, there is a gradual emergence of chorea following a drug dose, which reaches maximal severity simultaneously with the peak of drug effect. The chorea wanes as drug effect subsides (74). Over time, chorea may appear at shorter intervals after the onset of drug effect and may become more prolonged until it may occupy the entire duration of drug efficacy.

Diphasic chorea is less frequent and tends to affect younger, akinetic patients. It usually occurs after more prolonged treatment. This pattern of chorea consists of an initial postdose phase of chorea, followed by a period of improvement without chorea and then the reappearance of the movements as the drug effect wanes (75).

Dystonia

Dystonic postures in PD are more commonly associated with chronic dopaminergic treatment (76). There are two types of dystonia in PD patients. Withdrawal dystonia occurs as drug effect disappears, most frequently affecting the patient in the morning before the first dose of medication (7,76–78). The second type of dystonia occurs at the same time as drug-induced chorea, usually at peak dose or in a diphasic pattern (75). Dystonia can occur as the sole manifestation of dopaminergic-induced movement (79).

There is often a painful dystonic posturing of the feet and toes with an equinovarus deformity. The most severe posturing tends to occur on the side most affected by PD (78,80,81). In addition to foot dystonia, other types of dystonia including orofacial dystonia (82) and dystonic posturing of limbs, neck, and trunk have been reported (78,83).

Treatment-related dystonia tends to occur most frequently in young-onset PD (unpublished observation) (69). This is particularly true of diphasic dystonia (81,83).

Myoclonus and Asterixsis

L-dopa-induced myoclonus is characterized by brief, lightning-like involuntary jerks that are usually bilateral but may only affect one side. Two types of myoclonus are associated with chronic L-dopa use: nocturnal myoclonus and daytime myoclonus. Nocturnal myoclonus is more common and typically occurs during sleep, sometimes awakening the patient. Daytime myoclonus occurs less frequently. Although associated with prolonged dopaminergic treatment, both types of myoclonus appear to be independent of drug efficacy (84). The presence of nocturnal myoclonus has been suggested to predict the occurrence of drug-induced mental changes (10).

Asterixis may occur in association with a toxic delirium (85).

Basic Science

Chorea

Factors that appear to be important in the development of drug-induced chorea are the duration of disease, the duration of therapy (5), and the cumulative dose of L-dopa (6). It also appears that the age of PD onset plays an important role. Of those with onset less than 40 years, most will have abnormal movements by the end of six years (unpublished observation) (69). This group of young-onset patients tend to develop the more complex patterns of DD and often are affected by drug-induced dystonia (69).

The mechanism underlying drug-induced chorea is not known. However, the pharmacologic pathophysiology of choreic disorders in general is believed to involve striatal dopaminergic systems, reflecting a relative overactivity of dopamine. Some observations suggest that an abnormal nigrostriatal system may predispose to dopamine-induced chorea. L-dopa may exacerbate the chorea of Huntington's disease (8,70) and may produce a transient chorea in a third of those at risk for Huntington's disease (86). In 1-methyl-4-phenyl-1,2,3,6-tetrahydropyridine-induced parkinsonism, there is a selective degeneration of the substantia nigra (87,88). Chronic treatment of these patients with L-dopa results in movements similar to those found in treated idiopathic PD (89). In patients with hemiparkinsonism, drug-induced movements occur on the involved side and in those with thalamotomies, the side contralateral to the surgery is less affected, suggesting a protective influence of thalamotomy for these movements (73). Although these observations suggest that there may be a predisposition to drug-induced movements in those with abnormal dopaminergic pathways, there have been few normal subjects treated chronically with these drugs. Furthermore, tardive dyskinesia does occur in those with normal nigrostriatal pathways. Therefore, whether an altered anatomy is required for the production of L-dopa–induced movements remains unknown.

It is unlikely that a single process will explain the diverse clinical manifestations and motor fluctuations that occur. The fact that apomorphine, a direct-acting dopamine receptor agonist, and amphetamine, an indirect agonist, can result in movements identical to those occurring with L-dopa (91) suggests that the pathophysiology of drug-induced chorea involves the central dopamine receptors (92). Dopamine receptors are classically categorized as D_1 and D_2 receptors. The D_1 receptor is adenylate cyclase linked and is hypothesized to mediate drug-induced chorea (92). The D_2 receptors are adenylate cyclase independent and stimulation of these receptors is hypothesized to mediate drug-related improvement of PD symptoms. At least two other classes of dopamine receptors have been described by ligand binding techniques (93) but their function is unknown.

The role of denervation hypersensitivity in the pathogenesis of chorea is not clear. There is an elevated density of the D_2 dopamine receptors demonstrated in untreated PD patients by ligand binding using labeled apomorphine, haloperidol, and spiperone (94). This suggests that in untreated patients, chronic denervation may cause an increase in receptor number. In chronically treated patients, however, the receptor density does not differ from normal controls, suggesting that there is a reversal of the denervation related receptor changes with prolonged L-dopa treatment (93,95,96).

The current hypothesis is that the movements may be related to agonist-induced hypersensitivity. This hypothesis arose from the observation that in animals chronically pretreated with amphetamine or L-dopa there is a heightened sensitivity to apomorphine- and amphetamine-induced stereotyped behavior (97,98). This suggests that a postsynaptic dopaminergic hypersensitivity may develop in chronically treated animals. In support of this theory is the observation that plasma L-dopa levels have been found in humans to correlate with dyskinesias that occur at the time of maximal drug effect (75), suggesting that in this pattern of chorea there is a threshold L-dopa level above which the movements appear. This would be consistent with the hypothesis of a population of hypersensitive receptors. However, plasma L-dopa levels are not correlated with the occurrence of other patterns of dyskinesia (99). The diphasic movements occur as the plasma level of L-dopa is increasing and again as the level is decreasing, suggesting that in this pattern there is a critical L-dopa level at which the movements occur. Therefore, either plasma L-dopa levels do not reflect central dopaminergic activity or another mechanism is responsible.

Investigations into the role of dopamine metabolites, specifically 3-*O*-methyldopa, demonstrate that this metabolite is elevated in patients with diphasic dyskinesias and "on–off" (100–102). It is postulated that 3-*O*-methyldopa competes with L-dopa for central transport mechanisms and thus decreases the central availability of L-dopa, resulting in motor fluctuations. Other workers have argued that elevated 3-*O*-methyldopa is unlikely to have a significant effect on response fluctuations (103) and is merely the consequence of the higher doses of L-dopa used in treating those with more advanced disease. It may be that additional factors such as dietary protein or circadian elevations of large chain amino acids play a role in the more complex forms of movements by interfering with central availability of L-dopa (104,105). More information is needed before the pathogenesis of these movements is understood. Further investigations are in progress.

Dystonia

Drug withdrawal dystonia, which is the most common L-dopa-induced dystonia, appears to have a different mechanism than chorea. This hypothesis is based on pharmacologic observations. The parenteral administration of either anticholinergic or dopaminergic agents significantly improves L-dopa-induced early morning or off-period foot dystonia (83), whereas these drugs will often exacerbate chorea. Physostigmine, a centrally acting cholinergic drug, worsens this type of dystonia. Haloperidol, a dopamine receptor antagonist, while worsening parkinsonian symptoms, has little effect on dystonia but significantly improves chorea (7,83). At this time, the pathogenesis of the early morning dystonia is not known, but pharmacologic evidence suggests that the mechanism is distinct from that of chorea.

The mechanism underlying the dystonia occurring simultaneously with chorea may have a common pathogenesis. Little more is known at present.

Myoclonus

The mechanism underlying dopaminergic-induced myoclonus is postulated to involve alterations in serotonergic activity. This postulate is based on the observation that methysergide, a serotonin antagonist, has been reported to eliminate L-dopa-induced myoclonus (84).

Treament

Chorea

If chorea is the result of a relative overactivity of the striatal dopaminergic system, then reduction of central dopamine activity by reduction in dopaminergic drugs or by dopamine receptor antagonists should be successful in controlling chorea. This strategy, however, usually results in significant and often incapacitating reemergence of parkinsonian signs (106).

Fractionation of L-dopa dose by giving smaller doses at more frequent intervals can be of benefit primarily in peak dose dyskinesia (107) and perhaps in some patients with diphasic dyskinesias (108). This presumably works by avoiding large fluctuations in plasma L-dopa levels. Sustained release L-dopa preparations, when available, may serve the same function (109).

Dopamine agonists have been reported to cause less dyskinesias. Some have reported that bromocriptine alone can successfully treat the symptoms of PD with a decreased occurrence of dyskinesias (110). Others have observed that agonist therapy in low doses added to L-dopa early in the course of treatment is more effective in treating symptoms and avoiding dyskinesias (111,112). However, the efficacy of either of these options is limited.

Many clinicians attempt to delay the time of onset of dyskinesias by delaying the use of L-dopa. Evidence in support of this is provided by one series, which found a similar mean interval from time of L-dopa onset to the time of side effect, regardless of their age at PD onset (113). Many investigators now recommend that L-dopa therapy be delayed until postural reflex impairment occurs (114,115). In addition, when possible, the use of agents other than L-dopa, including anticholinergic drugs and amantadine (116), alone or in combination may forestall the initiation of L-dopa and therefore delay the occurrence of dyskinesias.

Dystonia

Withdrawal dystonia can significantly improve in some patients by the use of anticholinergic drugs. Dopamine agonists such as bromocriptine and pergolide mesylate may also be effective (77,81,117). Baclofen has also been reported to help some patients (79). In patients not responding to these drugs, lithium carbonate at therapeutic blood levels has been reported to be of use (118), although the potential for serious adverse effects with this drug must be considered.

All patterns of drug-induced dystonia respond to the discontinuation of dopaminergic therapy during DH. However, DH is least likely to benefit those with early morning and off-period dystonia. This type of dystonia tends to recur very early after the reintroduction of dopaminergic therapy (56).

Myoclonus

Myoclonus has been effectively treated with methysergide, although the side effects associated with chronic use limit long-term benefit (84). Periactin, with less associated toxic effects, may decrease myoclonus.

Drug Holiday

The procedure involved in DH has been previously described. In patients with disabling drug-induced dyskinesia, there may be an improvement of functional capacity with a decrease in abnormal movements for up to one year after DH.

REFERENCES

1. Hoehn M. Parkinson's disease: progression and mortality. Adv Neurol 1986;45:457–461.
2. Cotzias GC, Papaviliou PS, Gellene R. Modification of parkinsonism—chronic treatment with L-dopa. 1969;280:337–345.
3. Sweet RD, McDowell FH. Five years treatment of Parkinson's disease with levodopa: therapeutic results and survival of 100 patients. Ann Int Med 1975;83:456–463.
4. Barbeau A. Six years of high-level levodopa therapy in severely akinetic parkinsonian patients. Arch Neurol 1976;33:333–338.
5. Lesser RP, Fahn S, Snider SR, et al. Analysis of the clinical problems in parkinsonism and the complications of long-term levodopa therapy. Neurology 1979;29:1253–1260.
6. Rajput AH, Stern W, Laverty WH. Chronic low-dose levodopa therapy in Parkinson's disease: an argument for delaying levodopa therapy. Neurology 1984;34:991–996.
7. Peowe W, Lees A, Stern G. Foot dystonia in Parkinson's disease: clinical phenomenology and neuropharmacology. Adv Neurol 1986;45:357–360.
8. Markham CH, Treciokas LJ, Diamond SG. Parkinson's disease and levodopa— a five-year follow-up and review. West J Med 1974;121:188–206.
9. Bergman KJ, Mendoza MR, Yahr MD. Parkinson's disease and long-term levodopa therapy. Adv Neurol 1986;45:463–467.
10. Nausieda PA, Glantz R, Weber S, et al. Psychiatric complications of levodopa therapy of Parkinson's disease. Adv Neurol 1984;40:271–277.
11. Askenasy JJ, Yahr MD. Reversal of sleep disturbance in Parkinson's disease by antiparkinsonian therapy: a preliminary study. Neurology 1985;35:527–532.
12. Goetz CG, Wilson RS, Tanner CM, Garron DC. Relationships among pain, depression, and sleep alterations in Parkinson's disease. Adv Neurol 1986;45:345–347.
13. Sharf B, Moskovitz C, Lupton MD, Klawans HL. Dream phenomena induced by chronic levodopa therapy. J Neural Transm 1978;43:143–151.
14. Nausieda PA, Weiner WJ, Kaplan LR, et al. Sleep disruption in the course of chronic levodopa therapy; an early feature of the levodopa psychosis. Clin Neuropharmacol 1982;5:183–194.
15. Harper RW, Knothe BU. Coloured lilliputian hallucinations with amantadine. Med J Aust 1973;1:444–445.
16. Sweet RD, McDowell FH, Feigenson JS, et al. Mental symptoms in Parkinson's disease during chronic treatment with levodopa. Neurology 1976;26:305–310.
17. Moskovitz C, Moses H, Klawans H. Levodopa-induced psychosis: a kindling phenomenon. Am J Psychiatry 1982;139:494–497.
18. Gilbert GJ. Hallucinations from levodopa. J Am Med Assoc 1976;235:597.
19. Celesia GC, Barr AN. Psychosis and other psychiatric manifestations of levodopa therapy. Arch Neurol 1970;23:193–200.
20. Klawans HL. Behavioral alterations and the therapy of parkinsonism. Clin Neuropharm 1982;5(suppl 1):27–37.
21. Jenkins RB, Groh RH. Mental symptoms in parkinsonian patients treated with L-dopa. Lancet 1970;i:177–180.
22. Quinn NP, Toone B, Lang AE, et al. Dopa dose-dependent sexual deviation. Br J Psychiatry 1983;142:296–298.
23. Rondo P, de Recondo J, Coignet A, Ziegler M. Mental disorders in Parkinson's disease after treatment with L-dopa. Adv Neurol 1984;40:259–269.
24. Pollock M, Hornabrook RW. The prevalence, natural history and dementia of Parkinson's disease. Brain 1966;89:429–448.
25. Mindham RHS. Psychiatric symptoms in parkinsonism. J Neurol Neurosurg Psychiatry 1970;33:188–191.
26. Mindham RHS, Ahmed SWA, Clough CG. A controlled study of dementia in Parkinson's disease. J Neurol Neurosurg Psychiatry 1982;45:969–974.
27. Lieberman A, Dziatolowski M, Kupersmith M, et al. Dementia in Parkinson's disease. Ann Neurol 1979;6:355–359.
28. Newman RP, Weingartner H, Smallberg SA, Calne DB. Effortful and automatic memory: effects of dopamine. Neurology 1984;34:805–806.
29. Pullman SL, Watts RL, Juncos JL, et al. Dopaminergic effects on simple and choice reaction time performance in Parkinson's disease. Neurology 1988;38:249–254.
30. Lieberman AN. Parkinson's disease: a clinical review. Am J Med Sci 1974;267:66–80.
31. Dubois B, Danze F, Pillon B, et al. Cholinergic-dependent cognitive deficits in Parkinson's disease. Ann Neurol 1987;22:26–30.
32. DeSmet Y, Ruberg M, Serdaru M, et al. Confusion, dementia and anticholinergics in Parkinson's disease. J Neurol Neurosurg Psychiatry 1982;45:1161–1164.
33. Cianchetti C. Dopamine agonists and sleep in man. In: Wauquier A, ed. Sleep: Neurotransmitters and Neuromodulators. New York: Raven Press, 1985:121–134.
34. Gillin JC, Post RM, Wyatt RJ, et al. REM inhibitory effect of L-dopa infusion during human sleep. Electroencephalogr Clin Neurophysiol 1973;35:181–186.
35. Kales A, Ansel R, Markham C, et al. Effects of L-dopa administration on sleep in Parkinson's disease and control patients. Psychophysiology 1970;7:315.
36. Kales A, Ansel RD, Markham CH, et al. Sleep in patients with Parkinson's disease and normal subjects prior to and following levodopa administration. Clin Pharmacol Ther 1971;12:397–406.
37. Schmidt HS, Knopp W. Sleep in Parkinson's disease: the effect of L-dopa. Psychopathology 1972;9:88–89.
38. Greenberg R, Pearlman CA. L-Dopa, parkinsonism, and sleep. Psychophysiology 1970;7:314.
39. Monti JM. Mini review: catecholamines and the sleep–wake cycle: EEG and behavioural arousal. Life Sci 1982;30:1145–1157.
40. Monti JM. Mini review: catecholamines and the sleep–wake cycle: REM sleep. Life Sci 1983;32:1401–1415.
41. Everett GM, Borcherding JW. L-Dopa: effect on concentrations of dopamine, norepinephrine, and serotonin in the brains of mice. Science 1970;160:849–850.
42. Karobath M, Diaz J, Huttunen M. The effect of L-dopa on the concentrations of tryptophan, tyrosine, and serotonin in rat brains. Eur J Pharmacol 1971;14:393–396.
43. Fahn S, Snider S, Prasad ALN, et al. Normalization of brain serotonin by L-tryptophan in levodopa-treated rats. Neurology 1975;25:861–865.
44. Tanner CM, Vogel C, Goetz CG, Klawans HL. Hallucinations in Parkinson's disease: a population study. Ann Neurol 1983;14:136.
45. Jacobs B, Trulson M. Mechanisms of action of LSD. Am Sci 1979;67:394–404.
46. Goetz CG, Tanner CM, Klawans HL. Pharmacology of hallucinations induced by long-term drug therapy. Am J Psychiatry 1982;4:494–497.
47. Drachman DA, Leavitt J. Human memory and the cholinergic system: a relationship to aging? Arch Neurol 1974;30:113–121.
48. Drachman DA. Memory and cognitive function in man: does the cholinergic system have a specific role? Neurology 1977;27:783–790.
49. Caine ED, Weingartner H, Ludlow CL, et al. Qualitative analysis of scopalamine-induced amnesia. Psychopharmacology 1981;74:74–80.
50. Rabey JM, Vardi J, Askenazi JJ, Strifler M. L-Tryptophan in L-dopa-induced hallucinations in elderly parkinsonian patients. Gerontology 1977;23:438–444.
51. Miller EM, Nieburg HA. L-Tryptophan in the treatment of levodopa induced psychiatric disorders. Dis Nerv Syst 1974;35:20–23.
52. Beasley BL, Nutt JG, Davenport RW, Chase TN. Treatment with tryptophan of levodopa-associated psychiatric disturbances. Arch Neurol 1980;37:155–156.
53. Schwab RS, Poskanzer DC, England AC, Young RR. Amantadine in Parkinson's disease: review of more than two years experience. J Am Med Assoc 1972;222:792–795.
54. Postma J, Vantilburg W. Visual hallucinations and delirium during treatment with amantadine (Symmetrel). J Am Geriatr Soc 1975;23:212–215.
55. Fahn S, Craddock G, Kumen G. Acute toxic psychosis from suicidal overdosage of amantadine. Arch Neurol 1971;25:45–48.
56. Goetz CG, Tanner CM, Klawans HL. Drug holiday in the management of Parkinson's disease. Clin Neuropharm 1982;5:351–364.
57. Povlsen UJ, Noring U, Fog R, Geriach J. Tolerability and therapeutic effect of clozapine. Acta Psychiatr Scand 1985;71:176–185.
58. Friedman JH, Max J, Swift R. Idiopathic Parkinson's disease in a chronic schizophrenic patient: long-term treatment with clozapine and L-dopa. Clin Neuropharmacol 1987;10:470–475.
59. Scholz E, Dichgans J. Treatment of drug-induced exogenous psychosis in parkinsonism with clozapine and fluperlapine. Eur Arch Psychiatr Neurol Sci 1985;235:60–64.
60. Weiner W, Koller W, Perlik S, Nausieda P, Klawans HL. Drug holiday and the management of Parkinson's disease. Neurology 1980;30:1257–1261.
61. Koller W, Weiner W, Perlik S, et al. Complications of chronic levodopa therapy: long-term efficacy of drug holiday. Neurology 1981;31:473–476.
62. Bermejo F, Calandre L, Molina J, et al. Long-lasting drug holiday in Parkinson's disease. Adv Neurol 1986;45:503–506.
63. Tanner CM, Goetz C, Brandabur M, Klawans H. Drug holiday: duration of clinical improvement. Neurology 1987;37:(suppl 1):279.
64. Direnfeld L, Feldman R, Alexander M, Kelly-Hayes M. Is L-dopa holiday useful? Neurology 1980;30:785–788.
65. Mayeaux R, Stern Y, Mulvey K, Cote L. Reappraisal of temporary levodopa withdrawal ("drug holiday") in Parkinson's disease. N Engl J Med 1985;313:724–728.

66. Kofman O. Are levodopa "drug holidays" justified? Can J Neurol Sci 1984;11:206–209.
67. Feldman R, Kaye J, Lannon M. Parkinson's disease: follow-up after "drug holiday." J Clin Pharmacol 1986;26:662–667.
68. Keenan RE. The Eaton collaborative study of levodopa therapy in parkinsonism: a summary. Neurology 1970;20:46–59.
69. Quinn N, Critchley P, Marsden C. Young onset Parkinson's disease. Mov Disord 1987;2:73–91.
70. Barbeau A. L-Dopa therapy in Parkinson's disease: a critical review of nine years experience. Can Med Assoc J 1969;101:59–68.
71. Barbeau A, Mars H, Gillo-Joffroy L, Arsenault A. A proposed classification of dopa-induced dykinesias. In: Barbeau A, McDowell FH, eds. L-Dopa and Parkinsonism. New York: FA Davis, 1970:118–123.
72. Yahr MD. Abnormal involuntary movements induced by dopa: clinical aspects. In: Barbeau A, McDowell FH, eds. L-Dopa and Parkinsonism. New York: FA Davis, 1970:101–108.
73. Mones RJ, Elizan TS, Siegel GJ. Analysis of L-dopa induced dyskinesias in 51 patients with parkinsonism. J Neurol Neurosurg Psychiatry 1971;34:668–673.
74. Marsden CD, Parkes JD, Quinn N. Fluctuations of disability in Parkinson's disease—clinical aspects. In: Fahn S, Marsden CD, eds. Movement disorders. London: Butterworths, 1982:96–122.
75. Meunter MD, Sharpless NS, Tyce GM, Darley FL. Patterns of dystonia ("I-D-I" and "D-I-D") in response to L-dopa therapy for Parkinson's disease. Mayo Clin Proc 1977;52:163–174.
76. Melamed E. Early-morning dystonia, a late effect of long-term levodopa therapy in Parkinson's disease. Arch Neurol 1979;36:308–310.
77. Newman R, LeWitt P, Shults C, et al. Dystonia: treatment with bromocriptine. Clin Neuropharmacol 1985;8:328–333.
78. Kidron D, Melamed E. Forms of dystonia in patients with Parkinson's disease. Neurology 1987;37:1009–1011.
79. Parkes J, Bedard P, Marsden C. Chorea and torsion in parkinsonism. Lancet 1976;i:155.
80. Nausieda PA, Weiner WJ, Klawans HL. Dystonic foot response of parkinsonism. Arch Neurol 1980;37:132–136.
81. Ilson J, Fahn S, Cote L. Painful dystonic spasms in Parkinson's disease. Adv Neurol 1984;40:395–398.
82. Weiner W, Nausieda P. Meige's syndrome during long-term dopaminergic therapy in Parkinson's disease. Adv Neurol 1982;39:451–452.
83. Poewe WH, Lees AJ, Stern GM. Dystonia in Parkinson's disease: clinical and pharmacologic features. Ann Neurol 1988;23:73–78.
84. Klawans HL, Goetz CG, Bergen D. Levodopa-induced myoclonus. Arch Neurol 1975;32:331–334.
85. Glantz R, Weiner WJ, Goetz CG, et al. Drug-induced asterixes in Parkinson's disease. Neurology 1982;32:553–555.
86. Klawans HL, Paulson GW, Ringel SP, Barbeau A. The use of L-dopa in the detection of presymptomatic Huntington's chorea. N Engl J Med 1972;286:1332–1334.
87. Davis GC, Williams AC, Markey SP, et al. Chronic parkinsonism secondary to intravenous injection of meperidine analogues. Psychiatry Res 1979;1:249–254.
88. Burns RS, Chiueh CC, Markey SP, et al. A primate model of parkinsonism; selective destruction of dopaminergic neurons in the pars compacta of the substantia nigra by N-methyl-4-phenyl-1,2,3,6-tetrahydropyridine. Proc Natl Acad Sci 1983;80:4546–4550.
89. Langston JW. MPTP-induced parkinsonism; how good a model is it? In: Fahn S, ed. Recent developments in Parkinson's disease. New York: Raven, 1986:119–126.
90. Cotzias GC, Papavasiliou PS, Fehling K, et al. Similarities between neurologic effects of L-dopa and of apomorphine. N Engl J Med 1970;282:31–33.
91. Carlsson A. Biochemical implications of dopa-induced actions on the central nervous system, with particular reference to abnormal movements. In: Barbeau A, McDowell FH, eds. L-Dopa and Parkinsonism. Philadelphia: FA Davis 1970:205–213.
92. Calne D. Dopamine receptors in movement disorders. In: Marsden CD, Fahn S, eds. Movement disorders. London: Butterworths, 1982:348–355.
93. Jenner P, Marsden CD. Interpretation of radioactive ligand binding to cerebral dopamine receptors. In: Marsden CD, Fahn S, eds. Movement disorders. London: Butterworths, 1982:356–368.
94. Lee T, Seeman P, Rajput A, et al. Receptor basis for dopaminergic supersensitivity in Parkinson's disease. Nature 1978;273:59–61.
95. Guttman M, Seeman P. L-Dopa reverses the elevated density of D2 receptors in Parkinson's disease striatum. J Neural Transm 1985;64:93–103.
96. Guttman M, Seeman P, Reynolds GP, et al. Dopamine D2 receptor density remains constant in treated Parkinson's disease. Ann Neurol 1986;19:487–492.
97. Klawans HL, Margolin DI. Amphetamine-induced dopaminergic hypersensitivity in guinea pigs, implications in psychosis and human movement disorders. Arch Gen Psychiatry 1975;32:725–732.
98. Klawans HL, Goetz CG, Nausieda PA, Weiner WJ. Levodopa-induced dopamine receptor hypersensitivity. Ann Neurol 1977;2:125–129.
99. Meunter MD, Tyce GM. L-Dopa therapy of Parkinson's disease: plasma L-dopa concentration, therapeutic response and side effects. Mayo Clin Proc 1971;46:231–239.
100. Feurestein CL, Serre F, Gavend M, et al. Plasma O-methyldopa in levodopa-induced dyskinesias: a bioclinical investigation. Acta Neurol Scand 1977;56:508–524.
101. Reches A, Fahn S. O-methyldopa interferes with striatal utilization of levodopa. Ann Neurol 1981;10:94.
102. Mena MA, Muradas V, Bazan E, et al. Pharmacokinetics of L-dopa in patients with Parkinson's disease. Adv Neurol 1986;45:481–486.
103. Fabbrini G, Juncos JL, Mouradian MM, et al. 3-O-methyldopa and motor fluctuations in Parkinson's disease. Neurology 1987;37:856–859.
104. Fabbrini G, Juncos J, Mouradian MM, et al. Dietary influences on motor fluctuations in Parkinson's disease. Neurology 1987;37(suppl 1).
105. Nutt JG, Woodward WR, Hammerstad JP, et al. The "on–off" phenomenon in Parkinson's disease: relation to levodopa absorption and transport. N Engl J Med 1984;310:483–488.
106. Klawans HL, Weiner WJ. Attempted use of haloperidol in the treatment of L-dopa induced dyskinesias. J Neurol Neurosurg Psychiatry 1974;37:427–430.
107. Jankovic J. Management of motor side effects of chronic levodopa therapy. Clin Neuropharmacol 1982;5(suppl 1):19–28.
108. Lhermitte F, Agid Y, Signoret J. Onset and end-of-dose levodopa-induced dyskinesias: possible treatment by increasing the daily doses of levodopa. Arch Neurol 1978;35:261–263.
109. Chase T, Serrati C, Fabbrini G, Bruno G. Fluctuation in response to levodopa therapy: pathogenetic and therapeutic considerations. Adv Neurol 1986;45:477–480.
110. Lees AJ, Stern GM. Sustained bromocriptine therapy in previously untreated patients with Parkinson's disease. J Neurol Neurosurg Psychiatry 1981;44:1020–1023.
111. Rinne UK. Combined bromocriptine-levodopa therapy early in Parkinson's disease. Neurology 1985;35:1196–1198.
112. Rinne UK. Early combination of bromocriptine and levodopa in the treatment of Parkinson's disease: a five year follow-up. Neurology 1987;37:826–828.
113. Tanner CM, Kinori I, Goetz CG, et al. Age at onset and clinical outcome in idiopathic Parkinson's disease. Neurology 1985;35(suppl 1):276.
114. Melamed E. Initiation of levodopa therapy in parkinsonian patients should be delayed until the advanced stages of the disease. Arch Neurol 1986;43:402–405.
115. Fahn S, Bressman SB. Should levodopa therapy for parkinsonism be started early or late? Evidence against early treatment. Can J Neurol Sci 1984;11:200–205.
116. Timberlake WH, Vance MA. Four-year treatment of patients with parkinsonism using amantadine alone or with levodopa. Ann Neurol 1978;3:119–128.
117. Lieberman AN, Goldstein M. Treatment of advanced Parkinson's disease with dopamine agonists. In: Marsden CM, Fahn S, eds. Movement disorders. London: Butterworths, 1982:146–165.
118. Quinn N, Marsden CD. Lithium for painful dystonia in Parkinson's disease. Lancet 1986;i:1377.

Neural Transplants for the Movement Disorder of Parkinson's Disease

PHILIP A. STARR   CRAIG G. VAN HORNE

Animal experimentation with transplantation of neuronal tissues into the adult central nervous system began 100 years ago. However, the modern era of neuronal transplantation, culminating in clinical applications beginning in the 1980s, was heralded by two developments: the recognition that transplant survival is greatly enhanced by the use of fetal tissue as a graft source, and the development of animal models of neurologic disease in which physiologic and behavioral effects of transplantation could be carefully tested. Parkinson's disease (PD) is the neurodegenerative disorder most amenable to a transplantation paradigm, since it is characterized by a relatively specific deficiency in a neurotransmitter system, the dopaminergic system, in a focal brain region—the substantia nigra, pars compacta (SNC) and its projections. Since the major projection from SNC innervates the striatum, the strategy of all clinical transplantation efforts thus far has been to place dopamine-secreting tissue within the striatum.

EXPERIMENTAL MODELS OF PARKINSON'S DISEASE

Transplantation paradigms for PD are usually tested in two experimental models of PD: the 6-hydroxydopamine (6-OHDA) rat model and the 1-methyl-4-phenyl-1,2,3,6-tetrahydropyridine (MPTP) primate model.

Rat Model

In the rat, injection of 6-OHDA into the nigrostriatal pathway results in selective death of dopaminergic neurons within the SNC and subsequent loss of dopamine in the striatal projection. When injected with dopamine receptor agonists (apomorphine) or uptake blockers (amphetamine), a unilaterally lesioned rat rotates at a fairly consistent, reproducible, and quantifiable rate (1). The ability to diminish rotational behavior in this model has been used as the predominant screening test for many new potential Parkinson's disease treatments, including neuronal transplantation. However, drug-induced rotation, a behavioral manifestation of dopamine depletion, may not be the best physiologic correlate of human parkinsonism. Interventions that do not affect rat rotation in the 6-OHDA model may be highly beneficial to parkinsonian symptoms in primate models (2). Monitoring several spontaneous (non–drug-induced) behaviors in a dopamine-depleted animal may more accurately predict clinical efficacy (3). Thus, although the 6-OHDA rat model has provided much information, the excessive focus on drug-induced rotational behavior in this model, rather than spontaneous locomotive behaviors, has probably been misleading.

Primate Model

An excellent primate model of PD was developed following the discovery that the toxin MPTP causes parkinsonism in humans (4). When administered systemically to primates, MPTP produces a syndrome of tremor, rigidity, and bradykinesia (5). The syndrome is responsive to L-dopa, and resembles human Parkinson's disease in every way except that it is nonprogressive. MPTP can be administered unilaterally into the carotid artery, producing a hemiparkinsonian primate (6), which is often the preferred model since these animals are easier to care for and maintain long-term compared with bilaterally lesioned animals.

TRANSPLANTATION OF ADRENAL MEDULLA INTO STRIATUM

Transplantation of a nonneuronal dopamine-secreting tissue could theoretically prove effective for treatment of PD as long as graft reinnervation of host tissues is not critical in recovery. One such tissue source is the adrenal medulla. Although adrenal chromaffin cells in situ produce much more epinephrine than dopamine, denervated adrenal chromaffin cells grafted into the rat cerebrum produce more dopamine than epinephrine (7).

Autografting of chromaffin cells into the striatum in the 6-OHDA rat (8) or MPTP primate (9) models ameliorates motor abnormalities to some extent, though graft survival in the primate model is very limited (9). Nevertheless, adrenal medulla autografting entered clinical trials rapidly in the 1980s, prior to fetal tissue allografting, because the technique avoids the immunological and ethical issues associated with transplantation of nonautologous tissues. Although some early reports claimed significant benefit from this procedure (10,11), more careful studies showed only very modest improvement, along with significant surgical morbidity (12–15). Autopsy studies of patients who had received transplants revealed that the grafts did not survive (16,17). Animal studies have indicated that adrenal grafting, or even the creation of an inflammatory lesion, in the striatum can induce sprouting of dopaminergic fibers from the host ventral tegmental area, which is probably the mechanism underlying the modest degrees of improvement that were seen (18–20).

Adrenal chromaffin graft survival, and differentiation into a neuronal phenotype, is enhanced by treating the grafts with nerve growth factor after implantation (21). Based on this, one reported patient has undergone intrastriatal placement of an adrenal autograft, followed by a 23-day intraparenchymal infusion of nerve growth factor (NGF) into the region of the graft (22). Clinical improvements in this patient were longer lasting than in the same group's original effort with adrenal autografting (23), but were nevertheless modest. Several other patients have undergone cografting of adrenal medulla tissue with peripheral nerve as a source of NGF (24). Laboratory work continues in an effort to find or develop tissues that secrete NGF and survive following transplantation, to be used as possible cografts in enhancing survival of autologous adrenal chromaffin grafts (25,26).

TRANSPLANTATION OF FETAL MESENCEPHALON INTO STRIATUM

Animal Studies

In the developing mammalian fetus, the ventral mesencephalon (VM) contains the dopaminergic cell bodies that are the precursors of the mature SNC. In both rodent (27,28) and primate (29) models, intrastriatal grafts of fetal VM tissue have been shown to survive, reinnervate portions of the caudate and putamen, and correct abnormal motor behaviors. The mechanism of fetal VM graft function has been extensively studied in rats. Grafts of human fetal VM show spontaneous electrical activity (30) and are capable of releasing physiologically relevant levels of dopamine in response to depolarization (31).

Synaptically mediated graft-host interactions are probably important for graft function. Fetal VM can form ultrastructurally normal synapses onto denervated neurons of the host striatum (31–33). In addition, host cortical and striatal neurons appear to innervate the graft (33,34). Dopamine release from intrastriatal grafts can be increased by electrical stimulation of the host cortex (35) and by pharmacologic blockade of glutamate reuptake (36), as is true of normal striatal tissue in normal rats. Motor activities that increase striatal dopamine in normal rats, such as running on a treadmill, also increase striatal dopamine in grafted animals from which host dopaminergic innervation has been completely depleted (37). Thus, both anatomic and physiologic studies of intrastriatal fetal VM grafts suggest that synaptically mediated host-graft interactions occur and result in a more complex level of function than would be expected from implantation of an unregulated dopamine pump.

Clinical Trials of Human Fetal Tissue Transplants

Patient Characteristics and Clinical Outcomes

As of 1996, at least nine groups have reported at least 80 patients who have undergone transplantation of human fetal VM cells to the striatum for Parkinson's disease (38–48). All patients who received transplants suffered from idiopathic Parkinson's disease, except for 2 of the 6 patients in the Lund, Sweden, group, who suffered from MPTP-induced parkinsonism (39), and 1 of the 4 patients in the Yale group, who suffered from striatonigral degeneration, confirmed by autopsy (43,49). All patients had relatively advanced disease, with Hoehn and Yahr (H&Y) stages of about 3 when on and 4 to 5 when off. Most patients were 40 to 60 years old and had suffered from PD for 5 to 20 years prior to surgery. Patients were primarily symptomatic from bradykinesia and rigidity rather than from tremor.

Outcomes have been highly variable. Observations common to many studies were as follows: Improvements were rarely immediate but took several months. There was a worsening in many patient's motor symptoms during the first 4 to 6 weeks after surgery, and sometimes transient increased dyskinesias. There were several transient psychiatric complications, including hallucinations (42,44), panic attacks (43), and obsessive-compulsive disorder (44). There were several complications of immunosuppressive therapy that required its cessation (45). In most studies, there was modest benefit in most but not all patients, particularly in reduction of amount of time spent off, reduction in drug-induced dyskinesias (which may reflect lowering the dosage of medications), and some improvement in fine motor tasks. The majority of reported patients did not have a significant change in their H&Y functional status, and very few are off medication. The longest follow-up with documented graft survival that has been published is 3 years (40).

Types of Transplantation Protocols Used

All groups used human fetal tissue dissected from the ventral mesencephalon. All used tissue from elective abortions except for the Mexican group, who used tissue from spontaneous abortions (46,50). Treatment protocols differed widely with respect to several important variables: exact location of transplant (head of caudate, putamen, or both), surgical technique used (closed stereotactic injection or open craniotomy), unilateral versus bilateral implantation, age of fetal tissue used, number of fetuses used to provide donor tissue, and use of immunosuppressive therapy. Where immunosuppression was used, cyclosporine was the principal drug, though some groups added azathioprine and/or prednisone to the regimen. A summary of the treatment protocols is given in Table 33.1.

Processing of the fetal tissue varied among teams. Some protocols used solid pieces of ventral mesencephalon (42,43,45,48,50), others grafted strands or clumps of mechanically dissociated tissue (41,47,51), and others used chemically dissociated cells injected as a cell suspension (39,40,44). All groups performed the transplantation within 48 hours of tissue harvesting, except for the Yale group, who used cryopreserved tissue (43), and the University of Colorado group, who used tissue maintained in culture for

1 week (41). All but one (51) of the groups that implanted tissue using closed stereotactic techniques made multiple injections to distribute tissue at anatomically dispersed striatal sites.

Graft Survival: PET Scanning

Survival of grafted fetal dopaminergic cells can be assessed noninvasively using positron emission tomography (PET). A tracer of dopaminergic metabolic activity, such as 6-[^{18}F]fluoro-L-dopa (FD), is used as the positron-emitting source. The concentration of that positron source in the brain then reflects metabolic activity in dopaminergic cells. In Parkinson's disease, uptake of FD in the striatum is abnormally decreased compared with normal controls (52). Several groups have used PET to follow survival of fetal transplants in the striatum (39–44). In the patients followed for the longest time, from the Lund, Sweden, transplantation group, there is evidence for graft survival at 3 years (40). Tracer uptake by PET scanning cannot distinguish between survival of transplanted tissue and sprouting of host dopaminergic tissue, which is known to occur with lesioning of the striatum (53). However, short of autopsy studies, PET is currently the best method for following graft survival.

Graft Survival: Autopsy Studies

There have been three reports of autopsies on patients who have received fetal cell transplants for PD. Two studies, both

Table 33.1   Summary of Human Fetal Transplantation Protocols and Graft Survival Data

Group and Reference	No. of Patients	Target Nucleus	Surgical Technique	Graft Laterality	Tissue Age (weeks)	No. Fetuses per Side	Immunosuppression	Graft Survival (PET)	Graft Survival (autopsy)
Univ. of South Florida (42)	4	Put	Stereotactic	Bi	6.5–9	3–4	6 months	Yes, in all pts	Excellent
Univ. of Colorado (41)	7	Put or put + cau	Stereotactic	Uni or bi	6.5–8	1–2	None or perm	Yes, in 1 of 2 pts tested	
Yale (43)	4	Cau	Stereotactic	Uni	7–11	1	6 months	Yes, in 1 pt tested	Only non-TH + tissue
Lund, Sweden (38,40)	4	Put (pts 3,4)	Stereotactic	Uni	6–7	4	Perm	Yes, in pts 3 and 4 only	
Lund, Sweden (MPTP pts) (39)	2	Put + cau	Stereotactic	Bi	6–8	3–4	Perm	Yes, in both pts	
Créteil, France (44)	2	Put or put + cau	Stereotactic	Uni	6–9	2–3	Perm	Yes, in both pts	
Birmingham, England (47,51)	43	Put or cau	Stereotactic	Uni or bi	11–19	1	None	Not tested	Poor
Madrid, Spain (45)	10	Cau	Craniotomy	Uni	6–8	1	Perm	Not tested	
Havana, Cuba (48)	16	Put + cau	Stereotactic	Uni or bi	10.4 (avg)	1	Perm	Not tested	
Mexico City (46)	4	Cau	Craniotomy	Uni	12–14	1	Perm	Not tested	

pts = patients; put = putamen; cau = caudate head; avg = average; uni = unilateral; bi = bilateral; perm = permanent.

from patients receiving tissue of 11 weeks' gestational age or older, showed no survival of tyrosine hydroxylase (TH)-positive cells (49,54).

A patient from the University of South Florida group died 18 months after grafting, from a pulmonary embolism following orthopedic surgery (55). He had received bilateral grafts into the putamen of tissue from seven fetuses, aged 6.5 to 9 weeks. The patient had been immunosuppressed for 6 months after transplantation. Many TH-positive cells were observed in the grafts, up to 1000 per section, and they extended neuronal processes up to 7 mm into surrounding normal brain. There was no evidence of sprouting of TH-positive fibers from the host brain. This study demonstrated that human fetal tissue implanted in a human can survive and robustly reinnervate host tissues and that long-term immunosuppression (greater than 6 months after transplantation) may not be needed in human neural tissue transplants, even if multiple donors are used.

Which Transplantation Protocols Were Most Effective?

A small number of very well documented patients have had dramatic clinical benefit with good evidence of graft survival, and it is worth considering them individually. The fourth patient from the Swedish series of idiopathic PD patients has been followed for 3 years, and is the only reported patient now off all dopamimetic drugs (40). This patient's off periods have disappeared. Putamenal uptake of 5-fluorodopa has normalized on the operated side. Symptoms continued to improve during the second year after surgery, then remained stable. Two patients with MPTP-induced parkinsonism, also operated on by the Lund, Sweden, group, have also had great benefit, with 50-point decreases in Unified Parkinson's Disease Rating Scale (UPDRS) scores (both on and off) 2 years after transplantation, reductions in medications, elimination of drug-induced dyskinesias, and continued improvement during the second year (39). The four patients in the University of South Florida group (of whom one was the subject of an autopsy investigation described above) also had greater and better-documented improvement than most patients in other series, with a 22-point decrease in total UPDRS scores when off, reduction in percentage of off times from 30% to 12%, and reduction in the percentage of time on with dyskinesia from 44% to 3.8% (42).

Features common to the best-documented patients showing best results are use of younger (6–9 weeks' gestation) tissue, implantation of tissue from multiple fetal sources at multiple sites, implantation into the putamen or putamen and caudate rather than the caudate alone, and surgery using closed, stereotactically guided injection rather than open craniotomy. Although long-term immunosuppression may not be necessary for graft survival, most patients with the best clinical results had at least short-term (6 months post-surgery) immunosuppression.

Status of Human Fetal Cell Allotransplantation in 1996

In the evaluation of new treatments for Parkinson's disease, placebo effects and examiner bias frequently confound interpretation. In a study of pallidotomy for PD, for example, highly significant improvements in some categories, as rated by unblinded investigators, became statistically insignificant when the same ratings were performed by blinded investigators using videotapes (56). To better assess the benefit of fetal neural transplants for PD, a randomized, double-blind study has been sponsored by the National Institutes of Health (57) and is in progress as of 1996.

FUTURE DIRECTIONS IN CLINICAL TRANSPLANTATION

Several problems must be solved before cell transplantation becomes widely applicable in the treatment of PD. First, a source of tissue other than aborted human fetuses must be found; second, the transplantation procedure must be refined so as to produce more complete resolution of motor abnormalities in PD patients.

Alternative Tissue Sources

The most successful clinical transplantation protocols have also been the ones implanting the most tissue, often requiring six to eight fetuses per procedure. Each fetus must be obtained from an elective abortion taking place 6 to 8 weeks after conception. To harvest enough human fetal cells for a successful transplantation, all at the same specific, correct stage of development, is logistically difficult and ethically unsettling. Also, human fetuses are not raised in laboratory environments, and the medical histories of the biological parents of the aborted human fetuses are often unknown. Thus, quality control of the implanted tissue is more difficult than if the tissue source were produced in a controlled laboratory environment. Therefore, a variety of alternative tissue sources are being explored, including xenogeneic tissues and genetically engineered autografts that produce growth factors or L-dopa/dopamine.

Xenotransplantation: Induction of Host Tolerance

In the past, the main problem with using nonhuman tissues for transplantation (i.e., xenotransplantation) has been that the tissues are quickly rejected by the patient's own immune system. Transplant rejection is mediated mainly by major histocompatibility (MHC) antigens. One strategy to circumvent rejection is to use an antibody fragment directed against MHC antigens to induce tolerance of the foreign tissue in the host environment. Treating pancreatic and hepatic xenografts with the variable-region fragment F(ab')$_2$ of a monoclonal antibody against MHC antigens just prior to transplantation induces tolerance in the host that is long lasting, even though the transplant is treated only once (58).

By using antibody fragments from which the constant-region F(c) has been removed, activation of the complement cascade and antibody-mediated destruction is avoided while cellular immunity is modified. For the method to work, xenograft tissue must be treated and transplanted as a cell suspension rather than as solid tissue pieces.

This MHC masking technique has been applied to porcine neural xenografts. When pretreated with F(ab')$_2$ fragments of a monoclonal antibody against MHC-1 antigens, intrastriatal xenografts of porcine fetal VM survive in nonimmunosuppressed host rats as well as untreated xenografts survive in immunosuppressed (cyclosporine-treated) rats (59). Under standard cyclosporine immunosuppression, porcine fetal VM can survive, extend processes, and integrate into host tissue (60,61). In the primate MPTP model, transplants of porcine fetal VM restore motor function (62). In 1995, a clinical trial of xenotransplantation of porcine fetal VM for PD began, using F(ab')$_2$-treated xenografts without systemic immunosuppression in one branch of the study (Dr. John Dinsmore, Diacrin Inc., personal communication).

Xenotransplantation: Polymer Encapsulation of Grafts

Another strategy for sheltering xenografts from the host immune system is to encapsulate xenograft tissue within a synthetic biologically compatible polymer coating that allows diffusion of xenograft-produced molecules but prevents immune attack of the xenograft (63). In the hemiparkinsonian MPTP monkey, implantation of polymer-encapsulated PC12 cells, a dopamine-secreting cell line derived from a rat phenochromocytoma, is effective in ameliorating parkinsonian symptoms (64). A disadvantage of implanting encapsulated tissue is that graft-host synaptic interactions, which may be an important mechanism of behavioral recovery in fetal cell transplantation, are prevented.

Genetically Engineered Autologous Tissue

To completely circumvent the immunologic complexity of xeno- or allotransplantation, a patient's own tissues could be removed, genetically engineered to adopt a useful neuronal phenotype, then reimplanted into the host brain. Primary fibroblasts have been engineered to express tyrosine hydroxylase using retrovirus-mediated transfection; these cells then secrete L-dopa. Implantation of autologous L-dopa–secreting fibroblasts in the 6-OHDA model of PD results in behavioral improvement for at least 8 weeks after implantation, but the behavioral improvements decline after 2 weeks and the implanted fibroblasts show some signs of neoplasia (65). The use of plasmid-transfected primary cultured muscle cells in the same experimental paradigm has resulted in longer-term stable behavioral amelioration, with evidence of continued L-dopa secretion, up to 6 months posttransplant (66). As with polymer-encapsulated tissue, a disadvantage of using

nonneuronal tissues is that it is not possible for such tissues to form functional synapses with host tissue.

Enhancing Transplant Efficiency and Host Reinnervation

In the most successful human fetal transplantation protocols, less than 10% of implanted dopaminergic cells survive, and reinnervation of host structures occurs only over a few millimeters, necessitating the use of a large number of fetal cells and many passes of an injection needle. In the future, the efficiency of the procedure could be improved by providing transplanted tissue with a source of neurotrophic support and/or chemotactic guidance. In animals models, this has been achieved by cotransplanting fetal mesencephalon with fetal striatum (67) or by treating grafts in situ with glial-derived neurotrophic factor (GDNF) (68), which promotes survival and sprouting of dopaminergic neurons in culture (69) and in vivo (70).

Alternative Transplantation Sites

A basic assumption in previous clinical work on transplantation in PD is that depletion of striatal dopamine is fundamental to the pathophysiology of disordered movement, and thus that any transplantation strategy should seek to restore striatal dopamine levels. However, there are now a number of human recipients of transplantations who are documented to have robust dopaminergic reinnervation of the striatum (by PET or autopsy studies), yet whose recovery from the motor abnormalities of PD is only partial. This suggests that restoration of striatal dopaminergic innervation alone may not be sufficient for complete recovery from Parkinson's disease.

In addition to the long-distance nigrostriatal pathway, there are other, short-distance dopaminergic projections from the SNC that innervate neighboring mesencephalic structures and are also affected in Parkinson's disease. Such local circuits include a dopaminergic innervation of the substantia nigra, pars reticulata (SNR), a nucleus that neighbors the SNC and is physiologically homologous to the internal segment of the globus pallidus. Experiments have indicated that attention should be refocused on restoration of mesencephalic, rather than striatal, dopaminergic innervation. Transplantation of fetal dopaminergic cells directly into the lesioned SNC, without intrastriatal transplantation, can correct motor abnormalities in the 6-OHDA rat as long as cells are injected as a suspension and the SNC region, which is small, is meticulously targeted (71). Histologic evaluation showed that these grafts successfully reinnervated the neighboring SNR, but did not send long-distance projections to striatum. Additional evidence of the importance of short-distance SNC projections is provided by studies of GDNF in parkinsonian models. Intraparenchymal injection of GDNF in the hemiparkinsonian MPTP monkey results in substantial motor recovery, with sprouting of nigral dopaminergic fibers and restoration of nigral dopamine levels, but without restoration of dopaminergic innervation in the ipsilateral striatum (70).

These studies indicate that restoration of nigral dopamine levels plays an important role in the correction of parkinsonism in animal models. Future human transplantation protocols should test intranigral, or combined striatal and nigral, transplantation of dopaminergic tissue, rather than rely on intrastriatal transplantation alone. Surgical approaches to the nigral region in humans, once thought to be unacceptably dangerous, have now been developed using a combination of precise image-guided stereotaxis and electrophysiologic target confirmation (72).

CONCLUSIONS

To become an accepted treatment for PD, cell transplantation would have to show greater clinical efficacy than other invasive treatments for medically intractable PD. Posteroventral pallidotomy is an old surgical treatment for bradykinetic/rigid PD that has recently been refined and is undergoing careful study (56). Only a few patients undergoing fetal cell transplantation have experienced the degree of benefit provided by pallidotomy as performed at the best centers (56). Another surgical procedure for bradykinetic/rigid PD, subthalamic nucleus stimulation, shows promise, and, unlike pallidotomy, is a nonablative technique that may be safe to perform for bilateral disease (72). Intracerebral delivery of neurotrophins such as GDNF might, in the future, provide a logistically simple "restorative" therapy for PD, particularly in early stages before the SNC is fully depopulated.

It is still unclear which surgical procedure will ultimately prove most effective for PD. Nevertheless, transplantation in PD has the advantage of directly restoring a lost neuronal function without deliberate anatomic or physiologic brain lesioning. Human and animal studies have already shown that human fetal tissue, if transplanted fresh, at the correct gestational age, in sufficient quantity, and with minimal surgical trauma, can survive, reinnervate the host striatum, and partially correct abnormal motor function. In the future, more reliable tissue sources and the use of additional transplantation sites are likely to improve this procedure.

REFERENCES

1. Ungerstedt U. Striatal dopamine release after amphetamine or nerve degeneration revealed by rotational behavior. Acta Physiol Scand 1971;367(suppl):49–68.
2. Annett LE, Torres EM, Ridley RM, et al. A comparison of the behavioral effects of embryonic nigral grafts in the caudate nucleus and in the putamen of marmosets with unilateral 6-OHDA lesions. Exp Brain Res 1995;103:355–371.
3. Hoffman AF, van Horne CG, Gerhardt GA, Hoffer BJ. Deficits in spontaneous locomotor activity in the unilaterally 6-hydroxydopamine-lesioned rat. Soc Neurosci Abs 1995;21:225–6.
4. Davis CG, Williams AC, Markey SP, et al. Chronic parkinsonism secondary to intravenous injections of meperidine analogues. Psychiatry Res 1979;1:249–254.
5. Burns RS, Chiueh CC, Markey SP, et al. A primate model of parkinsonism: selective destruction of DA neurons in the pars compacta of the substantia nigra by n-methyl-1,2,3,6-tetrahydropyridine. Proc Natl Acad Sci USA 1983;80:4546–4550.
6. Bankiewicz KS, Oldfield EH, Chiueh CC, et al. Hemiparkinsonism in monkeys after unilateral internal carotid artery infusion of 1-methyl-4-phenyl-1,2,3,6-tetrahydropyridine (MPTP). Life Sci 1986;39:7–16.
7. Freed WJ, Farouk K, Spoor HE, et al. Catecholamine content of intracerebral adrenal medulla grafts. Brain Res 1983;269:184–189.
8. Freed WJ, Morihisa JM, Spoor E, et al. Transplanted adrenal chromaffin cells in rat brain reduce lesion-induced rotational behavior. Nature 1981;292:351–352.
9. Morihisa JM, Nakamura RK, Freed WJ, et al. Adrenal medulla grafts survive and exhibit catecholamine-specific fluorescence in the primate brain. Exp Neurol 1984;84:643–653.
10. Madrazo I, Drucker-Colín R, Díaz V, et al. Open microsurgical autograft of adrenal medulla to the right caudate nucleus in two patients with intractable Parkinson's disease. N Engl J Med 1987;316:831–834.
11. Jiao S, Ding Y, Zhang W, et al. Adrenal medullary autografts in patients with Parkinson's disease. N Engl J Med 1989;321:324–325. Letter.
12. Goetz CG, Olanow CW, Koller WC, et al. Multicenter study of autologous adrenal medullary transplantation to the corpus striatum in patients with advanced Parkinson's disease. N Engl J Med 1989;320:337–341.
13. Olanow CW, Koller W, Goetz CG, et al. Autologous transplantation of adrenal medulla in Parkinson's disease: 18 month results. Arch Neurol 1990;47:1286–1289.
14. Allen GS, Burns RS, Tulipan NB, Parker RA. Adrenal medullary transplantation to the caudate nucleus in Parkinson's disease. Arch Neurol 1989;46:487–491.
15. Apuzzo MLJ, Neal JH, Waters CH, et al. Utilization of unilateral and bilateral stereotactically placed adrenomedullary-striatal autografts in parkinsonian humans: rationale, techniques, and observations. Neurosurgery 1990;26:746–757.
16. Hurtig H, Joyce J, Sladek JR, Trojanowski JQ. Postmortem analysis of adrenal-medulla-to-caudate autograft in a patient with Parkinson's disease. Ann Neurol 1989;25:607–614.
17. Jankovic J. Adrenal medullary autografts in patients with Parkinson's disease. N Engl J Med 1989;321:325–326. Letter.
18. Bohn MC, Cupit L, Marciano F, Gash DM. Adrenal medulla grafts enhance recovery of striatal dopaminergic fibers. Science 1987;237:913–916.
19. Fiandaca MS, Kordower JH, Hansen JT. Adrenal medullary autografts into the basal ganglia of Cebus monkeys. Injury induced regeneration. Exp Neurol 1988;102:76–91.
20. Wang J, Bankiewicz K, Plunkett R, Oldfield E. Intrastriatal implantation of interleukin-1. Reduction of parkinsonism in rats by enhancing neuronal sprouting from residual dopaminergic neurons in the ventral tegmental area of the midbrain. J Neurosurg 1994;80:484–490.
21. Stromberg I, Herrera-Marschitz M, Ungerstedt U, et al. Chronic implants of chromaffin tissue into the dopamine-denervated striatum: effects of NGH on graft survival, fiber growth, and rotational behavior. Exp Brain Res 1985;60:335–349.
22. Olson L, Backlund EO, Ebendahl T, et al. Intraputaminal infusion of nerve growth factor to support adrenal meduallary autografts in Parkinson's disease. Arch Neurol 1991;48:373–381.
23. Backlund EO, Granberg PO, Hamberger B. Transplantation of adrenal medullary tissue to striatum in parkinsonsism. First clinical trials. J Neurosurg 1985;62:169–173.
24. Watts RL, Freeman A, Graham S, et al. Early experience with autologous intrastriatal adrenal medulla/nerve cografting in Parkinson's disease. J Neural Transplant Plast 1992;3:272–273.
25. Cunningham LA, Short MP, Breakefield OX, Bohn MC, Nerve growth factor released by transgenic astrocytes enhances the function of adrenal chromaffin cell grafts in a rat model of Parkinson's disease. Brain Res 1994;658:219–231.
26. Kordower JH, Fiandaca MS, Notter MFD, et al. NGF-like trophic support from peripheral nerve for grafted adrenal chromaffin cells. J Neurosurg 1990;73:418–428.
27. Perlow MJ, Freed WJ, Hoffer BJ, et al. Brain grafts reduce motor abnormalities produced by destruction of nigrostriatal dopamine system. Science 1979;204:643–647.
28. Bjorklund A, Steveni U. Reconstruction of the nigrostriatal pathway by intrastriatal nigral transplants. Brain Res 1979;177:555–560.
29. Taylor JR, Elsworth JD, Roth RH, et al. Grafting of fetal substantia nigra to striatum reverses behavioral deficits induced by MPTP in primates: a comparison with other types of grafts as controls. Exp Brain Res 1991;85:335–348.

30. van Horne CG, Mahalik T, Hoffer B, et al. Behavioral and electrophysiological correlates of human mesencephalic dopaminergic xenograft function in the rat striatum. Brain Res Bull 1990;25:325–334.

31. Stromberg I, Almqvist P, Bygdeman M, et al. Human fetal mesencephalic tissue grafted to dopamine-denervated striatum of athymic rats: light- and electron-microscopical histochemistry and in vivo chronoamperometric studies. J Neurosci 1989;9:614–624.

32. Clarke DJ, Brundin P, Strecker RE, et al. Human fetal dopamine neurons grafted in a rat model of Parkinson's disease: ultrastructural evidence for synapse formation using tyrosine hydroxylase immunocytochemistry. Exp Brain Res 1988;73:115–126.

33. Mahalik TJ, Finger TE, Stromberg I, Olson L. Substantia nigra transplants into denervated striatum of the rat: ultrastructure of graft and host interconnections. J Comp Neurol 1985;240:60–70.

34. Doucet G, Murata Y, Brundin P, et al. Host afferent into intrastriatal transplants of fetal ventral mesencephalon. Exp Neurol 1989;106:1–19.

35. Arbuthnott G, Dunnett S, MacLeod N. Electrophysiological properties of single units in dopamine-rich mesencephalic transplants in rat brain. Neurosci Lett 1985;57:205–210.

36. Kondoh T, Low WC. Glutamate uptake blockade induces striatal dopamine release in 6-hydroxydopamine rats with intrastriatal grafts: evidence for host modulation of transplanted dopamine neurons. Exp Neurol 1994;127:191–198.

37. Hattori S, Li QM, Matsui N, et al. Treadmill running combined with microdialysis evaluates motor deficits and improvement following dopaminergic grafts in 6-OHDA lesioned rats. Restor Neurol Neurosci 1992;4:165.

38. Lindvall O, Brundin P, Widner H, et al. Grafts of fetal dopamine neurons survive and improve motor function in Parkinson's disease. Science 1990;247:574–577.

39. Widner H, Tetrud J, Rehncrona S, et al. Bilateral fetal mesencephalic grafting in two patients with parkinsonism induced by 1-methyl-4-phenyl-1,2,3,6-tetrahydropyridine (MPTP). N Engl J Med 1992;22:1556–1563.

40. Lindvall O, Sawle G, Widner H, et al. Evidence for long-term survival and function of dopaminergic grafts in progressive Parkinson's disease. Ann Neurol 1994;35:172–180.

41. Freed CR, Breeze RE, Rosenberg NL, et al. Survival of implanted fetal dopamine cells and neurological improvement 12 to 46 months after transplantation for Parkinson's disease. N Engl J Med 1992;22:1549–1555.

42. Freeman TB, Olanow CW, Hauser RA, et al. Bilateral fetal nigral transplantation into the postcommissural putamen in Parkinson's disease. Ann Neurol 1995;38:379–388.

43. Spencer DD, Robbins RJ, Naftolin F, et al. Unilateral transplantation of human fetal mesencephalic tissue into the caudate nucleus of patients with Parkinson's disease. N Engl J Med 1992;22:1542–1548.

44. Peschanski M, Defer G, N'Guyen JP, et al. Bilateral motor improvement and alternation of L-dopa effect in two patients with Parkinson's disease following intrastriatal transplantation of foetal ventral mesencephalon. Brain 1994;117:487–499.

45. Lopez-Lozano JJ, Bravo B, Brera B, et al. Long-term follow-up in 10 Parkinson's disease patients subjected to fetal brain grafting into a cavity in the caudate nucleus: the Clinica Puerta de Hierro experience. Transplant Proc 1995;27:1395–1400.

46. Madrazo I, Franco-Bourland R, Ostrosky-Solis F, et al. Fetal homotransplants (ventral mesencephalon and adrenal tissue) to the striatum of Parkinson subjects. Arch Neurol 1990;47:1281–1285.

47. Hitchcock E. Current trends in neural transplantation. Neurol Res 1995;17:33–37.

48. Molina H, Quinones-Molina R, Munoz J, et al. Neurotranplantation in Parkinson's disease: from open microsurgery to bilateral stereotactic approach: first clinical trial using microelectrode recording technique. Stereotact Funct Neurosurg 1994;62:204–208.

49. Redmond DE, Leranth C, Spencer DD, et al. Fetal neural graft survival. Lancet 1990;336:820–822. Letter.

50. Madrazo I, Leon V, Torres C, et al. Transplantation of fetal substantia nigra and adrenal medulla to caudate nucleus in two patients with Parkinson's disease. N Engl J Med 1988;318:51. Letter.

51. Henderson BTH, Clough CG, Hughes RC, et al. Implantation of human fetal ventral mesencephalon to the right caudate nucleus in advanced Parkinson's disease. Arch Neurol 1991;48:822–827.

52. Vingerhoets FJG, Schulzer M, Snow BJ. Reproducibility of the fluorodopa PET indices in Parkinson's disease. Mov Disord 1994;9(suppl):119.

53. Bankiewicz KS, Plunkett RJ, Jacobowitz DM. Fetal nondopaminergic neural implants in parkinsonian primates. Histochemical and behavioral studies. J Neurosurg 1991;74:97–104.

54. Hitchcock EH, Whitwell HL, Sofroniew MV, Bankiewicz KS. Survival of TH-positive and neuromelanin-containing cells in patients with Parkinson's disease after intrastriatal grafting of fetal ventral mesencephalon. Exp Neurol 1994;129:3. Abstract.

55. Kordower JH, Freeman TB, Snow BJ, et al. Neuropathological evidence of graft survival and striatal reinnervation after the transplantation of fetal mesencephalic tissue in a patient with Parkinson's disease. N Engl J Med 1995;332:1118–1124.

56. Lozano AM, Lang AE, Galvez-Jimenez N, et al. Effects of GPi pallidotomy on motor function in Parkinsons's disease. Lancet 1995;346:1383–1387.

57. Cohen J. New fight over fetal tissue grafts. Science 1994;263:600–601. News and Comments.

58. Faustman D, Coe C. Prevention of xenograft rejection by masking donor HLA class I antigens. Science 1991;252:1700–1702.

59. Pakzaban P, Deacon TW, Burns LH, et al. A novel mode of immunoprotection of neural xenotransplants: masking of donor major histocompatibility complex class I enhances transplant survival in the central nervous system. Neuroscience 1995;65:983–996.

60. Isacson O, Deacon TW, Pakzaban P, et al. Transplanted xenogeneic neural cells in neurodegenerative disease models exhibit remarkable axonal target specificity and distinct growth patterns of glial and axonal fibres. Nat Med 1995;1:1189–1194.

61. Deacon TW, Pakzaban P, Burns LH, et al. Cytoarchitectonic development, axon-glia relationships, and long distance axon growth of porcine striatal xenografts in rats. Exp Neurol 1994;130:151–167.

62. Burns LH, Pakzaban P, Deacon T, et al. Xenotransplantation of porcine ventral mesencephalic neuroblasts restores function in primates with chronic MPTP-induced parkinsonism. Soc Neurosci Abs 1994;20:1330.

63. Aebischer P, Tresco PA, Winn SR, et al. Long-term cross-species brain transplantation of a polymer encapsulated dopamine-secreting cell line. Exp Neurol 1991;111:269–275.

64. Aebischer P, Goddard M, Signore AP, Timpson RL. Functional recovery in hemiparkinsonian primates transplanted with polymer-encapsulated PC12 cells. Exp Neurol 1994;126:151–158.

65. Fisher LJ, Jinnah HA, Kale LC, et al. Survival and function of intrastriatally grafted primary fibroblasts genetically modified to produce L-dopa. Neuron 1991;6:371–380.

66. Jiao S, Gurevich V, Wolff JA. Long-term correction of a rat model of Parkinson's disease by gene therapy. Nature 1993;362:450–453.

67. Yurek DM, Collier TJ, Sladek JR. Embryonic mesencephalic and striatal co-grafts: development of grafted dopamine neurons and functional recovery. Exp Neurol 1990;109:191–199.

68. Granholm AC, Mott JL, Hoffer BJ. Neurotrophic treatment of intraocular and intracranial fetal brain tissue transplants. Am Soc Neural Transplant Abs 1996;55. Abstract P-57.

69. Lin LF, Doherty DH, Lile JD, et al. GDNF: a glial cell line-derived neurotrophic factor for midbrain dopaminergic neurons. Science 1993;260:1130–1132.

70. Gash DM, Zhang Z, Ovadia A, et al. Functional recovery in parkinsonian monkeys treated with GDNF. Nature 1996;380:252–255.

71. Nikkhah G, Bentlage C, Cunningham MG, Bjorklund A. Intranigral fetal dopamine grafts induce behavioral compensation in the rat Parkinson model. J Neurosci 1994;14:3449–3461.

72. Limousin PL, Pollak P, Benazzouz A, et al. Effect on parkinsonian signs and symptoms of bilateral subthalamic nucleus stimulation. Lancet 1995;345:91–95.

Extrapyramidal Syndromes Sometimes Mistaken for Parkinson's Disease

Robert R. Young

INTRODUCTION

The majority of patients in any movement disorder clinic have Parkinson's disease (PD), as defined by tremor, rigidity, and/or bradykinesia plus a dramatic response to L-dopa therapy at some stage of the illness. If a postmortem examination is done, one finds cell loss in the substantia nigra (especially the pars compacta) and other pigmented brainstem nuclei (locus coeruleus and dorsal motor nucleus of the vagus), with Lewy body intraneuronal inclusions. Roughly 20% of patients who are initially thought to have PD because of gradually evolving rigidity and slowness of movement, however, fall into one of two other general categories: 1) those who do respond to L-dopa therapy but who also have dramatic symptoms and signs not usually considered to be part of PD (such as significant dementia, orthostatic hypotension, or incontinence of bowel and bladder function); and 2) those whose progressive rigidity, slowness of movement, and trouble walking have never responded adequately to L-dopa therapy. The former group are described as having PD plus—they appear to have PD, but one questions whether the extra difficulties are due to an additional illness or simply represent unusual exaggerations of symptoms and signs often present, subclinically perhaps, in patients with PD. The second group, on the other hand, can rather easily be differentiated from patients with PD by an experienced clinician. On careful examination, they clearly do not have PD, although they share certain rather nonspecific traits such as progressive difficulty in middle age with the motor system, characterized by slowness of movement, stiffness or dystonia (1), awkwardness, fixed postures (usually in flexion), and so on. Although the differential diagnosis of this sort of condition includes many more conditions, four idiopathic extrapyramidal syndromes

have been recognized among this group of patients; others presumably remain to be described.

If a patient thought to have PD does not respond dramatically to L-dopa therapy, consider one of these other extrapyramidal syndromes. It is often difficult to make a definite diagnosis early in the course of the illness, but the following symptoms should at least raise the possibilities of these alternate diagnoses. Ataxia and other cerebellar signs are seen in olivopontocerebellar atrophy (OPCA). Cortical sensory loss and profound apraxia suggest progressive apraxic rigidity (PAR), also known as corticobasal degeneration or, more appropriately, as cortical-basal ganglionic degeneration (CBGD). Rigid axial muscles with dystonic postures of the neck and difficulty looking down are hallmarks of progressive supranuclear palsy (PSP). Postural hypotension and other autonomic failure (affecting bladder function, potency, and sweating) characterize the Shy-Drager syndrome (SDS). Further details concerning these syndromes are to be found below and in Chapter 35.

Most of these symptoms may sometimes occur, to a minor degree, in patients with otherwise typical PD; the differential diagnosis between PD plus and one of the non-PD progressive degenerative disorders of late life is largely based on the presence or absence of L-dopa responsivity. Even though clinicopathologic correlations are not always clear-cut—for example, the typical neuropathologic findings in each of these syndromes are not always associated with the typical clinical picture—it is preferable to attempt to categorize each patient according to the schema outlined above. The alternative approach is to lump all such patients under the rubric of multiple-system atrophy or parkinsonism and acknowledge that different areas of the cerebral cortex, basal ganglia, cerebellum, brainstem, and so on, show variable degrees of degeneration or loss of neurons with reactive gliosis but no other distinctive features. This variable, non-homogeneous loss of neurons would account for cerebellar signs in some patients, ophthalmoplegia in others, and so on. Such an approach may appear to simplify the diagnostic dilemma but is ultimately unsatisfying because it deemphasizes understanding of the neurobiologic processes responsible for each of the symptom complexes in question, reduces one's ability to make an accurate prognosis, and makes the search for specific pathophysiologies appear less important.

OLIVOPONTOCEREBELLAR ATROPHY

Olivopontocerebellar atrophy is one of the hereditary ataxias that was formerly thought to be rare; typical cerebellar ataxia is not always evident in patients with OPCA, but studies of families with this disorder, computed tomography (CT), magnetic resonance imaging (MRI), and postmortem studies show it to be more frequent than was clinically suspected. The clinical picture associated with this condition is extremely variable, as is the hereditary pattern. Some examples of OPCA are dominantly inherited, some recessive, and others appear to be sporadic. Some patients have pure cerebellar ataxia, whereas others have mainly parkinsonian features and some have elements of both. Progressive dementia is common throughout, spasticity is not uncommon, and choreoathetosis may be seen. Occasional patients with Huntington's disease (as defined by a typical family history and the genetic abnormality on chromosome 4) have a clinical picture and autopsy findings much like those seen with OPCA. In OPCA one finds cerebellar cortical degeneration with resultant atrophy of the inferior olivary nuclei and degeneration of neurons in pontine nuclei with atrophy of their projections up the middle cerebellar peduncle. One may also see nonspecific loss of neurons in basal ganglia and the substantia nigra.

Autosomal dominant inheritance of OPCA involves mainly Portuguese families with Machado-Thomas-Joseph disease (see Chapter 39). Recessive inheritance (or sporadic occurrence or perhaps even what appears to be dominant inheritance) may be seen with glutamate dehydrogenase deficiency, raising the possibility that glutamate-associated excitotoxicity may account for progressive loss of certain neurons. Obviously, it has been difficult to define the boundaries of this syndrome, which leads some to suggest the use of the broader term multiple-system atrophy. One would then reserve the clinical term OPCA for those patients within the broader group who display a combination of cerebellar ataxia and parkinsonism resistant to L-dopa therapy. Certainly that definition of OPCA is suitable for the purposes of this chapter. For a more detailed review of OPCA in its widest context, see Duvoisin (2) and Harding (3), as well as Chapter 45.

Clinically, one should suspect OPCA when there is a scanning dysarthria (or sometimes a spastic dysphonia) early on, followed by difficulty walking due to an ataxic gait (legs may also be weak), nystagmus, oculomotor difficulties, and ataxia/dysmetria of the upper limbs together with extrapyramidal signs. In some patients, progressive cerebellar ataxia precedes the development of extrapyramidal signs, whereas more often, a parkinsonian picture develops first with later addition of cerebellar signs. L-Dopa therapy, although it does not alleviate the extrapyramidal signs, may produce facial dystonia. The presence of spasticity or dementia should not dissuade one from a diagnosis of OPCA. Both CT and MRI allow visualization of OPCA.

PROGRESSIVE APRAXIC RIGIDITY

Progressive apraxic rigidity, one of the corticobasal ganglionic degenerative diseases, is a recently described illness (4) that makes its appearance in middle life or later (fifth to seventh decades). Males are affected about twice as often as females. Onset is insidious, and progression is relentless; the patients become bedridden, and death results from pneumonia and inanition in 5 to 15 years. Initially, progressive rigidity, slowness of movement, masked facies, flexed posture, poor postural control with falls, and difficulty using the upper limbs constitute an asymmetric clinical picture that raises the question of PD. Careful examination, however, reveals abnormalities of sensation, grasping, and Babinski responses and striking apraxia, which, together with L-dopa unresponsiveness, make a diagnosis of PD untenable. Asymmetric sensory loss is of the cortical variety—that is, stereognosis, graphesthesia, touch localization, two-point discrimination, bilateral simultaneous stimulation, and often joint position sensation are clearly faulty early on. At the same time, asymmetric ideational/ideomotor apraxia is striking. Most of the loss of dexterity and disability with the limbs is due to inability to perform simple, well-practiced movements despite good strength, good primary sensation, absence of dysmetria, and good understanding of the request. This apractic disorder is profound at a time when there is little if any dementia. The latter is usually mild until 3 to 5 years after the illness begins. As noted by Riley et al (5), the affected upper limb often moves involuntarily and adopts unusual postures without the patient being aware of it or able to stop it. There may also be apraxia of eye movements that can look like that seen with PSP (see Chapter 35), except with PAR, horizontal and vertical eye movements are equally affected early on. After a year or two, rigidity becomes extreme; antagonistic muscle groups, which control elbow or wrist movement, for example, are strongly, simultaneously, and continuously contracted, rendering voluntary movement virtually impossible. A moderate-amplitude, rapid-action tremor (enhanced physiologic tremor) is associated with the strong muscle contractions. Because of this dystonia, which is sometimes painful, and the apraxia, patients soon become unable to carry out activities of daily living, become completely immobile and totally dependent on others after about 5 years, and then lead a bed-chair existence. The disorder eventually affects all four limbs, trunk, speech, and eye movements.

In more than half the patients, the electroencephalogram (EEG) shows sharp slowing over the hemisphere contralateral to the most affected upper limb. CT or MRI demonstrates asymmetric atrophy that is especially marked in the peri-Rolandic area contralateral to the more affected limb. Positron emission tomography scans show decreased metabolism and blood flow frontally worse on the more atrophic side, and cerebrospinal fluid somatostatin levels are low. Autopsy shows that medium to large pyramidal neurons are swollen, with poorly stained cytoplasm (achromasia); few neuritic plaques are seen. This typical neuronal change is particularly prominent in the paracentral regions, in layers II and III, and is more marked on the side contralateral to the worse limb. If routine autopsy (or biopsy) sections are taken from other areas of the cortex, neuronal achromasia may be missed. There is also severe loss of cortical neurons with reactive astrocytic gliosis plus neuronal loss and gliosis in the medial third of the substantia nigra, but inclusion bodies are very rarely seen (6). The etiology of this syndrome is unknown.

Apraxia should be sought when a patient with what appears to be PD has much more trouble using his or her limbs than can be accounted for by the rigidity. If pyramidal signs and cortical sensory loss are also present, PAR should be considered. For historical reasons (7), this syndrome is sometimes called corticodentatonigral degeneration or corticobasal ganglionic degeneration (5). The former term is not always inclusive, and the latter term applies equally well to many of these clinically disparate syndromes. Characteristic clinical aspects of this syndrome include the progressive apraxia and profound rigidity or dystonia.

PROGRESSIVE SUPRANUCLEAR PALSY

See Chapter 35 for a full description of this extrapyramidal syndrome.

SHY-DRAGER SYNDROME

In older men, a rare syndrome with progressive idiopathic autonomic failure may later be associated with symptoms of an extrapyramidal (or cerebellar) disorder. The dysautonomia is characterized by severe orthostatic hypotension (usually accompanied by hypertension when recumbent), a fixed pulse rate, anhidrosis, decreased tears and saliva, obstipation, bladder dysfunction (retention or incontinence), impotence, and reduced norepinephrine production at rest or during standing and exercise—a syndrome referred to in the older literature as idiopathic orthostatic hypotension and more recently and appropriately as primary autonomic insufficiency. Medical and pharmacologic causes of dysautonomia must be ruled out. If a patient with this idiopathic autonomic disorder later develops extrapyramidal or cerebellar symptoms and trouble speaking (stridor), he or she is

said to have SDS (8). The extrapyramidal features (particularly bradykinesia and rigidity) are the same as those seen in PD and may be relieved by L-dopa or dopamine agonists, but such relief is short-lived and partial at best. A history of preceding dysautonomia and findings of severe hypofunction of sympathetic and parasympathetic innervation easily differentiate SDS from PD. Patients who develop cerebellar symptoms may be thought to have OPCA.

Pathologically, one finds loss of cells in the intermediolateral column of the thoracic cord (and perhaps in peripheral autonomic ganglia) to account for the dysautonomia (9). In patients with SDS, there is also cell loss in the substantia nigra and other basal ganglia, with gliosis and, in some cases, Lewy bodies. As noted above, the term multiple-system atrophy is sometimes used to refer to all of these nonparkinsonian degenerative disorders or at other times to refer to only patients with SDS.

Ordinary neurodiagnostic tests are not particularly useful in the diagnosis of SDS, but MRI may show putamenal atrophy (10). Tests of autonomic function should be abnormal. For example, the heart rate should not vary with a Vasalva maneuver or with deep breathing and there should be no rise in blood pressure as a result of keeping a hand in ice water for several minutes.

SDS rarely affects females, begins in middle life, and becomes so disabling after 5 or 6 years that patients are bedridden, usually because of intractable postural hypotension. Initially, relief of postural lightheadedness can be obtained by expanding extracellular volume with a high-sodium diet plus fludrocortisone, avoiding loss of intravascular volume by sleeping with the head of the bed raised, and reducing fluid pooling in the legs with elastic stockings. Prostaglandin synthesis inhibitors such as indomethacin or ibuprofen may also help. Eventually, postural hypotension can no longer be avoided. Death usually follows in 8 or 10 years as a result of aspiration, sleep apnea, or an arrhythmia. See Polinsky (11) for a more detailed review.

SUMMARY

Patients whose apparent PD does not clearly respond to L-dopa or, in the case of those with SDS, in whom autonomic failure precedes the motor disorder can usually be categorized according to the scheme outlined above. Care must be taken to rule out another illness (such as a cerebellar or cortical neoplasm, brainstem infarct, or symptomatic dysautonomia) producing some of the symptoms mentioned above in patients with typical PD; PD does not preclude the development of another unrelated neurologic disorder.

REFERENCES

1. Rivest J, Quinn N, Marsden CD. Dystonia in Parkinson's disease, multiple system atrophy, and progressive supranuclear palsy. Neurology 1990;40:1571–1578.
2. Duvoisin RC. The olivopontocerebellar atrophies. In: Marsden CD, Fahn S, eds. Movement disorders. 2nd ed. London: Butterworths, 1987:249–269.

3. Harding AE. The hereditary ataxias and related disorders. Edinburgh: Churchill Livingstone, 1984.

4. Watts RL, Williams RS, Growdon JH, et al. Corticobasal ganglionic degeneration. Neurology 1985;35:178.

5. Riley DE, Lang AE, Lewis A, et al. Cortical-basal ganglionic degeneration. Neurology 1990;40:1203–1212.

6. Gibb WR, Luthert PJ, Marsden CD. Corticobasal degeneration. Brain 1989;112:1171–1192.

7. Rebeiz JJ, Kolodny EH, Richardson EP. Corticodentatonigral degeneration with neuronal achromasia. Arch Neurol 1968;18:20–33.

8. Shy GM, Drager GA. A neurological syndrome associated with orthostatic hypotension. Arch Neurol 1960;2:511–527.

9. Oppenheimer D. Neuropathology of progressive autonomic failure. In: Bannister R, ed. Autonomic failure. Oxford: Oxford University Press, 1983:267–283.

10. Pastakia P, Polinsky RJ, DiChiro G, et al. Multiple system atrophy (Shy-Drager syndrome): MR imaging. Radiology 1986;159:499–502.

11. Polinsky RJ, Shy-Drager syndrome. In: Jankovic J, Tolosa E, eds. Parkinson's disease and movement disorders. Baltimore: Urban & Schwarzenberg, 1988:153–166.

Progressive Supranuclear Palsy

KAREN SANTA CRUZ   RONALD C. KIM   ROBERT R. YOUNG

INTRODUCTION

The patient who initially kindled J. Clifford Richardson's interest in the condition that he later named progressive supranuclear palsy (PSP) presented with vague yet intriguing symptoms. He had given up playing the piano due to difficulty controlling his left hand. A year later he began to feel unsteady and clumsy at the office. By the third year, this successful business executive had difficulty thinking and was having trouble "seeing properly." Four years after onset, his symptoms and signs were distinctive enough to be recognized as what is now known as PSP.

PSP is a relentlessly progressive movement disorder beginning in late middle life, with abnormalities of gait, poor balance, frequent falls, masked facies, rigid axial musculature, slow movements, and soft speech, all of which sound parkinsonian. The patient's neck is usually stiff—dystonic in flexion or extension—but there is little dystonia of the limbs. The key diagnostic feature is difficulty looking down due to supranuclear palsy of vertical gaze. That is, the eyes move easily and fully to reflex inputs—vestibulo-ocular reflexes are preserved or hyperactive—whereas volitional eye movements are defective. In addition to this supranuclear ophthalmoplegia, primarily affecting vertical, especially downward, gaze (unfortunately for the diagnostician, abnormal eye movements are not always present, especially early in the disease), one finds pseudobulbar palsy with emotional liability, dystonic axial rigidity, frontal lobe signs, and mild dementia.

The original publication by Steele, Richardson, and Olszewski provided detailed clinical descriptions of nine patients and included extensive gross and histologic descriptions of neuropathology from four of these patients (1). The results of histologic examination of two more of these patients were published eight years later (2). Degenerative changes consisting of neuronal loss, gliosis, granulovacuolar degeneration, and, more important, neurofibrillary tangles were present bilaterally in basal ganglia and in brainstem and cerebellar nuclei. The subthalamic nucleus, globus pallidus, and substantia nigra were most consistently and heavily involved.

In retrospect, as many as 15 cases of probable PSP had been published prior to this original description. The earliest was credited to an American ophthalmologist, Campbell Posey, in 1904 (3). More recently, however, this assertion has been challenged by Siderowf et al, who reviewed the 1906 autopsy findings from this "earliest PSP patient" (4). The neuropathology best explaining the patient's clinical symptoms was a tumor, resembling a sarcoma or endothelioma, involving the right cerebral peduncle and periaqueductal area. They did not mention neurofibrillary tangles. Chavany et al published what is considered the first definite case of PSP in 1951 (5), and the number of publications describing PSP increased rapidly over the next 3 decades. Today, PSP is often considered in the differential diagnosis when a patient with atypical parkinsonian features fails to respond to L-dopa therapy, particularly when eye findings or mild dementia are present.

DIAGNOSIS

The clinical criteria for PSP set forth by Lees in 1987 (6) included one essential feature, supranuclear ophthalmoplegia, and two or more of the following additional features: postural instability, pseudobulbar palsy, bradykinesia and rigidity, frontal lobe signs, or axial dystonia and rigidity. Duvoisin considered five features essential for diagnosis: supranuclear palsy, rigidity, bradykinesia, onset after age 40, and a progressive course (7). Eight additional features were considered confirmatory: poor or absent response to L-dopa, severe bradyphrenia with frontal lobe features, axial dystonia, gait impairment, dysarthria and dysphagia, ocular fixation instability with macro square-wave jerks, apraxias of eyelid opening or closing or infrequent eye blink, and echolalia and palilalia.

In 1994, the National Institute of Neurological Disorders and Stroke (NINDS) and the Society for PSP published a set of diagnostic criteria based primarily on the histopathologic appearance of autopsy material (7). Another set of clinical criteria defining three degrees of certainty (possible, probable, and definite) for the diagnosis of PSP was proposed by the NINDS in 1996 (8). Mandatory exclusion criteria for possible or probable PSP have also been published by Litvan (9,10). These include a recent history of encephalitis or oculogyric crises, striking asymmetry of parkinsonian symptoms, tremor-dominant disease, marked or prolonged levodopa benefit, hallucinations and delusions unrelated to therapy, cortical dementia, prominent cerebellar symptomatology, dysautonomia, alien hand syndrome, and severe limb apraxia, to which we would add cortical sensory loss and spasticity. These criteria are designed to exclude diseases that may have clinical features in common with PSP, such as postencephalitic parkinsonism, Parkinson's disease, dementia with Lewy bodies, Alzheimer's disease, multiple-system atrophy, and corticobasal degeneration.

EPIDEMIOLOGY AND ETIOLOGY

Onset of symptoms in PSP usually occurs between 55 and 70 years of age. Onset before age 50 is distinctly rare. Death, from pneumonia or inanition, usually occurs within 5 to 10 years of diagnosis, and a median delay of approximately 4 years has been estimated to precede diagnosis. Patients seen in movement disorder clinics will have a significantly shortened delay to diagnosis. The originally described preponderance of male to female PSP patients of 2:1 was most likely due to sampling error; most neurologists now agree that the ratio of male to female patients approaches 1:1.

The etiology of PSP is unknown. It is not transmitted by inoculation, and no genetic, viral, toxic, medical, surgical, or personality associations have been described. Hypertension, smoking, and trauma are also unrelated to PSP. Golbe et al (11) noted that patients with PSP are less likely to have completed 12 years of school compared with age-matched controls. Poor early-life nutrition or exposure (occupational or residential) to some unknown toxin were proposed as possible explanations for this finding.

CLINICAL CHARACTERISTICS

Early manifestations of PSP may be quite subtle; this was true for most of the original patients presented by Steele, Richardson, and Olszewski. Common initial signs and symptoms include difficulty with balance and abrupt falls, dysphagia, dysarthria (and other speech irregularities such as slurring, stuttering, palilalia, and echolalia), and visual difficulties, particularly with downward gaze. Neurobehavioral findings such as an agitated depression, vague changes in personality, and apprehensiveness are also typically present early. Often, the patient denies problems even when his or her symptoms interfere with the patient's occupation or activities of daily living. Early signs may be difficult to assess, but as the disease progresses, horizontal eye movements are also affected, dysarthria worsens, and, after many months or several years, speech and voluntary eye movements become totally paralyzed. Although there are many similarities early on, PSP is more symmetric than early Parkinson's disease and has no clear-cut or striking response to L-dopa. The ophthalmoplegia or paresis itself is not specific for PSP (6), but it is difficult to be certain of the diagnosis without it. Before supranuclear downgaze paralysis becomes apparent, detailed ophthalmologic examination may reveal a loss of the fast component of nystagmus in caloric and otokinetic responses, with its replacement by tonic ocular deviations in the direction of the expected slow component (6). Similar tonic deviations can be elicited in the upward and downward directions by simultaneous hot and cold stimulation of both ears. Hesitancy in voluntary downgaze, with a tendency to flex the neck to look down, and poor suppression of the vertical vestibulo-ocular reflex may also be observed.

Eventually, the clinical presentation progresses to include the typical features of PSP. All voluntary vertical eye movements are lost. Bell's phenomenon and convergence are lost; the upper eyelids become retracted, imparting a surprised look. There is stiffening and extension or flexion of the neck and later some, but less, stiffening of the limbs, often with Babinski responses. Patients eventually develop prominent pseudobulbar palsy with masked, expressionless facies; the mouth may hang open. Slurred speech and difficulties with swallowing become prominent. Frontal signs include grasp responses and overfilling the mouth with food. The gait disturbance is often obvious, but difficult to assess. It is not entirely due to stiffening of the trunk and limbs and the inability to look down. Steps are awkward and tentative, with frequent falling, and the arms are often abducted at the shoulders and flexed at the elbows. There is mild ataxia of the limbs and a tendency to lean and fall backward. This toppling phenomenon has been likened to that seen with lateral medullary infarction. In late stages of the disease, the eyes become centrally fixed, the oculocephalic and vestibular reflexes are lost, and the patient becomes anarthric, immobile, and helpless. Dementia may remain mild to the end.

Unusual Presentations and Clinical Differential Diagnosis

Unusual presentations that make clinical diagnosis difficult, if not impossible, have been reported. We recently found frequent globose brainstem and basal ganglia neurofibrillary tangles with associated gliosis and cell loss in a patient who only had minimal difficulty with upgaze and dementia. Atypical presentations including palilalia and disturbances of vestibular function have been described. Ocular abnormalities may be absent; minimal or late trouble with eye movements and neuropathologically proven cases with pure akinesia and pure dementia have also been reported. Other unusual manifestations include cricopharyngeal dysfunction, abnormalities of respiratory rhythm, nontremulous involuntary movements, internuclear ophthalmoplegia, apraxia, and early severe dementia.

The clinical differential diagnosis may be extensive, considering the wide variety of reported atypical presentations. Akinetic rigid syndromes, such as Parkinson's disease, parkinsonian syndromes, multiple-system atrophy (including olivopontocerebellar atrophy, Shy-Drager syndrome, and striatonigral degeneration), and corticobasal degeneration (also known as progressive apraxic rigidity) should be considered. Dementia with Lewy bodies, Alzheimer's disease (AD), and cerebrovascular disease are often a consideration, as are other less common diseases such as prion disease, Whipple's disease, Pick's disease, and dentatorubropallidoluysial atrophy (DRPLA).

Imaging studies are of little help. On magnetic resonance imaging, in addition to nonspecific atrophic changes affecting the cerebral cortex and the ventricular system, the midbrain in PSP may also be unusually atrophic, but that can be difficult to be certain about and is not specific for PSP. Positron emission tomography (PET) scans (with either F-dopa or F-deoxyglucose) may help differentiate PSP from Parkinson's disease, but they are available primarily as research tools. Careful otoneurologic testing using Electronystagmography often documents the characteristic eye movement disorders even before they are clinically obvious.

GROSS AND MICROSCOPIC PATHOLOGY

Grossly, the brain in PSP may be normal or may show mild atrophy, particularly of the brainstem and cerebellum, with mild dilatation of the third and fourth ventricles and cerebral aqueduct. Both subcortical and cortical diffuse atrophy have been seen with imaging, but this is not well documented on postmortem examination. Mild atrophy of the motor cortex has been described as well. Atrophy of specific structures such as the globus pallidus, subthalamic nucleus, and superior colliculi, in addition to hypopigmentation of the substantia nigra and locus coeruleus, is often present. Histologic examination shows symmetrical bilateral loss of neurons and gliosis in the periaqueductal gray matter, superior colliculi, subthalamic nuclei, red nuclei, globus pallidus, dentate nuclei, pretectal and vestibular nuclei, and, to some extent, the oculomotor nuclei. In addition, loss of the medullated fiber bundles arising from these nuclei has been observed. Neurofibrillary tangles (NFT) and neuropil

threads (NT) constitute the histologic hallmark of PSP; they are seen in the basal ganglia (globus pallidus, subthalamic nucleus, and striatum), nucleus basalis of Meynert, brainstem (tegmentum, colliculi, periaqueductal gray matter, red nucleus, basis pontis, dorsal and median raphe nuclei, and inferior olives), and cerebellar nuclei (dentate nucleus) (Figs 35.1 to 35.3). A variety of other tau-immunoreactive structures have also been described, including three forms of astrocytic inclusions and coil-like structures (coiled bodies) within oligodendroglial cells (12). Neuritic plaques such as those seen in Alzheimer's disease are absent or extremely rare.

Specific histopathologic inclusionary and exclusionary criteria for the diagnosis of PSP were proposed at a National Institutes of Health workshop in 1994 (8). Minimal sections required for the diagnosis of typical, atypical, or combined PSP should include globus pallidus, putamen, caudate nucleus, subthalamic nucleus, midbrain, pons, medulla, and cerebellar dentate nucleus. To rule out other diseases that might be confused or associated with PSP, examination of the hippocampus, parahippocampal gyrus, and motor, frontal, and parietal cortices was recommended. Routine

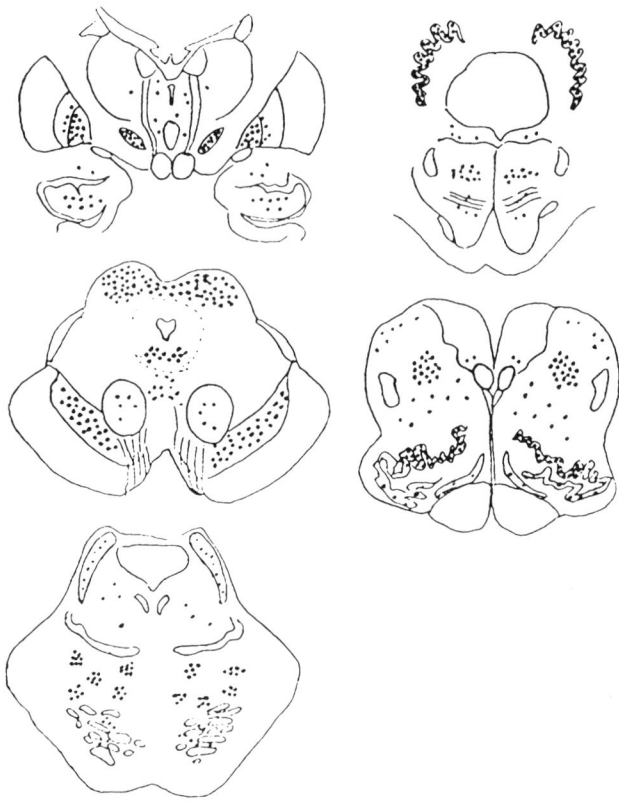

FIGURE 35.1   *Diagrammatic representation of the distribution of neurofibrillary tangles, as indicated by dots, in a case of progressive supranuclear palsy. Involvement is heaviest within the globus pallidus, subthalamic nucleus, superior colliculi, substantia nigra, superior cerebellar peduncles, nuclei basis pontis, medullary reticular formation, and inferior olivary nuclei.*

hematoxylin-eosin staining combined with either a silver-staining technique or tau and ubiquitin immunohistochemistry was considered essential. A high density of NFTs and NTs must be found in at least three of the following locations: pallidum, subthalamic nucleus, substantia nigra, and pons. In addition, lower numbers of NFTs and NTs must be seen in at least three of the following sites: striatum, oculomotor nuclear complex, medulla, and dentate nucleus. No strict criteria pertaining to the degree of cell loss and gliosis were proposed. Criteria for atypical PSP were less restrictive. Low-density NFTs and NTs in at least five of the following sites were considered supportive of that diagnosis: pallidum, subthalamic nucleus, substantia nigra, pons, medulla, and dentate nucleus.

The NFTs of PSP are primarily of the globose type, although occasional more typical (flame-shaped) tangles are present, primarily in the cerebral cortex. The pathogenesis of PSP may be related to abnormal metabolism of cytoskeletal components (neurofilaments) with accumulation of abnormal tau protein in neurons and glial cells. Tau proteins function in the polymerization of soluble tubulin to form microtubules. Abnormally phosphorylated tau is present in the NFTs of both PSP and AD, but ultrastructural examination reveals the NFTs of PSP to be composed primarily of straight (15-nm) fibrils, whereas those of AD consist of paired helical (10-nm) filaments. Conversely, the immunohistochemical profile of tau proteins is similar in AD and PSP. Abnormal phosphorylation of tau probably occurs early in PSP. Whether NFT formation precedes nerve cell loss and gliosis is less clear. Nerve cell loss and gliosis do not correlate with severity of tangle formation; rather, the cell loss appears to be related inversely to the number of NFTs.

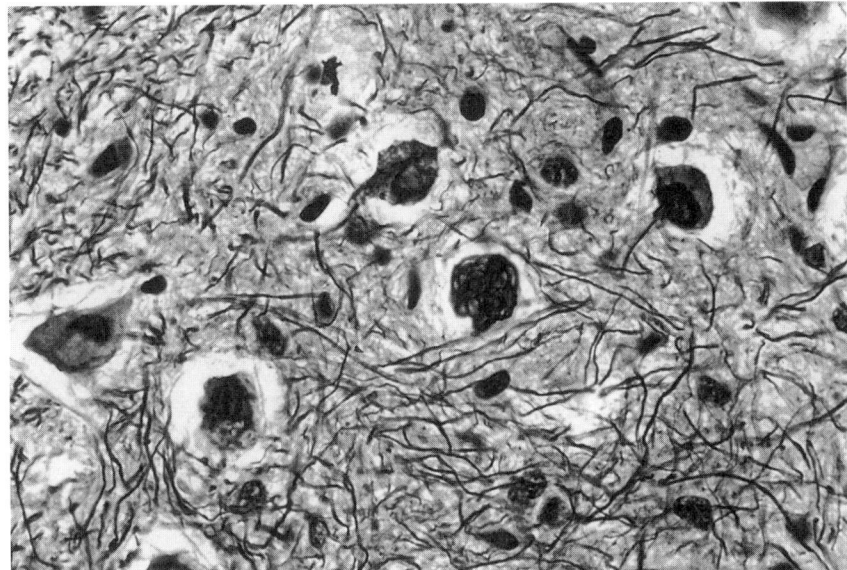

FIGURE 35.2   *Neurofibrillary degeneration within neurons of the basis pontis (Bodian stain, ×900).*

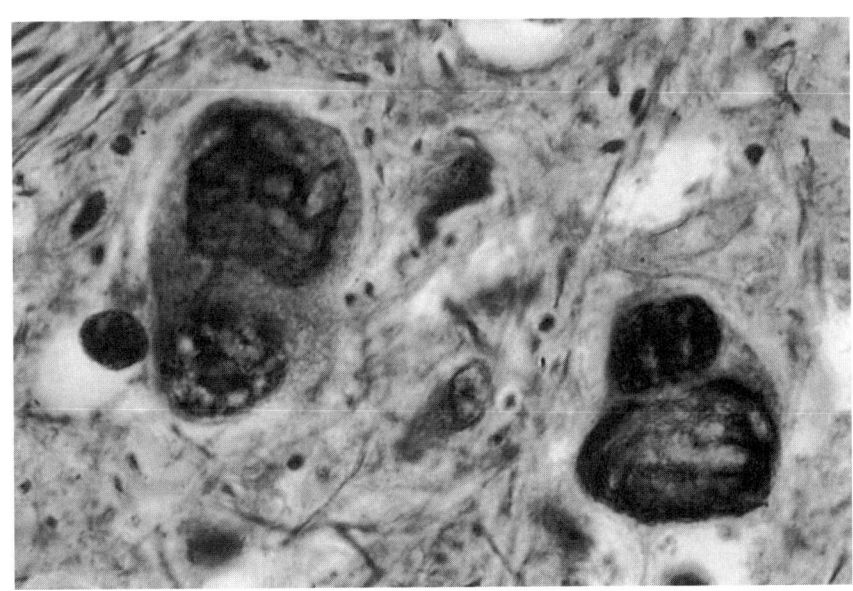

FIGURE 35.3   *Globose neurofibrillary tangles within neurons of the basis pontis (Bodian stain, ×1,500).*

Also, ghost tangles, such as those seen in the most heavily involved allocortical locations in AD, are not seen in PSP. These ghost tangles are thought to represent an end-stage form of NFT.

PATHOGENESIS

Two of the most consistent PET laboratory features of PSP are decreased oxygen utilization and blood flow, most prominent in the frontal lobes, and decreased striatal dopamine formation and storage. A possible explanation for the frontal cortex hypometabolism seen on PET scanning is that the heavily damaged subcortical nuclei have a reduced synaptic output to the frontal cortex (13). Levy et al (14) showed that GABAergic neurons in the basal ganglia are reduced in PSP. Neurons expressing GAD67 mRNA were reduced by as much as 43% to 68% in a variety of locations, including the caudate nucleus, putamen, and globus pallidus. Target neurons in the striatum also show reductions of choline acetyltransferase and glutamic acid decarboxylase activity, once again implying that output from this site is compromised. These findings provide an explanation not only for the motor and cognitive symptoms of PSP but also for the lack of responsiveness to L-dopa therapy.

HISTOLOGIC DIFFERENTIAL DIAGNOSIS

The histologic differential diagnosis is quite different from the clinical differential diagnosis. Histopathologic changes seen in DRPLA are similar but show few brainstem neurofibrillary tangles and relative sparing of the dentate nucleus. Postencephalitic parkinsonism (PEP) may also show similar histologic features, such as nerve cell loss and gliosis within the substantia nigra. However, the clinical history of encephalitis, early age of onset, absence of dementia, and slowly progressive course with good response to L-dopa are helpful in distinguishing PEP from PSP. In addition, histologic examination shows involvement of the periaqueductal gray matter and superior colliculi to be minimal or absent in PEP. The Guamanian amyotrophic lateral sclerosis–parkinsonism–dementia complex and multisystem atrophy (striatonigral degeneration, olivopontocerebellar atrophy, and Shy-Drager syndrome) show some degenerative changes similar to those seen in PSP but with different patterns of distribution. Dementia pugilistica and corticobasal degeneration also have histopathologic features in common with PSP. Fortunately, clinical features often help to distinguish these entities from PSP. In addition, amyloid 4 (A4) deposits, cortical contusions, and/or fenestration of the septum pellucidum are usually seen in dementia pugilistica. Achromatic neurons and neurons with basophilic inclusions are more common in corticobasal degeneration than in typical PSP.

Some have suggested that the diagnosis of atypical PSP may be made when the severity or distribution of neurofibrillary tangles is unusual. Others have used the term "combined PSP" when the clinical and histologic features of PSP were combined with those of another disease process such as Alzheimer's disease or multiple infarcts. When the validity and reliability of the preliminary NINDS neuropathologic criteria were investigated in 1996 (15), however, it was decided that differentiating between typical, atypical, and combined PSP was not possible without clinical information. Nor could PEP be separated from PSP strictly on the basis of pathologic findings. Conversely, Pick's disease and corticobasal degeneration could usually be distinguished histologically from PSP. It was therefore recommended that a supportive clinical history be required for diagnosis and that the term "atypical PSP" be avoided.

PATHOGENESIS OF DEMENTIA

Explanations for both the frontal lobe symptomatology and mild dementia of PSP have long been sought. The frontal lobe symptomatology may result from a reduction of output to the frontal lobes from the basal ganglia and thalamus, thereby leading to frontal deafferentation. Although the morphologic basis of the dementia is also unclear, the results of neuropsychological testing suggest that it is of subcortical origin. In addition to nerve cell loss and loss of dopamine in the putamen and substantia nigra, the caudate nucleus is often severely degenerated in PSP. This may contribute to the higher frequency of dementia in PSP as compared with Parkinson's disease. Reduced choline acetyltransferase activity and neuron loss within the nucleus basalis of Meynert have been described but do not appear to correlate with the severity of dementia. Braak et al (16) studied the histologic appearance of the entorhinal cortex in three demented PSP patients and found destructive changes within the allocortex that closely resembled those of AD. However, the subcortical or frontal lobe nature of the dementia seen in PSP is not fully explained by these changes.

TREATMENT AND SURVIVAL

A variety of therapeutic agents, including dopamine agonists, antidepressants, serotonin antagonists, cholinergic neurotransmitter enhancers, electroconvulsive therapy, and botulinum toxin-A (for rigidity), have been tried. However, the treatment of PSP is generally unsatisfactory. In a retrospective study of 87 patients, Nieforth and Golbe (17) found that 32% benefited from amitriptyline, 28% benefited from imipramine, and 38% benefited from levodopa/carbidopa. The best risk-benefit ratios were obtained with levodopa/carbidopa, amantadine, selegiline, and amitriptyline. In addition, single-drug therapy was more effective and better tolerated than multidrug therapy, but none of the benefits was striking or long lasting.

Litvan et al (18) examined a variety of clinical features and determined that the best predictors of shorter survival time were as follows: onset of falls during the first year, early dysphagia, and incontinence. Age, sex, early onset of dementia, and the presence of supranuclear palsy and axial rigidity did not influence prognosis. Pneumonia was the most common cause of death, possibly due to aspiration.

REFERENCES

1. Steele JC, Richardson JC, Olszewski J. Progressive supranuclear palsy. Arch Neurol 1964;10:333–359.
2. Steele JC. Progressive supranuclear palsy. Brain 1972;95:693–704.
3. Posey WC. Paralysis of the upward movements of the eyes. Ann Ophthalmol 1904;13:523–529.
4. Siderowf AD, Galetta SL, Hurtig HI, et al. Posey and Spiller and progressive supranuclear palsy: an incorrect attribution. Mov Disord 1998;13:170–174.
5. Chavany JA, van Bogaert L, Godlewski S. Sur un syndrome de rigidite a predominance axiale, avec perturbation des automatismes oculo-palpebraux d'origine encephalitique. Presse Med 1951;59:958–962.
6. Lees AJ. The Steele-Richardson-Olszewski syndrome (progressive supranuclear palsy). In: Marsden CD, Fahn S, eds. Movement disorders. 2nd ed. London: Butterworths, 1987:272–287.
7. Duvoisin RC. Clinical diagnosis. In: Litvan I, Yves A, eds. Progressive supranuclear palsy: clinical and research approaches. New York: Oxford University Press, 1992:17–19.
8. Hauw JJ, Daniel SE, Dickson D, et al. Preliminary NINDS neuropathological criteria for Steele-Richardson-Olszewski syndrome (progressive supranuclear palsy). Neurology 1994;44:2015–2019.
9. Litvan I, Agid Y, Calne D, et al. Clinical research criteria for the diagnosis of progressive supranuclear palsy (Steele-Richardson-Olszewski syndrome): report of the NINDS-SPSP International Workshop. Neurology 1996;47:1–9.
10. Litvan I. Clinical research criteria for the diagnosis of progressive supranuclear palsy. World Neurol 1997;12:6.
11. Golbe LI, Rubin RS, Cody RP, et al. Follow-up study of risk factors in progressive supranuclear palsy. Neurology 1996;47:148–154.
12. Nishimura T, Ikeda K, Akiyama H, et al. Immunohistochemical investigation of tau-positive structures in the cerebral cortex of patients with progressive supranuclear palsy. Neurosci Lett 1995;201:123–126.
13. Devebvre L, Destee A, Houdart P, Steinling M. Tomographic measurements of regional cerebral blood flow in progressive supranuclear palsy and Parkinson's disease. Acta Neurol Scand 1995;92:235–241.
14. Levy R, Ruberg M, Herrero MT, et al. Alterations of GABAergic neurons in the basal ganglia of patients with progressive supranuclear palsy: an in situ hybridization study of GAD67 messenger RNA. Neurology 1995;45:127–134.
15. Litvan I, Hauw JJ, Bartko JJ, et al. Validity and reliability of the preliminary NINDS neuropathologic criteria for progressive supranuclear palsy and related disorders. J Neuropathol Exp Neurol 1996;55:97–105.
16. Braak H, Jellinger K, Braak E, et al. Allocortical neurofibrillary changes in progressive supranuclear palsy. Acta Neuropathol 1992;84:478–483.
17. Nieforth KA, Golbe LI. Retrospective study of drug response in 87 patients with progressive supranuclear palsy. Clin Neuropharmacol 1993;16:338–346.
18. Litvan I, Mangone CA, McKee A, et al. Natural history of progressive supranuclear palsy (Steele-Richardson-Olszewski syndrome) and clinical predictors of survival: a clinicopathological study. J Neurol Neurosurg Psychiatry 1996;60:615–620.

Striopallidodentate Calcifications

ARMAND LOWENTHAL   PETER P. DE DEYN

INTRODUCTION

Striopallidodentate calcifications (SPDC), also known as basal ganglia calcifications or brain calcinosis, are still not well understood. The evolution of knowledge concerning SPDC is rather peculiar. It is illustrative of the tremendous developments in neurologic sciences because it encompasses the early period, which gave only an anatomic and clinical understanding, up to the present, in which more sophisticated techniques are applied. Despite the advances in the field, to which we had the opportunity to contribute, knowledge concerning SPDC is still fragmentary. It is hard to say when exactly SPDC were first described. To our knowledge, the first anatomicopathologic report describing stones in the basal ganglia dates from the nineteenth century.

The first physiopathologic association, which has been reviewed (1), suggested that these calcifications are related to a disturbance of the calcium metabolism, in particular, hypoparathyroidism. Later researchers tried to better understand the physiopathology of these calcifications by performing biochemical studies on the calcifications as such, as well as calcium metabolism studies in general. This permitted a better identification of the biochemical composition of these calcifications, at first by merely biochemical methods, later by much more complex techniques and by the association of these methods with newly developed morphologic approaches.

In the first edition of the *Handbook of Clinical Neurology* (2), a chapter was devoted to these calcifications, aiming to define the related clinical syndrome as well as the chemical composition of SPDC. In the second edition, published in 1986, this topic was covered again (3) and new observations were highlighted. It was recognized that computed tomography (CT) demonstrated SPDC to be much more frequent than previously thought, and that, clinically speaking,

these calcifications can be associated with an extremely broad variety of diseases. Since then, numerous new reports about SPDC have been issued. These reports highlighted many unresolved questions raised by the presence of these calcifications. Still, in a 1987 chapter devoted to Fahr's disease and to the calcifications of the gray central nuclei, published in the *Encyclopédie Medico-Chirurgicale* (4), it was stated that the very existence of these calcifications raises questions.

The bibliography of older papers can be consulted in the second edition of the *Handbook of Clinical Neurology* (3). In the light of recent publications, we will mainly discuss the following issues: the physiopathology underlying the formation of these calcifications, and the clinical aspects of these calcifications.

DEFINITION AND DENOMINATION OF THE CALCIFICATIONS OF THE BASAL GANGLIA

We consider it most important to define very precisely the entity that we will discuss. We will consider only macroscopic calcifications of the basal ganglia that detach from the nervous tissue during the anatomicopathologic examination. In other words, these calcifications fall out of the brain and leave a slice of nervous tissue that once was compared with a badly shaven beard, the "hairs" in fact being calcified vessels. These calcifications are always symmetric (Fig 36.1). The notion that these calcifications are macroscopically visible must be stressed. Calcifications that are only microscopically visible are not considered here. Moreover, SPDC are often accompanied by calcifications of the nucleus dentatus of the cerebellum. This aspect has been neglected in numerous publications. Microscopic examination reveals no involvement of other brain structures by a similar process. However, lesions of another type might be observed.

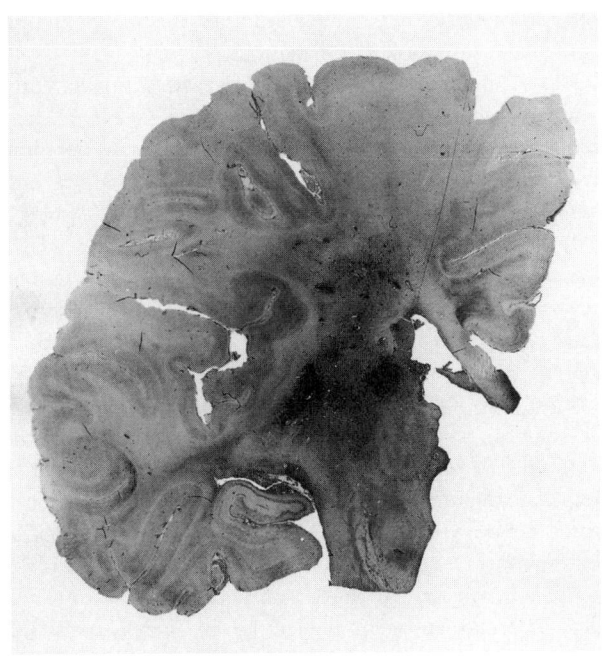

FIGURE 36.1 *Brain slice with calcification of the basal ganglia and the white matter.*

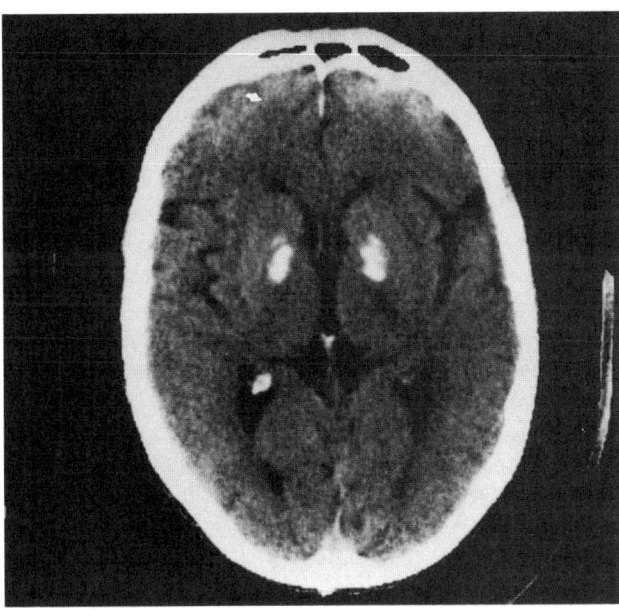

FIGURE 36.2 *CT scan illustrating symmetric calcification of the basal ganglia.*

Although originally the diagnosis of SPDC was exclusively an anatomicopathologic one, from 1935 on the diagnosis was made in vivo thanks to neuroradiologic examinations (5). Since the introduction of the CT scan (Fig 36.2), these calcifications in the basal ganglia as well as in the cerebellar dentate nuclei have been frequently diagnosed. CT scans demonstrated that the occurrence of these calcifications is much more frequent than originally thought: up to 1% of the patients examined exhibit them. A case of postoperative hypoparathyroidism with extensive calcifications shown on CT scan in the basal ganglia, the bifrontal periventricular white matter, the cerebellum, and even the brainstem has been described (6). An effort has even been made to define the evolutionary character of these lesions and to localize them more precisely by CT scan.

Controversy still exists concerning the diagnostic possibilities that magnetic resonance imaging (MRI) might yield. Theoretically, the calcifications would not be visualized by MRI. In a recent publication, however, Scotti et al (7) tentatively defined three different stages of degree of calcification, illustrating the possible diagnostic role of MRI. In our earlier-described and above-mentioned case of hypoparathyroidism, the white matter calcifications displayed a high signal intensity on MRI, probably due to a different stage of calcifying process in the white matter than in the basal ganglia (6). More recently, in large patient populations, MRI has been shown to yield abnormalities related to intracerebral calcifications, T2-weighted images being most sensitive (8). In one of our cases with post-

operative hypoparathyroidism, technetium-99m hexamethylpropyleneamine oxidase single-photon emission computed tomography (SPECT) findings were suggestive of hypoperfusion/hypometabolism in noncalcified brain regions, possibly due to a deafferentiation phenomenon (9). Uygur et al (10) used similar SPECT methodology and demonstrated decreased perfusion to the basal ganglia bilaterally as well as decreased perfusion to the cerebral cortices. Staffen et al (11) studied SPDC by PET and demonstrated anomalies of glucose metabolism only at the calcification sites.

One might wonder whether, in view of the given definition, it is accurate to call SPDC Fahr's disease. We have to remember that Fahr was not the first who described the disease. He did add the notion that the calcifications were nonatherosclerotic, despite the fact that it is a disease primarily of older persons. However, can one still retain this eponym in view of later discoveries and clinical correlations (which we will discuss later on)? We prefer the denomination of SPDC, provided that one remembers the notion that the calcifications under consideration are macroscopic and symmetric. Microscopic calcifications are excluded from this syndrome.

PHYSIOPATHOLOGY

Physiopathologic problems raised by these calcifications have been tackled by neuropathologists as well as by biochemists. Neuropathologists have described the macroscopic images and attempted histochemical studies. These studies, often using controversial histochemical techniques, demonstrated the anticipated presence of calcium as well as the existence of an organic matrix called pseudocalcium. It is hard to define exactly what corresponds with this pseudocalcium within the realm of neuropathology. Scanning electron microscopy revealed the presence of rather peculiar structures in these calcifications that could be illustrative of different types of calcifications (Fig 36.3) (12). Moreover, scanning electron microscopy links merely morphologic images with biochemical studies. There has been very little or no new development during the last few years related to studies carried out with scanning electron microscopy or research focusing on the biochemistry of SPDC.

Biochemical studies demonstrate that, besides calcium, these calcifications also contain PO_4 and CO_2 and that they probably are a mineral identified through totally different studies as being hydroxyapatite. Besides calcium phosphates and carbonates, other metals, such as iron, aluminium, zinc, manganese, and magnesium, have been found in these calcifications. In the recent literature, only one author elaborated on iron metabolism, studying patients showing ferritin increases and free serum iron modifications in SPDC (13). Probably these metals are only adsorbed to the calcifications without having physiopathologic importance. Kozik and Kulczycki (14) and Kuran et al (15) used laser analysis to confirm the previous findings concerning the mineral composition of these calcifications.

The organic matrix called pseudocalcium that is reportedly present in these calcifications, which led to the hypothesis that these calcifications are pseudocalcium, is much less well known. It has been claimed that mucopolysaccharides and glycoproteins constitute this matrix (16). However, we found large quantities of proteins containing an unidentified amino acid (12) in this matrix. Manyam et al (17) studied amino acids in the cerebrospinal fluid of patients with SPDC. They found increases of homocarnosine and

decreases of histidine. All these findings, including ours, are fragmentary and await confirmation.

The biochemical aspects of these calcifications have also been approached through metabolic studies. Neurologists and anatomicopathologists have put forth some quite curious hypotheses in this respect. For example, one considered hypo-oxygenation due to different factors (such as bradycardia) as a possible causative factor. Other researchers suggested arterial hypertension as playing a role. Also important was the notion that the calcifications were localized in so-called border zones or watershed areas at the junction of different vascular territories, resulting in an insufficient oxygenation that would give rise to the formation of stones. In our opinion it is more important to stress the fact that SPDC are frequently accompanied by clinical signs of an abnormal calcium metabolism such as hypoparathyroidism, pseudopseudohypoparathyroidism, or even hyperparathyroidism. It is, however, rather peculiar to emphasize that hypoparathyroidism with a diminution of circulating calcium would be accompanied by an increased calcium content of the basal ganglia and of the crystalline lens of the eye. The ideas are certainly not clear as yet in this respect.

Miyajima (18) related the genesis of the stones to a diminished enzymatic activity of apoceruloplasmine. A carbonic anhydrase II deficiency, which might underlie the formation of stones, has been described in familial cases of osteopetrosis with basal ganglia calcifications (19,20). Smits (21,22) devoted several papers to the hypothesis that another enzyme, adenylcyclase, might contribute to SPDC. His work is certainly interesting and important but has not been confirmed yet.

It can be concluded from these neuropathologic and biochemical studies that the calcifications are formed in an organic matrix whose origin and composition are unknown. The genesis of these calcifications can be related to a disturbance in the general calcium metabolism. Nevertheless, in many cases with calcifications discovered at autopsy or by neuroradiologic investigations, no metabolic or biochemical modifications are observed. The calcifications are believed to consist of hydroxyapatite with a rather particular structure that is different from other calcifications encountered in the central nervous system (23).

CLINICAL SYMPTOMS

Calcifications of the central nervous system are not always associated with symptoms ascribed to the basal ganglia or cerebellum and may be a chance discovery at autopsy or CT scan. Many reports, among them those of Rossi et al (24) and Avrahami et al (25), have demonstrated that similar SPDC may result in variable clinical syndromes. Förstl et al (26) investigated 166 patients with unilateral or bilateral basal ganglia calcifications on CT scan of the brain. In this population of patients with symmetrical and asymmetrical

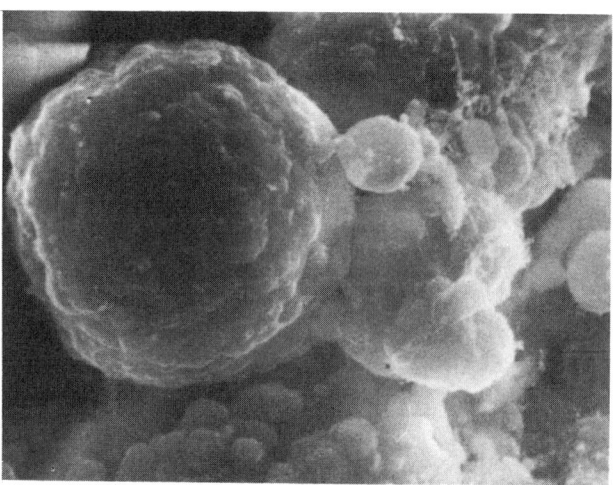

FIGURE 36.3 *Scanning electron microscopic picture of brain calcification.*

basal ganglia calcifications, they tested the significance of the neuroradiologic observation by statistical comparison of these patients' clinical disorders with the findings in a random sample of 622 patients without basal ganglia calcification. The odds for the most common neurologic disturbances were similar in patients with and without basal ganglia calcification. After adjustment for differences in age and brain atrophy, these authors indicated that there was no evidence of a significantly increased risk of dementia, cerebral infarction, epilepsy, vertigo, headache, or alcoholism.

However, a typical clinical symptomatology presents in a small percentage of patients with SPDC and is discovered on neuroradiologic examination. When and if symptoms are present, they form a syndrome that, despite its nonspecificity, shows sufficient constancy to arouse diagnostic suspicion. The clinical picture includes convulsive seizures (not to be confused with tetanic crises or carpopedal spasms), electroencephalographic abnormalities, mental deterioration and psychoses, papilledema, and endocrinologic symptoms as the main manifestations. Some of these patients unquestionably present signs and symptoms of parkinsonism or choreoathetosis (27). These patients, however, certainly do not represent the majority of cases. Some authors reported on the association of quite rare symptoms with SPDC, such as blepharospasms (28), supranuclear palsy (29), and choreoathetosis with hemiballism (30). We will not discuss the details of the clinical syndrome, as this has been done in a previous review (2). In fact, the diagnosis of SPDC is at present more of a neuroradiologic than a neurologic one (31).

In recent publications more attention has been paid to heredity (dominant autosomal trait) of cerebral calcifications (32). Heredity is only rarely described, mostly in young patients and even children, as shown by Goutières et al (33) and Ellie et al (34).

Currently, one can make an impressive list of diseases in which SPDC have been found without an established relation between the two. We would like to mention a certain number of these diseases in the following order: we will first discuss disturbances of the calcium metabolism, then we will examine the correlation between the prevalence of these calcifications and age. We will then focus on neurologic and muscular diseases associated with the calcifications. Next, we will consider associated cases of encephalitis and encephalopathy, and the relation between psychiatric symptomatology and SPDC, as well as the connection with epilepsy. Finally, the appearance of SPDC in nonneurologic diseases, such as diabetes or dermatologic diseases, will be discussed.

Abnormal Calcium Metabolism

We will not consider in detail the association of SPDC with hypoparathyroidism. The matter has been reviewed (28), and

this association has been described in an additional series of papers (31,35–41). Moriwaki et al (42) stressed the role played by hypoparathyroidism, and Bhimani et al (43) described the relation between SPDC and postsurgical hypoparathyroidism. Without doubt a relation exists between calcium metabolism and SPDC, although one certainly does not imply the other. Illum and Dupont (44) also considered this issue and in addition pointed out the association of the calcifications with pseudohypoparathyroidism. They also reported a rather important frequency of SPDC with pseudohypoparathyroidism. In recent publications, pseudohypoparathyroidism has been reported frequently (13). Margolin (45) and Siklos (46) described the calcifications in hyperparathyroidism as well.

Finally, one should not lose sight of the association with cases of bone disease, which has been known since 1972. Whyte (47) reconsidered this issue, describing three sisters presenting with osteopetrosis, renal tubular acidosis, and SPDC. Leone (48) described three more cases with this association. Sly et al (19) reported studies on 12 families displaying a comparable osteopetrosis syndrome with a carbonic anhydrase II deficiency. Again, the association is frequent—this time with a familial disease. Weisinger et al (49) tried to elucidate the mechanism of the formation of SPDC in a patient who also presented with a renal tubular defect; they concluded that the pathophysiology remains obscure. Bird et al (50) described a bone disease (lipomembranous polycystic osteodysplasia) with SPDC and dementia.

It can be concluded that there is a definite, though complex, relationship between disturbances of the calcium metabolism and SPDC.

Age-Related Incidence

All neuroradiologists agree that the frequency of SPDC, symptomatic or nonsymptomatic, increases with age. SPDC are certainly rare within pediatric populations. However, we would like to mention that in AIDS patients, especially in children, SPDC have been reported (32,51). Kauffman et al (52) found symmetrical basal ganglia calcifications in 10 of 29 children with perinatally transmitted HIV infection examined by CT. Kaya et al described a small series of children with calcifications of the basal ganglia related to basal ganglia ischemia (53). Stübgen and Lotz (54) described a case of membranous lipodystrophy with basal ganglia calcifications. This syndrome is usually characterized by presenile dementia, upper motor neuron involvement, myoclonus, and an aphasic-agnostic-apraxic syndrome. SPDC were also described in a 7-year-old patient with early-onset Cockayne's syndrome and chromosomal anomaly 47XXX (55). Brain calcifications, including symmetrical ones, were described in children treated with radiotherapy (56). This phenomenon is observed to be much less frequent in adults. Finally, Ou et al (57) described a case with dural arteriovenous malformations and SPDC, and Lera et al (58) reported on SPDC in cases of Leigh's disease.

Calcifications of the basal ganglia have also been seen in Down syndrome (59–61). Wisniewski et al (60) estimate that the calcifications are present in as many as 26.6% of cases of trisomy 21. One should not forget that, neuroradiologically speaking, similarities between the central nervous system involvement in Down syndrome and Alzheimer's disease have become apparent, with patients with Down syndrome being more prone to the development of Alzheimer's disease. In Alzheimer's disease, however, no increased frequency of SPDC has been observed, nor are there increased intracranial calcium depositions in the pineal gland or choroid plexus (62). Ikeda et al (63), however, published one case of atypical presenile dementia with basal ganglia calcifications. It is unclear whether this is also a coincidental association. Burns et al (64) described an association between basal ganglia calcifications on CT and extrapyramidal symptomatology in an Alzheimer population.

Neurologic Diseases

SPDC are found in other neurologic diseases, which we will divide into familial and nonfamilial categories.

Nonfamilial Neurologic Diseases

Constantinidis et al (65) described these calcifications not only in hypoparathyroidism but also in a case of frontal internal hyperostosis and in a case of Morell's nodular dysgenesis of the frontal cortex. Bruyn et al (66) described cerebral calcinosis in a patient with polycystic encephalopathy presenting with psychiatric problems. Morgante et al (67) described basal ganglia calcifications in patients who had disturbances of calcium metabolism and who had had meningoencephalitis in childhood. The relation between viral encephalitis and SPDC is surely not an accidental one. Eleopra et al (68) described a patient with motoneuron disease and extensive SPDC. One case of SPDC with astrocytic proliferation and astrocytoma has been published (69). Masson et al reported on the association between Rademaker-Garcin syndrome and SPDC (70). The work of Wannakrairot et al (71), who reported the frequent association between epilepsy and SPDC, and of Munir (72) and Kazis (73), who associated SPDC with psychiatric symptoms, completes this series of reports.

Familial Neurologic Syndromes

Hammerstein et al (74) reported the presence of symmetric SPDC in patients with a tapetoretinal degeneration. Lyon et al (75) reported similar calcifications combined with microcephaly and dwarfism in a case of leukodystrophy. Aicardi and Goutières (76) described a progressive familial infantile encephalopathy associated with calcifications of the basal ganglia and chronic cerebrospinal fluid lymphocytosis. Malat and Virapongse (77) reported a syndrome consisting

of gonadotropic hypogonadism, hyposmia, and sensorineural hearing loss in association with SPDC. Finally, Miyajima et al (18) associated these calcifications with an apoceruloplasmine deficiency. Hall (78) and Francis and Freeman (79,80) also found SPDC in patients presenting with familial schizophreniform psychosis. Singh et al (81) described a family in which two children with Möbius' disease (agenesis of the sixth and seventh cranial nerve nuclei) had cerebral involvement consisting of SPDC.

Muscular Diseases

Since 1975, a series of astonishing publications have been devoted to familial muscular diseases presented under different names but having SPDC in common. Shapira et al (82) and Markesbery (83) described a mitochondrial myopathy with calcifications of the basal ganglia and lactate acidemia. Pavlakis et al (84), Fuji et al (85), and Chiang et al (86) described a similar syndrome with additional stroke-like episodes. They reviewed the literature and pointed out the cases presenting SPDC. Grotemeyer et al (87) reconsidered the issue. Robertson et al (88) reported basal ganglia calcifications in a case of Kearns-Sayre syndrome. Carboni et al (89) observed the association of Kearn-Sayre syndrome with cerebral and cerebellar leukodystrophy and SPDC. Bastiaensen et al (90) and Yoda et al (91) described a similar syndrome. A rather close relation exists between certain rare muscular diseases, frequently accompanied by lactic acidosis, and SPDC. The frequency of these calcifications is perhaps higher than in hypoparathyroidism, but it seems premature to draw conclusions concerning the physiopathology.

Cutaneous Diseases

Calcifications have been reported in patients presenting with cutaneous diseases. Kotscher (92) described a case of lipoproteinosis with calcifications of the basal ganglia; Newton et al (93) described the same association. Copeland et al (94) reported SPDC in a mentally defective patient with hidrotic ectodermal dysplasia, and Matsuo et al (95) found the association in a patient with membranous lipodystrophy.

Miscellaneous

Sandfield et al (96) associated SPDC with diabetes. SPDC in association with white matter calcifications were described in a 15-year-old patient with juvenile rheumatoid arthritis (97). Nishiyama et al (98) reported on the association of pronounced SPDC and multiple myeloma in a 41-year-old woman with initial symptoms of dystonia and spasticity followed by gait disturbance, speech impairment, micrographia, and dementia. Midroni and Willinsky (99) described a case of SPDC in which the calcifications appeared within 17 days after cardiac arrest. Kolawole et al

(100) presented hypoxic-ischemic phenomena as a factor frequently underlying the pathophysiology of symmetrical calcifications in the basal ganglia. Beall et al (13) reported on the association of SPDC with late-onset porphyria.

CONCLUSIONS

For almost 50 years, we have been following the literature devoted to SPDC. At first it was thought that SPDC were only a manifestation of a disturbed calcium metabolism. Presently, this cannot always be confirmed, but alterations of calcium metabolism still remain frequent. It is impossible to define precise clinical syndromes associated with SPDC because the calcifications are found in an extensive number of diseases. Some diseases are familial, others are not. A considerable number of patients are even devoid of neurologic symptoms or signs. Generally, SPDC are CT scan findings. One wonders what would be the prevalence of these calcifications in a normal population. It is clear that the physiopathologic and clinical significance of SPDC await further clarification.

Finally, a word concerning therapeutic modalities. It has been reported before and recently confirmed by Salti et al (101), that one needs to try to correct the disturbance of the calcium metabolism, when present, in patients with SPDC. Treatments other than symptomatic therapy have not been proposed.

ACKNOWLEDGMENTS

We thank Dr B. Pickut for her editorial assistance. This work was supported by the Fonds voor Geneeskundig Wetenschappelijk Onderzoek (grants 3.0064.93 and G.0027.97), the Ministerie van Onderwijs, the University of Antwerp, the Born-Bunge Foundation, and the OCMW Medical Research Foundation.

REFERENCES

1. Lowenthal A. La calcification vasculaire intracérébrale non artérioscléreuse de Fahr est-elle la manifestation cérébrale d'une perturbation des fonctions parathyroïdiennes? Acta Neurol Belg 1948;48:613–631.
2. Lowenthal A, Bruyn GW. Calcification of the striopallidodentate system. In: Vinken PJ, Bruyn GW, eds. Handbook of clinical neurology. vol. 6, Diseases of the basal ganglia. Amsterdam: Elsevier, 1968:703–725.
3. Lowenthal A. Striopallidodentate calcifications. In: Vinken PJ, Bruyn GW, Klawans HL, eds. Handbook of clinical neurology. vol. 5, Extrapyramidal disorders. Amsterdam: Elsevier Science, 1986:417–436.
4. Fenelon G, Guillard A. Maladie de Fahr et calcifications des noyaux gris centraux. Encyclopédie médico-chirurgicale. Paris: Elsevier, 1987;10:1–5.
5. Appel L, Massart DL, Smeyers A, Lowenthal A. Aspects radiologiques et biochimiques des calcifications des noyaux de la base. J Belg Radiol 1973;56:283–290.
6. Jorens PG, Appel BJ, Hilte FA, et al. Basal ganglia calcifications in postoperative hypoparathyroidism: a case with unusual characteristics. Acta Neurol Scand 1991;83:137–140.
7. Scotti G, Scialfa G, Tampieri D, Landoni L. MR imaging in Fahr disease. J Comput Assist Tomogr 1985;9:790–792.
8. Schörner VW, Kunz D, Henkes H, et al. Nachweis von Verkalkungen in der Magnetresonanztomographie (MRT). Fortschr Röntgenstr 1991;154:430–437.
9. Dierckx R, Jorens PG, Appel B, et al. Tc-99 m HMPAO SPECT of the brain in a patient with striopallidodentate calcification. Clin Nucl Med 1991;16:439–440.
10. Uygur GA, Liu Y, Hellman RS, et al. Evaluation of regional cerebral blood flow in massive intracerebral calcifications. J Nucl Med 1995;36:610–612.
11. Staffen W, Karbe H, Rudolf J, et al. Functional significance of calcinosis of the basal ganglia via positron emission tomography. Fortschr Neurol Psychiatr 1994;62:119–124.
12. Smeyers-Verbeke J, Michotte Y, Pelsmaeckers J, et al. The chemical composition of idiopathic nonarteriosclerotic cerebral calcifications. Neurology 1975;25:48–57.
13. Beall SS, Patten BM, Mallette L, Jankovic J. Abnormal systemic metabolism of iron, porphyrin and calcium in Fahr's syndrome. Ann Neurol 1989;26:569–575.
14. Kozik M, Kulczycki J. Laser-spectographic analysis of the cation content in Fahr's syndrome. Arch Psychiatr Nervenkr 1978;225:135–142.
15. Kuran W, Kozik M, Kulczycki J. Laser analysis of pseudocalcium deposits in Fahr's syndrome. Neurol Neurochir Pol 1981;31:397–401.
16. Kobayashi S, Yamadori I, Miki H, Ohmori M. Idiopathic nonarteriosclerotic cerebral calcification (Fahr's disease): an electron microscopic study. Acta Neuropathol 1987;73:62–66.
17. Manyam BV, Bhatt MH, Moore WD, et al. Bilateral striopallidodentate calcinosis: cerebrospinal fluid, imaging and electrophysiological studies. Ann Neurol 1992;31:379–384.
18. Miyajima H, Nishimura Y, Sakamoto M, et al. Familial apoceruloplasmin deficiency with basal ganglia calcification. J Neurol 1985;232(suppl):149.
19. Sly WS, Whyte MP, Sundaram V, et al. Carbonic anhydrase II deficiency in 12 families with the autosomal recessive syndrome of osteopetrosis with renal tubular acidosis and cerebral calcification. N Engl J Med 1985;313:139–145.
20. Bejaoui M, Kamoun A, Baraket M, et al. Le syndrome associant: ostéopétrose, acidose tubulaire, retard mental et calcifications intracrâniennes par déficit en anhydrase carbonique II. Arch Fr Pediatr 1991;48:211–214.
21. Smits MG, Gabreëls FJM, Froeling PGA, et al. Calcium-phosphate metabolism in autosomal recessive idiopathic striopallidodentate calcinosis and Cockayne's syndrome. Clin Neurol Neurosurg 1983;85:145–153.
22. Smits MG. Familial strio-pallido-dentate calcinosis. Utrecht: Pressa Trajectina, 1984.
23. Michotte Y. Bijdrage tot de studie van biologische calcificaties. Ph.d. thesis, Free University, Brussels, 1976.
24. Rossi M, Morena M, Zanardi M. Calcificazione dei gangli della base e malattia di Fahr. Presentazione di due casi clinici e revisione della letteratura. Ital J Med 1993;84:192–198.
25. Avrahami E, Cohn DF, Feibel M, Tadmor R. MRI demonstration and CT correlation of the brain in patients with idiopathic intracerebral calcification. J Neurol 1994; 241:381–384.
26. Förstl H, Krumm B, Eden S, Kohlmeyer K. Neurological disorders in 166 patients with basal ganglia calcification: a statistical evaluation. J Neurol 1992;239:36–38.
27. Micheli F, Fernandez-Pardal MM, Casas-Parera I, Giannaula R. Sporadic paroxysmal dystonic choreoathetosis associated with basal ganglia calcifications. Ann Neurol 1986;20:750. Letter.
28. Blin O, Masson G, Serratrice G. Blepharospasm associated with pseudohypoparathyroidism and bilateral basal ganglia calcifications. Mov Disord 1991;6:379–383.
29. Saver JL, Liu GT, Charness ME. Idiopathic striopallidodentate calcification with prominent supranuclear abnormality of eye movement. J Neuroophthalmol 1994;14:29–33.
30. Goel A, Bhatnagar MK, Vashishta A, Verma NP. Hypoparathyroidism with extensive intracranial calcifications: a case report. Postgrad Med J 1994;70:913–915.
31. Vakaet A, Rubens R, de Reuck J, vander Eecken H. Intracranial bilateral symmetrical calcification on CT scanning. Clin Neurol Neurosurg 1985;87:103–111.
32. Fénelon G, Gray F, Paillard F, et al. A prospective study of patients with CT detected pallidal calcifications. J Neurol Neurosurg Psychiatry 1993;56:622–625.
33. Goutières F. Encéphalopathies familiales avec calcifications des noyaux gris centraux. Presse Med 1993;22:1948–1950.
34. Ellie E, Julien J, Ferrer X. Familial idiopathic striopallidodentate calcifications. Neurology 1989;39:381–385.
35. Garcia Urra D, Barquero Jimenez MS, Varela de Seijas E, Rico Lenza H. Calcificacion de los ganglios basales e hipoparatiroidismo: enfermedad de Fahr. Estudio de una familia. Arch Neurobiol 1990;53:18–22.

36. Cheek JC, Riggs JE, Lilly RL. Extensive brain calcification and progressive dysarthria and dysphagia associated with chronic hypoparathyroidism. Arch Neurol 1990;47:1038–1039.

37. Arias Mayorga J, Gonzalez Martin T, Escorial Miguel C, Maranon Cabello A. Calcificaciones intracraneales en el diagnostico diferencial de la enfermedad epileptica. Revista Clinica Espanola 1991;189:425–427.

38. Fulop M, Zeifer B. Case report: extensive brain calcification in hypoparathyroidism. Am J Med Sci 1991;302:292–295.

39. Vega MG, Alves de Sousa A, De Lucca F, et al. Sindrome extrapiramidal e hipoparatireoidismo. Arq Neuropsiquiatr 1994;52:419–426.

40. Polverosi R, Zambelli C, Sbeghen R. Calcification of the basal nuclei in hypoparathyroidism. The computed and magnetic resonance tomographic aspects. Radiol Med Torino 1994;87:12–15.

41. Kulczycki J, Boguslawska-Staniaszczyk R, Kozlowski P. The image of intracerebral calcification in CT and MR studies. A case report of Fahr syndrome. Neurol Neurochir Pol 1994;28:915–920.

42. Moriwaki Y, Matsui K, Yamamoto T, et al. Cerebral subcortical calcification and hypoparathyroidism, a case report and review of the literature. Jpn J Med 1985;24:53–56.

43. Bhimani S, Sarwar M, Virapongse C, et al. Computed tomography of cerebrovascular calcifications in post surgical hypoparathyroidism. J Comput Assist Tomogr 1985;9:121–124.

44. Illum F, Dupont E. Prevalences of CT-detected calcification in the basal ganglia in idiopathic hypoparathyroidism and pseudohypoparathyroidism. Neuroradiology 1985;27:32–38.

45. Margolin D. Intracranial calcification in hyperparathyroidism associated with gait apraxia and parkinsonism. Neurology 1980;30:1005–1007.

46. Siklos P. Basal ganglion calcification and hyperparathyroidism. Miner Electrolyte Metab 1982;7:166–168.

47. Whyte MP, Murphy WA, Fallon MD, et al. Osteopetrosis, renal tubular acidosis and basal ganglia calcification in three sisters. Am J Med 1980;69:64–74.

48. Leone G. Recessive osteopetrosis with cerebral calcifications. Report of three adults in two related families. Radiol Med 1982;68:373–378.

49. Weisinger JR, Mogollon A, Lander R, et al. Massive cerebral calcifications associated with increased renal phosphate reabsorption. Arch Intern Med 1986;146:473–477.

50. Bird TD, Koerker RM, Leaird BJ, et al. Lipomembranous polycystic osteodysplasia (brain, bone, and fat disease): a genetic cause of presenile dementia. Neurology 1983;33:81–86.

51. Belman AL, Lantos G, Horoupian D, et al. AIDS: calcification of the basal ganglia in infants and children. Neurology 1986;36:1192–1199.

52. Kauffman WM, Sivit CJ, Fitz CR, et al. CT and MR evaluation of intracranial involvement in pediatric HIV infection: a clinical-imaging correlation. AJNR 1992;13:949–957.

53. Kaya T, Özkan R, Bozoglu N, et al. Basal ganglia infarcts with calcifications in children. Eur J Radiol 1995;20:48–51.

54. Stübgen JP, Lotz BP. Membranous lipodystrophy. S Afr Med J 1992;81:620–622.

55. Hayashi M, Hayakawa K, Suzuki F, et al. A neuropathological study of early onset Cockayne syndrome with chromosomal anomaly 47XXX. Brain Dev 1992;14:63–67.

56. Fernandez-Bouzas A, Ramirez Jimenez H, Vazquez Zamudio J, et al. Brain calcifications and dementia in children treated with radiotherapy and intrathecal methotrexate. J Neurosurg Sci 1992;36:211–214.

57. Ou SF, Chi CS, Shian WJ, et al. Dural arteriovenous malformation with symmetrical calcification of the basal ganglia: a case report. Chung Hua I Hsueh Tsa Chih (Taipei) 1994;54:204–208.

58. Lera G, Bhatia K, Marsden CD. Dystonia as the major manifestation of Leigh's syndrome. Mov Disord 1994;9:642–649.

59. Jakab I. Basal ganglia calcification and psychosis in mongolism. Eur Neurol 1978;17:300–314.

60. Wisniewski KE, French JH, Rosen JF, et al. Basal ganglia calcification in Down's syndrome. Another manifestation of premature aging. Ann NY Acad Sci 1982;396:179–189.

61. Takashimas, Becker LE. Basal ganglia calcification in Down's syndrome. J Neurol Neurosurg Psychiatry 1985;48:61–64.

62. Friedland RP, Luxenberg JS, Koss E. A quantitative study of intracranial calcification in dementia of the Alzheimer type. Int Psychogeriatr 1990;2:37–43.

63. Ikeda M, Tanabe H, Mori T, et al. A case of atypical presenile dementia. Brain Nerve 1994;46:175–181.

64. Burns A, Jacoby R, Levy R. Neurological signs in Alzheimer's disease. Age Ageing 1991;20:45–51.

65. Constantinidis J, Aubert M, Tissot R. Contribution à l'étude des calcifications pallido-dentelées. Schweiz Arch Neurol Neurochir Psychiatr 1978;122:237–251.

66. Bruyn GW, Stam FC, Klawans HL Jr. Cerebral calcinosis with polycystic encephalopathy: an unusual case. Psychiatr Neurol Neurochir 1972;75:325–344.

67. Morgante L, Vita G, Meduri M, et al. Fahr's syndrome: local inflammatory factors in the pathogenesis of calcification. J Neurol 1986;233:19–22.

68. Eleopra R, Accurti I, Neri W, Bazzochi O. Unusual case of Fahr syndrome with motoneuron disease. Ital J Neurol Sci 1991;12:597–600.

69. Ang LC, Rozdilsky B, Alport EC, Tchang S. Fahr's disease associated with astrocytic proliferation and astrocytoma. Surg Neurol 1993;39:365–369.

70. Masson G, Blin O, Pouget J, Serratrice G. Syndrome de Rademaker et Garcin associé à des calcifications pallidales. Rev Neurol 1992;148:546–549.

71. Wannakrairot P, Suwangool P, Shuangshoti S. Symmetrical intracranial advanced pseudocalcium-calcium deposition associated with epilepsy (Fahr's disease): report of 2 cases. J Med Assoc Thai 1985;68:490–496.

72. Munir KM. The treatment of psychotic symptoms in Fahr's disease with lithium carbonate. J Clin Psychopharmacol 1986;6:36–38.

73. Kazis AD. Contribution of CT scan to the diagnosis of Fahr's syndrome. Acta Neurol Scand 1985;71:206–211.

74. Hammerstein W, Bischof G, Keck E. A tapetoretinal degeneration with symmetrical calcifications of the basal ganglia. Eur Neurol 1982;21:249–255.

75. Lyon G, Robain O, Philippart M, Sarlière L. Leucodystrophie avec calcifications strio-cérébelleuses, microcéphalie et nanisme. Rev Neurol 1968;119:197–210.

76. Aicardi J, Goutières F. A progressive familial encephalopathy in infancy with calcifications of the basal ganglia and chronic cerebrospinal fluid lymphocytosis. Ann Neurol 1984;15:49–54.

77. Malat J, Virapongse C. Brain calcification in Kallman's syndrome. Computed tomographic appearance. Pediatr Neurosci 1985–86;12:257–259.

78. Hall P. Calcification of the basal ganglia apparently presenting as a schizophreniform psychosis. Postgrad Med J 1972;48:636–639.

79. Francis AF. Familial basal ganglia calcification and schizophreniform psychosis. Br J Psychiatry 1979;135:360–362.

80. Francis AF, Freeman H. Psychiatric abnormality and brain calcification over four generations. J Nerv Ment Dis 1984;172:166–170.

81. Singh B, Shahwan SA, Singh P, et al. Mobius syndrome with basal ganglia calcification. Acta Neurol Scand 1992;85:436–438.

82. Shapira Y, Cederbaum SD, Cancilla PA, et al. Familial poliodystrophy, mitochondrial myopathy, and lactate acidemia. Neurology 1975;25:614–621.

83. Markesbery WR. Lactic acidemia, mitochondrial myopathy, and basal ganglia calcification. Neurology 1979;29:1057–1061.

84. Pavlakis SG, Phillips PC, DiMauro S, et al. Mitochondrial myopathy, encephalopathy, lactic acidosis, and stroke-like episodes: a distinctive clinical syndrome. Ann Neurol 1984;16:481–488.

85. Fuji H, Okuno T, Ito M, et al. 123 I-IMP SPECT findings in mitochondrial encephalomyopathies. Brain Dev 1995;17:89–94.

86. Chiang LM, Jong YJ, Huang SC, et al. Myopathy, encephalopathy, lactic acidosis and stroke-like episodes. J Formos Med Assoc 1995;94:42–47.

87. Grotemeyer KH, Lehmann HJ, Jorg J, et al. Familiare Stammganglienverkalkung, mitochondriale Myopathie und Epilepsie: folge einer einzigen Stoffwechselstorung? Nervenarzt 1984;55:202–207.

88. Robertson WC Jr, Viseskul C, Lee YE, Lloyd RV. Basal ganglia calcification in Kearns-Sayre syndrome. Arch Neurol 1979;36:711–713.

89. Carboni P, Giacanelli M, Porro G, et al. Kearns-Sayre syndrome. A case of the complete syndrome with encephalic leukodystrophy and calcification of basal ganglia. Ital J Neurol Sci 1981;2:263–268.

90. Bastiaensen LAK, Stadhouders AM, Ter Laak HJ, et al. Neuro-ophthalmology. vol. 4, Kearns-Sayre syndrome. Amsterdam: Aedus Press, 1984:55–63.

91. Yoda S, Terauchi A, Kitahara F, Akabane T. Neurologic deterioration with progressive CT changes in a child with Kearns-Shy syndrome. Brain Dev 1984;6:323–327.

92. Kotscher E. Familiäres Auftreten von endokraniellen Verkalkungen bei Lipoproteinose. Radiol Austr 1960;10:299–303.

93. Newton FH, Rosenberg RN, Lampert PW, O'Brien JS. Neurologic involvement in Urbach-Wiethe's disease (lipoid proteinosis). Neurology 1971;21:1205–1213.

94. Copeland DD, Lamb WA, Klintworth K. Calcification of basal ganglia and cerebellar roof nuclei in mentally defective patients with hydrotic ectodermal dysplasia. Neurology 1977;27:1029–1033.

95. Matsuo T, Suetsugu M, Eguchi M. Membranous lipodystrophy. A case report. Arch Psychiatr Nervenkr 1982;231:123–130.

96. Sandfield JA, Finkel J, Lewis S, Rosen SG. Alternating choreoathetosis associated with uncontrolled diabetes mellitus and basal ganglia calcification. Diabetes Care 1986;9:100–101. Letter.

97. Harada T, Ishizaki F, Ohshita T, et al. A case of Fahr's disease associated with juvenile rheumatoid arthritis. Brain Nerve 1991;43:957–963.

98. Nishiyama K, Honda E, Mizuno T, et al. A case of idiopathic, symmetrical non-arteriosclerotic, intracerebral calcification (Fahr's disease) associated with M-proteinemia, followed by multiple myeloma. Clin Neurol 1991;31:781–784.

99. Midroni G, Willinsky R. Rapid postanoxic calcification of the basal ganglia. Neurology 1992;42:2144–2146.

100. Kolawole TM, Patel PJ, Malabarey T, et al. Symmetrical lesions in the basal ganglia. Afr J Med Sci 1994;23:67–74.

101. Salti I, Faris A, Tannir N, Khouri K. Rapid correction by 1-alpha-hydroxycholecalciferol of hemichorea in surgical hypoparathyroidism. J Neurol Neurosurg Psychiatry 1982;45:89–90.

Dentatorubropallidoluysian Atrophy

Reiji Iizuka

INTRODUCTION

Dentatorubropallidoluysian atrophy (DRPLA) is an uncommon disease in which the dentatorubral and pallidoluysian segments of the extrapyramidal system degenerate simultaneously (1,2).

First described by Titica and van Bogaert (3) in 1946, this disease was only sporadically reported until Smith (4) reviewed and first named it in 1975. An increasing number of cases have been reported since then, especially in Japan (1), though some cases have been reported in the United States (5) and Germany (6).

The most important characteristic of this disease is that, despite relatively uniform pathologic findings, it shows, clinically, a complicated combination of movement disorders.

CLINICAL FEATURES

The main clinical symptoms of DRPLA are movement disorders. It is convenient to divide these disorders into three clinical forms, each named after the most prominent type of movement disorder:

1. the ataxochoreoathetoid type,
2. the pseudo-Huntington type, and
3. the myoclonus epilepsy type.

Ataxochoreoathetoid Type

In the early stage of the illness in ataxochoreoathetoid-type DRPLA, ataxia is the prominent clinical feature. It is more pronounced in the lower extremities and is not different from that seen in spinocerebellar degeneration. The age of onset varies from the lower teens to over 50. Most cases in the literature are sporadic, but some cases are considered

autosomal dominant or recessive. Then, as the degenerative process progresses, involuntary movements become more prominent. These movements have been described quite differently—for example, as "choreoathetoid," "dystonic," "choreiform and ballistic," "athetotic and hemiballistic," and "choreiform." Their appearance means that cerebellar symptoms are replaced by extrapyramidal symptoms.

Psychiatric symptoms are not prominent, but in the later stages of the disease the patients sometimes show an apathetic state accompanied by a slowing of the thought process that is identical with so-called subcortical dementia. Titica and van Bogaert (3) also reported psychiatric symptoms, such as personality changes, delusions, and dementia.

No myoclonus or myoclonus epilepsy has appeared at any time during the whole clinical course, except in one case reported by Neumann (7) that showed seizures of the grand mal type and myoclonus.

In the literature, many cases show disturbances of external ocular movements, such as upward gaze palsy with or without horizontal nystagmus. Many different expressions have been used to describe such eye movements, such as monocular nystagmus, opsoclonus, slow eye movements, and nystagmoid jerks. These eye movement disturbances are characteristic of this type of DRPLA. The duration of the disease is approximately 5 to 15 years.

Pseudo-Huntington Type

In this type, the cerebellar signs in the early stage are slight and short-lived; they are soon covered by typical choreic movements, which progress until the patient's death. This type of DRPLA has thus far been reported only from Japan. The age of onset of most cases is between 20 and 35, and the patients die after approximately 20 years. Most cases show an autosomal dominant type of inheritance.

In this type there is not only progressive chorea but also personality changes, such as emotional lability, delusions, and negativism, followed by severe dementia. Some authors have diagnosed these psychiatric symptoms as a "subcortical dementia" in nature. However, in the later stage the patients sometimes show severe dementia of the cortical type, with psychomotor excitement. Most cases of this type of DRPLA were misdiagnosed as Huntington's chorea before the computed tomography (CT) scan was available; this misdiagnosis was based on the choreic movement, the psychiatric symptoms developing into dementia, and inheritance of the autosomal dominant type. Seizures sometimes occur, though they are rare. No myoclonus or eye movement disturbances have been reported in this type of DRPLA.

Myoclonus Epilepsy Type

Takahata et al (8) and Naito and Oyanagi (9) have reported a degenerative form of myoclonus epilepsy that shows neuropathologic changes in DRPLA. Thereafter some other cases have been reported from Japan. All cases reported thus far are hereditary, usually of the autosomal dominant type. The onset of the disease is mainly in the late teens, younger than in the other types of DRPLA. Myoclonus and epileptic seizures appear, with progressive dementia, dysarthria, and ataxia developing subsequently. Clinically speaking, there is no difference between this type of DRPLA and the Ramsay Hunt's syndrome.

RADIOGRAPHIC FEATURES

In the CT scan, some cases of DRPLA show an atrophy of the tegmental portion of the lower brainstem without any atrophy of the ventral portion of the pons. In the future, more significant features will undoubtedly be found by the use of magnetic resonance imaging (MRI) (10).

NEUROPATHOLOGIC FEATURES

The nature of the histopathology of DRPLA is the same as that of other degenerative diseases of the nervous system—that is, neuronal loss and a glial reaction. The pathology of the DRPLA is fundamentally the same in all three clinical subtypes, except for the severe atrophy of the tegmentum of the lower brainstem in the choreoathetoid type.

It is, however, a unique point of DRPLA that, in spite of the relatively homogeneous brain lesion, it shows clinically different neurologic symptoms in the three clinical subtypes, as has been noted above.

The characteristic lesions in the central nervous system can be summarized as follows. In all cases reported, the dentate nucleus is constantly and severely involved, with intense neuronal cell loss and severe gliosis (Figs 37.1 and 37.2). "Grumose" degeneration has been frequently observed, most distinctly with silver staining, where it is observable as tiny granules surrounding the degenerative

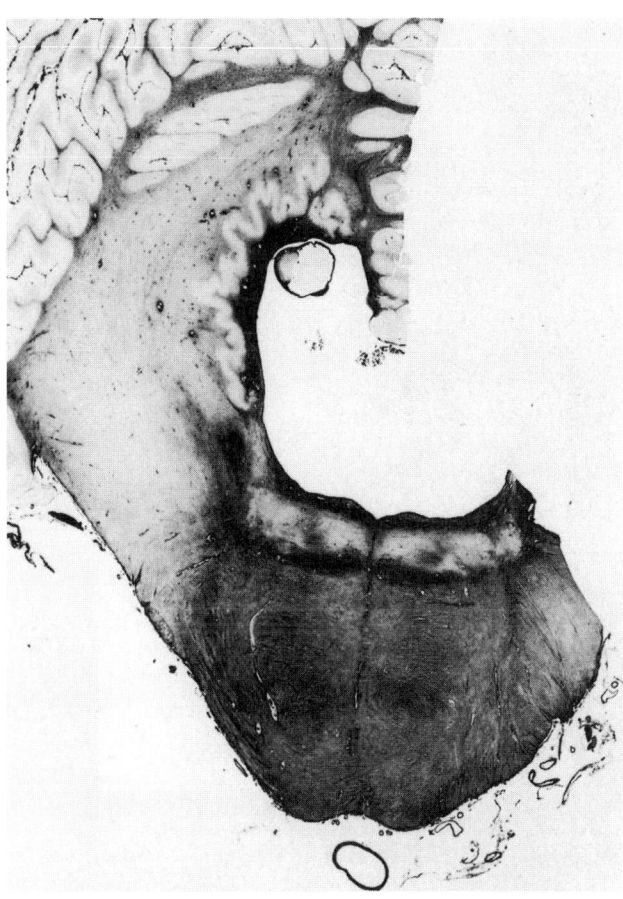

FIGURE 37.1 *Ataxochoreoathetoid type. Atrophy of the superior cerebellar peduncle and of the tegmentum, with gliosis. Gliosis of the medial longitudinal fasciculi and central tegmental tracts. Holzer stain. Original magnification ×2.3. Reproduced by permission from Iizuka R, Hirayama K. Dento-rubro-pallido-luysian atrophy. In: Vinken PJ, Bruyn GW, Klawans HL, eds. Handbook of clinical neurology. Vol. 5, Extrapyramidal disorders. Amsterdam: Elsevier Science, 1986.*

Purkinje cell and/or its dendrite. On the other hand, the pathologic changes in the pallidum are different in each case. The most typical form is severe nerve cell loss in the outer segment, with intensive cell and fiber gliosis (Figs 37.3 and 37.4). In some cases, the inner segment of the pallidum is more intensively affected than the outer segment. There are also cases in which the degenerative changes in the pallidum are rather slight.

The degenerative changes in the subthalamic nucleus also differ from case to case. Two different types of degeneration are observed: one is a severe cell gliosis, with relatively well-preserved nerve cells, whereas the other shows a spongy state, with marked nerve cell loss.

In the red nucleus, nerve cell loss accompanied by glial cell proliferation is a typical change, but sometimes this gliosis is difficult to distinguish from the associated gliosis of the degenerating ascending dentatothalamic fiber, which crosses at the level of the red nucleus.

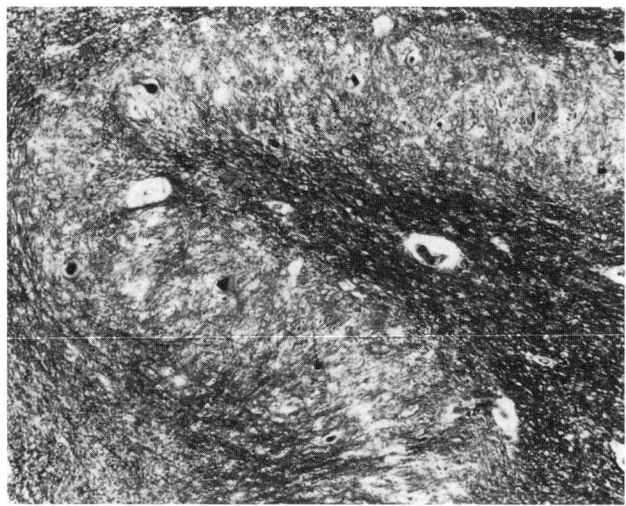

FIGURE 37.2 *Ataxochoreoathetoid type. The dentate nucleus shows marked loss of neurons. Klüver-Barrera stain ×130. Reproduced by permission from Iizuka R, Hirayama K. Dento-rubro-pallido-luysian atrophy. In: Vinken PJ, Bruyn GW, Klawans HL, eds. Handbook of clinical neurology. Vol. 5, Extrapyramidal disorders. Amsterdam: Elsevier Science, 1986.*

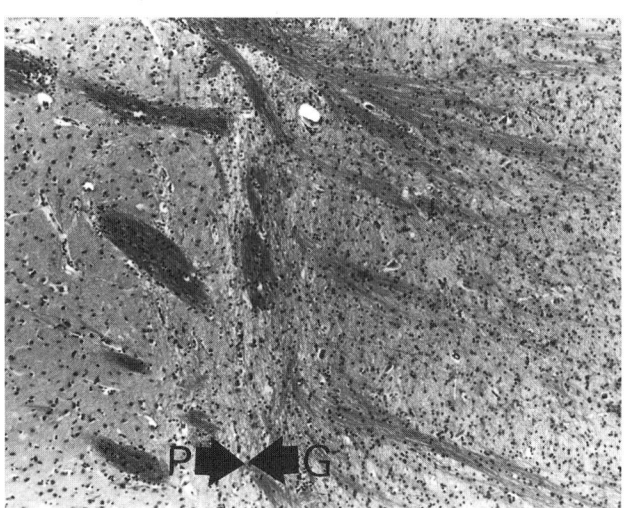

FIGURE 37.3 *Ataxochoreoathetoid type. The putamen (P) shows no marked change. The globus pallidus (G) shows almost complete neuronal loss, with severe gliosis and scattered pigment granules. Hematoxylin-eosin stain. Original magnification ×130. Reproduced by permission from Iizuka R, Hirayama K. Dento-rubro-pallido-luysian atrophy. In: Vinken PJ, Bruyn GW, Klawans HL, eds. Handbook of clinical neurology. Vol. 5, Extrapyramidal disorders. Amsterdam: Elsevier Science, 1986.*

Other extrapyramidal nuclei, such as the caudate nucleus, the putamen, and especially the substantia nigra, are not affected or degenerate only very slightly.

In the ataxochoreoathetoid form of DRPLA, significant tegmental atrophy is observed, caused by the degeneration of the superior colliculus, the central gray matter, and the

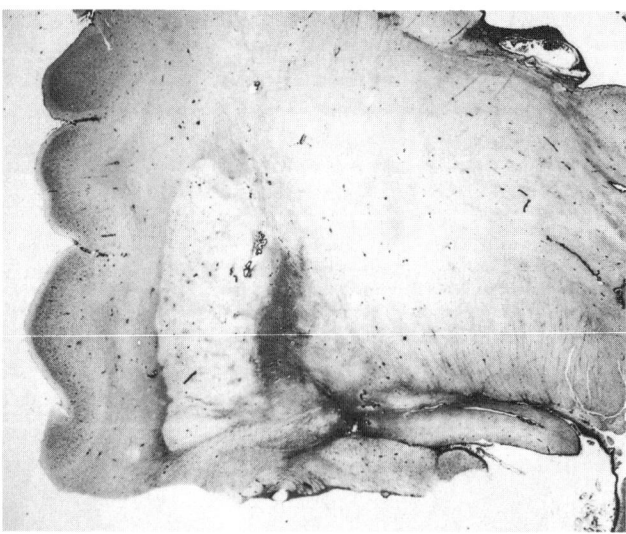

FIGURE 37.4 *Pseudo-Huntington type. Marked and circumscribed gliosis of the external segment of the globus pallidus. Original magnification ×1.3. Reproduced by permission from Iizuka R, Hirayama K. Dento-rubro-pallido-luysian atrophy. In: Vinken PJ, Bruyn GW, Klawans HL, eds. Handbook of clinical neurology. Vol. 5, Extrapyramidal disorders. Amsterdam: Elsevier Science, 1986.*

reticular formation at the midbrain level, and by that of the central segmental tracts and the reticular formation in the pons. These changes in the lower brainstem tegmentum are also found in the myoclonus epilepsy type of DRPLA, but not in the pseudo-Huntington type. This tegmental atrophy could be responsible for the disturbance of eye movements in DRPLA, mainly seen in the ataxochoreoathetoid type. In the pseudo-Huntington type, in which there is no disturbance of eye movements, there are no anatomic lesions in the tegmental portion of the lower brainstem.

The demyelination of the spinocerebellar tracts (1), of the posterior columns of the spinal cord (3), and of both (9,11) has also been reported. Only two cases (12,13) showed no spinal lesions. These pathologic changes in the spinal cord suggest a combination of DRPLA and Friedreich's ataxia. It is already known (14) that, in cases of Friedreich's ataxia, about 50% show degenerative changes not only in the spinal cord but also in the pallidum, in the subthalamic nucleus, and sometimes in the cerebellar dentate nuclei.

NEUROCHEMISTRY

The results of the neurochemical changes of DRPLA are still rare and obscure. The postmortem analysis of brains of patients with DRPLA has shown a very reduced level of γ-aminobutyric acid–related enzyme activity (15), whereas there was no decreased activity of the catecholamine-related enzymes (16). There is a clear-cut difference between olivopontocerebellar atrophy (OPCA) and DRPLA; thus, the cases with degeneration of the spinocerebellar system showing extrapyramidal symptoms could be separated into two subtypes, involving different mechanisms based on different metabolic changes.

DIFFERENTIAL DIAGNOSIS

Friedreich's Ataxia

Andre-Van Leeuwen and van Bogaert (17) described a case with pes cavus; the pathology in that case suggested a combination of DRPLA and Friedreich's ataxia. As has already been stated, many cases of DRPLA have lesions in the spinal cord, as with Friedreich's ataxia. It is quite possible that in the past some cases of DRPLA were reported as "Friedreich's ataxia, with atrophy of the dentate nucleus and brachium conjunctivum." Clinically, if the patient shows either choreic/choreoathetoid involuntary movement or myoclonus, accompanied by ataxia and other symptoms of Friedreich's ataxia, it is necessary to consider the possibility of DRPLA.

Ramsay Hunt's Syndrome

Since Hunt (18), progressive myoclonus and epilepsy with cerebellar ataxia have been well known. The dentatorubral atrophy is thought to be the most important change in the neuropathology of this syndrome (19). In the myoclonic form of DRPLA, the clinical features are just the same as in Ramsay Hunt's syndrome; the degeneration of the dentatorubral system is also common. Importantly, pallidoluysian atrophy could be proven in other cases reported as Ramsay Hunt's syndrome. On the other hand, the myoclonic form of DRPLA could account for some of the cases of so-called Ramsay Hunt's syndrome.

Joseph's Disease

Joseph's disease is a dominantly inherited disease that used to be said to appear only among people of Portuguese ancestry (20). However, some case reports of this disease have come from Japan (21). Joseph's disease has been divided into three types. In type I, the main neurologic features are pyramidal, but there are also extrapyramidal symptoms, such as dystonia and/or athetoid movements. In type II, cerebellar ataxia is the main symptom, sometimes accompanied by extrapyramidal symptoms. Type III shows cerebellar signs, with distal amyotrophy. All these symptoms are similar to those of DRPLA. Neuropathologically, however, a fundamental difference between DRPLA and Joseph's disease is seen in the substantia nigra; in the former it is well preserved, whereas in the latter it shows marked degeneration.

Mitochondrial Encephalomyelopathy

Fukuhara's disease, or myoclonus epilepsy with ragged-red fibers (MERRF) (22), is a subtype of mitochondrial encephalomyelopathy that shows myoclonus epilepsy, cerebellar ataxia, and hypotonia of the skeletal muscles, associated with progressive dementia. The rate of familial incidence is 50% of all patients. In some cases of MERRF, the differential diagnosis between this condition and the myoclonus type of DRPLA is quite difficult without muscle biopsy. There has been no DRPLA case with muscle biopsy; for an exact diagnosis of the myoclonus epilepsy type of DRPLA, therefore, it may be necessary to do muscle biopsy in the future.

OPCA

OPCA always affects the cerebellum and the brainstem, and very often the extrapyramidal system as well. The extrapyramidal signs of OPCA are the same as those of parkinsonism. In this point, they are clearly different from the extrapyramidal signs of DRPLA, which mostly show the choreic, choreoathetoid form of involuntary movements. In OPCA, no myoclonus or seizures take place. Thus, the differences in extrapyramidal signs between OPCA and DRPLA are clear-cut. These differences perhaps depend on the different biochemical changes in the two diseases (23).

TREATMENT

Because of the unknown etiology, there is still no reasonable and effective treatment.

DRPLA is a "disease" that is defined on the basis of clinical and neuropathologic data. In considering it as a disease, there may be two especially important points. One is the variety of clinical features with a relatively simple neuropathology, and the other is that the cases of spinocerebellar degeneration showing extrapyramidal symptoms can be divided into at least two separate subgroups, namely, OPCA with parkinsonism and DRPLA with choreic and/or myoclonic symptoms.

Whether or not DRPLA constitutes an independent disease entity may be clarified in the future through biochemical and genetic research into diseases with ataxia and extrapyramidal symptoms and into the occasional cases of degenerative forms of myoclonus epilepsy.

UPDATE: NEW DEVELOPMENTS

Recent studies have revealed molecular genetic changes in DRPLA (24,25). Comparative research on clinical pathology and molecular genetics should prove significant in the future.

REFERENCES

1. Iizuka R, Hirayama K, Maehara K. Dentato-rubro-pallido-luysian atrophy: a clinico-pathological study. J Neurol Neurosurg Psychiatry 1984;47:1288–1298.

2. Iizuka R, Hirayama K. Dentato-rubro-pallido-luysian atrophy. In: Vinken PJ, Bruyn GW, Klawans HL, eds. Handbook of clinical neurology. Vol. 5, Extrapyramidal disorders. Amsterdam: Elsevier, 1986.

3. Titica J, van Bogaert L. Heredo-degenerative hemiballismus—a contribution to the question of primary atrophy of the corpus Luysii. Brain 1946;69:251–263.

4. Smith JD. Dentatorubropallidoluysian atrophy. In: Vinken PJ, Bruyn GW, DeHong JMBV, eds. Handbook of clinical neurology. Vol. 21. Amsterdam: North-Holland, 1975:519–534.

5. Pfeiffer RF, McComb RD. Dentatorubro-pallidoluysian atrophy with posterior column degeneration. Neurology 1985;35(suppl 1):178.

6. Bergmann M, Gullota F, Gohler D. Dentatus-Ruber-Pallidum-Luys-Atrophie bei einem Säugling. Klin Padiatr 1990;202:1–4.

7. Neumann NA. Combined degeneration of globus pallidus and dentate nucleus and their projections. Neurology 1959;9:403–438.

8. Takahata N, Ito K, Yoshimura Y, et al. Familial chorea and myoclonus epilepsy. Neurology 1978;28:913–919.

9. Naito H, Oyanagi S. Familial myoclonus epilepsy and choreo-athetosis, hereditary dentatorubral pallidoluysian atrophy. Neurology 1982;32:798–807.

10. Iizuka R, Hirayama K. Dentato-rubro-pallido-luysian atrophy. In: Vinken PJ, Bruyn, GW, Klawans HL, eds. Handbook of clinical neurology. Vol. 16, Hereditary neuropathies and spinocerebellar atrophies. Amsterdam: North-Holland (in press).

11. Sasaki S, Uchiyama S, Aikawa T, et al. A sporadic case with degenerative changes, mainly in the dentate-rubral and the pallido-luysian systems. Clin Neurol 1980;20:863.

12. Verhaart WJC. Degeneration of the brainstem reticular formation, other parts of the brain stem and the cerebellum. An example of the heterogeneous systemic degeneration of the central nervous system. J Neuropathol Exp Neurol 1958;17:382–391.

13. Maeshiro H, Kato U, Nakamura S, et al. An unclassified case of degenerative disease of the central nervous system—with reference to hereditary pallidal and dentate system atrophy (Oyanagi). Psychiatr Neurol Jpn 1980;82:234–248.

14. Oppenheimer DR. Brain lesions in Friedreich's ataxia. Can J Neurol Sci 1979;6:173–176.

15. Kanazawa I. Regional distribution of markers for neurotransmitters in the basal ganglia of "choreic" disorders. Neurology. International Congress Series 568. Amsterdam: Excerpta Medica, 1982;4:220–232.

16. Nagatsu T, Kato T, Nagatsu I. Catecholamine-related enzymes in the brains of patients with parkinsonism and Wilson's disease. In: Poirier LJ, Sourkes TL, Bedard PJ, eds. Advances in neurology. Vol. 24. New York: Raven Press, 1979:283–292.

17. Andre-Van Leeuwen M, van Bogaert L. Hereditary ataxia with optic atrophy of the retrobulbar-neuritis type and latent pallido-luysian degeneration. Brain 1949;72:340–363.

18. Hunt R. Dyssynergia cerebellaris myoclonica—primary atrophy of the dentate system: a contribution to the pathology and symptomatology of the cerebellum. Brain 1921;44:490–538.

19. Bird TD, Shaw CM. Progressive myoclonus and epilepsy with dentato-rubral degeneration; a clinico-pathological study of the Ramsay Hunt syndrome. J Neurol Neurosurg Psychiatry 1978;41:140–149.

20. Rosenberg RN. Joseph's disease. In: Kark P, Rosenberg RN, Schut L, eds. Advances in neurology. Vol. 21, The inherited ataxias. New York: Raven Press, 1978:33–57.

21. Sakai T, Ohta M, Ishino H. Joseph's disease in a non-Portuguese family. Neurology 1983;33:74–80.

22. Fukuhara N, Tokiguchi S, Shirahama K, Tsubaki T. Myoclonus epilepsy associated with ragged-red fibers (mitochondrial abnormalities): disease entity or a syndrome? Light- and electronmicroscopic studies of two cases and a review of the literature. J Neurol Sci 1980;47:117–133.

23. Iizuka R, Hirayama K, Maehara K. A neuropathological observation of extrapyramidal components in cerebellar degeneration—a comparison of so-called dentato-rubro-pallido-luysian atrophy with OPCA. In: Sobue I, ed. Spinocerebellar degenerations. Tokyo: University of Tokyo Press, 1980:171–183.

24. Koide R, et al. Unstable expansion of CAG repeat in hereditary dentato-rubral-pallidoluysian atrophy (DRPLA). Nat Genet 1994;6:9–13.

25. Nagafuchi S, et al. Dentatorubral and pallidoluysian atrophy expansion of an unstable CAG trinucleotide on chromosome 12. Nat Genet 1994;6:14–19.

The Parkinsonian-Pyramidal Syndrome

P. NISIPEANU   AMOS D. KORCZYN

INTRODUCTION

Among the hypokinetic rigid disorders, Parkinson's disease is the most common. Other disorders with similar symptomatology, such as progressive supranuclear palsy (PSP) and multisystem atrophy (MSA), are distinguished by poor or absent response to levodopa and other dopaminergic drugs (1). On the other hand, some clinical syndromes have been delineated that consistently respond to dopaminergic medications. These include postencephalitic parkinsonism (2) and dopa-responsive dystonia (3). We here report our experience and review the literature of another clinical entity that belongs to this group, the parkinsonian-pyramidal syndrome (PPS), previously called pallido-pyramidal syndrome.

HISTORY AND DESCRIPTION

PPS is a rare disorder that associates parkinsonian features with pyramidal symptomatology. Its main clinical characteristics are as follows:

1. Onset occurs in young adulthood.
2. Extrapyramidal and pyramidal features emerge relatively slowly.
3. The onset may be unilateral, but the clinical disease evolves into a symmetric disorder.
4. The parkinsonian symptoms respond dramatically to levodopa therapy.
5. The response to levodopa is maintained for many years.

We review the symptomatology of PPS based on 18 reported patients, including 4 who we have personally followed for over two decades (4); we assume that case 2 of Remy et al (10) is the same patient described by Tranchant et al (8).

Davison was apparently the first to delineate the syndrome in 1954 (5). The first patient described (5) was 29 years old when evaluated at the Montefiore Home and Hospital in 1912 by Hunt (6) (case 2), where she was subsequently followed until her death more than 30 years later. She was born of consanguineous Jewish parents, but no other relevant familial data are available. This patient was apparently born following a normal pregnancy, developed normally, and was considered "bright" at school. At age 13, right-hand tremor appeared; tremor later involved the left hand as well. Gait difficulty appeared 2 years later, and by the time she was 20, the patient became unable to walk unaided. Dysarthria appeared when she was 23, together with dysphagia. The neurologic examination disclosed dysarthria, hypomimia with monotonous speech, and resting limb tremor of 4 to 6 Hz, more evident distally in the upper extremities. The tremor was somewhat enhanced at the beginning of a voluntary movement, but diminished during the movement, and Hunt was careful to emphasize that it was "in no sense an intentional tremor." Generalized rigidity, postural deformities, and hypokinesia were also present. The stretch reflexes were brisk; absent abdominal reflexes and bilateral Babinski signs were found later. The patient died of aspiration pneumonia at age 62.

Pathologic examination (5) showed mild shrinkage of the caudate nuclei, pallor of the pallidum, and thinning of the ansa lenticularis. Loss of neurons was found in the pallidum. The substantia nigra was "somewhat shrunken," with a reduced number of neurons, and many neurons showed hypopigmentation. There was no indication in the autopsy report of selective involvement of the pars reticulata or compacta, or of the existence of Lewy bodies. Pallor of the pyramids and swelling of myelin sheaths were noted in the medulla oblongata and extended into the spinal cord.

Because the main pathologic abnormality was found in the pallidum and in the pyramidal tracts, Davison termed this new syndrome "pallido-pyramidal" disease. He reported four other patients, all familial cases. Twenty years later, Horowitz and Greenberg (7) described two siblings and first reported the consistent and dramatic improvement of parkinsonism under levodopa therapy. In 1991, Tranchant et al (8) reported a sporadic case of a 13-year-old girl in whom spastic paraparesis was associated with extrapyramidal dopa-responsive symptoms. In 1994, we (4) reported two pairs of siblings belonging to two unrelated families who gradually developed parkinsonism and bilateral pyramidal symptomatology, with the extrapyramidal symptomatology again being very responsive to levodopa.

Al-Din et al (9) have described five somewhat different patients, who presented additional clinical features. These five siblings were affected not only by a parkinsonian and pyramidal syndrome but also by upgaze paresis and dementia. Quinn et al (11) described two first cousins with juvenile parkinsonism, bilateral pyramidal signs, mental retardation, and impaired upgaze. Because these patients have not definitely responded to levodopa, we did not include them in this review. Finally, Remy et al (10) reported two patients (one an 11-year-old boy born of consanguineous parents) who developed a mild cerebellar syndrome in association with bilateral pyramidal signs. Parkinsonian features apparently developed later and responded to levodopa therapy. Their second patient was probably one who had been described previously by Tranchant et al (8).

CLINICAL FEATURES

The onset of PPD is insidious, occurring between 7 and 24 years of age, with variable presenting symptoms. Sometimes the onset is vague; some patients were first examined and reported years after clinical onset. However, upper limb tremor and weakness of the legs or slowness of gait were the most frequently reported symptoms. When first examined, the patients exhibited extrapyramidal, pyramidal, and cerebellar signs in variable proportions, with rare upgaze paresis, nystagmus, and cognitive disturbances. Gait was impaired at the first examination in almost every case, described as "scissors-like," "spastic" without festination, or slow and without associated movements of the upper limbs. Walking was impossible for four patients (5,9).

Most patients were bradykinetic, and cogwheel rigidity involving all limbs was reported in approximately 80%. Rest tremor of the upper limbs—sometimes of the "pill-rolling" type—was present bilaterally in five patients and unilaterally in two; a few patients also had rest tremor of the legs. In a very few, the tremor was exacerbated by maintaining a posture. Hypomimia or amimia was present in more than one-third of the patients. Speech was described as slow and monotonous in less than half of them. Meyerson's sign was

reported in some. Postural deformities, including equinovarus and "striatal" toes (in the absence of any therapy) were sometimes noted.

The pyramidal symptomatology was present in all patients when first examined, except for the original case of Hunt and Davison. It consisted of bilateral Babinski signs in almost every patient and hyperactive stretch reflexes. Bilateral or unilateral ankle clonus were noted in some, and abdominal reflexes were absent. Spasticity was variable, generally restricted to the lower limbs. Strength and the ability to perform skilled movements were difficult to evaluate in many patients. However, loss of skilled movements of fingers was mentioned in a few patients, and mild or moderate paraparesis in more than half. Uncontrollable laughing spells were described in one patient, probably a reflection of pseudobulbar palsy. Moderate or severe dysarthria was present in at least eight patients.

Cerebellar symptomatology was reported in three patients (1,10). Bilateral hand intention tremor was found in two, in one case associated with rest tremor. Hypotonicity and hypometria were not observed, possibly due to coexistent pyramidal involvement. Supranuclear gaze paresis—usually upgaze—was reported, especially in the particular family described by Al-Din et al (9), in whom convergence paresis was also present. Horizontal or vertical upgaze nystagmus was seldom found. Few authors provided detailed cognitive evaluations. Mild dementia probably developed in four patients, and dementia without additional data was reported in two (5,9). None of our four patients had cognitive impairment.

Evolution

The single patient who did not have pyramidal signs at presentation (5) developed bilateral extensor plantar responses and absent superficial abdominal reflexes years later. Davison's patients became unable to walk unassisted after approximately 10 years of disease, whereas 16 years of disease elapsed from onset in one case (5) before the patient became wheelchair bound. The natural history of the extrapyramidal features in the remaining cases can be evaluated only prior to initiation of levodopa therapy. Horowitz and Greenberg's (7) two patients were probably at stage III (Hoehn and Yahr) parkinsonism, 10 and 13 years after the disease onset. Spasticity was relatively severe in one of them. Two patients described by us (4) were at stage III after less than 10 years of clinical evolution; two others were at stage II after 3 and 4 years of disease, at which point levodopa treatment was initiated. The pyramidal signs were considered to be moderate in one and mild in the remaining three. The patient reported by Tranchant et al (8) was relatively severely impaired, mostly due to spasticity, axial akinesia, and rest tremor; she was given levodopa after less than 2 years of progression. Severe akinesia was present in three of five patients reported by Al-Din et al (9); all three were bedridden after 3 to 20 years of evolution. These three patients were considered also to be demented. In this family the most aggressive evolution involved the extrapyramidal disturbances, the pyramidal symptoms being severe in only one patient after 20 years of disease. Finally, the patient reported by Remy et al (10) was probably at stage II 4 years after the onset, at which point levodopa was begun.

Horowitz and Greenberg's patient (7) continued to present pyramidal signs after 6 months of levodopa treatment. After a very long follow-up, our patients (4) had maintained the same pyramidal features without any worsening. Al-Din et al (9) and Remy et al (10) (first patient) also remarked that the pyramidal symptomatology was unchanged. However, the patient reported by Tranchant et al (8) continued to deteriorate and developed spastic paraplegia (10).

It seems, then, that PPS has an insidious evolution over several years, sometimes with different deterioration rates in the same family. Disability mainly reflects the extrapyramidal features, which respond well to levodopa. The spasticity contributes only mildly to the clinical disability and progresses only slightly over time.

GENETICS

Most cases were familial, and parental consanguinity was known to exist in all but three cases (see Table 38.1). Only one patient (8) did not belong to a consanguineous family and did not have another affected family member. Therefore, the mode of transmission seems to be autosomal recessive.

DIFFERENTIAL DIAGNOSIS

The presentation of PPS with slow onset of walking difficulty in young people may be difficult to distinguish from that of spastic paraparesis. Mild or moderate spasticity on examination, diminished or absent abdominal reflexes, brisk stretch reflexes, and extensor plantar responses, usually symmetric, in a patient with scissors-like gait may favor suspicion of spastic paraparesis. Nevertheless, the appearance of upper limb tremor and rigidity, bradykinesia, speech disturbances, and hypomimia at presentation or at follow-up examinations will exclude this possibility.

Dick and Stevenson (13) have reported hereditary spastic paraplegia in one family with later appearance of rigidity and hand rest tremor. However, the coexistence of choreoathetosis and dystonia, and the apparent dominant transmission, distinguishes this family from PPS.

The diagnosis of diplegic cerebral palsy will be excluded by a history of normal early development in the presence of a progressive neurologic deficit in the second or third decades of life.

The presentation of a child or young adult with parkinsonian features may suggest juvenile-onset parkinsonism or dopa-responsive dystonia (DRD). DRD usually starts with dystonia of gait, and may be very difficult to differentiate from juvenile-onset parkinsonism, in which focal dystonia is frequently an early feature. DRD onset is between 14 months and 12 years of age (3). The dystonic extension of the great toe ("striatal toe") may be interpreted erroneously as an extensor plantar response, and stretch reflexes are sometimes brisk. Parkinsonian symptoms may appear early, but typical rest tremor is unusual. The early-occurring tremor is usually postural. Diurnal variation is present in most of the patients, and "sleep benefit" was also described (3). Diurnal fluctuation was also sometimes reported in patients with juvenile parkinsonism, most of them familial cases (reviewed by Yamamura et al (15)). The key clinical feature of DRD may be provided by the striking improvement that occurs with levodopa, a response that may be obtained immediately and with small doses. This response seems to remain stable after many years of therapy, contributing a decisive clue differentiating DRD from juvenile parkinsonism (3). These diagnoses are excluded by the presence at onset or the later appearance of pyramidal symptoms or signs.

In familial cases of PPS, treatable diseases such as Wilson's disease must be considered. Other possibilities are early-onset inherited cerebellar ataxias, rigid-onset Huntington's disease, or Hallervorden-Spatz disease.

LABORATORY INVESTIGATIONS

Results of routine blood, cerebrospinal fluid, and urine examinations, and sometimes extensive metabolic work-ups, were normal in all PPS patients, as were results of slit-lamp examination and copper and ceruloplasmin studies. Results of electromyography and nerve conduction studies were normal in a small number of patients. The electroencephalogram (EEG) was normal in all patients, excepting Davison's case 4, whose EEG showed "intermittent electrical abnormalities affecting the posterior less than other areas," and Horowitz and Greenberg's case 2, whose EEG was reported as mildly abnormal.

Neuroimaging examinations (magnetic resonance imaging or computed tomography of the brain) were normal in five patients (4,8,10), but Al-Din et al (9) reported generalized brain atrophy, including the cerebellum and brainstem in some. Interestingly, two patients presented more selective atrophy of the lenticular nuclei and of the pyramids.

[18]F-fluorodeoxyglucose positron emission tomography (PET) was normal in one patient (4). ^{18}F-fluorodopa PET (^{18}F-DOPA PET) was used by Eidelberg et al (18) on the first patient reported by Horowitz and Greenberg (7) and by Remy et al in two patients (10). In all, ^{18}F-DOPA PET was consistent with a marked decrement in nigrostriatal function, comparable with the values obtained in severe Parkinson's disease, indicating dopaminergic nigrostriatal denervation.

RESPONSE TO LEVODOPA THERAPY

Except for the patients reported by Quinn et al (11), all others who were exposed to levodopa had a dramatic improvement at the institution of drug therapy, sometimes within 48 hours. Long-term follow-up is available for a few patients (4,10). The four patients followed by us for more than 20 years continue to respond to levodopa-carbidopa treatment. The dose was increased after years of stable response, reaching a mean total daily dose of levodopa of 750 mg. "Wearing-off" appeared in the last years of treatment. During "on" periods, patients are usually in stage II (Hoehn and Yahr). Patient 2 of Remy et al (10), who developed early peak-dose dyskinesias, was still very responsive to small doses of levodopa after 9 years of treatment. Patient 1 of Horowitz and Greenberg is currently wheelchair bound after failed adrenomedullary transplantation (D. Eidelberg, personal communication). Under levodopa therapy, it seems that in almost all patients the pyramidal syndrome did not change.

NOSOLOGICAL CONSIDERATIONS

Davison's patients were considered by Jellinger (19) to belong to the primary degeneration of the pallidum group whose pathologic hallmark was bilateral neuronal loss restricted to the globus pallidus or associated with degeneration of other systems, as was initially proposed by Hunt (19). According to Jellinger's review, pure pallidal atrophy seems to be extremely rare. The variable association with lesions of efferent pallidal fibers, with lesions of the subthalamic nucleus (pallidoluysian atrophy), with extension to the putamen, caudate, and substantia nigra ("extended form of pallidal degeneration"), or with lesions of other than extrapyramidal structures, including the corticospinal system, was also seldom reported (19). Since pathologic examinations are available only for Davison's cases, who has not described pathognomonic signs, it is not definitely clear that all cases indeed had the same disease.

Although the pathologic changes are still not defined, the group of patients with PPS seems to be clinically well characterized. The onset is at a young age and the parkinsonian-pyramidal features develop slowly; parkinsonian features respond dramatically and consistently to levodopa. Almost all were familial cases, born of normal parents who were frequently consaguineous, therefore suggesting autosomal recessive inheritance. Because the excellent levodopa responsiveness and F-DOPA PET results are more compatible with nigrostriatal denervation than with primary pallidal pathology, the term "parkinsonian-pyramidal syndrome" is a more representative description than "pallido-pyramidal syndrome."

REFERENCES

1. Jankovic J. Parkinsonian-plus syndromes. Mov Disord 1989;4:S95–S119.
2. Calne D, Stern GM, Laurence DR, et al. L-Dopa in postencephalitic parkinsonism. Lancet 1969;1:744–746.
3. Nygaard TG, Marsden CD, Fahn S. Dopa-responsive dystonia: long-term treatment response and prognosis. Neurology 1991;41:174–181.
4. Nisipeanu P, Kuritzki A, Korczyn AD. Familial levodopa responsive parkinsonian-pyramidal syndrome. Mov Disord 1994;9:673–675.
5. Davison C. Pallido-pyramidal disease. J Neuropathol Exp Neurol 1954;13:50–59.
6. Hunt R. Progressive atrophy of the globus pallidus (primary atrophy of the pallidal system). A system disease of the paralysis agitans type, characterized by atrophy of the motor cells of the corpus striatum. A contribution to the functions of the corpus striatum. Brain 1917;40:58–148.
7. Horowitz G, Greenberg J. Pallido-pyramidal syndrome treated with levodopa. J Neurol Neurosurg Psychiatry 1975;38:238–240.
8. Tranchant C, Boulay C, Warter JM. Le syndrome pallido-pyramidal: Une entité méconnue. Rev Neurol 1991;147:308–310.
9. Al-Din N, Wriekat A, Mubaidin A, et al. Pallido-pyramidal degeneration, supranuclear upgaze paresis and dementia: Kufor-Rakeb syndrome. Acta Neurol Scand 1994;89:347–352.
10. Remy P, Hosseini H, Degos JD, et al. Striatal dopaminergic denervation in pallido-pyramidal disease demonstrated in positron emission tomography. Ann Neurol 1995;38:954–956.
11. Quinn NP, Goadsby PJ, Lees AJ. Hereditary juvenile parkinsonism with pyramidal signs and mental retardation. Eur Neurol 1995;2:23–26.
12. Harding AE. Hereditary spastic paraplegias. Semin Neurol 1993;13:333–336.
13. Dick AP, Stevenson CY. Hereditary spastic paraplegia: report of a family with associated extrapyramidal signs. Lancet 1953;1:921–923.
14. Van Bogaert L. Contribution clinique et anatomique á l'étude de la paralysie agitante juvénile primitive. Rev Neurol 1930;2:315–326.
15. Yamamura Y, Sobue I, Ando K, et al. Paralysis agitans of early onset with marked diurnal fluctuation of symptoms. Neurology 1973;23:239–244.
16. Narabayashi H, Yokochi M, Iizuka R, Nagatsu T. Juvenile parkinsonism. In: Vinken PJ, Bruyn GW, Klawans HL, eds. Handbook of clinical neurology. Vol. 49 (revised series). Amsterdam: Elsevier Science Publishers, 1986:153–165.
17. Golbe L. Young-onset Parkinson's disease: a clinical review. Neurology 1991;41:168–173.
18. Eidelberg BD, Moeller JR, Dhawan V, et al. The metabolic anatomy of Parkinson's disease: complementary [18F] fluorodeoxyglucose and [18F] fluorodopa positron emission tomographic studies. Mov Disord 1990;5:202–213.
19. Jellinger K. Degenerations and exogenous lesions of the pallidum and striatum. In: Vinken PJ, Bruyn GW, eds. Handbook of clinical neurology. Vol. 6. Amsterdam: North Holland, 1969:632–693.

The Autosomal Dominant Spinocerebellar Ataxias: Clinicopathologic Findings and Genetic Mechanisms

BRYAN T. WOODS

For many years the major problems in classifying hereditary neuronal degenerative disorders were deciding how much to weight clinical manifestations relative to pathologic findings and how to deal with intrafamilial case-to-case variations in both. However, beginning with the localization of the genetic defect underlying Huntington's disease to chromosome 4, the results of molecular genetic studies have become more and more the final arbiters of classification. Thus, in the first edition of this book the argument that the spinocerebellar degeneration first described in several different Portuguese-American families from the Azores (1–4) was a distinct disease was made on clinicopathologic grounds. However, in the intervening few years detailed information has emerged on the genetic basis of this and several other spinocerebellar degenerations. Therefore it now seems more useful to discuss the Azorean disorder, which is also commonly known as Machado-Joseph disease (MJD), as part of a family of symptomatically and pathologically similar but genetically distinct disorders, and to discuss in some detail a new pathogenetic mechanism, trinucleotide repeat expansion, that has now been demonstrated to be the basis of not only this disorder but at least 11 other inherited neuronal degenerations.

CLASSIFICATION AND TERMINOLOGY

The concept of neuronal degeneration was developed at the end of the nineteenth century during the first flowering of neuropathology. Over time, classification of these disorders has taken into account six major features: neurological signs, neuropathologic changes, pattern of inheritance, age of onset, time course, and genetic localization (Table 39.1). The disorders to be discussed in this chapter are a subset of the hereditary spinocerebellar ataxias, a group of slowly progressive adult-onset dominantly inherited ataxias with pre-

dominant cell loss involving the cerebellum and/or its inflow and outflow nuclei and tracts in the brainstem and spinal cord. This group of disorders has been classified as autosomal dominant cerebellar ataxia, type 1 (ADCA1) by Harding (5). As different genetic loci for these disorders have been established, they have been labeled as spinocerebellar ataxias (SCAs) and assigned numbers in the order of their chromosomal localization. To date, the localizations of six SCAs have been established. The defect for SCA1 is localized to chromosome 6p, that for SCA2 to 12q, that for SCA3/MJD to 14q, that for SCA4 to 16q, that for SCA5 to centromeric 11, and, finally, that for SCA6 to 19p. (The genetic uniqueness of another disorder, SCA7, has also been established, but because it involves retinal degeneration as well as spinocerebellar ataxia it falls outside the overall ADCA1 category and will not be further discussed.)

Two other autosomal dominant adult-onset neuronal degenerations that sometimes manifest clinically in forms difficult to distinguish from SCA have also had their chromosomal loci established. Dentatorubropallidoluysian atrophy (DRPLA) has a locus on chromosome 12p (at the other end of the chromosome from SCA2), and autosomal dominant spastic paraplegia (SPG) has three separate loci: on 2p, on 14q (more centrally than the SCA3 defect), and on 15q.

In the first edition, this chapter took the position that descriptions of MJD in families of non-Azorean origin might be due to one or more different allelic defects affecting a single gene, but it is now clear that the genetic defect seen in both Azorean and non-Azorean patients showing the characteristic MJD clinical presentation and pathology is due to a single allelic defect consisting of excessive trinucleotide expansion at a single locus. Thus, the clinical and pathologic variations in the disorder are partially attributable to the *length* of the abnormal repeat at a single site rather than

Table 39.1   Bases for Classification of the
Neuronal Degenerations

I. Primary and Secondary Neurologic Signs
   A. Primary signs are those dominant findings that broadly characterize a
      group of disorders, and are sooner or later present in all patients with the
      diagnosis. The most common signs categorizing major groupings are
      dementia, choreoathetosis, extrapyramidal rigidity, ataxia, sensory loss,
      weakness with spasticity, weakness with muscle atrophy, and progressive
      blindness or deafness.
   B. Secondary signs are those which occur in some but not all patients in a
      primary category, for example, ataxia with retinal degeneration, ataxia
      with dementia, ataxia with extrapyramidal rigidity.
II. Neuropathologic Characteristics
   A. Anatomical sites of cell loss and tract degeneration. Almost any discrete
      structure or cell type within a structure may be affected in individual
      cases, but if the structure sooner or later shows cell loss or degeneration,
      in almost all patients diagnosed as having the disorder it is a primary
      characteristic; otherwise, it is secondary.
   B. Other pathologic markers, such as neuronal inclusions, gliosis,
      demyelination, or plaques.
III. Pattern of Inheritance
   A. Sporadic or familial. Within familial disorders there may be an autosomal
      dominant, autosomal recessive, or sex-linked pattern of transmission.
IV. Age of Onset
   A. Disorders may characteristically manifest in infancy, childhood/
      adolescence, young/middle-aged adulthood, or late life.
   B. Age of onset in familial disorders may show anticipation, that is,
      progressively earlier onset in succeeding generations.
V. Time Course
   A. Progression may be chronic (measured in years) or subacute (with
      changes discernible over a period of months).
   B. Degenerations occurring in utero may appear to be nonprogressive
      postnatally.
VI. Genetic Localization
   A. By chromosome and region (e.g., 12p).
   B. At the DNA codon level.

defects at different sites. However, it has also become evident from several large genetic surveys of patients from families with distinct SCAs that the clinical symptomatology and neuropathology of genetically distinct disorders can overlap with one another in specific individuals. It follows that one cannot clinically or neuropathologically differentiate the autosomal dominant spinocerebellar ataxias with complete reliability, and that genomic analysis is essential to establish the diagnosis.

HISTORY

The earliest hereditary ataxia to be clearly established as a separate genetic entity was that described by Friedreich in 1863. It has been found to be heterogeneous, with the commonest form due to a specific genetic defect on chromosome 9q that results in trinucleotide expansion (6), and a second form, with associated vitamin E deficiency, due to a

defect on chromosome 8q (7). Because Friedreich's ataxia is an autosomal recessive disorder that appears in childhood, it will not be discussed further.

SCA1

The first of the autosomal dominant ataxias was clearly described by Menzel in 1891, and in 1900 was given the name olivo-ponto-cerebellar atrophy (OPCA) by Dejerine and Thomas. Over the intervening years cases with both dominant and recessive patterns of inheritance have been described, as well as a number of clinicopathologically similar sporadic cases (8), but among the familial cases most show an autosomal dominant pattern. In 1974 it was reported that OPCA was genetically linked to the HLA locus on chromosome 6 (9), and a location on the short (p) arm of 6 has been subsequently confirmed. The disorder associated with this 6p defect was then termed SCA1. Its clinical features are outlined in Table 39.2.

In 1993 it was reported that the basic defect in SCA1 is an expansion of an exonic DNA trinucleotide repeat (CAG) that codes for polyglutamine (10). Normally this repeat ranges in length from 6 to 39 triplets, whereas in diseased patients the number of repeats ranged from 41 to 81 (10,11). The resulting abnormal protein has been named ataxin-1 (12).

SCA3/MJD

In 1969 Boller and Segarra described an autosomal dominant spinocerebellar degeneration in the "W" family that they termed spino-pontine degeneration (13). In 1971 Taniguchi and Konigsmark described a separate family, the "H" family, with a pathologically very similar pattern of abnormalities (14). The latter authors used the term spino-pontine atrophy, but suggested it was probably the same disorder as that described by Boller and Segarra. Further neuropathologic description of two afflicted patients from the "W" family was provided in 1978 (15).

In 1972 there appeared two independent reports of autosomal dominant spinocerebellar degenerative disorders found in two Portuguese-American families who had migrated to New England from the Azores, the Machado family (1) and the Thomas family (2). The disorders were both marked by gait ataxia but appeared to differ clinically from one another in that in the Machado family peripheral neuropathy was prominent, whereas in the Thomas family ophthalmoplegia, and extrapyramidal rigidity responsive to trihexyphenidyl, were salient characteristics. There were no neuropathologic data for the Machado family, but there were data from a complete neuropathologic examination of one member of the Thomas family. Based on differences in the neuropathologic findings, Woods and Schaumburg concluded that the disorder they termed nigro-spino-dentatal degeneration with nuclear ophthalmoplegia was probably distinct from other previously described spinocerebellar

Table 39.2 Clinical Characteristics of the Five Genetically Distinct Forms of Spinocerebellar Ataxia

	Disorder					
Abnormality	SCA1	SCA2	SCA3	SCA4	SCA5	SCA6
Gait ataxia	+++	+++	+++	+++	+++	+++
Limb ataxia	+	+++	+	+++	+++	+++
Dysarthria	+++	+++	++	++	+++	+++
Hyperreflexia	++	+	++	0	?	+
Babinski signs	++	+	++	+	?	+
Posterior column sensory loss	+	+	+	+++	?	++
Peripheral sensory loss	+	0	+	+++	?	+
Hyporeflexia/Areflexia	+	++	+	+++	?	++
Muscle wasting	+	+	+	+	?	0
Extrapyramidal rigidity	++	0	++	0	0	0/+
Hypotonia	0	++	0	?	?	+/++
Dystonia/Involuntary movements	++	+	++	0	0	+
Progressive Ext. Ophthalmoplegia	++	++	++	0	0	+
Bulging eyes	0	+	++	0	0	0
Dysphagia	+	+	+	0	+	0
Facial myokymia/Fasciculations	0	+	+	0	0	0
Incontinence	+	0	0	0	0	0/+
Dementia	++	0	0	0	0	0/+

ataxias, including spinopontine degeneration/spinopontine atrophy.

In 1976 an autosomal dominant spinocerebellar degenerative disorder was described in 13 members of the Joseph family, another Portuguese-American family from the Azores (4). The authors considered this family to have a unique disorder because of neuropathologic differences from the family described by Woods and Schaumburg, although this conclusion was disputed by a neuropathologist familiar with pathologic material from both families (16). A year later, spinocerebellar degeneration was described in still another Portuguese-American family of Azorean origin (17), and the suggestion was made that all three of the earlier reports, along with the current one, were descriptions of variants of the same disorder. In 1978 there appeared a clinical description of spinocerebellar degeneration in 40 patients from 15 families living in the Azores (18) and it was concluded that these patients also exemplified the disorder previously described in the emigrant families.

The disorder gradually became known as Machado-Joseph disease (MJD) since the Thomas family name had not been openly linked to the disorder at that time. There followed a number of reports of a clinically and pathologically similar disorder in families without a known link to the Azorean Portuguese. Families with the disorder were described not only in mainland Portugal (19) but also in France (20), in several large Japanese kindreds (21–23), and in African (24,25), Italian (26), and Sicilian (27) Americans. Finally, it was suggested in 1986 (28) that spinopontine degeneration/spinopontine atrophy (13–15) represents the

earliest description of the same disorder. In 1994 Kawaguchi et al reported that the genetic defect in Japanese families with MJD was localized to chromosome 14q and involved a CAG expansion (29). Subsequently, the same localization and abnormal triplet expansion were described in 16 Portuguese-Azorean families previously diagnosed with MJD (30).

In 1993, prior to the Kawaguchi study (29), there had been a report of seven French families with an autosomal dominant spinocerebellar ataxia thought to differ clinically from MJD, in which the genetic defect could be *excluded* from chromosomes 6 or 12 (31). This disorder was accordingly termed SCA3. In 1994 Stevanin et al (32) localized the SCA3 defect to 14q in two French families. There have been a number of subsequent reports addressing the issue of whether MJD and SCA3 are due to identical or allelic 14q defects. One study (33) reported that a family previously identified neuropathologically (34) as having spinopontine atrophy was genetically identified as having SCA3, and suggested that MJD and SCA3 are different alleles. Other observers have concluded that SCA3 and MJD are caused by an identical defect and that clinicopathologic variation is due to a combination of variations in repeat length and the modifying effects of variation in other genes (35,36).

As yet there are no published reports indicating whether either the "W" family (13) or the "H" family (14) actually have an expanded triplet repeat on 14q. If it should turn out that these families have the same defect as in MJD and SCA3, then credit for the initial description of the disorder should go to Boller and Segarra. If not, then MJD is a unique disorder and the families described by Boller and Segarra in 1969 and by Taniguchi and Konigsmark in 1971 have some other disorder. It should be pointed out that in several large surveys less than half of the families with clinically diagnosable autosomal dominant spinocerebellar ataxia actually had one of the five SCA genetic defects so far isolated (33,37,38).

The clinical features of SCA3 are also outlined in Table 39.2, along with those of SCA1, SCA2, and SCA4 through SCA6. Gait ataxia is the most prominent finding in SCA3, and as the table shows, none of the other clinical features commonly seen is unique to SCA3 (e.g., bulging eyes are also described in SCA2). Table 39.3 shows the pathologic features of SCA3 patients from three different geographic

origins (Azorean, Japanese, and European) and the original spinopontine atrophy/degeneration descriptions as well as the major pathologic features of SCA1, SCA2, and SCA6 for contrast. (As yet there are no pathologic studies available for SCA4 and SCA5.)

SCA2

An autosomal dominant spinocerebellar ataxia, described originally in a large kindred in Holguin in eastern Cuba (39–41), has been shown to result from a genetic defect on the long arm of chromosome 12 (42). A similar spinocerebellar ataxia with a 12q defect has been reported in an Italian family (43,44). This disorder was characterized as SCA2 because it was the second of the autosomal dominant

T a b l e 3 9 . 3   Pathologic Features of SCA1, SCA2, SCA6, and Four Subgroups of SCA3

| | SCA3 | | | | | | |
Structure	Azorean (n = 8)	Japanese (n = 3)	Other (n = 3)	SPA/SPD (n = 5)	SCA1	SCA2	SCA6
Somatic musculature	+	+	0	+	+		
Peripheral nerves	+	+	0	+	+	+	
Dorsal root ganglia	+	+	0	+	+	+	
Clarke's column	+++	+++	++	+++	++	++	0
Spinocerebellar tracts	++	+++	++	++	++	++	0
Anterior horn cells	+++	+++	++	++	++	++	0
Posterior columns	+	++	+	++	++	+++	0
Corticospinal tracts	+	0	+	0	+		0/+
Hypoglossal nucleus	++	0	0	0			
Vestibular nuclei	++	+	0	+			
Facial nerve nucleus	++	0	0	+			
Trigeminal nuclei	0	0	0	+			
Motor V nucleus	+	0	0	+			
Nuclei basis pontis	+++	++	++	++	+++	+++	0
Inferior olivary nucleus	0	0	+	+	+++	+++	++
Superior olivary nucleus	0	0	0	+	0		
Cerebellar granule cells	0	0	+	+	+++		++/+++
Purkinje cells	0	0	+	+	+++	+++	+++
Dentate nucleus	++	+++	++	+	+	0	0/+
Embol./Globose nuclei	0	0	0	+			
Abducens nucleus	+	0	0	0			
Trochlear nucleus	+	+	0	0			
Oculomotor nucleus	++	+++	++	0	+		
Locus ceruleus	+	+	+	0	+	+	
Medial long. fasciculus	+	0	0	0			
Nucleus ambiguus	+	0	0	+	+		
Nucleus ruber	+	++	+	+			0
Subthalamic nucleus	+	++	++	+	+		
Substantia nigra (PC)	+++	+++	+	+	++	+++	
Globus pallidus	+	++	+	++	+		0
Caudate/Putamen	+	0	0	+	+		0
Thalamic nuclei	0	0	0	+			0
Subcortical white matter	0	0	0	+			0
Cerebral cortex	0	0	0	0	+		0

spinocerebellar ataxias to be genetically localized, even though its initial clinical description came long after that of SCA3.

The combination of the phenomenon of anticipation in specific families with SCA2 and the tendency for severity and rate of progression to be associated with early onset suggested that an abnormal triplet repeat was also the underlying cause for this disorder (43). An expanded CAG repeat on 12q coding for polyglutamine has now been separately demonstrated by three independent groups of researchers (12).

SCA6

This disorder was not singled out as a genetically distinct entity until 1997 (45), but the initial report not only localized it to chromosome 19p but also identified the exact genetic defect responsible—a CAG triplet expansion in the α_{1A}-voltage–dependent calcium channel gene *CACNL1A4*. Remarkably, two other allelic defects in this same gene had been previously described, one of which is responsible for type 2 episodic ataxia (EA2), and the other of which causes familial hemiplegic migraine (46). SCA6 appears to be one of the most common of the SCAs in Japan (47,48), somewhat less common in a heterogeneous American study population (49), and distinctly uncommon in a Western European patient pool (50).

SCA4

The chromosomal localization for SCA4 is a defect on chromosome 16q found in a Utah kindred of Scandinavian origin (51,52). Characteristically this SCA presents in the fourth or fifth decade (range of age of onset: 19–59 years), but there is some suggestion of anticipation in later generations. There is no pathology yet reported, and the gene has not yet been cloned.

SCA5

The chromosomal localization in SCA5 families was reported in 1994 to localize to the centromeric region of chromosome 11 (53). In this family the disorder can be traced back to the grandparents of Abraham Lincoln. The age of onset is usually in the third to fourth decades, but it ranges from 10 to 68 years. There is as yet no published pathologic description. The gene has not yet been cloned, and it is not known whether it too will turn out to contain an expanded triplet in affected family members.

Other Overlapping Disorders

Recent genetic analyses of large numbers of individuals with autosomal dominant neuronal degenerations affecting the motor system have shown that occasional individuals thought on clinical grounds to have a disorder other than spinocerebellar ataxia turn out on analysis to have one of the SCA genetic defects. An example of this is a family with clinical features of dentatorubropallidoluysian atrophy found to have the 14q defect (54).

CLINICAL FEATURES

Table 39.2 shows the major clinical findings in the six genetically distinct spinocerebellar ataxias. By definition, ataxia of gait is present in all affected families with each of these disorders, and other cerebellar signs are prominent. There are differences both within and between groups as to whether there are prominent signs of involvement of peripheral nerves, spinal cord cell groups and tracts, cranial nerve nuclei, and basal ganglia. Cognitive functions are usually spared. (It should be noted that disorders that combine ataxia and retinal degeneration, such as SCA7, have been excluded by definition from this grouping.)

SCA1 is characterized by onset any time from infancy to late middle age, but the mean age of onset is about 30. The first observable abnormalities are usually gait and limb ataxia, often (but not always) followed by spasticity, extrapyramidal rigidity, impaired eye movements, and dementia. Sphincter disturbances and swallowing difficulties are also encountered in about a third of the patients (8).

SCA2 may vary in age of onset from early childhood to the seventh decade. As a rule the cases with early onset are more likely to show rapid progression and a severe course, with added features of slowing of saccadic eye movements and ophthalmoplegia, as well as dysphagia. Later-onset patients show a relatively pure cerebellar ataxia (41).

SCA3 has a similar range of ages of onset. Ataxia of gait is most likely to be an initial manifestation, whereas ataxia of the extremities is relatively minimal in most affected patients. Common but variable accompaniments during the course of illness are spasticity and hyperreflexia, extensor plantar responses, extrapyramidal rigidity, progressive external ophthalmoplegia of variable degree, and dysarthria. Less common accompaniments sometimes present are dystonic postures and choreoathetotic movements of the extremities, loss of either pain and temperature or posterior column sensation, and distal areflexia. Motor wasting, particularly of the distal extremities but also of the tongue, is increasingly commonly seen as the duration of illness lengthens (55), and facial muscle fasciculations may appear. Dysphagia when present is predominantly due to weakness of the bulbar musculature but may have a dystonic component to it. Some patients manifest bulging eyes, presumably due to weakness of the extraocular muscles (2). Interestingly, the dementia and affective disturbances that are so often seen in Huntington's disease and sometimes in SCA1 are notable by their absence.

Clinical subtyping has been proposed by several authors, basically dividing cases into those with extrapyramidal (both parkinsonian and dystonic) plus ataxic features, those with mainly ataxic features, and those with ataxic plus peripheral (both motor and sensory) features (18,55). Since it now seems likely that these distinctions are consequences of disease severity and duration, and that these in turn are strongly correlated with the length of the abnormal triplet repeat (see below), the subtyping is of undoubted heuristic value to researchers but not very relevant clinically.

In general, SCA6 tends have a later age of onset and to have symptomatology largely limited to truncal and limb ataxia, dysarthria, and horizontal and vertical gaze nystagmus (56); a minority of patients also have evidence of posterior column or peripheral sensory loss. Some patients with the identical 19p CAG expansion show only cerebellar signs and an age of onset over 50 years (49), which would have previously led to them being classified as Harding's type 3 ADCA (5). Furthermore, in one study a number of patients with apparently sporadic SCA also had the SCA6 genetic defect (47).

SCA4 presents with gait disturbance, incoordination, and dysarthria. Patients also show a peripheral neuropathy with pin, vibration, and joint-position sensation loss and absent knee and ankle jerks. Twenty percent showed extensor plantar reflexes as well (52).

SCA5 appears in general to be a milder disorder, with later-onset cases manifesting mainly with gait ataxia, limb incoordination, and slurred speech. Two early-onset cases also developed swallowing difficulties (53).

Because there is no clinical feature that is almost always present in one SCA and almost never present in the others, and because a number of apparently sporadic cases have been found to have a specific genetic defect (47), confident assignment of a patient to one group on clinical grounds alone is not possible, and genetic testing is a prerequisite for adequate diagnosis of patients with slowly progressive adult-onset ataxia.

PATHOLOGIC FEATURES

Table 39.3 shows the major neuropathologic findings in SCA1, SCA2, SCA3, and SCA6. The SCA1 data are taken with some modification from a review by Berciano (8), that for SCA2 from Orozco Diaz et al (40), and that for SCA6 from Gomez et al (56) and Ikeuchi et al (48). There are four separate SCA3 entries. Neuropathologic examinations of eight Azorean SCA patients (2–4,16,17,57,58) form the basis for one description. Non-Azorean SCA3 is shown as two separate categories: Japanese SCA3, with three neuropathologic cases (22,59), and Other SCA, also with three cases (60,61). On the assumption that spinopontine atrophy/spinopontine degeneration is also due to the SCA3 genetic defect, the early neuropathologic descriptions of that disorder, comprising five cases from two families (13–15), have been used to formulate the fourth category.

In SCA1 the major loss of neurons is seen in the cerebellar Purkinje cells, the basis pontis nuclei, and the inferior olives. Lesions are also seen frequently in the posterior columns, Clarke's columns, the anterior horn cells, the cor-

ticospinal tracts, the dentate nuclei, and the substantia nigra.

In SCA2, pathologic examination of 11 cases, 7 of which included the spinal cord, showed neuronal losses in the inferior olives, pons, cerebellum, and anterior horn cells, severe lesions of the posterior columns, and some degeneration of the spinocerebellar tracts.

In SCA3 there is almost always heavy involvement of Clarke's columns, the anterior horn cells, the nuclei of the basis pontis, the spinocerebellar tracts, and the substantia nigra. Other areas frequently involved are 1) the hypoglossal, facial, trigeminal motor, trochlear, and oculomotor nuclei; 2) the striatum, red nuclei, subthalamic nuclei, and globus pallidus; and 3) the posterior columns. The inferior olives and cerebellar granule and Purkinje cells are almost always spared. One can summarize by saying that this is primarily a disorder of lower motor neuron nuclei, cerebellar inputs and outflow (excluding olivocerebellar connections), and the substantia nigra.

The six autopsied cases of SCA6 have a relatively limited pathology that severely affects the Purkinje and granule cells of the cerebellum, moderately impacts the inferior olives, and occasionally involves the posterior columns and corticospinal tracts. Pathologically, SCA6 is almost the exact inverse of SCA3.

Figure 39.1 highlights the neuropathologic similarities and differences between SCA1 and a "consensus" SCA3. The numerical score assigned to each anatomic structure reflects both severity of lesions and frequency of occurrence. Level 3 implies marked abnormality *and* high frequency, level 2 implies either severe abnormalities with moderate frequency or moderate abnormalities with high frequency, and level 1 implies that the abnormality is moderate to severe but infrequent, or mild and frequent. The figure makes it clear that the abnormalities of SCA1 both overlap and extend beyond those of SCA3, so that the pathology of SCA3 is that of SCA1 minus involvement of the inferior olives and cerebellar parenchyma.

GENETIC MECHANISMS

In 1991 a new mechanism of genetic disease, expanded trinucleotide repeats, was described for two inherited neurologic disorders, X-linked spinobulbar muscular atrophy (62), and fragile X syndrome (63). Subsequently this mechanism has been found to be present in 11 distinct disorders, including Huntington's disease, Friedreich's ataxia, DRPLA, and SCAs 1 through 3 and 6. Those trinucleotide repeat expansions that are in the translated portions of genes (i.e., the exons) code for an excessively long chain of a single amino acid that is incorporated in the protein product of the gene. In the SCAs and several other disorders, the repeated triplet is CAG and the amino acid is glutamine.

It should be understood that the normal protein also contains a polyglutamine chain of variable length, so that it is not the presence of the chain that causes disease, but

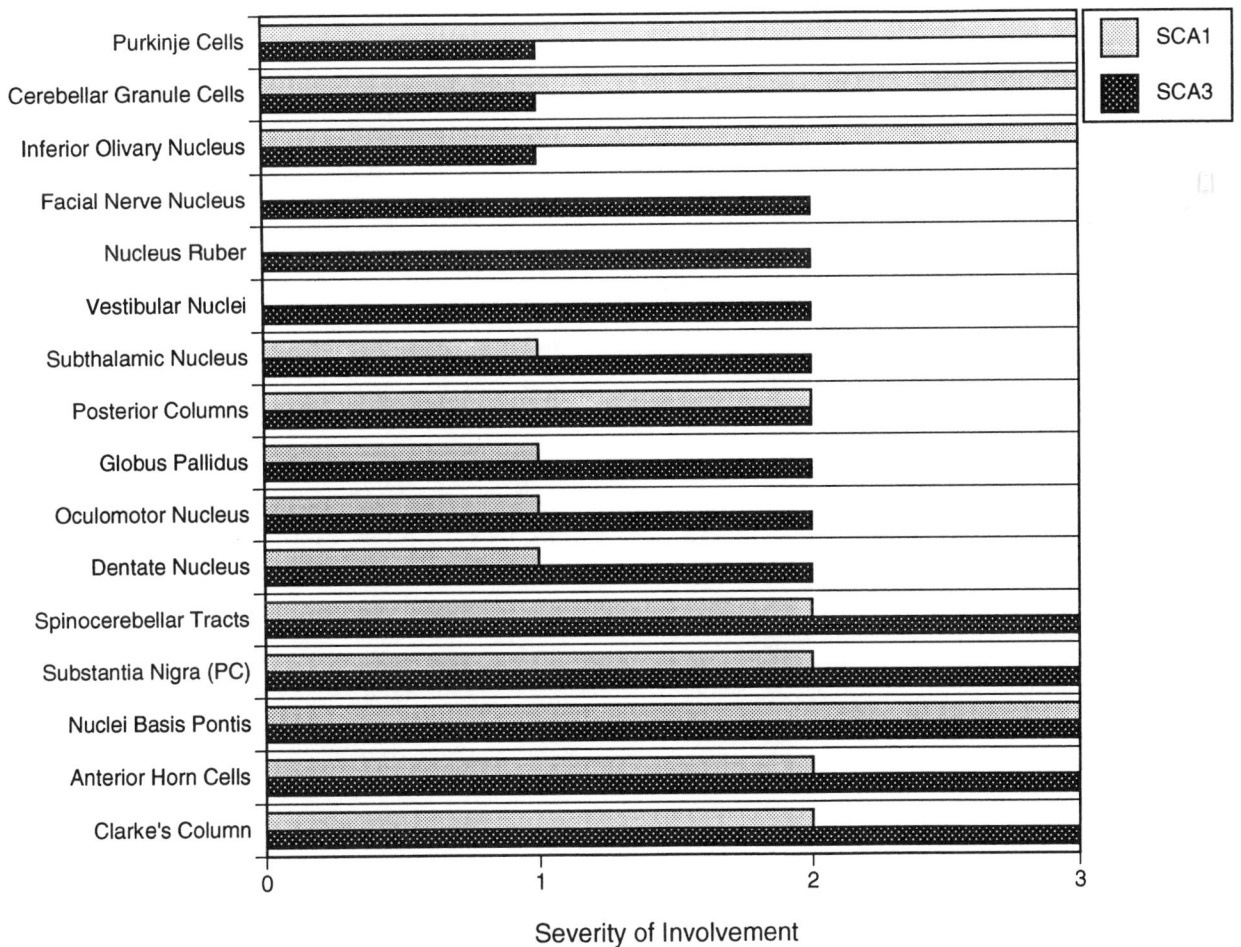

FIGURE 39.1 *Comparison of regions of primary cell loss and tract degeneration in SCA1 and SCA3. The levels assigned reflect both severity and frequency (see text for discussion).*

rather its excessive length. Because the presence of the expanded polyglutamine region on only one member of a chromosome pair is sufficient to cause disease, and because the defective gene product is expressed in the disease state, it has been suggested that these abnormal proteins result in a pathologic "gain of function" (64). One example of such gain of function could be the overactivity of a pathway regulating expression of other genes.

In several other disorders, the expanded trinucleotide sequences are located on portions of the gene that are not translated (i.e., the introns). In this case the mechanism of deleterious effects is certainly different in detail, though the net effect of disrupting a critical regulatory pathway might well be the same.

The disorders caused by excessive repeats in the exonic portions of genes differ in several important ways from those due to previously studied genetic defects (64):

1. Above the normal range of repeats, there tends to be a positive correlation between the number of excess repeats and the severity of the disease, and

an inverse correlation between the number of repeats and the age of onset of clinical symptomatology.

2. As the number of repeats at a locus on a chromosome increases, it becomes increasingly unstable during gametogenesis; that is, the number of repeats in gametes is increasingly likely to vary upward or downward (but more commonly upward) from that in the parental chromosomes as the parental repeat length increases. Thus, with each affected generation there is likely to be anticipation (i.e., earlier onset and more severe disease). In SCA6, in which the excessive repeat length (21–28) is less than that of the other SCAs, intergenerational stability of repeat numbers is the rule, but there is still at least some suggestion of anticipation (48).

3. Males show more repeat instability than females in their gametes, so children of affected fathers are usually more severely affected than children of affected mothers. In this context, this is referred to as *imprinting*.

4. Meiosis in affected men favors the allele with expanded repeats over that with normal repeat length, so the abnormal gametes have an increased chance of fertilizing an ovum relative to normal male gametes (65). Thus, there is a greater than 50% likelihood that an affected father who is heterozygous for the expansion will transmit it to each of his children.

5. Individuals with repeat numbers at the high end of the normal range will not develop disease themselves but are at increased risk for having children who will. This is because it is possible for the repeat number to expand into the pathologic range during oogenesis or spermatogenesis. Thus, a few patients with classic clinical presentations of one of the SCAs but no family history may nonetheless show the typical triplet expansion on DNA analysis.

6. Identical twins do not necessarily have the same number of repeats; thus, discordance for disease in identical twins is no longer prima facie evidence for an environmental role in disease causation (66).

SUMMARY

The autosomal dominant spinocerebellar ataxias have now been shown to result from a number of distinct genetic defects that nevertheless have overlapping clinical presentations and neuropathologic patterns of involvement. At the biochemical level, several of these disorders are the result of excessive expansions of repeating DNA triplets that code for proteins with abnormally long stretches of a single amino acid. Because reliable diagnostic discrimination between the different disorders is essentially impossible on clinical grounds alone, and uncertain even after neuropathologic examination, genetic testing is essential to precise diagnosis if one is confronted with a patient from an as-yet uncharacterized family.

At the moment there is no effective treatment to reverse or even halt the progression of any of the SCAs. Nevertheless, the careful clinical analysis of each newly encountered family with an SCA is important from the point of view of ultimate understanding of spinocerebellar system development; such an understanding in turn is likely to be a prerequisite for any future effective prevention or treatment. The new findings since 1993 already suggest a previously unsuspected complexity to the genetic control of the differentiation of specific components of the spinocerebellar system, and known genetic defects account for slightly more than half of all the familial cases of SCA. Thus, it is likely that a number of other genetic defects await discovery. In this context each new family that comes to clinical attention can potentially contribute one more piece to the puzzle.

REFERENCES

1. Nakano KK, Dawson DM, Spence A. Machado disease: a hereditary ataxia in Portuguese immigrants to Massachusetts. Neurology 1972;22:49–55.
2. Woods BT, Schaumburg HH. Nigro-spino-dentatal degeneration with nuclear ophthalmoplegia—a unique and partially treatable clinicopathological entity. J Neurol Sci 1972;17:149–166.
3. Woods BT, Schaumburg HH. Nigrospinodentatal degeneration with nuclear ophthalmoplegia. In: Vinkin PJ, Bruyn GW, eds. Handbook of clinical neurology. Vol. 22, System disorders and atrophies. Part II. Amsterdam: North Holland, 1975:157–176.
4. Rosenberg RN, Nyhan WL, Bay C, Shore P. Autosomal dominant striatonigral degeneration. Neurology 1976;26:703–714.
5. Harding AE. Clinical features and classification of inherited ataxias. In: Harding AE, Deufel T, eds. Advances in neurology. vol. 61. New York: Raven Press, 1993:1–14.
6. Campuzano V, Montermini L, Molto MD, et al. Friedreich's ataxia: autosomal recessive disease caused by an intronic GAA triplet repeat expansion. Science 1996;271:1423–1427.
7. Doerflinger N, Linder C, Ouahchi K, et al. Ataxia with vitamin E deficiency: refinement of genetic localization and analysis of linkage disequilibrium by using new markers in 14 families. Am J Hum Genet 1995;56:1116–1124.
8. Berciano J. Olivopontocerebellar atrophy. In: Jankovic J, Tolosa E, eds. Parkinson's disease and movement disorders. 2nd ed. Baltimore: Williams & Wilkins, 1993:163–189.
9. Yakura H, Wakisaka A, Fujimoto S, Itakura K. Hereditary ataxia and HL-A genotypes. N Engl J Med 1974;291:154–155.
10. Orr HT, Chung M-Y, Banti S, et al. Expansion of an unstable trinucleotide CAG repeat in spinocerebellar ataxia type 1. Nat Genet 1993;4:221–226.
11. Matilla T, Volpini V, Genis D, et al. Presymptomatic analysis of spinocerebellar ataxia type 1 (SCA1) via the expansion of the SCA1 CAG-repeat in a large pedigree displaying anticipation and parental male bias. Hum Mol Genet 1993;2:2123–2128.
12. Zoghbi HY. The expanding world of ataxins. Nat Genetics 1996;14:237–238.
13. Boller F, Segarra JM. Spino-pontine degeneration. Eur Neurol 1969;2:356–373.
14. Taniguchi R, Konigsmark BW. Dominant spino-pontine atrophy: report of a family through three generations. Brain 1971;94:349–358.
15. Pogacar S, Ambler M, Conklin WJ, et al. Dominant spinopontine atrophy. Arch Neurol 1978;35:156–162.
16. Nielsen SL. Striatonigral degeneration disputed in familial disorder. Neurology 1977;27:306.
17. Romanul FCA, Radvany J, Fowler HL, Tarsy D. Azorean disease of the nervous system. N Engl J Med 1977;296:1505–1508.
18. Coutinho P, Andrade C. Autosomal dominant system degeneration in Portuguese families of the Azores islands. Neurology 1978;28:703–709.
19. Lima L, Coutinho P. Clinical criteria for diagnosis of Machado-Joseph disease: report of a non-Azorean Portuguese family. Neurology 1980;30:319–322.
20. Chazot G, Knopp K, Barbeau A, et al. La maladie de Joseph (2 cas dans une familie Francaise). Rev Neurol 1983;139:228.
21. Sakai T, Ohta M, Ishino H. Joseph disease in a non-Portuguese family. Neurology 1983;33:74–80.
22. Yuasa T, Ohama E, Harayama H, et al. Joseph's disease: clinical and pathological studies in a Japanese family. Ann Neurol 1986;19:152–157.
23. Kitamura J, Kubuki Y, Tsurute K, et al. A new family with Joseph disease in Japan. Arch Neurol 1989;46:425–428.
24. Healton EB, Brust JCM, Kerr DL, et al. Presumably Azorean disease in a presumably non-Portuguese family. Neurology 1980;30:1084–1089.
25. Cooper J, Nakada T, Knight R, et al. Autosomal dominant motor system degeneration in a black family. Ann Neurol 1983;14:585–587.
26. Livingstone IR, Sequeiros J. Machado-Joseph disease in an American-Italian family. J Neurogenet 1984;1:185–188.
27. Suite NDA, Sequeiros J, McKhann GM. Machado-Joseph disease in a Sicilian-American family. J Neurogenet 1986;3:177–182.
28. Sequeiros J, Suite NDA. Spinopontine atrophy disputed as a separate entity: the first description of Machado-Joseph disease. Neurology 1986;36:1408. Letter.
29. Kawaguchi Y, Toshihiro O, Taniwaki M, et al. CAG expansions in a novel gene for Machado-Joseph disease at chromosome 14q32.1. Nat Genet 1994;8:221–228.
30. Sequeiros J, Silviera I, Maciel P, et al. Genetic linkage studies of Machado-Joseph disease with chromosome 14q STRPs in 16 Portuguese-Azorean kindreds. Genomics 1994;21:645–648.
31. Stevanin G, Chneiweiss H, Le Guern E, et al. Genetic heterogeneity of autosomal dominant cerebellar ataxia type 1: evidence for the existence of a third locus. Hum Mol Genet 1993;2:1483–1485.

32. Stevanin G, Le Guern E, Ravise N, et al. A third locus for autosomal dominant cerebellar ataxia type I maps to chromosome 14q24.3-qter: evidence for the existence of a fourth locus. Am J Hum Genet 1994;54:11–20.

33. Higgins JJ, Nee LE, Vasconcelos O, et al. Mutations in American families with spinocerebellar ataxia (SCA) type 3. Neurology 1996;46:208–213.

34. Bale AE, Bale SJ, Schlesinger SL, et al. Linkage analysis in spinopontine atrophy: correlation of HLA linkage with phenotypic findings in hereditary ataxia. Am J Hum Genet 1987;27:592–602.

35. Haberhausen G, Damian MS, Leweke F, Muller U. Spinocerebellar ataxia type 3 (SCA 3) is genetically identical to Machado-Joseph disease (MJD). J Neurol Sci 1995;132:71–75.

36. Matilla T, McCall A, Subramony SH, Zoghbi HY. Molecular and clinical correlations in spinocerebellar ataxia type 3 and Machado-Joseph disease. Ann Neurol 1995;38:68–72.

37. Ranum LPW, Lundgren JK, Schut LJ, et al. Spinocerebellar ataxia type I and Machado-Joseph disease: incidence of (CAG) expansions among adult-onset ataxia patients from 311 families with dominant, recessive and sporadic ataxia. Am J Hum Genet 1995;57:603–608.

38. Silviera I, Lopes-Cendes I, Kish S, et al. Frequency of spinocerebellar ataxia type 1, dentatorubropallidoluysian atrophy, and Machado-Joseph disease mutations in a large group of spinocerebellar ataxia patients. Neurology 1996;46:214–218.

39. Valles L, Estrada R, Basterrechea L. Algunas formas de heredo-ataxias en una region de Cuba. Rev Neurol 1978;6:163–187.

40. Orozco Diaz G, Estrada R, Perry TL, et al. Dominantly inherited olivo-ponto-cerebellar atrophy from eastern Cuba: clinical, neuropathological and biochemical findings. J Neurol Sci 1989;93:37–50.

41. Orozco Diaz G, Nodarse Fleites A, Cordoves Sagaz R, Auberger G. Autosomal dominant cerebellar ataxia: clinical analysis of 263 patients from a homogeneous popplution in Holguin, Cuba. Neurology 1990;40:1369–1375.

42. Gispert S, Twells R, Orozco G, et al. Chromosomal assignment of the second locus for autosomal dominant cerebellar ataxia (SCA2) to human chromosome 12q23–24.1. Nat Genet 1993;4:295–299.

43. Pulst SM, Nechiporuk A, Starkman S. Anticipation in spinocerebellar ataxia type 2. Nat Genet 1993;5:8–10.

44. Filla A, De Michelle G, Banfi S, et al. Is spinocerebellar ataxia type 2 a distinct phenotype? Genetic and clinical study of an Italian family. Neurology 1995;45:793–796.

45. Zhuchenko O, Bailey J, Bonnen P, et al. Autosomal dominant cerebellar ataxia (SCA6) associated with small polyglutamine expansions in the alpha1A-voltage–dependent calcium channel. Nat Genet 1997;15:62–69.

46. Ophoff RA, Terwindt GM, Vergouwe MN, et al. Familial hemiplegic migraine and episodic ataxia type-2 are caused by mutations in the Ca^{2+} channel gene CACNL1A4. Cell 1996;87:543–552.

47. Matsumura R, Futamura N, Fujimoto S, et al. Spinocerebellar ataxia type 6. Molecular and clinical features of 35 Japanese patients including one homozygous for the CAG repeat expansion. Neurology 1997;49:1238–1243.

48. Ikeuchi T, Takano H, Koide R, et al. Spinocerebellar ataxia type 6: CAG repeat expansion in α_{1A}-voltage–dependent calcium channel gene and clinical variations in Japanese population. Ann Neurol 1997;42:879–884.

49. Geschwind DH, Perlman S, Figueroa KP, et al. Spinocerebellar ataxia type 6: frequency of the mutation and genotype-phenotype correlations. Neurology 1997;49:1247–1251.

50. Stevanin G, Dürr A, David G, et al. Clinical and molecular features of spinocerebellar ataxia type 6. Neurology 1997;49:1243–1246.

51. Gardner K, Alderson K, Galster B, et al. Autosomal dominant spinocerebellar ataxia: clinical description of a distinct hereditary ataxia and genetic localization to chromosome 16 (SCA4) in a Utah kindred. Neurology 1994;44(suppl 2):A361.

52. Flanagan K, Gardner K, Alderson K, et al. Autosomal dominant spinocerebellar ataxia with sensory axonal neuropathy (SCA4): clinical description and genetic localization to chromosome 16q22.1. Am J Hum Genet 1996;59:392–399.

53. Ranum LPW, Schut LJ, Lundgren J, et al. Spinocerebellar ataxia type 5 in a family descended from the grandparents of President Lincoln maps to chromosome 11. Nat Genet 1994;8:280–284.

54. Cancel G, Abbas N, Stevanin G, et al. Marked phenotypic heterogeneity associated with expansion of a (CAG) repeat sequence at the spinocerebellar ataxia 3/Machado-Joseph disease locus. Am J Hum Genet 1995;57:809–816.

55. Barbeau A, Roy M, Cunha L, et al. The natural history of Machado-Joseph disease. Can J Neurol Sci 1984;11:510–525.

56. Gomez CM, Thompson RM, Gammack JT, et al. Spinocerebellar ataxia type 6: gaze-evoked and vertical nystagmus, Purkinje cell degeneration, and variable age of onset. Ann Neurol 1997;42:933–950.

57. Romanul FCA, Radvany J, Fowler HL, Tarsy D. Azorean disease of the nervous system: report of six additional families. Trans Am Neurol Assoc 1978;103:269–273.

58. Sachdev HS, Forno LS, Kane CA. Joseph disease: a multi-system degenerative disorder of the nervous system. Neurology 1982;32:192–195.

59. Sakai T, Ohta M, Ishino H. Joseph disease in a non-Portuguese family. Neurology 1983;33:74–80.

60. Durr A, Stevanin G, Cancel G, et al. Spinocerebellar ataxia 3 and Machado-Joseph disease: clinical, molecular, and neuropathological features. Ann Neurol 1996;39:490–499.

61. Lopes-Cendes I, Silviera I, Maciel P, et al. Limits of clinical assessment in the accurate diagnosis of Machado-Joseph disease. Arch Neurol 1996;53:1168–1174.

62. LaSpada AR, Wilson EM, Lubahn DB, et al. Androgen receptor gene mutations in X-linked spinal and bulbar muscular atrophy. Nature 1991;352:77–79.

63. Kremer EJ, Pritchard M, Lynch M, et al. Mapping of DNA instability at the fragile X to a trinucleotide repeat sequence p(CGG)n. Science 1991;252:1711–1714.

64. Paulson HI, Fischbeck KH. Trinucleotide repeats in neurogenetic disorders. Annu Rev Neurosci 1995:79–107.

65. Ikeuchi T, Igarashi S, Takiyama Y, et al. Non-Mendelian transmission in dentatorubral-pallidoluysian atrophy and Machado-Joseph disease: the mutant allele is preferentially transmitted in male meiosis. Am J Hum Genet 1996;58:730–733.

66. Roses AD. From genes to mechanisms to therapies: lessons to be learned from neurological disorders. Nat Med 1996;2:267–269.

Wilson's Disease (Hepatolenticular Degeneration)

John H. Menkes

Wilson's disease is an inborn error in copper metabolism that manifests itself by hepatic cirrhosis and degenerative changes in the basal ganglia.

During the second half of the nineteenth century, a condition termed "pseudosclerosis" was distinguished from multiple sclerosis by the lack of ocular signs. In 1902, Kayser (1) observed green corneal pigmentation in one such patient; in 1903, Fleischer commented on the association of the corneal rings with pseudosclerosis (2). In 1912, Wilson gave the classic description of the disease and its pathologic anatomy (3).

Because a derangement of copper homeostasis is one of the important features of this condition, it is pertinent to review briefly our present knowledge of the field (4). Copper homeostasis results from a balance between its absorption from dietary sources and its excretion in bile and, to a lesser extent, in urine.

The daily dietary intake of copper ranges between 1 and 5 mg. Healthy adults receiving a free diet absorb about 40% of dietary copper (5). The absorption site is probably in the proximal portion of the gastrointestinal tract. The processes involved in copper absorption are poorly understood, and there is no convincing evidence that metallothionein, a low-molecular-weight metal protein, is involved in regulating copper absorption (6).

An increased concentration of copper induces metallothionein biosynthesis. This leads to the sequestration of copper in cytoplasm and protects cellular constituents from damage by excess copper.

Following its intestinal uptake, copper enters plasma, where it is bound to the N-terminal tripeptide Asp-Ala-His of albumin in the form of cupric ion. Within 2 hours, the absorbed copper is incorporated into a liver protein. The concentration of the metal in normal liver ranges from 30 to 40 μg/gm dry weight. In the liver, copper is

either excreted into bile, stored in liver lysosomes in what is probably a polymeric form of metallothionein, or combined with apoceruloplasmin to form ceruloplasmin, which then enters the circulation. More than 95% of serum copper is in this form. Ceruloplasmin is an α-globulin with a single continuous polypeptide chain and a molecular weight of 132,000; it has six copper atoms per molecule (7,8).

The protein has multiple functions. Although it is not involved in copper transport from the intestine, it may be the major vehicle for the transport of the metal from the liver and contributes copper to cells and to intracellular copper proteins and enzymes (9). A ceruloplasmin receptor is believed to be involved in cellular copper uptake and in the formation of a variety of copper-containing enzymes. Ceruloplasmin also has ferrous oxidase activity. This is important for the oxidation of ferrous to ferric ion that controls the release of iron into plasma from cells, where the metal is stored in the form of ferritin. Ceruloplasmin is also the most prominent serum antioxidant and, as such, catalyzes the oxidation of ferrous ion to ferric ion and prevents the oxidation of polyunsaturated fatty acids and other similar substances. Finally, ceruloplasmin modulates the inflammatory response and may regulate the concentration of various serum biogenic amines (10).

The concentration of ceruloplasmin in plasma is normally between 30 to 40 mg/dl. It is elevated in a variety of circumstances, including pregnancy or other conditions with high estrogen concentrations, infections, cirrhosis, malignancies, hyperthyroidism, and myocardial infarction. The elevation described in autistic and schizophrenic patients is perhaps due to their poor nutrition and subsequent ascorbic acid deficiency. The concentration of ceruloplasmin is low in normal infants up to approximately 2 months of age and in children suffering from a combined iron and copper deficiency anemia. In the nephrotic syndrome, low levels are caused by the vast renal losses of ceruloplasmin. Ceruloplasmin is also reduced in kinky-hair disease (Menkes' disease), a sex-linked degenerative disorder in the distribution of copper that manifests itself by progressive gray matter degeneration.

Little is known regarding the intracellular transport of copper to the enzymes that require the metal for their activity.

Several other copper-containing proteins have been isolated from mammalian tissues. Most prominently these include the enzymes cytochrome C oxidase, lysyl oxidase, monoamine oxidase, dopamine-β-hydroxylase, superoxide dismutase, and tyrosinase. None of these is altered in Wilson's disease.

BIOCHEMICAL PATHOLOGY AND MOLECULAR GENETICS

Since dietary intake of copper far exceeds the daily trace amounts required by the body, and since the metal in its free form is extremely toxic to cells, it is vital that the intracellular content of the metal be regulated within narrow limits. Normally approximately 0.35 mg/day is lost from the skin surface, and urinary excretion averages 0.05 mg/day. An additional 0.2 mg/day is excreted via the bile and subsequently is lost in feces.

The processes involved in the hepatobiliary transport of copper are still unclear (11). In humans the most important pathway appears to be an ATP-dependent saturable copper-transporting system. It is this system that is defective in Wilson's disease (12).

Knowledge of disturbed copper metabolism in Wilson's disease lay dormant for more than three decades. In 1913, one year after Wilson's report, Rumpel found unusually large amounts of copper in the liver of a patient with hepatolenticular degeneration (13). Although this finding was confirmed, and an elevated copper concentration was also detected in the basal ganglia by Luthy (14), the implication of these reports went unrecognized until 1945, when Glazebrook demonstrated abnormally high copper levels in the serum, liver, and brain of a patient with this condition (15). In 1952, five years after the discovery of ceruloplasmin, several groups of workers simultaneously found it to be low or absent in patients with Wilson's disease. At first, it was thought that the condition represented a simple ceruloplasmin deficiency. However, this has not turned out to be the case. With the advent of genetic linkage analysis, the gene for Wilson's disease was localized to the long arm of chromosome 13 (13q14.3). By contrast, the gene that encodes ceruloplasmin was mapped to chromosome 3 (16,17). In 1993 three groups of workers identified the gene for Wilson's disease and demonstrated that it encoded a copper-transport protein with up to 76% amino acid homology with that encoded by the gene for kinky-hair disease (Menkes' disease) (18–21).

The gene whose mutation results in Wilson's disease contains 22 exons and covers a region of about 100 kb. It is expressed in liver and kidney (18) and encodes a protein of 1,411 amino acids, which functions as a P-type ATPase. The P-type ATPases are a large family of enzymes so named because of a phosphoaspartate intermediate in the ATP-driven cation transport cycle (22). These ATPases differ from one another with respect to cation specificity, and the direction of transport facilitated by them. The gene for the P-type ATPase is markedly conserved, and there is a high degree of homology with the bacterial metal resistance genes (22). In man, the copper-transporting ATPase is expressed in two forms: one is localized to the cellular trans-Golgi network, the other, probably representing a cleavage product, to mitochondria (22a).

A large number of mutations in this gene have been recognized in patients with Wilson's disease. Some are large delections that completely destroy gene function and result in early onset of symptoms. Others reduce but do not eliminate copper transport and are consistent with a late onset of symptoms (22b). Most patients are compound heterozygotes. A few of these mutations are common and population specific; the remainder are rare (23). In North America, the most common mutations are a point mutation and a frameshift mutation, seen in some 30% of patients (19). In Sardinian patients, a frameshift mutation that probably leads to a functionless copper-transport protein is the most common (23). The remainder of patients have mutations that are scattered throughout the gene.

The Long-Evans Cinnamon (LEC) rat, which shares many clinical and biochemical features with Wilson's disease, also has a deletion in the copper-transporting ATPase and serves as an experimental model for studying normal and pathologic copper transport (24).

Although the vast majority of Wilson's disease patients show markedly diminished ceruloplasmin concentrations, normal values have been recorded in about 5% of homozygotes. It appears likely that certain mutations in the Wilson's disease gene allow normal transport of copper into ceruloplasmin but prevent copper excretion. Recent work, however, questions whether the copper-transporting ATPase encoded by the Wilson's disease gene is directly involved in the incorporation of copper into ceruloplasmin apoprotein (25). Instead, a post-translational defect may be responsible for the absence of ceruloplasmin from bile and serum (25a). Raising the level of ceruloplasmin by giving estrogens or the purified copper protein fails to affect the course of the disease.

The finding that the gene for Wilson's disease encodes a copper-transport protein had already been suspected on the basis of physiologic studies of copper transport in patients with Wilson's disease.

Studies with radiosotopes have indicated that in patients with this condition the dynamic turnover of copper is disturbed, and the rate at which copper is incorporated into ceruloplasmin is markedly reduced (27). After intravenous administration of radiolabeled copper (Cu64) to a healthy person, there is a rapid rise in serum radioactivity, followed by an equally rapid fall. A secondary slow rise commences at about 6 hours, as ceruloplasmin enters plasma. In Wilson's disease, the initial rise is more extensive, the secondary rise is not observed, and no radioactivity enters the globulin fraction where ceruloplasmin is normally found. This phenomenon is also noted in patients who have nearly normal ceruloplasmin concentrations and in presymptomatic children with Wilson's disease. Because these abnormalities do not occur in biliary cirrhosis, a condition in which the copper pool is increased, they could not be explained on the basis of an increased size of the copper pool (28). The role of the copper-transport protein in the lysosomal-biliary excretory pathway is supported by the observation that biliary excretion of copper is reduced to between 20% and 40% of normal (29) and that fecal output of the metal is reduced (30).

In addition to these abnormalities, plasma levels of non-ceruloplasmin copper are increased to a level comparable with that seen in acute copper poisoning. Plasma ascorbic acid and uric acid are reduced, and allantoin, the oxidation product of uric acid, is increased. These changes are believed to reflect the oxidant stress and the free radical reactions that result from the elevation of non-ceruloplasmin-bound copper (31). The importance of free radical–induced DNA damage in the pathogenesis of hepatic and cerebral damage in Wilson's disease is being increasingly recognized (32,33).

A persistent aminoaciduria is generally accounted for by a damaging effect of copper on renal tubules. This abnormality has also been observed in a few asymptomatic patients and probably results from copper deposition in the kidney, the consequence of the defect in the renal expression of the copper-transport protein. Although the excretion of all amino acids is greater than normal, the greatest increase is observed in threonine and cystine (34).

PATHOLOGIC ANATOMY

The defect in the copper-transport protein results in the deposition in the metal in several tissues, most prominently liver, kidney, brain, and cornea.

Several stages of the disease have been recognized. Initially, there is an asymptomatic accumulation of copper in hepatocytes. At first, copper is spread diffusely within hepatic cytoplasm and firmly bound to copper proteins such as ceruloplasmin and superoxide dismutase, or it is in the cupric form complexed with monomeric metallothionein. Later in the course of the disease, the metal tends to be sequestered within lysosomes, which become increasingly sensitive to rupture (Fig 40.1) (35,36). Some hepatic cells are enlarged and contain fat droplets, intranuclear glycogen, and clumped pigment granules; other cells are necrotic, with regenerative changes in the surrounding parenchyma (Fig 40.2b, c) (37). When the hepatic copper load overwhelms

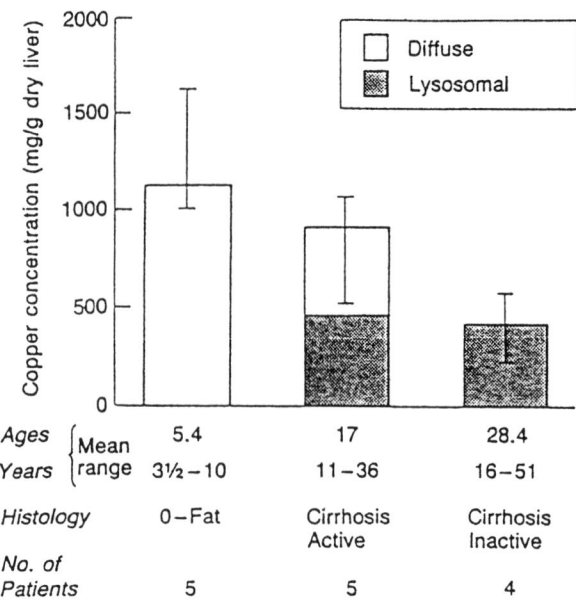

FIGURE 40.1   *Mean values and ranges of hepatic copper concentrations in patients with Wilson's disease grouped according to age and stage of disease. 1. Asymptomatic children with minimal histologic abnormalities. 2. Adolescents and young adults with active liver disease. 3. Adults with neurologic symptoms of Wilson's disease and inactive cirrhosis. The height of the bar graph indicates the concentration of copper in each group. There is a striking decrease with advancing age and progression of the disease, and the intracellular distribution of copper changes from its diffuse cytoplasmic distribution in the hepatocytes of children to its lysosomal concentration in the hepatocytes of patients with advanced disease. (Courtesy of Drs I.H. Scheinberg and I. Sternlieb, Albert Einstein College of Medicine, Bronx, New York. Reproduced by permission from Scheinberg IH and Sternlieb I. Wilson's disease. Philadelphia: WB Saunders, 1984.)*

the binding capacity of metallothionein, cytotoxic cupric copper is released, with ensuing damage to hepatocyte mitochondria and peroxisomes (38). Copper probably initiates and catalyzes peroxidation of the lysosomal membrane lipids, resulting in impaired mitochondrial respiration and changes in liposomal structure and function (33).

On a macroscopic level the liver shows a focal necrosis that progresses to a coarsely nodular, postnecrotic cirrhosis; the nodules vary in size and are separated by bands of fibrous tissues of different widths (Fig 40.2a).

After the hepatic storage capacity for copper is exceeded, the metal leaks from the liver into the blood, where it is taken up by other tissues, including kidney and brain. In kidney, the tubular epithelial cells degenerate, and their cytoplasm contains copper deposits (35). The observation that the copper-transporting ATPase that is defective in Wilson's disease is also expressed in the kidney suggests that the renal alterations reflect a primary copper deposition in that organ.

In brain, the largest proportion of copper is located in the subcellular soluble fraction, where it is bound not only

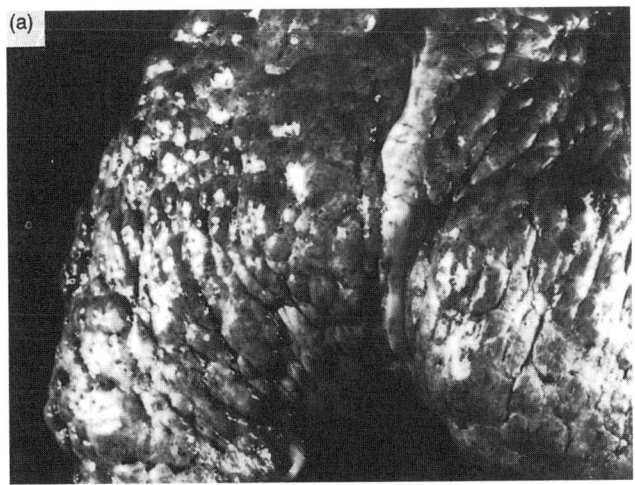

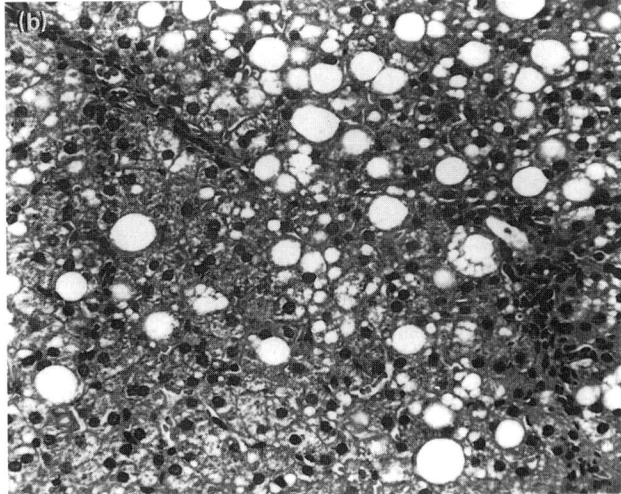

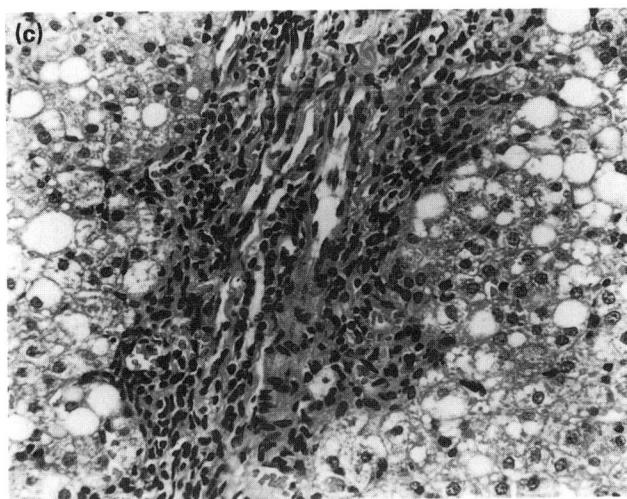

FIGURE 40.2 *Morphologic alterations in the liver in Wilson's disease. (a) Liver showing nodular cirrhosis typical of the end stages of this condition. (b) Some of the earliest pathologic findings visible by light microscopy include hepatocytes of irregular appearance, with lipid droplets of varying sizes, prominent Kupffer cells, moderate cellular infiltrates, and slender fibrous bands. Needle-biopsy specimen is from a 6-year-old asymptomatic boy. Liver copper: 1,158 µg/g dry weight (normal, 9 to 47 µg/g dry weight). (c) More pronounced cellular infiltrate in another portion of the liver biopsy specimen in b. (Courtesy of Drs I.H. Scheinberg and I. Sternlieb, Albert Einstein College of Medicine, Bronx, New York. Reproduced by permission from Scheinberg IH, Sternlieb I. Wilson's disease. Philadelphia: WB Saunders, 1984.)*

to cerebrocuprein but also to a number of other normal cerebral proteins.

On gross examination of the brain, particularly in patients whose symptoms commence prior to the onset of puberty, the basal ganglia show the most striking alterations. As a rule, the putamen is most affected, the globus pallidus and the caudate nucleus less so (Fig 40.3). These areas have a brick-red pigmentation. Spongy degeneration of the putamen frequently leads to the formation of small cavities (3). Microscopic studies reveal a loss of neurons, axonal degeneration, and large numbers of protoplasmic astrocytes, including giant forms termed Alzheimer's cells (Fig 40.4). These cells are not specific for Wilson's disease; they may also be seen in the brains of patients dying in hepatic coma or as a result of argininosuccinic aciduria. Opalski cells, also seen in Wilson's disease, are generally found in gray matter. They are large cells with a rounded contour and finely granular cytoplasm (Fig 40.5). They probably represent degenerating astrocytes.

In about 10% of patients, cortical gray and white matter is more affected than the basal ganglia. Here too there is extensive spongy degeneration and proliferation of astrocytes (39). Lesser degenerative changes are seen in the brainstem,

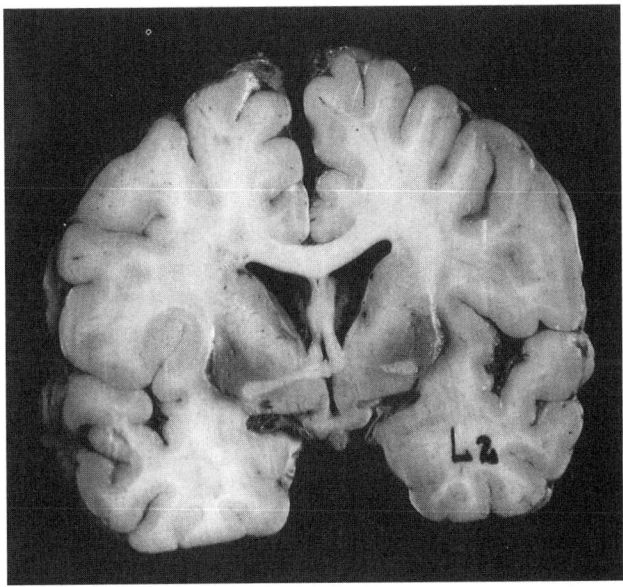

FIGURE 40.3 *Gross appearance of the brain in Wilson's disease.*

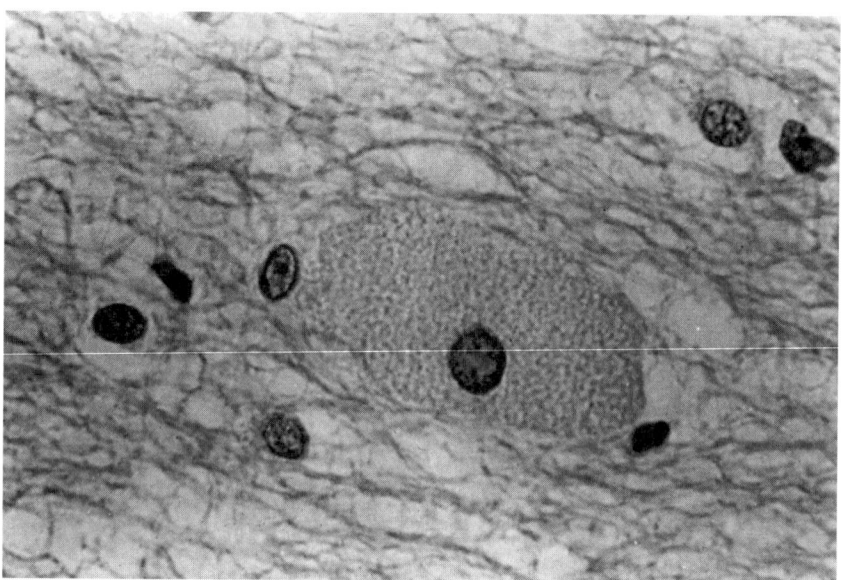

FIGURE 40.4   *Alzheimer's cells in Wilson's disease.*

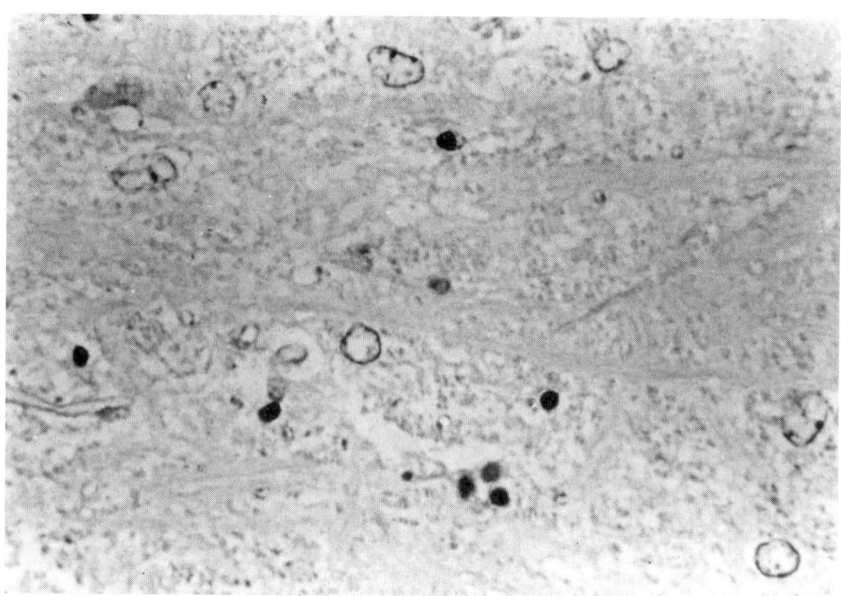

FIGURE 40.5   *Opalski cells in Wilson's disease.*

the dentate nucleus, the substantia nigra, and the convolutional white matter. Copper is deposited in the pericapillary area and within astrocytes, but it is uniformly absent from neurons and ground substance.

Copper is also found throughout the cornea, particularly the substantia propria, where it is deposited in an alcohol-soluble and probably chelated form. In the periphery, the metal appears in granular clumps close to the endothelial surface of the Descemet's membrane. Here the deposits are responsible for the appearance of the Kayser-Fleischer rings. The color of this ring varies from yellow to green to brown. Copper deposition in this area occurs in two or more layers, with particle size and distance between layers influencing the ultimate appearance of the ring (40).

CLINICAL MANIFESTATIONS

Untreated, Wilson's disease is a progressive condition with a tendency toward temporary clinical improvement and arrest. It is transmitted in an autosomal recessive manner; a high rate of consanguinity exists in parents of affected subjects. The condition occurs in all races, with a particularly high incidence in Eastern European Jews, in Italians from southern Italy, Sardinia, and Sicily, and in people from some of the smaller islands of Japan—groups in whom a high rate of inbreeding is known to exist. The worldwide prevalence of the disease is 30 per million, with a gene frequency of 1:180.

In most patients, symptoms begin between the ages of 11 and 25 years. Onset as early as age 2.5 years and as late as the fifth decade has been recorded (41). In reported cases, there is a slight preponderance of men.

About 40% of patients present with overt or subclinical evidence of liver disease. In a fair number of cases, primarily in young children, initial symptoms may take the form of an acute hepatitis with jaundice or portal hypertension, and the disease may be rapidly fatal without any detectable neurologic abnormalities (42,43). More commonly, the hepatitis has an acute onset but is self-limited. This course was seen in 24% of patients compiled by Scheinberg and Sternlieb (35). In about 10% to 25% of patients, psychiatric symptoms or a slowly progressive dementia is the initial presentation.

In about 40% of patients, the first clinical manifestation is neurologic. In essence, Wilson's disease is a disorder of motor function; despite often widespread cerebral atrophy, there are no sensory symptoms or reflex alterations. Scheinberg and Sternlieb have encountered eight modes of presentation (35). The most common of these has a picture of a resting or purposive tremor, dysarthria or hypophonic speech, drooling, clumsiness, and unsteadiness of gait. Less frequently the disease commences with rigidity, choreiform movements, or seizures.

In the past, texts have distinguished between pseudosclerotic and dystonic forms of the disease: the former dominated by tremor, the latter by rigidity and contractures. In actuality, most patients, if untreated, ultimately develop both types of symptoms. Symptoms at the onset of the disease are shown in Table 40.1.

As the disease evolves, symptoms of basal ganglia damage usually predominate, but cerebellar signs may be in the foreground. The tremor may be of the intention type, or it may resemble the alternating tremor of Parkinson's disease. More commonly, it is a bizarre tremor, localized to the arms and best described by the term "wing beating." This tremor is usually absent when the arms are at rest; it develops after a short latent period when the arms are extended. The beating movements may be confined to the muscles of the wrist, but it is more common for the arm to be thrown up and down in a wide arc. The movements increase in severity and may become so violent that the patient is thrown off balance. Changing the posture of the outstretched arms may alter the severity of the tremor. Although it may affect both arms, it usually is more severe in one. The tremor may occasionally be present even when the arm is at rest. Many patients have a fixed, open-mouth smile.

Rigidity and spasms of the muscles are often present. In some cases, a typical parkinsonian rigidity may involve all muscles. Torticollis, tortipelvis, and other dystonic movements are not uncommon. Dystonia of the laryngeal and pharyngeal muscles may lead to dysarthria and dysphagia. Drooping of the lower jaw and excess salivation are common. Progressive choreoathetosis and hemiplegia have also been described. Tendon reflexes are increased, but extensor plantar responses are exceptional. Somatosensory

Table 40.1   Clinical Manifestations at Onset of Wilson's Disease

Symptoms	Percentage
Hepatic or hematologic abnormalities	35
Behavioral abnormalities	25
Neurologic symptoms	40
Pseudosclerotic form	40
One or more of the following:	
Tremor, at rest or purposive	
Dysarthria or scanning speech	
Diminished dexterity or clumsiness	
Unsteady gait	
Tremor alone	33
Dysarthria alone	5
Dystonic form	60
One or more of the following:	
Hypophonic speech or mutism	
Drooling	
Rigid mouth, arms, or legs	
Seizures	1
Chorea or small-amplitude twitches	<1

Figures are approximate.
Table prepared with Drs I.H. Scheinberg and I. Sternlieb, Department of Medicine, Albert Einstein College of Medicine, Bronx, New York.

evoked potentials are abnormal in most patients with neurologic symptoms.

Wilson's disease may present with a variety of behavioral and psychiatric manifestations that antedate by years the appearance of a movement disorder, which at times is wrongly attributed to pharmacologic therapy for the psychiatric symptoms. Dementia may be severe in some patients, whereas other patients are merely emotionally labile. Subtle intellectual impairment is seen in many of the patients with neurologic symptoms (44,45).

Without treatment, death ensues within 1 to 3 years of the onset of dystonia and is usually a result of hepatic insufficiency.

The intracorneal ring-shaped pigmentation, first noted by Kayser (1) and Fleischer (2), may be evident to the naked eye or may only appear with slit lamp examination. The ring can be either complete or incomplete and is detected in 75% of patients who present with hepatic symptoms, and in all patients who present with cerebral symptoms or a combination of cerebral and hepatic symptoms. The Kayser-Fleischer ring may antedate overt symptoms of the disease and has been detected even in the presence of normal liver function. Less commonly, one sees "sunflower" cataracts (35).

Computed tomography (CT) scans usually reveal ventricular dilatation and diffuse atrophy of the cortex, cerebellum, and brainstem. In about half the patients, there are hypodense areas in the thalamus and basal ganglia. Increased density due to copper deposition is not observed. As a rule, magnetic resonance imaging (MRI) correlates better with clinical symptoms than CT. It demonstrates abnormal signals (hypointense on T1-weighted images, and hyperintense on T2-weighted images) in the lenticular, caudate, and dentate nuclei and thalamus. In a few subjects, there are focal white matter lesions (46,47) (Fig 40.6A). Positron emission tomography (PET) demonstrates a widespread depression of glucose metabolism, with the greatest focal hypometabolism in the lenticular nucleus. This abnormality precedes any alteration seen on CT scan (48).

Fluorodopa and methylspiperon PET scanning with dopaminergic agents indicates that both afferent and efferent projections are affected by the disease process. These defects persist despite prolonged penicillamine treatment (49–52).

DIAGNOSIS

The picture of Wilson's disease is fairly clear-cut when advanced. The important clinical features are the family history of hepatic or neurologic involvement, progressive extrapyramidal symptoms commencing during the second or third decade of life, abnormal liver function, aminoaciduria, cupriuria, and absent or decreased ceruloplasmin. The presence of a Kayser-Fleischer ring is the single most important diagnostic feature; its absence in a patient with neurologic symptoms rules out the diagnosis of Wilson's disease. The ring is not seen in the majority of presymptomatic patients, nor in 15% of children in whom Wilson's disease presents with hepatic symptoms (43).

Urinary copper is always elevated in symptomatic Wilson's disease, and a urinary copper excretion over 100 μg/day confirms the clinical diagnosis (44).

An absent or low serum ceruloplasmin level is of lesser diagnostic importance; some 5% of patients with Wilson's disease have normal levels of the copper protein. In affected families, the differential diagnosis between heterozygotes and presymptomatic homozygotes is of utmost importance, inasmuch as it is generally accepted that the latter should be treated preventively (35).

Low ceruloplasmin levels in an asymptomatic family member suggest the presymptomatic stage of the disease; however, some 5% of heterozygotes have ceruloplasmin levels below 15 mg/dL. An elevation of urinary copper is diagnostic of a presymptomatic patient, if the patient is age 15 years or older. When low ceruloplasmin levels are found on routine screening and are unaccompanied by any abnormality of hepatic function, the subject is most likely a heterozygote for Wilson's disease (35). Whenever the diagnosis remains unresolved, a liver biopsy must be performed to measure hepatic copper content. Copper levels over 250 μg/g dry weight are diagnostic of Wilson's disease (53).

Liver biopsy may also be required in patients who present with hepatic disease exclusively. In many of these patients Kayser-Fleischer rings are absent, and Wilson's disease hepatitis can raise serum ceruloplasmin levels (54).

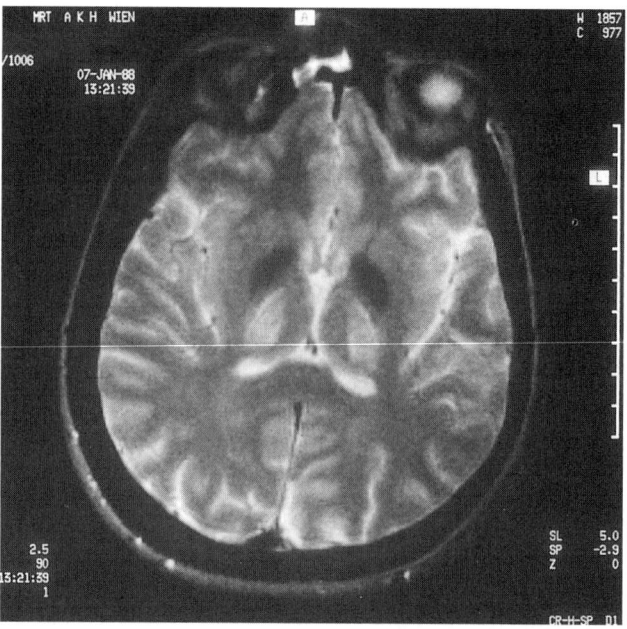

A

B

FIGURE 40.6   *Magnetic resonance imaging: Coronal T2-weighted images of a 22-year-old woman with Wilson's disease. A. Three months after the disease has been diagnosed and at start of penicillamine therapy. There are bilateral hyperintense thalamic lesions. These were hypointense on T1-weighted images. B. Same patient after 13 months of penicillamine therapy. There has been a significant regression of the thalamic lesions. Spin-echo sequences TR 2.5 msec, TE 90 msec, using Siemens Magnetom 63 operating at 1.5 Tesla. (Courtesy of Dr L. Prayer, Zentral Institut fur Radiodiagnose und Ludwig Boltzmann Institut, University of Vienna, Austria.)*

The measurement of urinary copper is a less satisfactory diagnostic procedure because in some asymptomatic homozygotes cupriuria is not significantly increased (55).

The presence of numerous mutations in the Wilson's disease gene, and the necessity of finding two mutant alleles to establish a diagnosis, preclude the use of DNA analysis for the diagnosis of a subject without affected family members. However, haplotype analysis does predict the presence of the disease in family members of a patient with Wilson's disease with nearly 100% accuracy (56).

Several variants of Wilson's disease have been described. One type begins in adolescence and is marked by progressive tremor, dysarthria, disturbed eye movements, and dementia. Biochemically it is characterized by low serum levels of copper and ceruloplasmin. Kayser-Fleischer rings are absent, and liver copper concentrations are low. Metabolic studies using labeled copper suggest a failure in copper absorption from the lower gut (57). In another type, the patient developed extrapyramidal movements but no liver disease. There were no Kayser-Fleischer rings. Blood copper levels were low, but hepatic copper was markedly elevated, with the metal stored in cytoplasm (58). The variants undoubtedly represent different mutations in the Wilson's disease gene.

Copper retention is also seen in any chronic interference with biliary excretion. This occurs in various forms of biliary cirrhosis, Indian childhood cirrhosis, and in the rare Aagenes syndrome (congenital lymphedema, recurrent cholestasis, and lenticular degeneration) (59).

TREATMENT

All patients with Wilson's disease, whether symptomatic or asymptomatic, require treatment. The aims of treatment are initially to remove the toxic amounts of copper and secondarily to prevent tissue reaccumulation of the metal.

Treatment can be divided into two phases: the initial phase, when toxic copper levels are brought under control; and maintenance therapy. Currently, there is no agreed on regimen for treatment of a new patient with neurologic or psychiatric symptoms. In the past, most centers relied on D-penicillamine (α-amino-β-mercaptoisovaleric acid) for forming a soluble complex with tissue copper. The drug is administered orally in divided doses: at least 0.5 g twice daily or 0.25 g in four divided doses for adults, 0.02 g/kg per day for children under ten years of age. The exact amount depends on the clinical response and copper excretion.

As a rule, the dosage of penicillamine is adjusted to allow copper losses of more than 2 mg/day at the start of therapy. Over the subsequent months, the excretion rate returns to normal; raising the penicillamine dosage can again cause a transient outpouring of the metal (4). Because of the antipyridoxine effect of penicillamine, the diet is usually supplemented with 25 mg/day of pyridoxine.

Although penicillamine effectively promotes urinary excretion of copper, adverse reactions during both the initial and the maintenance phase of treatment are seen in about 25% of patients. Other side effects of penicillamine include fever, gastrointestinal discomfort, rash, adenopathy, pyridox-

ine-responsive optic neuritis, nephrotic syndrome, pyridoxine deficiency, and, infrequently, thrombocytopenia and leukopenia. Penicillamine-induced myasthenia also has been observed on several occasions. During maintenance therapy, one may see polyneuropathy, polymyositis, and nephropathy. All of these symptoms improve with temporary interruption of therapy. Most importantly, within the first few weeks of penicillamine therapy there is a worsening of neurologic symptoms in up to 50% of patients that is frequently irreversible (60–62). This is believed to reflect mobilization of copper from tissues and redistribution to the brain. In the experience of Brewer and Yuzbasiyan-Gurkan, about 25% of patients developed significant long-term intolerance of penicillamine (41).

On the above regimen, there is a gradual improvement in neurologic symptoms. As a rule, this does not occur until 6 months after therapy has been started (44). The Kayser-Fleischer ring begins to fade within 6 to 10 weeks and disappears completely in a couple of years (63). Serial CT or MR imaging studies show regression of the lesions in the basal ganglia (Fig 40.6A, B) (64,65). As shown by successive biopsies, the amount of copper deposited in the liver decreases. Total serum copper and ceruloplasmin levels fall, and the aminoaciduria and phosphaturia diminish. As a rule, patients with the predominantly pseudosclerotic form of the disease fare better than those with dystonia as the main manifestation. In some dystonic patients, addition of L-dopa to the penicillamine regimen has been beneficial. Significant improvement after 2 years of therapy is unusual.

Because of the toxicity of penicillamine and the high incidence of adverse reactions, many institutions now advocate initial therapy with ammonium tetrathiomolybdate (67). It is given in doses of 60–300 mg/day in six divided doses (three with meals, three between meals) (44). This drug forms a complex with protein and copper and, when given with food, blocks the absorption of copper. Preliminary experience suggests it is effective without worsening pre-existing neurologic symptoms (44). The major drawback of this drug is that it still has not been approved for general use in this country.

Zinc acetate is the optimum drug for maintenance therapy and management of the presymptomatic patient (41). When given in doses of 50 mg three times daily, the metal induces the synthesis of intestinal metallothionein. This increases copper binding and produces a significant negative copper balance (68). Zinc is far less toxic than penicillamine but is much slower acting. The role of antioxidants in the treatment of Wilson's disease has not been explored, but since circulating levels of vitamin E are reduced by these drugs, I would recommend dietary supplementation with the vitamin.

Diet does not play an important role in the management of Wilson's disease, although liver and shellfish should be restricted during the first year of treatment.

Liver transplantation has been employed in patients with acute and potentially irreversible hepatic necrosis (69).

Neurosurgical procedures have been found ineffective for the relief of extrapyramidal symptoms.

When symptom-free patients with Wilson's disease discontinue chelation therapy, their hepatic function deteriorates within 9 months to 3 years, a rate that is far more rapid than that following birth (70). Scheinberg and coworkers postulate that penicillamine not only removes copper from tissue but also detoxifies the metal by forming a nontoxic copper–penicillamine complex or by inducing metallothionein synthesis and the formation of a metallothionein–copper complex (71).

REFERENCES

1. Kayser B. Ueber einen Fall von angeborener grünlicher Verfärbung der Cornea. Klin Monatsbl Augenheilkd 1902;40:22–25.
2. Fleischer B. Zwei weitere Fälle von grünlicher Verfärbung der Cornea. Klin Monatsbl Augenheilkd 1903;41:489–491.
3. Wilson SAK. Progressive lenticular degeneration: a familial nervous disease associated with cirrhosis of the liver. Brain 1912;34:295–509.
4. Danks DM. Of mice and men, metals and mutations. J Med Genet 1986;23:99–106.
5. Delves HT. Dietary sources of copper. Ciba Found Symp 1980;79:5–22.
6. Bremner I, Beattie JH. Copper and zinc metabolism in health and disease: speciation and interactions. Proc Nutr Soc 1995;54:489–499.
7. Moshkov KA, Lakatos S, Hajdu J, et al. Proteolysis of human ceruloplasmin—some peptide bonds are particularly susceptible to proteolytic attack. Eur J Biochem 1979;94:127–134.
8. Burnett D, Chandy KG. Evidence for a single-chain structure of native human ceruloplasmin using sodium dodecyl sulfate-polyacrylamide-crossed immunoelectrophoresis. Ann Biochem 1983;128:317–322.
9. Vulpe CD, Packman S. Cellular copper transport. Annu Rev Nutr 1995;15:293–322.
10. Frieden E. Caeruloplasmin: a multi-functional metalloprotein of vertebrate plasma. Ciba Found Symp 1980;79:93–124.
11. Dijkstra M, In't Veld G, van den Berg GJ, et al. Adenosine triphosphate-dependent copper transport in isolated rat liver plasma membranes. J Clin Invest 1995;95:412–416.
12. Lee NH, Hill GM, Sikha VKNM, et al. Pancreatobiliary secretion of zinc and copper in normal persons and patients with Wilson's disease. J Lab Clin Med 1990;116:283–288.
13. Rumpel A. Ueber das Wesen und die Bedeutung der Leberveränderungen und der Pigmentierungen bei den damit verbundenen Fällen von Pseudosklerose, zugleich ein Beitrag zur Lehre der Pseudosklerose (Westphal-Strümpell). Dtsch Z Nervenheilk 1913;49:54–73.
14. Luthy F. Ueber die hepato-lentikuläre Degeneration (Wilson-Westphal-Strumpell). Dtsch Z Nervenheilk 1931;123:101.
15. Glazebrook AJ. Wilson's disease. Edinburgh Med J 1945;52:83–87.
16. Frydman M, Bonne-Tamir B, Farrer LA, et al. Assignment of the gene for Wilson's disease to chromosome 13: linkage to the esterase D locus. Proc Natl Acad Sci USA 1985;82:1819–1821.
17. Bowcock AM, Farrer LA, Nebert JM, et al. Eight closely linked loci place the Wilson's disease locus within 13q14-q21. Am J Hum Genet 1988;43:664–674.
18. Bull PC, Thomas GR, Rommens JM, et al. The Wilson disease gene is a putative copper transporting P-type ATPase similar to the Menkes gene. Nat Genet 1993;5:327–337.
19. Petrukhin K, Fisher SG, Pirastu M, et al. Mapping, cloning and genetic characterization of the region containing the Wilson disease gene. Nat Genet 1993;5:338–343.
20. Tanzi RE, Petrukhin K, Chernov I, et al. The Wilson disease gene is a copper transporting ATPase with homology to the Menkes disease gene. Nat Genet 1993;5:344–350.
21. Yamaguchi Y, Heiny ME, Gitlin JD. Isolation and characterization of a human liver cDNA as a candidate gene for Wilson disease. Biochem Biophys Res Commun 1993;197:271–277.
22. Phung LT, Ajlani G, Haselkorn R. P-type ATPase from the cyanobacterium *Synechococcus* 7942 related to the human Menkes and Wilson disease gene products. Proc Natl Acad Sci USA 1994;91:9651–9654.
22a. Lutsenko S, Cooper MJ. Localization of the Wilson's disease protein product to mitochondria. Proc Natl Acad Sci USA 1998;95:6004–6009.
22b. Thomas GR, Forbes JR, Roberts EA, et al. The Wilson disease gene: spectrum of mutations and their consequences. Nat Genet 1995;9:210–217.
23. Figus A, Angius A, Loudianos G, et al. Molecular pathology and haplotype analysis of Wilson disease in Mediterranean populations. Am J Hum Genet 1995;57:1318–1324.
24. Wu J, Forbes JR, Chen HS, Cox DW. The LEC rat has a deletion in the copper transporting ATPase gene homologous to the Wilson disease gene. Nat Genet 1994;7:541–545.
25. Nakamura K, Enod F, Ueno T, et al. Excess copper and ceruloplasmin biosynthesis in long-term cultured hepatocytes from Long-Evans Cinnamon (LEC) rats, a model of Wilson disease. J Biol Chem 1995;270:7656–7660.
25a. Davis W, Chowrimootoo GF, Seymour CA. Defective biliary copper excretion in Wilson's disease: the role of ceruloplasmin. Eur J Clin Invest 1996;26:893–901.
26. Gitlin J. Aceruloplasminemia. Pediatr Res 1998;44:271–276.
27. Sass-Kortsak A, Cherniak M, Geiger DW, Slater RJ. Observations on ceruloplasmin in Wilson's disease. J Clin Invest 1959;38:1672–1682.
28. Gibbs K, Walshe JM. Studies with radioactive copper (64Cu and 67Cu); the incorporation of radioactive copper into caeruloplasmin in Wilson's disease and in primary biliary cirrhosis. Clin Sci Mol Med 1971;41:189–202.
29. Gibbs K, Walshe JM. Biliary excretion of copper in Wilson's disease. Lancet 1980;2:538–539.
30. Frommer DJ. Defective biliary excretion of copper in Wilson's disease. Gut 1974;15:125–129.
31. Ogihara H, Ogihara T, Miki M, et al. Plasma copper and antioxidant status in Wilson's disease. Pediatr Res 1995;37:219–226.
32. Carmichael PL, Hewer A, Osborne MR, et al. Detection of bulky DNA lesions in the liver of patients with Wilson's disease and primary haemochromatosis. Mutat Res 1995;326:235–243.
33. Britton RS, Brown KE. Genetic hemochromatosis and Wilson's disease: role for oxidant stress? Hepatology 1995;21:1195–1197.
34. Stein WH, Bearn AG, Moore S. Amino acids in Wilson's disease. J Clin Invest 1954;33:410–419.
35. Scheinberg IN, Sternlieb I. Wilson's disease. Philadelphia: WB Saunders, 1984.
36. Lindquist RR. Studies on the pathogenesis of hepatolenticular degeneration. Am J Pathol 1968;53:903–927.
37. Strohmeyer FW, Lshak NG. Histology of the liver in Wilson's disease: a study of 34 cases. Am J Clin Pathol 1980;73:12–24.
38. Elmes ME, Jasani B. Metallothionein and copper in liver disease. Lancet 1987;2:866.
39. Richter R. Pallial component in hepatolenticular degeneration. J Neuropathol Exp Neurol 1948;7:1–18.
40. Uzman LL, Jakus MA. The Kayser-Fleischer ring. Neurology 1957;7:341–355.
41. Brewer GJ, Yuzbasiyan-Gurkan V. Wilson disease. Medicine 1992;71:139–164.
42. Arima M, Takeshita K, Yoshino K, et al. Prognosis of Wilson's disease in childhood. Eur J Pediatr 1977;126:147–154.
43. Scott J, Gollan JL, Samourian S, Sherlock S. Wilson's disease, presenting as chronic active hepatitis. Gastroenterology 1978;74:645–651.
44. Brewer GJ. Practical recommendations and new therapies for Wilson's disease. Drugs 1995;50:240–249.
45. Medalia A, Isaacs-Glaberman K, Scheinberg IH. Neuropsychological impairment in Wilson's disease. Arch Neurol 1988;45:502–504.
46. Lang C, Mueller D, Claus D, et al. Neuropsychological findings in treated Wilson's disease. Acta Neurol Scand 1990;81:75–81.
47. Williams FJB, Walshe JM. Wilson's disease: an analysis of the cranial computerized tomographic appearances found in 60 patients and the changes in response to treatment with chelating agents. Brain 1981;104:735–752.
48. Lawler GA, Pennock JM, Steiner RE, et al. Nuclear-magnetic resonance imaging in Wilson's disease. J Comput Assist Tomogr 1983;7:1–8.
49. Hawkins RA, Mazziotta JC, Phelps ME. Wilson's disease studied with FDG and positron emission tomography. Neurology 1987;37:1707–1711.
50. Westermark K, Tedroff J, Thuomas KA, et al. Neurological Wilson's disease studied with magnetic resonance imaging and with positron emission tomography using dopaminergic markers. Mov Disord 1995;10:596–603.
51. Snow BJ, Bhatt M, Martin WR, Calne DB. The nigrostriatal dopaminergic pathway in Wilson's disease studied with positron emission tomography. J Neurol Neurosurg Psychiatry 1990;54:12–17.
52. Tatsch K, Schwarz J, Oertel WH, Kirsch C-M. SPECT imaging of dopamine D2 receptors with 123I-IBZM: initial experience in controls and patients with Parkinson's syndrome and Wilson's disease. Nucl Med Commun 1991;12:699–707.

53. Wilson's disease and copper-associated protein. Lancet 1981;1:644–646. Editorial.

54. Ludwig J, Moyer TP, Rakela J. The liver biopsy diagnosis of Wilson's disease. Am J Clin Pathol 1994;102:443–446.

55. Sternlieb I. Perspectives on Wilson's disease. Hepatology 1990;12:1234–1239.

56. Schilsky ML. Identification of the Wilson's disease gene: clues for disease pathogenesis and the potential for molecular diagnosis. Hepatology 1994;20:529–535.

57. Godwin-Austin RB, Robinson A, Evans K, Lascelles PT. An unusual neurological disorder of copper metabolism clinically resembling Wilson's disease but biochemically a distinct entity. J Neurol Sci 1978;39:85–98.

58. Neckman J, Saffer D. Abnormal copper metabolism: another "non-Wilson's" case. Neurology 1988;38:1493–1495.

59. Smith AL, Danks DM. Secondary copper accumulation with neurological damage in children with chronic liver disease. Br Med J 1978;2:1400–1401.

60. Danks DM. Hereditary disorders of copper metabolism. In: Stanbury JB, et al, eds. The metabolic basis of inherited disease. 5th ed. New York: McGraw-Hill, 1983:1251–1268.

61. Brewer GJ, Yuzbasiyan-Gurkan V, Lee DY. Use of zinc-copper metabolic interactions in the treatment of Wilson's disease. J Am Coll Nutr 1990;487–491.

62. Veen C, van den Hamer CJ, de Leeuw PW. Zinc sulphate therapy for Wilson's disease after acute deterioration during treatment with low-dose D-penicillamine. J Intern Med 1991;229:549–552.

63. Mitchell AM, Heller GL. Changes in Kayser-Fleischer ring during treatment of hepatolenticular degeneration. Arch Ophthalmol 1968;80:622–631.

64. van Wassenaer-van Hall HN, van den Heuvel AG, Algra A, et al. Wilson disease: findings at MR imaging and CT of the brain with clinical correlation. Radiology 1996;198:531–536.

65. Schwarz J, Antonini A, Kraft E, et al. Treatment with D-penicillamine improves dopamine D2-receptor binding and T2-signal intensity in de novo Wilson's disease. Neurology 1994;44:1079–1082.

66. Dahlman T, Hartvig P, Löfholm M, et al. Long-term treatment of Wilson's disease with triethylene tetramine dihydrochloride (Trientine). Q J Med 1995;88:609–616.

67. Brewer GJ, Dick RD, Yuzbasiyan-Gurkin V, et al. Initial therapy of patients with Wilson's disease with tetrathiomolybdate. Arch Neurol 1991;48:42–47.

68. Brewer GJ, Hill GM, Prasad AS, et al. The treatment of Wilson's disease with zinc. III. Prevention of reaccumulation of hepatic copper. J Lab Clin Med 1987;109:526–531.

69. Polson RJ, Rolles K, Calne RY, et al. Reversal of severe neurological manifestations of Wilson's disease following orthoptic liver transplantation. Q J Med 1987;64:685–692.

70. Walshe JM, Dixon AK. Dangers of non-compliance in Wilson's disease. Lancet 1986;1:845–847.

71. Scheinberg IH, Sternlieb I, Schilsky M, Stockert RJ. Penicillamine may detoxify copper in Wilson's disease. Lancet 1987;2:95.

Hallervorden-Spatz Disease

John H. Menkes

In 1922, Hallervorden and Spatz (1) described a rare familial disorder that began prior to age 10 years and was characterized by clubfoot deformity, gradually increasing stiffness of all limbs, impaired speech, and dementia. The genetic defect responsible for the condition has been mapped to the short arm of chromosome 20 (20p12.3-p13) (1a).

PATHOLOGY

The characteristic pathologic abnormalities are deposition of iron-containing pigments in the globus pallidus, the pars reticularis of the substantia nigra, and less often in the cerebral cortex; symmetric destruction of the globus pallidus and the pars reticularis of the substantia nigra; and axonal dystrophy. Axonal dystrophy is characterized by the presence of widely disseminated rounded structures, identified as swollen axons (axonal spheroids), and is seen with particular frequency in the basal ganglia, notably the pallidum (2).

Microscopically, the pigment is located within neurons and glial cells or may lie free in the neuropil, particularly around large blood vessels of affected areas. Histochemical and chemical analyses indicate that it contains iron and is related to neuromelanin. The cytoplasm of the renal tubules contains a brown granular pigment, similar in composition to that deposited in nerve tissues (3). In skeletal muscle there are subsarcolemmnal myeloid structures. Their presence indicates a nonspecific derangement of muscle metabolism (4).

It is not clear whether the disorder represents a lipofuscin storage disease with an iron-catalyzed pseudoperoxidation of lipofuscin to neuromelanin (5), or whether it is the result of an abnormality in axonal metabolism. If the latter is true, Hallervorden-Spatz disease is a specific form of primary axonal dystrophy with a predilection for the globus pallidus and substantia nigra, with the excess pigmentation resulting from lipid deposition. The condition would therefore be related to other types of primary axonal dystrophies, such as occur in normal aging humans, in cystic fibrosis, vitamin E deficiency, infantile neuroaxonal dystrophy, and poisoning with organic cyanides (6).

The biochemical defect is still unknown. No systemic abnormality of iron metabolism has been demonstrated. In 1985 Perry and co-workers reported the accumulation of cysteine and cystine and noted reduced activity of cysteine dioxygenase in the globus pallidus (7). Cysteine dioxygenase converts cysteine to L-cysteinesulfinic acid, the major catabolic product of cysteine. This observation of cysteine accumulation will need to be confirmed. It becomes particularly pertinent when one considers the parkinsonian symptoms of long-surviving patients with cystinosis.

CLINICAL MANIFESTATIONS

There is considerable variability in time of onset and in the major manifestations of Hallervorden-Spatz disease (8). The highlights of the classic form of the illness are progressive impairment of gait caused by pes equinovarus deformity of the feet and rigidity of the legs, slowing and diminution of all voluntary movements, dysarthria, and mental deterioration. About 50% of patients exhibit a choreiform and athetotic movement disorder. Spasticity has been evident in some cases, and atrophy of distal musculature or seizures in others. Retinitis pigmentosa and, less often, optic atrophy are commonly encountered. An associated acanthocytosis has been observed frequently (4,9). In other patients, bone marrow aspiration has disclosed the presence of sea-blue histiocytes (10). This phenomenon indicates the presence of complex lipids in histiocyte liposomes and is seen in a variety of other neurologic disorders. These include G_{M1}

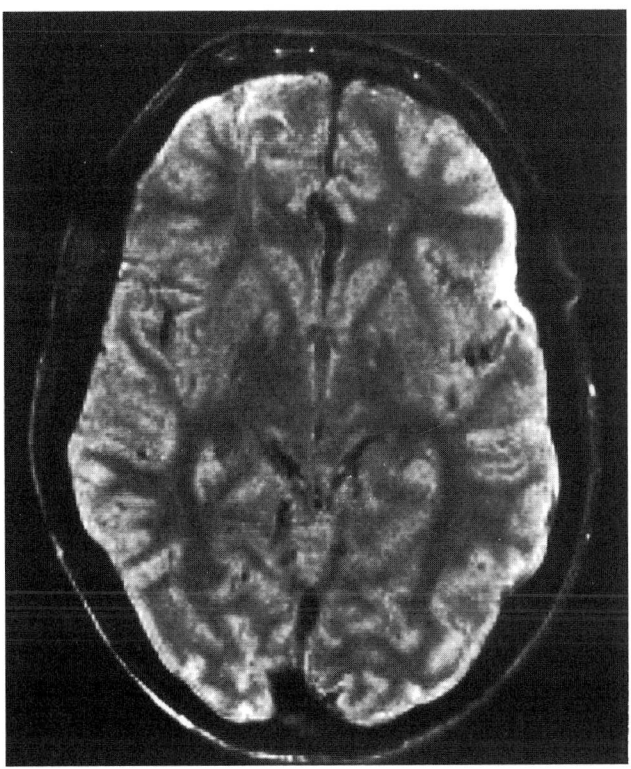

FIGURE 41.1   *Hallervorden-Spatz disease. Nuclear magnetic resonance scan of a previously developmentally delayed 14-year-old boy who experienced progressive dystonia and cognitive impairment. Scan demonstrates irregular areas of hypointensity in the globus pallidus on T2-weighted images.*

Neuroimaging studies are of considerable assistance in the diagnosis of the disease. The computed tomography scan shows bilateral high-density lesions within the globus pallidus (12). The presence of iron within the basal ganglia is best detected by magnetic resonance imaging using a T2-weighted spin-echo pulse sequence (Fig 41.1). Marked hypointensity of the globus pallidus has been observed in pathologically proven and several suspected cases (4,13,14). Iron chelation has not been successful, and at present there is no treatment for the disorder.

REFERENCES

1. Hallervorden J, Spatz H. Erkrankung im System mit besonderer Beteilung des Globus Pallidus und der Substantia Nigra. Z Gesamte Neurol Psychiat 1922;79:254–302.
1a. Taylor TD, Litt M, Kramer P, et al. Homozygosity mapping of Hallervorden-Spatz Syndrome to chromosome 20p12.3-p13. Nat Genet 1996;14:479–481.
2. Malandrini A, Cavallaro T, Fabrizi GM, et al. Ultrastructure and immunoreactivity of dystrophic axons indicate a different pathogenesis of Hallervorden-Spatz disease and infantile neuroaxonal dystrophy. Virchows Arch 1995;427:415–421.
3. Nakai H, Landing BH, Schubert WK. Seitelberger's spastic amaurotic axonal idiocy; report of a case in a 9-year-old boy with comment on visceral manifestations. Pediatrics 1960;25:441–449.
4. Malandrini A, Bonucccelli U, Parrotta E, et al. Myopathic involvement in two cases of Hallervorden-Spatz disease. Brain Dev 1995;17:286–290.
5. Park BE, Netsky MG, Betsill WL. Pathogenesis of pigment and spheroid formation in Hallervorden-Spatz syndrome and related disorders. Neurology 1975;25:1172–1178.
6. Vakili S, Drew AL, Von Schuching S, et al. Hallervorden-Spatz syndrome. Arch Neurol 1977;34:729–738.
7. Perry TL, Norman MG, Young VW, et al. Hallervorden-Spatz disease: cysteine accumulation and cysteine dioxygenase deficiency in the globus pallidus. Ann Neurol 1985;18:482–489.
8. Dooling EC, Schoene WC, Richardson EP Jr. Hallervorden-Spatz syndrome. Arch Neurol 1974;30:70–83.
9. Swisher CN, Menkes JH, Cancilla PA, Dodge PR. Coexistence of Hallervorden-Spatz disease with acanthocytosis. Trans Am Neurol Assoc 1972;97:212–216.
10. Swaiman KF, Smith SA, Trock GL, Siddiqui AR. Sea-blue histiocytes, lymphocytic cytosomes, movement disorder and Fe-uptake in basal ganglia: Hallervorden-Spatz disease or ceroid storage disease with abnormal isotope scan? Neurology 1983;33:301–305.
11. Eidelberg D, Sotrel A, Joachim C, et al. Adult onset Hallervorden-Spatz disease with neurofibrillary pathology. Brain 1987;110:993–1013.
12. Tennison MB, Bouldon TW, Whaley RA. Mineralization of the basal ganglia detected by CT in Hallervorden-Spatz syndrome. Neurology 1988;38:154–155.
13. Malandrini A, et al. Clinicopathologic study of familial late infantile Hallervorden-Spatz disease: a particular form of neuroacanthocytosis. Childs Nerv Syst 1996;12:155–160.
14. Tanfani G, Mascalchi M, Dal Pozzo GC, et al. MR imaging in a case of Hallervorden-Spatz disease. J Comput Assist Tomogr 1987;11:1057–1058.

gangliosidosis, Fabry's disease, Niemann–Pick disease, Tangier disease, and Wolman's disease. These cells are also found in chronic myelogenous leukemia, idiopathic thrombocytopenic purpura, and type I hyperlipoproteinemia.

Another variant of Hallervorden–Spatz disease manifests itself by dementia and progressive development of extrapyramidal dysfunction in previously retarded individuals. In these cases, the neuropathologic changes also include an abundance of neurofibrillary tangles, particularly evident in the basal forebrain and the hippocampus (11).

Gait Disorder in Normal-Pressure Hydrocephalus

PETER M. BLACK

INTRODUCTION

Normal-pressure hydrocephalus (NPH) is a clinical syndrome characterized by gait disturbance, memory loss, slowing of thought and action, and urinary incontinence in the setting of ventriculomegaly. It may be a manifestation of a brain tumor, may follow subarachnoid hemorrhage, brain surgery, or head trauma, or may appear without known cause (see below). Cerebrospinal fluid (CSF) pressure may be normal, low, or moderately high. The condition is often but not always helped by shunt placement.

GAIT DISORDER IN NPH

Gait disturbance is the most prominent symptom in NPH and is usually the earliest symptom; it is also the best prognostic indicator of a good response to shunting.

Characteristics

The typical NPH gait is characterized by wide base, slow speed, short steps, and vertical ataxia. Patients place their feet on the ground with variable force and sometimes feel as if their feet are "sticking to the ground" (3). They may describe feelings of weakness in their legs and may actually consume more energy in walking than normal persons because of increased extensor muscle activity compared with controls. The problems with walking can progress to complete inability to walk and in the extreme may result in the inability to stand or sit because of unsteadiness. Truncal ataxia or real "cerebellar" ataxia is not usually seen, however; the gait disorder appears to be more of a frontal gait apraxia with difficulty organizing a smooth gait rather than an actual ataxia. Cerebellar signs such as dysdiadochokinesis and heel-knee-shin ataxia are absent.

To emphasize the fact that this is not cerebellar ataxia, the same NPH patients with inability to walk may demonstrate unimpaired functioning of the legs when lying on their back (4). They may also have upper extremity involvement with tremor and deterioration of handwriting.

Differential Diagnosis

Gait disorders are regularly encountered in the elderly and NPH may only account for a minority of these cases; in one study, NPH was responsible for only 4% of gait problems in elderly patients (5). The following are some of the other conditions that can produce gait disorder.

In *high-pressure hydrocephalus*, the gait disorder may be exactly the same as that in NPH but develops more rapidly, over weeks rather than years, and is associated with other symptoms and signs. Headache is the most common associated complaint. It is usually bifrontal in location and worse in the morning. Nausea and vomiting accompany it and are also worse in the morning. There may also be visual changes including decreased visual acuity, diplopia, and an inability to look up. Changes in mental status include drowsiness, inattention, and memory loss.

Physical exam may reveal papilledema. Paralysis of upward gaze and accommodation result from pressure on the tectal plate.

Alzheimer patients may have a gait disorder but it tends to be shuffling and scuffing with a narrow base and very small steps. Patients have increased double support stride compared to NPH patients (4). The differential is made more complex, however, because the ventricular system may be enlarged in patients with Alzheimer's disease and may therefore resemble the ventricles of NPH. The gait disorder in Alzheimer's also tends to occur after cognitive deterioration and therefore the mental incapacity is often worse than in NPH patients; it may also be accompanied by aphasia and parietal lobe deficits.

Cerebellar ataxia must also be considered in the differential diagnosis. In cerebellar ataxia, movements of the legs are more variable in the transverse and sagittal planes compared to the evertical ataxia in NPH (3). Other evidence of cerebellar incoordination such as dysmetria, adiadochokinesis, and terminal tremor are not present in NPH.

Parkinson's disease is also characterized by a gait disorder and may be confused with NPH because both can display bradykinesia and increased tone. However, parkinsonian gait is hesitant, with festination, en bloc turning, flexed posture, and lack of accessory movements such as arm swinging (5). In addition, cogwheel rigidity and masked facies are distinguishing features of Parkinson's.

Patients with Binswanger's disease or *multi-infarct dementia* may also present with a gait disorder that is difficult to distinguish from NPH, although patients with NPH tend to present at a later age and have more frequent gait disturbance at onset (6).

OTHER CLINICAL FINDINGS IN NPH

A variety of mental changes have been described in NPH ranging from mild memory loss to severe dementia. Impairment of recent memory is the most frequent complaint. Tasks such as copying, drawing, and arranging objects may also be difficult.

A less well-known mental change in this disease is loss of initiative, spontaneity, and interest that may progress to apathy and abulia. Responses and voluntary movements are slow and delayed. This is so characteristic for NPH that it should be considered separately from the dementia, gait disturbance, and urinary incontinence as a fourth component of the syndrome.

This clinical picture of dementia is a subcortical type that may be frequently encountered in the elderly and may be difficult to distinguish from Alzheimer's, major depression, Binswanger's disease, and multi-infarct dementia. In Alzheimer's, aphasia, agnosia, and apraxia are frequently seen and frontal lobe release signs are common. The changes in mentation seen in Alzheimer's occur much earlier than the gait disturbance, which is usually a late symptom. In NPH, on the other hand, gait disorder usually precedes or occurs concurrently with changes in mentation. Major depression can present with memory loss, psychomotor retardation, and even pseudodementia. However, other neurovegetative symptoms and depressed mood should be present. Incontinence and gait disorder are generally not seen in depression. Binswanger's disease and multi-infarct dementia are similiar to NPH but generally do not have the gait disturbance as prominently displayed (6,7).

Urinary incontinence is the third part of the traditional NPH triad but is not seen with the same frequency as gait disorder and changes in mentation. It may occur as a late symptom. The incontinence ranges from a sense of urgency to a frontal lobe type of incontinence in which the appropriate awareness of the need to urinate is lost. Fecal incontinence is rare. Urinary incontinence can also be seen in Alzheimer's disease.

ETIOLOGY OF NPH

Almost all cases of hydrocephalus in adults are caused by an obstruction of flow through the ventricular system and subarachnoid pathways. This results in increased mean pulsatile pressures in the ventricular system and a consequent increase in ventricular size.

NPH can be caused by anything that results in low grade scarring or obstruction of the ventricular system or subarachnoid pathways. Some causes are listed in Table 42.1. Subarachnoid hemorrhage is the most common cause of NPH with a known etiology. Other causes include meningitis, partial obstruction of the CSF pathways by tumor, cranial radiation, and neurosurgery, particularly following a posterior fossa operation. NPH may follow trauma that causes a subarachnoid hemorrhage obstructing the basal cisterns or convexity subarachnoid space. Aqueductal stenosis, a congenital narrowing of the cerebral aqueduct, more frequently leads to high-pressure hydrocephalus but may cause NPH as well.

A significant number of cases of NPH may be idiopathic (4). Hakim and Adams have suggested that in this condition there is an initial rise in CSF pressure that leads to ventricular enlargement (8). This enlargement is maintained despite normal pressure because of Laplace's law in which pressure = force/area. Although the pressure is normal, the enlarged ventricular area reflects increased force on the ventricular wall. Even though the pressure appears normal most of the day, continuous intracranial pressure monitorings in some patients also show periods of increased intracranial pressure waves at night (9).

Table 42.1 Some Causes of Adult Normal-Pressure Hydrocephalus

Cause	Percent
Subarachnoid hemorrhage	34
Idiopathic (no known cause)	34
Head injury	11
Tumors	6
Prior surgery	5
Aqueduct stenosis	3
Meningitis	3
Others	4

Modified from Katzman R. Low pressure hydrocephalus. In Wells CE, ed. Dementia. Philadelphia: FA Davis, 1977.

DIAGNOSIS OF NPH

Because of the implications for treatment, the diagnosis of NPH is quite important in assessing a patient with a gait disorder. The first step is identifying the appropriate clinical tetrad. The next is a brain imaging study. This should be performed both with and without contrast; the unenhanced scan will demonstrate the ventricular contours, while contrast enhancement may reveal otherwise inapparent underlying lesions. Computerized tomography (CT) is usually the initial imaging study: the cardinal CT features of hydrocephalus include 1) enlargement of ventricles, with rounding of the ventricular contour, 2) prescence of periventricular lucencies, especially around the frontal horns, and 3) normal-sized subarachnoid space. Enlargement of the subarachnoid spaces and prominent cortical sulci are typically suggestive of atrophy but may also be present with hydrocephalus.

If CT scanning reveals ventricular enlargement characteristic of hydrocephalus and a clear etiologic lesion, further imaging is not needed. If there is no apparent cause, magnetic resonance imaging (MRI) is a useful adjunctive test. It is superior to CT in identifying underlying lesions, such as small periaqueductal or posterior fossa tumors. MRI is also the modality best equipped for assessing parenchymal disease seen with Binswanger's or multi-infarct dementia that may be difficult to distinguish from NPH on clinical grounds alone. Furthermore, sagittal imaging with MRI helps to distinguish hydrocephalus from atrophy by showing distinctive features of the former, such as thinning and bowing of the corpus callosum. Periventricular hypointensity on MRI is, however, less specific and can be seen in the setting of edema, ischemia, demyelination, and other disorders. Measurement of proton relaxation times of periventricular abnormalities may prove to be a technique for distinguishing these processes (10).

MRI also allows measurement of intracranial CSF volume, which may provide a sensitive volumetric index of ventricular size (11). In addition, quantification of the volumes of various intracranial compartments may prove to be of benefit in differentiation of hydrocephalus from other causes of ventriculomegaly (12).

In addition to volumetric determinations, MRI can image CSF flow patterns through the aqueduct of Sylvius. A variety of MRI techniques have been applied to establishing flow and pulsatility patterns through the aqueduct in patients with hydrocephalus (13–15). Recent reports suggest that these techniques may have value in identifying different types of hydrocephalus, although they are not yet clinically applicable.

Cisternography has been widely used in evaluating CSF dynamics in patients with ventricular enlargement and suspected NPH. It is performed by intrathecal injection of a radioactive isotope (isotope cisternography) or contrast material and serial CT scanning (CT cisternography). The passage of the isotope or contrast into the ventricles and subarachnoid space is visualized. A normal pattern shows flow over the convexities and not into the ventricles. A typical pattern of NPH is ventricular entry and stasis without ascent over the convexities. Most patients show a "mixed" pattern. The value of cisternography in diagnosis and prediction of shunt responsiveness has been brought into question. Recent reports indicate that cisternography provides no additional diagnostic accuracy over the combination of clinical and CT criteria (16,17).

Determination of CSF pressure by lumbar puncture should be done at some point in the management. An opening pressure of less than 180 mm H_2O suggests NPH. It is helpful to remove CSF to assess the effect of withdrawal. Clinical improvement, especially of gait, predicts a good response to shunting (18,19). Temporary lumbar drainage has also been suggested as a further maneuver to predict shunt responsiveness (20).

In many centers, overnight CSF pressure monitoring and lumboventricular perfusion may help establish CSF outflow blockade. Monitoring can be performed using a frontal ventricular catheter, lumbar catheter, or epidural transducer, all of which allow prolonged pressure recording over at least 24 hours. Increased baseline CSF pressure or pressure waves (A or B waves) can be used as criteria for shunt responsiveness (21). A more quantitative analysis of intracranial pressure (ICP) waves may allow greater accuracy in these determinations (22).

An adjunct to prolonged pressure recording is the use of infusion tests to assess resistance to CSF absorption. Lumbar infusion of normal saline has been shown to detect prolonged increases in ICP indicating deficits in CSF absorptive capacity (23,24). A well-proven technique involves measurement of CSF conductance by lumboventricular perfusion. Outflow resistance greater than 12.5 mL/mm/mm Hg has been correlated with improvement after shunting (25). These techniques may offer prognostic information for shunting in a selected group of individuals with idiopathic NPH in whom other less invasive testing has been unhelpful.

Functional tests such as single photon emission computed tomography (which shows patterns of cerebral blood flow), positron emission tomography (which demonstrates brain metabolism), and magnetic resonance spectroscopy (which measures ratios of chemical markers in the brain) have shown some evidence of being able to differentiate NPH from other causes of dementia and may also be of some predictive value in determining shunt responsiveness (26–29). These tests, however, are still being investigated and need further validation before they enter mainstream clinical practice. Electroencephalogram (EEG) and evoked responses have no utility in the diagnosis of hydrocephalus.

TREATMENT OF NPH

The definitive treatment for NPH is shunting, but marginal responses in some groups and the potential for complications must be considered in the decision to proceed with shunt placement.

When a clear etiology is present, such as recent subarachnoid hemmorhage, meningitis, evidence of aqueductal stenosis or obstructive tumor, shunting is the treatment of choice and is associated with good outcome.

For cases of idiopathic NPH the decision is more complex. Myriad clinical findings and tests have been advocated as predictors of shunt responsiveness. Many studies have addressed this issue (21,25,30–32). The following parameters have consistently proven to be good prognosticators for shunt response:

1. NPH of known etiology
2. shorter duration of symptoms, although long duration is not a contraindication
3. prominent gait disturbance
4. improvement after serial LPs
5. altered CSF dynamics as demonstrated by long-term monitoring or infusion testing, especially lumboventricular perfusion
6. CT scan demonstrating periventricular lucency

Studies of shunt responsiveness report response rates in the range of 30% to 80% (17,30,32). In our experience about 66% of patients improve and perhaps 5% worsen in some way with shunt placement. Differences in outcome may be due to differential selection for shunting.

Shunts

Shunt Systems

Currently the commonly employed systems for CSF shunting are ventriculoperitoneal (VP), ventriculoatrial (VA), ventriculopleural (VPl), and lumboperitoneal (LP) shunts. By far the most commonly used is the VP shunt.

The components of a typical CSF diversion system include the following:

1. Ventricular catheter. Ventricular catheters are inserted into the right frontal horn via a right frontal or right parieto-occipital burr hole. A lumbar catheter for lumbar CSF diversion is an option in communicating hydrocephalus and has the advantage of avoiding ventricular puncture and general anesthesia. Lumbar shunts, however, have a much greater tendency for obstruction, and have generally fallen out of favor.

2. Distal tubing. The silastic tubing is attached to the proximal catheter and tunneled subcutaneously to the distal site of entry, that is, the peritoneal cavity (VP and LP shunt), the right atrium via the common facial vein (VA shunt), or the pleural cavity (VPl shunt).

3. Valve. The valve is interposed between proximal and distal shunt components, usually near the site of the ventricular catheter. It regulates the pressure and prevents retrograde flow of shunted CSF. Several valve designs exist, including spring-loaded and slit valves, which vary by their mechanism of outflow regulation. More recently, variable

pressure valves have become available that allow percutaneous adjustment of pressure settings, offering the advantage of fine-tuning ICP in shunted patients without the need for reoperation (33,34). The ideal opening pressure of the valve for hydrocephalic patients is controversial. Low- and medium-pressure valves have been advocated in the past (35), but others have indicated the effectiveness of high-pressure systems (17). The utility of variable pressure valves is under investigation (33,34,36).

4. Ancillary components—ventricular reservoir and antisiphon device. Ventricular reservoirs are commonly placed in ventricular shunts, proximal to the valve system, and are generally palpable if present. They serve as a route for extracranial measurement of the ICP, CSF removal, and testing of the shunt system. Antisiphon devices are designed to prevent intraventricular pressure from falling below atmospheric pressure at the level of the antisiphon device, thus preventing overdrainage. When shunted patients are in an upright position the ICP may become subatmospheric leading to overdrainage.

Shunt-Related Complications

There are a variety of shunt-related complications. The most important include the following:

1. Shunt obstruction. Shunt obstruction can be of insidious, intermittent, or sudden onset, and usually presents with clinical deterioration. The ventricular catheter may become obstructed by debris, coagulum, or contact with choroid plexus or brain secondary to decreased size of the ventricles. Proximal catheter obstruction is the most common cause of shunt malfunction. The distal end may become blocked in VP shunts by omentum or peritoneal adhesions. Shunt blockage requires surgical exploration and revision.

2. Infection. The rate of shunt infections in adults is less than 5%, lower than rates in the pediatric population. Infection can manifest in several ways: wound infection at site of shunt insertion, ventriculitis and meningitis, or secondary infection of the vascular system including endocarditis (VA shunts) and peritoneal infection (VP shunts). Shunt infection most commonly presents insidiously as shunt malfunction, however, and typical findings of meningitis are generally not present.

The majority of infections present immediately or within a few months of shunt insertion and are commonly attributed to bacterial contamination during operation. Infection may also occur in the setting of systemic infection, such as pneumonia or urinary tract infection (UTI), even years after shunt placement. The most common pathogens are *S. epidermidis*, and less frequently *S. aureus, P. aeruginosa* and *Escherichia coli.* The general approach to shunt infection is to remove the entire shunt system and external ventricular drainage until there is a clearing of infection following a full course of IV antibiotics.

3. Subdural collections. There is a 5% to 10% likelihood of formation of a subdural hygroma or hematoma with

shunted hydrocephalus. A hygroma is a fluid collection that results from CSF accumulation into the subdural space; it is an effusion of high protein material perhaps caused by the pressure differentials associated with shunt placement. A subdural hematoma results from tearing of cortical bridging veins when the brain collapses around the shunt. The risk of subdural hematoma is increased with even minor head trauma. Use of higher pressure valves, or variable pressure valves that allow graded ventricular decompression, may decrease the incidence of this complication (33). For symptomatic collections, burr hole drainage is initially attempted. It may be necessary to temporarily tie off the shunt to allow brain expansion in order to occlude the subdural space.

4. Overdrainage. Symptoms of overdrainage often mimic those of underdrainage; they include headache, nausea, and vomiting. This may require an antisiphon device or a valve with higher opening pressure (37).

5. Mechanical failure. Disconnection of shunt components or fracture of the shunt tubing at stress points may occur, especially with head trauma. A shunt series, containing a selection of anterio-posterior (AP)/lateral skull films, AP/lateral chest films, and KUB/lateral abdominal films, can be helpful in determining the site of disconnection. Surgical exploration and revision will be required in cases of mechanical failure.

6. Shunt type-specific complications. Ventricular shunts carry a small risk (approximately 5%) of seizures; the incidence of this may be decreased with use of an occipital rather than frontal catheter. Prophylactic anticonvulsant medication is not indicated in routine management. VA shunts carry the unique risk of thromboembolic episodes such as pulmonary embolism; with the shunt materials currently in use, the risks are small. LP shunts commonly obstruct and have been associated with acquired tonsillar herniation (38).

Evaluation of a Patient with Suspected Shunt Malfunction

Shunt malfunction must be suspected in shunted patients presenting with recurrence of gait problems; regression of clinical improvement at any time after shunt placement should raise the question of shunt malfunction. The clinical deterioration is often stereotyped in any one patient (39). Palpation and compression of the valve suggests blockage of the ventricular catheter if the valve can be compressed but refills very slowly. Blockage within the valve or distally is likely if the valve is incompressible. A normally working shunt should allow easy valve emptying and refill within 5 to 30 seconds.

For determination of the CSF pressure, lumbar puncture (LP) or tapping of the shunt reservoir can be performed. LP is preferable if it can be performed safely, as shunt tapping carries a 1% risk of infection. A shunt tap should be considered an invasive procedure, requiring meticulous attention to sterility. Neurosurgical consultation prior to performing the procedure is warranted.

REFERENCES

1. Adams RD, Victor M. Principles of neurology. 5th ed. New York: McGraw Hill, 1993.
2. Black PM. Hydrocephalus and vasospasm following subarachnoid hemorrhage from ruptured intracranial aneurysm. Neurosurgery 1986;18:12.
3. Sorensen PS, Jansen EC, Gjerris F. Motor disturbance in normal-pressure hydrocephalus: special reference to stance and gait. Arch Neurol 1986;43:34.
4. Fisher CM. Hydrocephalus as a cause of disturbances of gait in the elderly. Neurology 1982;32:1358.
5. Sudarsky C, Ronthal M. Gait disorders among elderly patients: a survey study of fifty patients. Arch Neurol 1983;40:740.
6. Gallassi R, Morreale A, Montagna P, et al. Binswanger's disease and normal-pressure hydrocephalus: a clinical and neuropsychological comparison. Arch Neurol 1991;48:1156.
7. Roman GC. White matter lesions and normal-pressure hydrocephalus: Binswanger's disease or Hakim syndrome? AJNR Am J Neuroradiol 1991;12:40.
8. Hakim S, Adams RD. The special clinical problem of symptomatic hydrocephalus with normal cerebrospinal fluid pressure: observations on cerebrospinal fluid hydrodynamics. J Neurol Sci 1965;2:307.
9. Symon L, Dorsch NWC. Use of long-term intracranial pressure measurement to assess hydrocephalic patients prior to shunt surgery. J Neurosurg 1975;42:258.
10. Tamaki N, Nagashima T, Ehara K, et al. Hydrocephalic oedema in normal-pressure hydrocephalus. Acta Neurochir Suppl 1990;51:348.
11. Condon B, Patterson J, Wyper D, et al. Use of magnetic resonance imaging to measure intracranial cerebrospinal fluid volume. Lancet 1986;1:1355.
12. Matsumae M, Kikinis R, Lorenzo AV, et al. Intracranial compartments in patients with enlarged ventricles assessed by MRI based image processing. J Neurosurg 1996;84:972–981.
13. Mascalchi M, Ciraolo L, Bucciolini M, et al. Fast multiphase MR imaging of aqueductal CSF flow: 2. Study in patients with hydrocephalus. AJNR Am J Neuroradiol 1990;11:597.
14. Katayama S, Asari S, Ohmoto T. Quantitative measurement of normal and hydrocephalic cerebrospinal fluid flow using phase contrast cine MR imaging. Acta Med Okayama 1993;47(3):157.
15. Nitz WR, Bradley WG, Watanabe AS, et al. Flow dynamics of cerebrospinal fluid: assessment with phase-contrast velocity MR imaging performed with retrospective cardiac gating. Radiology 1992;183:395.
16. Vanneste J, Augustin P, Davies GAG, et al. Normal-pressure hydrocephalus. Is cisternography still useful in selecting patients for a shunt? Arch Neurol 1992;49:366.
17. Benzel EC, Pelletier AL, Levy PG. Communicating hydrocephalus in adults: prediction of outcome after ventricular shunting procedures. Neurosurgery 1990;26(4):655.
18. Wood JH, Bartlet D, James AE, Udvarhelyi GB. Normal-pressure hydrocephalus: diagnosis and patient selection for shunt surgery. Neurology 1974;24:517.
19. Wikkelso C, Andersson H, Bloomstrand C, Lindqvist G. The clinical effect of lumbar puncture in normal pressure hydrocephalus. J Neurol Neurosurg Psychiatry 1982;45:62.
20. Haan J, Thomeer RTWM. Predictive value of temporary external lumbar drainage in normal pressure hydrocephalus. Neurosurgery 1988;22(2):388.
21. Crockard HA, Hanlon K, Duda EE, Mullan JF. Hydrocephalus as a cause of dementia: evaluation by computerized tomography and intracranial pressure monitoring. J Neurol Neurosurg Psychiatry 1977;40:736.
22. Raftopoulos C, Chaskis C, Delecluse F, et al. Morphological quantitative analysis of intracranial pressure waves in normal pressure hydrocephalus. Neurol Res 1992;14:389.
23. Hussey F, Schanzer B, Katzman R. A simple constant-infusion manometric test for measurement of CSF absorption. II. Clinical studies. Neurology 1970;20:665.
24. Morgan MK, Johnston IH, Spittaler PJ. A ventricular infusion technique for the evaluation of treated and untreated hydrocephalus. Neurosurgery 1991;29:832.
25. Borgesen SE, Gjerris F. The predictive value of conductance to outflow of CSF in normal pressure hydrocephalus. Brain 1982;105:65.
26. Kamiya K, Yamashita N, Nagai H, Mizawa I. Investigation of normal pressure hydrocephalus by 123I-IMP SPECT. Neurol Med Chir 1991;31:503.
27. Waldemar G, Schmidt JF, Delecluse F, Andersen AR, et al. High resolution SPECT with 99MTc-d,1-HMPAO in normal pressure hydrocephalus before and after shunt operation. J Neurol Neurosurg Psychiatry 1993;56:655.

28. Jagust WJ, Friedland RP, Budinger TF. Positron emission tomography with [18F] Fluorodeoxyglucose differentiates normal pressure hydrocephalus from Alzheimer-type dementia. J Neurol Neurosurg Psychiatry 1985;48:1091.

29. Shiino A, Matsuda M, Morikawa S, et al. Proton magnetic resonance spectroscopy with dementia. Surg Neurol 1993;39:143.

30. Black PM, Ojemann RG, Tzouras A. CSF shunts for dementia, incontinence and gait disturbances. Clin Neurosurg 1985;32:632.

31. Larsson A, Wikkelso C, Bilting M, Stephensen H. Clinical parameters in 74 consecutive patients shunt operated for normal pressure hydrocephalus. Acta Neurol Scand 1991;84:475.

32. Vanneste J, Augutijn P, Dirven, et al. Shunting normal-pressure hydrocephalus: do the benefits outweigh the risks? A multicenter study and literature review. Neurology 1992;42:54.

33. Sindou M, Guyotat-Pelissou, Chidiac A, Goutelle A. Transcutaneous pressure adjustable valve for the treatment of hydrocephalus and arachnoid cysts in adults. Experience with 75 cases. Acta Neurochir (Wien) 1993;121:135.

34. Black PM, Hakim R, Olsen Bailey N. The use of the Codman-Medos programmable Hakim valve in the management of patients with hydrocephalus: illustrative cases. Neurosurgery 1994;34:1110–1113.

35. McQuarrie IG, Saint-Louis L, Scherer PB. Treatment of normal pressure hydrocephalus with low versus medium pressure cerebrospinal fluid shunts. Neurosurgery 1984;15:484.

36. Larsson A, Jensen C, Bilting M, et al. Does the shunt opening pressure influence the effect of shunt surgery in normal pressure hydrocephalus? Acta Neurochir (Wien) 1992;117:15.

37. Pudenz RH, Foltz EL. Hydrocephalus: overdrainage by ventricular shunts. A review and recommendations. Surg Neurol 1991;35:200.

38. Welch K, Shillito JS, Strand R, et al. Chiari I malformation—an acquired disorder? J Neurosurg 1981;55:604.

39. Puca A, Anile C, Maira G, Rossi G. Cerebrospinal fluid shunting for hydrocephalus in the adult: factors related to shunt revision. Neurosurgery 1991;29:822.

Wandering Behavior in Dementing Illness

GARY S. MOAK

INTRODUCTION

Wandering behavior represents a serious behavioral complication of dementing illness. While gait disorders and immobility account for significant disability in the advanced stages of dementing disorders, wandering ironically causes excess disability associated with intact locomotion. The wandering behavior of demented patients living at home poses a safety risk and burdens families and other caregivers. When unmanageable, wandering commonly leads to institutionalization.

Wandering also presents a difficult management problem in institutional settings. Nursing homes face additional liability for patients who wander from the facility and for those who are physically frail and unsteady of gait, for whom the risk of falling is great (1). Legal and ethical conflicts are raised when institutions must decide between respecting the freedom of movement of their residents and protecting their physical safety (2–4). Efforts to control this behavior commonly lead to the use of physical restraint or pharmacotherapy, interventions associated with morbidities of their own. Notwithstanding the prevalence of dementia and the difficulty of this problem, remarkably little has been written about its treatment.

Common sense suggests that wandering occurs as a non-specific concomitant of disorientation, memory impairment, and confused thinking. In fact, some data show that wanderers may be more cognitively impaired than nonwandering comparison groups (2,5,6). These findings have been interpreted to mean that wandering occurs as a function of severity of dementia.

While wandering may represent a nonspecific symptom of the dementia syndrome, it is unclear why this behavior does not occur in a larger percentage of patients with severe dementia. The prevalence of wandering among geriatric patients in long-term care facilities has been reported to be as low as 3.8% and as high as 75%, but most estimates fall between 5% and 25% (6–9). Why do some elderly demented patients wander while most do not? This question has prompted speculation that wandering represents a more specific or perhaps localizing syndrome (4,9). Wandering has been hypothesized to reflect the expression of lifelong styles of coping with stress through motor action (4) or a non-specific response to unmet needs for care (5).

While wandering is a disturbance of locomotion, it is not commonly classified as a movement disorder. For the purposes of this chapter, wandering will be defined as a tendency to move about either aimlessly or without an appropriate goal, due to dysregulation of initiation, direction, or termination of ambulation (i.e., movement), commonly occurring in the presence of dementia. It clearly is a problem related to the control of movement, and, therefore, may be classified as a movement disorder, broadly construed.

DIAGNOSIS

There is no accepted definition of wandering, and no diagnostic criteria have been established. Wandering is not a diagnosis *per se* but a heterogeneous behavioral syndrome.

Wandering is readily identified by caregivers who unambiguously report it when it occurs. Family members express concern to the physician after wandering has become persistent or has led the patient into dangerous predicaments. A typical history is that the patient has wandered into dangerous neighborhoods, local bars, heavy traffic, or onto highways. The patient may have wandered out of the house and gotten lost, only to be returned home by the police. Occasionally wanderers are found carrying large sums of money on their persons.

Aimless wandering may occur within the home in a manner that is disruptive to family life. This is endured by many families as long as the wanderer remains inside and responds to redirection. Some patients become agitated, hostile, or aggressive if redirected or restricted by family members. The caregivers may have placed locks on the doors and windows to prevent egress by the wanderer.

Patients who wander from nursing homes burden the staff with the task of search and retrieval, and require additional vigilance to prevent further egress. Wandering within institutional confines may lead to random intrusion into the space of other patients and to napping, urinating, or defecating in inappropriate places. This behavior can lead to aggressive conflicts between residents. The staff frequently are forced to confine the wanderer in a geriatric wheelchair; this can precipitate or aggravate agitation and combativeness, often necessitating the prescription of sedating medication.

Three subtypes of wandering have been described (3). Some patients may appear to be seeking a particular object. The patient reports that he or she is searching for something or someone (home, spouse, mother, etc.). Other wanderers report a need to pursue some industrious task (e.g., going to work). In these first two types, the patients exhibit varying amounts of affective pressure in association with their perceived objective. More intact patients may offer plausible confabulations that may be convincing to unfamiliar caregivers. Attempts to redirect the wanderer may precipitate agitation, hostility, or suspicious accusations. Overt confrontation may provoke assaultive behavior.

The third type of wandering appears aimless or random. The patient exhibits distractibility and rapid shifts of attention (3). Some of these patients appear to meander casually within the environment. Others exhibit an intense, driven quality that is nonetheless aimless. Such patients evince a "wind-up toy" appearance.

Wandering behavior requires a thorough neuropsychiatric evaluation. The diagnosis and severity of dementia must be established. Contributing problems such as sensory impairment, pain, incontinence, medication toxicity, and occult systemic illness must be recognized. The presence of concomitant neuropsychiatric symptoms, such as agitation, delusions, hallucinations, depression, and sleep disorders, which may be more prevalent among patients with wandering (8), should be evaluated. This permits differential diagnosis of various syndromes associated with dementia that may contribute to wandering behavior.

Careful cognitive assessment is necessary to identify more localizing neuropsychologic syndromes in which patients become disoriented and get lost. Patients with parietal lobe dysfunction have difficulty with navigation in the environment (10). Other patients with amnestic syndrome may forget their place or lose their way within unfamiliar surroundings (11). The disoriented, confused wandering of these patients may be qualitatively unlike the hyperactive locomotion of other patients.

Wandering behavior also should be distinguished clinically from pacing behavior (12). Pacing follows a repetitive, fixed path in contrast to the more random, aimless course of wandering. Wandering behavior may occur as a manifestation of neuroleptic-induced akathisia. This extrapyramidal side effect of neuroleptic drugs produces motor restlessness that may result in random ambulation in demented patients.

MANAGEMENT

A detailed discussion of the psychopharmacologic management of behavioral symptoms in demented patients is beyond the scope of this chapter. Unfortunately, there are no clinical research data upon which to base a rational approach to the pharmacologic treatment of wandering behavior. Neuroleptics and benzodiazepines commonly are prescribed for wandering behavior (13). Very low dose neuroleptics (e.g., haloperidol 0.5–1.0 mg, once or twice a day) may reduce excessive locomotion and blunt resistance to redirection by caregivers. If wandering subsequently becomes exacerbated by akathisia, it is generally best to reduce the dose or discontinue the offending drug.

A number of relatively simple behavioral and environmental measures may assist the home-dwelling wandering patient. A schedule of regular exercise, especially walking, may reduce wandering (2,3). Adult day care may reduce the burden on family members. The patient should wear an identifying bracelet or necklace, and neighbors, police, and local entrepreneurs should be alerted (4,12). Deadbolt locks can be installed on doors and windows to prevent egress when direct observation cannot be maintained. Under these circumstances, exclusive access to a protected area such as a fenced-in backyard is often satisfactory (13). When these measures are insufficient and institutionalization is threatened, pharmacotherapy should be considered.

Some nursing home units have been specially equipped for wandering patients. Exit alarms, selectively activated by wandering patients, enable the staff to prevent egress without having to maintain constant observation or use restraints (4,9). Electronically locked doors that require intact cognitive abilities to open obviate physical intervention by the staff to prevent escape, also reducing the need for restraint (9).

Intervention by caregivers to limit and contain wandering requires considerable behavioral management skill. Redirection is often effective for the casually meandering wanderer. Redirection of patients who exhibit an affect-laden goal, however, may precipitate agitation and aggressive behavior. Such patients should be engaged casually by the caregiver who subtly should attempt to redirect the focus of attention (12). One author has recommended a two-person approach for empathically engaging the wanderer in order to supportively manipulate return to a protected environment (4).

BASIC SCIENCE

Dementia is a heterogeneous syndrome with numerous and varied neurobehavioral manifestations (14). The possibility that various behavioral subsyndromes of dementia might reflect more focal and localizable brain dysfunction deserves consideration. The current paucity of research data permits only speculative hypotheses to be made regarding the neuropsychiatric basis of wandering. Some evidence, however, is suggestive of possible brain–behavior correlations for this behavior.

De Leon et al suggested that wandering might represent a specific manifestation of parietal lobe dysfunction in patients with senile dementia of the Alzheimer type (9). In their study of 21 ambulatory, demented patients in a nursing home, wanderers evinced greater impairment on neuro-psychologic tests of parietal lobe function compared with nonwanderers. The wanderers in this study, however, did not exhibit a greater degree of overall cognitive impairment, challenging the view that severity of dementia alone explains this phenomenon. Limitations of this study, however, were that wandering was defined operationally as a navigational disturbance (i.e., route-finding deficit); cases were identified by staff report without operationalized inclusion criteria; and quantitative levels of locomotion were not reported. It was thus unclear whether this sample exhibited aimless ambulation and hyperactivity, or simply a tendency to get lost.

In contrast, Snyder et al conducted a behavioral mapping study in a skilled nursing facility in which wanderers were found to be in motion considerably more than non-wanderers (32.5% versus 4.2%, respectively) (3). These data suggest that this sample of wanderers was hyperkinetic compared with nonwandering controls. In this study, unfortunately, neuropsychologic data were not reported. Hypermotility and aimless locomotion, however, are known concomitants of ablation of the prefrontal cortex in animals (15).

Hyperkinetic locomotion is a common symptom of attention deficit hyperactivity disorder (ADHD), a child-hood syndrome (16). As a result of inattention, distractibil-ity, impulsivity, and hyperkinesis, affected children sometimes move about their environment in a manner that resembles wandering. Frontal lobe dysfunction has been implicated in the pathophysiology of ADHD (17). Wandering behavior in dementia and hyperkinesis in ADHD may share a common pathophysiology of hyperactivity associated with frontal lobe dysfunction; the former in a degenerative context, the latter in a developmental context.

Catecholamine dysfunction has been implicated in the pathophysiology of ADHD (18) and alterations of cate-cholamine neurochemistry have been observed in Alz-heimer's disease (19). Catecholaminergic systems include major contributions from ascending dopaminergic pathways. The importance of the nigrostriatal dopaminergic system in the organization of movement and its role in the patho-physiology of extrapyramidal movement disorders is well-established. The ascending mesolimbic and mesocortical dopaminergic systems, on the other hand, may serve impor-tant roles in the control of locomotor activity (20–23). The extrapyramidal signs seen in some patients with Alzheimer's disease may signify a subgroup with greater involvement of the nigrostriatal dopaminergic system (24,25). Wandering behavior in demented patients may similarly delineate a subgroup with greater local dysfunction of the frontal and frontolimbic dopaminergic systems that mediate control of motor activity.

CONCLUSIONS

Wandering behavior is a source of excess disability for patients suffering with dementing illness. Notwithstanding the added burden of care imposed by this behavior, and the primitive state of the art with regard to treatment, wandering has been the subject of only a few research studies. Wandering probably subsumes a number of neu-robehavioral phenomena in which control of locomotion within the environment is impaired in the face of demen-tia. Careful phenomenologic description of wandering sub-types is needed, therefore, if productive treatment research is to begin. The observation that some demented patients wander while others do not poses an important theoretic question that leads to a number of testable neuropsychiatric hypotheses. The investigation of the neuronal systems integrating the control of locomotion and other aspects of behavior in demented wanderers would be of heuristic value. Such investigations hopefully will result in more sophisticated strategies for the treatment of this behavioral disturbance.

REFERENCES

1. Burnside IM. Wandering behavior in psychosocial nursing care and the aged. 2nd ed. New York: McGraw-Hill, 1980.
2. Cornbleth T. Effects of a protected hospital ward area on wandering and nonwandering geriatric patients. J Gerontol 1977;32:573–577.
3. Snyder LH, Rupprecht P, Pyrek J, Brekhus S, Moss T. Wandering. Gerontologist 1978;18:272–280.
4. Monsour N, Robb SS. Wandering behavior in old age: A psychosocial study. Social Work 1982;27:411–416.
5. Dawson P, Reid DW. Behavioral dimensions of patients at risk of wandering. Gerontologist 1987;27:104–107.
6. Rosin AJ. The physical and behavioral complex of dementia. Gerontology 1977;23:37–46.
7. Zimmer JG, Watson N, Treat A. Behavioral problems among patients in skilled nursing facilities. Am J Public Health 1984;74:1118–1121.
8. Rovner BW, Kafonek S, Filipp L, et al. Prevalence of mental illness in a community nursing home. Am J Psychiatry 1986;143:1446–1449.
9. de Leon MJ, Portegal M, Gurland B. Wandering and parietal signs in senile dementia of Alzheimer's type. Neuropsychobiology 1984;11:155–157.
10. Ratcliff G, Newcombe F. Spatial orientation in man: Effects of left, right, and bilateral posterior cerebral lesions. J Neurol Neurosurg Psychiatry 1973;36:448–454.
11. Kopelman MD. Amnesia: Organic and psychogenic. Br J Psychiatry 1987;150:428–442.
12. Heim KM. Wandering behavior. J Gerontol Nursing 1986;12:4–7.
13. Winograd CH, Jarvik LF. Physician management of the demented patient. J Geriatr Soc 1986;34:295–308.

14. Cummings JL, Benson DF. Dementia: a clinical approach. Boston: Butterworths, 1983.
15. Fuster JM. The prefrontal cortex. Anatomy, physiology, and neuropsychology of the frontal lobe. New York: Raven, 1980:58–65.
16. American Psychiatric Association. Diagnostic and statistical manual of mental disorders. 3rd ed, revised. Washington: American Psychiatric Association, 1987.
17. Lou HC, Henriksen L, Bruhn P. Focal cerebral hypoperfusion in children with dysphasia and/or attention deficit disorder. Arch Neurol 1984;41:825–829.
18. Zametkin AJ, Rapoport JL. The pathophysiology of attention deficit disorder with hyperactivity. In: Kazdin A, Lahey B, eds. Advances in clinical child psychology. New York: Plenum, 1986:177–216.
19. Sparks DL, Markesbery WR, Slevin JT. Alzheimer's disease: monoamines and spiperone binding reduced in nucleus basalis. Ann Neurol 1986;19:602–604.
20. Iverson SD, Koob GF. Behavioral implications of dopaminergic neurons in the mesolimbic system. Advances Biochem Psychopharmacol 1977;16:209–214.
21. Freed CR, Yamamoto BK. Regional brain dopamine metabolism: a marker for the speed, direction, and posture of moving animals. Science 1985;229:62–65.
22. Ungerstedt U, Ljungberg T. Behavioral patterns related to dopamine neurotransmission: Effect of acute and chronic antipsychotic drugs. Adv Biochem Psychopharmacol 1977;16:193–199.
23. Le Moal M, Galey D, Cardo B. Behavioral effects of local injection of 6-hydroxydopamine in the medial ventral tegmentum in the rat. Possible role of the mesolimbic dopaminergic system. Brain Res 1975;88:190–194.
24. Molsa PK, Marttila RJ, Rinne UK. Extrapyramidal signs in Alzheimer's disease. Neurology 1984;34:1114–1116.
25. Chui HC, Teng EL, Henderson VW, et al. Clinical subtypes of dementia of the Alzheimer type. Neurology 1985;35:1544–1550.

Senile Gait Disorders

NAGAGOPAL VENNA   THOMAS D. SABIN

INTRODUCTION

Although gait disorders in the elderly were clearly recognized over 50 years ago (1), it is only recently that they are beginning to be systematically studied (2–4). Persistent disturbances of gait are common in the elderly (5) and greatly affect the quality of their lives: the common fear of falling restricts physical activity and contributes to poor self-esteem, loneliness, depression, and social isolation. Falls, a frequent consequence of gait imbalance, only too regularly trigger a series of downhill events, such as fracture of osteoporotic femurs, enforced immobility, pulmonary embolism, pneumonia, subdural hematoma, and often a precipitous decline in the general function of the individual.

Such gait disorders are a heterogenous group of widely different etiologies. Some of them are peculiar to aging, others have predilection to old age, while still others affect a wide range of ages. The principal locus of pathology may be in the musculoskeletal system, peripheral nerves, spinal cord, cerebellum or cerebral hemispheres, but frequently multifocal abnormalities are encountered (Table 44.1). This chapter focuses on the idiopathic senile gait disorder (SGD) with briefer discussions of related conditions.

IDIOPATHIC SENILE GAIT DISORDER

A gait disorder without weakness, ataxia, or sensory loss in the limbs and peculiar to the elderly was identified in 1931 by Critchley in his comprehensive review of the neurology of old age (1). Subsequent sporadic studies of the condition have not particularly enlightened our understanding of the disorder. Within the last two decades, however, Sudarsky and Ronthal (2) made a systematic clinical and laboratory study of these gait disorders and defined several subgroups including one without identifiable cause that they termed "idio-

pathic SGD." Koller et al (3), in a clinical and brain computerized tomographic (CT) imaging study, further reinforced the concept of SGD as a distinct entity, but of unclear pathogenesis. Many hypotheses have been put forward to explain SGD but firm proof for its anatomic and physiologic basis has not been mustered. Innovations in therapy have been rudimentary.

CLINICAL PICTURE

The clinical spectrum extends from ill-defined instability of the body to total inability to walk. The difficulty in walking begins imperceptibly in people mostly over 65 years of age. Patients complain of a vague sense of instability while standing and walking. Fear of falling is often prominent and sometimes disabling in itself. Some patients complain of a tendency to fall back easily. The gait worsens gradually over several years so that patients may eventually be wheelchair bound. The course may be punctuated by abrupt and precipitous deterioration of gait by even brief immobility enforced by intercurrent illness such as a pneumonia or a fracture. Exposure to neuroactive drugs such as sedatives tend to readily impair the gait further. Urinary incontinence and limb paresthesias are not characteristic and most patients do not show accompanying cognitive decline.

On examination, patients demonstrate a reluctance to stand or walk, sometimes strikingly out of proportion to their actual ability to do so. The patients tend to steady themselves by grabbing the examiner and are unwilling to let go and may appear panicked. The base is wide and the steps short, slow, deliberate, and uncertain. Postural instability can be shown by the patient's tendency to fall back readily when gently pushed back but usually resist forward displacement well. There is often a flexed posture of trunk and decrease in arm swing while walking. There is no weak-

Table 44.1 Differential Diagnosis of SGD

Musculoskeletal diseases
Polymyalgia rheumatica
Proximal myopathies

Peripheral nerve disorders
Symmetric polyneuropathies
Diabetic amyotrophy
Lumbar spinal stenosis with claudication of cauda equina

Spinal cord syndromes
Compressive myelopathies
    Cervical spondylotic myelopathy
    Spinal cord tumors in the elderly
Noncompressive myelopathies
    Subacute combined degeneration due to vitamin B_{12} deficiency

Cerebral disorders
Idiopathic NPH
Aqueductal stenosis
Binswanger's subcortical arteriosclerotic encephalopathy
SDH
Multisensory gait disorder
Drug-induced gait disorders
Cerebellar syndrome
Extrapyramidal syndromes
Myxedema with ataxia
Idiopathic SGD

ness or ataxia of the lower limbs. Sensory examination may reveal only decrease in the perception of vibration of a tuning fork over the lower limbs. Ankle reflexes are often diminished or absent and occasionally plantar responses may be upgoing. Mental status examination usually does not reveal dementia.

There are no laboratory abnormalities that are specific to SGD. Brain CT and magnetic resonance imaging (MRI) reveal some enlargement of cerebral cortical sulci and of the lateral ventricles that overlap with changes seen in asymptomatic elderly persons. Laboratory tests are useful, chiefly to exclude other etiologies of gait disorders.

NEUROBIOLOGIC ASPECTS OF SGD

Firm anatomic basis for SGD has not been established beyond the fact that there are no gross abnormalities visible in the brain and spinal cord as imaged by CT and MRI. There are no comprehensive pathologicoanatomic studies of the central and peripheral neuromuscular apparatus in well-defined cases of idiopathic SGD especially to look for microscopic abnormalities of the motor systems. There have been no reports of physiologic brain imaging such as positron emission tomography (PET) in SGD. No neurochemical analyses have been published looking for deficiencies of neurotransmitters, such as dopamine in the different brain regions involved in motor function, akin to the Parkinson's disease model. Recently, vestibular function

was comprehensively investigated in 26 elderly persons with dysequilibrium of unknown etiology and age-matched controls. Seven patients had marked bilateral decrease of vestibular function, presumed to be due to age-related changes in the peripheral vestibular organs and in the vestibular nuclei. This indicates that in a subset of patients with SGD, vestibular abnormalities may play a significant role (6).

Most hypotheses regarding the mechanism of SGD have focused on cerebral derangements (7). The frontal lobes have often been implicated and SGD is frequently, if loosely, described as an example of "frontal ataxia." However, there is no convincing evidence to attribute SGD to frontal lobe dysfunction. Ataxia of gait in association with frontal lobe tumors was described by Bruns in 1892 (8). In these cases, however, it was difficult to separate the mass effect of the large tumors with many distant effects by distortion of other brain structures, such as the frontopontocerebellar networks. Furthermore, Meyer (9) found no gait disturbances in his thorough study of patients who underwent frontal leukotomies where frontopontine fibers were severed, thus casting doubt on the concept of frontal ataxia independent of mass effect.

Patients with other frontal lobe diseases affecting the premotor areas do develop a disorder of gait that has been called "gait apraxia" not explainable by any loss of elementary neurologic functions (10). However, the gait disorder in these instances is different from SGD. There is marked difficulty in starting to walk. There may be a burst of small steps starting off that has been described as "the slipping clutch syndrome." Once up, the patient appears glued to the floor and sways sideways to lift the foot off the floor and then takes a few small steps. With more walking, steps become longer. Gegenhalten, or "counter holding" in the limbs, palmar and plantar grasp reflexes, frontal lobe type of behavioral disinhibition, dementia, and abnormal bladder and bowel continence accompany these syndromes. Gegenhalten is a peculiar disturbance of muscle tone of the limbs: when the patient is instructed to let a limb become limp, the examiner notes normal resistance to passive movements of the joint. Soon, however, a resistance to the movement builds up in concert with the amount of force used by the examiner. When the examiner desists, the increased muscle tone melts away. This is often mistaken for uncooperativeness of the patient. Denny-Brown (11) attributed this form of frontal gait disorder to the release of the patient's foot grasp reflexes by contact with the floor, leading to a magnetic foot grasp response. These characteristics are absent in idiopathic SGD.

Fisher (12) felt that monosymptomatic SGD is indeed an early stage of normal-pressure hydrocephalus (NPH) based on his study of several patients by clinical and CT criteria and by the response to ventriculoperitoneal cerebrospinal fluid (CSF) shunting. This contention is controversial at present. Koller et al (3) do not agree with such formulation because ventriculomegaly was not found in most of their patients with SGD.

The extrapyramidal basal ganglionic structures were also implicated in SGD. Critchley attributed SGD to age-related dysfunction of the basal ganglia (1). Barbeau (13) considered age-related dopamine deficiency in the genesis of SGD, an idea suggested by sprinkling of postural changes and bradykinesia seen in SGD.

Sabin (4) proposed a novel pathogenesis for SGD emphasizing the role of a peripheral neuropathy of aging. He argued that the dampened or absent ankle reflexes and the diminished vibratory perception in the lower extremities in the aged are in fact signs of a peripheral neuropathy, with selective involvement of the large diameter fibers such as the IA muscle spindle afferents subserving the tendon reflex arc and proprioception. As most peripheral neuropathies affect the longest axons first, the axons to the muscles of the anterior tibial compartment that are much longer than those of the posterior tibial compartment would be affected earlier. This causes a differential denervation of the muscle spindles of the anterior compared with the posterior compartment muscles of the legs. This in turn leads to constantly varying erroneous proprioceptive input into the central nervous system from the muscle spindles of lower extremities and may cause the sense of imbalance experienced by the patient with SGD ("spindle vertigo"). The tonic relatively excessive spindle input from the posterior compartment muscles of the legs would also explain the patient's tendency to fall backwards.

From the above discussion, it is clear that a great deal of basic work needs to be done in understanding the anatomic as well as physiologic mechanisms of SGD.

DIFFERENTIAL DIAGNOSIS

In evaluating a patient with possible SGD, a wide differential diagnosis (Tables 44.1 and 44.2) needs to be considered because the clinical picture is not unique and there are no laboratory findings that unequivocally identify it.

Musculoskeletal Disorders

Skeletal and joint disorders such as severe spinal, hip, and knee osteoarthritis, which are common among the elderly, can impair gait and should be evident on physical examination. Incapacitating periarticular shoulder girdle and hip girdle pain and muscle tenderness and painful limitation of joint movements, accompanied by lassitude and anorexia characterize polymyalgia rheumatica (14), a disorder most commonly seen in the elderly. The resulting gait difficulty is subacute and painful. Careful examination will demonstrate that the proximal muscles are not weak though the muscle strength testing may be difficult because of pain. The erythrocyte sedimentation rate is markedly elevated, typically over 80 mm/h. Serum muscle enzymes and muscle biopsy are normal. This syndrome overlaps giant cell temporal arteritis, which causes subacute headaches and can lead to unilateral or bilateral visual loss. When occurring without

Table 44.2   Examinations Useful in the Evaluation of SGD

History
Neuroactive drug ingestion including over the counter medications and
    antivertiginous medications

Physical examination
Visual system
Musculoskeletal system
Neurologic system
Gait and balance

Mental status examination
Cognitive function
Behavioral changes

Blood tests
Complete blood count
Erythrocyte sedimentation rate
Serum vitamin B_{12}
Serum T4 and thyroid-stimulating hormone
Blood toxic screen for neuroactive drugs: e.g., benzodiazepines, barbiturates

Neuroimaging
Brain CT or MRI scans
Spinal MRI scan
Radioisotope cisternography

the component of temporal arteritis, polymyalgia rheumatica responds in a dramatic fashion to low-dose adrenal corticosteroids. In association with temporal arteritis high-dose corticosteroids are essential to prevent blindness.

Myopathy

Proximal myopathies, of many etiologies, can occur in the elderly and cause subacute or chronic gait disorders. Raising out of chairs and climbing stairs are particularly difficult. Symmetric weakness of hip girdle and shoulder girdle muscles are characteristic. Myopathic basis is confirmed by elevated serum creatine phosphokinase, electromyography, and muscle biopsy.

Peripheral Neuropathies and Proximal Neuropathies

Elderly patients with diabetes are prone to develop the subacute syndrome of diabetic amyotrophy (15,16) that can cause severe painful gait difficulty especially when it is bilateral. This is due to proximal neuropathy of the lower extremities. Often the diabetes is previously unrecognized and mild. Hip and thigh pain, usually unilateral but sometimes asymmetrically bilateral, is prominent. This is followed over days or weeks by wasting and weakness of gluteal and thigh muscles with depressed knee reflex and occasional Babinski response. When bilateral, these physical signs are asymmetric and can cause severe disability in walking because of the weakness of knee extensions and hip flexors and consequent inability to stabilize the knees. Marked weight loss may accompany this syndrome. Spontaneous recovery over six months to two years is the rule. Symmetric distal neuropathic syndromes of diverse etiologies can be recognized by symmetric stocking and glove pattern of sensory loss, loss of ankle and knee reflexes, and symmetric distal weakness, and can be confirmed by nerve conduction velocity measurements.

Another disorder, particularly relevant to the elderly that causes pain and difficulty in walking is the syndrome of lumbar spinal canal stenosis with neurogenic claudication (17). Degenerative changes of spondylosis affect multiple levels of the lumbar spine causing hypertrophy of facet joints, osteophytic overgrowth from vertebral bodies, and hypertrophy of ligamentum flavum. This leads to crowding of the lumbosacral nerve roots of the cauda equina. Elderly patients present with chronic history of months to years of deep pain and discomfort often asymmetric in gluteal and thigh regions, numbing paresthesias of the buttocks and lower extremities, and rubbery weakness of legs. These symptoms are characteristically induced by standing erect and walking (pseudoclaudication syndrome) and are relieved by lying down. Unlike aortofemoral occlusive disease, patients can bicycle bent forward without pain. Patients may accommodate to the pain by progressively decreasing their walking. Physical examination is often deceptively normal though root distribution sensory, motor, and reflex changes can be induced and symptoms reproduced by walking. Imaging of the spine by CT and MRI scans are diagnostic. Many patients obtain good relief of limb pain and experience increase in pain-free walking following multilevel lumbar spinal decompressive surgery.

Myelopathies

Several spinal cord syndromes cause major chronic abnormalities of gait. An unsteady gait may occur without actual weakness of the extremities. Myelopathic basis of the patient's gait disorder is recognized by spasticity, brisk tendon reflexes, Babinski responses, and upper motor neuron pattern of muscle weakness often combined with sensory abnormalities. Characteristic sensory changes are loss of proprioception to joint position sense and in more advanced cases impaired sensation to pinprick and transverse level on the trunk and bladder and bowel dyscontrol. In some patients this is combined with signs of peripheral neuropathy with absent ankle reflexes (neuromyelopathy).

Chronic compression of the spinal cord should be ruled out in this situation. Spinal cord pathology is generally neglected as a cause of SGD and treatable etiologies may be overlooked while attention is distracted by search for cerebral basis of gait difficulty. Sudarsky and Ronthal (2) found 16% of their patients with SGD had myelopathies. A common cause of this in the elderly is cervical spondylosis (18). However, in view of almost ubiquitous occurrence of spondylotic changes in cervical spine of the elderly on radi-

ography, other means are needed to establish the causal relationship between these and the myelopathy. The MRI now is being helpful in this by showing not only the bones and disc but also their mechanical effects of compression on the spinal cord.

An overlooked and unusual cause of chronic compressive myelopathy in the elderly is that due to meningiomas (19). These show a predilection to women and to the thoracic region and may masquerade as idiopathic SGD for many years with ataxic gait, without much weakness. These are eminently treatable by surgery even with signs of fairly advanced myelopathy. MRI of the spine and/or CT metrazamide myelography should readily identify these lesions.

The most important medical myelopathy in the elderly is subacute combined degeneration of the spinal cord due to vitamin B_{12} deficiency—a well-established clinicopathologic entity. It is characterized by demyelination affecting principally the cervical and thoracic dorsal and lateral columns, and sometimes the cerebral white matter. Symptoms evolve over months or several years with a preponderance of tingling, numbness paresthesias, often beginning in the hands. An ataxia of gait, which is worse in darkness, appears gradually and is due to impairment of proprioceptive input from lower limbs. Loss of joint position sense in distal extremities is a striking finding along with a sharply positive Romberg sign. Upper motor neuron signs of spasticity, Babinski reflexes, and peripheral neuropathic signs of absence of ankle reflexes may be superimposed along with a variety of changes in mental function from emotional instability to psychosis or dementia. Usually, the diagnosis is readily established by the presence of macrocytic anemia, megaloblastic change of the bone marrow, hypersegmented neutrophils in the peripheral blood smear, and a low plasma B_{12} level. However, occasionally anemia may be completely absent (20). Moreover, falsely normal serum B_{12} may be seen by radiodilution technique when in fact the active B_{12} is low. Thus when strongly suspected on clinical grounds, even in the presence of normal serum B_{12} levels, hematology consultation should be obtained to evaluate deficiency of B_{12} by the Schilling test, scrutiny of blood smear for hypersegmentation of neutrophils, and repeating of serum B_{12} levels by radiodilution using a purified intrinsic factor. Recently, the estimations of blood and urine levels of methylmalonic acid and homocystine have become widely available and appear to be sensitive biochemical markers of vitamin B_{12} deficiency; the elevated levels return to normal with therapy (20). As it is eminently treatable but full recovery depends on the duration of the disease, early diagnosis and early institution of therapy with parenteral B_{12} is essential.

CEREBRAL CAUSES OF SGD

In the elderly several well-defined disorders of the brain produce a syndrome in which a chronic gait disorder is a cardinal symptom, and thus need to be evaluated in consideration of SGD.

Hydrocephalic Syndromes

The syndrome of NPH is a well-recognized entity. In recent years a similar syndrome with chronic gait imbalance and bilateral upper motor neuron signs, variable occurrence of cognitive impairment, and urinary incontinence has been recognized due to nontumoral stenosis of the cerebral aqueduct (21). This presumably congenital abnormality may become symptomatic for the first time in the elderly (22), although the mechanism is uncertain. Brain CT images show prominent lateral and third ventricles with a normal fourth ventricle. Radioisotope cisternography reveals a normal pattern of absence of ventricular reflux, in contrast to the ventricular reflux and ventricular stasis of radioisotope NPH. MRI scan with sagittal views may reveal the narrowed aqueduct. Many patients respond to ventriculoperitoneal shunting or other modalities of CSF drainage.

Binswanger's Disease

Although first described briefly by Binswanger in 1894 (23) and established as a neuropathologic entity of Olszewski in 1962 (24), this disorder remained obscure until the last decade when it became increasingly recognized with the application of CT and especially MRI of the brain in elderly people. Pathologically there is widespread destruction of myelin and axons of the subcortical white matter of the cerebral hemispheres in the periventricular and supraventricular regions with only a few lacunar infarcts in basal ganglia; the cerebral cortical mantle is spared. The small arteries and arterioles perfusing the subcortical white matter show severe and widespread arteriosclerotic stenosis indicating an ischemic basis for this leukoencephalopathy.

The clinical picture (25) evolves against a background of chronic often unrecognized hypertension in the elderly, with a gradual gait deterioration (26) accompanied by a variety of mental status changes from mood disturbances to dementia and abulia. The course is often punctuated by step-like deteriorations with hemipareses or bulbar symptoms. The slow broadbased spastic gait is often accompanied by signs of hemiparesis and bilateral upper motor neuron signs. Extrapyramidal features such as bradykinesia may be an additional component. Lability of emotional expression with outbursts of crying, rarely laughing, and variable dementia are commonly seen. CT and especially MRI of the brain show striking confluent lucencies (hyperintensities on MRI) in the white matter surrounding and above the lateral ventricles of both cerebral hemispheres, often with lacunar infarcts in the basal ganglia. The radiologic changes above may occur with aging as well as with primary degenerative dementias in the elderly and are not specific for

Binswanger's disease. The term *leukoaraiosis* was coined for the radiographic finding by Hachinski et al to underline such a concept (27). Although no definite therapy is available at present, avoidance of very tight regulation of hypertension and prevention of postural hypotension seem to improve function and appear desirable in the elderly with this syndrome.

Subdural Hematoma (SDH)

Subacute and chronic intracranial SDH are well known to be particularly common in the elderly and often occur without history of head trauma. Subacute or chronic disturbance of gait with unsteadiness is one of the myriad presentations of this condition and has been described with unilateral as well as bilateral SDH (28,29). An unsteady gait, bilateral upper motor neuron signs often accompanied by some dementia and bradykinesia, mimick NPH syndrome, or cerebellar syndrome, or "gait apraxia" (29). The syndrome evolves over a few weeks to a few months and often is unassociated with evidence of increased intracranial pressure. Brain CT and MRI scans readily identify the lesions. However, in the subacute phase of SDH, when the lesions are bilateral, the hematomas may not be discerned by the CT scans because they are isodense with the brain. In fact the CT scan may appear "hypernormal" in the sense of showing small ventricles and small cortical sulci, while in the elderly we expect some dilation of the lateral ventricles and of the sulci. Gratifying improvement in gait and other abnormalities is the rule after evacuation of the SDH.

Multisensory Deficits

In their evaluation of 50 elderly patients with chronic gait disorders, Sudarsky and Ronthal (2) found 18% of patients in whom the gait disorder seemed to be due to a combination of sensory deprivations such as impaired vision, impaired vestibular function, and decreased proprioception in extremities due to peripheral neuropathy. It would appear that these deficits were insufficient to explain the gait imbalance singly, but together seemed to be responsible for the gait disturbance similar to those patients described by Drachman and Hart (30) in their paper on dizziness.

Cerebellar Syndromes

A variety of etiologies can cause cerebellar dysfunction. Cerebellar syndromes are recognized by broadbased unsteady gait, truncal instability demonstrated while sitting unsupported at the edge of the bed, and by the characteristic side-to-side leg tremor or heel-to-shin test. In some instances, similar incoordination is seen in upper limbs and may be accompanied by scanning dysarthria.

Extrapyramidal Syndromes

Gait disorder is a cardinal symptom of extrapyramidal syndromes many of which, such as Parkinson's disease and progressive supranuclear palsy, are predominantly diseases of the elderly. These are discussed in separate chapters. Limb, truncal and cervicofacial rigidity, bradykinesia, rest tremor, and ocular mobility abnormalities permit clinical identification of these entities.

Hypothyroidism and Gait Ataxia

A few cases of gait ataxia were described in association with myxedema (31), although this association does not seem to be unequivocally established. Ataxia is said to resolve with thyroxine replacement. In view of the prevalence of hypothyroidism in the elderly and the ease of treatment, it seems prudent to evaluate patients with SGD for hypothyroidism.

Drug-Induced Gait Disorders

The gait as well as mental functions of elderly patients are particularly susceptible to derangements by a variety of neuroactive drugs, often in doses that are not toxic to younger people. In view of the widespread use of neuroactive drugs in the elderly, particular attention needs to be paid to drug-related causes of SGD as they are eminently reversible (32).

Benzodiazepines (33), tricyclic antidepressant drugs, phenothiazines and antihypertensives, and barbiturates are often implicated in gait ataxia and falls in the elderly (34). Postural hypotension, extrapyramidal syndrome, and sedation related to the drugs indicate the gait disturbance in some patients. Salicylate intoxication and anticonvulsant drugs can also cause gait imbalance.

MANAGEMENT OF IDIOPATHIC SGD

At present there is no specific treatment for SGD, a state that reflects our ignorance of its pathophysiology and the lack of creative therapeutic trials.

Symptomatic treatments, however, are sometimes helpful. Gait training by physical therapists with particular interest in the elderly seem to be helpful when the patient is strongly motivated. The usefulness of such measures is supported by a recent study of multifactorial intervention in persons over the age of 70 with history of falls. The 301 people studied had different risk factors for falls that included sedative drugs and polypharmacy of lower limb dysfunction, and many had gait impairment. Adjustments of drugs were made and home physical therapy with gait training, teaching of transfer skills, and balance and limb strength exercises were given in comparison to a control group of usual health care and social visits. At the end of one year,

35% of the treated group experienced falls compared to 47% of the control group. The difference is even more marked when risk factors of gait and balance impairment were considered separately (35). Tai chi exercises are another strategy for improving balance in the elderly.

It is common clinical experience, however, that vigorous physical therapy is helpful in preventing the rapid gait deterioration that is seen in patients with SGD when they are restricted to bed or chair by intercurrent illness.

Correction of visual impairment seems sensible as visual input is of major importance in normal gait stability; a subject that has not been specifically studied in SGD.

Patients with SGD are especially susceptible to the ataxic effects of neuroactive drugs, even in small doses (33). Benzodiazepines, barbiturates, phenothiazines, tricyclic antidepressants, antihypertensive drugs, anticonvulsants, and antivertigo drugs are among those that can worsen SGD and should be avoided or used with extreme caution in patients to prevent worsening of gait ataxia and falls.

The role of CSF shunting in SGD is controversial. Fisher (12) felt that in his series of elderly patients with monosymptomatic gait disorder and associated enlargement of lateral ventricles that did not qualify as conventional cases of NPH syndrome, ventriculoperitoneal (VP) shunting improved gait in most patients. This recommendation remains controversial; others find that SGD is not specifically related to CT evident hydrocephalus and do not agree with the invasive procedure of VP shunting (3).

An alternative procedure that is less invasive and has fewer serious complications than shunting, is large volume lumbar punctures. Fisher (12) and others reported improvement of gait after 30–40 ml of CSF removal by lumbar puncture in patients with NPH and in patients with apparent SGD with equivocal hydrocephalus determined by CT. It seems a reasonable procedure for patients with a serious degree of SGD with equivocally large lateral ventricles. If improvement does occur it may well be feasible to perform repeated lumbar punctures in some patients. A study of this approach needs to be done prospectively. Intensive evaluation of the patients and their living environment by physical and occupational therapists can help minimize falls.

FUTURE DIRECTIONS

There is urgent need for careful microscopic and regional neurochemical analyses of cortical and peripheral neuromuscular systems including the innervation of the lower extremity muscle spindles of patients with well-defined SGD. Prospective studies of the natural history of the disease are needed.

Therapeutic trials with replacement of neurotransmitters, such as dopamine agonists would help determine if dopamine deficiency is significant in SGD.

Bioengineering techniques could be applied to the gait disorder to develop devices that would give an auditory signal when a dangerous degree of instability develops while walking, thus decreasing falls. Similar techniques can be applied to test the hypothesis of imbalanced propioceptive input from the anterior compared with the posterior compartment muscles of lower extremities by using a device that can equalize the large fiber proprioceptive input from these compartments.

A multidisciplinary approach is essential so that the combined expertise of neurologists, physical medicine rehabilitation specialists, gait analysts, and bioengineers interested in gait can be applied to this common and challenging problem of the elderly.

Another interesting concept that needs to be explored is that of prevention of SGD by regular exercise in the elderly. This is suggested by the observation that older men who have a physically active lifestyle with activities like jogging have reaction times and movement times that are no different from college age men who are not involved in regular physical exercise (36). Prospective studies are needed to test this hypothesis.

A recent study identifying a subgroup of elderly asymptomatic persons who subsequently went on to mobility-related and daily living impairments is of particular interest in this context. Among 1,122 nondisabled subjects older than 70, those with the lowest scores on certain physical performance measures were four times more likely to have disability at the four-year follow-up. The measures were readily tested at the bedside: assessment of standing balance, a timed eight-foot walk at normal pace, and a timed test of five repetitions of rising from a chair and sitting down. Such a group would be suitable for a prospective study of interventions such as exercise, a tai chi program, and gait and balance therapy (37).

REFERENCES

1. Critchley M. The neurology of old age. Lancet 1931;ii:1221–1230.
2. Sudarsky L, Ronthal M. Gait disorders in elderly patients. Arch Neurol 1983;40:740–743.
3. Koller WC, Glatt SL, Fox JH. Senile gait a distinct neurological entity. Clin Geriatr Med 1985;1:661–669.
4. Sabin T. Biological aspects of falls and mobility limitation in the elderly. J Am Geriatr Soc 1982;30:51–58.
5. Sixt E, Landahl S. Postural disturbances in a 75-year-old population. I. Prevalence and functional consequences. Age Ageing 1987;16:393–398.
6. Fife TD, Baloh RW. Disequilibrium of unknown cause in older people. Ann Neurol 1993;34:694–702.
7. Nutt JG, Marsden CD, Thompson PD. Human walking and higher level gait disorders, particularly in the elderly. Neurology 1993;43:268–279.
8. Bruns L. Uber storumgen des gleichgewichtes bei stirmhirmtumoven. Dtsch Med Wochenschr 1892;18:138.
9. Meyer R. The human fronto-pontine tract: functional insignificance of surgical interruption. Neurology 1951;1:341–356.
10. Gerstman J, Schilder P. Uber eine besondere gaugstorung bei stienhirnerkankungen. Wien Med Wochenschr 1926;76:97.
11. Denny-Brown D. The nature of apraxis. J Nerv Med Dis 1958;216:9.
12. Fisher CM. Hydrocephalus as a cause of disturbance of gait in the elderly. Neurology 1982;32:1358–1363.
13. Barbeau A. Aging and the extrapyramidal system. J Am Geriatr Soc 1973;21:1415–1419.
14. Healy LA, Wilski KR. Polymyalgia rheumatica and giant cell arteritis (medical progress). West J Med 1984;141:64–67.
15. Asbury AK. Proximal diabetic neuropathy. Ann Neurol 1977;2:179–180.
16. Chokroverty S, Reyes MG, Rubino FA, Tonaki H. The syndrome of diabetic amyotrophy. Ann Neurol 1977;2:181–194.
17. Hall S, Bartleso JD, Onofrio BM, et al. Lumbar spinal stenosis: clinical features, diagnostic procedures and results of surgical treatment in 68 patients. Ann Intern Med 1985;103:271–275.
18. Murray PK. Cervical spondylotic myelopathy: A cause of gait disturbance and urinary incontinence in older persons. J Am Geriatr Soc 1984;32:324–330.
19. Huang CY, Matheson J. Spinal cord tumors in the elderly. Aust NZ J Med 1979;9:538–544.
20. Lindenbaum J, Healton EB, Savage DG, et al. Neuropsychiatric disorders caused by cobalamin deficiency in the absence of anemia or macrocytosis. N Engl J Med 1988;318:1720–1728.
21. Vanneste V, Hyman R. Nontumoral aqueduct stenosis and normal pressure hydrocephalus in the elderly. J Neurol Neurosurg Psychiatry 1986;49:529–535.
22. Harrison MJG, Robert CM, Uttley D. Benign aqueductal stenosis in adults. J Neurol Psychiatry 1974;37:1322–1328.
23. Binswanger O. Die abgrenzung der allgemeinen progressiven paralyse. Berl Klin Wochenschr 1894;31:1103–1105, 1137–1139, 1180–1186.
24. Olszewski J. Subcortical arteriosclerotic encephalopathy. World Neurol 1965;3:359–374.
25. Caplan LR, Schoene WC. Clinical features of subcortical arteriosclerotic encephalopathy (Binswanger's disease). Neurology 1978;28:1206–1215.
26. Thompson PD, Marsden CD. Gait disorders of subcortical arteriosclerotic encephalopathy: Binswanger's Disease. Mov Disord 1987;2:1–8.
27. Hachinski VC, Potter P, Merskey H. Leuko-araiosis. Arch Neurol 1897;44:21–23.
28. Jacobson PL, Farmer TW. The "hypernormal" CT scan in dementia: Bilateral isodense subdural hematomas. Neurology 1979;29:1522–1524.
29. McLachlan RS, Bolton CF, Coates RK, Barnett HJM. Gait disturbance in chronic subdural hematoma. Can Med Assoc J 1981;125:865–868.
30. Drachman D, Hart C. An approach to the dizzy patient. Neurology 1972;22:323–334.
31. Price TR, Netsky MG. Myxedema and ataxia. Neurology 1966;16:957–962.
32. Macdonald JB. The role of drugs in falls in the elderly. Clin Geriatr Med 1985;1:621–636.
33. Salzman C. A primer on geriatric psychopharmacology. Am J Psychiatry 1982;139:67–74.
34. Dane JW, Blumenthal MD, Robinson-Hawkins S. A model of risk of falling for psychogeriatric patients. Arch Gen Psychiatry 1981;38:463–467.
35. Tinetti ME, Baker D, McAvay G, et al. A multifactorial intervention to reduce the risk of falling among elderly people living in the community. N Engl J Med 1994;331:821–827.
36. Spirduso WW. Physical fitness, aging and psychomotor speed: a review. J Gerontol 1980;35:850.
37. Guralnik JM, Ferrucci L, Simonsick E, et al. Lower extremity function in persons over the age of 70 years as a predictor of subsequent disability. N Engl J Med 1995;332:556–561.

Disorders of Movement Associated with Diseases of the Cerebellum

RAYMOND D. ADAMS   MARIA SALAM-ADAMS

INTRODUCTION

The function of the cerebellum has always been somewhat of an enigma. Perched astride the brainstem and constituting more than 10% of the human brain and serving as an integrating center for a vast array of sensory and motor systems, the effects of disease localized within it have been less than predictable. Not infrequently a developmental defect or a crude cerebellar lesion has been found in a patient who is said to have exhibited no disorder of motor function. In other instances, a cerebellar disease occasioned a lasting and severe disability or an acute destructive lesion has deranged function only temporarily, as though compensatory mechanisms had been capable of correcting the deficit.

There is good reason to believe that the cerebellum is an essential part of the motor system by the clinical evidence of derangements of stance, locomotion, ocular control, speech, and learned and planned movements of the extremities that result from disease. Uniformity of histologic structure suggests that whatever its function may be it is exercised uniformly on all of the musculature. But for a long time the specification of its contribution to movement proved to be elusive or at most esoteric. The classic anatomic studies by Larsell (1), Dow (2), and Brodal and Jansen (3) indicated a tripartite division in the distribution of its coordinating effects. And this has been borne out by the physiologic studies of Luciani (4), Moruzzi (5), Snider and Eldred (6), and Fulton (7) of animals whose cerebella had been partially or completely ablated. Always, however, there was uncertainty as to whether these anatomicophysiologic correlations, even those derived from studies of primates, were applicable to humans.

In comparatively recent times, advances in neurophysiologic methodology have begun to expose in both primates and humans the details of the functional disorders of movement resulting from diseases of different parts of the cerebellum. The articles and monographs by Gilman et al (8), Everts and Thach (9), Hallett et al (10), and Marsden et al (11) present the newest information on cerebellar function and describe also the many problems yet to be resolved. For an account of the historical development of our knowledge of the cerebellum, the reader should consult the monographs of Dow (2) and Larsell (1).

The focus of this chapter is on the degenerative diseases of the human cerebellum and the topic will be introduced by a brief review of the symptomatology of these diseases and their presumed anatomic and physiologic bases.

It is generally conceded that although the basic neuronal circuitry in all parts of the cerebellar cortex and central nuclei is the same, the functions of the flocculonodular lobe with its vestibular connections (vestibulocerebellum), the anterior and posterior vermis and anterior lobe with its spinocerebellar and cerebelloparietal lobe connections (spinocerebellum), and the lateral hemispheres with their corticopontoneocerebellar (cerebrocerebellum) connections are sufficiently different to justify separate consideration.

As would be expected, the main function of the vestibulocerebellum is to maintain equipoise or equilibrium of the body, that is, to coordinate the movements of head, neck, trunk, and limbs to maintain the body in three planes of space. Lesions limited to the nodulus and flocculi result in an ataxic gait while leaving limb movements properly coordinated. It appears that the axial musculature is then incapable of reacting to the influx of unconscious information coming from the proprioceptive apparatus, the utricles, sacculae, and semicircular canals. The medullablastoma, which tends to arise in the nodulus, is often cited as the prime example of a lesion more or less restricted to this part of the cerebellum.

In primates a unilateral lesion of the vestibulocerebellum results in the eyes being deviated slightly contralaterally and they cannot be held to the side of the lesion. Examples of such unilateral lesions confined to the vestibulocerebellum are rare in humans. Larger lesions also interfere with the maintenance of lateral gaze to the side of the lesion. There is, on such attempts, a tonic drift back to near the midline, which is compensated for by a lateral jerk (gaze–paretic nystagmus). This paresis of lateral gaze is due to a loss of the normal cerebellar inhibition of the ipsilateral medial vestibular nucleus in the lower brainstem. This tonic imbalance is also reflected in the Barany pointing test where the patient with eyes closed tends to miss touching a target toward the side of the lesion, and also in the inclination of the body to that side in standing or walking. It is believed also that the vestibulocerebellum via the fastigial nucleus exerts a tonic effect on and a coordination of eye and head movements, correcting them at all times according to incoming visual information coming to the cerebellum via the inferior olivary nucleus. Also quick movements of the eyes to the opposite side tend to overshoot the target (dysmetria) and slow pursuit movements are fragmented and jerky (microsaccades). Undamped microsaccades may appear on attempts at ocular fixation, leading to flutter of the eyes. Anterior vermian lesions are said to cause falling forward and posterior vermian lesions, falling backward. Thach (12) suggested that the physiologic disorder in ocular control with lesions of the vestibulocerebellum is comparable with disorder of limb movements with lesions of other parts of the cerebellum, which seems logical.

In summary, the vestibulocerebellum appears to be the central integrator of information coming from spindle fibers of ocular muscles, labyrinthine apparatus, receptors in neck and trunk muscles, and the gaze centers in the pons and midbrain. In human pathology, lesions of this part of the cerebellum nearly always have involved other parts of it as well.

Disturbances in the function of the spinocerebellum have been less perfectly delineated and there clearly is some overlap with those of the vestibulocerebellum. When lesions occur in the anterior vermis (lingula, central lobule, culmen) as in our cases of alcoholic cerebellar degeneration, in nearly all instances the anterior lobes and sometimes the nodulus and flocculus were also affected (13). Nevertheless, the syndrome differed from that attributed to pure vestibulocerebellar lesions. The most prominent abnormalities are those of stance, gait, and control of the legs. In the majority of the cases there is no nystagmus, dysarthria or incoordination of arm movements, and no complaint of vertigo. The patient stands with feet wide apart, trunk slightly pitched forward, arms held stiffly away from the sides, and trunk position unstable. Rhythmic tremor of head on the trunk is present in some of the patients. In walking there is slow progression by irregular steps, eyes fixed on the floor, and with unpredictable lurching in all directions. Hypotonia of the

limbs is difficult to discern though many of the patients have pendular knee jerks. When supine the legs are ataxic. This can be brought out in heel-to-knee-to-shin testing, tapping heel on knee, and in describing figures in the air with the foot and leg. Often a rhythmic tremor appears when the heel is poised on the kneecap. Visual input assists the patient in walking, as does contact, even a touch, with a reachable object such as an article of furniture.

Studies of primate conditioned movements by Thach and colleagues indicate that these spinocerebellar structures normally receive incoming information via spinocerebellar pathways from segmental spinal neurons, which enables the animal to modulate the ongoing movement. Yet lesions of the spinocerebellar tracts in the spinal cord and medulla have had uncertain effects. Both descending pathways and ascending ones to the thalamus and motor and sensory cortices are involved. Gilman (8) and Thach (12) discovered that the spinocerebellum becomes active only after movements are initiated, not in anticipation of movements. Thach (12) also observed that the globose and emboliform nuclei to which the spinocerebellum projects also have a normal dampening effect on inherent tremors or oscillations of the neuromuscular system. When damaged this effect is lost, allowing tremor to appear.

The cerebrocerebellum is believed to be most active in learned and skilled movements of the extremities and cranial musculature (ocular, lingual, laryngeal). In analyses of movements of trained monkeys, this neocerebellar cortex and dentate nucleus, which are connected to the premotor cortex through the ventral thalamic nuclei, become active a full 40 ms before the motor cortex. If the dentate nucleus is destroyed or paralyzed, there is a delay in the activation of the motor cortex. This is believed to account for the prolongation of the reaction time in initiating a movement, which was noted by Holmes in his study of human cerebellar disease, and also by Hallett et al (10). Holmes (14) and Hallett et al (10) also noted an abnormally slow build-up in the velocity of movement and a delay in the arresting of an ongoing movement; Holmes referred to this as "impaired deceleration." Hallett et al in an electromyographic (EMG) analysis of normal rapid voluntary movement (called "ballistic"), which is accomplished at a speed that does not allow for feedback control, described the existence of a characteristic "triphasic pattern"—first a burst of agonist activity (50–100 ms) then as the agonist falls silent an antagonist burst and finally resumption of agonist activity (15). The duration of the first EMG burst determines the distance and speed of the movement. In slow movements (called "ramp") prolonged EMG agonist bursts continue throughout the movement. With lesions of the cerebrocerebellum (and probably including spinocerebellum) the first agonist burst tends to be prolonged in both ballistic and ramp movements giving an abnormally long acceleration time, out of proportion to deceleration. This would explain the hypermetria and would also cause slowing of alternating or repeated reversals of movements (called adiadochokinesis). Beppu et al (16) in their study of visually guided slow movements in cerebellar disease confirmed the delayed reaction time, the difficulty in initiating the correct peak velocity, and the inaccuracy in deceleration at the target. In smooth tracking or pursuit movements, the EMG activity in agonist muscles was irregular and often interrupted by activity in antagonist muscles. This irregularity was less when vision was eliminated. This repetition of forward movements and arrests under visual control was called the "staircase tracking pattern."

Thus Hallett (10) concludes that cerebellar lesions impair both the planning as well as the execution of movements, quoting the findings of Sasacki et al (17) and Shibasaki et al (18) that in the cerebellar animal the premotor planning potential in the cerebral cortex is absent.

Still problematic are two other phenomena commonly ascribed to cerebellar disease: hypotonia and tremor. Beginning with Luciani (4), ablations of the cerebellum in animals was said to render the limbs unusually slack or hypotonic, which is most apparent during passive movement. Holmes (14), in his assessments of patients after receipt of gunshot wounds of the cerebellum, confirmed its presence. The examinations were for the most part made during the acute phases of the injury. With the passage of time the hypotonia lessens. Gilman (19) also found a hypotonia in recently operated monkeys, bilateral with complete cerebellectomy and ipsilateral in unilateral cerebellar ablation. Growden et al (20) obtained hypotonia after making lesions in the cerebellar nuclei of macaque. It has not been induced in dogs and cats for the reason that they tend to develop extensor rigidity that would mask any degree of hypotonia. Gilman (19) found at the spinal level a reduction in muscle spindle primary afferents, both in threshold of activation and in sensitivity to postural set and movement. This was believed to secondarily affect alpha motor neurons. Marsden et al (11) observed the short-latency stretch reflexes to be normal but the long-latency motor responses to be small and delayed. They concluded that this might explain acute hypotonia in humans. It has been our experience and that of others that hypotonia in the limb muscles of most patients with chronic cerebellar lesions is difficult to elicit except for that manifested by pendulous reflexes. In other words, the hypotonia is to a large extent of the nature of a shock phenomenon akin to spinal shock.

Tremor as a manifestation of cerebellar lesions has also been controversial. Animal physiologists and clinicians have identified three types of tremor in relation to cerebellar deficits. The most widely accepted form is a kinetic tremor that appears near the terminus of a projected or goal-directed voluntary movement. The hand moves more or less rhythmically from side-to-side, and once the goal is reached it becomes stable. This type of tremor, conjoined with ataxia and dysmetria, is a manifestation of disease of both the cerebrocerebellum and spinocerebellum. Holmes (21) suggested

that it was an expression of the basic fault in muscle tone and defective acceleration and deceleration. Sabra and Hallett (22) were inclined to relate it to dysmetria and remarked upon its correction under visual guidance. They pointed out that the tremor is nonrhythmic and that the alternating bursts of EMG activity are longer than 100 ms and quite variable in duration. They suggested that the term *serial dysmetria* be substituted for *intention tremor*. We agree with this interpretation but find in certain cases that the terminal tremor is so rhythmic as to suggest a true central disorder of rhythm control.

A static postural tremor, appearing in the outstretched arm (in proximal more than distal muscles) or in head and neck as titabation (when sitting upright) has also been attributed to cerebellar disease. When severe it may persist even during an attitude of repose and is greatly enhanced during a goal-directed movement. Holmes (21) suggested in 1906 that this combination of severe tremor, under conditions of both static postural and kinetic activities, is related to lesion of the red nucleus (rubral tremor). Since then its localization to this latter structure has been refuted. Carrera and Ferraro (23) claimed that lesions of either the brachium conjunctivum or the dentate nucleus would give rise to it. Gilman (19) localized the causative lesion in the ventral fibers in the brachium conjunctivum. Our own observations have tended to incriminate structures other than the red nucleus in the mesencephalon and subthalamus, perhaps involving the ascending dentatothalamic projection. Lesser degrees of the static postural tremor may only appear in an arm or leg after the part has been held in one position for several seconds. We observed it mainly in the leg in our cases of alcoholic cerebellar atrophy that involved the anterior vermis and adjacent anterior lobe (spinocerebellum).

The present authors find that to date the evidence for the attribution of the aforementioned symptoms to particular parts of the three major anatomic divisions of the cerebellum of humans is quite indefinite. But we are now in a period when, with the help of physiologists, each of the disorders of motor control can be more fully recorded and quantitated. The effects of vision, proprioception, and body posture on simple and complex movements will be determined over a period of time, especially with more chronic lesions, and with modern imaging techniques there can be much greater definition of the anatomy of cerebellar diseases than ever before. Nonetheless these data will still need to be supplemented by detailed single case studies and refined anatomic pathology.

CEREBELLAR DEGENERATIONS

One of the most interesting categories of cerebellar disease is commonly designated as "degenerative" or "heredodegenerative." These terms refer to a slow atrophy and eventual death of neurons, either of the cerebellum itself or of systems of neurons connected to it. It is assumed that the organ has been normally formed and functioned adequately up to a certain age when a disease process begins; and once started the latter advances slowly until death. The first of these attributes distinguish such a disease from the congenital or developmental anomalies, and the extremely slow pace of the degeneration of neurons separate it from some of the more acute and subacute diseases—viral, paraneoplastic, toxic, and so forth. The neurons destined to degenerate display no morphologic peculiarity and the rate of cell degeneration proceeds so slowly that there are no degeneration products left to excite a histocytic–vascular reaction. At most there is a replacement by fibrous astrocytes (replacement gliosis). Of course in the use of the term *degenerative* there must always be a caveat—that what is today an inexplicable "spontaneous" neuronal degeneration may tomorrow prove to be a recognizable biochemical fault.

A remarkable feature of the cerebellar degenerations is the systemic involvement of systems of neurons that are more or less linked anatomically and physiologically. Thus they stand in this respect alongside the motor system diseases and certain polyneuropathies. Not only is there a degeneration of neurons of the cerebellar cortex and central (roof) nuclei but also of the inferior olivary and pontine as well as reticular and vestibular nuclei of the brainstem and the Clarke columns, sensory ganglia, and posterior horn neurons in the spinal cord. This is manifested also in loss of axons in the spinocerebellar, posterior column, vestibulocerebellar, pontocerebellar, and dentatothalamic tracts. In part the extracerebellar nerve cell loss may be secondary to degeneration of axon terminals in the cerebellum, but it may at times appear to be a "chain reaction," a transsynaptic degeneration of neurons linked to degenerating ones. The idea of system degenerations implies biochemical and structural peculiarities of a neuronal system that renders all parts of it vulnerable to the same class of pathogenic agents. Unexplained by this hypothesis, however, are certain degenerative changes that sometimes occur in the retinas, optic nerves, auditory system, corticospinal tracts, and cerebral cortices.

From the time of the first description of progressive cerebellar ataxia by Friedreich (24) in 1861 to the familial ataxias of more recent discovery, there can be traced through all of them a hereditary tendency. In one family after another, one can find a pattern of inheritance conforming to that of a dominant, sex-linked, or recessive trait. As a rule the earlier-life onset cases conform to a mendelian recessive pattern and adult-onset cases to a dominant pattern. Even in sporadic cases one cannot always exclude an hereditary basis. These heredodegenerative cerebellar ataxias (a term given them by S.A.K. Wilson) have been assembled and analyzed by a number of prominent neurologists and neuropathologists. Two of the most informative references are those of Greenfield (25) and Harding (26).

Many workers have attempted to give some ordering to the cerebellar atrophies of genetic origin by devising a systematic classification, but none has proven to be all-inclusive and acceptable because of the diversity of non-cerebellar structural changes. Moreover, even within one family the age of onset and pattern of inheritance has not been the same in all members. Until more is known about cause and pathogenesis, we find the classification of Greenfield into predominantly spinal, spinocerebellar, and cerebellar (the latter including the pontocerebellar and parenchymatous or cortical) to be as useful as any. We concede, however, that the ultimate classification must combine the neuropathologic findings with the clinical phenotypes and genetic linkages. Results from a recent survey show that a purely genetic classification proves to be inadequate (27).

Why cerebellar neurons are disposed to degenerative diseases that leave other parts of the nervous system unscathed has always been a mystery. Saying the cause is genetic is only part of the explanation. One naturally searches for clues in the ways other diseases of known etiology act on the cerebellum. Aging itself proves to be a liability, for the Purkinje cell population undergoes a steady attenuation in late life. Victor et al (13) found a 20% loss between the early and late adult periods. Quantitative data are lacking for granule, basket, stellate, and Golgi cells and neurons of the dentate, globose, emboliform, and fastigial nuclei. In contrast Konigsmark and Weiner (28) detected no age attribution in the vestibular nuclei. One might suppose that this abiotrophic tendency in some cerebellar neuronal systems also predisposes them to genetic disease.

Hyperthermia of exogenous type appears to destroy Purkinje cells more completely than any other system of neurons. A protein derived from eosinophilic leukocytes has a selective effect on Purkinje cells and accounts for the rare cerebellar ataxia in some cases of ataxia with eosinophilia. Methyl mercury intoxication strikes the cerebellar cortex with singular regularity and results in a syndrome, a prominent feature of which is cerebellar ataxia. Cerebellar degeneration as part of a paraneoplastic syndrome has recently been traced to antibodies induced by tumor cells that cross-react with and destroy Purkinje cells. Such protean reactions of cerebellar neurons in pathologic process reactions suggest a number of investigations that have yet to be undertaken in the study of the heredodegenerative diseases of the cerebellum.

SPINOCEREBELLAR DEGENERATIONS

These are the disease states that most dramatically expose the contribution that the cerebellum makes to human motility. In their slow and inexorable progression, they are seen to gradually deprive the human organism of its capacity for locomotion and effective movement.

Friedreich's Ataxia

This was surely the first type of hereditary ataxia brought to medical attention, by Friedreich in 1861 and 1863. He had encountered six young individuals in two families living near Heidelberg who became ataxic during late childhood. Because at that time recessive mendelian inheritance was not known, the disease was called "familial." Friedreich studied the pathology of three cases and was impressed with the degeneration of the posterior roots and funiculi of the spinal cord.

Amplification of the neuropathology has been achieved by numerous workers (25) and it is now generally agreed that in many systems of neurons the cell loss is consequent to a dying-back of axons. The neurons themselves gradually fade into oblivion. Proven neuronal loss at the time of death involves the dorsal root ganglion cells, neurons of the posterior horns of the spinal cord and Clarke columns and accessory cuneate nuclei, gracilis and cuneate nuclei, and certain lower medullary nuclei. Purkinje cells in the superior parts of the cerebellum (in some cases only) and in the dentate nuclei as well as Betz cells in the cerebral cortex are also depleted. These cell losses account for the degeneration of the posterior roots, fasciculi of gracilus and cuneatus, spinocerebellar and corticospinal tracts, medial lemnisci, and superior cerebellar peduncles. Lesser degrees of cell loss are found, in the series reported by Oppenheimer (29), in the Gasserian ganglia, the vestibular nuclei, the external segment of the globus pallidus, and subthalamic nuclei. The optic tract and lateral geniculate bodies degenerate in some cases. Interstitial myocardiopathy has been the cause of death in the majority of cases and may add embolic cerebrovascular lesions to the above pathology.

It is evident from the neuropathology that this familial disease that usually begins in late childhood and nearly always before adult life is a spinocerebellar degeneration. Ataxia of gait is the first symptom, along with slight weakness and fatiguability of legs, and only months or years later are the arms involved. Dysarthria tends to appear late. Tendon reflexes are invariably absent because of the degeneration of muscle spindle afferents. The motor neurons of the spinal cord are preserved. Nystagmus, optic atrophy, and deafness are found in 20%, 8%, and 30%, respectively, of the 115 cases Harding (26) collected from the literature. Pes cavus deformity of the feet and kyphoscoliosis are variable, the foot deformity being an initial manifestation in some cases. The ataxia has been aptly termed "tabetocerebellar" by Charcot to emphasize a sensory defect (similar to that of tabes dorsalis) as well as the cerebellar. While Mollaret (30) considers the cerebellar element to be the more important, we have occasionally seen the opposite. Eventually walking becomes impossible. In attempts to stand the patient teeters and sways. Loss of vibratory and position senses and choreiform movements of the unsupported limbs (static ataxia of Friedreich) betray the loss of proprioceptive senses.

The clinical boundaries of Friedreich's ataxia are ill-defined and will remain so until the underlying biochemical abnormality is discovered. The abnormal gene is located on chromosome 9. The simultaneous involvement of peripheral and central nervous system, diabetes mellitus (10%), and the myocardium is indicative of an hereditary metabolic disorder. Oppenheimer (28) includes the Ramsay Hunt syndrome of dyssynergia cerebellaris myoclonica with degeneration of the dentate nuclei and superior cerebellar peduncles with the Friedreich syndrome. Cases have been described in which Charcot–Marie–Tooth peroneal muscular atrophy or Roussy–Lewy sensory neuropathy were combined with Friedreich's ataxia (25). Biemond (31) and Oppenheimer (29) report cases of hereditary posterior column ataxia identical with the spinal cord part of Friedreich's ataxia but without any cerebellar or corticospinal lesion. Other diseases that resemble the Friedreich phenotype are Friedreich's disease with retained reflexes, ataxia telangiectosia (Louis-Barr disease), Bossen-Kovusweig disease, Leigh's disease, and Refsum's disease (32).

Early life onset of cerebellar ataxia with retained tendon reflexes and lower frequency of pes cavas and kyphoscoliosis and with absence of myocardiopathy and diabetes mellitus is another recognized category of uncertain relationship to Friedreich's ataxia. Again, our impression of this latter group is that it represents a number of different diseases, some of which are clearly genetic while others, such as ataxia telangiectasia, are of uncertain origin but are probably an inherited immunologic defect leading to an obscure chronic viral infection. One of our recent cases, a six-year-old boy, began at the age of two years to become ataxic, to lose sight, to have the ability to turn the eyes laterally, to have other cranial nerve palsies (dysarthria, dysphagia) and an abnormal electroretinogram. The tendon reflexes were retained and the plantar responses were flexor. Elements of the syndrome had been noted in several antecedents on the maternal side of the family. The postmortem findings of global atrophy of the cerebellar cortex (molecular, Purkinje and granule layers) and dentate nuclei, spinocerebellar tract degeneration, degeneration of cranial nerve nuclei, and of retinal rods and cones did not conform exactly to any described type of cerebellar degeneration.

There is no treatment for this disorder. A form of 5-hydroxytryptophan is said to be helpful in alleviating the cerebellar ataxia.

Olivopontocerebellar Degenerations

Pure types and mixed forms of this cerebellar system degeneration are recognized. The anatomic pathology is so striking that diagnosis is now possible during life by the newer imaging techniques. The pons is extremely small owing to loss of pontine nuclei and degeneration of the pontocerebellar (middle) peduncles that lack myelinated fibers. In contrast the corticospinal and corticobulbar fibers are relatively intact. In the hereditary form described by Menzel in 1891 (33), the dentate neurons and superior cerebellar peduncles were preserved but there was loss of Purkinje and granule cells in the cerebellar hemispheres whereas the cerebellar cortex of the vermis and flocculus tended to be spared. The neurons of the inferior olivary nuclei are degenerated (probably secondary effect of cerebellar atrophy). In most cases the tracts of the spinal cord (corticospinal, columns of Goll and Burdach, spinocerebellar) are variably degenerated but not to the degree seen in Friedreich's ataxia. In the sporadically occurring cases described by Dejerine and Thomas (34) in 1900 there were no spinal lesions. In another series of cases, a striking degeneration of nigral cells and corpus striatum and substantia nigra coexisted and in a few of the cases there was a loss of lateral horn cells or a peripheral neuropathy.

Konigsmark and Weiner (27) attempted some ordering of the heterogeneous array of pathologies in the pontocerebellar degenerations by segregating them into five groups.

1. Menzel type—dominant inheritance of cerebellar ataxia with signs of sensory and upper motor neuron disorder.
2. Fickler–Winkler type—recessive inheritance of cerebellar ataxia, without sensory or corticospinal disorder.
3. Dominant inheritance of cerebellar ataxia with progressive visual failure due to retinal degeneration.
4. Schut–Haymaker type—dominant inheritance of cerebellar ataxia with multiple-system degeneration.
5. Dominant inheritance of cerebellar ataxia with parkinsonism, ophthalmoplegia, and dementia.

However, they found a number of cases in the literature that could not fit into this classification. Of the four cases described originally by Adams et al (35) as strionigral degeneration, one had a pontocerebellar degeneration. A typical Parkinson syndrome had been the dominant clinical finding until late in the course of the illness when elements of cerebellar ataxia were added. But other cases have now been described where the opposite sequence occurred—a progressive cerebellar ataxia complicated later by Parkinson symptoms. Degeneration of the lateral horn cells of the spinal cord, that is, the preganglionic sympathetic neurons (Shy–Drager syndrome), have been observed in about half of the reported cases.

A disease indigenous in the Portuguese population of the United States and of the Cape Verde islands (called Machado-Joseph disease) has been described. Adults over a period of years are overtaken by a progressive cerebellar ataxia with added features of extrapyramidal disorder. A subgroup presents mainly with a progressive polyneuropathy (36).

In all these conditions the core of the clinical syndrome is a cerebellar ataxia manifest by an unsteady gait that, as it worsens becomes reeling with unexpected lurches and falls. Ataxia of arms, dysarthria abnormalities of ocular movement, and nystagmus follow; static and kinetic tremors are prominent. Vertigo is rare as is dementia. The illness is slowly progressive over a period of years. Features suggestive of pontocerebellar atrophy are early affection of speech (scanning, "spastic dysphonia"), weakness of legs, extrapyramidal signs of parkinsonism, or dystonia. Polyneuropathy is frequent in the Portuguese population.

There are several other autosomal dominant phenotypes in which cerebellar ataxia is the principal finding. Giunti et al (27) subdivide them as follows: autosomal dominant cerebellar ataxia (type I) with ophthalmoplegia, pyramidal and extrapyramidal signs; type II with slow eye movements and slight pyramidal and extrapyramidal signs; type III with pure cerebellar ataxia; and type IV with sensory axonal neuropathy and pyramidal signs. The Machado-Joseph disease with parkinsonian symptoms and peripheral neuropathy fell into types I and III and had nucleotide CAG repeats on chromosome 6. Some were of olivopontocerebellar type, others were of cortical type.

Cerebellar Cortical Atrophy (Cerebello-Olivary Atrophy)

An atrophic degenerative process confined to the cerebellar cortex with progressive ataxia of gait and limb movements was first described by Holmes in 1907 (21). There was no sign of sensory defect. Nystagmus was present in some cases. The reflexes were normal and the disease had appeared in midadult life in three males and one female of a sibship; it was slowly progressive over a period of 15–20 years. By the time of the writing of Greenfield's monograph (25) in 1954, some 15 reports of additional cases of this type had been made, the most frequently quoted being that by Marie et al in 1922 (37). In the postmortem studies only the anterior and posterior vermis and anterior lobes and the flocculi were the site of severe neuronal loss, more of Purkinje than granule cells, with gliosis of Bergmann's layer. The topography of lesions in this group of cases corresponded to that of alcoholic nutritional cerebellar degeneration, according to Victor et al (13), but obviously the disease is of a genetic origin. We thought, as did Brouwer and Biemond (38), that these restricted parenchymatous atrophies should be distinguished from the more diffuse cortical atrophies. The latter are sporadic, of variable course, some subacute, some chronic; and often the more rapidly progressive ones are associated with carcinomatosis. Nonetheless, some cases are familial and fall into autosomal dominant group III.

The heredofamilial atrophies as a group are also variable. In some the dentate nuclei and superior cerebellar peduncles are also affected. Dysarthria, ocular palsies, vertigo, dementia, and Babinski signs are recorded in some cases. In a few an overlapping pathology includes olivopontocerebellar atrophy. Always, however, an ataxia extending from legs to arms and cranial musculature is the dominant abnormality. The age of onset is from 12 to over 50 years. Mendelian autosomal dominant inheritance is most frequent but there are many single cases. The Schut–Haymaker family is noteworthy in this respect (39). In the 47 affected members (of 343 examined individuals in five generations), the disease was observed to gradually differentiate into three syndromes, one resembling Friedreich's disease, another a pure cerebellar ataxia with normal reflexes, and a third with less ataxia and a prominent spastic paraparesis. Dysarthria and dysphagia were severe in all in the late stages of the disease. In the studies of the pathology of five cases Schut and Haymaker (39) found lesions resembling those of Friedreich's ataxia in two; an atrophy of the cerebellum in a third and of the spinocerebellar tracts and cerebellum in a fourth; and of pons, cerebellar white matter and dentate, and ambiguous nuclei in a fifth. The hypoglossal and olivary nuclei were involved in all five cases, accounting for the terminal dysphagia and loss of voice, linking the cases in the opinion of Greenfield (25) with Friedreich's ataxia.

To conclude, as a generalization one may say that the denominative marks of the heredogenerative cerebellar ataxias have been their extreme chronicity and progressivity. These qualities distinguish them from some of the acquired forms of cerebellar disease, such as the hyperthermic, alcoholic, and metal intoxicative, which, after an acute or subacute development, may allow long survival without progression. Any distinction to be drawn clinically between the spinocerebellar, olivopontocerebellar, and parenchymatous cortical cerebellar atrophies rests mostly on the finding of noncerebellar accompaniments. Sensory ataxia (Rombergism) areflexia, Babinski signs, and skeletal changes (pes cavus and kyphoscoliosis) characterize the spinocerebellar group. Myocardiopathy and cerebrovascular incidents are unique to Friedreich's ataxia. The olivopontocerebellar group are often accompanied by extrapyramidal signs, autonomic disorder, and a variety of hypothalamic and brainstem disorders. Only the parenchymatous cortical cerebellar atrophies present as a relatively pure ataxis and tremor. Myoclonus can occur in any of the groups and has no clear anatomic localization.

The cerebellar symptomatology as it presents in these degenerative diseases is not easily assigned to any one of the three anatomic physiologic divisions of the cerebellum. The presence of static and intention tremor tends to incriminate the dentate nuclei and their projections through the superior cerebellar peduncles to brainstem and thalamus. The peculiarities of stance, gait, and movement are common to all and are observed both with diseases affecting the vermis and anterior lobes as well as the cerebellar hemispheres. A pure vermian syndrome is rarely to be observed.

In recent publications, the role of the cerebellum in motor learning, formation of conditional reflexes, and cognition has received comment. These subjects, however, have not been adequately addressed in most of the articles on degenerative diseases of the cerebellum.

REFERENCES

1. Larsell O. The cerebellum. A review and interpretation. Arch Neurol Psychiatry 1937;38:580.
2. Dow RS. Effects of lesions in the vestibular part of the cerebellum in primates. Arch Neurol Psychiatry 1938;40:500.
3. Brodal A, Jansen J. The ponto-cerebellar projection in the rabbit and cat. Experimental investigations. J Comp Neurol 1946;84:31.
4. Luciani L. On the sensorial localizations in the cortex cerebri. Brain 1884;7:145–160.
5. Moruzzi G. Problems in cerebellar physiology. Springfield: Charles C Thomas, 1950.
6. Snider RS, Eldred E. Maintenance of spontaneous activity within the cerebellum. Proc Soc Exp Biol Med 1949;72:124.
7. Fulton JF. Cerebrum and cerebellum. In: Fulton J, ed. A textbook of physiology. Philadelphia: WB Saunders, 1949.
8. Gilman S, Bloedell J, Lechtenberg R. Disorders of the Cerebellum. Philadelphia: FA Davis, 1981.
9. Everts EV, Thach WT. Motor mechanisms of the cerebro-cerebellar interrelations. Annu Rev Physiol 1969;31:451–498.
10. Hallett M, Shahani RT, Young RR. EMG analysis of patients with cerebellar deficits. J Neurol Neurosurg Psychiatry 1975;38:1163–1169.
11. Marsden CD, Merlon PA, Morton HB, et al. Disorders of movement in cerebellar disease in man. In: Rose F, ed. The physiological aspects of clinical neurology. Oxford: Blackwell Scientific Publications, 1977.
12. Thach WT. The cerebellum. In: Mountcastle VB, ed. Medical physiology. 44th ed. St Louis: Mosby, 1978.
13. Victor M, Adams RD, Mancall EL. A restricted form of cerebellar cortical degeneration occurring in alcoholic patients. Arch Neurol 1959;1:577–688.
14. Holmes GM. The cerebellum of man. Brain 1939;62:1.
15. Hallett M, Marsden CD. Ballistic flexion movements of the human thumb. J Physiol 1979;294:33–50.
16. Beppu H, Suda M, Tanaka R. Analysis of cerebellar motor disorders by visually guided elbow tracking movement. Brain 1984;107:787–809 and 1987;110:1–18.
17. Sasaki K, Gamba H, Hashimoto S. Influences of cerebellar hemispherectomy on slow potentials in the motor cortex preceding self-paced hand movements in the monkey. Neurosci Lett 1979;15:23–28.
18. Shibasaki H, Barrett G, Neshiga R, et al. Volitional movement is not preceded by cortical slow negativity in cerebellar dentate lesion in man. Brain Res 1986;368:361–365.
19. Gilman S. The mechanism of cerebellar hypotonia. An experimental study in the monkey. Brain 1969;92:621–638.
20. Growden JH, Chambers WW, Liu CN. An experimental study of cerebellar dyskinesia in rhesus monkey. Brain 1967;90:603–637.
21. Holmes G. A form of familial degeneration of the cerebellum. Brain 1907;30:545–567.
22. Sabra AF, Hallett M. Action tremor with alternating activity in autoagonist muscles. Neurology 1984;34:151–156.
23. Carrera RMC, Ferraro FA. Function of the primate brachium conjunctivum and related structures. J Comp Neurol 1955;102:151.
24. Friedreich N. Ueber degenerative Atrophie der spinale Hinterstrange. Virchow's Archiv Pathol Anat Physiol 1863;26 and 27:391,433,1–26.
25. Greenfield JG. The Spinocerebellar Degenerations. Springfield: Charles C Thomas, 1954.
26. Harding AE. The hereditary ataxias and related disorders. London: Churchill Livingstone, 1984.
27. Giunti P, Sweeney MG, Harding AE. Detection of the Machado–Joseph disease shows cerebellar ataxia three trinucleotide repeat expansion in families with autosomal dominant motor disorders, including the Drew Family of Walworth. Brain 1995;118:1077–1085.
28. Konigsmark BW, Weiner LP. The olivopontocerebellar atrophies: a review. Medicine 1970;49:227–241.
29. Oppenheimer DR. Greenfield's neuropathology. 4th ed. New York: John Wiley, 1984.
30. Mollaret P. La maladie de Friedreich: etude physio-clinique. Paris: Legrand, 1929.
31. Biemond A. La forme radiculo-cordonnale posterieure des degenerescence spino-cerebelleuses. Rev Neurol 1954;91:3–21.
32. Iannacone ST, Rosenberg RN. Principles of molecular genetics and neurologic disease. In: Berg BO, ed. Principles of pediatric neurology. New York: McGraw Hill, 1996.

33. Menzel P. Beitrage zur Kenntris der hereditaren-ataxie and kleinatrophie. Arch Psychiatr Nervenkr 1891;22:160.
34. Dejerine J, Thomas A. L'atrophie olivo-ponto-cerebelleuse. Nouv Icon Salpetriere 1900;13:330.
35. Adams RD, van Bogaert L, Vander Eeken H. Striato-nigral degeneration. J Neuropathol Exp Neurol 1964;23:584–668.
36. Adams RD, Victor M. Principles of neurology. 4th ed. New York: McGraw-Hill, 1989.
37. Marie P, Foix C. Alajouanine T. De l'atrophie cerebelleuse tardive a predominance corticale. Rev Neurol 1922;38:849.
38. Brouwer B, Biemond A. Les affections parenchymateuses du cervelet et leur signification du point de vue de l'anatomie et de physiologie de cet organs. J Belge Neurol Pscyhiatry 1938;38:91.
39. Schut JW, Haymaker W. Hereditary ataxia: a pathologic study of five cases of common ancestry. J Neuropathol Clin Neurol 1951;1:183.

Mood and Movement

Disorders of Mood and Movement: An Overview

ANTHONY B. JOSEPH

INTRODUCTION

The observation that a nontrivial relationship exists between mood and movement is not new. As early as 1858 Sutherland was providing detailed descriptions of mania and depression in patients with seizures, paralysis, and other disturbances of movement. He related these clinically intertwined presentations to neuropathologic findings at autopsy (1). Sutherland also noted the relationship between pathophysiology, affective disorders, and motoric disturbance. Since his time these observations have been refined and it has become clear that there are four broad levels of analysis that can be used to understand the relationship between mood and movement: clinical, pathophysiologic, neuroanatomic, and neurophysiologic.

At the clinical level, many individual associations have been noted between disorders of mood and disorders of movement. Good examples are parkinsonism and depression, mania and hyperkinesis, depression and bradykinesis. The nature of these relationships is never certain. Are they fortuitous, causative, or associated presentations of a common pathology?

Once the pathophysiologies behind the clinical relationships are investigated, another level of understanding emerges. Instances abound in which a single disease process can cause both mood and motor disturbance. Stroke is a well-known example (2). Others are head injury and encephalitis (3,4). The conclusions that seem consistent with this general group of observations are 1) that it is not the disease process but the focal nature of the insult that causes the affective and motoric changes, and 2) that disorders of mood and movement often seem to occur together. These conclusions in turn suggest that the neural substrates for mood and movement are functionally interconnected, at least in part.

In support of this concept it can be said that neuroanatomically many areas of the brain seem to be important for the maintenance of both normal mood and movement (5–7). Some investigations have also raised the possibility that the lateralized functions of these areas are an important factor in their control (8,9). Also, at the level of neurophysiology, it has become clear that some of the specific neurochemical systems that are of importance in the control of mood and motor function have anatomically discrete distributions (10). When these localized neurotransmitter systems are perturbed by disease, disorders of both mood and movement can occur together (11,12).

Finally, it is interesting to note that the affective state of the individual is often expressed via motor system output. Tone, posture, activity level, and facial expression all change with mood. Actors use this knowledge to become adept at simulating different moods by adopting their accompanying motoric states.

In each of the sections that follow, a limited number of examples will be used to illustrate and assert some possible principles of the relationship between mood and movement. A full listing of these would be well beyond the scope of this chapter and cannot be undertaken here. Nevertheless, it is hoped that an overview of this topic can still be of use in considering this important problem at the interface of psychiatry and neurology.

CLINICAL RELATIONSHIPS BETWEEN MOOD AND MOVEMENT

It is a common clinical observation that there is a link between disorders of mood and disorders of movement. This observation seems to be valid at two levels. First, some disorders of mood and movement frequently occur together: parkinsonism and depression (13), mania and hyperkinesis

(14). Second, where there may not be a statistically demonstrable link between a disease state and disorders of both mood and movement, individual cases are seen in which profound affective disturbance is often accompanied by motor dysfunction, or vice versa. For example, in a study of secondary mania after focal brain injury it was found that mania is not a common presentation of focal brain injury; but when it does occur, motor dysfunction is a frequent accompaniment (15). Table 46.1 gives some other examples.

The mere observation that symptoms of disturbed mood and movement can occur together does little to explain why this should be so. In general there seem to be three types of relationship: 1) those of unknown type, 2) those in which a mood disorder causes a movement disorder, and 3) those in which a motor disorder causes a mood disorder. By far the majority of such relationships fall into the first category. It is simply not at all obvious why affective disorders should associate with tardive dyskinesia (16), or depressive spectrum disorders with compulsive movements (17).

Disorders of mood that at first glance seem to cause disorders of movement appear less mysterious. It is intuitively satisfactory that manics should be hyperkinetic and depressives hypokinetic. Thoughtful reflection, however, casts doubt on the possible simplicity of even these relationships. Perhaps manic hyperactivity has as much to do with neurochemistry as it does with a simple secondary motor expression of psychic agitation. Indeed, it is clinically possible to see patients with extreme psychic agitation, such as catatonics, who barely move at all.

The third category, in which disorders of movement seem to cause disorders of mood, is equally fascinating. Why

should akinesia induce anxiety and depression (18)? Why should akathisia do the same (19)?

It seems fair to conclude that clinical observations of related disorders of mood and movement can provide raw data from which to construct hypotheses, but not the hypotheses themselves.

PATHOPHYSIOLOGIC RELATIONSHIP BETWEEN MOOD AND MOVEMENT

There is an extensive literature on the various pathophysiologies that can cause disorders of both mood and movement. All types of data have been presented, and different effects have been seen. One study found that primary degenerative dementia caused both depression and psychomotor retardation (20). In another study of 100 consecutive patients attending a multiple sclerosis clinic, 42% had a lifetime history of depression and 13% of bipolar affective disorder (21); many of them had motor dysfunction. The lessons are not clear, however; a study of poststroke depressive disorders found that hemiparesis did not discriminate between depressed and nondepressed patients (2).

Although of great interest in documenting the different types of disease process that can cause secondary affective disorders both with and without motor dysfunction, these types of studies shed little further light on the relationship between mood and movement. For each new individual disease process that is shown to disorder both mood and movement, a gamut of useful questions must be answered. Incidence? Prevalence? Susceptible populations? Genetic vulnerability? Mechanism of the disease process? Even then, it seems to this author that little progress will have been

T a b l e 46.1 Postulated Relationships Between Mood and Movement Disorders

Unknown	Mood Disorder Causing Movement Disorder	Movement Disorder Causing Mood Disorder
Parkinsonism–depression	Mania–hyperkinesis	Akinesia–depression
Attention deficit disorder-mania–hyperactivity	Depression–bradykinesis	Restless legs–depression
Multiple sclerosis–affective disorders	Depression–hypophonia	Gelastic epilepsy–laughter
Stroke–depression	Anxiety–tremor	Dyscrastic epilepsy–crying
Stroke–mania	Anxiety–hyperkinesis	Sham mirth–false appearance of mirth
Neuroleptic malignant syndrome–bipolar disorder	Depression–lateralized motor "soft signs"	Sham rage–false appearance of rage
Catatonia–bipolar disorder	Mood disorder–corresponding state-dependent movement disorder	Subcortical movement disorders–depression
Tardive dyskinesia–affective disorders	Dysphoria–self-mutilation	Self-mutilation–euphoria
Spasmodic torticollis–depression	Dysphoria–aggressive behavior	"Addictive jogging"–euphoria
Compulsive movements–depressive spectrum disorders	Dysphoria–"addictive jogging"	
Narcolepsy–affective disorders	Dysphoria–repetitive pathologic movements	
Dementia–depression	PTSD–hyperstartle	
Oculogyric crises–anxiety	ADHD–hyperstartle	
Familial periodic paralysis–affective disorders		
Tourette's syndrome–anxiety		
Chronic motor tics–affective disorders		
Migraine coma–bipolar disorder		
Pseudobulbar palsy–emotional lability		

made toward defining the general relationship between movement and mood. Table 46.2 lists some pathophysiologies and diseases known to cause disorders of both mood and movement.

NEUROANATOMY OF MOOD AND MOVEMENT

Over several decades, there has been a burgeoning of interest in the behavioral neurology of affective disorders that has also shed light on their associated movement disorders (22). Several broad conclusions may be drawn from this work:

1. The frontal lobes and their interactions are important for the maintenance of normal mood (23).
2. The right hemisphere is important in emotional tone and emotional behavior (24).
3. The limbic system has important connections with the basal ganglia and hence the extrapyramidal system (7,10,25). This point may be of particular importance in understanding the relationship between mood and movement, and will be dealt with in more detail later.
4. The diencephalon and brainstem are profoundly important not only for emotional and neurovegetative functioning, but also for the integrated control of movement (7).

A further development is the possible role of the cerebellum in coordinating fundamental neurophysiological processes, not just in the domain of motor control but also of nonmotor functions. Projections have been described between the hypothalamus and cerebellum that could permit direct interactivity between areas of the brain that are important in motor, affect, and neuroendocrine control (26). When these observations are put together, it is fair to conclude that many of the brain subsystems important for movement are anatomically near those important for mood. It thus becomes reasonable to speculate that disease processes affecting one group of systems, such as motor control subsystems, could physically spill over and affect another such as mood control subsystems.

Less easy to understand are the role of the cerebellum, if any, in the unified control of mood and movement, or the exact nature of the structures that harmonize biorhythms, neuroendocrine homeostasis, mood, and movement.

A final consideration is that the anatomic sites that allow the integrated control of mood and movement may be widely distributed throughout the brain and be activated both sequentially and simultaneously depending on the task (27). Any disease that impairs these will also affect mood and movement simultaneously.

SOME NEUROPHYSIOLOGIC PRINCIPLES OF MOOD AND MOVEMENT CONTROL

So much work has been done in the various subareas of neurophysiology to explore the relationship between mood and movement that even an overview is far beyond the scope of this chapter. This section, then, will only address principles concerning some of the neurotransmitter systems involved in both, as it is at the level of clinical neurochemistry and psychopharmacology that perhaps what is the clearest and most fundamental view of the interrelationship between mood and movement is revealed. Table 46.3 lists a variety of psychopharmacologic observations concerning both mood and movement. It is interesting that when examined at the level of neurochemical systems, such as the dopaminergic system or the cholinergic system, many aspects of mood and movement are explainable, at least in an approximate manner. At this level of analysis, for example, it is reasonable to consider the hyperactivity of mania as a sympathetic phenomenon dependent on dopaminergic and noradrenergic function, and the depression and hypokinesia of parkinsonism as secondary to reduced central sympathetic activity.

The importance of using neurochemical and psychopharmacologic data to probe the relationship between mood and movement is well illustrated by the following generalizations:

1. Many factors that increase central sympathetic or noradrenergic tone or that reduce central parasympathetic or cholinergic tone also induce manic and hyperkinetic states (14,28).

T a b l e 4 6 . 2   Some Diseases and Pathophysiologies That Can Present with Disorders of Mood and Movement

Parkinson's disease	Intoxication
Huntington's disease	Extrapyramidal disorders
Wilson's disease	Head injury
Alzheimer's disease	Focal brain injury
Pick's disease	Cerebellar disorders
Fahr's disease	Hypothalamic disorders
Porphyria	Encephalitis
Neurosyphilis	Meningitis
Slow virus diseases	Toxic encephalopathy
Storage diseases	Metabolic encephalopathy
Deficiency states	Anoxic encephalopathy
Causes of mental retardation	Delirium
Autoimmune disorders	Raised intracranial pressure
The ataxias	Demyelination
Other neurodegenerative disorders	Myopathy
Psychiatric disorders	Epilepsy
Binswanger's disease	Migraine syndromes
Stroke	Arousal disorders
Dementia	Attentional disorders

Table 46.3   Some Neurochemical and Psychopharmacologic Observations Consistent with a Role for Central Dysautonomia in the Regulation of Mood and Movement

Observation	Possible Explanation			
	Central Sympathomimetic Effect	Central Sympatholytic Effect	Central Parasympathomimetic Effect	Central Parasympatholytic Effect
Hyperadrenergic signs in mania	+	—	—	+
Psychomotor acceleration in mania	+	—	—	+
Neurovegetative symptoms in depression	—	+	+	—
Psychomotor retardation in depression	—	+	+	—
Neuroleptic-induced akinesia, depression, suicidality	—	+	+	—
Reversal of above with anticholinergic drugs	—	—	—	+
Neuroleptic-induced parkinsonism	—	+	—	—
Reversal of above with anticholinergics	—	—	—	+
Hypokinesia and depression in parkinsonism	—	+	—	—
Reversal of above with anticholinergics	—	—	—	+
Cholinergically induced hypokinesia, depression, suicidality	—	—	+	—
Reversal of above with anticholinergics	—	—	—	+
Reserpine-induced depression and hypokinesia	—	+	—	—
Amphetamine-induced mania and hyperkinesis	+	—	—	—
Effective tricyclic antidepressant treatment	+	—	—	+
Monoamine oxidase inhibitor treatment of depression	+	—	—	—
Psychostimulant treatment of depression	+	—	—	—
Beta-blocker-induced depression	—	+	—	—
Alpha-methyldopa-induced depression	—	+	—	—
Tricyclic-induced mania	+	—	—	+
Monoamine oxidase inhibitor-induced mania	+	—	—	—
Psychostimulant-induced mania	+	—	—	—
Psychostimulant-induced involuntary movements	+	—	—	—
Electroconvulsive therapy treatment of depression	?	—	—	—
Electroconvulsive therapy treatment of mania	—	—	?	—
Reserpine treatment of mania	—	+	—	—
Beta-blocker treatment of mania	—	+	—	—
SSRI treatment of depression	+	—	—	—
SSRI-induced mania	+	—	—	—
SSRI-induced dysphorias	—	+	—	—
Dopaminergic-induced mania	+	—	—	—

2. Many factors that reduce central sympathetic or noradrenergic tone or that increase central parasympathetic or cholinergic tone increase depression and reduce movement (18,19,28).

Table 46.3 lists some clinical observations that support these hypotheses.

These conclusions are easily testable in a variety of ways. If correct, they are detailed enough to have useful predictive power. If incorrect, they are also detailed enough that disproving them would reveal useful new data. These factors will be examined again as they may pertain to a specific movement disorder, catatonia, in Chapter 48.

Another area of interest is the relationship between hormones, mood, and movement. Although no clear principles have yet emerged, it seems that neurohumoral effects on affective and motor functioning do exist and, as a further complication, that biorhythms are also fundamentally involved in these (29–31).

CONCLUSIONS

No final conclusions are possible about the relationship between mood and movement. Not enough is known. Some broad preliminary conclusions are justified, however, by the present state of knowledge.

Neurotransmitter systems are known to be important in both motor control and affective tone. These include, but are not limited to, the noradrenergic, dopaminergic, cholinergic, serotonergic, opioid, and gamma-aminobutyric acid systems. They are organized into discrete but interconnected neuroanatomic structures. Some of these structures, as already noted, are important in the control of both mood and movement, and they may be physically or functionally asymmetric (32–34). At a physiologic level, central sympathetic and parasympathetic balance may be important in the integrated control of both mood and movement.

It has also been proposed that the anatomic basis exists for massive functional interconnections between cortical areas, the limbic system, and the extrapyramidal system (35,36). The locus of this is the striatum, and it may be the physical link that connects and explains the observations from the various levels of analysis that have already been discussed. The detailed anatomy of the corticostriatolimbic circuitry is even consistent with a role for the basal ganglia in determining the basic neurophysiologic parameters that govern the initiation, development, and expression of both thought and movement (35,36). If this hypothesis is correct, then mood and movement disorders would become a special case of a larger class of cognition and movement disorders.

Future developments may confirm a role for the cerebellum in the integrated control of mood and movement, elucidate the nature and effects of endocrine influences, and explore the contribution of biorhythms.

This overview of motor and affective control systems is a parsimonious one. It is nontrivial because it has the advantage of predicting that pathophysiologic processes, of any etiology, can cause disorders of mood and movement in one of two ways: 1) by damaging the neuroanatomic structures that contain the relevant neurotransmitter systems, or 2) by perturbing the systems themselves in such a way as to prevent or disorder their normal physiologic functioning. It also predicts that not only are there unitary disorders of mood and unitary disorders of movement, but also disorders of both mood and movement together. What may be a specific example of this is discussed in Chapter 48.

REFERENCES

1. Sutherland AJ. Croonian lecture. On the pathology, morbid anatomy, and treatment of insanity. J Ment Sci 1861;7:1–19.
2. Robinson RG, Price TR. Post-stroke depressive disorders: A follow-up study of 103 patients. Stroke 1982;13:635–641.
3. Shukla S, Cook BL, Mukherjee S, et al. Mania following head trauma. Am J Psychiatry 1987;144:93–96.
4. Lishman WA. Organic psychiatry. Oxford: Blackwell Scientific, 1978.
5. Cummings JL. Clinical neuropsychiatry. Orlando, FL: Grune & Stratton, 1985.
6. Brazis PW, Masdeu JC, Biller J. Localization in clinical neurology. Boston: Little, Brown, 1985.
7. Brodal A. Neurological anatomy in relation to clinical medicine. 3rd ed. New York: Oxford University, 1981.
8. Flor-Henry P. Psychosis and temporal lobe epilepsy. A controlled investigation. Epilepsia 1969;10:363–395.
9. Geschwind N, Galaburda AM, eds. Cerebral dominance. The biological foundations. Cambridge, MA: Harvard University, 1984.
10. Nieuwenhuys R, Voogd J, Huijzen C. The human central nervous system. A synopsis and atlas. 2nd ed, revised. Berlin: Springer-Verlag, 1981.
11. Rogers D, Lees AJ, Smith E, et al. Bradyphrenia in Parkinson's disease and psychomotor retardation in depressive illness. Brain 1987;110:761–776.
12. Leonard BE. Neurochemical and neuropharmacological aspects of depression. Int Rev Neurobiol 1975;18:357–387.
13. Mayeux R, Williams JBW, Stern Y, Cote L. Depression and Parkinson's disease. Adv Neurol 1984;40:241–250.
14. Stasiek C, Zetin M. Organic manic disorders. Psychosomatics 1985;26:394–402.
15. Starkstein SE, Pearlson GD, Boston J, Robinson RG. Mania after brain injury. A controlled study of causative factors. Arch Neurol 1987;44:1069–1073.
16. Waddington JL. Tardive dyskinesia in schizophrenia and other disorders: associations with aging, cognitive dysfunction and structural brain pathology in relation to neuroleptic exposure. Hum Psychopharmacol 1987;2:11–22.
17. Pitman RK, Green RC, Jenike MA, Mesulam MM. Clinical comparison of Tourette's disorder and obsessive-compulsive disorder. Am J Psychiatry 1987;144:1166–1171.
18. Rifkin A, Quitkin F, Kane J, et al. Are prophylactic antiparkinson drugs necessary? A controlled study of procyclidine withdrawal. Arch Gen Psychiatry 1978;35:483–489.
19. Drake RE, Ehrlich J. Suicide attempts associated with akathisia. Am J Psychiatry 1985;142:499–501.
20. Lazarus LW, Newton N, Cohler B, et al. Frequency and presentation of depressive symptoms in patients with primary degenerative dementia. Am J Psychiatry 1987;144:41–45.
21. Joffe RT, Lippert GP, Gray TA, et al. Mood disorder and multiple sclerosis. Arch Neurol 1987;44:376–378.
22. Ross ED. Modulation of affect and nonverbal communication by the right hemisphere. In: Mesulam MM, ed. Principles of behavioral neurology. Philadelphia: FA Davis, 1985.
23. Joseph AB, O'Leary DH. Brain atrophy and interhemispheric fissure enlargement in Cotard's syndrome. J Clin Psychiatry 1986;47:518–520.
24. Ross ED, Rush AJ. Diagnosis and neuroanatomical correlates of depression in brain-damaged patients. Implications for a neurology of depression. Arch Gen Psychiatry 1981;38:1344–1354.
25. Marsden CD. The mysterious motor function of the basal ganglia: the Robert Wartenberg lecture. Neurology 1982;32:514–539.
26. Dietrichs E, Haines DE, Roste GK, Roste LS. Hypothalamocerebellar and cerebellohypothalamic projections—circuits for regulating nonsomatic cerebellar activity? Histol Histopathol 1994;9:603–614.
27. Schwartz AB. Distributed motor processing in cerebral cortex. Curr Opinion Neurobiol 1994;4:840–846.
28. Klein DF, Gittleman R, Quitkin F, Rifkin A. Diagnosis and drug treatment of psychiatric disorders: adults and children. 2nd ed. Baltimore: Williams & Wilkins, 1980.
29. Beckmann D, Hinckel P. Ontogenese der affekt regulation. Psychother Psychosom Med Psychol 1995;45:427–435.
30. Cushing BS, Marhenke S, McClure PA. Estradiol concentration and the regulation of locomotor activity. Physiol Behav 1995;58:953–957.
31. Rechlin T, Weis M, Kaschka WP. Is diurnal variation of mood associated with parasympathetic activity? Journ Affective Disord 1995;34:249–255.
32. Geschwind N, Galaburda AM. Cerebral lateralization I. Arch Neurol 1985;42:428–459.
33. Geschwind N, Galaburda AM. Cerebral lateralization II. Arch Neurol 1985;42:521–552.
34. Geschwind N, Galaburda AM. Cerebral lateralization III. Arch Neurol 1985;42:634–654.
35. Nauta WJH. Cross-roads of limbic, cortical and striatal circuitry. Typescript of a presentation at New Perspectives on Neuropsychiatry. University of California at San Francisco, February 1986.
36. Nauta WJH. Reciprocal links of the corpus striatum with the cerebral cortex and limbic system. A common substrate for movement and thought? In: Mueller J, Yingling C, Zegans L, eds. Neurology and psychiatry: a meeting of minds. Basel: Karger, 1989.

Laterality and Motility Disturbances in Psychopathology: A Theoretical Perspective

Pierre Flor-Henry

The fundamentally important motility disturbances invariably associated with the major psychopathologic syndromes are the agitation or psychomotor retardation of depression; the hypermotility of mania; the stereotypies and manneristic behaviors of schizophrenia; the excited or stuporous forms of catatonia; the compulsions of the obsessional syndrome; the spasms, jerkings, pseudoconvulsions, or functional paralyses of hysteria; and the motor tension of anxiety. These motility abnormalities are not secondary consequences of the psychopathologic syndromes with which they are associated but reflect, at the motor level, the disorganization of localized and lateralized cerebral systems of which the psychic symptom constellations and the motility abnormalities are the simultaneous expressions. Recent evidence suggesting that neurotransmitters are asymmetrically distributed in the brain—dopaminergic and cholinergic systems in the left and noradrenergic–serotoninergic systems in the right hemispheres (1)—can, as Tucker and Williamson (2) have proposed, be related to motility: motor readiness is subtended by dopaminergic activity in the left hemisphere and arousal by noradrenergic-dependent mediation in the right hemisphere. The corticopyramidal tracts and the bulbar pyramids have pronounced asymmetric patterns of decussation and the cortical regulation of motility is itself asymmetric. Yakovlev and Rakic (3), in a study of 130 fetal and neonatal autopsy material, found asymmetric patterns of decussation of the corticopyramidal tracts and bulbar pyramids: the decussating bundles of the left pyramids are larger than those of the right pyramid, more fibers of the left pyramid cross to the right side than vice versa, there are more ipsilateral corticospinal projections on the right side than on the left. Wyke (4), investigating the effects of right and left brain lesions on the rapidity of single and repetitive movements of the upper limbs, found that left hemisphere lesions produced both ipsilateral and contralateral

abnormalities, whereas right brain lesions had only contralateral effects. Goodale (5) reviewed more recent and very diverse evidence that indicate "that speech is but one example of a great number of different motor patterns mediated in part by neural systems within the so-called 'dominant' hemisphere." Thus the synchrony and sequencing of complex movements are determined by dominant hemisphere circuits. In its pure form the catatonic syndrome is paradigmatic of a functional dysregulation of the cerebral volitional controls of motility. Given the above organization one would, theoretically, therefore expect catatonic symptomatology to relate to the left hemisphere, more especially, left frontal pathology. There is evidence that this is the case. In their review of the literature on schizophrenic psychoses associated with organic disorders of the central nervous system, Davison and Bagley (6) found, in a subsample of 80 cases selected from their original 150 because of having circumscribed cerebral lesions, significant associations between catatonic features and left hemisphere and basal ganglia lesions. Luchins et al (7) reported a single case study of a schizoaffective patient subjected to a positron emission tomography (PET) examination during a catatonic episode. There was marked hemispheric asymmetry of regional glucose metabolism: 1.5 standard deviations above the whole brain average in the left basal ganglia and slightly below average on the right. Two weeks later, after the patient had been treated with lithium and become asymptomatic, the PET procedure was repeated. The left basal ganglia activity increased by 20%, but the right by 40%, thus eliminating the original asymmetry. These observations illustrate two important facts: the presence of frontostriatum and interhemispheric reciprocal relationships. There is an orderly topographic projection system from the frontal zone to the caudate nucleus and the left hemisphere, through transcallosal connections that are essentially inhibitory—in fact mirror image negative information transfer (8)—exercises a regulatory influence over emotional, aggressive, and sexual arousal functions, derivative of right hemispheric systems (9,10).

Denenberg (11) has shown how, formally, from a systems theory perspective, three principles are necessary, and sufficient, to account for a double brain system linked by a bridge: intrahemispheric activation, contralateral inhibition, and interhemispheric coupling. Given the fundamentally inhibitory nature of callosal transmission and given, as Cook (8) has pointed out, the fact that in the human brain there are approximately 250 million callosal fibers establishing contact with approximately 125 million cortical columns in each hemisphere, thus providing the neural infrastructure for reciprocal interhemispheric interactions—it is clear that in addition to the left brain inhibitory action on right brain functions described above, the right brain must, in turn, exercise a feedback control on the left hemisphere. This has been demonstrated in the elegant experiments of Renoux and Biziere (12), who showed that in the rodent, not only is the T-lymphocytic immunologic system and splenic killer phagocytic response dependent on the integrity of left brain functions but that, in addition, left brain ablations led to atrophy of the thymus, whereas right brain cortical lesions evoked hypertrophy of the thymus. This indicates that the regulatory influence of left brain systems is itself modulated by inhibitory influences originating in the right brain. A consideration of brain–psychopathologic interactions led to a similar representation (13). At a certain intensity of depression, psychomotor retardation, mutism, or even functional motor paralysis: depressive stupor—in effect—catatonic immobility supervenes. As negative emotions, dysphoric mood states, and depression are determined by right hemispheric events—more precisely, right frontolimbic events (14,15)—and if overall motor regulation hinges on left hemispheric functions, this suggests that with deepening of depression there is a progressive transcallosally mediated alteration of dominant hemispheric systems. A number of experimental approaches suggest that this is indeed the case.

1. The fact that in dextral depressives the degree of left hemisphere language competence is inversely correlated with depth of depression during intracarotid barbiturization (16).
2. The fact that depressions not responding to tricyclics but are electroconvulsive therapy (ECT)-responsive fail to show the expected right ear superiority to verbal stimuli on dichotic stimulation before treatment: it returns after treatment and with recovery (17).
3. The fact that in depression there is an increase in the acoustic threshold for the left ear (right hemisphere effect) that returns to normal after recovery (18). However, when psychomotor retardation supervenes in depression, the acoustic threshold for the right ear is increased (left hemisphere effect) (19).
4. Psychometric studies indicate a significant decrement of performance relative to verbal IQ in both psychotic depression and mania. The effect is stronger for mania than depression. Hence a functional disorganization of the right hemisphere, more pronounced in mania than depression, is implicated (20).
5. In both unipolar and bipolar depression the mean integrated amplitude of the electroencephalogram (EEG) over the left hemisphere is reduced compared with the right; the degree of this asymmetry is correlated with the severity of the depression (21,22).

In the bipolar psychoses, if one contrasts the symptomatology of the excited and inhibited forms of clinical presentation—the hypermotility, the speech acceleration, the euphoria, and the hypersexuality of mania—with the psychomotor retardation, paucity of speech/mutism, sadness, and hyposexuality of depression, it is clear that the two poles correspond to functional changes in the dominant hemisphere of opposite directionality, given the left hemisphere lateralization for speech, positive emotions, and motility regulation. With very deep depressions, patients no longer feel actual sadness but are subjectively empty, devoid of all emotions. An interesting point in the context of this argument, as Ross and Rush (23) have shown in the study of the modifications imposed by localized cerebrovascular accidents on depressive symptomatology in patients with prestroke depressive illnesses, is that with *left* temporoparietal lesions subjects were no longer aware of sadness, in spite of experiencing a typical recurrence of depression: the irritability, insomnia, and anorexia responding to tricyclic antidepressant therapy. Thus it would appear that, even though sadness is generated by right anterolimbic processes, its evaluation and monitoring is a function of dominant hemispheric systems. The changes in sexual functions can also be related to left brain activity as dopamine agonists promote sexual behaviors and have a left hemisphere preponderance, as opposed to serotonin, inhibiting sexual behaviors and right hemisphere preponderant and noradrenergic activity nonspecifically linked to sexual arousal (24).

Lohr and Caliguiri (25) studied the control of hand muscle force in schizophrenia and bipolar affective psychoses and found that they displayed opposite asymmetries. They investigated 23 schizophrenics, 13 patients with bipolar illness, and 50 controls assessing hand force stability with strain gauges to transduce fluctuations in steady-state force over time. The subjects attempt to maintain steady levels of isometric force by pressure on a lever with the index finger, the target being displayed on an oscilloscope where it could be viewed by the subjects. The schizophrenics had more right-hand dyscontrol and the bipolar patients greater left-hand dyscontrol. All subjects were right-handed and all patients were medicated. In a previous study of motor asymmetry in 15 never-medicated schizophrenics, the right-sided motor asymmetry was similar to that found in schizophrenics on neuroleptics.

The disturbance of dominance in hemispheric function in acute psychosis arising as a consequence of changes originating in the nondominant hemisphere is illustrated in the following single case study of psychotic depression presenting as acute schizophrenia.

Case Study

The patient was a 26-year-old with an illness of 6 to 12 months duration. He presented with the following symptoms: anxiety, auditory hallucinations, for example he heard "several voices, male and female, commenting on his thoughts and actions"; he said that his mind was influenced at a distance by both his mother and objects touching his head, for example hair brushes or shampoos; he experienced thought deprivation and thought insertion together with thought blocking; olfactory hallucinations, for example he believed that a foul smell emanated from his head. His mood was subjectively "empty" and objectively blunted. He had had intermittent thoughts of suicide but had made no suicidal attempts. Disturbances in sleep and appetite as well as impairment in concentration were present together with loss of sexual drive. There had been one previous episode four years earlier when he had "felt manic, high, full of energy" for several months, but this episode had not been associated with overspending, hypersexuality, grandiosity, or sleep disturbance, and no treatment had been required. In the family, one brother was on lithium. The patient was the second born (11 minutes after his brother) of twins, weighed 8 pounds at birth and had been an "easy child." He had completed high school successfully at the age of 19, and had a good work record in drilling and construction until the onset of his illness. He was single and had a heterosexual drive but had not dated or had any girlfriends after puberty.

He was treated with neuroleptics for the first eight weeks of hospitalization (40 mg/day trifluoperazine, then up to 1,000 mg/day chlorpromazine). He became progressively more thought disordered and clinical depression became evident. Extrapyramidal symptomatology was asymmetric: tremor and cogwheel rigidity left greater than the right. Neuroleptic therapy was stopped. There was remarkable improvement in his mental state one week after two bilateral ECT. After three weeks on lithium (0.8–1.2 mmol/L), he was completely asymptomatic and was discharged from hospital.

Neuropsychologic testing before treatment, when the clinical picture was of schizophrenia, revealed hemispheric dysfunction on the left side as compared with the right, even though the left hemispheric functions were essentially normal in absolute terms. When the patient became asymptomatic, that is after ECT and lithium, there was a reversal of hemispheric balance, with an improvement in left and a deficit in right hemispheric functions (Table 47.1, Figs 47.1 and

47.2). This revealed the underlying right hemispheric vulnerability that had been activated during the illness and that had evoked the schizophrenic symptomatology through contralateral disorganization. Power spectral EEG analysis before treatment had shown a pattern of diffuse right hemispheric and focal left temporal activation. The clinical EEG showed right temporal activity that disappeared after recovery (26).

Kinsbourne (15) has related emotions to motility, proposing that positive emotions are a correlate of approach and negative emotions of withdrawal behaviors. At the most fundamental level, biologic systems of minimal complexity are determined by their motility responses to environmental cues; hence the importance of motility–spatial cerebral processing interactions.

Emotions can be viewed as an extension of this interaction in brain evolution at a certain level of complexity. In

Table 47.1 Neuropsychologic Test Score Changes Expressed in Standard Deviation Units after Lithium Treatment

Neuropsychologic tests: improvement		
Williams verbal learning	+1.75	
Trail making B	+1.50	
Tactual performance—right hand	+0.80	
Tactual performance—memory	+0.80	Dominant (7)
Colored progressive matrices	+0.75	
Dynamometer—right hand	+0.60	
Speech sounds perception	+0.50	
Finger localization—left hand	+1.20	Nondominant (1)
Neuropsychologic tests: decrement		
Purdue pegboard—left hand	−1.10	
Purdue pegboard—both hands	−1.00	
Name writing—left hand	−1.00	
Trail making A	−0.75	Nondominant (6)
Seashore rhythm	−0.75	
Symbol digit—written	−1.00	
Purdue pegboard—right hand	−0.50	Dominant (2)
Finger tapping—right hand	−1.10	

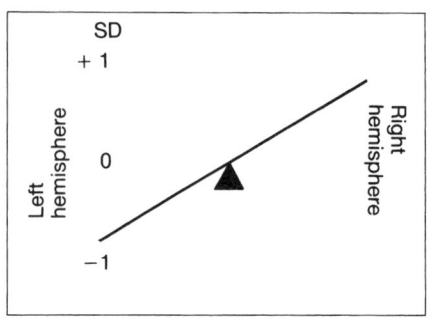

FIGURE 47.1 *Neuropsychologic evaluation pretreatment hemispheric relationships expressed in standard deviation (SD) units.*

more highly developed evolutionary forms, adaptation to either diurnal or nocturnal life has occurred. Neural organization, then, has become time-locked to circadian day/night alternations as well as to shorter and longer fluctuations such as seasonal ones. There is evidence that the consequent and complex biologic oscillations play an extremely important role in maintaining normal physical and psychologic state and that perturbation of the neural systems responsible for the synchronization of various biologic oscillations leads to certain types of mental disorders. Hence the periodic, or as is more frequently, the aperiodically periodic psychoses, catatonic, schizophrenic, schizodepressive, depressive, or manic. Seasonal affective disorders have recently been formally described.

Both neuropsychologic (27) and power spectral EEG parameters (28) indicate that the pattern of cerebral disorganization in mania and schizophrenia is very similar, although the severity of dysfunction is less in mania. In the majority of cases of symptomatic mania secondary to neurologic lesions (nonirritative) such as cerebral tumors or cerebrovascular accidents are statistically associated with right hemisphere localization (29–31).

Related phenomena are the euphoric emotional changes induced by intracarotid barbiturization of the nondominant hemisphere or by the euphoria or "transient hypomanic-like states" evoked by the electrical hemispheric inactivation of the nondominant hemisphere effected by unilateral ECT (32–34). A remarkably apposite animal model exists as Robinson (35) showed that in the rat, ligation of the right middle cerebral artery induced lasting hyperactivity of two or three weeks' duration accompanied by a 30% reduction of cortical noradrenaline and a 20% reduction of dopamine in the substantia nigra. Left brain infarcts had no behavioral consequences and produced no changes in catecholamines in any of the brain regions studied. The lateralized corticolimbic regulation of motility (hyperactivity) in the rat, however, is complex. Bradbury et al (36) found that infusion of dopamine in the amygdaloid produced hyperactivity only when the left amygdaloid was injected, provided the right hemisphere was dominant (preferentially turning

left in an open field). Further, even although it is well-established that in rats with unilateral striatal lesions the animals when engaged in circling behaviors rotate toward the less active side, that is, contralateral to the more active dopaminergic striatum, in the intact normal animal 3, 4-dihydroxy-phenyl acetic acid (DOPAC) concentrations are higher in the striata ipsilateral to the dominant direction of rotation: thus the rotation is toward the more active, not the less active side (37). Against this background should be situated two important observations that relate to amygdaloid dopamine asymmetry and abnormal circling behavior in schizophrenics. Reynolds (38) found a significant increase in dopamine concentration in the left amygdaloid of schizophrenic brains and Bracha (39) a significant excess of leftward circling behavior in 10 unmedicated schizophrenics—85 normal controls exhibiting no rotational asymmetry as a population. Contradicting earlier reports (40), Wilson et al (41) and Myslobodsky et al (42) showed that there is an equal incidence of right- and left-sided abnormal involuntary movements in unselected and diagnostically heterogeneous patients with tardive dyskinesia. It must be pointed out that in the study by Waziri (40) there was only one schizophrenic patient, in that by Wilson et al (41) there were 14, and in the Myslobodsky series, 7; the other diagnostic categories in all these studies consisting essentially of affective psychotics. Cumulating the schizophrenics in the three studies:

Lateralization of tardive dyskinesia in schizophrenia

Right (or R > L)	*Left* (or L > R)	*Bilateral and symmetric*
13	4	5

Thus there is a right-sided preponderance of neuroleptic-induced abnormal movements in schizophrenia, the right side implicated three times more frequently than the left in these patients, all of whom, except one, were dextral.

In a later study of schizophrenics with and without tardive dyskinesia, Myslobodsky et al (43) observed that 88% had complete lack of concern for their disability (anosognosia) and that the tardive dyskinesia subgroup had poorer recall of pictures presented in the right hemispatial field than the schizophrenics without abnormal movements. As both groups, naturally, were on neuroleptics, this suggests that in addition to a profound right hemisphere hypofunctional state (anosognosia) the tardive dyskinesia subjects, relative to those without dyskinesia, have a greater degree of left hemisphere deficit. Although tardive dyskinesia, in a subgroup of schizophrenics, particularly female, presumably with an underlying cerebral vulnerability, is in all probability a consequence of prolonged neuroleptic exposure, it must not be forgotten that the disorder was described in psychotics long before the discovery of neuroleptics. Furthermore, tardive dyskinesia is not always the permanent and static defect that is generally assumed. There are reports, of considerable theoretical importance, to indicate that in the manic–depressive

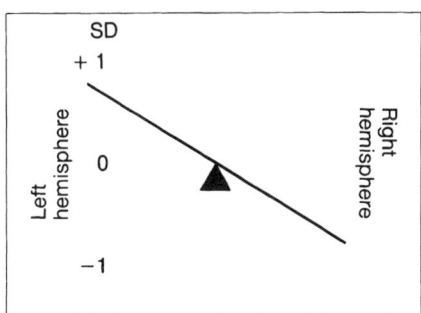

FIGURE 47.2 *Neuropsychologic evaluation posttreatment hemispheric relationships expressed in standard deviation (SD) units.*

syndrome tardive dyskinesia may be state-dependent: appearing during depressive episodes and disappearing in the manic phase (44,45). Very interestingly, similar oscillations have been described for obsessive–compulsive symptomatology where in patients with bipolar illness the compulsive symptomatology fluctuates regularly: disappearing during the manic phase and emerging during the depressive episodes (46). On a right hemisphere hypothesis for both mania and depression inducing either contralateral (left) functional inhibition (depression) or dysfunctional activation (mania) it would follow, assuming a left hemisphere origin for both tardive dyskinesia (90% of Broca aphasics have oral apraxia, a different but related disturbance (47)) and obsessive–compulsive symptomatology, that the induced abnormal left hemisphere activation underlying mania "overrides" the striatofrontal dysregulation common to both the obsessional syndrome and the tardive dyskinesias.

Of the major psychopathologic syndromes, two in which dysregulation of frontobasal ganglia, more especially of frontocaudate neural circuits, are prominent in the pathophysiology are the catatonic and obsessive–compulsive syndromes. I have already discussed in this chapter the evidence for the importance of dominant hemisphere lateralization in determining catatonic symptomatology. With respect to the obsessive–compulsive states, the evidence to date strongly points to bilateral frontobasal ganglia pathology on a variety of indicators: neuropsychologic, computerized tomography (CT) scan, neurometabolic studies (PET); however, superimposed on this evidence there are other investigations—spectral EEG, somatosensory and auditory evoked potential, and cliniconeuropathologic correlations—that all invariably implicate the left frontotemporal–left caudate axis (48).

The association of catatonic symptomatology with schizophrenia is well-known. On a left frontocaudate hypothesis for catatonia and obsessive–compulsive disorder, an association between catatonia and the obsessional syndrome would also be theoretically expected. It has in fact recently been described by Hermesh et al (49).

Laplane et al (50) described eight unusual patients with bilateral basal ganglia lesions, obsessive–compulsive disorder, a "frontal lobe-like" syndrome characterized by inertia, and loss of drive and paucity of thought. These patients were investigated in great detail with neuropsychologic, nuclear magnetic resonance imaging, and PET techniques. The lesions were restricted to the lentiform nuclei; frontal lobe dysfunction was indicated by the frequency of perseverative errors on the Wisconsin card sorting and also by the neurometabolic studies that revealed relative hypometabolism of the prefrontal cortex. They also had an absolute reduction of metabolic activity in the lentiform nuclei. The authors drew attention to the similarity existing between the akinesia and slowness seen in the major depressive syndromes. They concluded that their patients

were unable to inhibit some programs that were either purely mental, or both mental and motor . . . there

seems to be a continuity between the motor stereotypies, some resembling tics, the mental stereotypies and the obsessive–compulsive behaviors proper.

In this context, the postmortem neuropathologic study of Brown et al (51) is of interest. Comparing 41 schizophrenic and 29 patients with affective disorder, the schizophrenic group had a significant thinning of the left parahippocampal cortex. In the affective patients the right caudate nucleus was significantly smaller than the left. Localized neurometabolic pathology of the globus pallidus is also reported by Early et al (52) in the PET investigation of never-medicated schizophrenics. The only region significantly different from healthy controls was the left globus pallidus, with increased cerebral blood flow. Both authors relate their findings to the new knowledge about the detailed organization of the basal ganglia which, to quote Alexander et al (53) "has accumulated at a prodigious pace over the past decade, necessitating major revisions in our concepts of the structural and functional organization of these nuclei." Alexander and his collaborators reviewed the evidence from primates that indicates the presence of a series of "functionally segregated circuits linking basal ganglia and cortex," enumerating five: motor, oculomotor, dorsolateral prefrontal, lateral orbitofrontal, and anterior cingulate. Noteworthy is the fact that the supplementary motor area receives the output from the motor circuit, as the supplementary motor area plays a central role in the "programming, initiation and execution of movement . . . and it would appear that the basal ganglia and the supplementary motor area form part of a system involved in the programming and execution of complex movements." Nauta (54), in a detailed review of the new neuroanatomic evidence on the "reciprocal links of the corpus striatum with the cerebral cortex and the limbic system," suggested that these might be the common substrate for movement and thought. He emphasized the importance of limbic afferent into the striatum: from the hippocampal formation, the amygdala, and the cingulate cortex that then projects exclusively to the ventral pallidum, subsequently through the dorsomedial nucleus of the thalamus with "return loops" to the prefrontal cortex. Nauta drew attention to the parallel existing between limbic and nonlimbic transstriatal connections, both feeding back to the points of origin in the hemispheres. The "motor circuit": motor cortex . . . striatum . . . pallidum . . . thalamic ventroanterior–ventrolateral complex . . . premotor cortex . . . motor cortex, is balanced by its limbic equivalent: limbic system . . . striatum . . . ventral pallidum . . . dorsomedial nucleus of the thalamus . . . frontal and anterior limbic cortex. Nauta concluded with the hypothesis that the frontal limbic–striatal loop might play a regulatory role for cognitive processes comparable with that of the extrapyramidal motor loop in motility and movement regulation. Common to movement and ideation is "the need for propulsion and timing."

The central idea in this essay is that psychopathologic phenomena are intricately involved with disturbances of motility not because the one is secondary to the other, but because both are the simultaneous expressions of disorganized and lateralized corticolimbic systems. From an evolutionary perspective, motility and visual processing are the necessary conditions for biologic survival. With increasing complexity of central nervous system organization, increasing lateral hemispheric specialization occurred, *pari pasu* with increasing callosally mediated interhemispheric inhibitory capacity. On one side of the brain emotions, normal and pathologic, can be linked to motility mechanisms; on the other side, ideational representations, normal or pathologic, can be related to motility control: speech after all is only possible because of the extraordinary finely tuned control of the laryngeal apparatus by lateralized motor controlling hemispheric systems, and this in turn determines most of "subjective consciousness" normal or pathologic. The recent appreciation of the distinct corticostriatocortical loops in the motor system as well as in the limbic network—which are nevertheless to some extent overlapping at their striatal projections—again demonstrates the importance and the interrelatedness of cognitive–affective–motility states. Because the corticostriatocortical organization is a closed loop, the principles of lateral hemispheric specialization will necessarily apply subcortically as well as in the limbic–cortical regions. Further, lateralized corticofugal influences will be matched by equivalent striatocorticolimbic projected dysregulations. Thus it is not surprising that, with improving techniques with which to demonstrate regional cerebral pathology in psychopathology, lateralized striatal perturbation increasingly is being recognized.

REFERENCES

1. Flor-Henry P. Observations, reflections and speculations on the cerebral determinants of mood and on the bilaterally asymmetrical distributions of the major neurotransmitter systems. Acta Neurol Scand 1986;74(Suppl 109):75–89.
2. Tucker DM, Williamson PA. Asymmetric neural control systems in human self-regulation. Psychol Rev 1984;91:185–215.
3. Yakovlev P, Rakic P. Patterns of discussion of bulbar pyramids and distribution of pyramidal tracts on two sides of the spinal cord. Trans Am Neurol Assoc 1996;91:366–367.
4. Wyke M. Effect of brain lesions on the rapidity of arm movement. Neurology 1967;17:1113–1120.
5. Goodale MA. Hemispheric differences in motor control. Behav Brain Res 1988;30:203–214.
6. Davison K, Bagley CR. Schizophrenia-like psychoses associated with organic disorders of the central nervous system: a review of the literature. Br J Psychiatry 1969;4:113–184.
7. Luchins DJ, Metz JT, Marks RC, Cooper MD. Basal ganglia regional glucose metabolism asymmetry during a catatonic episode. Biol Psychiatry 1989;26:725–728.
8. Cook ND. The brain code. Mechanisms of information transfer and the role of the corpus callosum. London: Methuen, 1986.
9. Denenberg VH. Hemispheric laterality in animals and the effects of early experience. Behav Brain Sci 1981;4:1–19.
10. Denenberg VH. Brain laterality and behavioral asymmetry in the rat. In: Flor-Henry P, Gruzelier J, eds. Laterality and psychopathology. Amsterdam: Elsevier, 1983:29–34.
11. Denenberg VH. General systems theory, brain organization and early experiences. Am J Physiol 1980;238:R3–13.
12. Renoux G, Biziere K. Brain neocortex lateralized control of immune recognition. Integr Psychiatry 1986;4:32–40.
13. Flor-Henry P. The endogenous psychoses: a reflection of lateralized dysfunction of the anterior limbic system. In: Livingston KE, Hornykiewicz O, eds. Limbic mechanisms. New York, Plenum, 1978:389–404.
14. Flor-Henry P. Observations, reflections and speculations on the cerebral determinants of mood and on the bilaterally asymmetrical distributions of the major neurotransmitter systems. Acta Neurol Scand 1986;74(Suppl 109):75–89.
15. Kinsbourne M. Hemisphere interactions in depression. In: Kinsbourne M, ed. Cerebral hemisphere function in depression. Washington: American Psychiatric Association, 1988:135–162.
16. Hommes OR, Panhuysen LHHM. Bilateral intracarotid amytal injection. Psychiatry Neurol Neurochir 1970;73:447–459.
17. Moscovitch M, Strauss E, Olds J. Handedness in patients with unipolar endogenous depression who require electroconvulsive therapy. Am J Psychiatry 1981;138:988–990.
18. Sackeim HA, Epstein D, Decina P, et al. Auditory measures of lateralised activation imbalance in depression and effects of ECT. Presented at the VII World Congress of Psychiatry, Vienna. Ciba Geigy Switzerland, 1983;1124:243. Abstract.
19. Bruder G, Spring B, Yozawitz A, Sutton S. Auditory sensitivity in psychiatric patients and non-patients: monotic click detection. Psychol Med 1980;10:1338.
20. Flor-Henry P, Fromm-Auch D, Schopflocher D. Neuropsychological dimensions in psychopathology. In: Flor-Henry P, Gruzelier J, eds. Laterality and psychopathology. Amsterdam: Elsevier, 1983:59–82.
21. d'Elia G, Perris C. Cerebral functional dominance and depression. Acta Psychiatr Scand 1973;49:191–197.
22. Perris C. EEG techniques in the measurement of the severity of depressive syndromes. Neuropsychobiology 1975;1:16–25.
23. Ross E, Rush J. Diagnosis and neuroanatomical correlates of depression in brain damaged patients. Arch Gen Psychiatry 1981;38:1344–1354.
24. Flor-Henry P. On the cerebral neurophysiology and neurotransmitter determination of sexual deviation. Int Rev Psychiatry 1989;1:83–86.
25. Lohr JB, Caliguiri MP. Motor asymmetry, a neurobiologic abnormality in the major psychoses. Psychiatry Res 1995;57:279–282.
26. Flor-Henry P. The influence of laterality in psychopathology. In: Hamilton M, ed. Psychiatry in the 80s, ideas, research, practice. Amsterdam: Excerpta Medica, 1987:1–4.
27. Flor-Henry P. Cerebral basis of psychopathology. Boston: John Wright, 1983.
28. Flor-Henry P, Koles ZJ, Sussman PS. Multivariate EEG analysis of the endogenous psychoses. Adv Biol Psychiatry 1983;13:196–210.
29. Cohen MR, Niska RW. Localised right cerebral hemisphere dysfunction and recurrent mania. Am J Psychiatry 1980;137:847–848.
30. Cummings JL, Mendez MF. Secondary mania with focal cerebrovascular lesions. Am J Psychiatry 1984;141:1084–1087.
31. Starkstein SE, Robinson RG. Lateralized emotional response following stroke. In: Kinsbourne M, ed. Cerebral hemisphere function in depression. Washington: American Psychiatric Association, 1988:25–47.
32. Terzian H. Behavioral and EEG effects of intracarotid sodium amytal injection. Acta Neurochir 1964;12:230–239.
33. Rossi GE, Rosadini G. Experimental analysis of cerebral dominance in man. In: Darley FL, ed. Brain mechanisms underlying speech and language. New York: Grune & Stratton, 1967:167–184.
34. Deglin VL, Nikolaenko NN. Role of the dominant hemisphere in the regulation of emotional states. Hum Physiol 1975;1:394–402.
35. Robinson RG. Differential behavioral and biochemical effects of right and left hemispheric cerebral infarction in the rat. Science 1979;205:707–710.
36. Bradbury AJ, Costall B, Domeney AM, Naylor RJ. Laterality of dopamine function and neuroleptic action in the amygdala in the rat. Neuropharmacology 1985;24:1163–1170.
37. Jerussi TP, Taylor CA. Bilateral asymmetry in striatal dopamine metabolism: Implications for pharmacotherapy of schizophrenia. Brain Res 1982;246:71–75.
38. Reynolds GP. Increased concentrations and lateral asymmetry of amygdala dopamine in schizophrenia. Nature 1983;305:527–529.
39. Bracha HS. Asymmetric rotational (circling) behavior, a dopamine-related asymmetry: preliminary findings in unmedicated and never-medicated schizophrenic patients. Biol Psychiatry 1987;22:995–1003.
40. Waziri R. Lateralization of neuroleptic-induced dyskinesia indicates pharmacologic asymmetry in the brain. Psychopharmacology 1980;68:51–53.
41. Wilson RL, Waziri R, Nasrallah HA, McCalley-Whitters M. The lateralization of tardive dyskinesia. Biol Psychiatry 1984;19:629–635.
42. Myslobodsky MS, Holden T, Sandler R. Asymmetry of abnormal involuntary movements. A prevalence study. Biol Psychiatry 1984;19:623–628.
43. Myslobodsky MS, Tomer R, Holden T, et al. Cognitive impairment in patients with tardive dyskinesia. J Nerv Ment Dis 1985;173:156–160.

44. Cutler NR, Post RM, Rey AC, Bunney WE Jr. Depression-dependent dyskinesias in two cases of manic–depressive illness. N Engl J Med 1981;304:1088–1089.

45. de Potter RW, Linkowski P, Mendlewicz J. State-dependent tardive dyskinesia in manic–depressive illness. J Neurol Neurosurg Psychiatry 1983;46:666–668.

46. Gordon A, Rasmussen SA. Mood-related obsessive–compulsive symptoms in a patient with bipolar affective disorder. J Clin Psychiatry 1988;49:27–28.

47. Heilman KM, Gonzalez Rothi LJ. Apraxia. In: Heilman KM, Valenstein E, eds. Clinical neuropsychology. New York: Oxford University, 1985:131–150.

48. Flor-Henry P. Le syndrome obsessionel-compulsif: reflet d'un défaut de régulation fronto-caudée de l'hémisphère gauche? L'Encéphale 1990;xvi:325–329.

49. Hermesh H, Hoffnung RA, Aizenberg D, et al. Catatonic signs in severe obsessive–compulsive disorder. J Clin Psychiatry 1989;50:303–305.

50. Laplane D, Levasseur M, Pillon B, et al. Obsessive–compulsive and other behavioural changes with bilateral basal ganglia lesions. Brain 1989;112:699–725.

51. Brown R, Colter N, Corsellis JAN, et al. Postmortem evidence of structural brain changes in schizophrenia. Arch Gen Psychiatry 1986;43:36–42.

52. Early TS, Reiman EM, Raichle ME, Spitznagel EL. Left globus pallidus abnormality in never-medicated patients with schizophrenia. Proc Natl Acad Sci USA 1987;84:561–563.

53. Alexander GE, DeLong MR, Strick PL. Parallel organization of functionally segregated circuits linking basal ganglia and cortex. Ann Rev Neurosci 1986;9:357–381.

54. Nauta WJH. Reciprocal links of the corpus striatum with the cerebral cortex and limbic system: a common substrate for movement and thought? In: Mueller, ed. Neurology and psychiatry: a meeting of minds. Basel: Karger, 1989:43–63.

Catatonia

Anthony B. Joseph

INTRODUCTION

The concept of catatonia developed in the last century out of the confusion surrounding attempts to classify psychiatric illness. This confusion persists to the present, not least because even today there is no clear and universally accepted definition of catatonia.

It is generally accepted that the idea of a catatonic symptom complex was advanced in 1863 by the German psychiatrist Karl Kahlbaum in his *Grouping of Psychic Diseases*, and that the term itself was proposed the following year (1). The word *catatonia* is of Greek derivation and has been translated as "negative tension" or "cast down" (2). Kahlbaum's use of it seems to have arisen from his desire to differentiate diseases from syndromes. For him catatonia was a disease that passed through stages of melancholia, mania, stupor, confusion, and dementia, any of which might be absent in a given case.

Many of Kahlbaum's contemporaries disagreed and felt that catatonia was a syndrome rather than a disease, but the argument was more about classification than clinical course or presentation. By 1860 Morel had already used the term *demence precoce* regarding a group of young patients with chronic mental illness characterized by a deteriorating course. The question then, as now, was whether they suffered from a syndrome or a disease. The clinical science of the day limited the debate to this core group of patients. Their exact clinical characteristics, however, were never quite clear. The debate was thought to be important because an understanding of this group of patients could serve as a central paradigm applicable by neurology and psychiatry to other equally mysterious discreet groups of patients.

It was against this background that Kahlbaum brought forward the concept of catatonia. As the debate continued, Hecker, prompted by Kahlbaum, described the disease entity of hebephrenia, and catatonia was described by Schuele as "a hebephrenia in conjunction with tension neurosis" (1). Catatonia and hebephrenia still referred to similar groups of patients with chronic deteriorating psychoses. Etiologic questions were raised about the importance of heredity in the development of these diseases, their relationship to familial and idiopathic degenerations, and the need for the developmental prerequisite of "a defective brain." In 1891, Pick published on "simple deterioration" followed by Sommer in 1894. Sommer described the clinical picture of catatonia and classified hebephrenia as one of a group of primary dementias. Confusingly catatonia *per se* was described as separate from these dementias. In 1896, Kraepelin proposed that the "deteriorating psychoses" were part of a larger group of metabolic diseases. Dementia praecox corresponded to the hebephrenias and primary dementias. Primary catatonia was part of a different group of disorders. In 1899, Kraepelin reformulated his concepts and *dementia praecox* became the umbrella term for the hebephrenias, primary dementias, and catatonia. Bleuler later refined and also reformulated the concept of dementia praecox. For him it was schizophrenia, and catatonia was firmly established in his mind as a subtype.

This historical dualism perplexes us to the present day. It is ironic that the modern usage of the term *catatonia* is to describe a behavioral disorder that may be either primary or secondary, almost the same purpose for which the term was coined. In the development of psychiatry, however, it first became synonymous with schizophrenia and then with a subtype of schizophrenia. Both usages are still extant in the literature. Authors refer not only to catatonic schizophrenia as a synonym for catatonia, a disease, but also to catatonia as a neurobehavioral clinical presentation with a differential diagnosis including schizophrenia.

Since Bleuler there has been less interest in using catatonia as a stalking horse in the controversy between those who classify psychiatric illness into diseases and those who classify it into syndromes, and more attention has been paid to describing and trying to understand catatonic patients. As the century has progressed, several important enlargements have been made to the idea of catatonic schizophrenia. These include periodic catatonia, catatonic excitement, acute lethal catatonia, and catatonic-like syndromes in neurology. More recently observations on drug-induced catatonia, the relationship between catatonia and affective disorders, and the notion that catatonia and neuroleptic malignant syndrome may be indistinguishable have also become very important in expanding our understanding of this syndrome. Finally, in the current decade, it has seemed that catatonia the syndrome has become preeminent and catatonia the disease has been eclipsed, but the historical echoes of the great debate are still with us to influence both the modern categorization and conceptualization of this disorder.

DIAGNOSIS

As there is no clear definition of catatonia, diagnosis can be somewhat problematic. In this chapter, the position is taken that it is a behavioral syndrome. Although for many authors catatonia has been a psychiatric disorder marked by multiple possible motor and behavioral signs and symptoms (Table 48.1), much evidence supports the conclusion that it is frequently secondary to, or associated with, a number of primary disorders (3–5). Catatonia may therefore be primary and idiopathic or secondary to a known cause. The causes of secondary catatonia and the primary disorders associated with idiopathic catatonia are many and the differential diagnosis is significant (Tables 48.2 and 48.3).

The diagnosis is most clear when a patient presents with the triad of mutism or near mutism, akinesia or severe hpokinesia, and catalepsy or profound dystonia approximating catalepsy. In these cases, the diagnosis of catatonia is not in doubt although the cause may be. Some authorities do not require such a severe psychomotor disturbance, and for them accessory signs such as stereotypy, posturing, and automatic obedience are sufficient for diagnosis (6,7). This author views such cases as either partial forms of the syndrome or related phenomena in noncatatonic patients. In the case of catatonic excitement, extreme psychomotor excitement has been proposed as the only necessary presenting sign (8). In this chapter, the position is taken that catatonic excitement as described in the literature is usually an extreme and impressive form of mania or other excited state. These states can occur in patients with a past history of catatonia. This juxtaposition of past and present events, however, should not be regarded as sufficient a priori justification for classifying extreme psychomotor excitement as a form of catatonia.

Diagnosis, then, is made on the history, physical examination, and mental status examination. In the history it is important to differentiate a primary from a secondary catatonia. The practical differentiation is that a primary catatonia is either idiopathic or associated with some other primary psychiatric diagnosis and requires one of the standard approaches to management. A secondary catatonia is one in which a nonidiopathic cause can be diagnosed, which consequently requires a nonstandard intervention such as neurologic evaluation, discontinuation of a causative agent, or specific treatment of the cause.

It is important to note that a secondary catatonia can occur in any patient, even one with a previous history of primary catatonia. For example, a bipolar patient previously catatonic and maintained on lithium carbonate could be started on haloperidol and present with neuroleptic-induced secondary catatonia. This history would require initial treatment by discontinuation of haloperidol rather than by a course of medications used for primary catatonia. Historical evidence suggestive of primary catatonia includes previous episodes of primary catatonia; previous or concurrent major psychiatric illness, especially affective disorders; gradual onset; and family history of catatonia or affective disorder. Historical indices of a secondary catatonia are sudden or gradual onset complicated by sinister neurologic complaints; recent neuroleptic or other drug use; concurrent or recent toxic, metabolic, neurologic illness; simple, complex partial, grand mal, or absence seizures; and family history of seizure disorder or neurologic disease affecting movement.

The physical examination is less helpful in differentiating primary from secondary catatonia or catatonia from other states in which patients become mute, cataleptic, akinetic, and autonomically deranged.

Although it is not well-recorded in the literature, catatonic patients frequently have significant abnormalities on neurologic examination including lateralized reflex changes. They do not, however, have changes in the elementary sensory examination, or lateralized or focal weakness, unless related to an ictal or postictal state. If these signs are present, an emergent neurologic evaluation is indicated.

Frequent neurologic abnormalities found on physical examination are listed in Table 48.4.

MANAGEMENT

Management of catatonia may be divided into two parts: evaluation and treatment. The initial assessment provides grounds for dividing patients into those with an idiopathic or nonemergent secondary catatonia and those with an acute neurologic event presenting as catatonia. Management of the latter group should be that of the primary event. For the former, a number of further investigations may be performed. None of them are diagnostic, but all can help the

Table 48.1   Abnormal Signs in Catatonia

Motor	Speech and Language	Cognitive-Behavioral
Akinesia	Mutism	Extreme agitation (catatonic excitement)
Hypokinesia	Aphasia	Ganser's syndrome
Bradykinesia	Initiation difficulties	Leonhard's speech-prompt catatonia
Parkinsonism	Verbigeration	Combativeness
Tremor	Thought disorder	Denudativeness
Extrapyramidal dyskinesias	Confusion	Negativism
Stupor	Disorganized thinking	Posturing
Initiation difficulties	Echolalia	Grimacing
Catalepsy	Palilalia	Staring
Rigidity	Stuttering	Stereotypy
Gegenhalten		Psychosis
Positive limb placement		Depression
Other paratonias		Mania
Primitive reflexes		Impaired judgment
Abnormal deep tendon reflexes		Impaired insight
Abnormal Babinski response		Playfulness
Oculomotor disturbances		Withdrawal
Perseveration		Regression
Impulsivity		Mannerisms
Hyperkinesis		Rituals
Tics		Utilization behavior
		Imitation behavior
		Echopraxia
		Automatic obedience
		Impaired attention
		Obsessiveness
		Compulsiveness

Autonomic	End-Stage Signs	Laboratory Findings
Hypertension	Dehydration	Leucocytosis
Pyrexia	Acrocyanosis	Elevated epinephrine
Hyperpyrexia	Petechiae	Elevated norepinephrine
Diaphoresis	Circulatory collapse	Elevated creatine phosphokinase
Malignant hyperthermia	Respiratory collapse	Elevated aldolase
Tachycardia	Renal failure	Elevated ceruloplasmin
Tachypnea	Seizures	Abnormal brain computerized tomography
Pupillary dilation	Coma	Abnormal electroencephalogram
Autonomic instability	Death	Abnormal neuropsychological testing
Insomnia		Abnormal electrocardiogram
(?) Switch process		Abnormal echocardiogram
(?) Periodicity		

formulation of a case. Plain skull films are rarely useful. Computerized tomography, however, frequently reveals atrophic changes, particularly in the frontal lobes, cerebellar vermis, and brainstem (9). Their cause or meaning is unclear. It is not yet known whether magnetic resonance imaging, positron emission tomography, or single photon emission computerized tomography will be useful.

Plain electoencephalography may or may not show diffuse abnormalities or a spike focus. The results with brain electrical activity mapping are similar. Neuropsychologic testing often reveals a pattern of diffuse cerebral dysfunction, with the maximum impairment typically being anterior and bilateral. Finally, abnormalities of the electrocardiogram and echocardiogram have been reported, but their general significance is not clear (10).

Treatment has not been well worked out, and the literature on this is still sparse. A number of modalities do show promise, and these include benzodiazepines, anticonvulsants, amytal, lithium carbonate, and electroconvulsive therapy (11–15). Some experimental work suggests that

Table 48.2   Catatonias

Idiopathic catatonia
    Without brain atrophy
    With brain atrophy
    Associated with
        Bipolar disorder
        Major depressive disorder
        Other affective disorder
        Schizophrenia
        Other psychiatric disorder

Catatonia secondary to
    Temporal lobe epilepsy
    Other seizure disorder
    Brain tumor
    Brain trauma
    Encephalitis—postencephalitic state
    Central vascular disease
    Other causes of focal brain lesions
    Akinetic mutism
    Parkinsonism
    Toxic encephalopathy
    Metabolic encephalopathy
    Other medical disorders
    Neuroleptic malignant syndrome
    Neuroleptics
    Other prescribed psychotropics
    Illicit psychotropics

antidepressants, antihistamines, and narcotic antagonists could also be effective treatments (16–18).

Frequently, catatonic patients are presumed to be psychotic on the basis of their severe behavioral decompensation and are therefore given neuroleptics. It is then not uncommon for them to arrive at a tertiary treatment center stiff, cataleptic, and mute, with a history of neuroleptic exposure just prior to the maximum intensity of catatonic symptoms. Unless a careful history is taken, a mistaken diagnosis

Table 48.3   Differential Diagnosis of Catatonia

Idiopathic primary catatonia
Secondary catatonia
Lethal catatonia
Catatonic excitement
Neuroleptic malignant syndrome
Akinetic mutism
Acute neurologic event
Parkinsonian freezing
Akinetic epilepsy
Coma vigil
Coma
Extreme psychomotor retardation
Neuroleptic-induced akinesia
Serotonin syndrome

Table 48.4   Abnormalities of the Elementary Neurologic Examination in Uncomplicated Idiopathic Catatonia

			Fluctuating	
	Bilateral	Unilateral	Long Term/Slowly	Short Term/Rapidly
Elementary sensory deficits	−	−	−	−
Muscle atrophy/hypertrophy	−	−	−	−
Ictal or postictal weakness	+	+	−	+
Nonictal weakness	−	−	−	−
Ataxia			Rarely seen	
Aphasia			+	+
Gegenhalten	+	+	+	−
Positive limb placement	+	+	+	−
Cogwheeling	+	+	+	−
Catalepsy	+	+	+	−
Doll's eye reflex	+	+	+	−
Paresis of upgaze	+		+	−
Oculomotor paresis	+		+	−
Poor eye tracking	+		+	−
Lateral gaze impersistence	+		+	−
Positive glabellar response	+	+	+	−
Pout reflex			+	−
Grasp reflex	+	+	+	−
Utilization behavior	+	+	+	−
Imitation behavior			Rarely seen	
Environmental dependency syndrome			Expected to occur	

of neuroleptic-induced akinesia or catatonia will be made in autonomically compensated patients and of neuroleptic malignant syndrome in autonomically aroused ones. Often these patients are not and were not psychotic. If that is the case, neuroleptics should be discontinued in order to minimize further extrapyramidal symptoms. If the history reveals previous catatonic episodes unrelated to neuroleptic exposure, and with the same time course of onset and clinical presentation, then the diagnoses of neuroleptic-induced catatonia or neuroleptic malignant syndrome must be seriously in doubt, and special management is not required unless the patient fails to respond to conventional measures.

If patients have major concurrent psychiatric disorders, such as depression, mania, or psychosis, then treatment of these should be initiated.

Some special points remain. Electroconvulsive therapy can be an impressively rapid treatment of catatonia and should be used unhesitatingly in a life-threatening or treatment-unresponsive case. Intravenous lorazepam or diazepam can induce a remission in minutes. Unfortunately, these remissions do not seem to last and intramuscular and oral lorazepam and diazepam seem much less effective to this author. A recent report, however, demonstrated that very long-term treatment with lorazepam might be required for some patients (19).

When bipolar catatonic patients are given intravenous lorazepam or diazepam they may emerge from catatonia into depression, euthymia, or mania. This can be a dramatic phenomenon and may be the same as that observed with intravenous amytal during amytal interviews. The traditional advice with respect to amytal interviews is to always be prepared for the patient to become catatonically excited, and it seems prudent to repeat that advice here for the administration of any intravenous anticonvulsants to catatonic patients. This emergence into mania is another line of evidence suggesting that classic catatonic excitement is actually the same as mania in a previously catatonic patient.

A final caveat: Although it is unclear where catatonia with autonomic arousal ends and acute lethal catatonia begins and whether or not neuroleptic malignant syndrome is a variety of either of these or an independent entity, it is clear that any of these states in decompensated form can lead to death. Therefore, if a history of recent neuroleptic exposure exists and the patient is catatonic, autonomically decompensated, and hyperthermic, it is prudent and reasonable to proceed as if they had neuroleptic malignant syndrome, rather than be inappropriately diverted by an essentially academic debate over the precise diagnosis.

SCIENTIFIC BACKGROUND AND PRINCIPLES

At this time, catatonia is best described as a syndrome rather than a disease. This approach is parsimonious and has the advantage of allowing a rational classification of catatonia into primary and secondary types.

The neurophysiologic final common pathway that allows various diseases and brain insults to express themselves via the catatonic syndrome remains largely unexplored, and the natures of the individual causative diseases at the biochemical, neuropathologic, and genetic levels remain unelucidated. Epidemiologic data suggest that affective and seizure disorders are associated strongly with catatonia, but the natures of these associations are mysterious (3,4,20,21).

A number of different types of catatonia have already been described. There are others extant in the literature. The most prominent of these is periodic catatonia, which debatably is not a discrete entity but a recognition of the phenomenon of catatonia occurring in manic-depressive patients. To this author it seems that catatonia has a spectrum of presentations from mild to severe. At the mild end, the diagnosis may be missed or the presentation is only partial. At the other end of the spectrum, some cases may be called acute lethal catatonia, neuroleptic malignant syndrome, or severe catatonia with dysautonomia. Once this variation in severity and the distinction between primary and secondary cases is allowed for, it does not seem that significantly distinct subtypes occur.

The remainder of this discussion applies to catatonia as a whole. Early pathologic studies revealed macroscopic and microscopic changes in the brain and other organ systems, but patient selection and description make it difficult to be certain of their correct modern psychiatric diagnosis (22). A computerized tomographic study revealed frontal lobe, cerebellar, and vermian atrophy, but the sample size was small, and so far the study has not been repeated (9). One group reported increased serum ceruloplasmin in catatonia, a finding of unknown significance (23).

Clinically, the prominent features of catatonia are profound disturbances of posture, movement, muscle tone, speech or language, and autonomic function. Dysautonomia is particularly noticeable and clinically alarming in severe cases. In elementary terms, the neurologic abnormalities are consistent with extrapyramidal, frontal lobe, and cerebellar dysfunction (24–27). The dysautonomia raises the question of diencephalic and brainstem involvement.

Using a somewhat more complete neuroanatomic analysis, it is possible to speculate upon the relevance of lateralized brain dysfunction to catatonia. Current theories of affective disorders postulate that a balance between left and right anterior cerebral functioning is important in maintaining normal mood. If this balance is disturbed, affective disorders can result. This theory raises the possibility that the observed relationship between idiopathic catatonia and affective disorders may in some way be related to the lateralized cerebral dysfunction thought to be associated with affective disorders.

In the 1980s, a consensus began to develop that massive interconnections exist between the cortex, limbic system, and basal ganglia (28). The anatomic entrance for input from cortical and limbic areas to the extrapyramidal system is thought to be the striatum (28). The very existence of this system implies a need to somehow incorporate its presence into a fundamental model of catatonia. The connections described would allow a single lesion or abnormality to present with frontal lobe, basal ganglia, and limbic signs. Thus catatonia might represent a behavioral disorder for which corticolimbic-striatal circuitry is the final common pathway.

Animal work has suggested some other factors that may be important. Heath noted that catatonia could be induced in monkeys by antibrain antibody (29). Seizures in rats have also been shown to induce catatonia (30). Pharmacologic studies have suggested that naloxone, amantadine, diphenhydramine, monoamine oxidase inhibitors, and tricyclic antidepressants all have anticatatonic properties (16–18). Another interesting observation in animals is of the phenomenon of tonic immobility. This is a catatonic state that seems to be the behavioral manifestation of a fear response that has survival value for the animal (31).

Overall the animal work demonstrates possible significance for a number of neurotransmitter systems in catatonia. The existence of the tonic immobility response in animals raises the possibility that catatonia in humans is a pathologic version of the same response. A further observation in humans is of the "switch process" (32). This is a term used to describe a process in which depressed patients may suddenly become manic, manic patients depressed, or a catatonic patient either. Patients can also suddenly switch into catatonia.

Catatonia can also be considered from a neurochemical perspective. Depression may be conceptualized as a state in which depressed mood, bradykinesia, bradyphrenia, and neurovegetative disturbances occur. In mania the opposite happens. In general, depression could be thought of as a state of increased central parasympathetic-cholinergic activity. In mania, central sympathetic-adrenergic activity is increased. Numerous psychopharmacologic observations are consistent with this view and some were discussed in the previous chapter. Of particular note is that intravenous injection of cholinergic agents can lead to rapid onset of depression, hypokinesia, and suicidality in normal subjects. Anticholinergic agents relieve a similar syndrome induced by neuroleptics that themselves tend to be sympatholytic. Clinical experience supports the hypothesis that a balance between central sympathetic and parasympathetic tone is important in the maintenance of normal mood and motor activity. The association between affective disorders and catatonia is well-documented, and may indicate that when the balance between central sympathetic and parasympathetic activity is disturbed not only can disorders of mood occur but also profound disorders of movement such as bradykinesia, hyperkinesia, and catatonia. Some of these movement disorders may be mediated by or caused by disturbances in the corticolimbic-striatal system.

This hypothesis has the advantage of offering a unitary explanation for the range of disorders of mood and movement seen in catatonia, depression, and mania, as well as predicting the clinically different dysautonomias seen in these conditions. It is also consistent with attempts to lateralize and localize catatonia in terms of both anatomic structure and neurotransmitter systems. Central dysautonomia may be the final common mechanism for the development of catatonic states.

REFERENCES

1. Bleuler E. Dementia praecox or the group of schizophrenias. Zinkin J (trans). New York: International Universities, 1950.
2. Lohr JB, Wisniewski AA. Movement disorders. A neuropsychiatric approach. New York: Guilford, 1987.
3. Gelenberg AJ. The catatonic syndrome. Lancet 1976;i:1339–1341.
4. Catatonia. Lancet 1986;ii:954–955.
5. Riether AM, Stoudemire A, Anderson G. Catatonic syndromes in medicine and psychiatry. J Med Assoc Ga 1986;75:611–614.
6. Abrams R, Taylor MA. Catatonia. A prospective clinical study. Arch Gen Psychiatry 1976;33:579–581.
7. Taylor MA, Abrams R. Catatonia. Prevalence and importance in the manic phase of manic–depressive illness. Arch Gen Psychiatry 1977;34:1223–1225.
8. Morrison JR. Catatonia. Retarded and excited types. Arch Gen Psychiatry 1973;28:39–41.
9. Joseph AB, Anderson WH, O'Leary DH. Brainstem and vermis atrophy in catatonia. Am J Psychiatry 1985;142:352–354.
10. Boeve BF, Rummans TA, Philbrick KL, Callahan MJ. Electrocardiographic and echocardiographic changes associated with malignant catatonia. Mayo Clin Proceed 1994;69:645–650.
11. American Psychiatric Association. Task Force Report 14. Electroconvulsive therapy. Washington: American Psychiatric Association, 1978.
12. Linn L, McEvoy JP, Lohr JB. Intravenous sedatives and catatonia. Am J Psychiatry 1984;141:1135–1136.
13. Salam SA, Pillai AK, Beresford TP. Lorazepam for psychogenic catatonia. Am J Psychiatry 1987;144:1082–1083.
14. McEvoy JP, Lohr JB. Diazepam for catatonia. Am J Psychiatry 1984;141:284–285.
15. Singerman B, Raheja R. Malignant catatonia—a continuing reality. Ann Clin Psychiatry 1994;6:259–266.
16. Chopra YM, Dandiya PC. The mechanism of the potentiating effect of antidepressant drugs on the protective influence of diphenhydramine in experimental catatonia. The role of histamine. Pharmacology 1974;12:347–353.
17. Chopra YM, Dandiya PC. Potentiation of anticatatonic effect of antidepressants by amantadine. Indian J Med Res 1977;66:142–149.
18. Wilcox RE, Levitt RA. Naloxone reversal of morphine catatonia: Role of caudate and periaqueductal gray. Pharmacol Biochem Behav 1978;9:425–428.
19. Gaind GS, Rosebush PI, Mazurek MF. Lorazepam treatment of acute and chronic catatonia in two mentally retarded brothers. J Clin Psychiatry 1994;55:20–23.
20. Slater E, Roth M. Clinical psychiatry. 3rd ed. London: Bailliere Tindall, 1977.
21. Carroll BT, Boutros NN. Clinical electroencephalograms in patients with catatonic disorders. Clin Electroencephalography 1995;26:60–64.
22. Shulack NR. Exhaustion syndrome in excited psychotic patients. Am J Psychiatry 1946;102:466–475.
23. Alias AG, Vijayan N, Nair DS, Sukumaran M. Serum ceruloplasmin in schizophrenia: significant increase in acute cases especially in catatonia. Biol Psychiatry 1972;4:231–238.
24. Schneider RC, Crosby EC. The interplay between cerebral hemispheres and cerebellum in relation to tonus and movements. J Neurosurg 1963;20:188–198.
25. Roberts DR. Catatonia in the brain: A localization study. Int J Neuropsychiatry 1965;1:395–403.
26. Freund H-J, Hummelsheim H. Lesions of premotor cortex in man. Brain 1985;108:697–733.
27. Larochelle L, Bedard P, Poirier LJ, Sourkes TL. Correlative neuroanatomical and neuropharmacological study of tremor and catatonia in the monkey. Neuropharmacology 1971;10:273–288.
28. Nauta WJH. Reciprocal links of the corpus striatum with the cerebral cortex and limbic system. A common Substrate for movement and thought? In:

Mueller J, Yingling C, Zegans L, eds. Neurology and psychiatry: a meeting of minds. Basel: Karger, 1989.

29. Heath RG, Krupp IM. Catatonia induced in monkeys by antibrain antibody. Am J Psychiatry 1967;123:1499–1504.

30. Myslobodsky MS, Mintz M. Postictal behavioral arrest in the rat: "catalepsy" or "catatonia?" Life Sci 1981;28:2287–2293.

31. Peters RH, Hughes RA. Naloxone interactions with morphine- and shock-potentiated tonic immobility in chickens. Pharmacol Biochem Behav 1978;9:153–156.

32. Bunney WE. The switch process in manic–depressive psychosis. Ann Intern Med 1977;87:319–335.

Akinetic Mutism and Coma Vigil

D. Frank Benson

INTRODUCTION

The term *akinetic mutism* was introduced by Cairns et al in 1941 (1) to define the neurologic status of a patient with a mass lesion in the anterior portion of the third ventricle. A number of clinically similar cases have been described since that time (2–7), based on a variety of etiologies with locations in a number of separate but related anatomic sites.

While a considerable variation is acknowledged, the major clinical features are consistent; the patient usually lies with eyes closed, a state interrupted by irregular cycles of arousal that are most often independent of environmental stimuli; some patients present an appearance of vigilance because their eyes are open and move conjugately although they have little or no other movement or vocalization. Skeletal muscle movements, even when disagreeable or painful stimulations are given, range from minimal to nil. Both bowel and bladder incontinence is usual. Plum and Posner (8) posited two crucial factors for the diagnosis of akinetic mutism: 1) a seeming wakefulness without recognizable content, and 2) a relative paucity of signs implying significant damage to descending motor pathways to explain the immobile state. Despite the variations, akinetic mutism represents a recognizable neurologic state and a considerable number of confirmatory neuroanatomic/behavioral correlations have been gathered.

A resemblance between the neurologic disorder akinetic mutism and the psychiatric state called "catatonia" has been noted (9–11), but the absence of obvious neuroanatomic explanation and the far broader clinical picture of catatonia have maintained the two states as separate phenomena. In some instances, both diagnoses can be correct as is seen in the following case.

Case Study

A 31-year-old female was admitted to the neurology service at UCLA for evaluation of a slowly progressive state of unresponsiveness. Pertinent history included reports of long-standing emotional disturbance, moodiness, and abuse of both alcohol and drugs. Six years prior to admission she began to drink heavily, quit her job, and joined a motorcycle gang, eventually becoming a full-blown alcoholic. During this period, she made an unsuccessful attempt at suicide by slitting her wrist. Approximately 16 months prior to admission, she overdosed on benzodiazepine and alcohol, suffered a respiratory arrest, was hospitalized and remained in coma for seven days. Her subsequent hospital recuperation was complicated by infections and two tonic seizures. Within several weeks, however, she was said to be sufficiently alert to answer questions, could walk with encouragement, and could feed herself. Nocturnal urinary incontinence persisted. She was discharged to her mother's home where she originally could help with housework but showed a notable memory problem. She continually wandered from the house and finally had to be restrained, a tactic that produced anger and withdrawal. The family noticed a consistent, slow decline in other functions until she eventually quit walking and talking and required total care. A period of hospitalization about six months before the UCLA admission had led to a diagnosis of depression; treatment with antidepressant and psychotrophic drugs was without success. A computerized tomography scan done at that time showed only slightly greater atrophy than expected for her age, and an electroencephalogram (EEG) showed irregular posterior dominant rhythms with generalized slowing. A magnetic resonance imaging (MRI) scan several months later confirmed the general atrophy and also showed increased signal intensity in the basal ganglia bilaterally, suggesting old infarctions. At the time of the UCLA admission, she was both mute and unresponsive to verbal stimulation and was largely akinetic. She had lost 30 pounds and was doubly incontinent. Differential diagnosis at the time of admission to UCLA was akinetic mutism versus major depression with catatonic features.

The family history was positive for psychiatric disorder. A paternal uncle was known to have a manic–depressive disorder and the patient's father was a Skid Row alcoholic. An older brother had died of drug overdose, two paternal aunts and a paternal grandmother had psychiatric problems and had died in a psychiatric hospital.

On admission the patient was unresponsive, sitting in a slumped posture in a chair. General physical examination revealed no pertinent abnormalities. Examination of the cranial nerves was limited. She responded to threat bilaterally with eye blinking, but this was inconsistent and other extraocular movement and visual field tests could not be performed. Doll's eye movements were present in all directions. The corneal reflex was present bilaterally as was the gag reflex. Muscle tone and bulk appeared to be within normal limits in the upper extremities, but the tone was mildly increased in the lower extremities. No spontaneous movements were noted and if the patient was moved into a new position she tended to stay in that position (waxy flexibility). The reflexes were somewhat decreased but were present and symmetric bilaterally and the plantar responses were flexor bilaterally. Sensory examination was unsuccessful as she did not respond to pinprick, deep pain, or any other stimulus with any consistency.

On the neurology service, pharmacologic management included separate regimens of carbidopa–L-dopa and carbamazepine, each without any effect. At that time, a push-trial of lorazepam (Ativan) given intravenously produced a dramatic response. Some minutes after she received the intravenous (i.v.) injection she "work up," began to move and talk, eventually got out of her chair and walked with only slight assistance for balance. Her speech was dysarthric but she appeared to have a fairly bright affect. She could not give any account of recent events and did not appear to understand what had been happening to her. Approximately 10 or 12 hours later, she regressed to her original unresponsive state. The drug intervention was subsequently repeated, this time with EEG and television monitoring. No significant change was seen in the EEG pattern during or following the administration of lorazepam, but a positive clinical response was again noted; the improvement with the second trial was not as dramatic, however, and was considerably shorter in duration. Numerous related drugs were offered, utilizing alternate modes of presentation; all were without effect.

At this point she was transferred to an inpatient psychiatry unit with a proposed diagnosis of organic affective syndrome with catatonia. Again, a variety of drugs were attempted and all failed to produce alteration. A repeat trial of the i.v. lorazepam was given; this time there was no sig-

nificant response. Formal nursing observation on the psychiatric ward demonstrated that her attention waxed and waned during the day. She was always more responsive in the evenings than in the mornings, with the AM unresponsiveness interpreted at least by some of the staff as willful noncooperation.

Incontinence of urine and stool continued. Although she could swallow without difficulty, she seemed to tire quickly when solid foods were offered; in contrast, she could always handle liquids.

She was eventually discharged to the care of her mother and has been seen regularly on a follow-up basis. Many different drug regimens including stimulants, antidepressants, antipsychotics, benzodiazepines, and anticonvulsants have been offered, all producing limited or no alteration in her basic status. The patient continues to have waxing and waning of alertness but, even at her brightest, cannot ambulate, remains incontinent, often drifts off and does not appear to have memory function.

The above case presents an excellent example of the difficulties inherent in clinical definition. With her background and presenting behavioral pattern, the patient could certainly be described as catatonic. The family history of psychiatric abnormality includes both bipolar affective disorder and substance abuse. She had made one serious suicide attempt and was both a hard-core alcoholic and a drug abuser. The state in which she was brought to UCLA was described as a slowly progressive regression and, in the family's opinion, coincided with her increasing anger following the application of custodial procedures. In addition, a single i.v. dose of a diazepam produced a dramatic resolution of both the motor disturbance and the mutism, an alteration that was replicated at least once. A diagnosis of depression with catatonic features was fully acceptable.

On the other side of the coin, however, the patient showed the behavioral pattern and appropriate findings to be called "akinetic mute." While somnolent most of the time, on occasion her eyes would open and she appeared vigilant. Although she usually failed to respond when spoken to, she occasionally uttered words, phrases, or even sentences. Similarly, she did not move, even in response to strong noxious stimuli and yet, was seen to spontaneously move about. While the akinetic mute condition waxed and waned, the status varied only within a limited parameter. The history of respiratory arrest and prolonged coma plus the MRI suggestion of bilateral basal ganglia infarction is consistent with central nervous system damage as the cause of a behavior pattern considerably altered from that present prior to the incident. A diagnosis of akinetic mutism secondary to anoxic brain damage is fully reasonable.

It is obvious that the dividing line between catatonia, a motor complication of a number of psychiatric disturbances, and akinetic mutism, a status with limited verbal and physical response based on focal organic brain disease, is thin indeed. Either diagnosis is perfectly correct in this patient's case; although the two clinical syndromes are traditionally considered separately, they share crucial features. Catatonia has been discussed in the previous chapter as a phenomenon of psychiatric disorder; akinetic mutism and its variation called "coma vigil" will be discussed here.

REVIEW OF RELEVANT LITERATURE

Excellent reviews and discussions of akinetic mutism have been presented (12–14). Segarra and Angelo (13) define akinetic mutism as "a state of unresponsiveness to the environment with extreme reluctance to perform even elementary motor activities." The patient usually lies quietly in bed or in a slumped sitting posture, immobile except for occasional posture correcting movements. The patient most often appears sleepy but may be open-eyed and seemingly alert. The eyes may or may not follow the movements of the examiner but they do not react to the examiner's activities. The patient appears totally detached from the world but the expression in the eyes of some akinetic patients suggests an awakeness; a "stubborn refusal to cooperate" is often presumed by both medical and nursing personnel. Segarra and Angelo classify patients with this general picture into two broad categories—pseudoakinetic and true akinetic mutism (Table 49.1). Both clinical and pathologic differences underlie the distinction.

The first category, that of pseudoakinetic mutism, presents situations in which the individual fails to move or respond based on severe motor disturbance. Three types are to be considered.

1. *The locked-in syndrome.* A motionless mute state can result when severe paralysis interrupts all motor pathways descending to the spinal cord and lower cranial nerve motor nuclei. Only the ocular movements remain intact. The most common pathology in cases of locked-in syndrome is vascular, usually infarction involving the motor fibers running through the base of the pons. Kemper and Romanul (15) carefully described the state, including the pathologic cause, and the term *locked-in syndrome* was suggested by Plum and Posner (16). Additional well-described cases in the early literature include that of Fang and Palmer (17), Cravioto and Silberman (18), Feldman (19), Nordgren et al (20), and Karp and Hurtig (21). Improvements in life support available in the past several decades have made survival possible in this unfortunate state so the locked-in syndrome is not rare in current medical practice. The presence of severe motor paralysis (tetraplegia) easily distinguishes the locked-in syndrome from the akinetic mute state described above.

2. *Pallidal necrosis.* Under this term can be included a number of disorders in which damage in the territory of the basal ganglia has produced a rigidity (usually accompanied by at least some degree of paralysis) that inhibits both movement and vocalization. This clinical picture is a common end-state for all of the extrapyramidal motor disorders (e.g., Parkinson's disease, Huntington's disease) and can be seen following cerebrovascular accident or other conditions that produce bilateral destruction in putamen, caudate, or globus pallidus. Marinesco and Dragonesco (22) carefully described a case and Denny-Brown (23) thoroughly discussed the disorder. In the days when chemopallidectomy was performed as a treatment for Parkinson's disease, both mutism and akinesia were recognized as not infrequent complications (24). A mixture of rigidity, dysphagia, dyslalia, tongue paralysis, bilateral extensor plantar reflexes, and occasional outbursts of disinhibited (pseudobulbar) affect distinguishes this disorder from true akinetic mutism but the differentiation is not always obvious.

3. *Apallic state.* Destruction of the mantle zone of the hemispheric cortex can produce a clinical situation in which the patient is mute, immobile, and has wide open eyes that, at least in some cases, may follow the observer; the patient is otherwise unresponsive. A variety of disease states including anoxia, carbon monoxide poisoning, Creutzfeldt–Jakob disease, meningovascular syphilis, viral encephalitis, and increased intracranial pressure due to closed head trauma have been known to produce this state (25,26). The basic problem in these cases is injury to the sensorimotor areas of the cortex, destroying the neural substrate necessary for feeling, movement, and thought. The patient is both akinetic and mute but almost invariably will show marked alterations in muscle tone (spasticity and rigidity) and posture, extensor plantar responses, and considerable dysphagia. These features distinguish the apallic state from true akinetic mutism.

In all three pseudoakinetic conditions, the patient is rendered both akinetic and mute, although appearing to be awake. In each instance, however, the prime reason for both immobility and mutism is severe motor disturbance, either paralysis or rigidity, often coupled with some degree of sensory deafferentation. In some instances, most notably the locked-in syndrome, the patient may be acutely aware of environmental context; in others, particularly the apallic state, awareness is restricted. While not representing the true akinetic mute state and differing from catatonia by the presence of severe motor abnormality, these conditions deserve

Table 49.1   Varieties of Akinetic Mutism

Pseudoakinetic mutism
   Locked-in syndrome
   Pallidal necrosis
   Apallic state
True akinetic mutism
   Mesencephalic akinetic mutism
   Frontal akinetic mutism

Adapted from Segarra JM, Angelo JN. Anatomical determinants of behavioral change. In: Benton AL, ed. Behavioral change in cerebrovascular disease. New York: Harper & Row, 1970.

consideration in any individual who presents with decreased mobility and verbalization.

Segarra and Angelo (13) presented two variations of true akinetic mutism in their classification, also based on both anatomic and behavioral distinctions. While the two varieties are distinct, it must be recognized that most clinical presentations of "true" akinetic mutism are not so precisely differentiated. Combinations of the behavioral qualities of the two syndromes are the rule and imprecision in the anatomic site of the causative pathology must be accepted.

MESENCEPHALIC AKINETIC MUTISM

The most prominent component of akinetic mutism based on mesencephalic pathology concerns arousal abnormalities of the sleep/wake cycle and apparent hypersomnia are notable. In addition, oculomotor disturbances such as pupillary asymmetry, third nerve paralysis, upward gaze paralysis, and so forth are common and the presence of bilateral ptosis may increase the appearance of lethargy. A striking immobility is present. If given strong noxious stimuli (auditory, visual, or somesthetic), the patient may make slight protective movements and/or may vocalize, but the responses are inconsistent and pathetically limited in comparison with the severity of stimulus needed to evoke them. Incontinence is the rule. Dependent upon the extent of the causative lesion, additional factors such as a demented state, amnesia, or some degree of paresis may be present. In pure state, however, focal mesencephalic lesions can produce the full picture of akinetic mutism without any evidence of general motor paralysis. Not only is the degree of rigidity or paralysis insufficient to explain the immobility, but smoothly performed spontaneous movements do occur.

The differential diagnosis of an individual who is lethargic, has dysconjugate eye movements when the lids are lifted, who responds little to noxious stimuli and has no evidence of generalized paralysis or extrapyramidal motor disturbance is, of course, the differential diagnosis of coma. A patient chronically in this status but who does arouse on occasion to either move or vocalize or both, can be considered to be in a mesencephalic akinetic mute state. The dividing line between severe mesencephalic akinetic mutism and chronic coma (persistent vegetative state) is narrow, based only upon the occasional movements and/or vocalizations of the akinetic mute patient.

FRONTAL AKINETIC MUTISM

A number of cases with a clinical picture of akinetic mutism in which the pathology involves areas in the frontal lobes have been reported (27–33). Ackerman and Ziegler (14) contend that the frontal variety, based on impaired motor activation, is the only true akinetic mutism. Both the location and type of frontal lesions described varies considerably. Many of the early reports concerned cases with bilateral vascular abnormality involving the medial frontal regions, destroying cingulate cortex, supplementary motor areas, and additional supracallosal midline structures. In more recent reports, pathology in the frontal septal area has also been noted to produce the syndrome. The latter cases have been caused by either vascular infarction or tumor. When all case material is analyzed it appears that the site, not the etiology, is crucial to the development of the syndrome.

Clinically, patients with frontal akinetic mutism are best characterized as severely apathetic. They are immobile or only vaguely mobile and either mute or hypophonic with grossly decreased verbal output. They do not show, however, the eye findings characteristic of the mesencephalic group; their eyes are open and freely follow the examiner's movement; they are often described as vigilant in contrast to the somnolent akinetic state caused by the mesencephalic lesions (34). The term *coma vigil* vividly defines patients whose ocular movements suggest normal vigilance but who otherwise fail to respond in a normal manner.

Neighborhood signs frequently help define frontal akinetic mutism, particularly when the superior sagittal region is involved. Most characteristic and definitive is a crural paralysis, weakness affecting the contralateral lower extremity and shoulder musculature. In most cases with frontal akinetic mutism, however, bilateral medial frontal destruction has occurred; the resulting bilateral paralysis may make it difficult to differentiate these individuals from those with the locked-in state. Two clinical features help separate the two states. First, the spastic paralysis is largely confined to the lower extremities and shoulders in the frontal cases leaving the arms, hands, neck, and vocal apparatus relatively normal in tone. A second striking differential point reflecting this freedom from universal spasticity is in the relative clarity of vocalization occasionally heard in the frontal akinetic mutes in comparison with the severely dysarthric output of patients with the locked-in syndrome.

THE NEURAL BASIS OF AKINETIC MUTISM

On the basis of the reported cases and the clinical/anatomic correlations, a neural basis for awakeness (consciousness) and movement has been suggested. Since the initial work of Moruzzi and Magoun (35) and subsequent studies (36–38), a correlation between the degree of awakeness and the intactness of the mesencephalic reticular area has been consistently accepted. Mesencephalic akinetic mutism correlates directly with these laboratory demonstrations. Damage to the mesencephalic reticular system disrupts the arousal system; in addition, dependent upon the exact location of pathology in the mesencephalic tegmentum, damage to the nuclei or along the course of the third cranial nerve is likely, leading to disorders of extraocular movement. The clinical characteristics of the mesencephalic akinetic mute state follow damage or malfunction in a relatively restricted neuroanatomic area.

Lesions that involve frontal midline structures in any locus from the septal region around the genu of the corpus callosum and upward into the superior sagittal regions including cingulate cortex and supplementary motor area can produce a disturbance in activation (39–41). An akinetic mute state without the extraoculomotor component results; in fact, the impression of alertness conveyed by the eyes has suggested the term *coma vigil*.

Two areas—the upper mesencephalic reticular area and a circular system of midline frontal structures beginning with the septal cortex and running around the genu of the corpus callosum into the medial sagittal frontal area—appear to be involved in akinetic mutism. When it is recognized that the mesencephalic nucleus and the septal nuclei are closely related, both in location and function, and are directly connected via the median forebrain bundle, it can be suggested that this is a single functional system, crucial for the awakeness, arousal, alertness, attention, and response aspects of human mental function. Damage along this functional axis produces akinetic mutism with variations in the degree of awakeness and eye movement disturbance based on the degree of damage and the caudal–rostral locus of the damage.

RELATIONSHIP OF AKINETIC MUTISM TO CATATONIA

The relationship between catatonic and akinetic mutism discussed at the beginning of this chapter deserves further attention. The clinical picture of the two disorders is strikingly similar if not identical. The etiology, however, often appears different. Those cases presenting with immobility and mutism not based on primary motor disturbance but with evidence of focal cerebral damage deserve classification as akinetic mutism. Those without focal damage, however, can well be considered under the broader heading of catatonia. It would appear that one form of catatonia, as illustrated by the case of repeated carbon monoxide poisoning (42) and the patient presented at the beginning of this chapter, may follow organic pathology affecting crucial neural areas but not demonstrable by current imaging techniques. In such instances, catatonia and akinetic mutism appear to be different names for the same problem. Even in those cases in which catatonia appears in well-established "functional" psychotic disorders such as schizophrenia, the immobility and mutism may well represent neurotransmitter dysfunction affecting areas where structural damage is known to produce the akinetic mute state. Response to "psychotropic" pharmacologic agents in such cases would support a neurotransmitter dysfunction, not a psychogenic etiology. Future research into the causes, effects, and treatment of catatonia should benefit from the model of akinetic mutism.

REFERENCES

1. Cairns H, Oldfield RC, Pennybacker JB, Whitteridge D. Akinetic mutism with an epidermoid cyst of III ventricle. Brain 1941;64:273–290.
2. Cairns H. Disturbances of consciousness with lesions of the brain stem and diencephalon. Brain 1952;75:109–146.
3. Devinsky O, Lemann W, Evans AC, et al. Akinetic mutism in a bone marrow transplant recipient following total-body irradiation and amphotericin-B chemoprophylaxis. Arch Neurol 1987;44:414–417.
4. Segarra JM. Cerebral vascular disease and behavior. I. The syndrome of the mesencephalic artery (basilar artery bifurcation). Arch Neurol 1970;22:408–418.
5. Smith S. An investigation and survey of 27 cases of akinesis with mutism (stupor). J Ment Sci 1959;105:1088–1094.
6. Scott TF, Lang D, Gingis M, Price T. Prolonged akinetic mutism due to multiple sclerosis. J Neuropsychiatry Clin Neurosci 1995;7:90–92.
7. Gutling E, Landis T, Kleiner P. Akinetic mutism in bilateral necrotizing leucoencephalopathy after radiation and chemotherapy. J Neurol 1992;293:125–128.
8. Plum F, Posner JB. The diagnosis of stupor and coma. 2nd ed. Philadelphia: FA Davis, 1972.
9. Sours JA. Akinetic mutism simulating catatonic states. Am J Psychiatry 1962;119:451–455.
10. Gelenberg AJ. The catatonic syndrome. Lancet 1976;i:1339–1341.
11. Taylor MA. Catatonia: a review of a behavioral neurologic syndrome. Neuropsychiatry Neuropsychol Behav Neurol 1990;3:48–72.
12. Klee A. Akinetic mutism. J Nerv Ment Dis 1961;133:536–553.
13. Segarra JM, Angelo JN. Anatomical determinants of behavioral change. In: Benton AL, ed. Behavioral change in cerebrovascular disease. New York: Harper & Row, 1970:3.
14. Ackerman H, Ziegler W. Akinetischer motismus—eine literaturubersicht. Fortschr Neurol Psychiatr 1995;63:59–67.
15. Kemper TL, Romanul FC. State resembling akinetic mutism in basilar artery occlusion. Neurology 1967;17:74–80.
16. Plum F, Posner JB. The diagnosis of stupor and coma. Philadelphia: FA Davis, 1966.
17. Fang HCH, Palmer JJ. Vascular phenomena involving brainstem structures: a clinical and pathologic correlation study. Neurology 1956;6:402–419.
18. Cravioto H, Silberman J. A clinical and pathologic study of akinetic mutism. Neurology 1960;10:10–21.
19. Feldman MH. Physiological observations in a chronic case of "locked-in" syndrome. Neurology 1971;21:459–478.
20. Nordgren RE, Markesbery WR, Fukuda K, Reeves AG. Seven cases of cerebromedullospinal disconnection: The "locked-in" syndrome. Neurology 1971;21:1140–1148.
21. Karp JS, Hurtig HI. "Locked-in" state with bilateral mid-brain infarcts. Arch Neurol 1974;30:176–178.
22. Marinesco G, Dragonesco S. Contribution anatomo-clinique a l'etude du syndrome de Foerster. Encéphale 1929;24:685–699.
23. Denny-Brown D. The basal ganglia and their relation to disorders of movement. London: Oxford University, 1962.
24. Riklan M, Levita E. Psychological studies of thalamic lesions in humans. J Nerv Ment Dis 1970;150:251–265.
25. French JD. Brain lesions associated with prolonged unconsciousness. Arch Neurol Psychiatry 1952;68:727–747.
26. Jellinger K, Gerstenbrand F, Pateisky K. Die protahierte form der posttraumatischen Encephalopathie. Nervenartz 1963;34:145–159.
27. Aymes EW, Neilsen JM. Clinicopathologic study of vascular lesions of the anterior cingulate region. Bull Los Angeles Neurol Soc 1955;20:112–130.
28. Barris RW, Schuman HR. Bilateral anterior cingulate gyrus lesions. Syndrome of the anterior cingulate gyri. Neurology 1953;3:44–52.
29. Damasio AR, Van Hoesen GW. Emotional disturbances associated with focal lesions of the limbic frontal lobe. In: Heilman KM, Satz P, eds. Neuropsychology of human emotion. New York: Guilford, 1983:85–110.
30. Faris AA. Limbic system infarction. J Neuropathol Exp Neurol 1967;26:174.
31. Freemon FR. Akinetic mutism and bilateral anterior cerebral artery occlusion. J Neurol Neurosurg Psychiatry 1971;34:693–698.
32. Nielsen JM, Jacobs LL. Bilateral lesions of the anterior cingulate gyri: Report of a case. Bull Los Angeles Neurol Soc 1951;16:231–234.
33. Ross ED, Stewart RM. Akinetic mutism from hypothalamic damage: successful treatment with dopamine agonists. Neurology 1981;31:1435–1439.
34. Yakovlev PI. Personal communication as quoted by Segarra JM, Angelo JN. In: Benton AL, ed. Behavioral change in cerebrovascular disease. New York: Harper & Row, 1970:7.

35. Moruzzi G, Magoun HW. Brain stem reticular formation and activation of the EEG. Electroencephalogr Clin Neurophysiol 1949;1:455–473.

36. Magoun HW. The waking brain. Springfield: Charles C Thomas, 1963.

37. Rossi GF, Zanchetti A. The brain stem reticular formation: anatomy and physiology. Arch Ital Biol 1957;95:199–435.

38. Scheibel A. Anatomical and physiological substrates of arousal—a view from the bridge. In: Hobson JA, Brazier MA, eds. Reticular formation revisited. New York: Raven, 1980:55–66.

39. Botez MI, Barbeau A. Role of subcortical structures and particularly the thalamus in the mechanisms of speech and language. Int J Neurol 1971;8:300–320.

40. Freedman M, Alexander MP, Naeser MA. The anatomical basis of transcortical motor aphasia. Neurology 1984;34:409–417.

41. Stuss DT, Benson DF. The frontal lobes. New York: Raven, 1986.

42. Smith JS, Brierly H, Brandon S. Akinetic mutism with recovery after repeated carbon monoxide poisoning. Psychol Med 1971;1:172–177.

Motor and Motivational Disorders in Limbic–Paralimbic Lesions

MICHEL H. HABIB   ALBERT M. GALABURDA

INTRODUCTION

The role of the limbic system in motor processes is not well-understood, which may reflect a host of unique anatomic and functional features. First, the anatomic constituents of the limbic system (1) are rather heterogenous and are grouped together because of their apparently common phylogenetic origin. Second, unlike the more easily explorable instrumental functions of the neocortex, the archaic limbic structures appear to underlie a number of operationally ill-defined and incoherent functions, such as memory, emotion, motivation, and attention. However, that these structures also have a role to play in motor function is suggested by some recent and old experimental and clinical evidence that we will develop in the present chapter.

ANATOMIC BASES

The term *limbic system* refers to a group of brain structures that includes limbic allocortex proper (hippocampal formation, piriform cortex) and corticoid regions (septal region, substantia innominata, amygdaloid complex), paralimbic areas [mesocortex, proisocortex (2)] including the insula, and a cortical belt ("the great limbic lobe" of Broca) around the isthmus of the hemisphere (parahippocampal and cingulate gyri as well as caudal orbitofrontal cortex), and some subcortical structures comprising part of the basal ganglia (ventral striatum and pallidum) and part of the thalamic nuclei (3).

Cortical Structures

One major step toward understanding the role of the limbic cortex in motor function may be derived from the com-

parative cytoarchitectonic work of Friedrich Sanides (2).★ According to Sanides, and based on the early work of Abbie [cited in Sanides (2)], the primitive vertebrate forebrain contains two types of allocortex: the archipallium (hippocampal primordium), found medially, and the paleopallium (olfactory/piriform primordium), laterally. Sanides proposed, on architectonic grounds, that the evolutionarily more recent neocortex (isocortex), characterized by a six-layered architecture, is derived from these archicortical and paleocortical moieties. In turn, each portion of the neocortex retains some structural features of the allocortex from which it was derived, and, thus, two morphologic trends can be discerned even within the primate neocortex. One of these trends, relating to the archicortical root, is characterized by a relative wealth of pyramidal neurons; the other, reflecting the influence of the paleocortex, exhibits a strong granular cell development. The archicortical influence reaches its apogee in the dorsal portion of gigantopyramidal area 4 and in the pericingulate supplementary motor area (SMA). The granular influence is most richly illustrated first by the primary sensory (konio) cortices and second by their association (parakoniocortical) belt areas most closely associated with the perisylvian regions. In the human brain, the lines of influence abut one another at the inferior frontal (principal sulcus in the monkey), the intraparietal, and the inferior temporal sulci. Thus, the two regions of the primate cortical mantle consist of (a) a dorsomesial part, which includes the cingulate cortex, pericingulate motor and sensory supplementary areas, the medial portion and roughly the dorsal half of the frontal and parietal lobes, and the inferior and

---

★ The Sanides concept described here reflects in part the written record cited as well as private discussions between one of us (A.M.G.) and Professor Sanides during his sabbatical leave at Harvard University in 1977.

medial portions of the temporal lobe; and (b) a ventrolateral part, which includes the perisylvian cortices, the opercula, the occipital pole, the temporal convexity, the insula, and the orbitofrontal cortex.

Within these two spheres of influence, Sanides described successive stages of architectonic differentiation, named according to phylogenetic criteria, starting with the archaic allocortices—not truly layered and present in fishes and amphibians, proceeding through the periallocortical and proisocortical stages—not yet sporting six layers and present together with the former in reptiles—and culminating in the true six-layered isocortex seen together with the former two stages only in mammals and in some turtles. These successive stages are represented in the primate brain, respectively, by the allocortical and periallocortical hippocampal formation, piriform cortex, septal region, substantia innominata, and amygdaloid complex, the proisocortical anterior insula and anterior cingulate gyrus, the caudally lying orbitofrontal cortex, and temporopolar cortex, and the neocortex, which occupies the dorsocaudal insula and opercular, pericingulate, posterior cingulate, retrosplenial, mesiotemporal, and convexity sites (4,5). As stated, each of the two cortical influences in the primate brain contains each stage of cortical differentiation.

An application of this duality of brain to motor function has recently been suggested in a comprehensive review by Goldberg (6). From multiple anatomic connectional, neurophysiologic, and pathologic evidence, Goldberg proposed a concept of opposing forces between the "mesial motor system" (MMS), which corresponds to Sanides's archicortical trend, and the "lateral motor system," which corresponds to the paleocortical trend. The MMS, which is connected cortically mainly with the superior parietal lobule and the pericingulate supplementary sensory area (SSA) and subcortically with the basal ganglia, acts in a projectional, self-initiated mode (we believe through its afferents from the reticular formation and hypothalamus), and may subserve the control of internally motivated movements. On the other hand, the lateral system, the connections of which include, in the cortex, the inferior parietal lobule, the peri-insular secondary sensory area processing somesthetic information, and the superior two temporal gyri and intervening superior temporal sulcus processing visual and auditory information, and subcortically the thalamus and cerebellum, is rather specialized for responsive, externally bounded movements. One of the main differences between these two systems lies in their subcortical efferent projections: while the lateral system possesses largely contralateral efferents, the mesial system projects more bilaterally to motor effectors on both sides of the body, which may account for the finding that the motor disturbance of a unilateral mesial lesion is generally less severe and of shorter duration than that of a comparable lesion affecting the lateral cortex. This holds true also for language disturbances following mesial lesions (see below), which never reach the same degree of severity of lesions of the classic (perisylvian, lateral) language areas.

Generally, the most lateralized of brain functions are linked to the lateral system, while functions subserved by parts of the mesial system tend to be represented in both hemispheres.

Subcortical Structures

Significant additional knowledge about motor function has been derived from anatomic studies on the link between the basal ganglia and the limbic system. Thus, Nauta et al (7–9) have described in detail the limbic innervation of the rat striatum. They contrast the dorsal part of the striatum with the ventral part—limbic striatum—which includes the nucleus accumbens and olfactory tubercle. Whereas the former receives nigral dopaminergic afferents and is mainly connected with the sensorimotor cortex, the latter receives its dopaminergic innervation from the ventral tegmental area (VTA) as well as projections from limbic structures (hippocampus, amygdala, cingulate cortex) and the prefrontal cortex (Fig 50.1). This dual nature of the striatum is also reflected in its pallidal projections; the nucleus accumbens, for instance, does not project to the main mass of the pallidum but to the smaller ventral pallidum, which in turn projects specifically to several limbic structures: the amygdala, the habenular nucleus, and the mediodorsal nucleus of the thalamus (Fig 50.1).

Mogenson et al (10) have postulated that the ventral striatopallidal system realizes a "motor interface" between the limbic system and the strictly motor basal ganglia, and hence represents a good candidate for subserving the function of

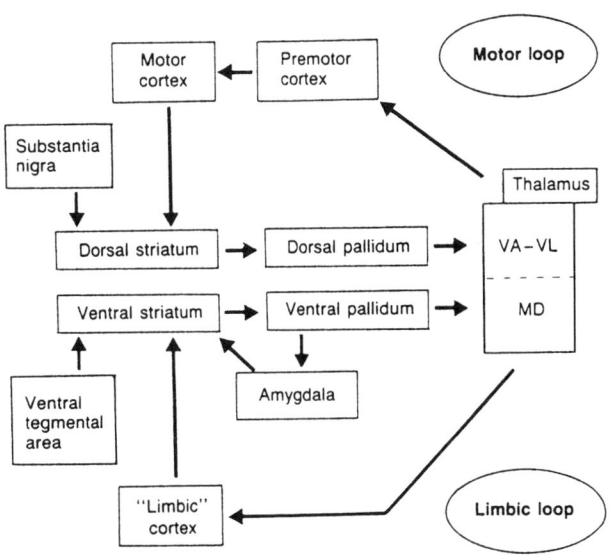

FIGURE 50.1 *The dual nature of the striatum: schematic representation of the two corticosubcortical loops. (Adapted from Nauta WJH. Circuitous connections linking cerebral cortex, limbic system, and corpus striatum. In Doane BK, Livingston KE, eds. The limbic system: functional organization and clinical disorders. New York: Raven, 1986:43–54.)*

translating internal drives into motor acts. This view is not inconsistent with the model hypothesized by Panksepp (11) of a specific "foraging system," including the dopaminergic fibers of the medial forebrain bundle and their striatolimbic projections, which subserves behaviors such as "interest–curiosity–expectancy."★

IMPAIRMENTS OF MOTOR FUNCTION AND MOTIVATION IN LIMBIC CORTICAL DAMAGE

The effects of lesions of the cortical component of the limbic system have been occasionally described in the past decades but were only rarely considered with regard to motor functions. Among the various cortical structures included under the heading of limbic cortex (3), we shall consider three main cortical regions: mesial frontal, insular, and orbitofrontal cortex.

Effects of Cingulate Lesions

Cingulate lesions usually affect both the cortex (anterior cingulate area 24 and/or subcallosal region) and the cingulum bundle (subcortical fibers coursing just underneath the cingulate cortex). MacLean (12) recently summarized the effects of cingulate lesions as disrupting the "[three] forms of behavior that characterize the evolutionary transition from reptiles to mammals: (a) nursing and maternal care; (b) audiovocal communication; and (c) playful behavior." In humans, bilateral damage to the cingulate gyrus has been mainly associated with states of akinetic mutism (13,14). In such cases, this akinetic state is often associated with severe vegetative disorders leading to coma and death after a few days (15). Buge et al (16) reported three clinicopathologic observations of bicingulate softening and discussed the notion of akinetic mutism in the light of their patients' behavior. They proposed to single out an "anterior and wakeful" variety of akinetic mutism, in contrast to that caused by diencephalic and mesencephalic injury, which is generally associated with a diminished level of consciousness. Laplane et al (17) reported a single case of bilateral infarction of the anterior cingulate region without reduction of motor or speech activities but considerable behavioral changes that included attentional disturbance, severe amnesia, compulsive use of objects, emotional indifference (apathy), docility, and abulia. Left 24 hours without food, the patient did not complain or show any evidence of hunger. Her spontaneous speech was not absent but only reduced

and totally incoherent. Postmortem findings showed that the lesion, grossly bilaterally symmetric, involved the anterior third of the cingulate gyrus, including the portion of the gyrus lying anterior to and beneath the genu of the corpus callosum, leaving undamaged the caudal part of area 24 and most of the mesial portion of premotor cortex (area 6 and the SMA).

Bilateral excisions of the same areas have been performed for the surgical management of some psychiatric states or intractable pain: besides a diminution of anxiety and agitation, such cingulectomies resulted in docility, indifference, and loss of general interest. However, these symptoms were reported to resolve rapidly and spontaneously. It thus seems probable that the akinetic mutism in massive, spontaneously occurring lesions is related to the size of the lesions and/or the concomitant involvement of adjacent premotor areas and the SMA.

In a more recent case report (18), a bilateral, asymmetrical lesion involving the cingulate on one side and the head of caudate nucleus in the other hemisphere was responsible for profound mental changes, with apathy and unusual tameness not unlike patients described in the next section of this chapter with bistriatal lesions, associated with additional signs of frontal dysfunction (grasping and utilization behaviors, confabulatory amnestic syndrome).

Overall, both lesion studies and data from epileptic patients (19) concur to demonstrate that the human cingulate plays a crucial role in initiation, motivation, and goal-directed behavior whereas its more rostral part is involved in modulating autonomic activity and internal emotional responses. Such a complex role is compatible with preliminary data obtained to date with modern functional imaging techniques showing activation in the cingulate areas during a large number of motor or nonmotor situations (20,21).

Effects of Unilateral Damage to the SMA

The SMA, as primarily described by Penfield and Welch (22,23) is a cortical area situated on the premotor area 6 (Brodmann) portion of the mesial aspect of the frontal lobe, just anterior to the inferior limb representation of the primary motor area 4. Actually, its definition, functional rather than anatomic, is that of a cortical region the stimulation of which induces (typically bilateral) motor phenomena. Unlike the unilateral destruction of the anterior cingulate area, which has not been specifically studied to our knowledge, the effect of unilaterally destroying the SMA has been reported in surgical cases in epileptic patients (24). Postoperatively, patients developed global akinesia, more prominent contralaterally, and mutism. An interesting sign reported by these authors was "emotional" or "reversed" facial palsy, whereby the facial weakness became evident only during spontaneous smiling and not during grimacing to command. A few days later, recovery occurred to the point that the patients were again able to answer questions, although very scantily, and to move ipsilateral but not

---

★ More recently, this model has been refined from two points of view (63–64): First, from anatomic studies in primates, it has been suggested that the connections between basal ganglia and cortical structures are organized in five parallel circuits, two of them connecting limbic components of the basal ganglia to paralimbic cortical areas; moreover, it has been proposed, at least for the "motor" loop, an additional "indirect" pathway from the striatum to output nuclei, passing first to the external segment of the globus pallidus, then to the subthalamic nucleus, before reaching the internal portion of the globus pallidus. However, this demarcation of direct and indirect striatopallidal pathways would not be as clear-cut for the limbic as for the motor circuits (64,85). Finally, these refinements remain compatible with the model presented in Figure 50.1.

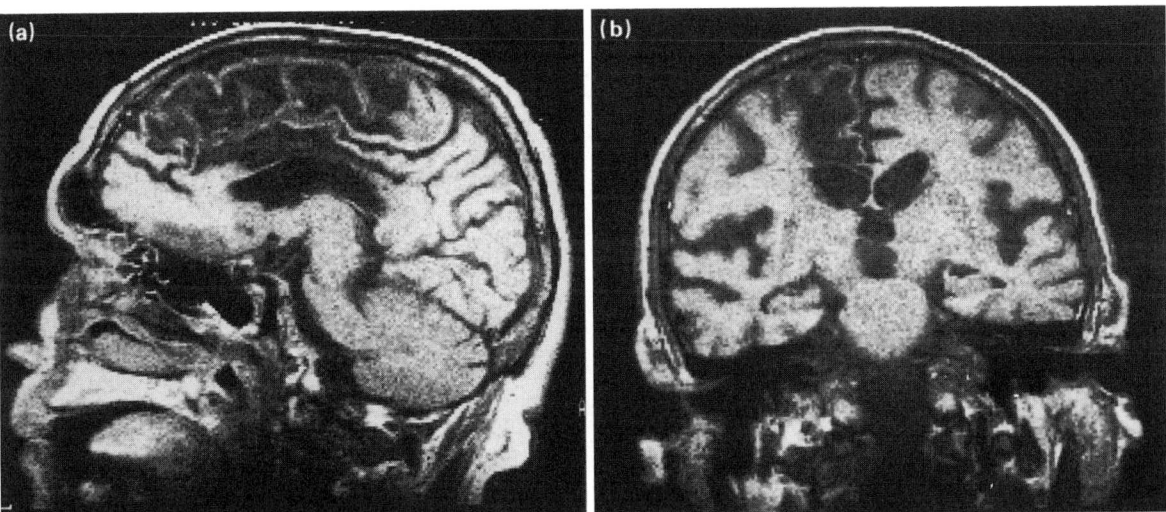

FIGURE 50.2   *MRI images on sagittal (a) and coronal (b) sections in a case of right anterior cerebral artery infarct. The lesion involves the anterior cingulate, a large part of the mesial motor cortex, including the SMA and adjacent dorsal area 6, as well as underlying white matter. The foot representation of primary motor area 4 is also involved, as well as part of the corpus callosum. Accordingly, the patient, one year after onset, had severe left leg and shoulder paresis, Babinski sign, forced grasping reaction of the left hand, decreased speech spontaneity and fluency, and an intermanual behavior close to the alien hand sign (see text).*

contralateral limbs on command. Spontaneous speech and movements returned to a nearly normal level within one to eight months postoperatively.

Effects of Unilateral Cingulate and SMA Lesions

This is by far the commonest clinical occurrence, as the most usual spontaneous injury to this region, produced by ischemic infarcts in the territory of the anterior cerebral artery, usually involve both the supplementary motor and cingulate areas (Fig 50.2). The clinical features usually include, after a short period of total akinesia and mutism, a paresis of the contralateral inferior limb with a Babinski sign, a grasp reflex and forced grasping of the hand, akinesia or hypokinesia of the upper limb with moderate to severe proximal weakness of the shoulder. Fine alternating movements of the fingers or the hand usually appear disturbed in both hands, but more so on the contralateral side, in which the hand could seem paralyzed were it not for the presence of a forced grasp.

Besides these motor symptoms, patients may develop a particular form of speech disorder much akin to the syndrome of "transcortical motor aphasia" (TCMA). This syndrome consists of a lack of spontaneous speech, difficulty initiating speech, intact comprehension, and well-preserved ability to repeat words and sentences (25–29). These features often follow a period of complete mutism lasting days to weeks. Damasio and Van Hoesen (30) reported the following case.

Case Study
A 35-year-old woman suffered an ischemic infarct in the left mesial frontal lobe. During the first few days postonset, there

was complete absence of spontaneous speech and she gave no reply whatsoever to questions posed to her. Moreover, she gave no evidence of attempting to mouth words or to compensate with gestures for her verbal deficit. In contrast to the absence of spontaneous language, however, repetition was carried out albeit slowly. Three days postonset, she could produce occasional one-word answers to questions, but only after delays of a minute or longer. Three weeks later, she was able to use short sentences but her speech remained poorly informative. Her performance on a test of verbal fluency—such as the controlled oral word association, in which the patient is required to provide as many words belonging to a given semantic category or beginning with a particular letter as possible—was severely impaired. Interestingly, when questioned about the reasons for her mutism during the early period, she answered she had "nothing to say" and felt "no will to reply."

One may wish to ask whether the disorder presently under discussion represents a form of TCMA. Most reports (25,28,29,31,32) refer to such disturbances as TCMA. Damasio's view (33) is that such lesions interfere with speech motor control but not linguistic processing itself. Freedman et al (34), suggest that TCMA may result either from 1) lesions limited to the SMA, or 2) destruction of fibers from the SMA to Broca's inferior premotor and prefrontal areas. They thus consider the disorder to be a consequence of suppressing the speech "starter mechanism" in the former case or disconnection of this mechanism from perisylvian cortical motor speech centers in the latter. Stuss and Benson (35) (pp. 166–167) prefer to consider the "SMA language disturbance" as merely the linguistic aspect of a broader motor disorder affecting all voluntary movements, differently from an instance of TCMA attributed to the separation of the SMA from Broca's area. Whichever term or explanation is used, the facts are in good agreement with the role generally proposed for the SMA as a "supramotor area" or "energizer unit" necessary for initiating movements according to internal needs and drives (6,36,37). Such a role, for language as well as for other voluntary motor acts, would include the activation of preestablished motor subroutines—for instance, speech utterances and fine-finger manipulative movements.

One important question concerning speech control from mesial frontal cortex is whether this control is lateralized. Most descriptions of transcortical motor aphasia after anterior cerebral artery territory infarcts refer to left-sided lesions. This could suggest left hemisphere lateralization of speech control by the mesial system, similar to that of left perisylvian language areas. Damasio (33,38), however, states that "there is no evidence that the side of lesion plays a major role here, and dominant as well as nondominant lesions cause much the same result." In fact, at least two individual cases of speech disorders have been reported after right-sided mesial frontal lesions (29,39). In both patients, language disturbances were not significantly different from those of left-hemisphere cases. In our experience, some features of TCMA, especially reduced fluency and delay in initiating responses, may be encountered in both left and right mesial frontal lesions, which is consistent with the notion that archicortically derived cortex is less lateralized than paleocortically derived cortex (see above).

Penfield and Roberts (40) reported that electrical stimulation of either SMA can produce speech phenomena. These included speech arrest, vocalization, hesitation, and distortion. On the other hand, truly aphasic disturbances were elicited from stimulation of the lateral left cortical areas only. Neither did Bancaud and Talairach (41) find hemispheric differences in speech phenomena induced by SMA stimulation, nor did the studies of Larsen et al (42) on cerebral blood flow during language tasks show any lateral differences in activation of the SMA during speech. Finally, corticectomy involving either right or left SMA produced similar language disturbances (24).

Both SMA appear to be active in normal language processing, as evidenced by stimulation and cerebral blood flow studies. Rapid improvement and predictable recovery of language function in unilateral SMA damage may result from compensation by the contralateral SMA. Such compensation, however, may be easier for the left SMA in right-lesioned cases than the reverse, this being possibly related to asymmetries in contralateral connections (6). We believe that as lesions of the SMA are likely to involve fibers decussating in the corpus callosum, or the vascular insult that leads to SMA injury can also injure the callosum directly, asymmetry of effect between left and right SMA lesions relates to the fact that a left SMA lesion can disconnect the dominant Broca's area from both SMA, thus impeding one likely mechanism for compensation; a right SMA lesion, on the

other hand, leaves ipsilateral connections within the left hemisphere intact, thus permitting compensation. Alternatively, the left SMA may be in fact specialized in language control; if so, it remains obvious that the degree of lateralization of this cortical region is far less than that of the perisylvian language areas.

Further asymmetric functioning of the mesial frontal cortex has been recently suspected for unimanual gestural activity. Goldberg et al (43) first reported a particular behavior of interhemispheric conflict, termed "alien hand sign," in two patients with left mesial frontal infarction (and a classic SMA speech syndrome). In both cases, the right hand could be seen to involve itself in activities apparently out of control of the subject's conscious self. Moreover, bimanual conflict was noted on some occasions, with the right hand uncontrollably hindering goal-directed movements of the left. As the authors noted, such behavior is often present in split-brain subjects, but only for the left arm (44,45).* The phenomenon could result from the combination of callosal and mesial cortical damage contralateral to the "alien" hand (35,43), and in a more recent account, Goldberg (46) hypothesizes that the upper limb contralateral to a mesial frontal lesion may function under two different modes: an "alien" mode, in which the hand behaves independently of conscious volition, and a "volitional" mode, where distal movements are clumsy and hypometric (Fig 50.3).

Also intriguing are the findings of Watson and collaborators of differential control of movements by the right and left SMA (47,48). On the basis of two cases of left mesial lesion with ideomotor apraxia and one case of right mesial lesion with hypokinesia and hypometria, these authors suggested that the left SMA is involved in sequencing the primary motor programs and translating spatial and temporal representations of gestures into motor programs, while the right SMA is critical for setting the activational level for motor output. Although attractive, this view needs further empiric support, as most other reports of left SMA lesions did not describe apraxic behavior, even when specifically searched for (30,32). In our own experience, the only instances of apraxia from mesial lesions are illustrated by the presence of left unilateral ("sympathetic") apraxia related to associated callosal damage and bilateral melokinetic apraxia (35), but never true bilateral ideomotor apraxia such as reported by Watson et al (47). However, it is conceivable, in some cases of callosal apraxia, to suspect a contribution of the medial frontal damage to the severity, if not to the nature, of the apraxia (49). Also, hypokinesia as measured by reaction time to accomplish a movement does not appear to be significantly more severe in right than left mesial

---

* It must be pointed out that the term *signe de la main étrangère* first proposed by Brion and Jedynak, originally referred specifically to a tactile delusional phenomenon, the patient being unable tactually to acknowledge his own hand as belonging to him.

(a)

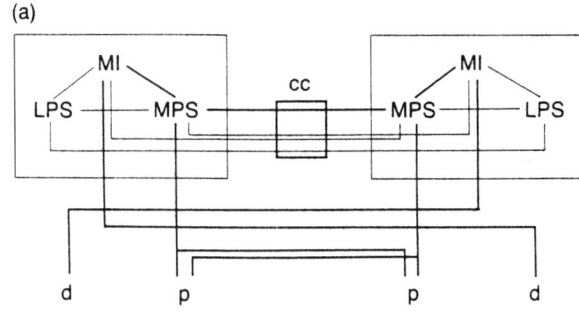

(b)

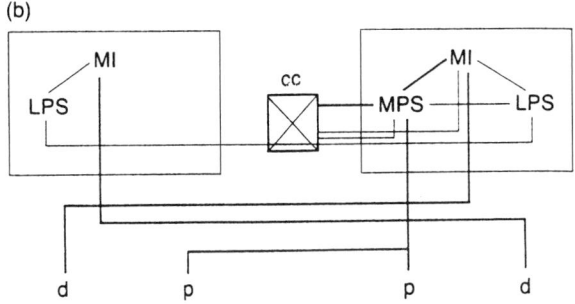

FIGURE 50.3   *(a) Normal connections between the mesial premotor system (MPS), including the SMA, the lateral premotor areas (LPS) and the primary motor area (MI). Outputs from MI are strictly contralateral and concern distal movements. (b) In case of mesial frontal lesion with callosal damage, the hand contralateral to the MPS lesion may function either in an "alien" mode (when controlled by contralateral MI) or in "volitional" mode (when controlled by ipsilateral MPS). (Redrawn from Goldberg G. Premotor systems, motor learning, and ipsilateral control. Behav Brain Sci 1987;10:323–329.)*

lesions (J. Massion, personal communication).* Finally, it may be worthwhile to consider that the same distinction that exists between volitional grimacing and spontaneous smiling may exist for hand movements, in terms of emotional expression by the hands and volitional hand control. In that case, the right SMA may be slightly more dominant for the former function, just as the left is slightly dominant for the latter. Unilateral and/or callosal injury may thus lead to conflict between these two functions.

Effects of Insular Lesions

The behavioral role of the insular cortex in humans is still unclear. Besides evidence of its implication in gustatory functions and in the control of some visceral mechanisms, the insula has been very rarely investigated from a neuropsychologic point of view. Anatomically, the insula derives from the olfactory portion of the limbic system and its major connections involve, in addition to other limbic stuctures (amygdala, orbitofrontal cortex, cingulate cortex), neighboring cortical regions such as the opercular sensorimotor region and the auditory zones in the superior temporal gyrus.

One of us has recently reported a very unusual case of bilateral lesions almost exclusively limited to the insular cortex (50), thus providing the unique opportunity of a new insight to the role of this mysterious region. The patient, a young woman recently operated on for a mitral valvulopa-

thy, suffered within one week postsurgery two consecutive embolic accidents that resulted in profound behavioral changes including total mutism, hyperactivity with continuous tendency to manipulate objects, distractibility, and a total inaptitude to communicate. Seated in front of the examiner, she behaved exactly as if she were alone, exploring visually the examination room without apparent affect, showing no tendency to communicate verbally or nonverbally, neither spontaneously nor in response to questions. When re-examined two months later, her speech abilities had gradually recovered and she was again able to communicate almost normally. She was then shown the videotape taken during the earlier interview and questioned about her mutism. Very surprisingly, she replied that she was totally conscious of what happened and understood everything perfectly, and that she was convinced at the time that she had been answering all questions posed to her. This behavior was therefore clearly different from a "nonwillingness" to communicate, suggesting rather attentional and emotional disturbances specifically interfering with social interaction and communicative abilities. This interpretation is consistent with the anatomic characteristics of the insula, at the interface between brain structures controlling verbal communication (auditory areas and buccofacial projection in the sensorimotor zone) and those subserving emotional behavior and social interactions (amygdala and orbitofrontal cortex).

Effects of Orbitofrontal Lesions

Behavioral and emotional disturbances resulting from lesions occurring in the frontal lobes have been described for a long time. These subjects have been variously characterized as childish, facetious, rude, careless, irresponsible, impulsive, irascible, egotist, seeking immediate rewards, feeling no remorse, and so on. Such a terminological diversity actually masks the extraordinary complexity of the underlying

---

* Another interesting issue is the subjective emotional experience of the patient with unilateral cingulate and SMA lesions. Patients are generally reported to show decreased emotional expression or indifference. In some cases, they are also said to display flattened affect, but these evaluations are based on the subjects' apparent behavior, and do not provide insight into the patients' subjective emotions. In fact, emotional experience may often be largely spared in this condition. Thus, when specifically investigated, it appears that patients experience a whole range of appropriate emotions. In particular, when faced with their motor deficits, they often show verbal or nonverbal evidence of vexation or frustration.

mechanisms. Blumer and Benson (51) referred to these traits as "pseudopsychopathic" and related them to lesions located in the orbital region.

In rhesus monkeys, orbitofrontal lesions provoke aversion toward social contact, with decreased tendency to interact with their mates and decreased aggressive behavior. Single-neuron recording experiments tend to show that orbitofrontal cortex is involved in a complex manner in the process leading to adapt responses to external stimuli previously associated with a reward (reinforcing stimulus). Globally (52), the specificity of orbitofrontal neurons is to signal whether or not an expected reward is being obtained, thus probably allowing the modification of an ongoing behavior whenever a response becomes inappropriate.

Behavioral changes due to orbitofrontal lesions in humans have recently been reformulated by Damasio (53,54), in light of two prototypic observations, one from the classical medical literature (the famous Phineas Gage), the other from his own records [case EVR (55)]. In these two cases, a lesion involving the orbitofrontal regions had provoked considerable behavioral changes without significant impairment in cognitive functioning and intelligence. From the analysis of certain aspects of these patients' behavior, which he proposed to refer to under the term *acquired sociopathy*, Damasio elaborated a theory known as the "somatic marker" hypothesis. This hypothesis supposes that decisions whose outcome could be potentially harmful or potentially advantageous, and are made in circumstances similar to previous experience, prompt a somatic response involving autonomic, endocrine, visceral, and musculoskeletal expressions. This somatic response acts as a "marker" used by the organism to signal the potential danger or advantage of a given situation or action, and will be reactivated, more or less consciously, upon each new occurrence of the same situation. As evidence for this theory, EVR and other patients with similar lesions were submitted to a skin conductance experiment (56). Whereas elementary stimuli, such as an intense noise, produced normal visceral responses, "emotionally or socially significant stimuli" failed to do so, suggesting that, unlike controls with frontal lesions outside the orbital region, orbitofrontal patients would be unable to elicit somatic states previously associated to specific social situations.

A more direct evaluation of this hypothesis derives from the "gambling experiment" (57). Subjects are presented with four decks of cards and are asked to pick a card from one deck at a time. Certain decks, unknown to the subjects, are associated with a high probability of important monetary loss and a low probability of important monetary reward. The other decks are associated with low monetary reward but also low probability of loss. Normal subjects learn after a few trials that low-risk decks are more profitable, and will soon stop drawing from the other high-risk decks. On the contrary, orbitofrontal subjects will continue to prefer the more onerous condition, in spite of the fact that they explicitly realize their irretrievable losses. In addi-

tion, subjects have been submitted to skin conductance recordings while engaged in the gambling task. Whereas normal controls showed large visceral responses in anticipation of choosing a card from the "risky" decks, patients showed no anticipatory response, suggesting that their aberrant behavior may be related to the failure of the ongoing action to elicit appropriate somatic states apt to modulate their choice.

Thus, according to Damasio, there exists in the orbital regions of the frontal lobes, a system able to ascribe and retrieve the somatic sensations corresponding to the previously learned valence of a given social situation. This function of the orbital cortex would be possible owing to its connections with other limbic structures (amygdala and hypothalamus), which trigger the visceral responses and with sensory association cortices, which convey informations about the contextual significance of the situation via the dorsolateral frontal cortex.

Finally, another very intriguing behavioral consequence of orbitofrontal lesions is the fact that such patients may be impaired not only in their decisions, their actions, or behaviors but also in the way they can judge their own or somebody else's acts, especially by reference to moral standards. There are a few instances in the literature reporting impaired "moral reasoning" in patients with frontal lobe damage (58,59), with an analysis of "moral dilemmas" reflecting an arrest at an early stage of moral development. Accordingly, it appears from these reports that only frontal lesions occurring during childhood—during a period when the frontal lobe has nor yet reached complete maturation— are likely to alter moral reasoning. Patients sustaining frontal lesions during adulthood usually demonstrate an intact judgment of their socially deviant behaviors. Patient EVR, for instance, scored at a superior level on a questionnaire of moral reasoning. One of us (M.H.) has examined a young man who, two years after severe head trauma, was dismissed from his job, had divorced his spouse, and lost all his friends due to antisocial behavior. He also had committed futile thefts, which he recognized was very unusual for him. Moreover, he reported that, in several instances, he felt unable to decide "whether an act was good or bad" and had repeatedly manifested the need to ask someone else "which was the right way to act" since "he could no longer feel it by himself." Unlike patients with developmental frontal lobe lesions, however, his discussion of moral dilemmas was good, as if he could not use in everyday life moral concepts yet intellectually available to him. Brain MRI in this patient showed bilateral orbitofrontal abnormal signals corresponding to traumatic injury sequelae (Fig 50.4). Such observations are in good agreement with Damasio's concept of a "somatic marker," extending the notion of autonomic control of behaviors to that of moral judgment and suggesting that the visceral signaling role of the orbitofrontal cortex is important not only for adapting one's acts to socially relevant context but also as a basis for personal morality.

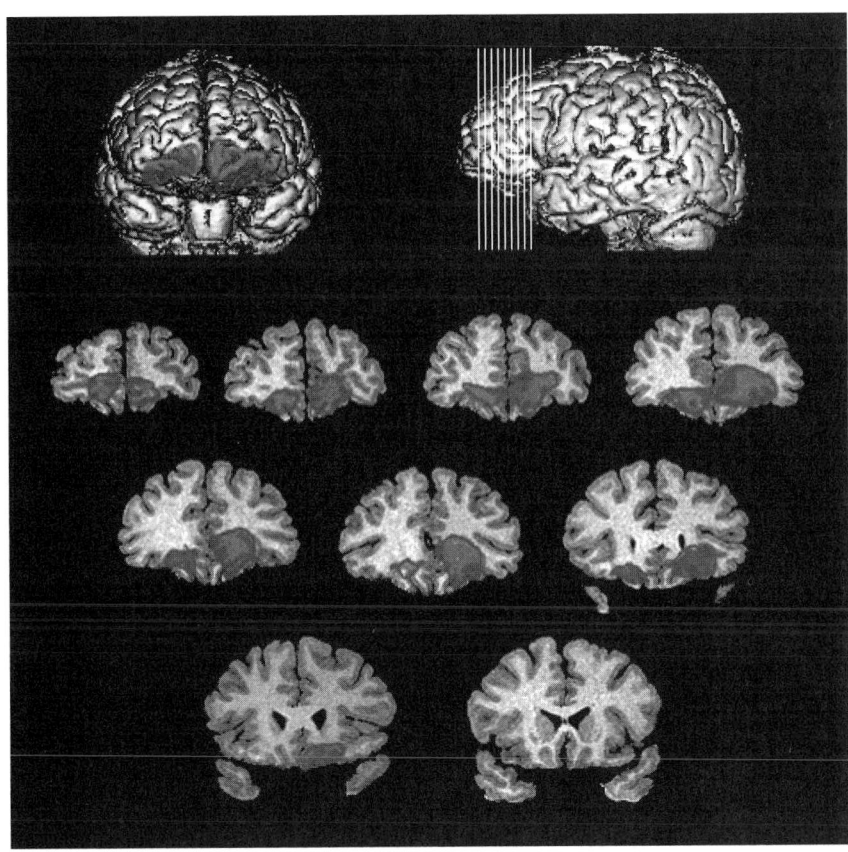

FIGURE 50.4 *Schematic representation of lesion in a case of "acquired sociopathy" due to traumatic injury of orbitofrontal regions.*

APATHY ("ATHYMHORMIA") IN LESIONS OF THE BASAL GANGLIA

This section deals with a group of behavioral disorders that have been referred to in the early neurologic literature variously as "placidity" or "abulia" (60), and that were often considered as a milder form of akinetic mutism (61). This position, which was dominant in North American neurologic writings, has probably obscured the real nature of these disorders and of their anatomical substrate, the only suggested pathophysiology being an interruption of frontothalamic connections. One interesting approach, however, has been that of some psychiatrists trying to group under the term *apathy* certain behavioral traits shared by both some psychiatric and neurologic patients. Marin (62) thus defined apathy as "absence or lack of feeling, emotions, interest, or concern," and proposed that it "refers primarily to lack of motivation," clearly suggesting that human motivation, as one aspect of emotional life, may be the object of clinica investigation. Marin, however, made no attempt at defining its neural substrate.

In this section, we will demonstrate how a series of clinical observations (Table 50.1) mainly published over the past 15 years in the French neurologic literature under the terms *loss of psychic autoactivation* (63), *pure psychic akinesia* (64), or, probably more accurately and usefully, *athymhormic syndrome* (65) has provided significant improvement to our

understanding of the role of the basal ganglia in human motivation.

Our purpose in the last part of this chapter will be 1) to summarize the clinical features of these observations and to show how, put altogether, these features may be viewed as a distinct neurobehavioral syndrome, 2) to provide arguments suggesting that this syndrome results from the disruption of a specific brain system and to delineate, on the basis of radio-anatomical/behavioral correlations, the structural organization of this brain system, and 3) to propose a tentative neuroanatomical and psychodynamic model of human motivation.

Lenticular Nucleus Lesions

The first reports of this syndrome relate to patients with bilateral lesions of the lenticular nucleus, particularly the globus pallidus, primarily following carbon monoxide poisoning or wasp sting. After an initial period of coma, patients showed persistent abulia—dramatically reduced activity and disturbed affect. The full extent of the syndrome emerged from descriptions by family members: patients spent their days doing nothing, apparently without thinking or showing any sign of mental activity; they rested motionless all day long, either in their beds or in a chair, unless strongly urged or stimulated by the relatives; one remarkable characteristic of their behavior was the discrepancy between spontaneous

Table 50.1   Isolated Disturbances of Motivation and Action Following Damage to the Basal Ganglia

Authors	Number of Cases	Age	Lesion Location	Lesion Type
Laplane et al (63,64,67)	8	53	Pallido-striatal, bilateral	Wasp sting
		23	Pallidal, bilateral	Carbon monoxide (CO) intoxication
		59	Pallidal, bilateral	CO
		52	Pallido-striatal, bilateral	Disulfiram intoxication
		27	Pallidal, bilateral	Anoxia
		?	Pallido-striatal, bilateral	Anoxia
		31	Pallidal, bilateral	CO
		22	Pallidal, bilateral	CO
Ali-Chérif et al (66)	2	39	Pallidal, bilateral	CO
		18	Pallidal, bilateral	CO
Habib & Poncet (65)	2	64	Caudate, bilateral	Ischemic (lacunes)
		60	Caudate, bilateral	Ischemic (lacunes)
Strub (90)	1	60	Pallidal, bilateral	Ischemic/anoxic
Trillet et al (70)	3	54	Caudate, bilateral	Ischemic infarcts, hemorrhage
		56	Caudate, bilateral	Ischemic infarcts
		59	Caudate, bilateral	Ischemic infarcts
Danel et al (91)	1	72		Ischemic (lacunes)
Milandre et al (73)	1	49	Caudate, left Pallidal, right	Ischemic (Moya Moya syndrome)
Bellmann & Assal (74)	1	30	Caudate, left Pallidal, right	Ischemic infarcts

activity, which was nearly absent, and the strictly normal motor function that occurred on command. Thus, patients could remain motionless and speechless before a friend or relative for one hour, but would answer promptly and accurately any question posed to them. When questioned about the content of their thoughts, patients systematically answered that they thought about nothing, or that their minds were empty.

Besides decreased spontaneous motor and mental activity patients with bipallidal lesions showed loss of interest and curiosity and apparent flattening of affect. They did not demonstrate any desire or drive; neither hunger nor the need to smoke, not even pain, seemed capable of eliciting appropriate motor behavior. One patient [(66), case 2], stayed several hours in the sun without moving until her parents came and took her away with second-degree burns. The same patient walked without complaining in shoes too small for her until her mother noticed a bleeding blister on her toe. Interestingly, this extreme loss of drive and affect was not accompanied by loss of intellectual function, except for some memory deficit.

In all cases, computerized tomography scan or MRI showed bilateral involvement of the globus pallidus only (Fig 50.5), and positron emission tomography scans done on some indicated reduced striatal but normal cortical glucose utilization (67). The authors only report a relative frontal

hypometabolism, which they explain as a deafferentiation of the prefrontal cortex. The mild nature of the cortical metabolic abnormalities, however, as compared with the dramatic behavioral changes, leads one to attribute the latter to the subcortical deficits. Finally, in some—but not all—of these patients, authors describe an associated obsessive–compulsive behavior, a symptom discussed in other chapters of the present book.

Thus, it appears from these observations of impaired motor and mental activity following lenticular damage that this region of the human brain must play a special role in the regulation of affective behavior. Actually, more recent observations have shown that the crucial structure, in this regard, is the medial pallidal nucleus, since brain MRI is now apt to demonstrate very accurately lesions restricted to this small (but obviously crucial) region of the basal ganglia (see Fig 50.5(b)). Accordingly, a recent review of behavioral consequences of basal ganglia damage (68) has shown that putaminal lesions by themselves do not result in similar mental changes (69).

Striatal Lesions

One important advance in the understanding of this syndrome has come from the observation that behavioral changes very similar to those resulting from bipallidal lesions

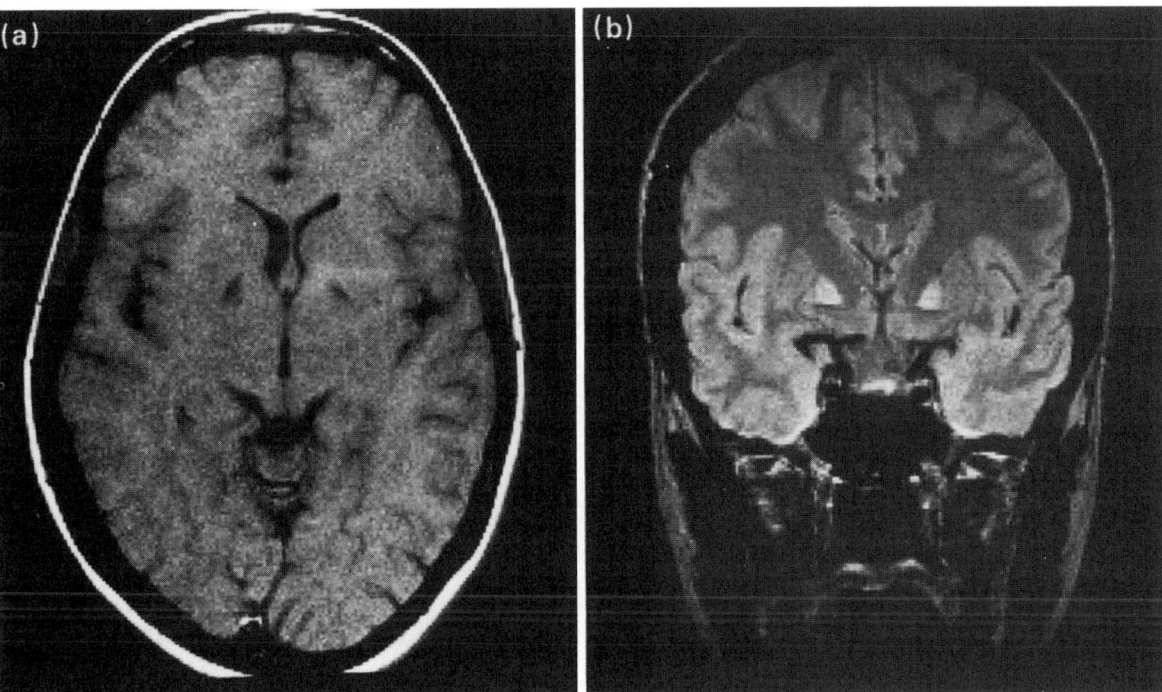

FIGURE 50.5 *MRI images [(a) axial section, partial recovery; (b) coronal section, T2-weighted spin-echo] in a case of bipallidal lesions due to carbon monoxide poisoning. This 26-year-old female displayed the typical "athymhormia syndrome" (see text), persisting unchanged eight years after the initial accident. Note that the area of abnormal signal involves only the mesial part of the globus pallidus, sparing in particular the striatum (including the nucleus accumbens) and surrounding white matter. Courtesy of Dr A. Alicherif.*

may occur from lesions located in another distinct part of the basal ganglia, namely, the head of the caudate, especially in cases of small lacunar infarcts restricted to this region (65). Patients—usually hypertensive—were reported to show, often abruptly, radical personality changes.

Case Study

The patient, previously very active, quick-tempered, and authoritarian, became "gentle as a lamb" and unable to take any initiative. His only daily activity was watching TV, but only if his wife would turn the set on; otherwise, he never asked for it. He never spoke unless questioned, but was perfectly able to give answers on current events. He never asked for food, but ate with apparent appetite when food was presented; however, he did not show any of the food preferences he had before. He seemed indifferent to emotionally loaded events or stimuli, and never fell into fits of anger, as had usually been the case in comparable situations prior to his illness. If questioned about his mood, he answered he was not sad, and always exhibited an impassive smile. Neuropsychologic assessments showed normal language, praxis, and constructions. The Wechsler memory quotient was 98 and he scored 93 in the full-scale IQ of the Wechsler adult intelligence scale. Here again, it was possible to assert that the patient was neither demented nor depressed. Magnetic resonance imaging (MRI) (Fig 50.6) showed multiple, subcortical small lesions, mainly involving bilaterally the striatum (caudate and putamen), as well as surrounding white matter.

Notably, the frontal lobes and the pallidum were spared. The site of white matter involvement made it possible to interpret the syndrome, at least in part, as relating to bilateral disconnection of the medial cortices from perisylvian and subcortical targets, as the fibers involved in this connection hug the lateral ventricles and travel just lateral to the head of the caudate nucleus.

It seems then that a second locus other than the globus pallidus is involved in the impaired process, strongly suggesting that the neural substrate of this function includes bilaterally two separate subcortical loci, most probably linked through a specific network. This was later confirmed by the report (70) of three new cases of pure athymhormic syndrome after focal—ischemic or hemorrhagic—lesions of the head of the caudate [Fig 50.7 and (72)]. Accordingly, in their meta-analysis of isolated basal ganglia lesions, Bhatia and Marsden (68) have found that abulia is even more frequent in caudate (25%) than in pallidal (20%) lesions. Finally, one particularly interesting circumstance is the occurrence of asymmetrical basal ganglia lesions involving the caudate head on one side and the medial globus pallidus on the other side (74) (Fig 50.8). These observations clearly indicate that the syndrome under consideration is indeed the consequence of lesions located at either site of a subcortical network. In the following section, we will show that this subcortical network is likely part of the limbic loop depicted in Figure 50.1 and suggest a crucial role for this loop in

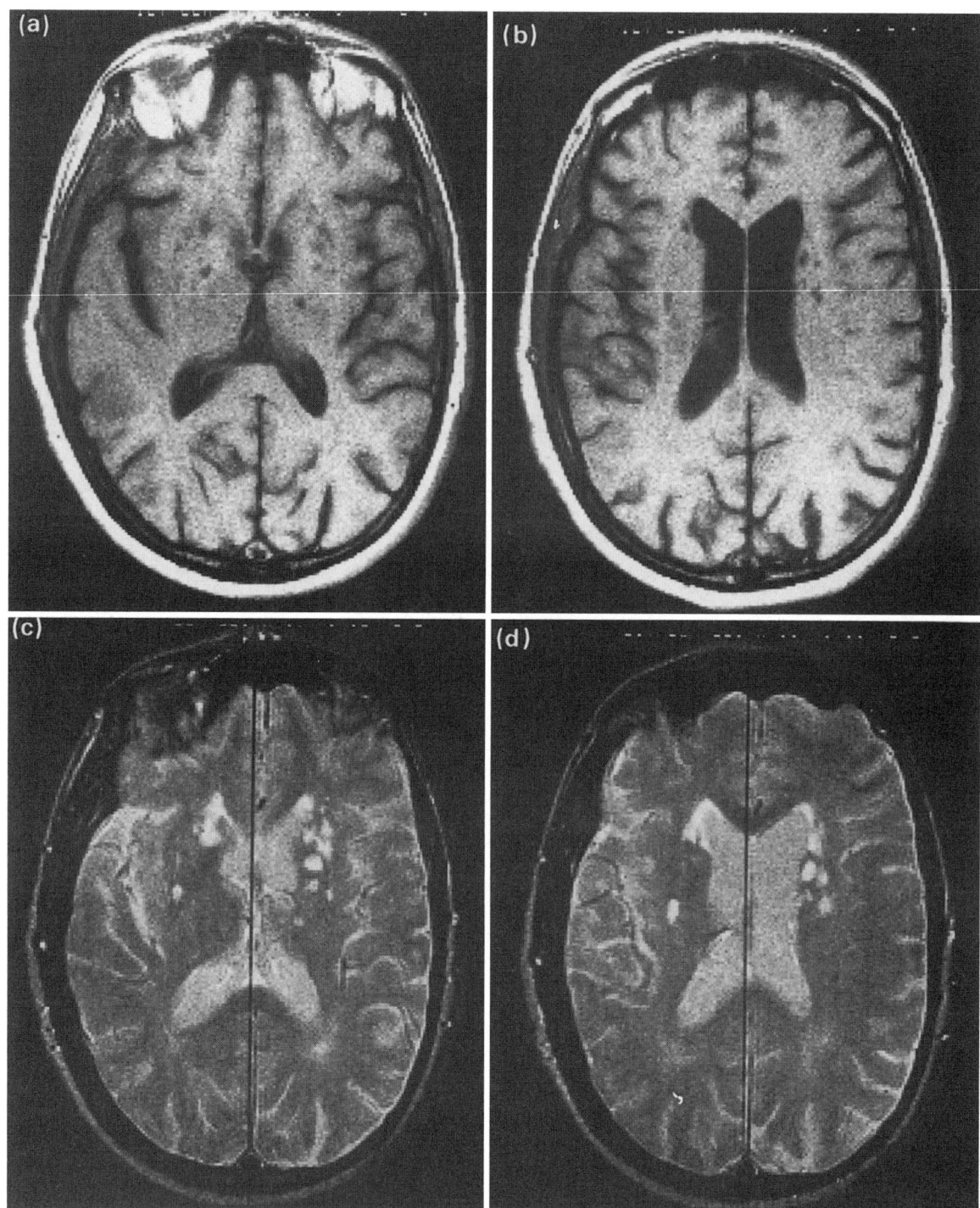

FIGURE 50.6   *MRI images obtained with partial recovery (a,b) and T2-weighted (c,d) spin-echo, showing multiple small areas of decreased signal suggesting lacunar microinfarcts involving the caudate, lenticular nuclei and adjacent white matter. Note the relatively intact frontal white matter.*

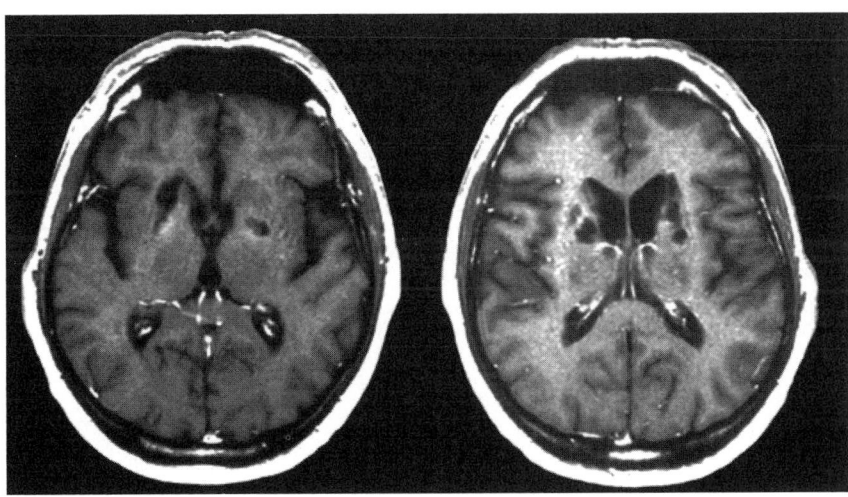

FIGURE 50.7   *Brain MRI scan in a patient with athymhormic syndrome (apathy) due to bilateral striatal ischemic infarcts.*

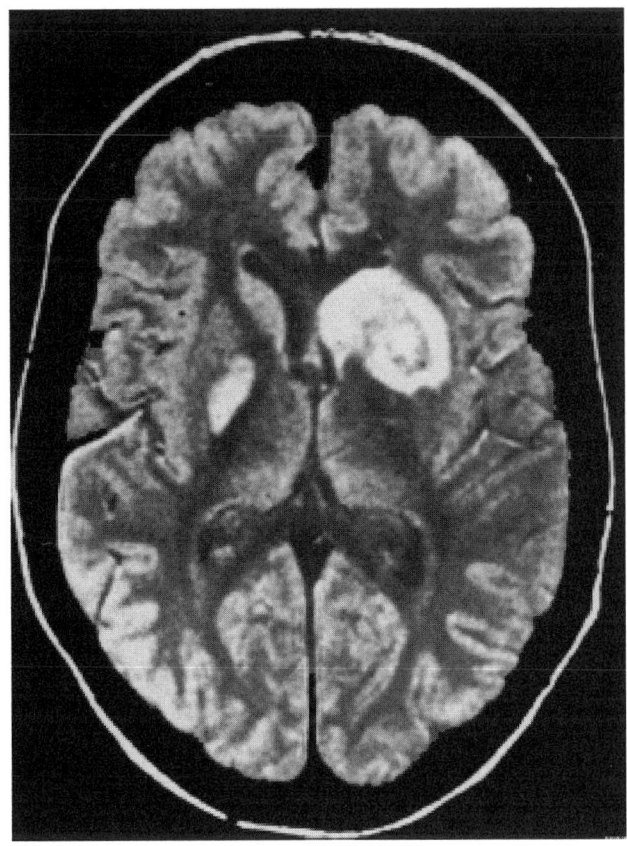

FIGURE 50.8   *Asymmetric basal ganglia lesions in a case of athymhormic syndrome. Lesion involves the caudate head on the left and the medial globus pallidus on the right hemisphere, suggesting that these two structures are part of a bilateral network involved in motivated behavior. (Reproduced with permission from Bellmann A, Assal G. Les multiples propos d'une athymhormique. Rev Neuropsychol 1996;6:101–120.)*

brain mechanisms "engaged in the neuronal integration of motivational processes into behavioral output" (75).

TOWARD A NEUROANATOMIC MODEL OF HUMAN MOTIVATION

Consistent with the role of this limbic loop is evidence showing that lesions disrupting bilaterally the loop at other sites than the above-mentioned basal ganglia are also apt to provoke very similar symptoms, although the clinical picture may be obscured by associated cognitive impairments. This is the case, in particular, of frontal and thalamic lesions, two important stages in the loop, whose lesions usually result in memory, attentional, and other behavioral changes.

Frontal Lesions

Classic descriptions of patients with frontal lobe tumors or frontal leukotomies often include symptoms such as apathy, apragmatism, loss of interest and drive, and impoverished affective life (35,76). Associated intellectual deficits expand this syndrome beyond the purely affective realm. In their report of case EVR, besides the above-mentioned behavioral changes, Eslinger and Damasio (55) also mentioned a loss of spontaneous motivation to action that may be related to bilateral damage to the mesial frontal cortex.

More recently, Laplane et al (77) studied a case of post-traumatic bifrontal lesions involving periventricular white matter. Behavioral changes were, here again, very similar to bistriatal or bipallidal cases, including loss of interest, drive, and mental activity. Once again, neuropsychologic testing was dramatically preserved. A similar explanation to that for the striatal lesions, that is mesocortical disconnection (see above), could be invoked to account for the present deficits.

Other Brain Lesions

Apathy, loss of volition, and lack of spontaneity were reported in one case of basal forebrain infarction (78). Like the aforementioned cases, this patient had no spontaneous speech but was alert and responsive when directly addressed. His affect was reported as "very impassive." He also showed a classic memory defect and postmortem brain examination disclosed basal forebrain infarction involving various cholinergic cell groups, which was thought to account for the memory disorder. Emotional and personality changes were ascribed to damage to the basal ganglia, especially to the nucleus accumbens and rostroventral pallidal areas.

Still another similar syndrome was also reported by Katz et al (79) in several cases of bilateral lesions of the median thalamic nuclei, such as from involvement of the paramedian thalamic artery. Again, these patients were reported to show lack of motivation, apathy, and flattened affect. In these cases, however, the symptoms were but a part of a more global impairment—presenting as a dementia syndrome—that included loss of intellectual function. Finally, Bogousslavsky et al (80) reported a very pure clinical picture of athymhormic syndrome in two cases of bilateral paramedian thalamic infarcts. Both patients "became apathetic, aspontaneous, indifferent, and seemed to have lost motor and affective drive, as well as the need itself for any psychic activity," making them "resemble robots." Interestingly, metabolic investigation with SPECT showed remote frontomesial hypoperfusion. However, this metabolic aspect may not be regarded as implicating the frontal cortex in the observed semeiology since frontal blood flow has been found nearly normal in cases of bipallidal apathetic patients (67).

Integrating Clinical Data into a Pathophysiologic Model

Taken together, these clinicoanatomic correlations strongly point to a specific anatomic network subserving one specific set of behavioral capacities. In 1922, Dide and Guiraud (81) coined the term *athymhormia* (from the Greek roots *thymos*, meaning mood or affect, and *hormè*, meaning ardor, spirit, elan) to refer to the defect in "thymic" and instinctual vital dynamism present in some cases of schizophrenia. Disruption of the so-called hormothymic system, according to these authors, located in subcortical brain structures, resulted in loss of affect, interest, and *élan vital*. Behavioral changes in all the neurologic patients mentioned in this section fit this description closely and may be usefully referred to as displaying the "athymhormia syndrome" (65). Thus, these patients exhibit both "thymic" (specific subjective affective) symptoms and "hormic" (lacking any tendency to satisfy primary needs or to search for socially gratifying situations) signs. Lesions associated with this syndrome all act bilaterally to disrupt a subcortical pathway that involves periventricular frontal white matter, neostriatum, pallidum, and medial dorsal nucleus of the thalamus.

As reported in the first section of this chapter, the periventricular frontal white matter, neostriatum, pallidum, and medial dorsal nucleus of the thalamus are parts of the limbic loop described in Figure 50.1, centered on the striatal and pallidal ventral (limbic) segment. These deep structures probably extend in primates to include more widespread regions of the caudate nucleus (7,82) and represent the nonmotor dopaminergic component of the basal ganglia, considered by Nauta and Domesick (8) as "the interface between motivational and motor aspects of movement."

Figure 50.9 summarizes a tentative model of the brain mechanisms subserving motivation in humans. In the light of theories derived from animal research, motivation may be seen as the behavioral consequence of processes leading to the establishment of an association between a stimulus and its affective significance for the animal, namely, the potentially rewarding nature of the stimulus (52,75). Not unlike classical conditioning in the pavlovian sense, repetition over time of such associations would result in a kind of conditioning that determines a goal-directed behavior from the animal. It is usual to distinguish, among these stimuli, primary rewards, whose motivational value is innately determined for the species and whose role is to restore homeostatic balance, and secondary reinforcers that acquire their motivational value by repeated association with primary reinforcers. In the latter group, one may consider anticipation as the key process, since the animal must possess some kind of mental representation of the result of its action. The situation would probably be much more complex in humans, since most of our behaviors may depend on more or less conscious actualization of the goal to be reached, but the basic underlying mechanism would not be fundamentally different.

From an anatomic point of view, there is strong evidence that the amygdala is the structural site of association between stimulus and reward (7–11,52). The dense projections from the amygdala to the limbic striatum and connections between limbic and motor parts of the striatum may give to this region a role in converting affective representations contained in the amygdala into motor programs.

Considering the specific functioning of the frontostriatal connections as parallel interconnected loops (83–85), the three major loops may be conceived as articulated gears turning together, the motor and associative loops being driven by the limbic one, with "energy" being provided by their respective dopaminergic input. According to this representation, damage to the limbic loop, while leaving intact the other two, would result in impaired spontaneous cognitive and motor activity, giving rise to the characteristic symptoms of athymhormia: lack of spontaneous action (but intact motor functioning), blunting of emotional expression (but possible preservation of emotional experience), and poverty of spontaneous thinking (but relatively preserved intellectual capacities).

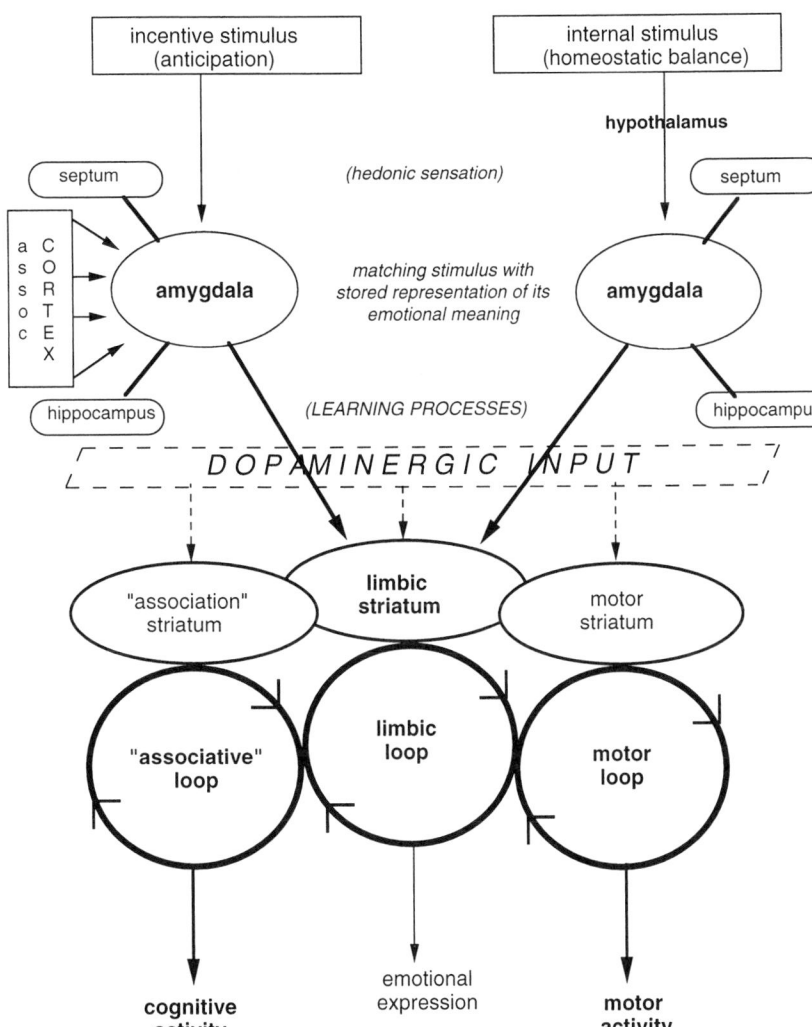

FIGURE 50.9 *An integrative neuroanatomical model of the brain substrate of human motivation. This model accounts for the major symptoms composing the athymhormic syndrome: lack of spontaneous motor and mental activity (with preserved motor abilities) and blunting of emotional expression (with preserved emotional experience).*

CONCLUDING REMARKS

It is of great interest that, while "athymhormia" was initially described for schizophrenic patients, recent evidence in the psychiatric literature points to basal ganglia involvement in this disease, for example, increase in caudate dopaminergic, dopamine type 2 (D_2) receptors (86), regional blood flow abnormality in the globus pallidus (87), and considerable other clinical and experimental evidence [summarized, for instance, in (88)]. In particular, type II schizophrenics, characterized by negative symptoms such as flat affect and poverty of speech (as opposed to type I with predominantly positive symptoms such as delusions and hallucinations), may have a specific deficit in D_2 receptors (89). Interestingly, in their recent attempt at unifying several psychiatric diseases into a neurologic model, Swerdlow and Koob proposed a hypothesis according to which a number of symptoms of psychotic illness can be thought to arise from dysfunction of a complex corticostriatopallidothalamic circuit converging on the nucleus accumbens. Although different in several respects, the neurologic and the psychiatric approaches are strikingly convergent in several aspects, in particular for the suggestion that the role of the basal ganglia in emotional behavior is probably of critical importance and deserves special consideration in future studies.

Finally, it appears from the different pieces of evidence presented in this chapter, that lesions at various sites of the so-called limbic system, either cortical or subcortical, are likely to impair some special features of motor function. They concern specifically a preparatory stage leading to movement or action, in that lesions result in loss of drive or incitement to move, while the realization of the movement itself remains intact. However, cortical and subcortical lesions seem to predict for different deficits—cortical lesions involving the cingulate and SMA bilaterally provoke the most severe disorder, the syndrome of akinetic mutism, with nearly total loss of voluntary movement, speech, and even movement on command. With lesions at subcortical sites the picture is one of loss of spontaneous activity, while commands still elicit movement; but in this case, the subjective experience of interest and desire, or the search for satisfaction, also seems to be completely abolished, giving rise to the syndrome of athymhormia. However, isolated bicingulate lesions seem to lead to a relatively pure form of athymhormia.

This dual clinical picture—abolition of spontaneous movement and loss of subjective desire—can be related to the double pathway postulated in Figure 50.1: athymhormia results from lesions of the "limbic" loop, including the cingulate cortex; akinetic mutism is seen when the lesion also involves the SMA, an area connected to the "motor" extrapyramidal loop. It is conceivable, then, that the system comprises a double interface between limbic and motor mechanisms: the "limbic" basal ganglia (8,10) comprise the first interface, translating inner needs and desires into a general drive to act. The SMA, closely connected with the anterior cingulate cortex, on the one hand, and the primary motor cortex, on the other, represents the next stage of initiation of action—a conscious will to move and/or communicate. Finally, the perisylvian cortices, of paleocortical origin, translate the will to move and communicate into specific, often learned, motor programs.

ACKNOWLEDGMENTS

The writing of this chapter was supported, in part, by NIH grants HD 20806, HD 19819, a grant from the Carl W. Herzog Foundation, a grant from the Research Division of the Orton Dyslexia Society to AMG, and by INSERM CJF and CNRS-APHM PRA grants to M. Habib.

REFERENCES

1. MacLean PD. Some psychiatric implications of physiological studies on fronto-temporal portions of limbic system ("visceral brain"). Electroencephalogr Clin Neurophysiol 1952;4:407–418.
2. Sanides F. Representation of the cerebral cortex and its areal lamination patterns. In: Bourne GH, ed. The structure and function of the nervous tissue. Vol. 5. New York: Academic, 1972:329–353.
3. Mesulam M-M. Patterns in behavioral anatomy: association areas, the limbic system, and hemispheric specialization. In: Mesulam M-M, ed. Principles of behavioral neurology. Philadelphia: Davis, 1985:1–40.
4. Galaburda AM, Pandya DN. Role of architectonics and connections in the study of primate brain evolution. In: Armstrong E, Falk D, eds. Primate Brain Evolution: Methods and Concepts. New York: Plenum, 1982:203–216.
5. Galaburda AM. The anatomy of language: lessons from comparative anatomy. In: Caplan D, Lecours AR, Smith A, eds. Biological perspectives in language. Cambridge, MA: MIT, 1984:290–302.
6. Goldberg G. Supplementary motor area structure and function: review and hypotheses. Behav Brain Sci 1985;8:567–616.
7. Kelley AE, Domesik VB, Nauta WJH. The amygdalostriatal projection in the rat—an anatomical study by anterograde and retrograde tracing methods. Neuroscience 1982;7:615–630.
8. Nauta WJH, Domesick VB. Afferent and efferent relationships of the basal ganglia. In: Functions of the basal ganglia. Ciba Foundation Symposium. London: Pitman, 1984:3–29.
9. Nauta WJH. Circuitous connections linking cerebral cortex, limbic system, and corpus striatum. In: Doane BK, Livingston KE, eds. The limbic system: functional organization and clinical disorders. New York: Raven, 1986:43–54.
10. Mogenson GJ, Jones DL, Yim CJ. From motivation to action: functional interface between the limbic system and the motor system. Prog Neurobiol 1980;14:69–97.
11. Panksepp J. The anatomy of emotions. In: Plutchik R, Kellerman H, eds. Emotion: theory, research and experience. Vol. 3, Biological foundations of emotions. Orlando: Academic, 1986:91–124.
12. MacLean PD. Culminating developments in the evolution of the limbic system: the thalamo-cingulate division. In: Doane BK, Livingston KE, eds. The limbic system: functional organization and clinical disorders. New York: Raven, 1986:1–28.
13. Nielsen JM, Jacobs LL. Bilateral lesions of the anterior cingulate gyri—report of a case. Bull Los Angeles Neurol Soc 1951;18:48–51.
14. Barris WR, Schuman HR. Bilateral anterior cingulate gyrus lesions. Syndrome of the anterior cingulate gyri. Neurology 1953;3:44–52.
15. Amyes EW, Nielsen JM. Clinico-pathologic study of vascular lesions of the anterior cingulate region. Bull Los Angeles Neurol Soc 1955;20:112–130.
16. Buge A, Escourolle R, Rancurel G, Poisson M. Mutisme akinétique et ramollissement bicingulaire. 3 observations anatomo-cliniques. Rev Neurol 1975;131:121–137.
17. Laplane D, Degos JD, Baulac M, Gray F. Bilateral infarction of the anterior cingulate gyri and of the fornices. J Neurol Sci 1981;51:289–300.
18. Degos JD, da Fonseca N, Gray F. Severe frontal syndrome associated with infarcts of the left anterior cingulate gyrus and the head of the right caudate nucleus. Brain 1993;116:1541–1548.
19. Devinsky O, Morrell MJ, Vogt BA. Contributions of anterior cingulate cortex to behaviour. Brain 1995;118:279–306.
20. Frith CD, Friston KJ, Liddle PF, Frackowiak RSJ. Willed action and the prefrontal cortex in man: a study with PET. Proc R Soc Lond B Biol Sci 1991;244:241–246.
21. George MS, Ketter TA, Parekh PI, et al. Brain activity during transient sadness and happiness in healthy women. Am J Psychiatry 1995;152:3, 341–351.
22. Penfield W, Welch K. The supplementary motor area in the cerebral cortex of man. Trans Am Neurol Assoc 1949;74:179–184.
23. Penfield W, Welch K. The supplementary motor area of the cerebral cortex. Arch Neurol Psychiatry 1951;66:289–317.
24. Laplane D, Talairach J, Meininger V, Bancaud J, Orgogozo JM. Clinical consequences of corticectomies involving the supplementary motor area in man. J Neurol Sci 1977;34:301–314.
25. Rubens AB. Aphasia with infarction in the territory of the anterior cerebral artery. Cortex 1975;11:239–250.
26. Racy A, Janotta FS, Lehner LH. Aphasia resulting from occlusion of the left anterior cerebral artery. Arch Neurol 1979;36:221–224.
27. Masdeu JC. Aphasia after infarction of the left supplementary motor area. Neurology 1980;30:359.
28. Alexander MP, Schmitt MA. The aphasia syndrome of stroke in the left anterior cerebral artery territory. Arch Neurol 1980;37:97–100.
29. Gelmers HJ. Non-paralytic motor disturbances and speech disorders: the role of the supplementary motor area. J Neurol Neurosurg Psychiatr 1983;46:1052–1054.
30. Damasio AR, Van Hoesen GW. Emotional disturbances associated with focal lesions of the limbic frontal lobe. In: Heilman KM, Satz P, eds. Neuropsychology of human emotion. New York: Guilford, 1983:85–110.
31. Masdeu JC, Schoene WC, Funkenstein H. Aphasia following infarction of the left supplementary motor area. Neurology 1978;28:1220–1223.
32. Bogousslavsky J, Assal G, Regli F. Infarctus du territoire de l'artère cérébrale antérieure gauche. II. Troubles du language. Rev Neurol 1987;143:121–127.
33. Damasio AR. The frontal lobes. In: Heilman KM, Valenstein E, eds. Clinical neuropsychology. New York: Oxford University, 1985:339–375.
34. Freedman M, Alexander MP, Naeser MA. Anatomic basis of transcortical motor aphasia. Neurology 1984;34:409–417.
35. Stuss DT, Benson DF. The frontal lobes. New York: Raven, 1986.
36. Orgogozo JM, Larsen B. Activation of the supplementary motor area during voluntary movement in man suggests it works as a supramotor area. Science 1979;206:847–850.
37. Damasio AR, Van Hoesen GW. Structure and function of the supplementary motor area. Neurology 1980;30:359.
38. Damasio AR. Understanding the mind's will. Behav Brain Sci 1985;8:589.
39. Brust JCM, Plank C, Burke A, et al. Language disorder in a right-hander after occlusion of the right anterior cerebral artery. Neurology 1982;32:492–497.
40. Penfield W, Roberts L. Speech and brain mechanisms. Princeton, NJ: Princeton University, 1959.
41. Bancaud J, Talairach J. Organisation fonctionnelle de l'aire motrice supplémentaire. Neurochirurgie 1967;13:343–356.
42. Larsen B, Skinhøj E, Lassen NA. Variations in regional cerebral blood flow in the right and left hemispheres during automatic speech. Brain 1978;101:193–209.
43. Goldberg G, Mayer NH, Toglia JU. Medial frontal cortex infarction and the alien hand sign. Arch Neurol 1981;38:683–686.

44. Brion S, Jedynak CP. Trouble du transfert interhémisphérique à propos de 3 observations de tumeurs du corps calleux: le signe de la main étrangère. Rev Neurol 1972;126:257–266.

45. Bogen JE. The callosal syndrome. In: Heilman KM, Valenstein E, eds. Clinical neuropsychology. New York: Oxford University, 1979:308–359.

46. Goldberg G. Premotor systems, motor learning, and ipsilateral control. Behav Brain Sci 1987;10:323–329.

47. Watson RT, Fleet S, Gonzalez-Rothi L, Heilman KM. Apraxia and the supplementary motor area. Arch Neurol 1986;43:787–792.

48. Meador KJ, Watson RT, Bowers D, Heilman KM. Hypometria with hemispatial and limb motor neglect. Brain 1986;109:293–305.

49. Goldenberg G, Wimmer A, Holzner F, Wessely P. Apraxia of the left limbs in a case of callosal disconnection: the contribution of medial frontal lobe damage. Cortex 1985;21:135–148.

50. Habib M, Daquin G, Milandre L, Royère ML, Rey M, Lantéri A, Salamon G, Khalil R. Mutism and auditory agnosia due to bilateral insular damage. Role of the insula in human communication. Neuropsychologia 1995;33:327–339.

51. Blumer D, Benson DF. Personality changes with frontal and temporal lobe lesions. In: Benson DF, Blumer D, eds. Psychiatric aspects of neurologic disease. New York: Grune & Stratton, 1975:151–170.

52. Rolls ET. A theory of emotion and consciousness, and its application to understanding the neural basis of emotion. In: Gazzaniga MS, ed. The cognitive neurosciences. Cambridge, MA: MIT, 1995:1091–1106.

53. Damasio AR. Toward a neurobiology of emotion and feeling: operational concepts and hypotheses. Neuroscientist 1995;1:19–25.

54. Damasio AR. Descartes' error: emotion, reason, and the human brain. New York: Grosset/Putnam, 1994.

55. Eslinger PJ, Damasio AR. Severe disturbance of higher cognition after bilateral frontal lobe ablation: patient EVR. Neurology 1985;35:1731–1741.

56. Damasio AR, Tranel D, Damasio H. Individuals with sociopathic behavior caused by frontal damage fail to respond autonomically to social stimuli. Behav Brain Res 1990;41:81–94.

57. Bechara A, Damasio AR, Damasio H, Anderson S. Insensitivity to future consequences following damage to human prefrontal cortex. Cognition 1994;50:7–12.

58. Price BH, Daffner KR, Stowe RM, Mesulam M-M. The comportmental learning disabilities of frontal lobe damage. Brain 1990;113:1383–1394.

59. Eslinger PE, Grattant LM, Damasio H, Damasio AR. Developmental consequences of childhood frontal lobe damage. Arch Neurol 1992;49:764–769.

60. Adams RD, Victor M. Principles of neurology. New York: McGraw-Hill, 1985:388.

61. Fischer CM. Abulia minor vs. agitated behavior. Clin Neurosurg 1983;31:9–31.

62. Marin RS. Differential diagnosis and classification of apathy. Am J Psychiatry 1990;147:22–30.

63. Laplane D, Baulac M, Pillon B. Panayatopoulou-Achimastos I. Perte de l'autoactivation psychique. Activité compulsive d'allure obsessionnelle. Lésion lenticulaire bilatérale. Rev Neurol 1982;138:137–141.

64. Laplane D, Baulac M, Widlöcher D, Dubois B. Pure psychic akinesia with bilateral lesions of basal ganglia. J Neurol Neurosurg Psychiatry 1984;47:377–385.

65. Habib M, Poncet M. Loss of drive, interest, and affect ("athymhormia syndrome") with lacunar lesions of the striatum. Rev Neurol 1988;144:571–577.

66. Ali-Chérif A, Royère ML, Gosset A, Poncet M, Salamon G, Khalil R. Troubles du comportement et de l'activité mentale après intoxication oxycarbonée. Lésions pallidales bilatérales. Rev Neurol 1984;140:401–405.

67. Laplane D, Levasseur M, Pillon B, et al. Obsessive–compulsive and other behavioural changes with bilateral basal ganglia lesions. A neuropsychological,

magnetic resonance imaging and positron tomography study. Brain 1989;112:699–725.

68. Bhatia KP, Marsden D. The behavioural and motor consequences of focal lesions of the basal ganglia in man. Brain 1994;117:859–876.

69. Pelletier J, Habib M, Khalil R, et al. Putaminal necrosis after methanol intoxication [letter]. J Neurol Neurosurg Psychiatr 1992;55:234–235.

70. Trillet M, Croisile B, Tourniaire D, Schott B. Perturbations de l'activité motrice volontaire et lésions du noyau caudé. Rev Neurol (Paris) 1990;146:338–344.

71. Richfield EK, Twyman R, Berent S. Neurological syndrome following bilateral damage to the head of the caudate nuclei. Ann Neurol 1987;22:768–771.

72. Mendez MF, Adams NL, Lewandowski KS. Neurobehavioral changes associated with caudate lesions. Neurology 1989;39:349–354.

73. Milandre L, Habib M, Royere ML, et al. Syndrome athymhormique par infarctus striato-capsulaire bilatéral. Maladie de Moya-Moya de l'adulte. Rev Neurol (Paris) 1995;151:383–387.

74. Bellmann A, Assal G. Les multiples propos d'une athymhormique. Rev Neuropsychol 1996;6:101–120.

75. Apicella P, Ljundberg T, Scarnati E, Schultz W. Responses to reward in monkey dorsal and ventral striatum. Exp Brain Res 1991;85:491–500.

76. Stuss DT, Benson DF. Emotional concomitants of psychosurgery. In: Heilman KM, Satz P, eds. Neuropsychology of human emotion. New York: Guilford, 1983:111–140.

77. Laplane D, Dubois B, Pillon B, Baulac M. Perte d'autoactivation psychique et activité mentale stéréotypée par lésion frontale. Rev Neurol 1988;144:564–570.

78. Phillips S, Sangalang V, Sterns G. Basal forebrain infarction: a clinicopathologic correlation. Arch Neurol 1987;44:1134–1138.

79. Katz DI, Alexander MP, Mandell AM. Dementia following strokes in the mesencephalon and diencephalon. Arch Neurol 1987;44:1127–1133.

80. Bogousslavsky J, Delayote-Bischof A, Assal G. Loss of psychic self-activation with bithalamic infarction: neurobehavioural, CT, MRI and SPECT correlates. Acta Neurol Scand 1991;83:309–316.

81. Dide M, Guiraud P. Psychiatrie du médecin praticien. Paris: Masson, 1922.

82. Kelley AE. Dopamine and mental illness: Phenomenological and anatomical considerations. Behav Brain Sci 1987;10:219–220.

83. Alexander GE, De Long MR, Strick PL. Parallel organization of functionally segregated circuits linking basal ganglia and cortex. Ann Rev Neurosci 1986;9:357–381.

84. Alexander GE, Crutcher MD. Functional architecture of basal ganglia circuits: neural substrates of parallel processing. Trends Neurosci 1990;13:266–271.

85. Cummings JL. Frontal-subcortical circuits and human behavior. Arch Neurol 1993;50:873–880.

86. Wong DF. Positron emission tomography reveals elevated D2 dopamine receptors in drug-naive schizophrenics. Science 1986;234:1558.

87. Early TS, Reiman EM, Raichle ME, Spitznagel EL. Left globus pallidus abnormality in never-medicated patients with schizophrenia. Proc Natl Acad Sci USA 1987;84:561–563.

88. Swerdlow NR, Koob GF. Dopamine, schizophrenia, mania, and depression: Toward a unified hypothesis of corticostriato-pallido-thalamic function. Behav Brain Sci 1987;10:197–245.

89. Crow TJ. Two syndromes in schizophrenia? Trends Neurosci 1982;5:351–354.

90. Strub RL. Frontal lobe syndrome in a patient with bilateral globus pallidus lesions. Arch Neurol 1989;46:1024–1027.

91. Danel T, Goudemand M, Ghawche F, et al. Mélancolie délirante et lacunes multiples des noyaux gris centraux. Rev Neurol (Paris) 1991;147:60–62.

The Stiff-Man Syndrome

ROBERT H. BROWN

INTRODUCTION

Chronic, continuous stiffness of muscles is an unusual complaint. While numerous neurologic disorders cause intermittent muscle hyperactivity or rhythmic abnormalities of muscle tone such as tremors, few produce constant muscle stiffness in both the resting and active states. In the central nervous system, disorders of the corticospinal system and basal ganglia, respectively, may produce spasticity and extrapyramidal rigidity. In both types of disorders, however, the muscles at rest are generally slack, although enhanced tone may be evident on passive testing of motor tone. By contrast, two disorders cause marked muscle stiffness during activity and at rest. These conditions, stiff-man syndrome and Isaacs' disease or neuromyotonia, are disabling yet potentially treatable. This chapter outlines the major features of the stiff-man syndrome and its differentiation from Isaac's disease.

CLINICAL SYNDROME

As first reported by Moersch and Woltman (1), the stiff-man syndrome is characterized by chronic, progressive, continuous muscle stiffness. This usually begins in the fifth decade or so but may occur in children (2). While most cases are sporadic, some clearly arise on a familial basis (3–6) with an autosomal dominant inheritance pattern. In these families, the disorder may be congenitally present. Indeed, in some cases, fetal movements are thought to be hyperactive; fetal muscle stiffness may necessitate cesarean section (6). Children with congenital muscle stiffness may be normal by the third or fourth year. Whether inherited or sporadic, stiff-man syndrome affects both males and females. In recent reviews,

the male-female ratio has been unity (7) or has slightly favored females (8). In many patients the syndrome is associated with adult-onset, insulin-dependent diabetes mellitus (IDDM) (9). Other associated conditions have included spinal cord lesions (10), encephalomyelitis (11), hyperthyroidism (12), dementia (13), and other disorders affecting the central nervous system (14).

Examination of stiff-man patients reveals symmetric muscle rigidity, which initially affects neck and axial truncal muscles but spreads over several months to the proximal limb muscles. The face and distal limb muscles are usually spared, although facial involvement is documented (15,16). Sustained hyperactivity of the truncal muscles, particularly the extensor muscles of the back, produces lordosis and an uplifting of the shoulders, a diagnostic posture. The combined back extension and limb stiffness may produce difficulty walking. In advanced cases, the entire torso and proximal limbs are moved en bloc. Such stiffness may be severely disabling; falling is common. Superimposed on the chronic stiffness are intermittent but sustained spasms of muscle hyperactivity, lasting from several minutes to hours. These are provoked by sensory stimuli such as loud noises or abrupt jarring and can be painfully forceful, causing the patient to cry out. Patients often sweat profusely during these episodes. In some individuals, fixed skeletal deformities result from fractures secondary to massive muscle contraction. Spasms may develop focally in the larynx, esophagus, or diaphragm and accessory respiratory muscles. Restricted diaphragmatic involvement has produced dyspnea and restrictive ventilatory insufficiency (3). Despite excessive muscle rigidity, there is usually no frank weakness. Sensory function is normal. Deep tendon reflexes may be hyperactive and rarely the Babinski reflex may be upgoing. Hyporeflexia is unusual.

Routine laboratory studies are normal. By contrast, electrophysiologic studies are distinctively abnormal in stiff-man patients. The essential electromyographic (EMG) feature is constant motor unit activity correlating with the unvarying hypertonicity (1,3,7,17). Attempts at relaxation do not diminish the hyperactivity. Unlike patients with spasticity due to suprasegmental reflex disinhibition, stiff-man patients cannot diminish the electrical hyperactivity by relaxing the muscles. Removal of all sensory stimuli, which may quiet overactive muscle in spastic states, also fails to reduce the abnormal electrical activity. On the other hand, the constituent compound muscle action potentials are normal; there is no consistent suggestion either of myopathic or neuropathic features. As noted below, pharmacologic studies suggest the primary problem is at the segmental or suprasegmental level within the spinal cord or brainstem.

The muscle biopsy in stiff-man syndrome is largely normal (1,2,15,16,18). Some authors have described a slight muscle inflammation (19). Others have noted subtle manifestations of muscle degeneration and regeneration (19,20), possibly attributable to recurrent muscle ischemia caused by the intense, constant muscle contractions (3,21).

DIAGNOSTIC CRITERIA

In an excellent recent review of experience at the Mayo Clinic (7), seven diagnostic criteria were suggested:

1. prodrome of axial muscle rigidity
2. progressive spread of stiffness to the proximal limb muscles
3. fixed spinal lordosis
4. superimposed spasms lasting many seconds to several minutes, triggered by sensory stimuli
5. normal motor and sensory examination
6. normal intelligence
7. characteristic EMG findings as above

PHARMACOLOGY AND PATHOGENESIS

Pharmacologic studies suggest the disease originates within the central nervous system. The muscle hyperactivity is diminished or blocked by the following: 1) neuromuscular junction blockade using succinylcholine (14), tubocurarine (22), or curare (16); 2) direct neural block using local anesthesia (3,14); 3) general anesthesia (3,15); 4) diazepam (13,23,24); 5) sleep (2,3,15); and 6) the association of the syndrome with other diseases involving the central nervous system (11,13,14,25).

As recently reviewed (7), while these data implicate the central nervous system in the genesis of this disease, the precise mechanisms remain unclear. Early hypotheses implicated defective Renshaw collateral inhibition on motor neurons (23,24) or abnormal gamma motor neuron activity (3). It was subsequently suggested that there is either an increase in catecholaminergic tone or a decrease in gamma-aminobutyric acid (GABA)-ergic tone within the spinal cord. Agents that augment catecholamine levels in the spinal cord worsen muscle stiffness in this syndrome (26). Some patients with stiff-man syndrome secrete elevated levels of norepinephrine metabolites in the urine (27).

More recently, evidence for direct involvement of the GABA-ergic system was reported by Solimena et al who described a single patient with stiff-man syndrome, epilepsy, and IDDM with autoantibodies to GABA-ergic nerve terminals in both cerebrospinal fluid and serum (9). Studies suggested the target antigen was the GABA-synthesizing enzyme glutamic acid decarboxylase (GAD). Of considerable interest was the observation that the antibodies also reacted with GAD in pancreatic beta cells. In a later study, these investigators reported detecting this pattern of antibody reactivity in 20 of 33 patients with stiff-man syndrome (8). Of the 20 with antibodies against GABA-ergic neurons, 19 were tested for anti-islet cell antibodies and 18 of 19 were positive. About one-third of these patients had IDDM. By contrast, none of the 13 patients without anti-GABA-ergic neuron antibodies had either anti-islet cell antibodies or IDDM. In 218 control (normal and other diseases) sera, 57 and 4 patients had antibodies, respectively, against pancreatic islet cells and GABA-ergic neurons.

The finding that two-thirds of stiff-man patients have an autoantibody with a high degree of specificity for GABA-ergic neurons suggests the antibodies may primarily trigger an autoimmune disturbance of GABA function in the central nervous system. The observation that one HLA type is overrepresented in stiff-man patients lends support to this hypothesis (28). The autoimmune hypothesis predicts that stiff-man patients with elevated antibody titers should respond to immunosuppressive therapy. While this has been reported (29), it is not universally true (30), perhaps because the disorder is heterogeneous. It should now be possible to correlate response to anti-immune therapy with the titers of the offending antibodies before and after treatment. A corollary of the autoimmunity hypothesis is the prediction that one should be able to produce animal models of the illness either by immunization with GAD or by passive transfer from human patients. Neither model has yet been reported.

TREATMENT

Unfortunately, few drugs effectively treat stiff-man syndrome. The mainstay of diazepam may be dramatically effective, albeit in relatively large and frequent doses (23). Another benzodiazepine, clonazepam, may also be effective as may drugs such as clonidine that act centrally to diminish catecholaminergic tone (26). In some patients, valproate is beneficial, perhaps by augmenting GABA-ergic tone (31). Baclofen (32) and cortisol (33) are sometimes therapeutic. Phenytoin has not been effective. L-Dopa exacerbates both the baseline and the paroxysmal muscle hyperactivity (34).

DIFFERENTIAL DIAGNOSIS

The major differential considerations in the diagnosis of the stiff-man syndrome have been well reviewed elsewhere (3,7). Table 51.1 summarizes the salient features of diseases resembling stiff-man syndrome. Perhaps most confusing is Isaacs' syndrome, also designated "neuromyotonia" or "myokymia" or, rarely, "quantal squander" (35,36). Clinically, this is characterized by muscle rigidity that is either generalized or focal and that, by contrast with the stiff-man syndrome, may commonly involve the face, hands, and feet. Focal laryngeal involvement has been reported as has isolated ocular myotonia, particularly after radiation therapy to the brainstem and hypothalamus (37,38). Unlike the stiff-man syndrome, sleep and general anesthesia do not abolish motor hyperactivity in Isaacs' syndrome. Isaacs' disease may begin in adulthood or childhood; in the latter instance, there may be regression of symptoms after several years (39). Data suggest the hyperactivity in neuromyotonia may arise in the distal motor nerve, by contrast with the central origin of

hyperactivity in stiff-man syndrome (40). Thus, while neuromuscular junction blockade terminates stiffness in Isaacs' syndrome, proximal nerve root blockade and general anesthesia do not. The hypothesis that Isaacs' disease originates in abnormal distal peripheral nerves is underscored by familial cases in which affected individuals have a frankly neuropathic appearance with distal limb wasting reminiscent of Charcot–Marie–Tooth disease (40). Although such familial cases of Isaacs' disease are likely to be genetic in origin, many cases are sporadic, suggesting an exogenous etiology. Case reports have occasionally incriminated specific toxic substances, including penicillamine (41) and insecticides (42,43). The pharmacotherapy of stiff-man syndrome and Isaacs' disease also differ. Isaacs' syndrome responds well to phenytoin but not to diazepam (36,42,44); the converse is true of the stiff-man syndrome (36).

There are several reports of Isaacs' disease or neuromyotonia occurring in association with carcinoma (45–48); by contrast, we have been unable to find reports of stiff-man syndrome with cancer. It must be cautioned that the phys-

T a b l e 5 1 . 1   Clinical Features of the Stiff-Man Syndrome and Related Disorders

	Disease					
Features	Stiff-Man Syndrome	Isaac's Disease	Myotonia	Tetanus	Parkinson's Disease	Spasticity
Clinical						
Onset	Slow	Slow	Slow	Abrupt	Slow	Slow
Muscles involved						
Axial	+	+/−	−	+	+/−	+/−
Facial	−	+/−	+	+	+	+/−
Eyes	−	+	+/−	−	+/−	−
Myotonia	−	−	+	−	−	−
Reflexes	++	N	N	++	N	+++
Atrophy	−	+/−	+/−	−	−	−
Hypertrophy	−	+/−	−	−	−	−
Sensory Sx	+/−[a]	+/−[a]	−	−	−	−
Superimposed spasms	+++[b]	+[c]	++[c]	+++[c]	−	−
Abolished by sleep	+	−	+	+	+	+
Family Hx	+/−	+/−	+	−	+/−	+/−
Laboratory						
Resting EMG	Active	Active	Quiet	Quiet	Quiet	Quiet
Creatine phosphokinase	N	N/H	N	N	N	N
Drug therapy[d]						
Diazepam	+++	−	+/−	+	−	+/−
Phenytoin	−	+++	+/−	+	−	+/−.
Nerve block	+++	+++	−	+++	+++	+++
NMJ block	+++	+++	−	+++	+++	+++

[a] Muscle pain.
[b] Very prolonged.
[c] Relatively brief.
[d] +, improved; −, no change.
N, normal; H, high; NMJ, neuromuscular junction.

iologic details in the reports of paraneoplastic Isaacs' syndrome do not always allow a clear exclusion of the diagnosis of stiff-man syndrome.

Continuous muscle activity is encountered in chondrodystrophic myotonica or Schwartz–Jampel disease (49). However, the short stature and peculiar facial appearance of children with Schwartz–Jampel disease clearly distinguishes them from patients with either Isaacs' disease or stiff-man syndrome. In Schwartz–Jampel children, neuromuscular blockade with curare eliminates muscle irritability, suggesting the hyperactivity is derived from the motor nerve or its terminals (50); in this sense, the pathophysiology of Schwartz–Jampel may be closer to Isaacs' disease than either myotonia or stiff-man syndrome.

By the same token, myotonia should not be confused with stiff-man syndrome. Myotonia is a form of muscle hyperactivity arising from electrical irritability of the muscle cell membrane. Unlike stiff-man syndrome or Schwartz–Jampel disease, it persists after nerve or myoneural junction block. Moreover, individuals with the two major forms of myotonia are usually clinically distinctive. Thus, in typical myotonic dystrophy, the complex of distal atrophy and multisystem disorders (frontal balding, cataracts, testicular atrophy, atypical diabetes) are diagnostic as is diffuse muscle hypertrophy in myotonia congenita. In myotonia congenita, forceful volitional movements may produce sustained and sometimes painful muscle stiffness lasting usually no more than several seconds. However, this is unlike the paroxysms of muscle tightness induced in stiff-man syndrome by sensory stimuli.

The rigidity in neuroleptic malignant syndrome and malignant hyperthermia are unlike that in stiff-man syndrome, primarily because of the clear correlation with use of an offending anesthetic or major tranquilizer and, in most instances, the presence of fever.

The diagnosis of stiff-man syndrome has been entertained in occasional patients with myoclonic spasms. As discussed by Lorish et al, myoclonic spasms are usually quite brief in duration; they may be preceded by electroencephalographic (EEG) bursts (7). On the other hand, the spasms in stiff-man syndrome are very long-lasting (up to minutes or even hours) and are not accompanied by EEG abnormalities. The sustained, slow time course of the stiff-man paroxysms helps distinguish episodes of rigidity from other forms of stimulus-induced muscle contractions. Thus, in patients with pathologically exaggerated startle responses [e.g., "hyperexplexia" (51) or "latah," "myriachit," and the "jumping Frenchmen of Maine" (52)], the profoundly enhanced and abnormal reflexive startle lasts a mere few seconds.

Acute and chronic tetanus should be considered in the differential diagnosis of stiff-man syndrome but do not usually pose a significant diagnostic problem. The temporal profile of acute tetanus, which develops fulminantly and typically resolves over time, is distinctly unlike that in stiff-man disease. Chronic tetanus may be more difficult to exclude but its self-limiting nature is unlike the progressive nature of the stiff-man syndrome. In tetanus it may be possible to elicit a history of a preceding wound, presumably the portal of entry for the offending clostridial pathogen. In either form of tetanus there may be facial spasms or trismus; this is precedented but unusual in the stiff-man syndrome.

REFERENCES

1. Moersch FP, Woltman HW. Progressive fluctuating muscular rigidity and spasm "stiff-man syndrome": report of a case and some observations on 13 other cases. Proc Staff Meet Mayo Clin 1956;31:421–427.
2. Bowler D. The stiff-man syndrome in a boy. Arch Dis Child 1960;35:289–292.
3. Gordon EE, Januszko DM, Kaufman L. Review: a critical survey of stiff-man syndrome. Am J Med 1967;42:582–599.
4. Klein R, Haddon JE, DeLuca C. Familial disorders resembling stiff-man syndrome. Am J Dis Child 1972;124:730–731.
5. Negri S, Caraceni T, Boiardi A. Neuromyotonia: report of a case. Eur Neurol 1977;16:35–41.
6. Sander JE, Layzer RB, Goldsobel AB. Congenital stiff-man syndrome. Ann Neurol 1979;8:195–197.
7. Lorish TR, Thorsteinsson G, Howard FM Jr. Stiff-man syndrome updated. Mayo Clin Proc 1989;64:629–636.
8. Solimena M, Folli F, Aparisi R, et al. Autoantibodies to GABA-ergic neurons and pancreatic beta cells in stiff-man syndrome. N Engl J Med 1990;322:1555–1560.
9. Solimena M, Folli F, Denis-Donini S, et al. Autoantibodies to glutamic acid decarboxylase in a patient with stiff-man syndrome, epilepsy, and type I diabetes mellitus. N Engl J Med 1988;318:1012–1020.
10. Nakamura N, Fujiya S, Yahara O, et al. Stiff-man syndrome with spinal cord lesion. Clin Neuropathol 1986;5:40–46.
11. Kasperek S, Zebrowski S. Stiff-man syndrome and encephalomyelitis: report of a case. Arch Neurol 1971;24:22–30.
12. Werk CE Jr, Sheldon LJ, Marnell RT. The stiff-man syndrome and hyperthyroidism. Am J Med 1961;31:647–653.
13. Drake ME Jr. The stiff-man syndrome and dementia. Am J Med 1983;74:1085–1087.
14. Werk EE Jr, Sholiton LJ, Marnell RT. The "stiff-man" syndrome with central and peripheral nervous manifestations. J Neurol 1961;219:171–176.
15. Price TM, Allott EH. The stiff-man syndrome. Br Med J 1958;1:682–685.
16. Brage D. The stiff-man syndrome. Rev Clin Exp 1959;72:30.
17. Ricker K, Mertens HG. EMG phenomena in the "stiff-man" syndrome. Electroencephalogr Clin Neurophysiol 1968;25:413. Abstract.
18. Trethowan WH, Allsop JL, Turner B. The "stiff-man syndrome": a report of two further cases. Arch Neurol 1960;3:448–456.
19. Asher R. A woman with the stiff-man syndrome. Br Med J 1958;1:265–266.
20. Ornstein AM. Chronic generalized fibromyositis. Ann Surg 1935;101:237.
21. Barcroft H, Miller JLE. Blood flow through muscle during sustained contraction. J Physiol 1930;97:17–31.
22. Stuart FS, Henry M, Holly HL. The stiff-man syndrome: report of a case. Arthritis Rheum 1960;3:229.
23. Howard FM Jr. A new and effective drug in the treatment of the stiff-man syndrome: preliminary report. Proc Staff Meet Mayo Clin 1963;39:131–144.
24. Olafson RA, Mulder DW, Howard FM. "Stiff-man" syndrome: a review of the literature, report of three additional cases and discussion of pathophysiology and therapy. Proc Staff Meet Mayo Clin 1964;39:131–144.
25. Heiligman R, Paulson MJ. The stiff-man syndrome: a psychiatric disease? Int J Psychiatr Med 1976–77;7:363–371.
26. Meinck H-M, Ricker K, Conrad B. The stiff-man syndrome: new pathophysiological aspects from abnormal exteroceptive reflexes and the response to clomipramine, clonidine, and tizanide. J Neurol Neurosurg Psychiatry 1984;47:280–287.
27. Schmidt RT, Stahl SM, Spehlman R. A pharmacological study of the stiff-man syndrome. Correlation of clinical symptoms with urinary 3-methoxy-4-hydroxy-phenyl glycol excretion. Neurology 1975;25:622–626.
28. Williams AC, Nutt JG, Hare T. Autoimmunity in stiff-man syndrome. Lancet 1988;ii:222.

29. Vicari AM, Fooli F, Pozza G, et al. Plasmapheresis in the treatment of stiff-man syndrome. N Engl J Med 1989;320:1499.

30. Harding AE, Thompson PD, Kocen RS, et al. Plasma exchange and immunosuppression in the stiff-man syndrome. Lancet 1989;ii:915.

31. Spehlman R, Norcross K, Rasmus SC, Schlageter NL. Improvement of stiff-man syndrome with sodium valproate. Neurology 1961;31:1162–1163.

32. Miller F, Korsvik H. Baclofen in the treatment of stiff-man syndrome. Ann Neurol 1981;9:511–512.

33. George TM, Burke JM, Sobotka PA, et al. Resolution of stiff-man syndrome with cortisol replacement in a patient with deficiencies of ACTH, growth hormone, and prolactin. N Engl J Med 1984;310:1511–1513.

34. Guilleminault C, Sigwald J, Castaigne P. Sleep studies and therapeutic trials with L-dopa in a case of stiff-man syndrome. Eur Neurol 1973;10:89–96.

35. Isaacs H. A syndrome of continuous muscle-fibre activity. J Neurol Neurosurg Psychiatry 1961;24:319–325.

36. Brown TJ. Isaacs' syndrome. Arch Phys Med Rehabil 1984;65:27–29.

37. Lessell S, Lessell IM, Rizzo JF. Ocular neuromyotonia after radiation therapy. Am J Ophthalmol 1986;102:766–770.

38. Shults WT, Hoyt WF, Behrens M, et al. Ocular neuromyotonia: a clinical description of six patients. Arch Ophthalmol 1986;104:1028–1034.

39. Isaacs H, Heffron JJA. The syndrome of "continuous muscle-fibre activity" cured: further studies. J Neurol Neurosurg Psychiatry 1974;37:1231–1235.

40. Lance JW, Burke DE, Pollard J. Hyperexcitability of motor and sensory neurons in neuromyotonia. Ann Neurol 1978;5:523–532.

41. Reeback J, Benton S, Swash M, Schwartz M. Penicillamine-induced neuromyotonia. Br Med J 1979;1:1464–1465.

42. Wallis WE, Poznak AV, Plum F. Generalized muscle stiffness, fasciculations, and myokymia of peripheral nerve origin. Arch Neurol 1970;22:430–439.

43. Black JT, Garcia-Muller R, Good E, Brown S. Muscle rigidity in a newborn due to continuous peripheral nerve hyperactivity. Arch Neurol 1972;27:413–425.

44. Zisfein J, Sivak M, Aron AM, Bender AN. Isaacs' syndrome with muscle hypertrophy reversed by phenytoin therapy. Arch Neurol 1983;40:241–242.

45. Waerness E. Neuromyotonia and bronchial carcinoma. Electromyogr Clin Neurophysiol 1974;14:527–535.

46. Humphrey JG, Hill ME, Gordon AS, Kalow W. Myotonia associated with a small cell carcinoma of the lung. Excerpta Medica Int Congress Series, 1974;334:154 pp.

47. Walsh JC. Neuromyotonia: an unusual presentation of intrathoracic malignancy. J Neurol Neurosurg Psychiatry 1976;39:1086–1091.

48. Partanen VSJ, Soininen H, Saksa M, Riekkinen P. Electromyographic and nerve conduction findings in a patient with neuromyotonia, normocalcemic tetany and small-cell lung cancer. Acta Neurol Scand 1980;61:216–226.

49. Schwartz O, Jampel RS. Congenital blepharophimosis associated with a unique generalized myopathy. Arch Ophthalmol 1962;68:52–57.

50. Taylor RG, Layzer R, Davis HS, Fowler WM Jr. Continuous muscle fiber activity in the Schwartz–Jampel syndrome. Electroencephalogr Clin Neurophysiol 1972;33:497–509.

51. Andermann F, Keene DL, Andermann E, Quesney LF. Startle disease or hyperexplexia: further delineation of the syndrome. Brain 1980;103:985–997.

52. Saint-Hilaire M-H, Saint-Hilaire J-M, Granger L. Jumping Frenchmen of Maine. Neurology 1986;36:1269–1271.

Bipolar Disorder and Dyskinesias

Jonathan M. Himmelhoch

This very circumstance that answers come so slowly . . . shows that in this patient we have not to deal with indifference; shows that in this patient we have not to deal with a fear of expressing himself, but with some obstacle to utterance of speech. . . . [U]nder these circumstances, it will be permissible here to speak of an impediment of volition.

Kraepelin, *Lectures on Clinical Psychiatry* (1)

The reader of this excerpt could hardly be criticized if he thought Kraepelin were speaking of Parkinson's disease. And it will be the premise of this chapter that Kraepelin's fundamental concept of "impediment of volition" is closely related to the dyskinesia–akinesia axis of Parkinson's syndrome. First Beigel and Murphy (2) and then, in far more detail, Himmelhoch and the University of Pittsburgh group (3–7) have explicated the volitional inhibition and motor retardation typical of the depressed phase of most bipolar depression (circa 70% in bipolar I, 90% in bipolar II). These investigators have subjected more than 2,000 subjects to analysis, using both clinical observation and pharmacologic probes. The repeated upshot of their analysis is that bipolar depression is, as Kraepelin originally insisted, most often a motor-retarded and volitionally impeded state.

There is potentially a close relationship between the volitional inhibition of bipolar depression and the akinesia of parkinsonism (8), especially since the "paralysis of will" in bipolar depression is invariably accompanied by marked decreases in instrumental motor behavior and slowness of cognition. Indeed, most bipolar depressives undergoing their first or second episode report little or no anhedonia. They simply express bewilderment at their lack of "get-up and go." Although bipolar depressives eventually become equally suicidal to unipolar depressives, their suicidality is not present early in the course of their illness. Moreover, even

after repeated episodes of volitional inhibition kindle dangerous suicidality (9–11), suicide intent develops late in the course of a given episode, when motor and volitional inhibition become self-attributed (11) as laziness, incompetence, helplessness, and hopelessness. Suicide is an omnipresent threat in unipolar illness, equally or more intense early in an episode. Moreover, repeated episodes do not have the same lethal kindling effect. Anergia and volitional inhibition are the primary link between bipolar depression and extrapyramidal illness.

But there are other parallels equally important. Parkinsonism is an illness of balancing pathologies, tremor, and agitation on the one hard and, on the other, akinesia (12). Akinesia is sufficiently puzzling to the medical observer to often be confused with depression, slowed cognition, and constipated thinking. Nauta, in his definitive and elegant anatomic studies, does not fail to notice that motor akinesia and "freezing episodes" (10,13) include impediments of cognition parallel to those of movement. Moreover, when treated, parkinsonism presents a teeter-totter between tremor on the one hand and akinesia on the other. Over enthusiastic treatment with L-dopa or L-dopa plus amino acid decarboxylase can activate tremor (14), paranoia (15), anxious depression, and, most striking, hypomania or mania (16).

Even more important are the parallels between the switch phase of bipolar disease and the "on-off" phenomenon of parkinsonism, which is defined as "a severe movement disorder characterized by alternating states of akinesia and choreoathetotic dyskinesias" (17,18). The relationship of "on-off" mechanisms to the switch state of severe, unidirectional (19) bipolar I illness (psychotic mania alternating rapidly with anergic depression or mixed presentations) is uncanny. The "on-off" phenomenon has been attributed to a mixture of factors:

1. Alternating states of postsynaptic dopamine (DA) receptor supersensitivity and hyposensitivity (20).
2. Fluctuations of serum and cellular levels of L-dopa (21). Both serum and intraneuronal concentrations are substantially altered by a high-protein diet (22) that counteracts L-dopa through competing amino acid precursors and pyridoxine, all of which block L-dopa activity.

The "on–off" phenomenology expressed in Parkinson's disease has mirror similarities with the pathology and pathophysiology of the switch states and oscillating, mixed episodes found in severe cases of bipolar I illness (17,18,23–26). Both the "on-off" phenomenon and the "mixed state" are markers of severe, often end-stage illness (27). In both, supersensitivity and kindling (10) have been invoked as mechanisms of clinical deterioration. Difficulties in attaining therapeutic blood levels, L-dopa in Parkinson's disease and lithium in bipolar I illness, compound treatment resistance; both are markers of severe end-stage illness and, consequently, are closely associated with the aging process.

Early investigators including Kraepelin (1), Schule (28), and Mendel (29) were convinced that the natural course of manic–depressive illness inevitably followed the following pattern:

1. gradual change to shallower, more rapidly occurring episodes;
2. the onset of chronic mania (or, in rarer cases, chronic anergic depression);
3. increasing dementia; and finally,
4. the onset of fatal senescence perhaps of an Alzheimer type, but equally likely to be atherosclerotic or induced by Creutzfeldt–Jakob etiologies.

This neuronal deterioration pattern is precisely that surmised for those severe parkinsonians with the "on-off" phenomenon. First, they develop decreasing response to L-dopa, Sinemet, deprenyl, bromocriptine, or other DA agonists; then they show the "on-off" response, reflecting the development of postsynaptic receptor supersensitivity, decreasing serum and intracellular levels of administered medication, and plain cellular depletion in the substantia nigra. In parkinsonism, this treatment refractoriness gradually appears, just as in bipolar illness, and is followed by the necessity for synergistic medications—in bipolar illness carbamazepine, or clonazepam or valproate; in parkinsonism deprenyl, carbidopa, bromocriptine, and so on. Next switch phenomena are manifested—rapid cycling in bipolar illness; the "on-off" phenomenon in Parkinsonism. Then a chronic pathologic state appears, either chronic mania (more common) or depression in bipolar disease, and severe akinesia or disabling positive symptoms (tremor, festination) in parkinsonism. Finally there is terminal dementia in bipolar disease, and end-stage akinesia and dementia in parkinsonism. The par-

allels are more than coincidental and Walle Nauta's work shows the anatomic substrate of these changes, forging the critical link between severe psychiatric disease and deteriorating neurologic illness. Nauta has produced seminal data that will drive both clinical fields in new and productive directions.

Kraepelin's and Schule's hypothesis has probably turned out to be wrong. There is no doubt that there is a strong linkage between chronic mania and dementia, but recent investigation by Himmelhoch and others into the relationship of aging to lithium response has uncovered a complex yet different effect of dementia and/or motor disorder (either naturally occurring or a tardive syndrome from neuroleptic treatment) on bipolar illness. Age has little connection with poor lithium response and the development of neurotoxicity. But as shown in Tables 52.1 to 52.3, the presence of interepisodic dementia and particularly of motor disorders have profound effects on outcome. Every patient who developed chronic mania (19 of 81) experienced interepisodic dementia and/or motor disease before the onset of their chronic mania and often before the acceleration in frequency of their mood swings. Motor disease was absolutely devastating. Every subject with parkinsonism not only failed to respond to lithium salts but became severely neurotoxic when it was administered, even at very low doses. Perhaps it is not so surprising that this Kraepelinian

T a b l e 5 2 . 1   Dementia versus Involuntary Motor Disease and Lithium Response in Aging Bipolar Patients

Extrapyramidal Syndrome (EPS) and Interepisodic Dementia (ID)	Lithium Response		
	Good	Poor	Total
EPS[a]	0	15	15
ID without EPS[b]	2	8	10
Neither	54	2	56
Total	56	25	81

$\chi^2 = 64.46; p < 0.001$.
[a] Fourteen of fifteen patients with EPS developed chronic mania.
[b] Five of ten patients with dementia developed chronic mania.

T a b l e 5 2 . 2   Effects of Dementia versus Involuntary Motor Disease on Lithium Response in Aging Bipolar Patients

Extrapyramidal Syndrome (EPS) and Interepisodic Dementia (ID)	Lithium Response		
	Good	Poor	Total
EPS	0	15	15
ID without EPS	2	8	10
Total	2	23	25

$\chi^2 = 3.26; p < 0.10$.

Table 52.3 The Evolution of Chronic Mania

Extrapyramidal Syndrome (EPS) and Interepisodic Dementia (ID)	Type of Poor Outcome		
	Chronic Mania	Other	Total
EPS	14	1	15
ID	5	5	10
Total	19	6	25

$\chi^2 = 6.17; p < 0.01.$

outcome is connected with dementia, but the even more powerful linkage with motor disorders makes the observations of Nauta (and of Kraepelin himself) critical to our understanding.

Wittigenstein (30) in his epistemologic investigations into aesthetics noted the intertwinings of thought and movement in the development of language. He demonstrated that unsophisticated expressions or aesthetic pleasure are mere interjection, purely *motor* expression. True aesthetic understanding involves extensively developed cognition. The differences almost exactly parallel Piaget's (31) cognitive stages of operational (motor) versus abstract development. Nauta (13) has traced the motor–cognitive connections that form the basis for the parallel motor and cognitive aspects of mood, so confusing to clinical investigators in the past. His degenerative staining of meticulously dissected pathways at the crossroads of limbic and striatal pathways, and his horseradish peroxidase staining and proline-leucine autoradiography have shown the anatomical links between the akinesia of Parkinson's disease and the paralyses of thought that occur both in Parkinson's disease and in all forms of bipolar illness.

Tracing these anatomic connection backward, they begin with the hippocampus of the limbic system and proceed by means of the medial forebrain bundle to the critical nuclei of the lateral hypothalamus, the tegmentum, periaqueductal gray matter, and finally to the striatum of the basal ganglia; linkage is made with the putamen and globus pallidus and then outflow proceeds to the midbrain via the ansa lentricularis, forming connections with the nucleus tegmenti, the pontine pediculae and the pars compacta of the substantia nigra, and, finally, with the thalamus, then proceeding to the voluntary motor cortex and the pryamidal system. These elegant anatomical dissections and staining make clear the close anatomical relationship between akinesia and anergic depression.

This relationship can also show clinically, strengthening these hypotheses considerably. First and most convincing are those dramatic cases of mood-contingent motor disorder. Second, there is the well-demonstrated worsening of neuroleptic-induced motor disorders by lithium salts (32). It has been demonstrated again and again that the addition of lithium makes both tardive dyskinesia (TD) and

neuroleptic-induced parkinsonism worse (ironically pretreatment with lithium salts prevents the onset of parkinsonism and/or TD) (33). In the mood-contingent motor disorders, bipolar patients, when depressed, show worsening of any akinesia present; but when manic, buccolingual dyskinesias and choreoathetoid movements suddenly appear, and the motor disorders appear or disappear as mood reverses or returns to normal.

The observation of a pathophysiologic and a clinical relationship between bipolar disease and basal ganglia dysfunction has been reinforced many times since the first edition of this book. Parkinson's disease remains the most-often mentioned, but other diseases of the involuntary motor system have also shown a relationship to mood swings, some occurring in reaction to treatment with lithium and others preceding the onset of bipolar illness as triggers for secondary manic–depressive episodes. Most investigators have posited that DA function forms the basis for these pathophysiologic relationships, although not only DA receptor blockade, but DA receptor supersensitivity and DA receptor downtuning would each have to be invoked if all neostriatal–mood relationships are to be explained. In all, Parkinson's, pseudoparkinson's, idiopathic dystonia, choreoathetosis, hemiballismus, and Tourette's each has been seen to occur either in direct relationship to bipolar illness or in the wake of lithium treatment. These relationships are the focus of Chapter 19 (Special Lithium-Induced Movement Disorders) and of this chapter. Two cases follow that demonstrate the close relationship between bipolar depression and akinesia during mood swings, reflecting the close interaction between motor and cognitive function in determining normal mood.

Case Studies

1. M.P. is a 39-year-old white woman with manic–depressive illness since age 18. She had been well maintained on lithium carbonate for four years when she had a manic relapse and was admitted. During her inpatient stay she was kept on lithium and received two 25 mg shots of fluphenazine decanoate, after which she became hypokinetic and developed mask-like facies. She was discharged. Her pseudoparkinsonian syndrome lasted 102 days after the second depot injection. During this time she was also depressed. Lithium was increased, but her motor disorder worsened, so it was stopped. Her parkinsonism lessened, but did not disappear. Tranylcypromine was introduced. In eight days her depression and parkinsonism simultaneously lysed.

2. W.J. is a 58-year-old white male who presented in the depressed phase of manic–depressive illness. For seven years, he had been treated with large doses of chlorpromazine, but had been off neuroleptics for two years. He was started on lithium salts. As his mood elevated, a mild facial dyskinesia became evident. A manic episode ensued, and his facial dyskinesia became florid. When his mania diminished so did his dyskinesia. Since then, the severity of his dyskinesia has been consistently linked to the level of his mood.

It is of particular interest that each of these examples shows a very different mood-contingent relationship: akinesia with increasing anergic depression in the first case and TD manifesting itself parallel to elevating mood in the second. On the surface, these differences are readily explained: DA receptor blockage worsened by depression in the first; DA receptor supersensitivity worsened by increasing hypomania in the second. But recent literature has considerably muddled these straightforward relationships and has created considerable controversy at the same time. Yazici et al (34) have observed the spontaneous improvement of two cases of TD during mania. Scappa et al (35), in a letter to the Canadian Journal of Psychiatry, have made similar observations and have gone so far to propose that a hypothesized DA excess occurring during mania explains their cases and those of Yazici as well. However, Northcott, Lunn, and Yatham (36), in reply to Scappa's letter, quite appropriately made the following points:

1. If the DA excess theory were correct, one would expect the DA-deficient state of parkinsonism to invariably improve with the onset of mania.
2. Tardive dyskinesia, on the other had, with its proposed DA receptor supersensitivity, should evolve by first worsening and then improving when mania produces DA excess: worsening because exposure of supersensitive receptors to excess DA should cause TD to intensify; improving because eventually DA excess would lead to downtuning of the same receptors.
3. Finally, they then actually report a 66-year-old white, male bipolar patient whose Parkinson's disease worsens during his manic episodes in direct contradiction to Scappa et al (35). Bhugra and Baker (37) further complicate the question with their study.

The upshot of these varying observations is that although there is evidently a relationship between mood in bipolar disorder and various neostriatal motor disorders, this relationship is unpredictable. Parkinsonism can worsen during depression or during mania; TD can also worsen during depression or during mania. Simple theories of neurotransmitter concentration for explaining mood or motor disorder or their connection, therefore, break down. Nor is there any reason they should not. There are at least five postsynaptic DA receptors; there are an unknown number of inhibitory, presynaptic DA receptors; these receptors can be blocked, made supersensitive, and/or down-tuned, all of which adds up to many permutations and combinations of effects. Moreover, as if the above were not sufficient, TD has been reported to vary according to melatonin concentrations and even according to the presence of enlarged calcified pineal glands (38,39). There *are* some well-established

clinical principles: the bipolar–TD relationship intensifies with worsening cognitive impairments, with prolonged clinical course, and with an increasing number of recurrent bipolar episodes.

The incidence of TD occurring in bipolar subjects ranges between 19% and 23% (40,41)—a much greater incidence than associated with any other neuroleptic-treated disorder. The presence of TD and/or Parkinson's disease has considerable negative impact on outcome. In his series of 81 geriatric bipolar patients, Himmelhoch et al (8) showed that the presence of a significant motor disorder had an 80% association with mild to moderate dementia and a devastating effect on outcome. No patient with a motor disorder responded to treatment; all developed lithium neurotoxicity at low doses and blood levels of lithium. Moreover, chronic mania/hypomania—felt by Kraepelin (1) to be an inevitable development for bipolar patients, followed quickly by dementia and death—developed in 19 of 21 patients with motor disorders; chronic depression was the outcome in the other two.

Tardive dyskinesia has some surprisingly specific correlations with bipolar affective disorder and its treatment. Most interesting is the different impact of orofacial dyskinesias versus limb-axial dyskinesia on electroconvulsive therapy (ECT) responsiveness (42). Patients with orofacial TD are responsive to ECT, but those with limb-axial involvement are totally refractory to ECT and most other antidepressant interventions.

To summarize the conclusions thus far, the clinical, physiologic, and pathologic relationship between bipolar mood states, particularly anergic depression, and motor disorders is undeniable. It is not merely provocative clinical anecdotes that show this relationship, first brought to light by Kraepelin himself, but there is powerful and carefully analyzed anatomic and pharmacologic evidence. These data, the anatomic side developed by Walle Nauta and the pharmacologic aspects by Himmelhoch and his group, have created elegant anatomic and pharmacologic probes into these related pathologies. Nauta has shown clearly, using elegant radioactive and enzymatic staining techniques, the palintropic interaction of unconscious, basal ganglial activity with cognition and emotion.

Coffey et al (27) have pharmacologically explained the notorious "on-off" phenomenon in Parkinson's disease, which has startling parallels with the switch phase, rapid cycling, and the mixed manias of bipolar illness. Keshavan et al (43) have reported a patient with idiopathic Parkinson's disease where the "on-off" phenomenon showed a consistent relationship with mood. The "on" phase (dyskinetic) coincided with manic symptomatology and the "off" (akinetic) phase with depression. Moreover, there are now various reports that lithium salts significantly diminish "on-off" effects in deteriorating Parkinson's patients.

Not only do the bipolar disorders (bipolar I and bipolar II) seem to manifest greater vulnerability to the onset of basal ganglia syndromes, it has recently been observed with increasing frequency that specific basal ganglial syndromes can trigger significant secondary manias and secondary bipolar syndromes. Starkstein et al (44) have carefully observed the relationship of secondary mania and of newly occurring bipolar mood swings to head injury or to stroke. In both instances, a combination of nondominant cortical injury and small subcortical lesions had to be simultaneously produced in order for secondary bipolar syndromes to appear.

Kim et al (45) described two patients with longstanding idiopathic Parkinson's disease without family history of bipolar disease who both developed bipolar mood disorders late in the course of their illness. In the first patient, a 59-year-old female with an 11-year history of Parkinson's, lithium proved effective; but in the second, a 60-year-old male with a 14-year history of Parkinson's, neither lithium nor the atypical antipsychotic, clozapine could stop worsening cycling. It is noteworthy that both patients were at that stage of Parkinson's disease where neuronal death in the substantia nigra produces "on-off" phenomenon.

In the investigation by Scappa et al (35) already mentioned, the authors reported three patients whose rapid-cycling bipolar disorder had once been treated with neuroleptics and who eventually developed a pattern where first severe parkinsonism and then TD, occurring in rapid succession, signaled the onset of a switch into depression. While TD worsened during depression, all motor symptoms disappeared when the patient cycled into hypomania then mania.

In each of these examples, either the onset or the worsening of bipolar cycling is associated with decreasing neuronal mass in subcortical gray matter, most probably the basal ganglia. It is just such a situation in which receptor supersensitivity can occur or become worsened. Dopamine efficacy can be ravaged by neuroleptic blockade or by neuronal dropout or a combination of both. Steiner et al (46) have hypothesized that DA supersensitivity can produce TD when it occurs in the neostriatum and acute schizophrenic psychosis when it occurs in mesolimbic dopaminergic cells. The same investigators have reported supersensitivity psychosis in patients with bipolar affective disorder who had been sufficiently exposed to neuroleptics. This psychosis theoretically associates with supersensitivity in both neostriatal and mesolimbic DA receptors. However, attempts to demonstrate decreased basal ganglial volume and increased white matter hyperintensities in bipolars when compared to normal controls by means of magnetic resonance imaging have failed.

Still, other cases of secondary bipolar episodes occurring after other specific diseases of the basal ganglia continue to be reported. Kulisevsky et al (47) describe an 81-year-old white right-handed woman who developed hemiballismus and a disinhibition syndrome very like secondary mania after a small right thalamic infarction. The patient's behavioral disinhibition disappeared after she was treated with low doses of butyrophenone. Lauterbach, Spears, and Price (48)

have reported five cases of bipolar disorder occurring in five patients with idiopathic dystonia. All five manifested rapid cycling and mixed episodes. In three patients, this secondary bipolar disorder developed soon after the onset of cervico-cranial dystonia. The following case, treated in consultation by our Research Affective Disorders Clinic at the University of Pittsburgh School of Medicine, demonstrates many of the atypical features often seen in such secondary bipolar patients.

Case Study
The author was asked to consult on a 26-year-old single male who had been hospitalized four times in a nine-month period with either irritable hypomania or with depression complicated by severe panic attacks. His initial psychiatric illness was generalized anxiety disorder (GAD) that had begun when he was 14 years old and that he self-treated with excessive alcohol and street "downers." He was hospitalized at age 15 and when given two oral doses of butyrophenone totaling 5mg developed a cervicocranial dystonia that was neither recognized nor treated. This dystonia never completely remitted and he suffered chronic dystonia in his left cervical cranial area with acute attacks from that time on. Six weeks after his acute dystonia he became hypomanic. The episode lasted six weeks, after which he became depressed for ten weeks. He has cycled at nearly this rate for 11 years.

Both hypomania and depression are atypical. When hypomanic, expansiveness, talkativeness, and excess spending are rapidly replaced by pure sleepless irritability. Over these 11 years, the patient has constantly been in legal difficulties for physically abusing girlfriends and female relatives while hypomanic. His depressions are also sleepless, colored by chronic anxiety, which often intensifies into panic. He has been resistant to lithium salts, which also make his dystonia worse. The patient is partially controlled on divalproex and phenelzine. Low doses of clozapine are being considered for his irritability and pervasive anxiety.

There has also been a growing awareness of a relationship between Tourette's syndrome and youth-onset mania. Kerbeshian and Burd (49) reported in 1989 three boys with an early history of attention deficit disorder with hyperactivity who then developed Tourette's syndrome. At the respective ages of 13, 12, and 8, all three met the Diagnostic and Statistical Manual-III criteria for either a manic episode or bipolar disorder. All three had families with multiple cases of affective or bipolar affective disorders. All three stabilized on lithium carbonate given at the rather high maintenance range of 0.8–1.2mEq/L; two showed improvement of their Tourette's syndrome. The author's experience with bipolar disorder occurring with Tourette's syndrome is much more foreboding. Few such patients respond to lithium; most suffer worsening of their Tourette's. In the past two years, better results have been obtained with divalproex sodium–selective serotonin reuptake inhibitor (SSRI) combinations. Consider, however, the following example of abject treatment failure.

Case Study

A 17-year-old boy from West Virginia was referred to our clinic's outreach program in Wheeling, West Virginia. The young man suffered from serious Tourette's disorder, obsessive-compulsive symptoms, and mood swings. His tics, gesticulations, and vocalizations became intrusive at age 13, but he responded nicely to 4 mg daily pimozide. Over time, however, he developed chronic anergia and was left between the Scylla of tics with socially intrusive behaviors and the Charybdis of depression (neuroleptics are notorious for inducing episodes of bipolar depression, as would be deduced from principles evinced in this chapter). The young man had become a charming, attractive neighborhood favorite once his Tourette's was controlled. When we identified his mood swings, his pimozide was lowered to 3 mg per day and first 600 mg lithium then 30 mg tranylcypromine were added. Results were striking—first in terms of recovery, then in terms of manic breakthrough. The young man disappeared into the artist's colony on Wheeling Island and became a very successful male prostitute. His mania, his income, and his rich array of colorful associates reinforced his desire to avoid treatment of his hypomania, which he first sustained by a pharmacist's generous handing out of two years' unprescribed refills of tranylcypromine; eventually, once his pharmacist's largesse had been replaced by common sense, he sustained his energetic, sexual impulsivity by street stimulants including both crystal ice and cocaine. He was lost to treatment and to his family.

We are now aware that Tourette's signals the most complicated bipolar disorder, always mixed and often rapid cycling. In our group of 73 adolescent (less than 18 years) bipolars, four Tourette's have appeared and all required the most complex polypharmaceutical regimens to cover their variety of clinical pathology—antikindling anticonvulsants, low-dose lithium, SSRIs, bupropion or monoamine oxidase (MAO) inhibitors, low-dose neuroleptics (most often pimozide), hypermetabolic thyroid supplementation in female patients, and trazodone (or appropriate benzodiazepines) for sleep.

Recently, Kerbeshian et al (50) have done a standard epidemiologic study of the comorbidity of Tourette's with bipolar I and bipolar II disorders. They conclude that

comorbidity between Tourette's disorder and bipolar disorder does not appear to be due to chance co-occurrence of the two disorders. Although a genetic mechanism may play a casual role, in the absence of family studies an explanatory model involving the concept of canalization of basal-ganglia mediated dysfunction is offered. In such a construct, Tourette's disorder would be a likely accompaniment to other conditions including bipolar disorder[s] whose patho-

genic determinants might channel through neural pathways involving the basal ganglia.

Finally, there are the paradoxical effects of lithium salts on neuroleptic-related parkinsonism and TD. Pert et al (33) have shown *pretreatment* with lithium salts blocks the occurrence of these severe motor diseases. On the other hand, *posttreatment* with lithium worsens them in every case. The excellent membrane investigations of Mallinger et al (51), where the phloretin-sensitive lithium countertransport system produces electrogenically active sodium efflux from red blood cells (and presumably neurons) altering membrane permeability and electric transmissibility, may provide an explanation for these phase opposite behaviors. In any case, the relationship between bipolar disease (particularly bipolar I) and varying basal ganglial pathologies (particularly parkinsonism and TD) is powerful. Indeed, bipolar I illness may be more closely related to Parkinson's disease than it is to unipolar depressive illness.

The upshot of recent research and clinical study is that there is now abundant evidence to suggest the following:

1. Bipolar I and bipolar II disorders involve the basal ganglia, which are structures central to its pathophysiology. Neostriatal loci and their afferent and efferent projections to the reticular activating system, to the mesolimbic area, to the hypothalamic nuclei, and to the frontal cortex are abundantly clear not just from the excruciatingly refined anatomy of Nauta (13) but from the way the bipolar syndromes unroll their natural course, from the effects of pharmacologic agents (especially lithium and neuroleptics), and from those secondary bipolar syndromes that occur in the wake of specific basal ganglial syndromes including Parkinson's disease, TD, hemiballismus, choreoathetosis, idiopathic dystonia, and Tourette's disorder.

2. It is clear that any clinical insult that decreases dopaminergic receptor density, either by pharmacologic blockade or by apoptosis and/or cell death, can reciprocally set off bipolar disorder or specific basal ganglial pathology, and that these events can follow according to any sequence.

3. These above interrelationships bespeak a particular "target organ" type vulnerability to infectious agents, trauma, vascular accident, drugs of abuse, and psychopharmacologic agents—particularly those with dopaminergic effects. Most studies, with one exception (52), show a greater propensity to develop TD in affective patients, even more marked in bipolar affective patients. Bipolar I patients can develop catatonia within the natural parameters of their illness. Therefore, it readily follows that the bipolar patient is very vulnerable to neuroleptic malignant syndrome in the context of catatonia. Raja et al (53) describe three patients whose catatonia was premonitory of neuroleptic malignant syndrome. This dangerous turn of events has also been described as occurring in a patient simply on amitriptyline and lithium carbonate (54). Another patient with a bipolar psychotic depression secondary to schizencephaly developed catatonia and neuroleptic malignant syndrome on

imipramine (55). Finally there are the classic reports of haldol/lithium combinations given in a careless fashion with similar outcome. But the vulnerability is not a pharmacologic one; it is a built-in genetic variation in neostriatal function that leaves the patient vulnerable to both catatonia and neuroleptic malignant syndrome. One would project that there are at least some elderly bipolar patients who can spontaneously develop a catatonic state in every way similar to that seen in neuroleptic malignant syndrome.

In Chapter 19, lithium's unusual ability to uncover ancient neurologic insults and motor pathology is discussed, along with the membrane physiology behind these changes.

REFERENCES

1. Kraepelin E. Lectures on clinical psychiatry. Johnstone T, ed. New York: Hafner, 1968.
2. Beigel A, Murphy DL. Unipolar and bipolar affective illness. Arch Gen Psychiatry 1971;24:215–220.
3. Detre T, Himmelhoch JM, Swartzburg M, et al. Hypersomnia and manic-depressive disease. Am J Psychiatry 1972;128:123–125.
4. Kupfer DJ, Himmelhoch JM, Swartzburg M, et al. Hypersomnia in manic-depressive disease: a preliminary report. Dis Nerv Sys 1972;33:720–724.
5. Himmelhoch JM, Fuchs CZ, Symons BJ. A double-blind study of tranylcypromine treatment of major anergic depression. J Nerv Ment Dis 1982;170:628–634.
6. Kupfer DJ, Pickar D, Himmelhoch JM, Detre TP. Are there two types of unipolar depression? Arch Gen Psychiatry 1975;32:866–871.
7. Himmelhoch JM, Coble P, Kupfer DJ, Ingenito J. Agitated psychotic depression associated with severe hypomanic episodes: a rare syndrome. Am J Psychiatry 1976;133:765–771.
8. Himmelhoch JM, Neil JF, May SJ, et al. Age, dementia, dyskinesias, and lithium response. Am J Psychiatry 1980;137:941–945.
9. Post RM, Kopanda RT. Cocaine, kindling, and psychosis. Am J Psychiatry 1976;133:627–634.
10. Himmelhoch JM. What destroys our restraints against suicide? J Clin Psychiatry 1988;49(suppl):46–52.
11. Himmelhoch JM. Lest treatment abet suicide. J Clin Psychiatry 1987;48(suppl):44–54.
12. Lee T, Seeman P, Rajput A, et al. Receptor basis for dopaminergic supersensitivity in Parkinson's disease. Nature 1978;273:59–61.
13. Nauta WJH. Crossroads of limbic and striatal circuitry. Presented at Western Psychiatric Institute & Clinic (WPIC) Guest Lecture Series, Pittsburgh, PA. WPIC Library Tape #399, 1979.
14. Christensen AV, Nielsen IM. Dopaminergic supersensitivity: influence of dopaminergic agonists, cholinergics, anticholinergics and drugs used for the treatment of tardive dyskinesia. Psychopharmacology 1979;62:111–116.
15. Friedhoff AJ, Bonnet K, Rosengarten H. Reversal of two manifestations of dopamine receptor supersensitivity by administration of L-dopa. Res Commun Chem Pathol Pharmacol 1977;16:411–423.
16. Himmelhoch JM. Mania: the dual nature of elation. In: Giannini AJ, ed. The biological foundations of clinical psychiatry. New York: Medical Examination, 1986:116–130.
17. Fabbrini G, Mouradian MM, Juncos JL, et al. Motor fluctuations in Parkinson's disease: central pathophysiological mechanisms—part I. Ann Neurol 1988;24:372–378.
18. Mouradian MM, Juncos JL, Fabbrini G, et al. Motor fluctuations in Parkinson's disease: central pathophysiological mechanism—part II. Ann Neurol 1988;24:372–378.
19. Court J. The continuum model as a resolution of paradoxes in manic–depressive psychosis. Br J Psychiatry 1972;120:133–141.
20. Wooten GF. Progress in understanding the pathophysiology of treatment-related fluctuations in Parkinson's disease. Ann Neurol 1988;24:363–365.
21. Leenders KL, Palmer AG, Quinn N, et al. Brain dopamine metabolism in patients with Parkinson's disease measured with positron emission tomography. J Neurol Neurosurg Psychiatry 1986;49:853–860.
22. Fahn S. "On–off" phenomenon with levodopa therapy in parkinsonism. Clinical and pharmacologic correlations and the effect of intramuscular pyridoxine. Neurology 1974;24:431–441.
23. Himmelhoch JM, Mulla D, Neil JF, et al. Incidence and significance of mixed affective states in a bipolar population. Arch Gen Psychiatry 1976;33:1062–1066.
24. Himmelhoch JM, Garfinkel ME. Sources of lithium resistance in mixed mania. Psychopharmacol Bul 1986;22:613–620.
25. Himmelhoch JM. Major mood disorders related to epileptic changes. In: Blumer D, ed. Psychiatric aspects of epilepsy. Washington: American Psychiatric, 1984:271–294.
26. Himmelhoch JM, Thase ME. The vagaries of the concept atypical depression. In: Howells JG, ed. Modern perspectives in the psychiatric of affective disorders. New York: Brunner/Mazel, 1989:223–242.
27. Coffey CE, Ross DR, Ferren EL, et al. Treatment of the "on–off" phenomenon in parkinsonism with lithium carbonate. Ann Neurol 1982;12:375–379.
28. Schule H. Klinische Psychiatrie. Leipzig: FCW Vogel, 1886.
29. Mendel E. Die Manie. Vienna: Urban & Schwarzenberg, 1881.
30. Wittgenstein L. Lectures & Conversations. Barrett C, ed. Los Angeles: University of California, 1983.
31. Piaget J. Biologie et connaissance. Paris: Gallimard, 1967.
32. Addonizio G, Roth DS, Stokes PE, Stoll PM. Increased extrapyramidal symptoms with addition of lithium to neuroleptics. J Nerv Ment Dis 1988;176:682–685.
33. Pert A, Rosenblatt JE, Sivit C, et al. Long-term treatment with lithium prevents the developments of dopamine receptor supersensitivity. Science 1978;201:171–173.
34. Yazici O, Kantemir E, Tastaban Y, et al. Spontaneous improvement of tardive dystonia during mania. Br J Psychiatry 1991;158:847–850.
35. Scappa S, Teverbaugh P, Ananth J. Episodic tardive dyskinesia and parkinsonism in bipolar disorder patients. Can J Psychiatry 1993;38:633–634.
36. Northcott C, Lunn V, Yatham LN. Parkinsonism and bipolar affective disorder. Can J Psychiatry 1995;40:159–160.
37. Bhugra D, Baker S. State-dependent tardive dyskinesia. J Nerv Ment Dis 1990;178:720.
38. Sandyk R. The relationship of pineal calcification to subtypes of tardive dyskinesia in bipolar patients. Int J Neurosci 1990;54:307–313.
39. Sandyk R. Tardive dyskinesia associated with depression in a bipolar patient: possible role of melatonin. Int J Neurosci 1990;52:79–83.
40. Hunt N, Silverstone T. Tardive dyskinesia in bipolar affective disorder: a catchment area study. Int Clin Psychopharmacol 1991;6:45–50.
41. Dinan TG, Kohen D. Tardive dyskinesia in bipolar affective disorder: relationship to lithium therapy. Br J Psychiatry 1989;155:55–57.
42. Sandyk R. The relationship between ECT responsiveness and subtypes of tardive dyskinesia in bipolar patients. Int J Neurosci 1990;54:315–319.
43. Keshavan MS, David AS, Narayanen HS, Satish P. "On–off" phenomena and manic–depressive mood shifts: case report. J Clin Psychiatry 1986;47:93–94.
44. Starkstein SE, Pearlson GD, Boston J, Robinson RG. Mania after brain injury: a controlled study of causative factors. Arch Neurol 1987;44:1069–1073.
45. Kim E, Zwil AS, McAllister TW, et al. Treatment of organic bipolar mood disorders in Parkinson's disease. J Neuropsychiatry Clin Neurosci 1994;6:181–184.
46. Steiner W, Laporta M, Chouinard G. Neuroleptic-induced supersensitivity psychosis in patients with bipolar affective disorder. Acta Psychiatr Scand 1990;81:437–440.
47. Kulisevsky J, Berthier ML, Pujol J. Hemiballismus and secondary mania following a right thalamic infarction. Neurology 1993;43:1422–1424.
48. Lauterbach EC, Spears TE, Price ST. Bipolar disorder in idiopathic dystonia: clinical features and possible neurobiology. J Neuropsychiatry Clin Neurosci 1992;4:435–439.
49. Kerbeshian J, Burd L. Tourette disorder and bipolar symptomatology in childhood and adolescence. Can J Psychiatry 1989;34:230–233.
50. Kerbeshian J, Burd L, Klug MG. Comorbid Tourette's disorder and bipolar disorder: an etiologic perspective. Am J Psychiatry 1995;152:1646–1651.
51. Mallinger AG, Hanin I, Himmelhoch JM, et al. Stimulation of cell membrane sodium transport activity by lithium: possible relationship to therapeutic action. Psychiatry Res 1987;22:49–59.
52. Remington GJ, Voineskos G, Pollock B, et al. Prevalence of neuroleptic-induced dystonia in mania and schizophrenia. Am J Psychiatry 1990;147:1231–1233.
53. Raja M, Altavista MC, Cavallari S, Lubich L. Neuroleptic malignant syndrome and catatonia. A report of three cases. Eur Arch Psychiatry Clin Neurosci 1994;243:299–303.
54. Fava S, Galizia AC. Neuroleptic malignant syndrome and lithium carbonate. J Psychiatry Neurosci 1995;20:305–306.
55. Black KJ, Kilzieh N. Severe imipramine-induced myoclonus in a patient with psychotic bipolar depression, catatonia, and schizencephaly. Ann Clin Psychiatry 1994;6:45–49.

Pathologic Crying

RONALD L. GREEN   JAMES L. BERNAT

INTRODUCTION

Pathologic laughing and crying are a class of behaviors in which a neurologically impaired patient exhibits a motor pattern ostensibly indistinguishable from normal emotional expression. These displays are unlike normal emotional displays, however, in that they are uncontrollable and commonly do not reflect the subjective emotional experience of the patient. They can be caused by a variety of neurologic illnesses. The phenomenon will be referred to in this chapter as "pathologic laughing or crying," or PLC, as suggested by Panzer and Mellow (1). This chapter will focus chiefly on pathologic crying. Pathologic laughing is discussed in Chapter 54.

The literature on this subject dates to the latter half of the nineteenth century and consists primarily of clinico-pathologic correlations of the distribution and type of lesions that are found in patients with PLC. In 1912, Tinley and Morrison (2) culled prior literature on pseudobulbar palsy, then thought to be the underlying condition in most cases of PLC. They found 173 cases of bilateral cortical and brainstem motor tract lesions and added 5 cases of their own. About 50% had PLC. Wilson in 1924 (3), in a largely theoretical paper that included an analysis of 6 of his own cases, and Davison and Kelman (4) in 1939, reporting 53 patients, offered the first systematic observations of PLC and documented the various loci and types of lesions that can produce it. Wilson postulated pyramidal voluntary and nonpyramidal involuntary pathways to a "center" in the pons linking the nuclei controlling the facial and respiratory muscles involved in emotional expression, and opined that interruption, especially bilaterally, of the voluntary pathways caused PLC. Davison and Kelman (4), on the other hand, emphasized the hypothalamus as the key region of interest in PLC.

Poeck and Pilleri (5) contributed the modern classic paper on PLC in 1963. They analyzed autopsy findings in 223 confirmed cases of PLC in the literature and 8 of their own. A summary of their findings was published in English in 1969 (6) and again in 1985 (7). They concluded that motor system involvement is necessary in PLC, that the internal capsule and extrapyramidal structures are most frequently involved, and that both bilateral and unilateral lesions can cause the disorder.

In 1967, Brown (8) drew together prior literature on PLC in an effort to generate hypotheses about the phylogeny and physiology of emotional expressions. In this regard, he stressed the importance of a rostral mid-brain region, previously identified by Kelly et al (9), that subserves the motor coordination of faciovocal activities. He presumed this region to be capable of orchestrating emotional displays such as those seen in PLC when stimulated to do so by upstream lesions that activate or disinhibit the region.

In 1982, Sackheim et al (10) reported data bearing on the cerebral lateralization of PLC mechanisms. They analyzed 119 cases of PLC, 103 cases of epilepsy in which laughing or crying were the ictal events, and 19 cases of hemispherectomy associated with PLC. They found that left-sided irritative or right-sided destructive lesions were more likely to produce pathologic crying, and that the converse was true for pathologic laughing.

Ross and Stewart (11) also reviewed the variety of brain disturbances that can produce PLC. They identified two mechanisms: bilateral lesions that produce pseudobulbar palsy, and unilateral or bilateral lesions that involve the basal forebrain, medial temporal lobe, diencephalon, or tegmentum and do not cause pseudobulbar palsy. To these they added a third mechanism based on two of their own cases in which PLC occurred as a consequence of right inferior frontal lobe lesions in conjunction with major depressive disorder. House et al (12) observed that left frontal lesions, large brain lesions, and significant cognitive impairment all correlate with PLC.

DIAGNOSIS

Definitions

Crying refers to the familiar behavioral constellation of rhythmic vocalizations, clonic heaving respirations, pained facial expressions, and lacrimation with rhinorrhea that occurs episodically throughout life. Crying is termed normal when it occurs in response to an appropriately sad affect or emotional state and serves to release inner tensions and feelings. Pathologic crying (known also as forced crying, spasmodic crying, or emotionalism) refers to sudden attacks of involuntary crying behavior resulting from central nervous system disease that are not necessarily indicative of affect and serve no cathartic function (13). Poeck (6,7) defined four operational criteria for pathologic crying:

1. Response to a nonspecific stimulus
2. Lack of a relationship between affect and expression
3. Absence of voluntary control of the extent and duration of facial expressions
4. Absence of a change in mood as the result of the crying

Pathologic laughter (known also as forced laughter) is a related disorder in which paroxysmal bouts of involuntary laughter occur independent of affective state. Pathologic laughter is rarer than pathologic crying, but both are caused by similar lesions and are seen in similar neurologic disorders (see Chapter 54) (14).

Epidemiology

The incidence and prevalence of pathologic crying resulting from specific disease processes have been measured in several studies. Pathologic crying is seen most commonly following stroke, amyotrophic lateral sclerosis, multiple sclerosis, traumatic brain injury, Alzheimer's disease and other causes of dementia, and various causes of delirium. Rarer causes include bilateral brainstem lesions resulting from central pontine myelinolysis (15), brainstem arteriovenous malformations (16), and neoplasms of the posterior fossa (17).

Because of the great prevalence of stroke, pathologic crying is encountered most frequently in clinical practice in the patient who has suffered a stroke. In one series of stroke patients, pathologic crying was reported in 13 (15%) of 89 patients at 1 month, 19 (21%) at 6 months, and 10 (11%) at 1 year following the stroke (12). In a second series of 211 stroke patients, pathologic crying was reported in 30 (14%) at 1 month, 21 (10%) at 6 months, and 23 (11%) at 1 year following the stroke (18).

In a series of patients with Alzheimer's disease, after the administration of a specific "pathological laughter and crying scale," 40 (39%) of 103 patients showed pathologic affect, 26 (25%) demonstrated crying episodes, and 14 (14%) showed mixed laughing and crying episodes (19). In a series of 73 patients with amyotrophic lateral sclerosis with onset over 45 years of age, 36 (49%) experienced episodes of pathologic laughter and/or crying, 20 (27%) had both laughing and crying, 9 (12%) had only crying episodes, and 7 (10%) had only laughing episodes (20).

The prevalence of PLC in multiple sclerosis has varied greatly in reported series, from 7% to 95%, depending on the severity of the disease and, in particular, on the presence and severity of dementia (21). In unselected patients with multiple sclerosis seen in general practice, pathologic crying is observed in approximately 10% of patients (21).

In an effort to learn how often, in medically or surgically hospitalized patients, crying is caused by a brain disorder, Green et al (22) studied 47 medically or surgically hospitalized patients referred for psychiatric consultation because of crying. Only 9 (19%) had purely psychiatric disorders underlying the crying. The rest had a variety of focal and diffuse brain disorders.

History

Evaluation of the patient with frequent crying centers on the setting of the crying and whether the motor manifestations of the crying are appropriate for the patient's underlying affect. Inquiry should be made concerning the stimuli that trigger crying. Pathologic crying often is triggered by nonspecific or emotionally neutral stimuli, such as startle from hearing a door slam. Is the crying accompanied by sadness? This question is complicated by the fact that many patients will assume they are sad (even when they are not) merely because they are crying. Does the crying start and stop suddenly and uncontrollably? Paroxysmal attacks are characteristic of pathologic crying. Is there embarrassment from the crying? Patients with pathologic crying are frequently very embarrassed by their outbursts of crying, whereas depressed patients appear less concerned.

Physicians should inquire about the patient's past crying characteristics to determine whether the current symptoms are distinct. Past medical history questioning should attempt to identify symptoms of diseases of the nervous system associated with pathologic crying, especially multiple sclerosis, motor neuron disease, cerebrovascular disease, dementia, and brain trauma.

Most important, the physician should attempt to determine if the patient has historical features to suggest the diagnosis of depression or of a neurologic disorder. Depression and neurologic disease are not independent, however. Some patients with both have pathologic as well as normal crying (18). One group of investigators has devised a semistructured interview to precisely measure the quality, quantity, and frequency of pathologic crying and its distinction from other types of crying (23,24). Two groups independently developed a "pathological laughter and crying scale" to quantify severity and measure response to therapy (25,26).

Examination

A complete neurologic and mental status examination should be performed. The clinician should pay particular attention to evidence of signs of bilateral corticobulbar tract lesions producing the syndrome of pseudobulbar palsy (27). Pseudobulbar palsy is the classic setting for pathologic crying and occurs most commonly from cerebrovascular disease, motor neuron disease, multiple sclerosis, and diffuse brain trauma. Patients with classic pseudobulbar palsy have spastic dysphonia, dysarthria, and dysphagia, and have hyperactive gag and jaw reflexes. They may or may not have pyramidal signs in their extremities. One case of pathologic crying has been reported, however, resulting from bilateral brainstem involvement by an arteriovenous malformation without specific signs of pseudobulbar palsy (16).

Pathologic crying also may be seen in patients with bilateral hemispheric strokes without fully developed pseudobulbar palsy (22). In addition to looking for pyramidal and long tract sensory signs, the clinician should test for signs of bilateral hemispheric dysfunction, which are often positive in such patients. These include the frontal release signs (regressive reflexes) such as the suck, snout, grasp, glabellar, and palmomental reflexes, as well as the presence of paratonia, limitation of upward gaze, limb holding, and errors on the cognitive portion of the mental status examination (28).

Crying in patients with delirium and dementia is classically attributed to their emotional lability. Because some of these patients demonstrate true pathologic crying, however, the mental status examination should be directed to the demonstration of signs of delirium and dementia (22).

If the clinician is fortunate enough to observe the patient's crying behavior, he or she should look for the typical signs of pathologic crying. The pattern of pathologic crying differs from normal crying in several respects (13,22): 1) pathologic crying can be induced by a seemingly trivial stimulus, even one without an obvious emotional context; 2) the crying occurs without a concomitant affect of sadness; 3) the crying starts and stops suddenly and paroxysmally (pushbutton crying); 4) the crying tends to occur as an all-or-none phenomenon, and not as a graded emotional response; 5) the crying cannot be controlled by the patient; 6) the crying is stereotyped, so that each episode resembles the others; 7) the patients make a facial display that is characteristic of crying but often with little audible vocalization and few tears; 8) pathologic crying may rapidly convert to pathologic laughter and back again; and 9) there is considerable embarrassment from the episodes and a fear that they will recur.

Pathologic crying is exceedingly distressing and embarrassing to patients. If severe, it may lead to social withdrawal and interference with rehabilitation. The fear provoked in a patient by his uncontrollable paroxysms of pathologic crying was well described by a patient with motor neuron disease reported by Lieberman and Benson (29):

> I am mortally afraid of squealing bawls. They destroy me—they weaken and crumble me . . . those deep debilitating agonizing episodes. You have no idea how terrible it is when the crying is fully triggered and takes hold like a seizure. I can't control any of it. I simply disintegrate and it isn't only emotionally horrible with me, it is physically painful and debilitating.

Laboratory Assessment

The appropriate laboratory investigations will depend on the clinical situation. In the patient with pathologic crying due to hemispheric strokes, diffuse brain trauma, dementia, or multiple sclerosis, brain scanning by computed tomography or magnetic resonance will often document the causative lesions. The patient with pathologic crying due to motor neuron disease usually requires no imaging techniques to establish the diagnosis. In patients suspected of delirium, the usual laboratory screening survey, including electroencephalography, should be performed (30).

Differential Diagnosis

The diagnosis of pathologic crying can be made when the characteristic features are present, as described above. Other states of abnormal emotional expression that need to be considered in the patient suspected of pathologic crying include emotional lability, *witzelsucht*, essential crying, and dacrystic epilepsy. Crying from depression must always be considered. There is a positive correlation between depression and pathologic crying after stroke because both may result from the same brain lesions (18).

Emotional lability is a related disorder in which easy laughing and crying occur, generally in states of bilateral hemispheric dysfunction. Here, however, there is no dissociation of motor function from affect but merely an amplification of affect. Thus, states of mild sadness can generate an inappropriately large amount of crying behavior. The emotionally labile patient does not show the typical motor characteristics of pathologic crying discussed above. In patients with bilateral hemispheric dysfunction there is probably a continuum between pathologic crying and emotional lability.

A characteristic type of euphoria and facetiousness known as *witzelsucht* is seen in diffuse disorders of white matter, particularly in multiple sclerosis and frontal lobe diseases. Here the patient does not have emotional lability so much as a persistently and inappropriately elevated affect in which everything strikes him or her as genuinely funny. Here again, the motor behavior is appropriate for the affect; it is the affect that is inappropriate for the situation.

Essential crying is a term that we coined in 1987 to refer to certain patients with a lifelong and hereditary propensity to easy crying (22). Such patients cry very frequently but always with an appropriate affect. It is as if their crying threshold were congenitally lower than the average person. Crying thresholds probably have both genetic and cultural determinants.

Certain rare epileptic disorders can produce involuntary crying and laughter. Dacrystic epilepsy features ictal crying and sobbing (31). Gelastic epilepsy is characterized by ictal laughter, often with pleasure of a sexual nature (32,33). Patients with these disorders have markedly altered states of consciousness during their seizures, and the diagnosis of epilepsy is usually not difficult.

The most common and important distinction is between pathologic crying and normal crying due to depressive disease. Patients need to be carefully assessed for the presence of underlying depression whenever crying occurs. Even in the patient with obvious pathologic crying, there may be depressive disease that requires treatment (18). In a series of patients believed to have purely unilateral hemispheric lesions of the inferior right frontal lobe, pathologic crying was found to be a marker for depression (11,34).

MANAGEMENT

Psychological Intervention

The treatment of the patient with pathologic crying begins with a careful explanation to the patient and the family of the physiologic basis for the crying. Patients and families need to be reassured that the crying is a frequent sequel to the brain damage and thus in this circumstance is quite expected behavior. Families should be counseled that the crying is not necessarily indicative of sadness or depression, so the patient need not be comforted each time it occurs. It takes time for families to realize that the crying is not evidence of sadness. Patients and families can be told that the impairment in controlling emotion parallels the impairment in controlling paralyzed limbs (23). Ignoring the crying is often the best coping strategy because too much attention serves only to worsen the crying. Another coping strategy is to attempt to distract the patient.

The physician should attempt to identify those factors that may provoke the crying paroxysms. This may not be possible because nonspecific stimuli are often sufficient to provoke the episodes. Yet if specific inciting stimuli can be identified, these can be minimized or avoided. The physician should always maintain a high index of suspicion for the presence of depression in patients with pathologic crying, particularly in poststroke patients, who have been found to show a high incidence of depression (18,35).

Drug Therapy

A number of pharmacologic agents have been used with limited success to treat pathologic crying. Tricyclic antidepressant agents, including amitriptyline, imipramine, nortriptyline, and desipramine, have been shown to be of some value in reversing the pathologic crying of patients with multiple sclerosis and other disorders (1,25,36–38). In such patients, the benefits are believed to be exerted by potentiating dopaminergic and serotonergic pathways in the damaged corticobulbar tracts. The efficacy of tricyclic antidepressants has been shown to be independent of reversing concomitant depression. Doses of amitriptyline or imipramine need not exceed 75 mg daily (39).

Selective serotonin reuptake inhibitor (SSRI) antidepressants have also been shown to be effective. In controlled trials and uncontrolled reports, fluoxetine, sertraline, and citalopram significantly reduced episodes of pathologic crying from stroke and other disorders (19,40–44). The SSRI agents are used in their ordinary antidepressant dosages and can reduce the frequency of pathologic crying by approximately 50%. The mechanism for the efficacy of SSRIs may be to increase the availability of serotonin in those serotonergic pathways known to be damaged in patients with pathologic crying (45).

Enhancement of dopaminergic pathways by L-dopa and amantadine has had some success in reducing pathologic crying (46,47). Lithium carbonate and methylphenidate also have been reported to be of benefit in isolated cases (48,49).

BASIC MECHANISMS

The neural mechanisms underlying PLC have not been clearly determined. The wide variety of neuropathologic entities and the diverse location of causative lesions, extending from pons to cortex, have made it difficult to establish any simple or unitary hypotheses. In 1985, Poeck (7) summarized the extent of what can be stated confidently about basic mechanism: "PLC are probably produced by the interruption of a control system, the details of which are as yet unknown." Nevertheless, certain clinical observations and conceptual advances have provided clues about the pathogenesis of this disorder.

An interesting point of departure is the observation of Poeck and Pilleri (5), Gamper (50), and Monnier and Willi (51) that anencephalic infants (in some cases with few intact structures rostral to the pons) display seemingly normal crying behavior. Thus, the caudal brainstem appears to contain sufficient neural apparatus to elaborate the motor manifestations of crying. Consistent with this view is Brown's (8) speculation that pathologic crying may be more like other stereotyped and phylogenetically more primitive motor behaviors organized by the brainstem (such as retching or coughing) than the nuances of more voluntary aspects of human emotional behavior. The subtleties and flexibility of human emotional behavior were presumably made possible as limbic and neocortical regions evolved the capacity to modulate previously reflex-like behaviors in response to environmental and intrapsychic demands.

Early concepts of the mechanisms underlying pathologic crying were based on this phylogenetic and hierarchical view that "lower centers" orchestrated these pathologic affects and that these "centers" were subject to higher-level control. Related to this view and also central to early hypotheses was the observation that emotional expression is subserved by anatomically distinct voluntary and involuntary pathways. Kahn (52) and Monrad-Krohn (53), for example, reported several patients who showed either paresis of voluntary emotional expression with preserved involuntary expression or the converse. Figure 53.1, from Monrad-Krohn's paper (53), vividly demonstrates the former. This 20-year-old patient suffered an acute traumatic injury to the left hemisphere, causing confluent aphasia and spastic right hemiparesis that included the right lower face. The figure shows the findings at examination 6 months postinjury. There remains paresis of voluntary facial expression in the right lower face, but preserved involuntary (spontaneous) smiling.

A more recent report (54) illustrates the reverse situation: preserved voluntary emotional expression and concomitant paresis of involuntary expression. Figure 53.2 shows a patient with temporal lobe epilepsy and a right temporal focus on electroencephalography. The photograph to the left shows the neutral face, the middle photograph shows intact voluntary movements of both sides of the face, and the photograph to the right shows impairment of left facial movement on spontaneous smiling. Collectively, these reports provide strong evidence that facial movements can be controlled by both voluntary and involuntary mechanisms. Further, the pathways are anatomically separable. The voluntary pathway is the anteriorly placed pyramidal system. The involuntary pathways originate in more posterior temporolimbic regions.

Over 50 years ago, Wilson (3) speculated that the voluntary corticobulbar pathways normally served to inhibit involuntary expressions of emotion. Destruction of these pathways, particularly when bilateral, could lead to disinhibition of the involuntary pathways or lower "centers," with resultant spontaneous and inappropriate laughing and crying. The concepts of inhibition and disinhibition as organizing principles in the central nervous system had been elaborated as early as the latter nineteenth century by Jackson (55). The so-called regressive reflexes are examples

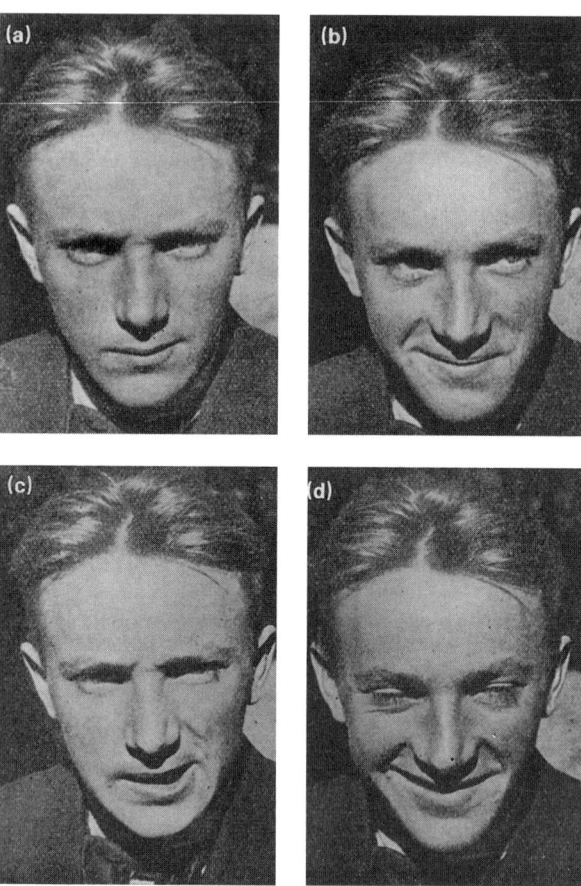

FIGURE 53.1   *Paresis of voluntary smiling. (a) Patient's face at rest. (b) Beginning of a spontaneous smile. (c) Patient tries to show his teeth. (d) Fully developed spontaneous smile. (Reproduced from Monrad-Krohn G. On the dissociation of voluntary and emotional innervation in facial paresis of central origin. Brain 1924;47:22–35.)*

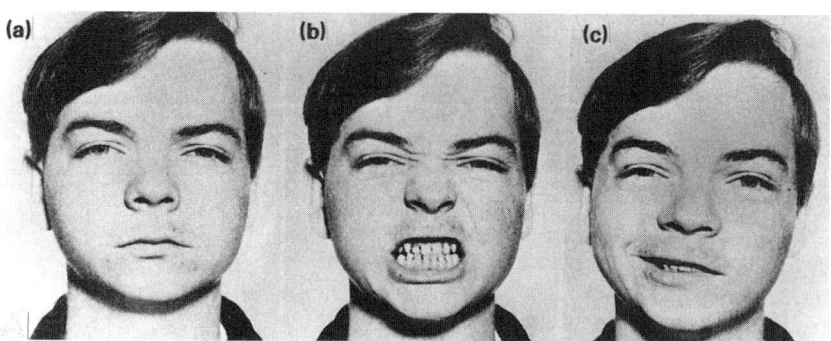

FIGURE 53.2   *Paresis of involuntary smiling. (a) Patient's face at rest. (b) Patient showing his teeth. (c) Spontaneous smile. (Reproduced from Remillard G, Andermann F, Rhi-Sausi A, Robbins N. Facial asymmetry in patients with temporal lobe epilepsy. Neurology 1977;27:109–114.)*

of disinhibition (28). The cerebral cortex is thought to exert a tonic inhibitory influence on these reflexes; in the presence of bilateral cerebral disease, these reflexes can be released from inhibition. This reasoning was extended by Wilson (3) to explain PLC. The disinhibition hypothesis of pathologic crying has been challenged by Brown (56), as discussed below, but has not been supplanted.

Over the ensuing decades, numerous case reports and series, most notably by Davison and Kelman (4) and Poeck and Pilleri (5–7), documented, through clinicopathologic correlation, the various lesions and their loci associated with PLC. The lesions may be unilateral or bilateral and are distributed throughout the brain from medulla to cortex. Poeck (7) emphasized motor system involvement, either pyramidal or extrapyramidal. Exceptions are reports implicating the basal forebrain, temporolimbic regions, diencephalon, and midbrain tegmentum (11). These reports do not shed much light on basic mechanisms.

In 1967, Brown (8) summarized and integrated the prior literature on pathologic laughing, crying, and rage and offered a hypothesis for the neuroanatomic substrate of the expression of these emotions. He proposed an "isolable mechanism" for these expressions in the rostal midbrain, where the periaqueductal gray matter (PAG) can exert an excitatory effect on the adjacent tegmentum, which, in turn, is capable of orchestrating a full emotional display. Because of its reciprocal connections with a number of limbic regions, the PAG is well situated to serve as an effector mechanism for these behaviors. There are, for example, connections to forebrain and temporolimbic regions (57) to provide input from and feedback to regions thought to play a role in elaborating subjective emotional states. Connections with the hypothalamus allow integration of autonomic responses with motor displays of affect. Connections with somatic motor systems allow synchronized coordination of the motor aspects of these expressions, which have facial, vocal, respiratory, and sometimes truncal components. Brown proposed that PLC can result from either disinhibition of the PAG excitatory system or "by enhancement of the sensory evocation of the display." In a later publication (56), he argued that PLC occurs not as a disinhibition phenomenon but rather as a consequence of some kind of "recognition" of these emotions in forebrain or temporolimbic regions, perhaps cued by some environmental or intrapsychic event.

Additional clues to the brain mechanisms of pathologic crying may be found by considering the anatomic substrates of vocal expression in animals. This information may be relevant because vocalization is usually a prominent feature of pathologic and normal crying. One type of vocalization, the separation call, may be directly analogous to human crying, as discussed by MacLean (58). Ploog (59) has summarized animal vocalization findings. Based on depth electrode stimulation experiments, particularly in the squirrel monkey, Ploog noted that vocal expressions are organized at four levels of the brain:

1. The lower brainstem, where motor execution of calls is orchestrated
2. The PAG and nearby midbrain tegmentum, where motivational states may be linked to mechanisms elaborating appropriate vocal patterns
3. Certain temporolimbic and diencephalic regions, which generate the motivational states that underlie the calls
4. The anterior cingulate region, thought to be a cortical site for regulation of vocalization in primates (see below)

Ploog asserts that in humans the cingulate cortex may have a role in voluntary vocalization and may have the capacity, independent of motivational stimuli, to facilitate or inhibit the PAG's effect on the tegmentum. MacLean (58) has opined that the anterior cingulate cortex in mammals subserves the separation call.

These findings suggest that control systems for emotional expression are likely hierarchically organized and may be described in terms of stages of information processing. For example, a feeling of sadness may be elaborated by forebrain and limbic regions in response to environmental events that can access these regions by communication to and from unimodal and heteromodal sensory association cortices, or in response to emergence of emotionally charged memories accessed via the hippocampus/amygdala or from the prefrontal cortex (60). Furthermore, there may be temporolimbic regions that, through some unknown mechanism, instruct the PAG-tegmentum ensemble to orchestrate an episode of crying. Temporolimbic regions have access to the PAG via Nauta's limbic-midbrain continuum (61). Finally, midbrain mechanisms coordinate the activation of the necessary motor nuclei and autonomic components to produce the full orchestration of crying. Voluntary mechanisms, perhaps in the cingulate cortex or pyramidal or extrapyramidal systems, normally exert a modulatory control over the midbrain effector circuits, as suggested by Brown (8) and Ploog (59).

This model hypothesizes that normal crying may occur under the following conditions:

1. By a forced voluntary effort even in the absence of a concomitant appropriate subjective emotional state. Actors and actresses strive to develop this capacity.
2. Sadness or some other emotion elaborated in temporolimbic regions, in response to external or internal cues, activates midbrain mechanisms to bring about crying. Voluntary inhibitory effort may be overwhelmed by the intensity of the emotion, or the inhibitory efforts may be voluntarily relaxed, for example, allowing oneself to relax and be emotionally affected by music, poetry, or the like (19,40,43).

Pathologic crying, on the other hand, may be caused by neurologic disorders in the following ways: (1) the voluntary inhibitory pathways may be interrupted by lesions, "releasing" the involuntary pathways; and (2) disease may activate the involuntary pathways directly. Dacrystic epilepsy (31), in which crying is the ictal event, is an example in which temporolimbic discharge may activate midbrain mechanisms. A third possible mechanism, mentioned earlier, has been suggested by Ross and Stewart (11). They reported two patients who were clinically depressed, then began to display pathologic crying when they suffered acute right inferior frontal lobe brain damage. They concluded that this cortical area may normally help to inhibit temporolimbic activation of pathologic crying. They also discussed possible lateralization effects in the elaboration of pathologic crying. Although there is some evidence (10) of a lateralization effect, further confirmation is needed.

These mechanisms cannot explain all reported instances of pathologic crying. A unilateral pontine lesion (62), for example, does not fit easily with a disinhibition or temporolimbic excess discharge hypothesis. Clarification of mechanisms of pathologic crying depends on further elucidation of the motor systems that subserve emotional expression. More also needs to be known about the nature of hemispheric specialization for emotion and emotional expression. Increased understanding of the neurochemistry of limbic and motor systems is also necessary. In this regard, a report that ascending endorphin pathways inhibit distress vocalization in guinea pigs is interesting (63), as is the capacity of psychopharmacologic agents to reduce pathologic crying (36–39,46–49).

REFERENCES

1. Panzer MJ, Mellow AM. Antidepressant treatment of pathologic laughing or crying in elderly stroke patients. J Geriatr Psychiatry Neurol 1992;5:195–199.
2. Tinley F, Morrison J. Pseudo-bulbar palsy, clinically and pathologically considered, with the clinical report of five cases. J Nerv Ment Dis 1912;39:505–534.
3. Wilson S. Some problems in neurology: pathological laughing and crying. J Neurol Psychopathol 1924;4:299–333.
4. Davison C, Kelman H. Pathologic laughing and crying. Arch Neurol Psychiatry 1939;42:595–643.
5. Poeck K, Pilleri G. Pathologisches lachen und weinen. Schweiz Arch Neurol Neurochir Psychiatr 1963;92:323–370.
6. Poeck K. Disorders of higher nervous activity. In: Vinken P, Bruyn G, eds. Handbook of clinical neurology. Vol. 3. New York: John Wiley, 1969:343–367.
7. Poeck K. Pathological laughter and crying. In: Vinken P, Bruyn G, eds. Handbook of clinical neurology. Vol. 45. Amsterdam: Elsevier, 1985:219–225.
8. Brown J. Physiology and phylogenesis of emotional expression. Brain Res 1967;5:1–14.
9. Kelly A, Beaton L, Magoun H. A midbrain mechanism for facio-vocal activity. J Neurophysiol 1946;9:181–189.
10. Sackheim H, Greenberg M, Weiman A, et al. Hemispheric asymmetry in the expression of positive and negative emotions. Arch Neurol 1982;39:210–218.
11. Ross ED, Stewart RS. Pathological display of affect in patients with depression and right frontal brain damage: an alternative mechanism. J Nerv Ment Dis 1987;175:165–172.
12. House A, Dennis M, Molyneux A, et al. Emotionalism after stroke. Br Med J 1989;298:991–994.
13. Allman P, Hope T, Fairburn CG. Crying following stroke: a report on 30 cases. Gen Hosp Psychiatry 1992;14:315–321.
14. Black D. Pathological laughter: a review of the literature. J Nerv Ment Dis 1982;170:67–71.
15. Van Hilten J, Buruma O, Kessing P, Vlasveld L. Pathologic crying as a prominent behavioral manifestation of central pontine myelinolysis. Arch Neurol 1988;45:936.
16. Asfora WT, DeSalles AAF, Masamitsu A, Kjellberg RN. Is the syndrome of pathological laughing and crying a manifestation of pseudobulbar palsy? J Neurol Neurosurg Psychiatry 1989;52:523–525.
17. Cantu R, Drew J. Pathological laughing and crying associated with a tumor ventral to the pons. J Neurosurg 1966;24:1024–1026.
18. Andersen G, Vestergaard K, Ingemen-Nielsen M. Post-stroke pathological crying: frequency and correlation to depression. Eur J Neurol 1995;2:45–50.
19. Seliger GM, Hornstein A, Flax J, et al. Fluoxetine improves emotional incontinence. Brain Inj 1992;6:267–270.
20. Gallagher JP. Pathologic laughter and crying in ALS: a search for their origin. Acta Neurol Scand 1989;80:114–117.
21. Minden SL, Schiffer RB. Affective disorders in multiple sclerosis. Arch Neurol 1990;47:98–104.
22. Green R, McAllister T, Bernat J. A study of crying in medically and surgically hospitalized patients. Am J Psychiatry 1987;144:442–447.
23. Allman P. Emotionalism following brain damage. Behav Neurol 1991;4:57–62.
24. Allman P, Hope P, Marshall M, Fairbur C. Emotionalism following stroke: development and reliability of a semi-structured interview. Int J Meth Psychiatr Res 1992;2:125–131.
25. Robinson RG, Parikh RM, Lipsey JR, et al. Pathological laughing and crying following stroke: validation of a measurement scale and a double-blind treatment study. Am J Psychiatry 1993;150:286–293.
26. Starkstein SE, Migliorelli R, Teson A, et al. Prevalence and clinical correlates of pathological affective display in Alzheimer's disease. J Neurol Neurosurg Psychiatry 1995;59:55–60.
27. Langworthy O, Hesser F. Syndrome of pseudobulbar palsy: an anatomic and physiologic analysis. Arch Intern Med 1940;65:106–121.
28. Jenkyn J, Reeves A. Signs of cortical disinhibition in neuropsychiatric disorders. Psychiatr Med 1984;1:389–446.
29. Lieberman A, Benson D. Control of emotional expression in pseudobulbar palsy: a personal experience. Arch Neurol 1977;34:717–719.
30. Lipowski Z. Delirium (acute confusional state). JAMA 1987;258:1789–1792.
31. Offen M, Davidoff R, Troost B, et al. Dacrystic epilepsy. J Neurol Neurosurg Psychiatry 1976;39:829–834.
32. Gascon G, Lombrosco C. Epileptic (gelastic) laughter. Epilepsia 1971;12:63–76.
33. Loisseau P, Cohadon F, Cohadon S. Gelastic epilespy. Epilepsia 1971;12:313–323.
34. Ross E, Rush A. Diagnosis and neuroanatomical correlates of depression in brain-damaged patients: implications for a neurology of depression. Arch Gen Psychiatry 1981;38:1344–1354.
35. Starkstein S, Robinson R, Price T. Comparison of cortical and subcortical lesions in the production of post-stroke mood disorders. Brain 1987;110:1045–1059.
36. Schiffer R, Cash J, Herndon R. Treatment of emotional lability with low-dose tricyclic antidepressants. Psychosomatics 1983;24:1094–1096.
37. Schiffer R, Herndon R, Rudick R. Treatment of pathologic laughing and weeping with amitriptyline. N Engl J Med 1985;312:1480–1482.
38. Lawson I, MacLeod R. The use of imipramine ("Tofranil") and other psychotic drugs in organic emotionalism. Br J Psychiatry 1969;115:281–285.
39. Caroscio J, Cohen J, Cudesblatt M. Amitriptyline in amyotrophic lateral sclerosis. N Engl J Med 1985;313:1478.
40. Sloan RL, Brown KW, Pentland B. Fluoxetine as a treatment for emotional lability after brain injury. Brain Inj 1992;6:315–319.
41. Seliger GM, Hornstein A. Serotonin, fluoxetine, and pseudobulbar affect. Neurology 1989;39:1400.
42. Benedek DM, Peterson KA. Sertraline for treatment of pathological crying. Am J Psychiatry 1995;152:953–954.
43. Andersen G, Vestergaard K, Riis JO. Citalopram for post-stroke pathological crying. Lancet 1993;342:837–839.
44. van Gijn J. Treating uncontrolled crying after stroke. Lancet 1993;342:816–817.
45. Andersen G, Ingeman-Nielsen M, Vestergaard K, Riis JO. Pathoanatomic correlation between poststroke pathological crying and damage to brain areas involved in serotonergic neurotransmission. Stroke: J Cereb Circulation 1994;25:1050–1052.
46. Wolf J, Santana H, Thorpy M. Treatement of "emotional incontinence" with levodopa. Neurology 1979;29:1435–1436.
47. Udaka F, Yamao S, Nagata H, et al. Pathologic laughing and crying treated with levodopa. Arch Neurol 1984;41:1095–1096.
48. Massey E, Lowe S. Lithium carbonate in pseudobulbar palsy. Ann Neurol 1981;9:97.
49. Jankovic J. Amitriptyline in amyotrophic lateral sclerosis. N Engl J Med 1985;313:1478–1479.

50. Gamper E. Bau und Leistungen eines menschlichen Mittelhirnswesens. Neurology 1926;102:154–235.

51. Monnier M, Willi H. Die integrative Tatigkeit des Nervensystems beim Meso-Rhombo-Spinalen Anencephalus (Mittelhirnwesen). Mechr Psychiatr Neurol 1953;126:239–273.

52. Kahn E. On facial expression. In: Shillito J, Cotter W, Flanigan S, et al, eds. Clinical neurosurgery. Proceedings of the Congress of Neurological Surgeons. Baltimore: Williams and Wilkins, 1966:9–22.

53. Monrad-Krohn G. On the dissociation of voluntary and emotional innervation in facial paresis of central origin. Brain 1924;47:22–35.

54. Remillard G, Andermann F, Rhi-Sausi A, Robbins N. Facial asymmetry in patients with temporal lobe epilepsy. Neurology 1977;27:109–114.

55. Jackson JH. Discussions at the Neurological Society on muscular hypertonicity in paralysis. In: Taylor J, ed. Selected writings of John Hughlings Jackson. London: Hodder and Stoughton, 1932:472–476.

56. Brown J. Affect: mind, brain and consciousness. New York: Academic Press, 1977:126–135.

57. Nieuwenhuys R, Voogd J, van Huijzen C. The human central nervous system. 3rd rev. ed. New York: Springer-Verlag, 1981.

58. MacLean P. Brain evolution relating to family, play and the separation call. Arch Gen Psychiatry 1985;42:405–417.

59. Ploog D. Biological foundations of the vocal expressions of emotions. In: Plutchik R, Kellerman H, eds. Emotion theory, research and experience. Orlando: Academic Press, 1986:173–197.

60. Mesulam M. Principles of behavioral neurology. Philadelphia: FA Davis, 1985:1–70.

61. Nauta W. The central visceromotor system: a general survey. In: Hockman C, ed. Limbic system mechanics and autonomic function. Springfield: Charles C. Thomas, 1972:21–38.

62. Tatemichi T, Nichols F, Mohr J. Pathological crying: a pontine pseudobulbar syndrome. Ann Neurol 1987;22:133. Abstract.

63. Herman B, Panksepp J. Ascending endorphin inhibition of distress vocalization. Science 1981;211:1060–1062.

Pathologic Laughter

SAMUEL F. BERKOVIC   FREDERICK ANDERMANN

Splen turmidus nocet, risum tamen addit ineptum.
(People with swollen spleens have foolish laughter.)
—Q. Serenus Samonicus, 250 AD

INTRODUCTION

Laughter is a complex yet intimately familiar phenomenon whose occurrence as a symptom of disease has long fascinated physicians. An individual's laugh is often regarded as an integral part of his or her personality and, thus, its perversion by illness frequently causes dismay and bewilderment in patients and relatives.

The ancient Greeks believed that the spleen produced laughter by cleansing the black bile, and this view persisted until at least 1000 years ago. Laughter as an expression of neurologic disease was not generally appreciated until the end of the nineteenth century.

Trousseau in 1873 clearly recognized laughter as an occasional epileptic manifestation (1), although, according to Temkin, Erastus (1581) should be given priority (2). Féré in 1903 described the remarkable phenomenon of *le fou rire prodromique*, referring to inappropriate bouts of laughter as the prodrome to an attack of hemiplegia (3). The pathologic substrate for abnormal laughter was first explored by Oppenheim and Siemerling (1886), by Brissaud (1895), and by Nothnagel (1889), but it was the 1924 contribution of Wilson that stands as the early landmark of clarification in this complex field (4–7).

DIAGNOSIS

Normal laughter occurring in an appropriate social context is associated with an emotional feeling of mirth and is expressed as a characteristic motor pattern. Pathologic laughter is deceptively difficult to define, and the term has been used in different ways by various authors.

Poeck adopts the strictest and narrowest definition, demanding that four criteria be met. First, that the laughter occurs in response to nonspecific stimuli. Second, that there is no corresponding change in affect. Third, that there is no voluntary control of the extent and duration of the change in facial expression. Finally, that there is no corresponding change in mood lasting beyond the actual laughter and no relief after the laughter (8).

This definition excludes emotional lability in diffuse organic brain diseases, where the patient is overcome by emotional responses. These attacks are regarded as abnormalities of emotion rather than of the expression of same. Similarly, *witzelsucht* is regarded as an abnormality of an excessive emotional oscillation rather than an abnormality of the laughter mechanism itself (8). For clinical purposes, however, it is appropriate to include these phenomena under the broad rubric of pathologic laughter.

Laughter in epileptic seizures is particularly difficult to define. The presence of a change in affect or mood and the patient's subjective appreciation of the phenomenon usually cannot be determined, as consciousness is often impaired. We rely simply on the sounds that are made. At times epileptic laughter may have the features of typical infectious laughter that resembles the patient's normal laugh. More often, however, the character of the laughter varies and it is difficult to determine its precise resemblance to the patient's normal laugh.

It is a common human experience to observe somebody in an obvious emotional state and to be uncertain as to whether they are laughing or crying. Similarly, when hearing sounds and not observing the person, this difficulty may be compounded. There seems to be no definable characteristics to the sound that identifies laughter in its normal or pathologic forms. We will therefore use pathologic laughter in its broader sense, which perhaps can be best encapsulated as "in the ear of the beholder."

The types of pathologic laughter will now be described under the headings of nonepileptic laughter and epileptic laughter.

NONEPILEPTIC LAUGHTER

Le Fou Rire Prodromique

This is a spectacular but rare clinical event characterized by prolonged laughing, with preserved consciousness, prior to an apoplectic event such as hemiplegia, sometimes culminating in death. First described by Féré (3), a small number of subsequent cases have been described (9–12); the most remarkable, reported by Martin, bears repetition.

Case Study
A man aged 25 years had his first attack of uncontrollable laughter while attending his mother's funeral. He was admitted to hospital and had one or two more attacks, without any apparent cause for hilarity and was distressed by these attacks. A few days later he was found dead in bed and at postmortem a large ruptured aneurysm was found in the interpeduncular space, compressing the mammillary bodies and elevating the anterior part of the third ventricle (11).

Other cases have been described that progressed to hemiplegia, but not death, sometimes due to a proven cerebral hemorrhage (11,12). This remarkable syndrome is excessively rare and probably more so now with better control of hypertension.

Pseudobulbar Palsy

Pseudobulbar palsy is the commonest cause of pathologic laughter. It is due to bilateral lesions of the corticobulbar connections, which may be interrupted anywhere from the cortex itself to the lower brainstem. Pseudobulbar palsy is nearly always caused by multiple or diffuse lesions, but rarely may occur with a single strategically placed pontine lesion (11–16). Rarely, pontine lesions may cause pathologic laughing and crying without clinical features of pseudobulbar palsy. Such exceptional cases may represent lesions of the putative faciorespiratory control center (see "Basic Science," below) that may have a modulating influence on the corticobulbar tracts (17).

The usual causes of pseudobulbar palsy are motor neuron disease, advanced multiple sclerosis, and bilateral vascular lesions. Bilateral vascular lesions anywhere along the corticobulbar pathway may be responsible, but the classic cause is multiple lacunar infarcts in the internal capsule (état lacunaire). Rarer causes include progressive supranuclear palsy, head injury, and neoplastic, vascular, or inflammatory disorders of the brainstem (11–17).

These patients typically have bilateral upper motor neuron paresis of the bulbar and facial muscles. The face is mask-like with a paucity of expression. There is an explosive "Donald Duck" dysarthria, dysphagia, regurgitation, and drooling. The tongue appears small and spastic and cannot be protruded beyond the lips. The palatal reflexes and jaw jerk are exaggerated, and pyramidal signs are usually evident in the limbs (16).

Superimposed on this state of facial and bulbar immobility are periods of forced pathologic laughter. These may be provoked by attempts to speak, excitement or emotions of any kind, or may appear spontaneously. The patient is usually aware that the laughter is inappropriate, and this may cause severe embarrassment if laughter occurs when a patient is informed of sad news such as the death of a relative (8,12–16).

According to Ironside, such pathologic laughter can also occur with exclusively bulbar nuclear lesions (12). He based this conclusion on a clinicopathologic study of motor neuron disease. Although there was said to be no supranuclear involvement, the jaw jerk was exaggerated in his cases. Nuclear bulbar paralysis is not, however, generally accepted as a cause of pathologic laughter.

Single Cerebral Lesions

Although the majority of cases of nonepileptic pathologic laughter have bilateral lesions, Poeck and Pilleri assembled a small autopsy series from the literature with single lesions (8,18). Supratentorial lesions usually involved both the anterior limb of the internal capsule and the adjacent deep gray matter. Single cortical lesions cannot produce the phenomenon (8,18). Swash reported a well-studied clinical case of temporal lobe infarction with pathologic laughter, but the extent of the lesion was not known, nor was a subclinical contralateral lesion excluded (19). As noted above, single unilateral supranuclear brainstem lesions may also rarely cause pathologic laughter with or without features of pseudobulbar palsy.

Diffuse Cerebral Disease and *Witzelsucht*

Pathologic laughter can be a feature of a wide variety of dementias with diffuse cerebral abnormalities. It is well known in Alzheimer's disease and other common dementias, but is also regarded as a characteristic feature of tertiary syphilis and of kuru. Unlike the forced laughter of pseudobulbar palsy, the patient laughs excessively, or more commonly cries, in response to a minor but appropriate stimuli (*Affekt-Inkontinenz*). The patient cannot suppress the laughter, but it can be interrupted if his or her attention is diverted. Mood is altered in parallel with the emotional expression and, as pointed out by Poeck, the phenomenon is strictly a disorder of mood, rather than one of laughter itself (8).

More persistent elevations of mood, with or without marked mood swings, may also occur in diffuse cerebral disorders. *Witzelsucht* is a peculiar form of self-parody, classically described as a feature of tertiary syphilis. The patient is inappropriately euphoric and makes remarks, which he or she regards as humorous, directed at his or her own actions or words (20).

Miscellaneous

Psychiatric disorders are important causes of abnormal laughter. Kraepelin himself (1883) emphasized abnormal laughter as a symptom of schizophrenia, as did Bleuler in 1911. Laughter can be a feature of hysteria, and even of epidemic hysteria (15). Inappropriate laughter can also be seen as an effect of intoxicants and hallucinogens.

Pathologic laughter, of uncertain mechanism, occurs in the rare "happy puppet" syndrome of Angelman (21). Puppet children have severe developmental delay, microcephaly, protruding tongues, ataxic gait, puppet-like arm movements, and paroxysms of laughter (20,21).

EPILEPTIC LAUGHTER

Laughter as a part of epileptic seizures is uncommon, but it has created an unusual amount of interest (1,2,22–36). Presumably this is because of the incongruity of the expression of hilarity occurring in an event as serious as an epileptic seizure. The term gelastic epilepsy (*gelan*, to laugh; Greek) has been used (22). It must be emphasized, however, that laughing seizures do not constitute a specific epileptic disorder (24).

Epileptic laughter can occur as a feature of a variety of epileptic syndromes, both focal and generalized, but two causes of epileptic laughter account for the majority of cases. The commoner type occurs as a manifestation of temporal lobe epilepsy, and the other as part of a peculiar epileptic syndrome associated with hypothalamic hamartomas.

Temporal Lobe Epilepsy

Temporal lobe epilepsy is the usual cause of laughing seizures (22–28). Vocalization is a common feature of complex partial seizures of temporal lobe origin, but it usually involves nondescript utterances such as grunts, squeaks, or cries, occasionally understandable words, and rarely laughter. The presence of laughter does not strongly correlate with the cause, lateralization, electroencephalographic (EEG) characteristics, or associated clinical features of the temporal lobe seizures. It is our impression, however, both from personal cases and the literature, that laughter is a more common feature of temporal lobe seizures in children than in adults. This may reflect the fact that the observer may be more likely to interpret repetitive high-pitched vocalizations as laughter in a child.

Laughter in temporal lobe seizures usually occurs when the patient is unconscious. There may or may not be a preceding aura, and there generally is no recollection of the event. More rarely, the patient may be partially or completely aware of the sounds, but usually they do not feel amused. Fear is the typical affective accompaniment of temporal lobe seizures, and laughing seizures arising from the temporal lobe are no exception. Nevertheless, the observer may be impressed by the mirthful and infectious quality of the laughter and the apparently amused expression of the patient. Relatives may be able to distinguish the patient's natural laughter from the laughing seizures.

The manifestations of complex partial seizures often gradually vary in patients with chronic temporal lobe epilepsy. In some patients, laughing seizures may be reported for a few months or years and then disappear or be replaced by other vocalizations that do not resemble laughter.

Diagnosis is usually not difficult. The patient may report an aura suggestive of temporal lobe seizures, but, more important, eyewitnesses will describe the typical components of a complex partial seizure. The EEG will often show focal temporal interictal epileptiform discharges (22–28).

Hypothalamic Hamartomas

Hypothalamic hamartomas usually take the form of nodules attached to the tuber cinereum or mammillary bodies. They may be asymptomatic throughout life or they may be associated with precocious puberty, with a peculiar epileptic syndrome, or with both. The epileptic syndrome is a generalized epileptic encephalopathy with laughing seizures (26,29–35).

Laughing seizures characteristically begin in infancy, sometimes within the neonatal period. The laughter is brief, frequent, and usually not associated with any discernible loss of consciousness. Often the diagnosis is delayed; one of our patients won a "happy baby" competition. Psychomotor development is usually normal in the preschool years, although the seizures may become a little longer and be associated with loss of awareness, facial jerking, and, rarely, running (26,30,32,34,35).

The disorder enters a more ominous phase in the later half of the first decade. Tonic, atonic, and tonic-clonic seizures develop, cognitive impairment is evident, and the EEG shows generalized slow spike-and-wave discharges—the typical electroclinical picture of a severe secondary generalized epilepsy. Laughing attacks continue and may usher in the other forms of seizure. Behavior difficulties are common, and rage attacks may occur. Seizures continue through adolescence and adult life, although laughter may be less prominent (34,35).

The laughter in this disorder is characteristically mirthless, noninfectious, and mechanical. Certainly, the patients never feel amused. Gascon and Lombroso observed that the character of laughter in this disorder was quite different from that seen in temporal lobe epilepsy, with the latter having more of an affective component (26). Although we partially agree with this view, the laughing attacks of hypothalamic hamartomas in early childhood can be difficult to distinguish from normal laughter, and the attacks in temporal lobe epilepsy can certainly be mirthless and non-infectious.

Diagnosis of this disorder is often delayed, probably because it is not widely known. The clinical picture is highly characteristic, the association of laughing seizures and precocious puberty being pathognomonic (34). Even when precocious puberty is absent, a careful history usually reveals laughing seizures from very early life. Although a neonatal onset of temporal lobe laughing seizures has been reported (36), this is extremely rare, and laughing seizures dating from infancy virtually always indicate a hypothalamic hamartoma. The lesions can sometimes be difficult to visualize with computed tomography scanning, but are well shown by magnetic resonance imaging (34).

Rarer Causes of Epileptic Laughter

Complex partial seizures associated with laughter usually originate from the temporal lobe, but may rarely begin in the frontal lobes (24). Laughing seizures in frontal lobe epilepsy do not appear to have any distinguishing features.

Exceptionally, lesions in the hypothalamic area that are not hamartomas are associated with epileptic laughter (29,37). Usually these are gangliogliomas, although the pathologic distinction between hamartoma and ganglioglioma is not clear-cut. Conventional hypothalamic gliomas rarely, if ever, cause epileptic laughter.

Laughter-like vocalizations have also been described in infantile spasms and occasionally as components of generalized myoclonic or tonic seizures (23,24). The latter have been noted especially in association with generalized epileptic encephalopathies due to encephalitis or to storage disorders such as Tay-Sachs and Niemann-Pick diseases (23–25). Care must be taken to distinguish brief laughing seizures with atonia from laughter-induced cataplexy, which is not an epileptic phenomenon (38).

MANAGEMENT

Pseudobulbar Palsy

Treatment of pathologic laughter in pseudobulbar palsy is difficult. The underlying disease processes are usually progressive and untreatable, although some spontaneous improvement can be expected following an acute stroke that has resulted in the syndrome. Stimuli known to provoke outbursts of laughter or crying in the individual patient should be avoided if possible.

Pharmacologic treatment may be beneficial (39–43), although brain-damaged patients may be quite sensitive to side effects of psychotropic medication. L-Dopa and amantadine have been used in stroke patients and reported as effective in open trials (40,41). Stronger evidence supports the use of tricyclic antidepressants, especially amitriptyline, in pseudobulbar palsy due to stroke and multiple sclerosis (39,42). Fluoxetine, a serotonin reuptake inhibitor, has been used successfully in a stroke patient who failed to respond to amitriptyline (43).

Epileptic Laughter

Laughing seizures due to temporal lobe epilepsy respond to the same measures used for temporal lobe epilepsy in general. Carbamazepine is the drug of choice, with phenytoin, the barbiturates, and benzodiazepines being second-line drugs. Approximately one-third of chronic cases will be refractory despite optimal medical therapy, and surgical treatment by temporal lobectomy may be considered. The presence of laughing seizures does not alter the principles of presurgical evaluation or the surgical success rate (44).

Treatment of laughing seizures associated with hypothalamic hamartomas is extremely difficult. Anticonvulsants have little or no effect on the laughing seizures, although there may be some benefit with respect to the more disabling associated tonic, atonic, and tonic-clonic seizures. Excision of the hamartoma does not influence the seizure disorder (34).

BASIC SCIENCE

Laughter Centers

In 1924 Wilson (7) proposed an anatomic model for the expression and control of laughter, based on Jacksonian principles of cerebral organization. He postulated a supranuclear pontobulbar center controlling input to the facial nerve nucleus, nucleus ambiguus, and anterior horn cells in the upper cervical cord that subserves the phrenic nerve. This center coordinates the facial and respiratory movements that constitute the motor aspects of laughter and is under both voluntary and involuntary control from higher centers. The voluntary and involuntary control systems utilize different anatomic pathways. These aspects of Wilson's model are generally accepted, based essentially on clinical evidence (8,45). However, the exact routes of the voluntary and involuntary control pathways through the brainstem and the anatomic correlate of Wilson's faciorespiratory center remain unknown. Pathologic laughter in pseudobulbar palsy is easily explained by this model as a "release phenomenon" due to lesions of the voluntary pathway.

Wilson also suggested that there was an integrative center in the region of the medial thalamus, subthalamus, and hypothalamus (7). The presence of such a deep midline laughter center is supported by clinical cases of laughter associated with lesions in this region, particularly of the hypothalamus, but the critical anatomic structures in the diencephalon are not known. Clinical data includes remarkable descriptions of mechanical stimulation of the floor of the third ventricle under local anesthesia in humans producing laughter (46). Second, apoplectic events associated with *le fou rire prodromique* typically involve hemorrhages in the deep midline gray matter structures (3,11). Finally, the ictal laughter associated with hypothalamic hamartomas strongly supports the importance of this region in the genesis of laughter. The mechanism of laughter in this syndrome is unclear. Ictal EEG recordings from the scalp may show no change, generalized desynchronization, or generalized epileptic discharges. It is unclear whether these laughing attacks are true hypothalamic seizures or if they represent an automatism or release phenomenon due to more widespread epileptic activity (34).

Cortical Control

Laughter induced by lesions in the hypothalamus and brainstem typically lacks subjective and objective qualities of mirth. Indeed, Martin used the term "sham mirth" to highlight this (11). It seems that the affective qualities of laughter require the involvement of other structures of the limbic system and of the cerebral cortex. Appreciation of humor and the emotion of mirth must involve these "higher" centers. Thus, the motor and affective components of normal laughter are generated in the cortex and processed in the deep midline structures in and around the hypothalamus, and the final motor output is coordinated in Wilson's putative pontine faciorespiratory center.

Little is known about the cortical structures crucial for appreciation of humor and for laughter generation. The importance of the limbic cortical structures in emotion has been known since Papez's seminal paper (47). The fact that laughing seizures most often are associated with temporal lobe epilepsy supports the importance of the temporal lobe structures in the generation of laughter. The frontal lobes are also likely to be important as they are most often implicated as the major focus of disease in pseudobulbar palsy.

Attempts have been made to lateralize the cortical structures for appreciation of humor and for regulation of emotion. There is considerable evidence supporting the preeminent role of the right hemisphere in the appreciation and modulation of emotion (48,49). Retrospective reviews have suggested that destructive lesions causing nonepileptic laughter or euphoric mood are predominantly right sided, whereas epileptic laughter more often arises in the left temporal lobe than the right. These data are open to question because of their retrospective method of collection, although they are broadly in agreement with certain other data regarding the lateralization of emotional regulation (28,48,49). Unfortunately, the correlation with laterality is insufficiently strong to be of any use in clinical lateralization. Indeed, the relative weakness of the correlation urges caution in the speculative interpretation of these findings with respect to models of the cortical organization of emotion.

Virtually nothing is known about the neurotransmitters involved in the generation of laughter. However, the therapeutic effect of tricyclic antidepressants and of fluoxetine in pseudobulbar palsy (see above) argues for a role of the monoaminergic systems.

ACKNOWLEDGMENTS

Dr Berkovic was supported by the National Health and Medical Research Council of Australia.

REFERENCES

1. Trousseau A. Clinique Médicale de l'Hôtel-Dieu de Paris. 4th ed. Paris: Baillière, 1873:409.
2. Temkin O. The falling sickness. Baltimore: Johns Hopkins Press, 1971: 190–191.
3. Féré C. Le fou rire prodromique. Rev Neurol 1903;11:353–358.
4. Oppenheim H, Siemerling E. Mittheilungen über Pseudobulbärparalyse und acute Bulbärparalyse. Berl Klin Wochenschr 1886;23:791–794.
5. Brissaud E. Lecons sur les maladies nerveuses (Salpètrière, 1893–94). Paris: Masson, 1895.
6. Nothnagel H. Zur Diagnose der Schügelerkrakungen. Z Klin Med 1889;16:424–430.
7. Wilson SAK. Some problems in neurology. No II. Pathological laughing and crying. J Neurol Psychopathol 1924;4:299–333.
8. Poeck K. Pathological laughter and crying. In: Vinken PJ, Bruyn GW, Klawans HL, eds. Handbook of clinical neurology. vol. 45. Amsterdam: Elsevier, 1985:219–225.
9. Andersen C. Crise de rire spasmodique avant décès: hémorragie thalamique double. J Belge Neurol Psychiatr 1936;36:223–227.
10. Badt B. Lachen als erstes Symptom eines apoplektischen Insultes. Z Neurol Psychiatrie 1927;110:297–300.
11. Martin JP. Fits of laughter (sham-mirth) in organic cerebral disease. Brain 1950;73:453–464.
12. Ironside R. Disorders of laughter due to brain lesions. Brain 1956;79:589–609.
13. Davison C, Kelman H. Pathologic laughing and crying. Arch Neurol Psychiatry 1939;42:595–632.
14. Poeck K. Pathophysiology of emotional disorders associated with brain damage. In: Vinken PJ, Bruyn GW, eds. Handbook of clinical neurology. vol. 3. Amsterdam: North Holland, 1969:343–367.
15. Black DW. Pathological laughter: a review of the literature. J Nerv Ment Dis 1982;170:67–71.
16. DeJong RN. The neurologic examination. 4th ed. Hagerstown, MD: Harper & Row, 1979:264–265.
17. Asfora WT, De Salles AAF, Abe N, Kjellberg RN. Is the syndrome of pathological laughing and crying a manifestation of pseudobulbar palsy? J Neurol Neurosurg Psychiatry 1989;52:523–525.
18. Poeck K, Pilleri G. Pathologisches lachen uno weinen. Schweiz Arch Neurol Psychiatr 1963;92:323–370.
19. Swash M. Released involuntary laughter after temporal lobe infarction. J Neurol Neurosurg Psychiatry 1972;35:108–113.
20. Duchowny MS. Pathological disorders of laughter. In: McGhee PE, Goldstein JH, eds. Handbook of humour research. vol. II. New York: Springer-Verlag, 1983:89–108.
21. Angelman H. Puppet children: a report on three cases. Dev Med Child Neurol 1965;7:681–688.
22. Daly DD, Mulder DW. Gelastic epilepsy. Neurology 1957;7:189–192.
23. Druckman R, Chao D. Laughter in epilepsy. Neurology 1957;7:26–36.
24. Loiseau P, Cohadon F, Cohadon S. Gelastic epilepsy; a review and report of five cases. Epilepsia 1971;12:313–323.
25. Chen RC, Forster FM. Cursive epilepsy and gelastic epilepsy. Neurology 1973;23:1019–1029.

26. Gascon GG, Lombroso CT. Epileptic (gelastic) laughter. Epilepsia 1971;12:63–76.
27. Yamada H, Yoshida H. Laughing attack: a review and report of nine cases. Folia Psychiatr Neurol Jpn 1977;31:129–137.
28. Myslobodsky MS. Epileptic laughter. In: Myslobodsky MS, ed. Hemisyndromes: psychobiology, neurology, psychiatry. New York: Academic Press, 1983:239–263.
29. List CF, Dowman CE, Bagchi BK, Bebin J. Posterior hypothalamic hamartomas and gangliogliomas causing precocious puberty. Neurology 1958;8:164–174.
30. Sher PK, Brown SB. Gelastic epilepsy; onset in neonatal period. Am J Dis Child 1976;130:1126–1131.
31. Diebler C, Ponsot G. Hamartomas of the tuber cinereum. Neuroradiology 1983;25:93–101.
32. Ponsot G, Diebler C, Plouin P, et al. Hamartomes hypothalamiques et crises de rire. Arch Fr Pediatr 1983;40:757–761.
33. Breningstall GN. Gelastic seizures, precocious puberty, and hypothalamic hamartoma. Neurology 1985;35:1180–1183.
34. Berkovic SF, Andermann F, Melanson D, et al. Hypothalamic hamartomas and associated ictal laughter: evolution of the characteristic epileptic syndrome and diagnostic value of magnetic resonance imaging. Ann Neurol 1988;23:429–439.
35. Andermann F, Berkovic S. Secondary generalized epilepsy in patients with hypothalamic hamartoma, precocious puberty, and laughing attacks: a study of five patients. In: Niedermeyer E, Degen R, eds. The Lennox-Gastaut syndrome. New York: AR Liss, 1988:433–446.
36. Mutani R, Agnetti V, Durelli L, et al. Epileptic laughter: electroclinical and cinefilm report of a case. J Neurol 1979;220:215–222.
37. Dott NM. Surgical aspects of the hypothalamus. In: Le Gros Clark WE, Beattie J, Riddoch G, Dott NM, eds. The hypothalamus: morphological, functional, clinical and surgical aspects. Edinburgh: Oliver and Boyd, 1938:131–185.
38. Duchowny MS, Deray MJ, Papazian O. Narcolepsy-cataplexy and gelastic-atonic seizures. Neurology 1985;35:775–776.
39. Lawson IR, MacLeod RDM. The use of imipramine ("Tofranil") and other psychotropic drugs in organic emotionalism. Br J Psychiatry 1969;115:281–285.
40. Wolf JK, Santana HB, Thorpy M. Treatment of "emotional incontinence" with levodopa. Neurology 1979;29:1435–1436.
41. Udaka F, Yamao S, Nagata H, et al. Pathologic laughing and crying treated with levodopa. Arch Neurol 1984;41:1095–1096.
42. Schiffer RB, Herndon RM, Rudick RA. Treatment of pathologic laughing and weeping with amitriptyline. N Engl J Med 1985;312:1480–1482.
43. Seliger GM, Hornstein A. Serotonin, fluoxetine and pseudobulbar affect. Neurology 1989;39:1400.
44. Engel J Jr, ed. Surgical treatment of the Epilepsies. New York: Raven Press, 1987:707.
45. Monrad-Kohn GH. On facial dissociation. Acta Psychiatr Neurol 1939;14:557–566.
46. Foerster O, Gagel O. Ein Fall von Ependymcyste des III Ventrikels: Ein Beitrag zur Frage der Beziehungen psychischer. Störungen zum Hirnstamm. Z Neurol Psychiatr 1933;149:312–344.
47. Papez JW. A proposed mechanism of emotion. Arch Neurol Psychiatry 1937;38:725–743.
48. Sackhiem HA, Greenberg MS, Weiman AL, et al. Hemispheric asymmetry in the expression of positive and negative emotions. Arch Neurol 1982;39:210–218.
49. Bear DM. Hemispheric specialization and the neurology of emotion. Arch Neurol 1982;40:195–202.

Disturbances in Language Initiation: Mutism and Its Lesser Forms

Michael P. Alexander

INTRODUCTION

Initiation of language production is impaired in a variety of neurologic and psychiatric conditions. In some disorders mutism is the overwhelming clinical manifestation, for instance, in patients with infarction in the distal portions of the left anterior cerebral artery territory (1). In other disorders, the impaired initiation is commensurate with widespread signs of delayed motor initiation, for instance, patients with Parkinson's disease (2). Delayed initiation of language may also be embedded in a general poverty and slowness of mental operations, often called abulia (3); large prefrontal tumors or moderately advanced Alzheimer's disease would be examples. So too, from a different perspective might be profound depression (4) and the "negative sign" schizophrenias (5).

This review will highlight five aspects of delayed initiation of language.

1. It must be recognized that there are major and minor forms of the problem.
2. Delayed initiation of language can be seen after lesions in several brain regions. Analysis of the array of possible lesion sites in the context of animal investigations on relevant anatomic connections suggests that it may be possible to define broadly the systems that are involved in language initiation as afferent or efferent. These systems share the supplementary motor areas and the anterior cingulate gyri.
3. Available evidence supports the conclusion that part of the afferent system is dopaminergic.
4. The afferent system may not have any lateralized dominance, but the efferent system is partially lateralized to the left hemisphere.

5. There are several dimensions in which this system of language initiation may be important in clinical psychiatry.

FORMS OF THE DEFICIT IN LANGUAGE INITIATION

The most severe impairment is the inability to produce language at all despite normal, or at least adequate, attention and nonverbal responsiveness. Differential diagnosis also demands exclusion of cases with profound motor disturbances and anarthria, on either a brainstem or an upper motor neuron basis. The specific inability to produce speech is customarily referred to as mutism, although it might be logically consistent to label this behavior as akinesia for language. In milder forms, the patient is not entirely mute but has various lesser forms of disordered production. These might include long delays in production or simplification of utterances (6). The patient might assume a generally terse and laconic style of response. There may be initially normal production but progressively briefer and less elaborated utterances over time until responses cease altogether (3). These disturbances could all be considered hypokinesia for language. Standard terminology fails clinical observation at this point, but there is no evidence from clinical or animal studies that there is anything but a smooth continuum of deficits in the recruitment of language. For this review all references to mutism should be understood to refer as well to all of the less profound impairments. Likewise, all references to hypokinesia, delays, long latencies, or terseness should be understood to refer to lesser forms of mutism.

A second important point about the impairment in initiation is that it is independent of the content of language.

Many patients with mutism are not aphasic; when they do speak, the structure and form may be normal (7). Some patients with aphasia are transiently mute and/or have persistent delays in the initiation of whatever language that they can produce (6,8). Lesions that result in many of the anterior aphasias also damage the efferent system of language initiation (see below). In these aphasic profiles, delayed initiation may be a portion of the communication deficit, but the initiation system can be damaged without any disturbance in the form or content of language. Initiation refers to *why* we talk; aphasia refers to myriads of types of deficits in *how* we talk.

A final point about the clinical manifestations of mutism concerns the accompanying deficits. The prototypical syndrome is akinetic mutism. Patients have global akinesia and apathy (3). Cognitive impairments are uniformly observed, and they are usually of a profile that is considered "frontal" (9,10)—psychomotor retardation, poor reasoning, poor abstract thinking, poor mental flexibility, and forgetfulness, if not frank amnesia. In milder cases or after partial recovery, the mental impairment may be subtle—slight slowness in solving complex problems, mildly reduced verbal fluency, etc. With some lesion types, the dementia is so profound that special focus on the overall mental state is required. The cognitive deficits of akinetic mutism are not the topic of this chapter, but in all cases to be described below (except the deep left lateral frontal lesions) this profile of mental impairments at some level of severity can be assumed to accompany the poor language initiation.

LESIONS PRODUCING MUTISM: IMPLICATIONS FOR ORGANIZATION OF LANGUAGE INITIATION

Evidence for specific anatomic substrates of mutism comes from many sources. In 1941, Cairns et al (11) described a young woman with akinetic mutism associated with a craniopharyngioma impinging on the region of the anterior third ventricle. Decompression of the cyst produced prompt resolution of mutism; shunting of the associated hydrocephalus did not affect the clinical state. There have been other reports confirming the correlation between this region and akinetic mutism. Ross and Stewart (12) described a patient with akinetic mutism after removal of a cystic craniopharyngioma at the anterior margin of the third ventricle; computed tomography (CT) demonstrated extensive injury to the region immediately anterior and inferior to the third ventricle. This case is of particular importance because the investigators were able to demonstrate specific neuropharmacologic mechanisms of mutism (see the discussion below).

There are numerous reports of akinetic mutism after bilateral damage to the anterior portions of the cingulate gyri (13–17). Very few of these cases, perhaps cases 1 and 3 of Buge et al (16), have had small discrete lesions of the anterior cingulate. Most have also had considerable damage

in the medial superior frontal gyrus, the deep frontal white matter, or the heads of the caudate nuclei. The very small lesions of surgical cingulectomy have not, on the other hand, been associated with persistent mutism (18), but some variation upon diminished responsiveness to emotional and painful stimuli has been used to account for the favorable, at least transiently, effect of cingulotomy on obsessive states and chronic pain states.

Damage to the supplementary motor area (SMA), the medial and premotor portion of the superior frontal gyrus, has often been reported as a cause of mutism (1,6,8,19). The vast majority of the cases reported have been unilateral left-sided injury, but isolated right SMA injury may also produce mutism (20,21). The majority of cases with SMA lesions of either side have initially had global akinesia with evolution over days to weeks to only contralateral akinesia. Small unilateral left lesions may cause only brief mutism (19). Larger left prefrontal lesions, including the cingulate, produce very long-lasting mutism and permanent reduction in ease of initiation and elaboration of discourse (8).

Lesions in the deep left frontal white matter adjacent to and immediately superior to the anterior frontal horn of the lateral ventricle also produce transient mutism (6,22). It is an issue of controversy in aphasia studies whether cases with either purely SMA damage, extensive medial frontal damage including SMA, or deep anterior periventricular white matter damage should be considered aphasic (6). The syndrome of transcortical motor aphasia (TCMA) is characterized by effortful, delayed utterances that are usually truncated and grammatically incomplete (23). Comprehension and repetition are normal. With recovery, the patients may not seem overtly aphasic beyond minor naming problems, but they remain impaired on all tests of spontaneous, extended language generation. Freedman et al (6) suggested that TCMA includes impaired initiation as one, but only one, of its features. It is the extension of lesion into the deep anterior, superior periventricular white matter that generates that one feature.

Damage to the putamen (bilateral or left sided alone) may cause transient mutism (24–26). The course of recovery often includes a period of reduced spontaneous language. Other abnormalities associated with extrapyramidal motor impairments may be observed during recovery—rapid rate, hypophonia (presumably hypokinesia of voicing), and articulatory imprecision (presumably hypokinesia of articulation). Although less frequently reported, damage to the globus pallidus bilaterally may result in a very similar profile of mutism with global akinesia and apathy (27).

Damage to the thalamus has often been reported to produce mutism, usually with global akinesia. A literature based on very precise CT and magnetic resonance imaging (MRI) localization within the thalamus has developed in recent years (28–32), but two factors continue to limit the certainty of clinicoanatomic correlations. First, the variety of lesion locations within the thalamus associated with mutism simply precludes any unitary explanation of the role of the thalamus. Second, the most revealing cases are those with discrete infarctions, and the vascular territories of the thalamus are sufficiently unpredictable (29) that many cases have idiosyncratic lesion profiles that subtend numerous structures within the thalamus.

Bilateral damage to the paramedian thalamic (and rostral midbrain) regions, including the lateral dorsomedial (DM) nuclei, the centromedian (CM) nuclei, and the intralaminar (IL) nuclei, has been one commonly reported lesion profile (29,31,33–36). Most of these patients have had dramatic memory disorders and global attentional deficits. Persistent global akinesia has only occasionally been described (33), but remarkable mental apathy (abulia) and absence of spontaneous speech have been prominent (29,31,34–36). The much less commonly reported unilateral infarct of the left (37), but not the right, CM and ventrolateral nuclei may also produce transient mutism (or at least aspontaneity) with sparse, slow, underelaborated output.

Unilateral damage to the left, but not the right, lateral thalamic territory, including the ventrolateral nucleus, the anterior nucleus, and the ventroanterior nucleus, has also been reported to produce transient mutism (29,31,38,39). With recovery, these patients are often unequivocally aphasic, ranging from mild anomic aphasia (29) to severe transcortical sensory aphasia (38,39). In addition, many meet *Diagnostic and Statistical Manual of Mental Disorders, Revised Fourth Edition* criteria for dementia (40). But whatever the cognitive and language profile, the reduction in spontaneous vocalization is very prominent.

There are numerous reports concerning the effects on speech of thalamic tumors (41), thalamic hemorrhages (24,42), and thalamic surgery (43). The specific intrathalamic location of lesions is impossible to specify in many of the tumor and hemorrhage cases, but mutism is prominent. In the tumor cases, mutism has evolved as attention and overall responsiveness have declined (41). In hemorrhage cases, mutism has been essentially restricted to left-sided cases (24,42). In survivors, once mutism clears, a variety of aphasic profiles may emerge. The main literature on thalamic surgery comes from stereotactic procedures for Parkinson's disease (43). Patients with bilateral damage (or occasionally with solely left-sided surgery) to the ventrolateral nuclei were reported to show markedly reduced language output and hypophonia.

Finally, Botez and Barbeau (7) have summarized a number of disparate observations supporting the possibility that bilateral damage to the periaqueductal gray matter may result in prolonged mutism in humans. Most case material is impossible to interpret because of alterations in consciousness or severe bilateral elemental motor disturbances. Even the case with postmortem study cited by Botez and Barbeau had lesions extending down into the ventral tegmental area, a region of potential relevance to mutism to be discussed below. A more recent case with convincing periaqueductal damage also had bilateral paramedian diencephalic damage (44).

ANATOMIC INVESTIGATIONS IN ANIMALS

Jürgens (45) completed an examination of the afferent and efferent connections of the SMA in squirrel monkeys. These are summarized in Table 55.1. Most connections are bidirectional, but there are only afferent connections from the basal forebrain, the amygdala, the hypothalamus, and the reticular activating system in the brainstem. There are only efferent connections to the striatum. The dorsolateral frontal cortex, including all regions commonly considered to be motor (Brodmann's areas 4, 6, 44, and 8), is highly connected with the SMA through pathways that probably run over the anterior, superior margin of the lateral ventricle. Thalamic connections are particularly rich to and from the ventrolateral (VL), ventroanterior (VA), and DM nuclei. This anatomic placement between the limbic afferents is shared by the anterior cingulate (see below), to which the SMA is developmentally related (46).

Numerous behavioral studies in primates of the effects of lesions of the SMA have demonstrated a role in motor control and programming. It is well established that the SMA has bilateral motor system connections (47–49), and that lesions in SMA impair integration of bimanual activities (50) and impair initiation of motor activities (51). Impairments are more marked for behaviors that are difficult, volitional (that is, spontaneous and not simple responses to environmental stimuli), and that require concentration and effort. It has been demonstrated, for instance, that squirrel monkeys with bilateral SMA ablations have severely reduced free volitional vocalizations (52). Jürgens has interpreted the behavioral and anatomic literature to reflect a role for the SMA in the "initiation of global motor programs," including those for vocalization.

The connections of the anterior cingulate have been elaborated by Baleydier and Mauguiere (53). They are summarized in Figure 14 of that report and are briefly summarized here in Figure 55.1. Note again that most connections are bidirectional, the most striking exceptions being the purely efferent relationship with the striatum (including the nucleus accumbens) and the amygdala. The outflow to

Table 55.1 Connections of the Supplementary Motor Area

Afferent Connections	Efferent Connections
Frontal convexity (areas 9, 8, 6, 44, 4)	Frontal convexity
Parietal convexity (areas 2, 5, 7)	Parietal convexity
Superior temporal cortex	Anterior cingulate
Insular cortex	Putamen, caudate
Anterior cingulate	Thalamus (VA, VL, DM, CM)
Basal forebrain	Reticular activating system
Amygdala	
Thalamus (VA, VL, LP, PUL)	
Hypothalamus	
Reticular activating system	
Locus coerulus	

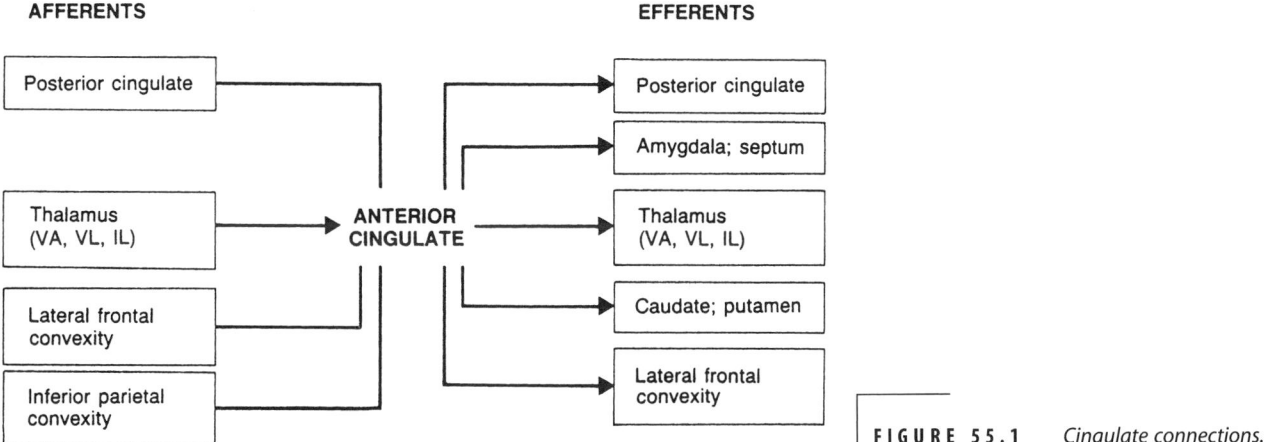

FIGURE 55.1   *Cingulate connections.*

the dorsal striatum is particularly rich, making up the subcallosal fasciculus (54), a major white matter bundle that lies just along the anterior, superior edge of the lateral ventricle. This structure may be particularly critical for speech and language initiation (55), and damage to this structure may account for the high frequency of impaired initiation with frontal periventricular lesions (6). There are rich afferent connections from the lateral frontal association cortex, the inferior parietal region, and the posterior cingulate, which is itself a polysensory convergence area. The thalamic connections are primarily to the ventroanterior, DM, and IL nuclei.

Other investigators had demonstrated that the hemispatial neglect induced in monkeys by lesions of the anterior cingulate was actually hemiakinesia (56). Bilateral lesions could be interpreted as bilateral or global akinesia. Baleydier and Mauguiere interpreted the anatomic and behavioral studies to suggest a role for the anterior cingulate "as a highly specialized motor area" primarily serving to initiate and organize (presumably volitionally) motor programs in response to emotional stimuli.

Regarding lesions of the midbrain, highly focused lesions in the periaqueductal gray matter may not result in akinetic mutism (57). It is possible, however, that there is a specific ascending mesencephalic system that is important in language initiation. There is evidence from animals (58) and from postmortem studies of humans with Parkinson's disease (59) that there are several related ascending dopaminergic systems. The substantia nigra is the origin of pathways that terminate in the striatum and perhaps the cingulum. The ventral tegmental area is the origin of pathways to the medial frontal cortex (58). Javoy-Agid and Agid and Ruberg et al have defined the separation of clinical effects of lesions in the various dopaminergic systems in Parkinson's disease (59) and progressive supranuclear palsy (60).

Lindvall et al (58) demonstrated that the route of the mesocortical pathways was through the medial forebrain bundle via the lateral hypothalamus rising through the deep medial frontal white matter to the medial frontal cortex. Global akinesia may be secondary to damage to either of these systems, whereas reduced language initiation and psychomotor retardation (abulia) may be more specifically related to damage to the mesocortical system. In this regard the patient of Ross and Stewart (12) is particularly revealing. This patient had had decompression of a cystic craniopharyngioma with postoperative akinetic mutism. Despite lack of any clinically significant response to methylphenidate or to L-dopa, the patient had dramatic amelioration of signs with high doses of bromocriptine, a direct dopaminergic agonist.

The findings in human lesion studies and animal anatomic and behavioral studies taken together suggest the following summary. There are at least three ascending afferent systems that are involved in triggering language initiation as well as motor programs of all types. One system originates in the mesencephalic tegmentum. The portion that terminates in the medial frontal cortex arises in the ventral tegmental area. The system is dopaminergic. A second system originates in the upper reticular formation, particularly the IL portions of the thalamus. It projects diffusely to the cortex, but more cogently to the topic of this report, to the anterior cingulate and SMA. A third system originates in limbic circuitry and via connections from the amygdala to the medial DM nucleus of the thalamus projects to the prefrontal association cortex. These systems may all be fairly symmetrically arrayed in the two hemispheres, and the available evidence suggests that the pathways are located in the periventricular white matter of the frontal lobe.

The outflow for these systems of initiation is at several levels of the nervous system. From SMA the important projections are to cortical motor and language systems, and for language the critical systems are in the left hemisphere. These projections to the left motor and language cortex are from the SMA of both hemispheres. In addition, there are key connections to the striatum, anterior cingulate, and ventrolateral nucleus of the thalamus. These pathways run in the immediate periventricular white matter near the anterior frontal horn of the lateral ventricle. This creates an efferent loop of SMA to dorsal striatum to dorsal globus pallidus to ventrolateral thalamus to SMA (61).

From the anterior cingulate, much the same set of loops is seen as for the SMA, but there are a few differences. The anterior cingulate also has outflow to the amygdala, the nucleus accumbens (ventral striatum), and the IL thalamus. So in addition to contributing to the loop defined above, a second loop is created of anterior cingulate to ventral striatum to ventral globus pallidus to lateral DM thalamus to medial frontal cortex to anterior cingulate (62). For the subcortical elements of this loop, it is not clear that there is any important lateralization to the left hemisphere.

All of these afferent and efferent loops contribute to the initiation and maintenance of a variety of activities, from the purely motor (speech) to the cognitive (language) to the behavioral (motivation). The SMA and anterior cingulate are particularly critical intersections of ascending mechanisms, including limbic ones, and efferent mechanisms, including those that loop back to the limbic system. The thalamus includes several nuclei that have different, if not exactly independent, roles in these loops, thus the overwhelming frequency of thalamic lesions in the literature of mutism. The striatum is also an important crossroads, with potentially different roles for the dorsal striatum (motor) and the ventral striatum (motivational/limbic).

CLINICAL IMPORTANCE IN PSYCHIATRY

The relevance to clinical psychiatry is threefold. First, it is essential to recognize these disorders for what they are. Patients may appear depressed, with their terse and delayed responses overlaying an emotionless mien, with forgetfulness and inattention, and loss of interest in pleasurable activities. But these patients are not depressed; many of them seem to have lost the capacity to become depressed. Their level of spontaneous involvement in their environment is very low. Mental activities—including language—are underactivated. Recent reports from France seem to capture this disorder perfectly, referring to *"perte de l'élan vital, de l'intérêt et de l'affectivité"* (26) or *"perte d'autoactivation psychique"* (27).

The treatment of psychiatric disorders may be an inadvertent mechanism for the production of akinetic mutism. Akinesia is often a part of neuroleptic-induced extrapyramidal disorder, but it is less well recognized that neuroleptics can produce a virtually pure akinesia (63). Prominent symptoms are delayed initiation of speech and reduced spontaneous speech and gesture. The mechanism is presumably dopaminergic blockade of the medial frontal and/or striatal dopamine systems. Other medications that decrease dopaminergic activity may have a similar effect. These include some antidepressants (64) and monoaminedepleting antihypertensives.

A third important factor for clinical psychiatry is the illumination provided on possible neurologic bases of important signs in psychiatric diagnoses. It would be presumptuous to assume that superficial similarities between the signs of very different diseases necessarily means that the basic neuropathologic processes are the same, but there are

at least two of interest for this paper. Schizophrenia is a disorder that has eluded pathophysiologic explanations. Some patients have a disorder that is labeled schizophrenia, but without the prominent hallucinatory/delusional state. This is variously considered "chronic" (40) or "negative" (5) schizophrenia. The prominent findings in these cases include poverty of thought, poverty of speech, apathy, and "loss of volition" (65). These signs are not successfully treated with neuroleptics (66), and it is even possible that this complex is related to a reduced dopaminergic state (65).

The second arena of psychiatry that might be illuminated by the clinicoanatomic bases of mutism is depression. A diagnosis of depression can be entertained in the presence of markedly diminished interests, hypersomnia, psychomotor retardation, and diminished concentration plus one more major criterion (40). This presumes exclusion of neurologic processes, of course, and it is unlikely that a patient with a large left frontal stroke would be mistaken for having primary affective disorder. But at least a portion of the signs of depression may be due to reduction of dopaminergic activity. Patients with depression can experience psychomotor activation with L-dopa treatment without improvement of mood (67). It is plausible, then, that some of the signs of psychiatric disorders may be due to dysfunction in one of the ascending afferent systems described above, perhaps the dopaminergic one.

The sign of impaired initiation of speech—mutism—has distinct neuropathologic bases. The function of initiating speech and language seems to be embedded in a complex afferent and efferent brain network. The afferent side is bilaterally represented in the brain and may be amenable to neurochemical manipulation (12). The efferent side has increasing lateralization to left-sided dominance as it moves from subcortical and medial structures to lateral cortical ones. Neurochemical treatment may be less effective on this side, but cognitive strategies that facilitate psychomotor activation may have a role (9,68).

REFERENCES

1. Alexander MP, Schmitt MA. The aphasia syndrome of stroke in the left anterior cerebral artery territory. Arch Neurol 1980;37:97–100.
2. McDowell FH, Lee JE, Sweet RD. Extrapyramidal diseases. In: Baker AB, Joynt RJ, eds. Clinical neurology. Philadelphia: Harper & Row, 1985.
3. Fisher CM. Honored guest presentation: abulia minor vs. agitated behavior. Clin Neurosurg 1985;31:9–31.
4. Cohen RM, Weingartner H, Smallberg SA, et al. Effort and cognition in depression. Arch Gen Psychiatry 1982;39:593–597.
5. Andreasen NC. Negative symptoms in schizophrenia. Arch Gen Psychiatry 1982;39:784–788.
6. Freedman M, Alexander MP, Naeser MA. Anatomical basis of transcortical motor aphasia. Neurology 1984;34:409–417.
7. Botez MI, Barbeau A. Role of subcortical structures, and particularly the thalamus, in the mechanisms of speech and language. Int J Neurol 1971;8:300–320.
8. Rubens AR. Transcortical motor aphasia. Stud Neurolinguistics 1976;1:293–306.
9. Luria AR, Tsvetkova LS. Towards the mechanisms of "dynamic aphasia." Acta Neurol Psychiatr Belg 1967;67:1045–1067.
10. Stuss DS, Benson DF. The frontal lobes. New York: Raven Press, 1985.

11. Cairns H, Oldfield RC, Pennybacker JB, Whitteridge D. Akinetic mutism with an epidermoid cyst of the third ventricle. Brain 1941;64:273–290.

12. Ross ED, Stewart RM. Akinetic mutism from hypothalamic damage: successful treatment with dopamine agonists. Neurology 1981;31:1435–1439.

13. Nielsen JM, Jacobs LL. Bilateral lesions of the anterior cingulate gyri. Bull Los Angeles Neurol Soc 1951;16:231–234.

14. Amyes EW, Nielsen JM. Clinicopathological study of vascular lesions of the anterior cingulate region. Bull Los Angeles Neurol Soc 1955;20:112–130.

15. Barris RW, Schuman HR. Bilateral anterior cingulate lesions. Syndrome of the anterior cingulate gyri. Neurology 1953;3:44–52.

16. Buge A, Escourolle R, Rancurel G, Poisson M. "Mutisme akinétique" et ramollissement bicingulaire. Rev Neurol 1975;131:121–137.

17. Freemon FR. Akinetic mutism and bilateral anterior cerebral artery occlusion. J Neurol Neurosurg Psychiatry 1971;34:693–698.

18. Ballantine HT, Cassidy WL, Flanagan NB, Marino R. Stereotaxic anterior cingulotomy for neuropsychiatric illness and intractable pain. J Neurosurg 1967;26:488–495.

19. Damasio AR, Kassel NF. Transcortical motor aphasia in relation to lesions of the supplementary motor area. Neurology 1980;28:396 Abstract.

20. Laplane D, Talairach J, Meininger V, et al. Clinical consequences of corticectomies involving the supplementary motor area in man. J Neurol Sci 1977;34:301–314.

21. Gelmers HJ. Non-paralytic motor disturbances and speech disorders: the role of the supplementary motor area. J Neurol Neurosurg Psychiatry 1983;46:1052–1054.

22. Von Stockert TR. Aphasia sine aphasia. Brain Lang 1974;1:277–282.

23. Goodglass H, Kaplan E. Assessment of aphasia and related disorders. 2nd ed. Philadelphia: Lea & Febiger, 1983.

24. Alexander MP, Lo Verme SR. Aphasia after left intracerebral hemorrhage. Neurology 1980;30:1193–1202.

25. Levin HS, Madison CF, Bailey CB, et al. Mutism after closed head injury. Arch Neurol 1983;40:601–606.

26. Habib M, Ponçet M. Perte d'élan vital, ce l'intérêt et de l'affectivité (syndrome athymormique) au cours de lésions lacunaires des corps striés. Rev Neurol 1988;144:571–577.

27. Laplane D, Baulac M, Widlocher D, Dubois B. Pure psychic akinesia with bilateral lesions of basal ganglia. J Neurol Neurosurg Psychiatry 1984;47:377–385.

28. Archer CP, Ilinski IA, Goldfader PR, Smith KR. Aphasia in thalamic stroke: CT stereotactic localization. J Comput Assist Tomogr 1981;5:427–432.

29. Graff-Radford NR, Damasio H, Yamada T, et al. Nonhaemorrhagic thalamic infarction: clinical, neuropsychological, electrophysiological findings in four anatomical groups defined by computerized tomography. Brain 1985;108:485–516.

30. Mori E, Yamadori A, Mitani Y. Left thalamic infarction and disturbance of verbal memory: a clinicoanatomical study with a new method of computed tomographic lesion localization. Ann Neurol 1986;20:671–676.

31. Bogousslavsky J, Regli F, Uske A. Thalamic infarcts: clinical syndromes, etiology, and prognosis. Neurology 1988;38:837–848.

32. Von Cramon DY, Hebel N, Schuri U. A contribution to the anatomical basis of thalamic amnesia. Brain 1985;108:993–1008.

33. Segarra JM. Cerebral vascular disease and behavior: the syndrome of the mesencephalic artery (basilar artery bifurcation). Arch Neurol 1970;22:408–418.

34. Castaigne P, Lhermitte F, Buge A, et al. Paramedian thalamic and midbrain infarcts: clinical and neuropathological study. Ann Neurol 1981;10:127–148.

35. Guberman A, Stuss DS. The syndrome of bilateral paramedian thalamic infarction. Neurology 1983;33:540–546.

36. Katz DI, Alexander MP, Mandell AM. Dementia following strokes in the mesencephalon and diencephalon. Arch Neurol 1987;44:1127–1133.

37. Davous P, Bjanco C, Duval-Lota AM, et al. Aphasie par infarctus thalamique paramedian gauche. Rev Neurol 1984;140:711–719.

38. McFarling D, Rothi LJ, Heilman KM. Transcortical aphasia from ischaemic infarcts of the thalamus: a report of two cases. J Neurol Neurosurg Psychiatry 1982;45:107–112.

39. Gorelick PB, Hier DB, Benevuto L, et al. Aphasia after left thalamic infarction. Arch Neurol 1984;41:1296–1298.

40. American Psychiatric Association. Diagnostic and statistical manual of mental disorders. 4th rev. ed. Washington, DC: American Psychiatric Association, 1996.

41. Cheek WR, Taveras JM. Thalamic tumors. J Neurosurg 1966;24:505–513.

42. Puel M, Cardebat D, Demonet JF, et al. La rôle du thalamus dans les aphasies sous-corticales. Rev Neurol 1986;142:431–440.

43. Bell DS. Speech functions of the thalamus inferred from the effects of thalamotomy. Brain 1968;91:619–638.

44. Hegedüs K, Németh G. Fibromuscular dysplasia of the basilar artery: case report with autopsy verification. Arch Neurol 1984;41:440–442.

45. Jürgens U. The efferent and afferent connections of the supplementary motor area. Brain Res 1984;300:63–81.

46. Sanides F. Functional architecture of motor and sensory cortices on primates in light of a new concept of neocortex evolution. In: Noback C, Montagna W, eds. The primate brain. New York: Appleton-Century-Crofts, 1970;137–208.

47. Travis AM. Neurological deficiencies following supplementary motor area lesions in *Macaca mulatta*. Brain 1955;78:174–201.

48. Pandya DN, Vignolo LA. Intra- and interhemispheric projections of the precentral, premotor and arcuate areas in the Rhesus monkey. Brain Res 1971;26:217–233.

49. Muakkassa KF, Strick PL. Frontal lobe inputs to primate motor cortex: evidence for four somatotopically organized "premotor" areas. Brain Res 1979;177:176–182.

50. Brinkman C. Supplementary motor area of the monkey's cerebral cortex: short- and long-term deficits after unilateral ablation and the effects of subsequent callosal section. J Neurosci 1984;4:918–929.

51. Smith AM, Bourbonnais D, Blanchette G. Interaction between forced grasping and a learned precision grip after ablation of the supplementary motor area. Brain Res 1981;222:395–400.

52. Kirzinger A, Jürgens U. Cortical lesion effects and vocalization in the squirrel monkey. Brain Res 1982;223:299–315.

53. Baleydier C, Mauguiere F. The duality of the cingulate gyrus in monkey: neuroanatomical study and functional hypothesis. Brain 1980;103:525–554.

54. Yakolev PI, Locke S. Limbic nuclei of thalamus and connections of limbic cortex. Arch Neurol 1961;5:364–400.

55. Naeser MA, Palumbo CL, Helm-Estabrook N, et al. Severe nonfluency in aphasia: role of the medial subcallosal fasciculus plus other white matter pathways in recovery of spontaneous speech. Brain 1989;11:211–239.

56. Watson RT, Heilman KM, Cauthen JC, King FA. Neglect after cingulotomy. Neurology 1973;23:1003–1007.

57. Skultety FM. Clinical and experimental aspects of akinetic mutism: report of a case. Arch Neurol 1968;19:1–14.

58. Lindvall O, Bjorkland A, Moore RY, Stenevi U. Mesencephalic dopamine neurons projecting to neocortex. Brain Res 1974;81:325–331.

59. Javoy-Agid F, Agid Y. Is the mesocortical dopaminergic system involved in Parkinson's disease? Neurology 1980;30:1326–1330.

60. Ruberg M, Javoy-Agid F, Hirsch E, et al. Dopaminergic and cholinergic lesions in progressive supranuclear palsy. Ann Neurol 1985;18:523–529.

61. Schell GR, Strick PL. The origin of thalamic inputs to the arcuate premotor and supplementary motor areas. J Neurosci 1984;4:539–560.

62. Haber SN, Groenewegen HJ, Grove EA, Nauta WJH. Efferent connections of the ventral pallidum in the rat: evidence of a dual striatopallidofugal pathway. J Comp Neurol 1985;238:322–335.

63. Rifkin A, Quitkin F, Klein DF. Akinesia: a poorly recognized drug-induced extrapyramidal behavioral disorder. Arch Gen Psychiatry 1975;32:672–674.

64. Gammon GD, Hansen C. A case of akinesia induced by amoxapine. Am J Psychiatry 1984;141:283–284.

65. Crow TJ. Positive and negative schizophrenia symptoms and the role of dopamine, part 2. Br J Psychiatry 1980;137:383–386.

66. Angrist B, Rotrosen J, Gershon S. Differential effects of neuroleptics on negative versus positive symptoms in schizophrenia. Psychopharmacology 1980;72:17–19.

67. Goodwin FK, Murphy DL, Brodie HKH, Bunney WE. L-Dopa, catecholamines and behavior: a clinical and biochemical study in depressed patients. Biol Psychiatry 1970;2:341–357.

68. Sparks R, Helm N, Albert ML. Aphasia rehabilitation resulting from melodic intonation therapy. Cortex 1974;10:303–316.

Restless Legs Syndrome

Daniel Tarsy

Restless legs syndrome (RLS) is a symptom complex characterized by subjective lower extremity discomfort relieved by movement. Originally described by Thomas Willis in 1685, it received little attention until a series of articles written by Ekbom beginning in the 1940s (1–3), following which it became known as Ekbom's syndrome. In recent years there has been increasing interest in the neurophysiologic and neuropharmacologic aspects of RLS.

CLINICAL FEATURES

RLS is a clinical syndrome the diagnosis of which is based on a group of characteristic symptoms and the absence of abnormal physical findings. The condition is a relatively common cause of insomnia and, unfortunately, often goes undiagnosed in milder cases. The hallmark of the condition is unpleasant discomfort of the lower extremities at rest that is characteristically relieved by movement. The abnormal sensations are typically deep seated and usually localized to the lower legs. Distribution is usually bilateral, although some asymmetry may occur and the upper extremities are occasionally involved. The discomfort is typically difficult for patients to describe but is distinguished from pain. A variety of descriptive terms are used, such as crawling, creeping, pulling, itching, drawing, or stretching sensations typically localized to deep structures such as muscles, tendons, or bones. Characteristic is the fact that the discomfort occurs only when the patient is at rest and is promptly relieved with physical activity. The symptoms become worse late in the day and evening and become maximal at night when the patient is in bed. In severe cases the discomfort may occur earlier in the day while the patient is seated, but in most cases the most disturbing symptoms occur at night, within 15 or 30 minutes of assuming a recumbent position. In milder cases patients will fidget, move, and kick their legs

or massage them for relief, whereas patients with more severe symptoms are forced to pace the floor. Relief is usually temporary, with eventual return of symptoms when the patient is once again recumbent. Sudden jerking movements of the legs (nocturnal myoclonus) are sometimes described by the patient but more often mentioned by the patient's spouse because in most cases the jerking movements associated with RLS occur while the patient is asleep. Sleep laboratory studies have demonstrated that nearly all patients with RLS have characteristic periodic leg movements during sleep (PMS) (4,5). These sudden jerking movements of the legs were not emphasized by Ekbom (1–3) but have been recognized for some time (6). Some occur while the patient is awake, whereas others will awaken a patient from a sound sleep and can be a major cause of insomnia and excessive daytime drowsiness. Originally the sudden movements were thought to represent myoclonus (5). However, sleep laboratory studies have shown that they consist of slower, nonmyoclonic dorsiflexion movements of the foot, extension of the large toe, and sometimes flexion of the knee and hip lasting between 1.5 and 2.5 seconds each (5). They are characteristically periodic and recur on a fairly regular basis every 30 seconds for prolonged periods during stages 1 and 2 of non-REM sleep (4).

The diagnosis of RLS is based on the presence of lower extremity discomfort relieved by movement of the legs in the absence of other neurologic symptoms and with normal results from neurologic and physical examinations (7). Similar symptoms may be produced by peripheral neuropathies such as those associated with uremia, diabetes, and thiamine deficiency. These should be identifiable by the presence of sensory paresthesias such as burning feet, objective sensory deficit, loss of tendon reflexes, and abnormality of electromyography and nerve conduction tests. Nocturnal cramp disorders are characterized by severe pain and contraction of calf muscles; fasciculations and myokymic muscle contractions should be evident on examination and are unlikely to cause the unique desire to move characteristic of RLS. A much rarer syndrome of "painful legs and moving toes" has been described (8–10), which is characterized by pain in the legs and feet associated with dystonic movements of the toes and an abnormal electromyographic examination. This syndrome is often associated with lumbosacral root abnormalities. Akathisia can strongly resemble RLS in producing subjective feelings of discomfort in the legs with a need to move, but is typically constant throughout the day, is more generalized in distribution with less in the way of localized leg discomfort, is associated with more subjective anxiety, and is confined to patients receiving neuroleptic drugs and occasional patients with Parkinson's disease (11). When PMS are clinically prominent, differentiation from sleep startles and nocturnal myoclonus associated with an underlying seizure disorder is based on the more generalized distribution of the latter movements. PMS may occur in the absence of RLS in a variety of other conditions, including narcolepsy, sleep apnea, and other disorders of sleep (4).

EPIDEMIOLOGY AND PATHOPHYSIOLOGY

The cause and underlying mechanism of RLS are unknown. If mild cases elicited by patient surveys are included, the condition is relatively common, with an estimated prevalence of approximately 5% (2,7,12). Onset occurs at any age but is reportedly more common in older age groups. A family history consistent with dominant inheritance is present in 25% to 50% of cases (13), with an equal sex distribution. A pattern of inheritance consistent with an autosomal dominant trait has been documented in two families who manifested both RLS and PMS (14,15).

Ekbom (1–3) emphasized an association between RLS and a variety of underlying medical conditions, including iron deficiency, other anemias, vitamin deficiencies, pregnancy, uremia, diabetes, gastric resection, and malabsorption, and suggested the possibility of a vascular basis, for which no proof has ever emerged. More recent surveys of associated conditions include chronic pulmonary disease, carcinoma, amyloidosis, infectious disease, and rheumatoid arthritis (16–18). Since many of these conditions may be associated with a painful sensory peripheral neuropathy, it may be that at least some cases should be considered secondary forms of RLS, to be distinguished from the vast majority of primary familial or sporadic cases unassociated with peripheral neuropathy. Although it the past primary cases of RLS have shown no pathologic abnormalities in peripheral nerve or muscle (19), a recent study of eight patients with RLS without clinical signs of neuropathy showed a high incidence of electrophysiologic or morphometric abnormalities of peripheral nerve (20).

Clinical neurophysiologic studies have begun to demonstrate objective abnormalities in patients with RLS. As already mentioned, nearly all patients with RLS can be shown to have a well-defined pattern of PMS with nocturnal sleep recordings (4,5,14,15,21). These may be associated with electroencephalographic changes associated with sleep arousal (16). Resemblance of PMS to the triple flexion reflex and Babinski sign associated with pyramidal tract pathology and other neurophysiologic features have suggested a locus of physiologic abnormality in the spinal cord or brainstem (16,21,22). Patients with PMS have been shown to have a pattern of abnormal blink reflexes and long latency responses, suggesting that increased excitability of segmental reflexes in the central nervous system may be responsible for PMS (23).

NEUROPHARMACOLOGY AND TREATMENT

There is no uniformly and persistently effective therapy for RLS; as a result, most patients are treated with large numbers of medications in rotating fashion (17). The large variety of proposed treatments for RLS have only occasionally been subjected to critical study. Since the natural history of RLS is characterized by spontaneous fluctuations (6,24), double-blind controlled studies are necessary to assess the effects of drugs or other treatments in this condition. Early reports described a beneficial effect of iron (2,24), vasodilators (2,3), and vitamins (16) in RLS, but controlled studies were lacking and the degree of improvement poorly defined. In some cases a response to iron or vitamin treatment occurred in the absence of preexisting anemia or vitamin deficiency. Drugs that have been reportedly effective include a wide variety of agents, among them benzodiazepines, baclofen, L-dopa, bromocriptine, clonidine, and several opioids. Walters and Hening have divided reportedly effective drugs by their effects on GABAergic, dopaminergic, adrenergic, and endogenous opiate systems (16).

Benzodiazepines taken before sleep have been widely used for treatment of RLS for many years. These drugs are believed to exert a γ-aminobutyric acid (GABA) agonist action at benzodiazepine binding sites within the GABA receptor. In uncontrolled studies diazepam (5–15 mg nightly) was believed to be more effective than iron or vasodilator therapy (25). Clonazepam in doses of 1–4 mg nightly has been reportedly effective in patients with RLS as well as PMS (26–29), but most studies have not been placebo controlled. Studies in patients with PMS indicated reduction in the number of PMS with improved sleep in patients with or without associated RLS (16). RLS associated with uremia has also been successfully treated with clonazepam (30). Baclofen, a putative GABAergic agent by virtue of its effect on presynaptic GABA-B receptors (31), was associated with a reduction in amplitude and increase in frequency of PMS in five patients with PMS and sleep disorder who had no subjective manifestations of RLS.

Dopaminergic drugs appear to be more effective than benzodiazepines for RLS (32). Akpinar (33) reported complete disappearance of RLS in 5 of 5 patients treated with

L-dopa in an open trial. Bromocriptine, a dopamine agonist, was similarly effective in 3 of 3 cases, whereas pimozide, a dopamine antagonist, worsened symptoms. In a follow-up double-blind, placebo-controlled crossover study by the same investigator, L-dopa (200 mg nightly) plus bensarazide produced a statistically significant reduction in the number of awakenings and duration of waking periods among 13 patients with RLS (34). In an open study of 7 patients, L-dopa (50–200 mg nightly) plus bensarazide improved RLS, improved sleep, and reduced daytime fatigue in all patients (35). Sleep laboratory studies of these patients showed reduction of PMS in the first third of the night and a rebound increase of PMS in the last third (35). In two studies heredofamilial cases required higher doses of L-dopa for relief (33,35). A double-blind trial showed L-dopa to be effective in both idiopathic and uremic restless legs syndrome (36). Tachyphylaxis to L-dopa and emergence of withdrawal-induced exacerbation of symptoms in the early morning often occurs and results in gradual escalation of L-dopa dosage requirements (37). L-Dopa drug holidays and temporary treatment with alternative agents may be useful in this situation.

A variety of opiates, including codeine, morphine, oxycodone, methadone, and propoxyphene, have been reported in uncontrolled experience to be effective in RLS (2,16,32,33,35,38). Hening et al (39) have shown that several opioid drugs reduced restlessness, dysesthesia, myoclonus, and PMS, which could be reversed with naloxone. The various opioid drugs that have been used all act at the mu opioid receptor subtype, which is distributed in basal ganglia, brainstem, and spinal cord. In a double-blind crossover study, oxycodone produced significant improvement in symptoms of RLS and frequency of nocturnal PMS compared with placebo (40). It has recently been suggested that iron, which has been reported to improve the symptoms of RLS (2), may act by virtue of its interaction with dopamine and opiate receptors (41).

Other miscellaneous medications that have been reported to be effective in RLS include carbamazepine (42), clonidine (43,44), precursors of serotonin, such as 5-hydroxytryptophan (45) and L-tryptophan (46), and gabapentin (47).

CONCLUSION

In summary, RLS is a clinical syndrome characterized by severe lower extremity discomfort with a need to move the legs for relief. It is nearly always associated with characteristic triple flexion movements of the legs during sleep known as PMS. The condition is relatively common but in most cases does not lead to medical attention. Most cases are idiopathic and many are familial. Evaluation should include neurologic examination and electromyographic studies to rule out peripheral neuropathy, as well as appropriate medical evaluation and laboratory studies to rule out uremia, diabetes, anemia, chronic pulmonary disease, rheumatologic disorders, vitamin deficiency states, and pregnancy. Treatment should include management of underlying medical disorders and trials of benzodiazepines, L-dopa, dopamine agonists, and opioids.

REFERENCES

1. Ekbom KA. Restless legs. Acta Med Scand 1945;158(suppl):1–123.
2. Ekbom KA. Restless legs syndrome. Neurology 1960;10:868–873.
3. Ekbom KA. Restless legs. In: Vinken PJ, Bruyn GW, eds. Handbook of clinical neurology. vol 18. Amsterdam: North Holland, 1970:311–320.
4. Coleman RM, Pollak CP, Weitzman ED. Periodic movements in sleep (nocturnal myoclonus): relation to sleep disorder. Ann Neurol 1980;8:416–421.
5. Lugaresi E, Cirignotta F, Coccagna G, Montagna P. Nocturnal myoclonus and restless legs syndrome. In: Fahn S, Marsden CD, Van Woert MH, eds. Myoclonus. New York: Raven Press, 1986:295–307.
6. Behrman S. Disturbed relaxation of the limbs. Br Med J 1958;1:1454–1457.
7. Gibb WRG, Lees AJ. The restless legs syndrome. Postgrad Med J 1986;62:329–333.
8. Nathan PW. Painful legs and moving toes: evidence on the site of the lesion. J Neurol Neurosurg Psychiatry 1978;41:934–939.
9. Schoenen J, Gonce M, Delwaide PJ. Painful legs and moving toes: a syndrome with different physiopathologic mechanisms. Neurology 1984;34:1108–1112.
10. Dressler D, Thompson PD, Gledhill FR, Marsden CD. The syndrome of painful legs and moving toes. Mov Disord 1994;9:13–21.
11. Blom S, Ekbom KA. Comparison between akathisia developing on treatment with phenothiazine derivatives and the restless legs syndrome. Acta Med Scand 1961;170:689–694.
12. Feest T, Read D. Clonazepam: effective treatment for restless legs syndrome in uraemia. Br Med J 1982;284:510.
13. Godbout R, Montplaisir J, Poirier G. Epidemiological data in familial restless legs syndrome. Sleep Res 1987;16:228.
14. Boghen D, Peyronnard JM. Myoclonus in familial restless legs syndrome. Arch Neurol 1976;33:368–370.
15. Montplaisir J, Godbout R, Boghen D, et al. Familial restless legs with periodic movements in sleep: electrophysiologic, biochemical, and pharmacologic study. Neurology 1985;35:130–134.
16. Walters AS, Hening W. Clinical presentation and neuropharmacology of restless legs syndrome. Clin Neuropharmacol 1987;10:225–237.
17. Clough C. Restless legs syndrome. Br Med J 1987;294:262–263.
18. Salih AM, Gray RES, Mills KR, Webley M. A clinical, serological, and neurophysiological study of restless legs syndrome in rheumatoid arthritis. Br J Rheumatol 1994;33:60–63.
19. Harriman DGF, Taverner D, Woolf AL. Ekbom's syndrome and burning paresthesiae. Brain 1970;93:393–406.
20. Iannaccone S, Zucconi M, Marchettini P, et al. Evidence of peripheral axonal neuropathy in primary restless legs syndrome. Mov Disord 1996;10:2–9.
21. Trenkwalder C, Bucher SF, Oertel WH. Electrophysiological pattern of involuntary limb movements in the restless legs syndrome. Muscle Nerve 1996;19:155–162.
22. Smith RC. Relationship of periodic movements in sleep (nocturnal myoclonus) and the Babinski sign. Sleep 1985;8:239–243.
23. Wechsler LR, Stakes JW, Shahani BT, Busis NA. Periodic leg movements of sleep (nocturnal myoclonus): an electrophysiologic study. Ann Neurol 1986;19:168–173.
24. Nordlander NB. Therapy in restless legs. Acta Med Scand 1953;145:453–457.
25. Morgan LK. Restless limbs: a commonly overlooked syndrome controlled by valium. Med J Aust 1967;2:589–594.
26. Matthews WB. Treatment of restless leg syndrome with clonazepam. Br Med J 1979;1:751.
27. Boghen D. Successful treatment of restless legs with clonazepam. Ann Neurol 1981;8:341.
28. Montagna P, Sassoli de Bianchi L, Zucconi M, et al. Clonazepam and vibration in restless legs syndrome. Acta Neurol Scand 1984;69:428–430.
29. Ohanna N, Peled R, Rubin AE, et al. Periodic leg movements in sleep: effect of clonazepam treatment. Neurology 1985;35:408–411.
30. Read DJ, Feest TG, Nassim MA. Clonazepam: effective treatment for restless legs in uraemia. Br Med J 1981;283:885–886.
31. Guilleminault C, Flagg W. Effect of baclofen on sleep-related periodic leg movements. Ann Neurol 1984;15:234–239.

32. Montplaisir J, Lapierre O, Warnes H, Pelletier G. The treatment of the restless leg syndrome with or without periodic leg movements in sleep. Sleep 1992;15:391–395.

33. Akpinar S. Treatment of restless legs syndrome with levodopa plus benserazide. Arch Neurol 1982;39:739.

34. Akpinar S. Restless legs syndrome treatment with dopaminergic drugs. Clin Neuropharmacol 1987;10:69–79.

35. Montplaisir J, Godbout R, Poirier G, Bedard MA. Restless legs syndrome and periodic movements in sleep: physiopathology and treatment with L-dopa. Clin Neuropharmacol 1986;9:456–463.

36. Trenkwalder C, Stiasny K, Pollmacher TH, et al. L-Dopa therapy of uremic and idiopathic restless legs syndrome: a double-blind, crossover trial. Sleep 1995;18:681–688.

37. Guilleminault C, Cetel M, Philip P. Dopaminergic treatment of restless legs and rebound phenomenon. Neurology 1993;43:445.

38. Trzepacz PT, Violette EJ, Sateia MJ. Response to opioids in three patients with restless legs syndrome. Am J Psychiatry 1984;141:993–995.

39. Hening WA, Walters A, Kavey N, et al. Dyskinesias while awake and periodic movements in sleep in restless legs syndrome: treatment with opioids. Neurology 1986;36:1363–1366.

40. Walters AS, Wagner ML, Hening WA, et al. Successful treatment of the idiopathic restless legs syndrome in a randomized double-blind trial of oxycodone versus placebo. Sleep 1993;16:327–332.

41. Pall HS, Williams AC, Fonseca A, Blake DR. Restless legs syndrome. Neurology 1987;37:1436.

42. Telstad W, Sorensen O, Larsen S, et al. Treatment of the restless leg syndrome with carbamazepine: a double blind study. Br Med J 1984;288:444–446.

43. Handwerker JV Jr, Palmer RF. Clonidine and the treatment of "restless legs syndrome." N Engl J Med 1985;313:1228–1229.

44. Wagner ML, Walters AS, Coleman R, et al. A double-blind study of clonidine in restless legs syndrome. Neurology 1994;44(suppl 2):A218.

45. Billiard M, Besset A, Passouant P, et al. Treatment of chronic insomnia: long-term follow-up. Sleep Res 1978;7:210.

46. Sandyk R. L-Tryptophan in the treatment of restless legs syndrome. Am J Psychiatry 1986;143:554–555.

47. Mellick G, Mellick L. Successful treatment of restless leg syndrome with gabapentin. Neurology 1995;45(suppl 4):285–286.

Mood-Dependent Tardive Dyskinesia

Daniel E. Casey

HISTORICAL INTRODUCTION

Tardive dyskinesia, a potentially irreversible neuroleptic drug–induced neurologic syndrome of abnormal involuntary movements, is primarily characterized by orofacial dyskinesias but may also include limb and truncal choreoathetosis. It occurs in predisposed individuals, though it is not possible prior to the onset of symptoms to predict who is at risk (1,2). Although tardive dyskinesia was initially reported in 1957, it did not become more widely recognized until the late 1960s and 1970s. The search for risk factors has identified increasing age and female sex as important predisposing elements (1,2). Later, cumulative total exposure to neuroleptic drugs was also clearly demonstrated as a risk factor in prospective studies (3,4).

Only in the late 1970s and early 1980s did it become clear that affective disorders may also be a significant risk factor for tardive dyskinesia (5,6). Developments from two lines of research support this conclusion. First, patients with histories of mood disorders, primarily depression, are overrepresented in groups of patients with tardive dyskinesia. Second, though uncommonly reported, a few patients exhibited striking changes in tardive dyskinesia with fluctuations in mood. This latter group is characterized as mood-dependent or affective state–dependent tardive dyskinesia (5,6).

DIAGNOSIS

Clinical Description

The clinical phenomenology of mood-dependent tardive dyskinesia is similar to all other types of symptoms seen in typical tardive dyskinesia. Some reports suggest that mood-dependent tardive dyskinesia patients may have more frequent symptoms of tardive dystonia. However, this perspective is confounded with the observation that tardive dystonia occurs more often in younger patients, who also have psychiatric diagnoses other than schizophrenia. To accurately diagnose mood-dependent dyskinesias it is necessary to follow symptoms over a sufficient time period to observe the course of dyskinesia through at least one, and preferably several, mood cycles, whether they be unipolar or bipolar episodes.

Affective Disorder as a Tardive Dyskinesia Risk Factor

Epidemiological evidence supports the conclusion that affective disorders are a risk factor for developing tardive dyskinesia. In a long-term prospective study there was an increased incidence of tardive dyskinesia in affective disorder patients compared with those with schizophrenia (3). Additionally, there is a higher prevalence of tardive dyskinesia in retrospective studies correlating mood disorders with neuroleptic-induced motor side effects. These latter data show a clear pattern of depression being more common than mania in those patients with tardive dyskinesia and affective disorders (5–22).

Data from treatment studies also identify an association between affective disorders and tardive dyskinesia. When the underlying mood disorder is adequately treated, tardive dyskinesia may decrease or, in rare cases, subside. Examples of this relationship include treatment with pharmacotherapy (excluding neuroleptics) for either depression or mania, as well as electroconvulsive therapy (ECT) (5,6,23,24).

Mood-Dependent Tardive Dyskinesia as a Distinct Subtype

A small series of reports clearly identifies a subgroup of patients who have tardive dyskinesia that greatly fluctuates with changes in mood. These cases appear to be rare, and quite different in the degree of mood-related change compared with that seen in most patients with tardive dyskinesia. Although uncommon, when it occurs it is unforgettably striking and appropriately deserves the label of mood- or affective state–dependent tardive dyskinesia.

This syndrome was first reported in 1981 (12), and was followed by a succession of case reports (13,16,17,19,21,22). The large majority of these patients suffered from rapid-cycling bipolar manic-depressive illness (5,6). They all shared the common characteristic of improved or resolved tardive dyskinesia during mania, and most patients had tardive dyskinesia worsen during depression. Euthymia had a variable association with tardive dyskinesia symptoms.

When the time course of these coexisting disorders was tracked, the change in tardive dyskinesia *preceded* the changes in mood by one to a few days. This suggests that both syndromes have some mechanisms in common, and that tardive dyskinesia may have a lower threshold for expressing the underlying changes. Thus, it may be a useful indicator of impending mood alterations. Unfortunately, too few patients are described to conclude whether other risk factors for the onset of tardive dyskinesia (e.g., sex, total drug exposure) or the outcome of tardive dyskinesia are specifically associated with these mood-dependent dyskinesias.

MANAGEMENT

Clinical management strategies for patients with tardive dyskinesia who have affective disorders alone or in combination with mood-dependent dyskinesia are the same as for patients with tardive dyskinesia and other psychiatric diagnoses. The treatment guidelines of the American Psychiatric Association (APA) Task Force on Tardive Dyskinesia are the first lines of treatment strategy (2). These include a high vigilance for early detection of tardive dyskinesia, reducing or discontinuing neuroleptics when possible, and using neuroleptics in the lowest effective dosage in patients who need and benefit from these agents.

Schizophrenia is the only disorder for which the long-term use of neuroleptic drugs has been convincingly demonstrated. Using neuroleptics in affective disorders must depend on clinical judgment because of a lack of rigorous data in this area to guide treatment decisions. Indications for short-term use (defined as approximately 6 months or less) are tailored to manage acute psychotic symptoms effectively. Since tardive dyskinesia rarely occurs within this relatively brief time, the risk is minimized. The primary indications for short-term use of neuroleptic drugs are 1) acute psychotic episodes, 2) acute reduction of manic excitement when the onset of lithium's effect is too slow, and 3) adjunc-

tive therapy for psychotic depression when antidepressants or ECT alone may not be successful.

The long-term use of neuroleptic drugs in affective disorders is controversial. None of the recommended primary indications for the appropriate extended use of these drugs, as indicated by the APA Task Force on Tardive Dyskinesia, is related to affective disorders. One of the justified secondary indications is extremely unstable manic-depressive psychosis. The Task Force acknowledges under the category of questionable indications that these drugs are used in regard to mood disorders, but neither the efficacy nor the safety of this approach has been adequately demonstrated in controlled studies. The absence of adequate research notwithstanding, however, clinical experience shows that there are some patients with affective disorders who require neuroleptics for long-term management (25).

Risks and benefits of continued or discontinued neuroleptic treatment should be reviewed with the patient and a concerned family member if possible. Periodic efforts to decrease or discontinue neuroleptics in these patients are indicated, though it is clear that some patients will require extended neuroleptic therapy. Whether continued neuroleptic treatment uniquely affects the long-term outcome of tardive dyskinesia in affective disorder patients is unknown, though the vast majority of data on the long-term outcome of tardive dyskinesia indicates that continued neuroleptic treatment does not inevitably aggravate tardive dyskinesia. Indeed, approximately half of the patients over long-term follow-up studies show significant improvement or complete resolution of tardive dyskinesia (5,26,27).

BASIC SCIENCE

To adequately address the interrelationships between tardive dyskinesia and affective disorders, a parsimonious explanation has to involve at least partially overlapping mechanisms that address the pathogenesis and/or pathophysiology of these disorders. Since both disorders are incompletely understood, any such hypothesis must be considered tentative and oversimplified (5,6). Decreased aminergic activity (serotonin, norepinephrine, dopamine) has been proposed as the fundamental neurotransmitter alteration underlying depression. Reduced neurotransmitter tone could result in altered postsynaptic sensitivity. Neuroleptic drugs that preferentially block dopamine receptors but also influence other amines could similarly lead to a state of postsynaptic altered sensitivity. Thus, treating depressed patients with neuroleptic drugs could produce a combined neurotransmitter or synaptic sensitivity that might increase the vulnerability to tardive dyskinesia.

Extending this concept to mania, the hypothesized increased influence of norepinephrine, serotonin, or possibly dopamine could lead to a decreased receptor sensitivity. Thus, neuroleptic treatment at this time would be less likely to produce increased sensitivity because of the offsetting increased and decreased neuronal effects. Carrying this model further, antidepressant treatment, which also theoretically decreases receptor sensitivity, may be able to compensate, at least in part, for the neuroleptic drug–induced increased sensitivity. Lithium, whose mechanism is incompletely understood but perhaps works by membrane stabilization, may be able to maintain homeostatic processes to reduce both mood swings and possibly the risk of psychopharmacologically induced central nervous system changes in sensitivity (5).

This schematic approach implies that using neuroleptic drugs during depression would be more likely to produce tardive dyskinesia that using neuroleptics in acute mania. It is also possible to understand that patients with unipolar depressive syndromes may be at greater risk for tardive dyskinesia if they receive neuroleptics, whereas bipolar mood changes or unipolar mania may have less associated tardive dyskinesia risk.

A separate mechanism of cycling mood states as represented by the kindling model also might explain the increased risk of tardive dyskinesia in affective disorders. The repeated cycling of moods could lead to—or perhaps is only reflective of—increased central nervous system instability or liability and therefore increase the vulnerability either to disease- or treatment-induced receptor or neurotransmitter alterations. Until data bear out any of these hypothetical explanations, it is necessary to carefully balance the potential benefits and risks of neuroleptic drugs for extended periods in the control of depression and/or mania.

Biochemical explanations for the dramatic mood-dependent dyskinesias are even more difficult. These dyskinesias appear to change in ways that conflict with what might be expected from the mechanisms proposed above. According to the classic hypothesis, mania, which is associated with a relative increase in amine activity, should further activate the oversensitive mechanism underlying tardive dyskinesia, and thus produce more dyskinetic symptoms. Conversely, depression should lead to a decrease in tardive dyskinesia because of reduced amine availability. The findings of the mood-dependent dyskinesias obviously do not conform to this framework. Instead, the clinical observations are the opposite of the predicted effects.

However, it must be recognized that the vast majority of patients with affective disorders and tardive dyskinesia are not characterized by these dramatic mood-dependent dyskinesias. Thus, these patients may be the exception rather than the rule to a proposed interaction between affective disorders and tardive dyskinesia. Whatever the ultimate explanation, the clinical observations identify a subgroup of patients (i.e., rapid cyclers, poor responders to treatment, patients with mood-dependent dyskinesias) who may provide important data about the pathophysiologic mechanisms underlying these disorders.

In summary, affective disorders, particularly depression, are likely risk factors for the onset of neuroleptic-induced tardive dyskinesia. An uncommon, though striking, mood-dependent tardive dyskinesia syndrome illustrates the complex interactions among mechanisms underlying these two disorders. A hypothesis of how these processes of disease state and drug action may have compounding or offsetting effects has been offered, though it must be considered highly tentative. Until it is possible to determine in advance the risks and benefits of neuroleptics in patients with affective disorders, using the lowest effective dose for the shortest duration is the preferred clinical strategy.

ACKNOWLEDGMENTS

This work was supported in part by funds from the Veterans Affairs Research Program, NIMH grant MH 36657, and core grant RP00163. The typescript was prepared by Crystal Berger.

REFERENCES

1. Casey DE. Tardive dyskinesia. In: Meltzer HY, ed. Psychopharmacology: the third generation of progress. New York: Raven Press, 1987:1411–1419.
2. Baldessarini RJ, Cole JO, Davis JM, et al. Tardive dyskinesia: a task force report. Washington, DC: American Psychiatric Association, 1980.
3. Kane JM, Woerner M, Weinhold P, et al. Incidence and severity of tardive dyskinesia in affective illness. In: Gardos G, Casey DE, eds. Tardive dyskinesia and affective disorders. Washington, DC: American Psychiatric Press, 1984:22–28.
4. Kane JM, Woerner M, Sarantakos S, et al. Do low-dose neuroleptics prevent or ameliorate tardive dyskinesia? In: Casey DE, Gardos G, eds. Tardive dyskinesia and neuroleptics: from dogma to reason. Washington, DC: American Psychiatric Press, 1986:100–107.
5. Casey DE. Tardive dyskinesia and affective disorders. In: Gardos G, Casey DE, eds. Tardive dyskinesia and affective disorders. Washington, DC: American Psychiatric Press, 1984:1–20.
6. Casey DE. Affective disorders and tardive dyskinesia. Encephale 1988;14:221–226.
7. Davis KL, Berger PA, Hollister LE. Tardive dyskinesia and depressive illness. Psychopharmacol Commun 1976;2:125–130.
8. Rosenbaum AH, Niven RG, Hanson NP, et al. Tardive dyskinesia: relationship with a primary affective disorder. Dis Nerv Syst 1977;38:423–427.
9. Kane J, Struve FA, Weinhold P, et al. Strategy for the study of patients at high risk for tardive dyskinesia. Am J Psychiatry 1980;137:1265–1267.
10. Rosenbaum AH, Maruta T, Duane DD, et al. Tardive dyskinesia in depressed patients: successful therapy with antidepressants and lithium. Psychosomatics 1980;21:715–719.
11. Rosenbaum AH, O'Connor MK, Duane DD, et al. Treatment of tardive dyskinesia in an agitated, depressed patient. Psychosomatics 1980;21:765–766.
12. Cutler NR, Post RM, Rey A, et al. Depression-dependent dyskinesias in two cases of manic-depressive illness. N Engl J Med 1981;304:1088–1089.
13. Applebaum PS. Dyskinesia and unipolar depression. Am J Psychiatry 1982;139:140–141.
14. Cutler NR, Post RM. State-related cyclical dyskinesias in manic-depressive illness. J Clin Psychopharmacol 1982;2:350–354.
15. Rush M, Diamond F, Alpert M. Depression as a risk factor in tardive dyskinesia. Biol Psychiatry 1982;17:387–392.
16. Weiner WJ, Werner TR. Mania-induced remission of tardive dyskinesia in manic-depressive illness. Ann Neurol 1982;12:229–230.
17. DePotter RW, Linkowski P, Mendlewicz J. State-dependent tardive dyskinesia in manic-depressive illness. J Neurol Neurosurg Psychiatry 1983;46:666–668.
18. Hamra BJ, Nasrallah HA, Clancy J, et al. Psychiatric diagnosis and risk for tardive dyskinesia. Arch Gen Psychiatry 1983;40:346–347.
19. Linnoila M, Karoum F, Cutler NR, et al. Psychiatric diagnosis and risk for tardive dyskinesia. Biol Psychiatry 1983;18:513–516.
20. Yassa R, Ghadirian AM, Schwartz G. Prevalence of tardive dyskinesia in affective disorder patients. J Clin Psychiatry 1983;44:410–412.
21. Lal KP, Saxena S, Mohan D. Tardive dystonia alternating with mania. Biol Psychiatry 1988;23:312–316.
22. Wessely S, Feinstein A, Trimble MR. State-dependent movement disorder. Biol Psychiatry 1988;24:945.

23. Asnis GM, Leopold MA. A single-blind study of ECT in patients with tardive dyskinesia. Am J Psychiatry 1978;135:1235–1237.

24. Price TRP, Levin R. The effects of electroconvulsive therapy on tardive dyskinesia. Am J Psychiatry 1978;135:991.

25. Gardos G, Cole JO. Neuroleptics and tardive dyskinesia in nonschizophrenic patients. In: Casey DE, Gardos G, eds. Tardive dyskinesia and neuroleptics: from dogma to reason. Washington, DC: American Psychiatric Press, 1986:56–74.

26. Casey DE, Gerlach J. Tardive dyskinesia: what is the long-term outcome? In: Casey DE, Gardos G, eds. Tardive dyskinesia and neuroleptics: from dogma to reason. Washington, DC: American Psychiatric Press, 1986: 76–97.

27. Casey DE, Gardos G, Gerlach J. The long-term outcome of tardive dyskinesia. Proc Am Psychiatric Assoc 1989:41D.

Other Psychiatric Disorders

Movement Disorders in Schizophrenia

Mark T. Wright   William C. Wirshing   Jeffrey L. Cummings

INTRODUCTION

Aberrant movements and other neurologic abnormalities have been consistently observed in unmedicated individuals with schizophrenia. Catatonic phenomena, parkinsonism and dyskinesia, oculomotor disturbances, and soft neurologic signs have been noted (Table 58.1). In this chapter, these abnormalities are described and are distinguished from movement abnormalities associated with treatment with neuroleptic medications.

The preneuroleptic-era schizophrenia literature provides one method understanding the movement and other neurologic abnormalities that are inherent in schizophrenia. Several problems arise when using this approach, however. A significant number of the patients included in earlier schizophrenia studies may have had illnesses other than schizophrenia as it is currently conceived. A lack of modern diagnostic refinement probably led to the inclusion of patients with mood disorders, patients with neurologic diseases such as Huntington's disease, and patients with diseases now rarely seen, such as encephalitis lethargica and general paresis of the insane. All of these illnesses can produce psychosis and abnormal movements. Additionally, the widespread use of neuroleptics in recent years has given rise to a host of drug-induced movement disorders that have made verification of the early findings difficult. Despite these limitations, the detailed, rich case reports of early observers allow tentative conclusions to be drawn regarding the intrinsic movement and other neurologic abnormalities of schizophrenia. Contemporary studies of neuroleptic-naive schizophrenic patients supplement the earlier studies.

DIAGNOSIS

Catatonic Phenomena

A number of phenomena comprise the syndrome of catatonia. Some catatonic phenomena occur spontaneously, whereas others are seen only with interpersonal interaction (1). Spontaneous catatonic phenomena include mannerisms (goal-directed activities carried out in exaggerated or unusual ways), stereotypies (purposeless actions performed repetitiously), and a tendency to assume bizarre postures. Spontaneous catatonic movements reported in schizophrenic patients include nose wrinkling, lip pouting and puckering, grimacing, grinning, tongue protrusion and clicking, head shaking and nodding, hand wringing, arm flinging, hair twining, shrugging, back arching, hopping, skipping, jerky leg movements, and marionette-like motions (2–4). Evoked catatonic phenomena include automatic obedience phenomena such as waxy flexibility, echolalia, echopraxia, *mitmachen* (abnormal cooperation and passivity), and *mitgehen* (a tendency for the patient to allow himself or herself to be moved by light touch) as well as oppositional phenomena such as aversion, negativism, mutism, and *gegenhalten* (resistance to movement of body parts by others) (2).

The syndrome of catatonia was first described by Kahlbaum in 1873 (5). Although the work of subsequent investigators strongly associated catatonia with schizophrenia, catatonia also is seen with other psychiatric disorders (e.g., mood disorders) as well as a variety of medical illnesses and intoxications (Table 58.2) (6).

Catatonia may be overlooked if it is not properly sought. Patients should first be observed while they are engaged in routine activities: this allows conclusions to be drawn

Table 58.1 Abnormal Movements and Other Neurologic Abnormalities Seen in Schizophrenia

Catatonic Phenomena
Mannerisms
Stereotypies
Bizarre postures
Waxy flexibility
Echolalia, echopraxia
Mitmachen, mitgehen
Aversion, negativism
Mutism
Gegenhalten

Parkinsonism and Dyskinesia
Tremor
Rigidity
Bradykinesia

Oculomotor Disturbances
Smooth pursuit disturbances
Saccadic abnormalities
Blinking aberrations
Visual fixation abnormalities
Visual scanning defects

Soft Neurologic Signs
Poor repetition of tongue twisters
Head movement with lateral glances
Motor impersistence
Pseudoathetoid movements
Agraphesthesia, astereognosis
Minor reflex asymmetries
Posturing with stress maneuvers
Poor balance
Poor coordination
Mirror movements

Table 58.2 Some Causes of Catatonic Phenomena

Psychiatric
Schizophrenia
Mood disorders
Dissociative disorders
Conversion disorder

Neurologic
Frontal lobe lesions
Temporal lobe lesions
Limbic system lesions
Basal ganglia lesions (e.g., globus pallidus)
Diencephalic lesions (e.g., region of the third ventricle; thalamus)
Traumatic brain injury
Epilepsy
Infection (e.g., syphilitic)
Wernicke's encephalopathy
Narcolepsy
Tuberous sclerosis

Medical
Hypercalcemia
Diabetic ketoacidosis
Hepatic encephalopathy
Membranous glomerulonephritis
Pellagra
Acute intermittent porphyria
Homocystinuria

Drugs and Toxins
Aspirin
Neuroleptics
Adrenocorticotropin (ACTH)
Ethanol
Amphetamine
Mescaline
Phencyclidine (PCP)

SOURCE: Gelenberg AJ. The catatonic syndrome. Lancet 1976;1:1339–1341.

regarding spontaneous movements such as abnormal mannerisms, stereotypies, posturing, and gait abnormalities. On mental status and physical examination, signs of negativism such as averting the gaze, turning away from the examiner, mutism, resistance to tone testing, and refusal to participate may be seen. Alternatively, some catatonic patients may let their limbs go flaccid, maintain postures chosen by the examiner, or allow themselves to be moved by the pressure of a single finger, even after instructions to the contrary.

Considerable debate has arisen concerning the relationship between these movements and neuroleptic-induced tardive dyskinesia (TD). Some investigators have asserted that the tardive movements seen with neuroleptic treatment are similar if not identical to catatonic movements seen in untreated schizophrenic patients and that the emphasis on the tendency for neuroleptics to produce movement abnormalities is too strong or misguided (7–9). Preneuroleptic-era descriptions of abnormal movements in psychotic patients, however, offer little support for this view. While movements of the face and hands resembling those seen in TD were mentioned, more complex movements were also described.

Griesinger (10), for example, described tooth-grinding and choreiform movements but also noted postural and gait abnormalities not seen in TD. Kahlbaum (5) noted a "snout cramp" resembling movements occurring in TD, but he also noted odd movements such as nose grasping and wrapping of the arms around the head that go well beyond a simple choreiform disorder. Kraepelin (11) thought the movements of schizophrenia closely resembled chorea, but the behavioral complex he described included hair winding, "contortionist" movements, and postural and gait changes not seen in TD or other choreas. Finally, Bleuler (12) believed that the movements he observed were not choreic in nature and emphasized their abrupt, complex, and bizarre nature (Table 58.3).

Other features commonly seen in TD and uncommon in catatonia may allow more confident differentiation of the two syndromes. The typical movements of TD are seen at rest and in the orobuccal structures and distal extremities

Table 58.3   Descriptions of Abnormal Spontaneous Motor Activity in Schizophrenic Patients Observed Before the Advent of Neuroleptics

Author (year)	Description of Motor Activity
Griesinger (1867) (10)	Difficulty of movement of the whole body; statue-like cataleptic rigidity; muscular rigidity, moderate and of short duration; automatic grimacing; painful convulsions of the muscles of the neck; confused convulsive movements of the extremities which cause the patient often to walk irregularly or to progress in short leaps; constant trembling; grinding of teeth; chorea-like symptoms; automatic circular movements; walking backward.
Kahlbaum (1873) (5)	Grasps the tip of his nose; turns his arms horizontally around his head and ends this movement by jerking his hands away; made arm and hand movements similar to those executed during spinning; rolling a piece of cloth in the shape of a sausage; frequent grimacing; spasmodic pursing of the lips ("snout cramp"); choreiform convulsions of the face and extremities; waxen flexibility.
Bleuler (1911) (12)	Walk about in a very special fashion, tapping a certain spot with their feet, dancing around; nodding their heads; perform the same somersaults; tear their hair out by the roots; keep their finger stuck in their ani or smear feces in certain designs; pull and knot their clothing; . . . stereotyped yelling, screaming, roaring or squeaking; . . . pursing of the lips (*Schnauzkrampf*); grimaces of all kinds; peculiar ways of shrugging, extraordinary movements of tongue, lips, finger play, sudden involuntary gestures; . . . all these peculiarities are the reason why some authors have spoken of choreic or tetanic movements in catatonia, quite mistakenly though; choreal, athetotic, and tetanic phenomena are entirely different from the motor symptoms which accompany schizophrenia.
Kraepelin (1919) (11)	Repetition of the same movements or actions; twitching movements; "contortionist movements," waving with the hands, touching definite parts of their bodies; conspicuous clearing of their throats, smacking of their lips, snorting; almost uninterrupted series of senseless movements; begin and end jerkily and appear therefore stiff, wooden, and angular; face is distorted by spasmodic grimacing; peculiar attitudes and deportment, balance themselves on one leg, put their heads between their legs, lie on the edge of the bed, spread out their arms in cruciform attitude; wrinkling of the forehead, distortion of the mouth, irregular movements of the tongue and lips, twisting of the eyes, opening them wide and shutting them tight; . . . they remind one of the corresponding disorders of choreic patients; rhythmical movements of the body, odd movements of arm and finger, wringing of the hands, picking and pulling the fingers, running up and down; making faces; whimsical ways of shaking hands; threatening flourishes, senseless shaking and nodding of the head; monotonous crying, crowing, yodeling, clicking, spitting like a cat; lips are often pursed forward like a snout ("snout cramp") and show now and then lightning or rhythmic twitchings; grinning, sudden laughter, and making faces are common; single movements are stiff, slow, forced, or they are done jerkily and then often as quick as lightning.

more than other body regions. The movements of TD are accentuated by distraction and stress and are ameliorated by calling attention to the movements, asking the patient to suppress the movements, and activity in the involved area. Patients are usually unaware of the movements (2). These features are not common in catatonia. Table 58.4 contrasts the cardinal characteristics of TD with those of catatonic movements.

Parkinsonism and Dyskinesia

Parkinsonism also has been noted in unmedicated schizophrenic patients. Caligiuri and colleagues (13), in a controlled study of 24 neuroleptic-naive schizophrenic patients, found tremor, rigidity, and bradykinesia in a significant proportion of their patients and found that these signs did not correlate with the patients' psychiatric symptoms. Right-sided signs were more common than left-sided abnormalities. In a study of 89 first-episode, neuroleptic-naive schizophrenic and schizoaffective patients, Chatterjee and colleagues (14) found a 16.9% frequency (15/89) of extrapyramidal signs (plastic rigidity, cogwheel rigidity, and bradykinesia). These signs did not correlate with patients' ages or ages at onset of illness, positive symptoms or formal thought disorder, or a family history of parkinsonism; they did, however, correlate positively with negative symptoms.

Some modern studies have suggested that isolated dyskinetic movements resembling those seen in TD can be seen

Table 58.4   Clinical Features of Tardive Dyskinesia and Catatonic Movements

Characteristic	Tardive Dyskinesia	Catatonic Movements
Distribution		
Upper face	Usually spared	Usually involved
Lower face	Involved	Involved
Limbs	Primarily distal	Distal and proximal
Timing	Resting movements	Resting and action
Response to activity	Decreased	Little consistent effect
Voluntary control	Present	Inconsistent response to requests to stop
Response to distraction	Increased	Inconsistent effect
Awareness of motion	Little awareness	Aware

in neuroleptic-naive schizophrenic patients. These movements, however, are probably rare (14–16). Spontaneous dyskinetic movements are more common in older patients, women (16), and patients with prominent negative symptoms. They may portend a poor outcome (17).

Oculomotor Disturbances

Smooth pursuit eye movement (SPEM) disturbances, saccadic abnormalities, blinking aberrations, visual fixation abnormalities, and visual scanning defects are some of the oculomotor disturbances that have been observed in schizophrenic patients.

SPEM abnormalities are reported in 50% to 80% of patients with schizophrenia but in only 8% of nonschizophrenic individuals (18–20). Two specific abnormalities are noted when schizophrenic patients' pursuit movements are examined: abnormally low gain (i.e., reduced ratio of eye velocity to target velocity; differences between patients with schizophrenia and control subjects increase with increasing target speed) and an increase in the frequency of saccadic intrusions (21,22). Pursuit abnormalities are most severe in patients who become ill late in life and in patients with few positive psychotic symptoms (i.e., delusions, hallucinations) (23–25).

Other saccadic abnormalities observed in schizophrenic patients include abnormal staring, lateral glances, and rapid to-and-fro ocular movements (26–28). Bursts of saccadic movements are observed more commonly in patients with schizophrenia than in nonschizophrenic control subjects (29,30). Patients with schizophrenia also have been noted to perform more poorly on the antisaccade task (i.e., voluntary, immediate looking away from a visual stimulus) than nonschizophrenic controls (31). Stevens and colleagues (32) were unable to demonstrate a consistent relationship between saccadic abnormalities and perceptual abnormalities or behavioral disturbances in schizophrenic patients.

The rate of blinking is abnormal in patients with schizophrenia: they have a mean blink frequency of 31/minute, whereas the blink frequency in nonschizophrenic individuals is about 23/minute (33,34). This difference is most pronounced when blink rates are measured during visual fixation (35). The blink frequency also is greater in patients with schizophrenia than in patients with other psychotic illnesses (33). Stevens (27) found that schizophrenic patients had paroxysms of rapid blinking associated with hallucinations, delusions, and impulsive acts.

A decrease in the ability to fixate on a visual stimulus has been described in patients with schizophrenia. Visual fixation abnormalities correlate only moderately with SPEM abnormalities (36).

A limited range of gaze has been noted in studies of schizophrenic patients' exploratory/scanning eye movements (37,38). Schizophrenic individuals perform poorly on controlled tasks dependent on visual exploration, such as the Wechsler Adult Intelligence Scale (WAIS) picture completion subtest (39). Kurachi and colleagues (38) suggested that this poor performance stems from inefficient visual searching (i.e., schizophrenic patients do detailed local analyses rather than beginning with an initial global scan and then proceeding to examine the details).

Soft Neurologic Signs

Soft, or subtle, signs are neurologic examination abnormalities that do not reflect regional brain dysfunction. Discussions of soft signs have focused mostly on signs reflecting problems with motor coordination, sensory integration, and sequencing of complex motor tasks (40). Some specific examples of soft signs include impaired repetition of tongue twisters, head movements that accompany lateral glances, motor impersistence, small-amplitude choreiform movements with extension of the arms, agraphesthesia, astereognosis, minor reflex asymmetries, dystonic posturing with heel or toe walking, and imbalance with standing or hopping on one leg (41).

Soft neurologic signs are found in 60% to 90% of patients with schizophrenia; these signs are noted much less frequently in patients with other psychiatric disorders and in normal control subjects (42–45). Several studies have sought to explore the relationship between soft neurologic signs and other dimensions of the schizophrenia syndrome. Soft signs correlate positively with thought disorder (46,47), negative symptoms (48), and cognitive impairment (44,49). Soft signs do not distinguish paranoid from nonparanoid schizophrenic patients and do not correlate with electroencephalographic abnormalities. Whether soft signs are consistently lateralized is unclear, and the relationships between soft signs and premorbid asociality, cerebral ventricular enlargement, and chronicity of illness also are uncertain (50–57).

TREATMENT

The neurologic abnormalities seen in schizophrenia are rarely the principal targets of therapy. Psychotic symptoms and behavioral problems are usually the main determinants of treatment type and dosage.

The fact that catatonic phenomena are now rarely encountered in patients with schizophrenia suggests that neuroleptics prevent, or reduce the intensity of, these motor abnormalities. Benzodiazepines can ameliorate catatonia, but the effect of these drugs is usually short-lived (58). Significantly impaired (e.g., not eating) catatonic patients who do not respond adequately to benzodiazepines should be treated with electroconvulsive therapy (ECT). ECT effectively treats catatonia regardless of the underlying etiology (59). Schizophrenic patients who manifest catatonic phenomena may be more treatment resistant than patients without these signs (60–62).

Schizophrenic patients with spontaneous parkinsonism may develop significant parkinsonism early in a course of neuroleptic treatment. Patients with spontaneous parkinsonism may be at increased risk for developing TD and treatment outcomes in these patients may be poorer than those in patients without spontaneous extrapyramidal dysfunction (14).

Several lines of evidence suggest that SPEM abnormalities are not caused by neuroleptic treatment (63). These abnormalities are neither worsened nor improved by treatment with typical neuroleptics; a reduction of SPEM gain and increased numbers of "catch-up" saccades have, however, been noted in schizophrenic patients treated with the atypical neuroleptic clozapine (21,23,64). SPEM appear to be the same in schizophrenic patients with and without TD (65). Some saccadic abnormalities may be responsive to treatment with neuroleptic agents: Karson (26) reported that abnormal staring was noted in 69% of unmedicated and 59% of medicated schizophrenic patients and that abnormal glancing was observed in 62% of unmedicated and 36% of medicated patients. Performance on the antisaccade task is not affected by neuroleptics (66). A positive correlation between saccadic distractibility (i.e., failure to inhibit inappropriate saccades toward distracting stimuli) and TD has been reported (65). Blinking abnormalities are probably not caused by neuroleptic treatment (35). The increased blink rate observed in schizophrenic patients is diminished by neuroleptics, except in patients with lateral ventricular enlargement (33,67,68). Visual fixation abnormalities are not changed by neuroleptics (69) and do not correlate with TD (65).

Gupta and colleagues (70) suggested that while neuroleptics probably do not cause soft neurologic signs they may increase the prevalence of these signs. Patients with soft signs may be predisposed to the development of TD (71,72).

BASIC SCIENCE

Catatonic Phenomena

Several lines of evidence suggest that catatonia is associated with dopaminergic dysfunction. Amphetamine, a drug that increases synaptic concentrations of dopamine (and norepinephrine), can cause the appearance of stereotyped behaviors when a large dose is injected into the striatum of an animal (73). This effect can be blocked by the administration of neuroleptics and by lesioning the caudate nucleus (74,75). Amphetamine also can induce stereotyped behaviors in humans (76), and neuroleptics may forestall the appearance of stereotypies and other catatonic movements in patients with schizophrenia. Pedro and colleagues (77) found that striatal dopamine D_2 receptor binding asymmetry (left greater than right) correlated positively with a standardized measure of stereotypy in patients with schizophrenia.

Dopaminergic dysfunction may be neither necessary nor sufficient to explain catatonic phenomena. Preneuroleptic-era descriptions of catatonic behaviors in schizophrenic patients strongly suggest that these movements are neither parkinsonian nor choreiform in nature. Catatonia is seen in other illnesses where dopaminergic dysfunction is less apparent (Table 58.2). These observations suggest that catatonic phenomena are not primary movement disorders stemming directly from alterations in dopaminergic neurotransmission. The association of catatonic phenomena with neurologic illnesses affecting the frontal lobes or the limbic system (2) suggests that the frontolimbic-subcortical axis may be the primary site of dysfunction.

Catatonic movements correlate positively with affective flattening, language deterioration, thought disorder, and soft neurologic signs in patients with schizophrenia. Positive symptoms such as delusions correlate poorly with these movements (78,79). These facts suggest that affect, language coherency, orderliness of thought, and movement have common neurophysiologic determinants.

One model of motor functioning suggests that a decision to act results when historically determined internal states and current environmental contingencies trigger the synthesis of motor programs according to an executive motor plan (80). Motor abnormalities thus can be seen with problems at the perceptual, planning, synthetic, and executive levels. The evidence described above suggests that catatonic phenomena in schizophrenia stem from a breakdown of motor act planning, although disturbances at other levels may coexist.

Parkinsonism and Dyskinesia

Parkinsonism is usually attributed to reduced nigrostriatal dopaminergic activity. The appearance of spontaneous parkinsonism in schizophrenia, an illness whose positive symptoms have been ascribed to excessive mesolimbic dopaminergic activity, seems contradictory. Experimental evidence, however, suggests that schizophrenia is not a purely hyperdopaminergic illness. Negative symptoms correlate with decreased dopaminergic activity in the frontal cortex; this frontal abnormality may lead to excessive mesolimbic dopaminergic activity and positive symptoms (81). The parkinsonism that can be seen in untreated schizophrenic patients may arise out of a compensatory response to increased mesolimbic dopaminergic activity (13). Alternatively, the general frontal deficiency seen in schizophrenia may result in diminished descending stimulative input to the striatum.

Oculomotor Disturbances

Oculomotor abnormalities seen in diseases affecting the basal ganglia and with treatment with neuroleptics suggest that staring, blinking, and extraocular movements are governed partially or wholly by dopaminergic systems. Parkinson's disease and progressive supranuclear palsy, two diseases associated with marked dopaminergic dysfunction, produce widened palpebral fissures, diminished blinking, and abnormalities of voluntary and pursuit gaze (33). Treatment with neuroleptics likewise results in an increase in palpebral fissure width, decreased blinking, and abnormal staring (67,82). These facts suggest that dopamine plays an important role in oculomotor functions and that the oculomotor abnormalities of schizophrenia are related to dopaminergic disturbances.

About 40% of schizophrenic patients' nonschizophrenic first-degree relatives demonstrate SPEM abnormalities (20). Abnormal pursuit is significantly concordant in monozygotic twins discordant for schizophrenia and less so in dizygotic twins discordant for the illness (83). These observations indicate that SPEM abnormalities may be genetically determined. The fact that SPEM performance correlates positively with Wisconsin Card Sorting Test (WCST) performance in schizophrenic patients (84) suggests that frontal lobe dysfunction may play a role in their pursuit abnormalities. Abnormal functioning of the frontal eye fields (and related subcortical structures) may lead to both the abnormal gain (85) and the inappropriate saccades (86) seen with schizophrenic patients' tracking eye movements.

Frontal lobe dysfunction also may cause antisaccade task abnormalities. Performance on this task correlates positively with WCST performance in schizophrenic patients (66), and one study (31) showed a correlation between poor antisaccade task performance and frontal lobe atrophy on computed tomography scans in schizophrenic patients.

The impulses that generate blinks arise in the pontine reticular formation and are transmitted to the lateral geniculate bodies of the thalamus. A circuit in which tectal (e.g., superior colliculus) structures and the substantia nigra facilitate blinking and the cerebellum and occipital cortex inhibit blinking has been proposed and posited to be abnormal in patients with schizophrenia (35).

A high rate of visual fixation abnormalities has been noted among nonschizophrenic first-degree relatives of schizophrenic patients. Animal studies suggest that visual fixation abnormalities may stem from dysfunction of the superior colliculus and/or dorsomedial frontal cortex (36). Visual search abnormalities may also be related to frontal dysfunction (38).

Soft Neurologic Signs

Low birth weights and neonatal problems correlate with soft signs in schizophrenic patients (87). Soft signs are found in the parents, siblings, and offspring of schizophrenic patients, and a family history of psychosis predicts the presence of soft signs (88–91). Minor neurologic abnormalities are more common in the affected members of twin pairs discordant for schizophrenia (92). This information suggests that soft neurologic signs may be inherited or acquired and that they are associated with a predisposition to schizophrenia.

Soft signs have also been observed in developmentally delayed children, individuals with learning disorders and other psychiatric illnesses, and after traumatic or vascular brain insults.

Problems with motor coordination, sensory integration, and sequencing of complex motor acts suggest the presence of pathologic abnormalities in systems involving the frontal

cortex, parietal cortex, basal ganglia, limbic system, and/or cerebellum (40).

REFERENCES

1. Hamilton M. Fish's schizophrenia. 3rd ed. London: Wright-PSG, 1984.
2. Cummings JL. Clinical neuropsychiatry. New York: Grune & Stratton, 1985.
3. Jones H. Observations on schizophrenic stereotypies. Compr Psychiatry 1965;6:323–335.
4. Marsden CD, Tarsy D, Baldessarini RJ. Spontaneous and drug-induced movement disorders in psychotic patients. In: Benson DF, Blumer D, eds. Psychiatric aspects of neurologic disease. New York: Grune & Stratton, 1975:219–265.
5. Kahlbaum KL. Catatonia. (Originally published 1873.) Mora G, trans. Baltimore, MD: The Johns Hopkins University Press, 1973.
6. Gelenberg AJ. The catatonic syndrome. Lancet 1976;1:1339–1341.
7. Rogers D. The motor disorders of severe psychiatric illness: a conflict of paradigms. Br J Psychiatry 1985;147:221–232.
8. Owens DGC, Johnstone EC, Frith CD. Spontaneous involuntary disorders of movement. Arch Gen Psychiatry 1982;39:452–461.
9. Crow TJ, Cross AJ, Johnstone EC, et al. Abnormal involuntary movements in schizophrenia: are they related to the disease process or its treatment? Are they associated with changes in dopamine receptors? J Clin Psychopharmacol 1982;2:336–340.
10. Griesinger W. Mental pathology and therapeutics. 2nd ed. (Originally published 1867.) Robertson CL, Rutherford J, trans. New York: Hafner Publishing, 1965.
11. Kraepelin E. Dementia praecox and paraphrenia. (Originally published 1919.) Barclay RM, trans. New York: Robert E. Krieger Publishing, 1971.
12. Bleuler E. Dementia praecox or the group of schizophrenias. (Originally published 1911.) Zinkin J, trans. New York: International Universities Press, 1950.
13. Caligiuri MP, Lohr JB, Jeste DV. Parkinsonism in neuroleptic-naive schizophrenic patients. Am J Psychiatry 1993;150:1343–1348.
14. Chatterjee A, Chakos M, Koreen A, et al. Prevalence and clinical correlates of extrapyramidal signs and spontaneous dyskinesia in never-medicated schizophrenic patients. Am J Psychiatry 1995;152:1724–1729.
15. McCreadie RG, Ohaeri JU. Movement disorder in never and minimally treated Nigerian schizophrenic patients. Br J Psychiatry 1994;164:184–189.
16. Casey DE, Hansen TE. Spontaneous dyskinesias. In: Jeste DV, Wyatt RJ, eds. Neuropsychiatric movement disorders. Washington, DC: American Psychiatric Press, 1984:68–95.
17. Fenton WS, Wyatt RJ, McGlashan TH. Risk factors for spontaneous dyskinesia in schizophrenia. Arch Gen Psychiatry 1994;51:643–650.
18. Diefendorf AR, Dodge R. An experimental study of the ocular reactions of the insane from photographic records. Brain 1908;31:451–489.
19. Holzman PS, Proctor LR, Hughes DW. Eye-tracking patterns in schizophrenia. Science 1973;181:179–181.
20. Holzman PS, Proctor LR, Levy DL, et al. Eye-tracking dysfunctions in schizophrenics and their relatives. Arch Gen Psychiatry 1974;31:143–151.
21. Litman RE, Hommer DW, Radant A, et al. Quantitative effects of typical and atypical neuroleptics on smooth pursuit eye tracking in schizophrenia. Schizophr Res 1994;12:107–120.
22. Abel LA, Friedman L, Jesberger J, et al. Quantitative assessment of smooth pursuit gain and catch-up saccades in schizophrenia and affective disorders. Biol Psychiatry 1991;29:1063–1072.
23. Shagrass C, Amadeo M, Overton DA. Eye-tracking performance in psychiatric patients. Biol Psychiatry 1974;9:245–260.
24. Bartfai A, Levander SE, Sedvall G. Smooth pursuit eye movements, clinical symptoms, CSF metabolites, and skin conductance habituation in schizophrenic patients. Biol Psychiatry 1983;18:971–986.
25. Levy DL, Dorus E, Shaughnessy R, et al. Pharmacologic evidence for specificity of pursuit dysfunction to schizophrenia. Arch Gen Psychiatry 1985;42:335–341.
26. Karson CN. Oculomotor signs in a psychiatric population: a preliminary report. Am J Psychiatry 1979;136:1057–1060.
27. Stevens JR. Disturbances of ocular movements and blinking in schizophrenia. J Neurol Neurosurg Psychiatry 1978;41:1024–1030.
28. Wallach MB, Wallach SS. Involuntary eye movements in certain schizophrenics. Arch Gen Psychiatry 1969;11:71–73.
29. Cegalis JA, Sweeney JA. Eye movements in schizophrenia: a quantitative analysis. Biol Psychiatry 1979;14:13–26.

30. Matsue Y, Okuma T, Saito H, et al. Saccadic eye movements in tracking, fixation, and rest in schizophrenic and normal subjects. Biol Psychiatry 1986;21:382–389.

31. Fukushima J, Fukushima K, Chiba T, et al. Disturbances of voluntary control of saccadic eye movements in schizophrenic patients. Biol Psychiatry 1988;23:670–677.

32. Stevens JR, Bigelow L, Denney D, et al. Telemetered EEG-EOG during psychotic behaviors of schizophrenia. Arch Gen Psychiatry 1979;36: 251–262.

33. Karson CN. Spontaneous eye-blink rates and dopaminergic systems. Brain 1983;106:643–653.

34. Helms PM, Godwin CD. Abnormalities of blink rate in psychoses: a preliminary report. Biol Psychiatry 1985;20:94–119.

35. Karson CN, Dykman RA, Paige SR. Blink rates in schizophrenia. Schizophr Bull 1990;16:345–354.

36. Amador XF, Malaspina D, Sackeim HA, et al. Visual fixation and smooth pursuit eye movement abnormalities in patients with schizophrenia and their relatives. J Neuropsychiatry Clin Neurosci 1995;7:197–206.

37. Moriya H, Ando K, Kojima T, Shimazono Y. Eye movements during perception of pictures in chronic schizophrenia. Folia Psychiatr Neurol Jpn 1972;26:189–199.

38. Kurachi M, Matsui M, Kiba K, et al. Limited visual search on the WAIS picture completion test in patients with schizophrenia. Schizophr Res 1994;12:75–80.

39. Wechsler D. The measurement and appraisal of adult intelligence. 4th ed. Baltimore, MD: Williams & Wilkins, 1958.

40. Heinrichs DW, Buchanan RW. Significance and meaning of neurological signs in schizophrenia. Am J Psychiatry 1988;145:11–18.

41. Tupper DE. The issues with "soft signs." In: Tupper DE, ed. Soft neurological signs. New York: Grune & Stratton, 1987:1–16.

42. Cox SM, Ludwig AM. Neurological soft signs and psychopathology. Can J Psychiatry 1979;24:668–673.

43. Manschreck TC, Ames D. Neurologic features and psychopathology in schizophrenic disorders. Biol Psychiatry 1984;19:703–719.

44. Tucker GJ, Campion EW, Silberfarb PM. Sensorimotor functions and cognitive disturbance in psychiatric patients. Am J Psychiatry 1975;132:17–21.

45. Woods BT, Kinney DK, Yurgelun-Todd D. Neurologic abnormalities in schizophrenic patients and their families. I. Comparison of schizophrenic, bipolar, and substance abuse patients and normal controls. Arch Gen Psychiatry 1986;43:657–663.

46. Manschreck TC, Maher BA, Ader DN. Formal thought disorder, the type-token ratio, and disturbed voluntary motor movement in schizophrenia. Br J Psychiatry 1981;139:7–15.

47. Tucker GJ, Campion EW, Kelleher PA, Silberfarb PM. The relationship of subtle neurologic impairments to disturbances of thinking. Psychother Psychosom 1974;24:165–169.

48. Merriam AE, Kay SR, Opler LA, et al. Neurological signs and the positive-negative dimension in schizophrenia. Biol Psychiatry 1990;28:181–192.

49. Liddle PF. Schizophrenic syndromes, cognitive performance and neurological dysfunction. Psychol Med 1987;17:49–57.

50. Torrey EF. Neurological abnormalities in schizophrenic patients. Biol Psychiatry 1980;15:381–388.

51. Walker E, Green M. Soft signs of neurological dysfunction in schizophrenia: an investigation of lateral performance. Biol Psychiatry 1982;17:381–386.

52. Kolakowska T, Williams AO, Ardern M, et al. Schizophrenia with good and poor outcome. I. Early clinical features, response to neuroleptics and signs of organic dysfunction. Br J Psychiatry 1985;146:229–239.

53. Nasrallah HA, Tippen J, McCalley-Whitters M, Kuperman S. Neurological differences between paranoid and nonparanoid schizophrenia. III. Neurological soft signs. J Clin Psychiatry 1982;43:310–312.

54. Williams AO, Reveley MA, Kolakowska T, et al. Schizophrenia with good and poor outcome. II. Cerebral ventricular size and its clinical significance. Br J Psychiatry 1985;146:229–246.

55. Quitkin F, Rifkin A, Klein DF. Neurologic soft signs in schizophrenia and character disorders. Arch Gen Psychiatry 1976;33:845–853.

56. Weinberger DR, Wyatt RJ. Cerebral ventricular size: a biological marker for subtyping chronic schizophrenia. In: Usdin E, Hanin I, eds. Biological markers in psychiatry and neurology. New York: Pergamon Press, 1982.

57. Johnstone EC, Macmillan JF, Frith CD, et al. Further investigation of the predictors of outcome following first schizophrenic episodes. Br J Psychiatry 1990;157:182–189.

58. Rosebush PI, Hildebrand AM, Furlong BG, Mazurek MF. Catatonic syndrome in a general psychiatric inpatient population: frequency, clinical presentation, and response to lorazepam. J Clin Psychiatry 1990;51:357–362.

59. Rohland BM, Carroll BT, Jacoby RG. ECT in the treatment of the catatonic syndrome. J Affect Disord 1993;29:255–261.

60. Abrams R, Taylor MA. Catatonia: prediction of response to somatic treatments. Am J Psychiatry 1977;134:78–80.

61. Guggenheim FG, Babigan HM. Catatonic schizophrenia: epidemiology and clinical course. J Nerv Ment Dis 1974;158:291–305.

62. Yarden PE, Discipio WJ. Abnormal movements and prognosis in schizophrenia. Am J Psychiatry 1971;128:317–323.

63. Holzman PS. Eye movement dysfunctions and psychosis. Int Rev Neurobiol 1985;27:179–205.

64. Levy DL, Lipton RB, Holzman PS, Davis JM. Eye tracking dysfunction unrelated to clinical state and treatment with haloperidol. Biol Psychiatry 1983;18:813–819.

65. Thaker GK, Nguyen JA, Tamminga CA. Saccadic distractibility in schizophrenic patients with tardive dyskinesia. Arch Gen Psychiatry 1989;46:755–756. Letter.

66. Rosse RB, Schwartz BL, Kim SY, Deutsch SI. Correlation between antisaccade and Wisconsin Card Sorting Test performance in schizophrenia. Am J Psychiatry 1993;150:333–335.

67. Karson C, Freed WJ, Kleinman JE, et al. Neuroleptics decrease blinking in schizophrenic subjects. Biol Psychiatry 1981;16:679–682.

68. Kleinman JE, Karson CN, Weinberger DR, et al. Eye-blinking and cerebral ventricular size in chronic schizophrenic patients. Am J Psychiatry 1984;141:1430–1432.

69. Amador XF, Sackeim HA, Mukherjee S, et al. Specificity of smooth pursuit eye movement and visual fixation abnormalities in schizophrenia: comparison to mania and normal controls. Schizophr Res 1991;5:135–144.

70. Gupta S, Andreasen NC, Arndt S, et al. Neurological soft signs in neuroleptic-naive and neuroleptic-treated schizophrenic patients and in normal comparison subjects. Am J Psychiatry 1995;152:191–196.

71. King DJ, Wilson A, Cooper SJ, Waddington JL. The clinical correlates of neurological soft signs in chronic schizophrenia. Br J Psychiatry 1991;158:770–775.

72. Youssef HA, Waddington JL. Primitive (developmental) reflexes and diffuse cerebral dysfunction in schizophrenia and bipolar affective disorder: overrepresentation in patients with tardive dyskinesia. Biol Psychiatry 1988;23:791–796.

73. Randrup A, Munkvad I. Pharmacology and physiology of stereotyped behaviour. J Psychiatr Res 1974;11:1–10.

74. Fog R. On stereotypy and catalepsy: studies on the effect of amphetamines and neuroleptics in rats. Acta Neurol Scand 1972;48(suppl. 50):1–64.

75. Asher IM, Aghajanian GK. 6-Hydroxydopamine lesions of olfactory tubercles and caudate nuclei: effect on amphetamine-inducd stereotyped behaviour in rats. Brain Res 1974;82:1–2.

76. Connell PH. Amphetamine psychosis. Oxford: Oxford University Press, 1958.

77. Pedro BM, Pilowsky LS, Costa DC, et al. Stereotypy, schizophrenia and dopamine D2 receptor binding in the basal ganglia. Psychol Med 1994;24:423–429.

78. Manschreck TC. Motor abnormalities in schizophrenia. In: Nasrallah HA, Weinberger DR, eds. The neurology of schizophrenia. New York: Elsevier, 1986:65–96.

79. Manschreck TC, Maher BA, Rucklos ME, Vereen DR. Disturbed voluntary motor activity in schizophrenic disorder. Psychol Med 1982;12:73–84.

80. Marsden CD. The mysterious motor function of the basal ganglia: the Robert Wartenberg lectures. Neurology 1982;32:514–539.

81. Davis KL, Kahn RS, Ko G, Davidson M. Dopamine in schizophrenia: a review and reconceptualization. Am J Psychiatry 1991;148:1474–1486.

82. Karson CN, Bigelow LB, Kleinman JE, et al. Haloperidol-induced changes in blink rates correlate with changes in BPRS score. Br J Psychiatry 1982;140:503–507.

83. Holzman PS, Kringlen E, Levy DL, et al. Abnormal-pursuit eye movements in schizophrenia. Arch Gen Psychiatry 1977;34:802–805.

84. Litman RE, Hommer DW, Clem T, et al. Correlation of Wisconsin Card Sorting Test performance with eye tracking in schizophrenia. Am J Psychiatry 1991;148:1580–1582.

85. Lynch JC. Frontal eye field lesions in monkeys disrupt visual pursuit. Exp Brain Res 1987;68:437–441.

86. Levin S. Frontal lobe dysfunctions in schizophrenia. I. Eye movement impairments. J Psychiatr Res 1984;18:27–55.

87. Pollin W, Stabenau JR, Mosher L, Tupin J. Life history differences in identical twins discordant for schizophrenia. Am J Orthopsychiatry 1966;36:492–509.

88. Kinney DK, Woods BT, Yurgelun-Todd D. Neurologic abnormalities in schizophrenic patients and their families. II. Neurologic and psychiatric findings in relatives. Arch Gen Psychiatry 1986;43:665–668.

89. Walker E, Shaye J. Familial schizophrenia. A predictor of neuromotor and attentional abnormalities in schizophrenia. Arch Gen Psychiatry 1982;39:1153–1156.

90. Woods BT, Yurgelun-Todd D, Kinney DK. Relationship of neurological abnormalities in schizophrenics to family psychopathology. Biol Psychiatry 1987;21:325–331.

91. Rieder RO, Nichols PL. Offspring of schizophrenics. III. Hyperactivity and neurological soft signs. Arch Gen Psychiatry 1979;36:665–674.

92. Mosher LR, Pollin W, Stabenau JR. Identical twins discordant for schizophrenia. Arch Gen Psychiatry 1971;24:422–430.

Oculomotor Disorders in Schizophrenia

Craig N. Karson

INTRODUCTION

Oculomotor disorders were recognized in schizophrenia even as this illness was being defined. Impaired visual pursuit, the earliest oculomotor disorder described in schizophrenia, stands today as one of the few firmly established neurobiologic dysfunctions in the disorder (1,2). More recently, increased blink rate has drawn sustained interest in schizophrenia research (3,4).

Much is known about the neural control of saccadic movements, and there is an emerging body of data about the neurobiologic factors that are involved in the regulation of blink rate (see below). Hence, ease of measurement and some comprehension of neurobiologic control suggest that the oculomotor disorders may provide useful information about the pathophysiology of schizophrenia.

SMOOTH PURSUIT IMPAIRMENT IN SCHIZOPHRENIA

Physiologic and Neuroanatomic Control

Pursuit is the slow movement of the eyes fixed on a moving target: latency is 125 ms and the maximum velocity is 30° to 50° per second, with the eye movements being smooth and conjugate (5). Pursuit is initiated by the signal of conjugate retinal error velocity to the cortex, which forwards the decision for eye movement to the pontine paramedian reticular formation (PPRF). Motor commands are then passed from the PPRF to the oculomotor nuclei (OMN) and subsequently to the extraocular muscles (EOM) (5). Positron emission tomography (PET) studies of normal controls during saccadic eye movements find regional blood flow increased in the frontal eye fields, supplementary eye fields, insula, lenticular nucleus, thalamus, and cerebellar vermis (6).

Methodology

Early studies employed an oscillating pendulum in front of the subject (2). Normal following generated a sine wave electro-oculographic (EOG) tracing; the intrusion of rapid saccadic movements or asymmetries and inconsistencies of frequency and amplitude distorted this sine wave pattern. Today's studies use a target with changing characteristics (to reduce the effects of inattention) projected on a screen and record signals using infrared reflectometry (7–9).

Eye tracking can be disrupted in healthy control subjects by single doses of sedatives and other medications (10). The high prevalence of pursuit abnormalities in first-break patients with schizophrenia, in first-degree relatives of schizophrenic patients, and in untreated patients with schizotypal personality disorder suggests, however, that schizophrenia rather than drug treatment is associated with the deficits in smooth pursuit (8,9). Moreover, smooth pursuit dysfunction in schizophrenia was described before the introduction of neuroleptic medications (1).

Smooth Pursuit Eye-Tracking Performance in Schizophrenia

The neuroanatomic basis of schizophrenia remains unresolved, though sound evidence exists for structural changes in multiple cortical and subcortical regions. Many brain areas implicated in schizophrenia are also relevant to oculomotor function. These areas include the prefrontal cortex, thalamus, and mesopontine tegmentum. Most commonly it has been suggested that impaired tracking reflects dysfunction of the frontal lobe in the disorder (10–12). Using delayed response tasks (DRT) to survey spatial working memory in schizophrenic patients and their first-degree relatives, Park et al (13) found impairments in both patients and relatives, asserting a strong association between DRT performance and the function of the prefrontal cortex. But a comprehensive study of brain structure and eye tracking in first-break patients with schizophrenia found that 31% (22/70) of these patients had structural brain abnormalities with little relationship between any structural changes and pursuit dysfunction (8). Neural network dysfunction in schizophrenia could explain some of this complexity, as different elements of the oculomotor network may be dysfunctional in the disorder (14,15).

Neurogenetics

Genetics were made relevant by the study in which eye-tracking impairment was found in 45% of the first-degree relatives of patients with chronic schizophrenia compared with 7% of nonschizophrenic control subjects (10). Holzman continued his genetic argument through studies of mono- and dizygotic twin pairs with schizophrenic probands (16). Mono- and dizygotic twin pairs were equally concordant for poor eye tracking; five of seven pairs were concordant for pursuit impairment. Coupled with the observation of good tracking in some schizophrenic probands with poor tracking in the nonschizophrenic twin, the "latent-trait" model emerged (17), which hypothesized that a latent trait could cause schizophrenia or eye-tracking impairment. Because bad tracking is more common than schizophrenia, the transmitted disease is more likely to invade the smooth pursuit system than systems involved in the causation of schizophrenia. Insofar as schizophrenia may be a spectrum of disorders, support for this view comes from the study of the putative mild spectrum disorders, such as schizoid personality. Qualitatively poorer tracking in schizotypal patients and an association of the impairment with the deficit-like symptoms suggest a dysfunction linked to neurobiologic parameters of the deficit state rather than schizophrenia itself (9).

At this writing, however, it is not clear that such findings will make a meaningful contribution to our understanding of the neurogenetics of schizophrenia. This may reflect weak genetic influences in schizophrenia, although there is still optimism about the contributions of identifiable genes, most recently on chromosome 6 (18).

BLINK RATES IN SCHIZOPHRENIA

Normal Blinking: What Is the Function?

Spontaneous eye blinking is a universal mammalian phenomenon that occurs spontaneously and as a reflex. In the quiet resting human, the average rate is about 20 blinks per minute (bpm) (4). A blink rate of only 2 to 4 bpm should prevent corneal drying, which begins to occur 15 to 30 seconds after a blink (19). It has been suggested that spontaneous blinks (and saccadic eye movements) may serve to clean the visual slate by erasing the neural traces of past fix-

ation and thereby promote the shifting of gaze from point to point (20).

Ponder and Kennedy were the first to study human blinking (21). The enormous variability of blink rate caused them to speculate that blink rate depended on both the cognitive and emotional state of the individual. It is now known that tasks requiring speech or memory increase blinking, whereas tasks requiring visual fixation, such as reading, reduce blinking (4,22). Blink rate can be voluntarily suppressed or enhanced for limited time periods, with men being able to suppress blinking longer than women (80 $\pm$ 86 seconds versus 15 $\pm$ 15 seconds) and voluntarily increase their rate to a greater speed than women (220 $\pm$ 27 bpm versus 153 $\pm$ 47 bpm).

Blount observed blinking in several animal species and found that nocturnal animals such as rodents, cats, and dogs had low blink rates (<3 bpm) in contrast to primates (approximately 10 bpm at rest) (23). Stevens and Livermore replicated these results studying animals housed in zoos and preserves (24). Since nocturnal animals demonstrated slow blink rates and diurnal animals relatively fast rates, a photic pulsing function for blinking was proposed. Slowly blinking nocturnal animals may maximize their ocular and central exposure to light. In contrast, diurnal animals exposed to greater amounts of light may blink more frequently to reduce ocular and central light exposure.

Neurochemical Regulation

Animals

Conclusive evidence now exists that treatment with mixed dopamine agonists or those specific to the D_1 or D_2 type receptors increases the blink rate of nonhuman primates and that these effects can be blocked by dopamine receptor antagonists (4,26,27). A subcutaneous dose of the rapid-acting dopamine agonist apomorphine (0.36 mg/kg) produces a peak effect 30 minutes after injection, with the median blink rate increasing from 8 to 37 bpm (4). Recent studies using specific D_1 and D_2 agonists and antagonists provide evidence that stimulation of both receptor classes corresponds to increased blink rate in an independent fashion (25). Lawrence and Redmond (26) also confirmed that treatment with the neurotoxin 1-methyl-4-phenyl-1,2,3,6-tetrahydropyridine (MPTP) (2.0 mg/kg IM divided over 5 days) substantially reduced blink rate measured 2 to 6 months later. Moreover, blink rate in these animals was highly and inversely correlated to the degree of parkinsonism produced ($r = -0.80$).

Healthy Volunteers

In their seminal study, Ponder and Kennedy also conducted the first neuropharmacologic study of blink rate, demonstrating that alcohol diminished blinking, with large doses virtually eliminating blinks (21). Nearly 50 years later, in the context of studying drug effects on contingent variation, Tecce et al (27) studied the effects of dextroamphetamine in 20 student volunteers. In the light of finding no obvious effect in schizophrenic patients receiving neuroleptic medications, these investigators concluded that an exacerbation of negative hedonic states was associated with increased blink rate.

A more recent study finds that apomorphine treatment significantly increases blink rate in young controls (28). Eight healthy male volunteers, ranging in age from 21 to 27 years, were given subcutaneous injections of placebo or apomorphine at doses of 0.5, 1.0, and 2.0 mg/kg at 48-hour intervals. Placebo had no effect on blink rate. Beginning at 15 minutes after injection and continuing to 30 minutes after injection, apomorphine treatment at each dose increased blinking. The mean increase of the 1.0 mg/kg dose at 15 and 20 minutes after injection equaled or exceeded 5 bpm.

In summary, a new series of neuropharmacologic investigations of blink rate find that dopamine agonists increase blinking in nonhuman primates and healthy controls.

Neuroanatomy of Blinking

A proposed anatomy of blink rate involves a neural circuit with its origins in the pontine reticular formation rostral to cranial nerve VII and includes the cerebellum, substantia nigra, midbrain tectum, lateral geniculate body (LGB), and the occipital cortex (14). Although pontine involvement is assumed, Cohen and Feldman conducted an eloquent set of electrophysiologic investigations that specifically implicated the PPRF and LGB (29). Studying juvenile rhesus monkeys implanted with electrodes, they found that approximately 20 milliseconds prior to blinks (and other rapid eye movements), triphasic discharges occurred in the PPRF. Nearly 50 milliseconds after these discharges, discharges were also noted in the LGB. These investigators concluded that the pontine eye movement potentials probably reflected activity in neurons that generated blinks and rapid eye movements, and that some of these neurons were responsible for activity that ascended to the LGB.

A second study demonstrated a possible inhibitory role for the cerebellum in rat blink rate, as cerebellectomy increased the mean rate ($\pm$SD) from 2 ± 0 bpm in unlesioned rats to 7 ± 1 bpm in lesioned rats (30). Some characteristics of blink rate in rats, including the very slow rate and the relatively high frequency of unilateral "winks," make it difficult to generalize these results to diurnal primates, including humans.

Finally, blinks have been elicited by stimulation of the posterior parietal association cortex in subhuman primates, suggesting a role in blink regulation for cortical areas involved in visual processing (31).

Brain Stem Involvement:
Relationship to EEG Alpha Rhythm

Prior to a blink, the peak frequency of electroencephalographic (EEG) alpha rhythm increases nearly 1 Hz, a phenomenon known as alpha squeak (14). The disruption of alpha rhythm and increased blink rate in schizophrenia, coupled with the phenomenon of alpha squeak, led Karson et al to propose a blink-alpha neurocircuit (BANC) that was especially disrupted in schizophrenia (14). Additional evidence in support of the BANC has been forthcoming in two recent studies. Blink rates and alpha rhythm were measured in smokers, 13 of whom were medicated patients with schizophrenia and 13 of whom were age-matched non-schizophrenic controls (32). Measurements were obtained during several mental tasks after the subject had abstained from cigarette smoking for 2 hours. Then the procedure was repeated 6 minutes after smoking a cigarette. Essentially, few differences were found between patients and controls, which is to be expected in medicated schizophrenic patients. However, for the entire subject group, blink rate and alpha frequency were increased after smoking and the blink rate was highly correlated with average daily cigarette consumption, particularly after smoking. Moreover, there were parallel changes between blink rate and alpha power during the mental tasks. Taking another tack, Barbatto et al (33) measured blink rate and alpha power in a group of eight sleep-deprived healthy subjects. Sleep deprivation increased blink rate and decreased alpha power, particularly in the low alpha range. This study and others from this group also suggest that the light-pulsing function of blinking may be relevant in human subjects as well as in nocturnal and diurnal mammals.

Nearly 50 years after Moruzzi and Magoun (34) first suggested that reticular formation stimulation produced activation of the EEG, there is convincing evidence regarding how this occurs. The reticular thalamus and thalamocortical nuclei are now understood to be the generators and promulgators of large-wave synchronous brain electrical activity such as alpha activity and some electrical patterns seen in sleep. Input from the mesopontine tegmentum, particularly from mesopontine cholinergic cell groups such as the pedunculopontine nucleus (PPN) and the lateral dorsal tegmental nucleus (LDT), disrupts this synchrony and produces activation (in sleep this is rapid eye movement sleep) (35). Hence, alpha squeak could result from isolated blink-generating electrical events in or near the PPN and LDT, which, in turn, are transmitted to thalamocortical neurons, yielding a brief increase in alpha frequency (the increase in peak alpha frequency would represent a form fruste of desynchronization). The results from Barbatto et al (33) could suggest that the increase in alpha frequency related to blinking is actually a relative decrease in the amount of slow alpha power.

Parkinsonism

Decreased blink rate was first reported in patients with post-encephalitic parkinsonism and later in a more diverse group of untreated parkinsonian patients, most with idiopathic parkinsonism (4). In untreated patients, those with mild signs and symptoms had a rate of 15 ± 9 bpm compared with only 6 ± 9 bpm ($p < 0.02$) in more symptomatic patients

(4). In levadopa-treated patients, similar results were obtained for those who did not have levodopa-induced dyskinesia. Levadopa-induced dyskinesia was associated with a 200% to 300% increase in blink rate (4). These data suggest that blink rate changes could alert the clinician to a worsening of Parkinson's disease (decreased blinking) or the presence of dyskinesia (increased blinking).

Progressive Supranuclear Palsy

An even more profound reduction of blink rate has been reported in patients with progressive supranuclear palsy (PSP), even in the face of treatment with dopamine agonists (4). This implicates structures in addition to the substantia nigra in the modulation of blink rate, because in PSP there is a bilateral loss of neurons and gliosis found in the periaqueductal gray matter, superior colliculus, subthalamic nucleus of Luys, red nucleus, pallidum, and several other nuclei (36). In this regard, patients with mass lesions in the area of the sylvian aqueduct can have either increased or decreased blinking depending on the exact location of the lesion (37). The superior colliculus may be of specific interest because of its integrative role in visual function, receiving innervation from the basal ganglia, from structures involved in other eye movement, and from cortical visual centers.

Cortical Involvement

With regard to cortical involvement, a patient with bilateral lesions of the parieto-occipital cortex (Balint's syndrome) had markedly reduced blink rate, and another report illustrates the return of the visual percept in this syndrome after a voluntary blink (38,39). These reports echo results that stimulation of the association areas of the parietal cortex elicits a blink in subhuman primates (31) and suggest that blinking relates to visual reorientation activity in the visual association cortex. The linkage between cortical activation and blinking might be reciprocal, as suggested by a case study of a 6-year-old boy in whom central midtemporal spikes were triggered by blinks (40).

Summary of Neuroregulation of Blink Rate

Blink rate is regulated by a complex set of neural structures at and rostral to the level of the PPRF. Within this neural network, the most obvious neurochemical control for blinking is exerted by dopamine.

Blink Rate in Schizophrenia

It is now clear that an increase in mean blink rates can be seen not only in schizophrenic patients who have been withdrawn from medications but also in patients who are naive to treatment with antipsychotic medications (4,41,42). There may well be developmental issues in pathology to explain the finding that blink rates are not different from controls in childhood schizophrenia (43). Still open is the question of rapid eye blink rate in seasonal affective disorder and periodic psychoses (44–46).

Neuroleptic treatment normalizes blink rate in schizophrenia (4) except in those patients with enlarged cerebral ventricles (47). Reduction in positive symptoms during haloperidol treatment correlates with the reduction in blinking (48). A significant reduction in blink rate (mean approximately 6 bpm) occurs 4 hours after an IM injection of 5 mg of haloperidol; in the small minority of subjects in whom haloperidol does not reduce blink rate (3/15), the medication does not prove to be effective in treating the signs and symptoms of schizophrenia (49).

Other evidence that provoking a blink rate response via dopaminergic-acting drugs may serve as a useful clinical indicator of treatment response in schizophrenia comes from the studies of Lieberman et al, who administered an acute infusion of methylphenidate, an indirect dopamine agonist, to patients with schizophrenia (50). They found that blink rates increased to a greater degree in medication-free patients. More important, patients whose blink rates increased by more than 7 bpm during the infusion had a reduced interval to relapse (23 versus 45 weeks to relapse, $p < 0.06$). Whether these two examples of hyporesponsiveness to dopaminergic agents in poorly responding schizophrenic patients relate to a variable such as cerebral ventricular enlargement remains an open question (51).

SUMMARY AND CONCLUSIONS

Smooth pursuit eye movements and spontaneous eye blink rate combine clinical simplicity (easy to measure) with heuristic complexity (neurocircuits, neurotransmitters, and neurogenetics), making them intriguing research tools in the battle against this devastating and poorly understood brain disorder. If smooth pursuit breaks can provide a classification for subjects in neurogenetic studies, especially at the edges of the schizophrenia spectrum, then smooth pursuit should remain a vibrant area of study in schizophrenia research.

This viability question notwithstanding, the presence of saccadic intrusions during pursuit in many schizophrenic patients suggests an affected neural circuit in the disorder extending as far caudal as the PPRF, an area now implicated in schizophrenia (52,53) (Figure 59.1).

Changes of spontaneous eye blink rate may be the best sign of the state of central dopamine activity in individuals receiving dopaminergic drugs. The increased rate in schizophrenia does support the dopamine hypothesis, but the considerable overlap of blink rates in groups of schizophrenic patients with the normal blink rate and the other factors that can change blinking call for some resistance to simplistic interpretation. Not surprisingly, a neural network with many elements in common with the network for smooth pursuit is involved in blink rate, and, as our under-

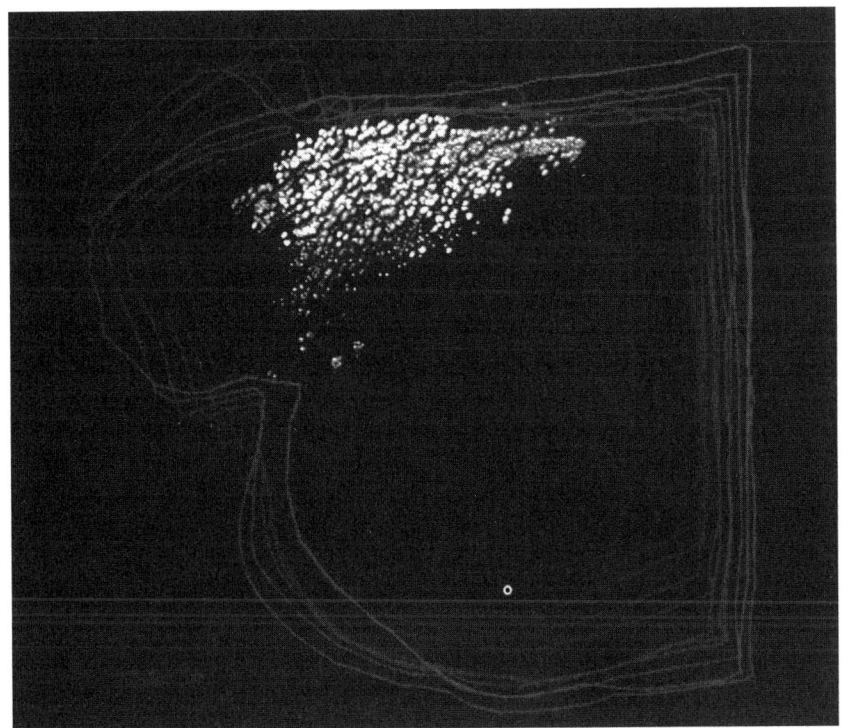

FIGURE 59.1   *New morphometric and molecular methods now make possible detailed study of the mesopontine regions that regulate oculomotor function. This is a three-dimensional reconstruction of a human mesopons. The lines represent the outlines of sagittal sections. The superior and inferior colliculi are at the top left, and the fourth ventricle is at the top. The view is from medial to lateral so that outlines showing the cerebral aqueduct (top left, ventral to the colliculi) are foremost. Laterodorsal tegmental cholinergic neurons are shown in as the medialmost cell group. Noradrenergic locus coeruleus neurons are the most lateral cell group, and the cholinergic pedunculopontine nucleus is the large remaining cell group. Each 100-μm sphere denotes the location of an individual neuron. Patients with schizophrenia have increases in the number of nitric oxide synthase–positive pedunculopontine nucleus neurons, which are excitatory to midbrain dopaminergic nuclei and regulate the flow of sensory information from thalamus to cortex (52).*

standing of the anatomy of schizophrenia grows, the oculomotor network seems harder to differentiate from that implicated in schizophrenia. After nearly a century of study, these two oculomotor signs may yet inform us about where schizophrenia affects the brain and which neurochemical systems are involved.

REFERENCES

1. Diefendorf AR, Dodge R. An experimental study of ocular reactions of the insane. Brain 1908;31:474.
2. Holzman PZ, Proctor LR, Hughes DW. Eye tracking patterns in schizophrenia. Science 1973;181:179–181.
3. Stevens JR. Eye blink and schizophrenia: psychosis or tardive dyskinesia? Am J Psychiatry 1978;133:223–225.
4. Karson CN. Spontaneous eye-blinks and dopaminergic systems. Brain 1983;106:643–653.
5. Glaser JS. Neuroophthalmology. Hagerstown, MD: Harper & Row, 1978.
6. Fox PT, Fox JM, Raichle ME, Burde RM. The role of cerebral cortex in the generation of voluntary saccades: a positron emission tomographic study. J Neurophysiol 1985;54:348–369.
7. Levin S, Jones A, Stark L, et al. Identification of abnormal patterns in eye movements of schizophrenic patients. Arch Gen Psychiatry 1982;39:1125–1130.
8. Lieberman J, Jody D, Alvir J, et al. Brain morphology, dopamine and eye tracking abnormalities in first-episode schizophrenia. Arch Psychiatry 1993;50:357–368.
9. Siever LJ, et al. Eye movement impairment and schizotypal psychopathology. Am J Psychiatry 1994;15:1209–1215.
10. Holzman PS. Recent studies of psychophysiology in schizophrenia. Schizophr Bull 1987;13:49–75.
11. Ingvar DR, Franzen G. Distribution of cerebral activity in chronic schizophrenia. Lancet 1974;ii:1484–1486.
12. Weinberger DR, Berman KF, Zec RF. Physiologic dysfunction of dorsolateral prefrontal cortex in schizophrenia. I. Regional cerebral blood flow evidence. Arch Gen Psychiatry 1986;43:114–124.
13. Park S, Holzman P, Goldman-Rakic P. Spatial working memory deficits in the relatives of schizophrenic patients. Arch Gen Psychiatry 1995;52:821–828.
14. Karson CN, Dykman RA, Paige SR. Blink rates in schizophrenia. Schizophr Bull 1990;16:345–354.
15. Watson S, Meador-Woodruff J. Neocortical abnormalities in schizophrenia. Arch Gen Psychiatry 1995;52:819–820.
16. Holzman PS, Kringlen E, Levy DL, et al. Abnormal pursuit eye movements in schizophrenia: evidence for a genetic marker. Arch Gen Psychiatry 1977;34:802–805.
17. Matthysse S, Holzman PS. Genetic latent structure models: implication for research on schizophrenia. Psychol Med 1987;17:271–274. Editorial.
18. Buckley P, Buchanan R, Schulz SC, Tamminga C. Catching up on schizophrenia research. Arch Gen Psychiatry 1996;53:456–462.
19. Doane MG. Interaction of eyelid and tears in corneal wetting and the dynamics of the normal eyeblink. Am J Ophthalmol 1980;89:507–516.
20. Evinger C, Manning K, Pellegrini J, et al. Not looking while leaping: the linkage of blinking and saccadic gaze shifts. Exp Brain Res 1994;100:337–344.
21. Ponder E, Kennedy WP. On the act of blinking. Q J Exp Physiol 1928;18:89–119.
22. Hall A. The origin and purposes of blinking. Br J Ophthalmol 1945;29:445–467.
23. Blount WP. Studies of the movements of the eyelids of animals: blinking. Q J Exp Physiol 1928;18:111–125.
24. Stevens JR, Livermore A. Eye blinking and rapid eye movement: pulsed photic stimulation of the brain. Exp Neurol 1978;60:541–546.
25. Elsworth J, et al. D_1 and D_2 dopamine receptors independently regulate spontaneous blink rate in the vervet monkey. J Pharmacol Exp Ther 1996;259:595–600.
26. Lawrence MS, Redmond DE. MPTP lesions and dopaminergic drugs alter eye blink rate in African green monkeys. Pharmacol Biochem Behav 1991;38:869–874.
27. Tecce J, Savignano-Bowman J, Cole JO. Drug effects on contingent negative variation and eyeblinks: the distraction-arousal hypothesis. In: Lipton MA, Dimascio A, Killam KF, eds. Psychopharmacology: a generation of progress. New York: Raven Press, 1978:745–758.
28. Blin G. Apomorphine-induced blinking and yawning in healthy volunteers. Br J Clin Pharm 1990;30:769–773.
29. Cohen B, Feldman M. Relationship of electrical activity in the pontine reticular formation and lateral geniculate body to rapid eye movements. J Physiol 1968;31:806–817.
30. Freed WJ, Karson CN, Kleinman JE, Wyatt RJ. Increased spontaneous eye-blinks in cerebellectomized rats. Biol Psychiatry 1981;16:789–792.
31. Shibvitami H, Sakata H, Hyvarinen J. Saccade and blinking evoked by microstimulation of the posterior parietal association cortex of monkey. Exp Brain Res 1984;55:1–8.

32. Klein C, Andreson B, Thom E. Blinking, alpha brain waves and smoking in schizophrenia. Acta Psychiatr Scand 1993;87:172–178.

33. Barbatto G, Ficca G, Beatrice M, et al. Effects of sleep deprivation on spontaneous eye blink rate and alpha EEG power. Biol Psychiatry 1995;88:340–341.

34. Moruzzi G, Magoun HW. Brain stem reticular formation and the activation of the EEG. Electroencephalogr Clin Neurophysiol 1949;1:455–473.

35. Garcia-Rill E. The pedunculopontine nucleus. Prog Neurobiol 1991;36:363–389.

36. Adams RD, Victor M. Principles of neurology. 2nd ed. New York: McGraw-Hill, 1981.

37. Smith JL, Zieper I, Gay AJ, Cogan DG. Nystagmus retractorius. Arch Ophthalmol 1959;62:156–159.

38. Watson R, Rapcoak S. Loss of spontaneous blinking in a patient with Balint's syndrome. Arch Neurol 1989;46:567–570.

39. Gottlieb D, Calvino R, Levine DN. Reappearance of the visual percept after intentional blinking in a patient with Balint's syndrome. J Clin Neuroophthalmol 1991;11:62–65.

40. Nadkarni M, Postolache V, Gold A, Labar D. Central mid-temporal spikes triggered by blinking. Electroencephalogr Clin Neurophysiol 1994;90:36–39.

41. Karson CN, Goldbert T, Leleszi JP. Increased blink rate in adolescent patients with psychosis. Psychiatr Res 1986;17:195–198.

42. Mackert A, Woyth C, Fletchner K, Volz H. Increased blink rate in drug-naive acute schizophrenia patients. Biol Psychiatry 1990;27:1197–1202.

43. Caplan R, Guthrie D. Blink rate in childhood schizophrenia spectrum disorder. Biol Psychiatry 1994;35:228–234.

44. Depue RA, Arbisi P, Krauss S, et al. Seasonal independence of low prolactin concentration and high spontaneous eye blink rates in unipolar and bipolar II seasonal affective disorder. Arch Gen Psychiatry 1990;47:356–364.

45. Karson CN. In the blink of an eye. Biol Psychiatry 1992;32:467–468.

46. Lovestone S. Periodic psychosis associated with the menstrual cycle and increased blink rate. Br J Psychiatry 1992;161:402–404.

47. Kleinman JE, Karson CN, Weinberger DR, et al. Eye-blinking in chronic schizophrenic patients grouped by ventricular brain rations. Am J Psychiatry 1984;141:1430–1431.

48. Karson CN, Bigelow LB, Kleinman JE, et al. Haloperidol induced changes in blink rates correlate with changes in BPRS score. Br J Psychiatry 1982;140:503–507.

49. Bartko G, Herczeg I, Zador G. Blink rate responses to haloperidol as possible predictor of therapeutic outcome. Biol Psychiatry 1990;17:113–115.

50. Lieberman JA, Kane JM, Sarantakos S, et al. Prediction of relapse in schizophrenia. Arch Gen Psychiatry 1987;44:597–603.

51. Weinberger DR, Bigelow LB, Kleinman JE, et al. Cerebral ventricular enlargement in chronic schizophrenia: an association with poor response to treatment. Arch Gen Psychiatry 1980;37:11–13.

52. Garcia-Rill E, Karson CN, Mrak RE, et al. Mesopontine neurons in schizophrenia. Neuroscience 1995;66:321–335.

53. Karson CN, Casanova MF, Kleinman JL, Griffin WST. Choline acetyltransferase in schizophrenia. Am J Psychiatry 1993;147:1646–1649.

Conversion Symptoms

Frank W. Putnam

INTRODUCTION

Conversion symptoms are among the most fascinating of neuropsychiatric conditions, demonstrating the power of psychological processes to deprive an individual of motor and sensory functions. Classic conversion symptoms typically suggest neurologic conditions such as paralysis, seizures, movement disorders, aphonia, anesthesias, and blindness. Symptoms such as pain, vomiting, fainting, and pseudocyesis have been reported. Their acceptance as conversion symptoms, however, is a matter of controversy (1). Although many theories on the psychodynamics of conversion symptoms have been advanced over the years, little is actually known about the neurobiologic mechanisms responsible for the alterations in sensory and motor function characteristic of these symptoms.

HISTORICAL REVIEW

Conversion symptoms have long been closely associated with the notion of hysteria. Some have pronounced hysteria to be an extinct or nonexistent disorder; however, it demonstrates a resiliency that has sustained it through two and a half millennia of Western medicine (1). The term "conversio" was used in the Middle Ages to describe disorders in women characterized by a crisis and thought to result from "suffocation of the womb" (2). In the 1770s, English physician John Ferriar introduced the term "hysterical conversion." Modern views of hysteria date to Briquet's *Treatise on Hysteria*, published in 1859, though classic clinical descriptions extend back to the *Corpus Hippocraticum*. Briquet's original study of 430 cases seen over a 10-year period in Paris included many conversion symptoms such as hyperesthesia, spasms, anesthesias, convulsions, and paral-

yses (3). Medical interest in hysteria and conversion symptoms was further stimulated by the work of Jean-Martin Charcot (4) and Pierre Janet (5) at the Salpêtrière hospital in Paris around the turn of the century.

Following a century of disuse, Breuer and Freud reintroduced the term hysterical conversion in the 1890s (2,6). Freud conceptualized hysterical conversion as a psychological defense involving the separation of an affect from an incompatible idea, resulting in the "conversion" of unresolved psychological conflicts and unassimilated emotions into physical symptoms (2). Freud lost interest in hysteria and conversion symptoms after 1900, and the diagnosis fell out of favor shortly thereafter (7). In recent times, however, the concept of hysteria or Briquet's syndrome has been reexamined by several investigators, most notably the St. Louis group led by Samuel Guze and his colleagues at Washington University (8).

DIAGNOSIS

DSM-IV Criteria

The complaint has been raised that psychiatry has assumed responsibility for the definition of conversion disorder but rarely for its treatment (9). Conversion disorder patients are more likely followed by a neurologist or internist than by a psychiatrist. The *Diagnostic and Statistical Manual of Mental Disorders, Fourth Edition* (DSM-IV) divides the classic manifestations of conversion into three syndromes (10). Conversion disorder is characterized by the loss or alteration of a physical function that suggests a physical disorder but which has a psychological basis. In pain disorder, individuals suffer from severe and prolonged pain that appears to have a significant psychological component. Somatization disorder is characterized by multiple recurrent somatic symptoms for which medical attention has been sought, but which are not due to any physical disorder or which exceed the social or occupational impairment that is expected from the history, physical examination, or laboratory findings. Somatization disorder must begin before age 30 and the individual must suffer from a minimum number of symptoms (four pain symptoms plus two gastrointestinal symptoms plus one sexual symptom plus one pseudoneurologic symptom— usually a conversion symptom). The diagnosis of somatization disorder takes precedence when conversion symptoms are part of the somatization. In practice, these three disorders often overlap, and no study has, as yet, demonstrated the discriminant validity of the DSM criteria.

The DSM-IV requires that conversion disorders satisfy the following criteria (10):

1. The patient has one or more symptoms or deficits affecting voluntary motor or sensory function that suggest a neurologic or other general medical condition.
2. Psychological factors are judged to be associated with the symptom or deficit because the initiation or exacerbation of the symptom or deficit is preceded by conflicts or other stressors.
3. The symptom or deficit is not intentionally produced or feigned (as in factitious disorder or malingering), but it may be maintained by secondary gain.
4. The symptom or deficit cannot, after appropriate investigation, be fully explained by a general medical condition, or by the direct effects of a substance, or as a culturally sanctioned behavior or experience.
5. The symptom or deficit causes clinically significant distress or impairment in social, occupational, or other important areas of functioning or warrants medical evaluation.
6. The symptom or deficit is not limited to pain or sexual dysfunction, does not occur exclusively during the course of somatization disorder, and is not better accounted for by another mental disorder.

For the purposes of this chapter, we will focus on conversion symptoms per se irrespective of whether they occur in the context of conversion disorder, somatization disorder, or other psychiatric or neurologic disorders. Conversion symptoms are the relatively persistent losses or alterations of motor or sensory functions that cannot be explained by known physical symptoms or pathophysiologic mechanisms (11). Common examples include paralysis, abnormal movements, blindness, deafness, and pseudoseizures.

History, Examination, and Assessment

The diagnosis of a conversion symptom/disorder can only be made when it is established that the symptom/disorder cannot be accounted for by a neurologic or medical condition. This diagnosis is most easily established for pseudoneurologic symptoms where the individual's understanding of the condition does not fit with neuroanatomic pathways. It can be very difficult to establish for some medical symptoms. Individuals with conversion symptoms may present with a relative lack of concern about their symptom (*la belle indifférence*) or with a histrionic display. However, neither of these presentations is pathognomonic, and either may occur in some individuals with medical conditions.

History should include the chronicity of the symptoms, their number, and the degree of limitation of function. Family, work, and other stressors occurring proximal to the onset should be inquired about. Possible secondary gain should be explored in an indirect fashion, for example, by asking about special arrangements that have had to be made to accommodate the individual since the onset of the symptom. It is recommended that the medical review of systems be conducted during the physical examination rather than in the context of taking the chief complaint, to minimize their future association with the primary symptom (12).

No psychological test can definitively establish the presence of a conversion disorder. Laboratory studies that are inconsistent with the symptom in question are useful to support the diagnosis of conversion. However, laboratory findings consistent with an organic etiology do not necessarily rule out conversion disorder because the DSM-IV only requires that the symptom is not fully explained by the medical condition. Specific procedures have been devised for sensory and motor pseudoneurologic conversion symptoms (13,14) and for pseudoseizures (15). The use of sodium amobarbital or similar hypnosedative to interview the patient and test the symptom has also been reported to be useful in some cases (16,17). A videotape of this interview may prove helpful in later psychotherapy (16).

Incidence and Prevalence

The incidence of conversion symptoms varies widely according to the population under study. Engel estimates that among patients in a general medical service about 20% have had conversion symptoms at some time in their lives (18). In a sample of 500 psychiatric outpatients, 120 (24%) had at least one conversion symptom (19). Farley et al found rates as high as 33% in their sample of psychiatric patients (20). In contrast, Trimble (21) and Marsden (22) found rates of approximately 1% of admissions to neurologic services. Although few systematic data exist, many investigators believe that conversion symptoms are more common in rural areas or lower socioeconomic classes, in the military during wartime, and in certain ethnic populations (11).

Sex

Several studies report a higher incidence of conversion symptoms in women (11,20,23,24). Some authorities, however, suggest that there is either an equal incidence or a bias against diagnosing male cases (7,25).

Age

Conversion symptoms typically first occur in adolescence or early adulthood. Onset is rare before age 5 years or after age 35 years. The mean age in samples of adult patients is typically in the mid-20s to early 30s (18,23).

Family History

There has been much speculation but few studies on family psychopathology and possible genetic contributions to conversion and hysterical symptoms (26). Ljungberg's study (26) of Swedish probands treated for conversion symptoms found an increased risk in relatives, but Shields' reanalysis of these data suggests that biosocial factors may be responsible (27). Small-sample studies by Slater and others have found no evidence of concordance for conversion symptoms in monozygotic twins (28,29). At present, there are no detectable genetic contributions to hysterical or conversion symptoms.

Child and Adolescent Presentations

As with adults, the incidence and prevalence of conversion disorders in children and adolescents are not well known. Estimates vary widely from 0.5% to 20% of pediatric cases (12,30,31). Incidence appears to increase substantially during adolescence. Girls are typically diagnosed three to five times more often than boys (12,30). Family problems and situational stressors are frequently identified in child and adolescent cases (31–33). A model of illness in a family member bearing similarities to the child's presentation is common (33). The modal presentation differs across reviews and case series, but physical problems suggestive of a neurologic disorder are the most common form. These typically include gait disturbances, weakness and paralysis, seizure-like behaviors, syncope, stupor, aphonia, deafness, ocular fixation, anesthesias, and paresthesias. Respiratory problems (dyspnea, choking, sneezing, and cough), gastrointestinal symptoms (dysphagia, globus, abdominal pain, or abnormal sensations), and cardiac symptoms (chest pain, palpitations, and orthopnea) are also frequent pediatric presentations.

Concurrent Psychopathology and Organic Illness

All investigators have found high rates of concomitant psychopathology in patients with conversion symptoms. It is often assumed that conversion symptoms are confined to the hysterical personality type. This does not seem to be the case, however, as most studies report that hysterical personality features are found in fewer than half of patients with conversion symptoms (23,34,35). Depression and antisocial personality disorder are the most commonly reported psychiatric diagnoses in patients with conversion symptoms

(19,23,36,37). Patients with dissociative disorders have high rates of conversion symptoms (38).

Several studies find high rates of concurrent neurologic and medical illness in patients with conversion symptoms (11,25,39). McKegney found that half of his sample of patients with conversion disorders had coexisting organic disease (23). Head injury or other physical trauma and certain neurologic diseases such as multiple sclerosis and focal abnormalities of the temporal lobe are thought to predispose to the development of conversion symptoms (25,40).

False Positive Diagnoses

Concerns about a false positive diagnosis of conversion disorder haunt clinicians evaluating these patients. Whitlock reported a 62% incidence of organic disease appearing within 6 months of the supposed conversion symptoms (39). Slater and Glithero describe a 48% incidence of false positive conversion diagnoses on 7- to 11-year follow-up (41). However, the most systematic study, a 10-year follow-up by Watson and Buranen (42) comparing 40 male veterans diagnosed as conversion reactions with a matched group of patients with nonhysteric neurotic diagnoses, found only a 25% incidence of false positives. The most common organic disorders in the false positive group were degenerative diseases and structural conditions affecting the spinal cord, peripheral nerves, bones, joints, and muscles (42). To date, efforts to develop a definitive psychological profile for identification of conversion patients have been unsuccessful.

MANAGEMENT

General Principles

The literature on treatment is replete with single case reports and small-sample case series, but lacks controlled clinical trials for any modality. Psychotherapy, supportive and psychodynamic, is probably used most often, but a number of studies report significant success with behavioral modification approaches (15,43). Irrespective of the therapeutic approach, goals of treatment include diminishing or eliminating the symptoms, facilitating healthier patterns of adaptation to stress, and preventing unnecessary procedures or treatments, including medications and surgery.

Virtually all authorities agree that directly confronting the patient about the psychological nature of the symptom is counterproductive and only serves to reinforce resistance and denial (11,44). Conversion symptoms should neither be trivialized nor reinforced. Attention and praise should be paid to improvement of function. Medical evaluations should include other health issues and minimize the focus on the conversion symptom. Results of examinations and laboratory and other tests should be discussed with the patient, particularly as they demonstrate the minimal organic nature of the symptom. These findings can be used to create the expectation of recovery in the patient and in the family (44).

Silver (44) suggests that the patient be educated about the psychological nature of the symptoms in a stepwise fashion. First discuss the process at the level of the brain, as if it were a separate entity; for example, "The signal from your brain to your muscles is temporarily blocked" (p. 135). Once there is some acceptance of this level of explanation, the concept of the mind, perhaps using the concept of a mental block, can be introduced.

Psychotherapy

Brief psychotherapy has been found to be useful in some cases (7,45). A nonpsychoanalytic, noninterpretative, non-confrontational approach that develops an alliance with the patient and shifts the focus from the physical symptom to the psychological environment is preferable.

Behavioral Management

Behavior therapy interventions are directed at the symptom and the environmental antecedents and consequences that are thought to sustain the symptom. Typically the sustaining reinforcers are thought to be social attention or escape from a noxious activity and are similar to the concepts of primary and secondary gain discussed below. Behavior therapy seeks to systematically reduce the reinforcement of the symptom and to reinforce more adaptive social, emotional, and task-oriented behaviors (46,47).

Hypnosis and Abreactive Therapy

A number of case reports suggest that hypnosis, relaxation, or drug-induced altered states of consciousness are beneficial for patients with acute conversion symptoms (48–50). Hafeiz described a study comparing the pairing of a suggestion that the symptom would disappear with four randomly assigned treatment protocols (51). He found that briefly applied faradic stimulation to the limbs, relaxation produced by an electrosleep machine, and methedrine were equivalent, with success rates of 80% to 90%. In most cases the removal of the symptom was "usually accompanied by emotionally charged scenes with sighing, tears or shaking" (p. 548). These treatments probably all worked through the common principle of abreaction long noted to be of value in traumatically induced symptoms (38).

Medication

With the exception of drug-induced abreaction, medication appears to be singularly ineffective in the treatment of conversion symptoms. Benzodiazepines are contraindicated because of a high rate of abuse in these patients, and inca-pacitating side effects from neuroleptics and antidepressants are common (45).

Milieu and Family Therapy

Clinicians can often trace the onset or maintenance of conversion symptoms to family or environmental dynamics. Consequently, family therapy and other environmental interventions are often tried and reported to sometimes be of value in treatment (46,48). Helping families to express previously blocked feelings and modifying family dynamics that reinforce the conversion symptom are common interventions.

Prognosis

The prognosis for a given conversion symptom appears to be associated with a number of factors. Symptoms with an acute and recent onset generally have a good prognosis (11,45,51). The precipitation of the symptom by an identifiable stressful event, good premorbid health, and the absence of concomitant organic or psychiatric illness are favorable factors (11). Improvement is most consistently related to recent symptom onset, fewer symptoms, and the absence of significant psychiatric comorbidity. Relapse rates are correlated with the duration of the symptom and are low for intervals of less than 30 days but increase dramatically for symptoms present for a year or longer (45,51). Motor disturbances and aphonia appear to have better prognoses than pseudoseizures and psychogenic blindness (51). A study by Couprie et al found that about 59% of conversion disorder patients had fully recovered on follow-up (52). Volkmar et al note that children who have experienced conversion symptoms associated with sexually stressful events have a poor prognosis (33).

Lateralization of Conversion Symptoms

In adults, conversion symptoms appear most often on the nondominant side of the body (53–55). This observation has led to speculations about the role of the right cerebral hemisphere in mediating affectively laden somatic symptoms. Attempts to document right hemisphere involvement have found, at best, mixed results (56). Regan and LaBarbara found, however, that conversion symptoms in children are more likely to occur on the dominant side of the body (57). They suggest that this is due to an incomplete lateralization of the hemispheres in children. Further research is needed to clarify the role of hemispheric specialization and the apparent lateralization of conversion symptoms.

The Role of Trauma

Battlefield psychiatrists have long noted a high incidence of conversion symptoms and dissociative states occasioned by acute stress (7,58). While many have speculated that these symptoms function to remove the patient from combat (7), Slater and others have pointed out that by impeding critical motor or sensory functions, conversion symptoms are often life-threatening on the battlefield (58).

In peacetime, conversion symptoms are often preceded by an acute stress (11,55). Raskin et al (59) and Whitlock (39) found that an identifiable stressor preceded the onset of conversion symptoms in 54% to 93% of patients. A specific form of conversion symptom, pseudoseizures, in children and adolescents has been closely linked to a history of sexual abuse (60). Loewenstein has cogently reviewed the evidence that somatoform disorders in general are strongly associated with a history of childhood abuse (60).

Psychodynamic Theories

Psychodynamic theories of conversion symptoms have received wide acceptance in North America (7,25). For the most part, they are derived from Freud's early explanation that conversion represents a substitution of physical symptoms for repressed instinctual impulses and that the physical symptom contains a symbolic representation of the repressed impulses (7). The conversion symptom binds the individual's anxiety by preventing activities that may lead to the expression of the repressed impulse, for example, limb paralysis preventing the acting out of sexual impulses.

Behavioral Theories

A second commonly held theory is derived from Charcot's theory of the legitimization of the sick role as a way in which an individual communicates his or her emotional distress through the socially acceptable device of a physical symptom (7,25). The sick role is adopted whenever its advantages outweigh the disadvantages. An individual's threshold for adoption of the sick role is dependent on personality and constitutional factors. For some the sick role is preferable most of the time; for others it is attractive only in times of great stress, such as in soldiers at war (61). The high incidence of conversion symptoms in the young is, according to this theory, explained by their relative immaturity and greater dependency so that the adoption of a role in which one is dependent and cared for comes more easily. Others have used similar rationale to explain the apparently high incidence of conversion symptoms in women (61,62).

Primary and Secondary Gain

The concepts of primary and secondary gain are invoked by both psychodynamic and behavioral theories of conversion. In primary gain, the conversion symptom serves to keep an internal conflict or need out of conscious awareness. In such cases, the conversion symptom is thought to be symbolically related to the conflict and usually occurs in close temporal proximity to an environmental event that activates the conflict or need. In secondary gain, the conversion symptom allows the patient to avoid an activity or situation that is noxious to him or her.

Altered States of Consciousness

Charcot and Marie believed that hysteria and conversion symptoms were the results of a special state of consciousness (4). Breuer and Freud emphasized the role of a particular type of altered state, the hypnoid state, in the production of hysterical symptoms (6). Modern theorists and clinicians continue to identify the operation of special or altered states of consciousness in the creation of hysterical and conversion symptoms (63).

Clinically, conversion symptoms share a number of general properties associated with state-specific alterations in consciousness. Altered states of consciousness are discrete constellations of physiologic and behavioral variables that repeat themselves, are self-organizing and self-perpetuating, and relatively stable (64). Transitions between states of consciousness (switches) are associated with discontinuous changes in state-defining variables; for example, there are nonlinear changes in variables such as affect, motor behavior, access to memory, attention and cognition, regulatory physiology, and sense of self (64). Switches between states of consciousness are rapid and abrupt in state-related psychiatric syndromes, for example, panic attacks, catatonic states, affective state shifts in bipolar illness, and the onset/offset of dissociative states (64). There is state-specific access to memory, so that memories and knowledge available to an individual in one state of consciousness are not as available in another state (64). States of consciousness, particularly affective and anxiety states, are communicable to others and play an important role in nonverbal communication.

Most conversion symptoms, for example, pseudoseizures and limb paralysis, have abrupt onsets and offsets with a time course consistent with switching between states of consciousness (64,65). Major alterations in motor behavior are characteristic of shifts in states of consciousness (64,65) and typically occur in conversion symptoms. A disturbance in access to specific memories and an altered sense of self are often reported in conversion symptoms and allied dissociative states (40,58,63,66). Stress, conflict, and trauma are important precipitants of conversion symptoms and have long been identified as triggers for altered states of consciousness (64). Conversion symptoms are communicable or contagious in a manner similar to the transmission of anxiety and affective states. Epidemic hysteria and conversion symptoms typically have an explosive onset, are associated with anxiety or dissociative states, and serve to abreact group trauma or conflict (67).

There is surprisingly little data on the psychophysiology of conversion symptoms, but current data are consistent with the hypothesis that conversion symptoms show alterations in regulatory physiology similar to those observed with altered states of consciousness. Several small-scale studies indicate that conversion symptoms are associated with alterations in sweat gland activity, heart rate, and muscle activity (68). Evoked potential studies of conversion sensory deficits, for example, hysterical anesthesias, blindness, and deafness, have yielded conflicting results (68). In most instances, no clear alterations in normal psychophysiology have been identified; some research centers use these measures as standard procedures for detecting hysterical symptoms.

REFERENCES

1. Lewis A. The survival of hysteria. In: Roy A, ed. Hysteria. Chichester: John Wiley, 1982:21–26.
2. Mace C. Hysterical conversion. I. A history. Br J Psychiatry 1992;161: 369–377.
3. Mai F, Merskey H. Briquet's treatise on hysteria. Arch Gen Psychiatry 1980;37:1401–1405.
4. Charcot J. Hysteria. In: Tuke E, ed. Dictionary of psychological medicine. Philadelphia: Blakiston, 1892:621–735.
5. Janet P. The major symptoms of hysteria. New York: Macmillan, 1907.
6. Breuer J, Freud S. Studies on hysteria. 1895. Reprint, New York: Basic Books, 1957.
7. Chodoff P. The diagnosis of hysteria: an overview. Am J Psychiatry 1974;131:1073–1078.
8. Guze S, Perley M. Observations on the natural history of hysteria. Am J Psychiatry 1963;119:960–965.
9. Mace C. Hysterical conversion. II. A critique. Br J Psychiatry 1992;161:378–389.
10. American Psychiatric Association. Diagnostic and statistical manual of mental disorders. 4th ed. Washington, DC: American Psychiatric Association, 1994.
11. Lazare A. Current concepts in psychiatry. N Engl J Med 1981;305:745–748.
12. Hodgman C. Conversion and somatization in pediatrics. Pediatr Rev 1995;16:29–34.
13. Wilbourn AJ. The electrodiagnostic examination with hysteria-conversion reaction and malingering. Neurol Clin 1995;13:385–404.
14. Morota N, Deletis V, Kiprovski K, et al. The use of motor evoked potentials in the diagnosis of psychogenic quadriparesis. A case study. Pediatr Neurosurg 1994;20:203–206.
15. Slater JD, Brown MC, Jacobs W, Ramsay RE. Induction of pseudoseizures with intravenous saline placebo. Epilepsia 1995;36:580–585.
16. Bradley RH, Zonia CL, Caputo SJ. The amobarbital sodium interview in conversion disorders: use of video feedback in therapy. J Am Osteopath Assoc 1995;95:122–125.
17. Hyatt M, Braun N, Briscoe G, Dickson L. The use of midazolam for hypnosedative interviews. Gen Hosp Psychiatry 1993;15:260–262.
18. Engel G. Conversion symptoms. In: MacBryde C, Blacklow R, eds. Signs and symptoms: applied and pathologic physiology and clinical interpretation. Philadelphia: JB Lippincott, 1970:223–234.
19. Guze S, Woodruff R, Clayton P. A study of conversion symptoms in psychiatric patients. Am J Psychiatry 1971;128:643–646.
20. Farley J, Woodruff R, Guze S. The prevalence of hysteria and conversion reactions. Br J Psychiatry 1968;114:1121–1125.
21. Trimble M. Neuropsychiatry. Chichester: John Wiley, 1974.
22. Marsden C. Hysteria—a neurologist's view. Psychol Med 1986;16:277–288.
23. McKegney E. The incidence and characteristics of patients with conversion reactions. 1. A general hospital consultation service sample. Am J Psychiatry 1967;124:128–131.
24. Woodruff R, Dayton P, Guse S. Hysteria. Br J Psychiatry 1969;128:1243–1248.
25. Klerman G. Hysteria and depression. In: Roy A, ed. Hysteria. Chichester: John Wiley, 1982:211–228.
26. Ljungberg L. Hysteria: a clinical, prognostic and genetic study. Acta Psychiatr Neurol Scand 1957;32(suppl 112):1–13.
27. Shields J. Genetical studies of hysterical disorders. In: Roy A, ed. Hysteria. Chichester: John Wiley, 1982:41–58.
28. Slater E. The thirty-fifth Maudsley lecture "Hysteria 311." J Ment Sci 1961;107:359–381.
29. Inouye E. Genetic aspects of neurosis. Int J Ment Health 1972;1:359–381.
30. Gold M, Friedman S. Conversion reactions in adolescents. Pediatr Ann 1995;24:296–306.
31. Goodyer I. Hysterical conversion reactions in childhood. J Child Psychol Psychiatry 1981;22:179–188.
32. Maloney M. Diagnosing hysterical conversion reactions in children. J Pediatr 1980;97:1016–1020.
33. Volkmar F, Poll J, Lewis M. Conversion reactions in childhood and adolescence. J Am Acad Child Psychiatry 1984;23:424–430.
34. Stephens J, Kamp M. On some aspects of hysteria: clinical study. J Nerv Ment Dis 1962;134:205–215.
35. Chodoff P, Lyons H. Hysteria, the hysterical personality and hysterical conversion. Am J Psychiatry 1958;114:734–740.
36. Cloninger S, Guze S. Psychiatric illness and female criminality. Am J Psychiatry 1970;127:303–311.
37. Blumer D, Montouris G, Hermann B. Psychiatric morbidity in seizure patients on a neurodiagnostic monitoring unit. J Neuropsychiatry Clin Neurosci 1995;7:445–456.
38. Putnam F. Diagnosis and treatment of multiple personality disorder. New York: Guilford Press, 1989.
39. Whitlock F. The etiology of hysteria. Acta Psychiatr Scand 1967;43:144–162.
40. Pincus J. Hysteria presenting to the neurologist. In: Roy A, ed. Hysteria. Chichester: John Wiley, 1982:131–144.
41. Slater J, Glithero E. A follow-up of patients diagnosed as suffering from hysteria. J Psychosom Res 1965;9:9–13.
42. Watson C, Buranen C. The frequency and identification of false positive conversion reactions. J Nerv Ment Dis 1979;167:243–247.
43. Fishbain D, Goldberg M, Khalil T, et al. The utility of electromyographic biofeedback in the treatment of conversion disorder. Am J Psychiatry 1988;145:1572–1575.
44. Silver F. Management of conversion disorder. Am J Phys Med Rehabil 1996;75:134–140.
45. The Quality Assurance Project. Treatment outlines for the management of the somatoform disorders. Aust N Z J Psychiatry 1985;19:397–407.
46. Munford P, Liberman R. Behavior therapy of hysterical disorders. In: Roy A, ed. Hysteria. Chichester: John Wiley, 1982:287–304.
47. Speed J. Behavioral management of conversion disorder: retrospective study. Arch Phys Med Rehabil 1996;77:147–154.
48. Brooksbank D. Management of conversion reaction in five adolescent girls. J Adolesc 1984;7:359–376.
49. Caldwell T, Steward R. Hysterical seizures and hypnotherapy. Am J Clin Hypn 1981;23:294–297.
50. Williams D, Spiegel H, Mostosfsky D. Neurogenic and hysterical seizures in children and adolescents: differential diagnostic and therapeutic considerations. Am J Psychiatry 1978;135:82–86.
51. Hafeiz H. Hysterical conversion: a prognostic study. Br J Psychiatry 1980;136:548–551.
52. Couprie W, Wijdicks E, Rooijmans H, van Gijn J. Outcome in conversion disorder: a follow-up study. J Neurol Neurosurg Psychiatry 1995;58:750–752.
53. Galin D, Diamond R, Braff D. Lateralization of conversion symptoms: more frequent on the left. Am J Psychiatry 1977;134:578–580.
54. Stern D. Handedness and the lateral distribution of conversion reactions. J Nerv Ment Dis 1977;164:122–128.
55. Ford C, Folks D. Conversion disorders: an overview. Psychosomatics 1985;71:380–383.
56. Drake M. Conversion hysteria and dominant hemisphere lesions. Psychosomatics 1993;34:524–530.
57. Regan J, LaBarbara J. Lateralization of conversion symptoms in children and adolescents. Am J Psychiatry 1984;141:1279–1280.
58. Slater E. What is hysteria? In: Roy A, ed. Hysteria. Chichester: John Wiley, 1982:37–40.
59. Raskin M, Talbott J, Myerson A. Diagnosed conversion reactions: predictive value of psychiatric criteria. JAMA 1966;197:530–534.
60. Loewenstein F. Somatoform disorders in victims of incest. In: Kluft R, ed. Incest-related syndromes of adult psychopathology. Washington, Dc: American Psychiatric Press, 1990:75–112.
61. Kendall R. A new look at hysteria. In: Roy A, ed. Hysteria. Chichester: John Wiley, 1982:27–36.
62. Hollender M. Conversion hysteria: a post-Freudian reinterpretation of 19th century psychosocial data. Arch Gen Psychiatry 1972;26:311–314.

63. Fenton G. Hysterical alterations in consciousness. In: Roy A, ed. Hysteria. Chichester: John Wiley, 1982:229–246.

64. Putnam F. The switch process in multiple personality disorder and other state-change disorders. Dissociation 1988;1:24–32.

65. Pincus J, Tucker G. Behavioral neurology. 2nd ed. New York: Oxford University Press, 1978.

66. Ludwig A. Hysteria: a neurobiological theory. Arch Gen Psychiatry 1972;27:771–777.

67. Sirois F. Epidemic hysteria. In: Roy A, ed. Hysteria. Chichester: John Wiley, 1982:101–116.

68. Lader M. The psychophysiology of hysteria. In: Roy A, ed. Hysteria. Chichester: John Wiley, 1982:81–86.

Neurologic Soft Signs in Psychiatric Disorders

BRYAN T. WOODS

HISTORICAL DEVELOPMENT OF THE CONCEPT OF SOFT SIGNS

Before one can review the topic of soft signs in psychiatry it is necessary to devote considerable attention to definitions and to the evolution of the concept. This is so because over the 40 years since the beginnings of the whole idea, studies of soft signs have been more notable for their differences than their similarities in both the signs they include and those they exclude. Because of this imprecision the very term "soft signs" was once derided as a symptom of soft thinking. Nevertheless, if soft signs are viewed in the broader context of the essentially probabilistic nature of diagnostic methodology in neurology, their value can be better appreciated.

The original development of the concept of soft signs occurred in pediatric neurology in the context of the diagnosis of minimal brain damage (MBD) (1). The idea of MBD emerged from the observation that in children who were suspected of having suffered perinatal brain insults, one might see a disorder with both neurologic symptoms and behavioral symptoms, but without any of the hallmarks of classic neurologic disease, either in terms of localizing lesions or other fixed characteristics. The behavioral abnormalities first noted were particularly related to hyperactivity, while the neurologic signs included an excess of associated (or overflow) movements, choreiform movements, incoordination and clumsiness, and persistence of immature (primitive) reflexes and motor patterns. In 1962 Prechtl and Stemmer (2) described the choreiform syndrome, stating that it was characterized neurologically by fluctuating and shifting jerky movements and twitches of the extremities and the head and was associated behaviorally with hyperactivity and difficulties with concentration and learning. However, it soon became evident that although such signs as choreiform

movements were more common in children with a history of behavioral difficulties, they were also present in a considerable number of otherwise apparently normal children, particularly boys (3,4).

Even though the specificity of the choreiform syndrome could not be established by these replication studies (3,4), the general observation of an increased association in some children among relatively minor abnormalities of motor function, behavioral disturbances, and learning difficulties was well established. The original notion that these children had actual brain damage was modified to the less specific term "minimal brain dysfunction." Nevertheless, the underlying assumption that such dysfunction might be related to brain insults suffered during pregnancy, delivery, or the perinatal period persisted. As an outgrowth of this work, several batteries of neurologic examinations that emphasized soft signs were developed and published. In 1970 Touwen and Prechtl (5) published *The Neurological Examination of the Child with Minor Nervous System Dysfunction*, which emphasized assessments of posture, spontaneous motility, muscle power, resistance to passive movements, plantar responses, standing posture, and involuntary movements such as choreiform movements, athetosis, tremor, diadochokinesis, and associated movements. They also included observation of walking and variations in eye movements such as strabismus and altered optokinetic nystagmus in their recommended examination.

In 1975 Peters et al (6) described their standardized neurologic examination of children with learning disabilities. Much of it is similar to the Touwen and Prechtl battery (5), but it also includes certain other items of higher cerebral function, such as tests for right-left confusion, speech, writing, spelling, and finger gnosis. Items of cortical sensory examination were also introduced by the inclusion of two-point discrimination. Subsequently, other tests of cortical sensory function, including graphesthesia, double simultaneous stimulation (both visual and tactile), and stereognosis have been added to the evolving repertoire of soft signs. Most recently, tests of motor sequencing intended to look at frontal lobe function, some taken from the work of Luria in adult patients (7), have been added to soft sign examinations (8).

A move in the opposite direction, to be more restrictive in the soft sign examination, is embodied in the 1985 revision (9) of the original physical and neurologic examination for soft signs (10). Items eliminated from the original by this revised battery include eye-tracking tests, stereognosis, tactile double simultaneous stimulation, and other sensory items; it is redesignated as an examination for subtle (rather than soft) signs. This latest version then becomes similar to the early soft signs inventories in primarily emphasizing motor function: gait, coordination, balance, alternating movement, and overflow movements.

As the range of abnormalities encompassed by the term "soft signs" extended far beyond the original emphasis in the early pediatric studies, the defining characteristic came to be the nonlocalizing character of these signs (11), that is, their lack of clear association with a focal neurologic lesion. Even this defining criterion tends to break down, however, because many of the soft signs are certainly localizable to a specific system (such as the extrapyramidal system or sensory association areas), even though, if the system is anatomically widely distributed, the sign is not diagnostic of a lesion in a single specific location.

Table 61.1 categorizes the different neurologic examination items that various authors have used in looking for soft signs. The first category, developmental motor functions, includes most of the classic soft sign items. The items in 1(a) have in common an assessment of simple motor performance, both in terms of smoothness and rapidity of intended movements and suppression or inhibition of simultaneous unintended movements. These abilities increase with nervous system maturation, so that what is normal at age 5 may be abnormal at age 10—hence the characterization of the signs as developmental, and the original postulation that soft signs were evidence of nervous system immaturity (12,13). The items of category 1(b), tests for primitive reflexes, look for persistence of responses that normally disappear within the first 2 years of life. They are also developmental, but differ from the 1(a) signs in being essentially all-or-none phenomena, whereas most of the items in 1(a) have gradations.

Category 2 of Table 61.1, tests of motor system symmetry, assesses what might be better termed subtle signs, since such asymmetries are localizing to a degree (though it is not always easy to decide whether the defect is central or peripheral, or even whether the asymmetry results from "too much" on one side or "too little" on the other). The inclusion of extraocular movement and skeletal growth asymmetry in this group of signs seems justified because asymmetries of both are frequently seen along with

T a b l e   6 1 . 1   Categories of Soft Neurologic Signs

1. Developmental Motor Functions
    (a) Items that assess speed and coordination of simple intentional movements along with the inhibition of unintended (associated) movements
        (i) Alternating movements of tongue, hands and fingers, or feet
        (ii) Maintenance of fixed posture without instability; e.g., holding extended arms supine and fingers spread with no pronation choreiform movements, or impersistence
        (iii) Balance: Romberg's sign, hopping on one foot
        (iv) Gait: balance plus inhibition of associated movements plus coordination
            —Heel and toe walking; varus and valgus walking
            —Tandem walking
        (v) Sitting quietly
        (vi) Mouth opening, finger spreading
    (b) Persistence of primitive reflexes
        (i) Babinski reflexes
        (ii) Grasp reflexes
        (iii) Tonic neck reflexes, changes in motor tone or posture
        (iv) Palmomental reflexes
        (v) Snout reflex
        (vi) Glabellar reflex
2. Tests of Motor Systems Symmetry
    (a) Deep tendon reflex symmetry
        (i) Lateral
        (ii) Upper versus lower extremities
    (b) Motor strength and tone symmetry
    (c) Facial symmetry
    (d) Oculomotor symmetry
    (e) Body part (skeletal) size symmetry
3. Laterality Measures (Hand, Foot, Eye Preference)
    (a) Inconsistency of laterality and motor dexterity
    (b) Inconsistency of eye, hand, and foot preferences
4. Cortical Functions
    (a) Sensory
        (i) Stereognosis
        (ii) Graphesthesia
        (iii) Two-point discrimination
        (iv) Extinction to visual or tactile double simultaneous stimulation
        (v) Cutaneous localization
        (vi) Matching patterns across sensory modalities
    (b) Spatial orientation
        (i) Left-right confusion
        (ii) Finger gnosis
    (c) Language functions
        (i) Stuttering, dysarthria
        (ii) Dysphasia
        (iii) Dysgraphia
        (iv) Dyslexia
        (v) Dyscalculia
        (vi) Constructional apraxia
    (d) Motor functions
        (i) Alternating motor sequences
        (ii) Tests of skilled motor programs
        (iii) Facial praxis
        (iv) Motor persistence

other signs of unilateral early-life nervous system injury (14).

Category 3, laterality assessment, is included as a separate category of sign because hand, eye, or foot preferences may be pathologically determined and an excess of left handedness has been considered a soft sign in group studies, even though it cannot be so considered as such in any given individual. Inconsistencies of preference and performance, such as the right hander who does alternating movements better with the left hand, may be significant signs even at the individual level.

Category 4 comprises the cortical soft signs. These too are an extension of the learning disability items utilized in the early MBD studies, but they have also been influenced by adult behavioral neurology and neuropsychology. These signs, which in many cases *are* of localizing value in adult neurology, are not consistent with the notion of soft signs as nonlocalizing. Furthermore, because some of them require quantitation for interpretation, they begin to overlap with neuropsychologic test batteries. They continue to be labeled soft signs in the literature, however, and thus are included here for historical reasons and for the sake of completeness.

Although all the items in Table 61.1 have been described in the literature as soft signs, it is not an exhaustive list; even so, it is evident how difficult it is to come up with an all-encompassing definition. Historically, the signs in 1(a) have been the core of the concept, and these may be defined as signs of a nonlocalizing motor system dysfunction marked by slowness, incoordination, and disinhibition inconsistent with developmental age. The question is whether such a narrow definition is more useful than one that would encompass the other categories of soft signs as well. The case for a narrow definition would be stronger if it resulted in the delimitation of a specific clinical entity or even if the narrowly defined signs had a specific clinicoanatomic or pathophysiologic correlate. Unfortunately, they do not. A good example is provided by mirror movements. These movements, which are induced on one side by intentional movements on the opposite side, had been noted clinically as early as 1842 (15). They are one of the central group of classic soft signs, and the responsible defects can be tentatively localized at different levels of the nervous system (Table 61.2). Thus, given this heterogeneity of both causation and localization in a well-studied classic soft sign, it seems that when one is looking for evidence of subtle brain injury or dysfunction there is little justification for restrictiveness; a reasonable case can be made for the clinical use of signs belonging to any of the categories listed in Table 61.1, as long as one has due regard for their varying methodologic limitations.

The second question about soft signs implied at the outset was that of their utility in research and clinical neurology; that is, what it is possible to infer from soft sign abnormalities (16). As critics of the soft signs concept have pointed out, these signs are nonspecific as to disorder, often

Table 61.2   Types of Mirror Movement

1. Normal developmental. Maximal in preschool children; declines steadily up to ages 10 to 12; may still be seen in adults under conditions of fatigue or exertion. Can be suppressed with conscious effort.
2. Congenital pathologic. Associated with structural brain deficits present during prenatal development, e.g., Klippel-Feil syndrome, Kallman's syndrome. Probably due to uncrossed corticospinal tracts; obligatory (nonsuppressable).
3. Hereditary. Seen as an isolated abnormality with an autosomal dominant pattern of inheritance; obligatory. Not associated with behavioral disorders.
4. Delayed maturational. Excessive for age; suppressable; strong statistical association with learning disabilities, hyperactivity, and impulsivity.
5. Hemiparetic/hemianesthetic. Acquired hemiparesis, especially of early onset, results in mirroring in the "good" hand. Hemianesthesia less commonly can lead to mirroring in the "bad" hand.

nonlocalizing (or, more correctly, localized to a major system that is distributed over many brain regions), variable from examination to examination and over individual developmental stages, subject to examiner bias and variation in threshold sensitivity, and at times present in otherwise apparently normal individuals. In fact, however, qualitatively similar criticisms can be made about any neurologic sign, not excluding upgoing toes. The above limitations are in essence reflections of the probabilistic nature of neurologic diagnosis based on physical examination. The experienced clinician does not depend to any large degree on the presence or absence of pathognomonic signs of disease in making a diagnosis, but rather uses knowledge and experience to weight not only individual signs but patterns of signs, along with similarly weighted historical and laboratory data. If one looks at the neurologic examination in this framework, one can then characterize soft signs as differing quantitatively from hard signs in that less diagnostic weight can ordinarily be given to them on an individual basis, but as not differing qualitatively from any other portion of the examination. Denckla (9) has called them subtle signs, which implies something of the same notion. Although Denckla's subtle-signs battery (9) is actually quite closely limited to the traditional soft signs listed in 1(a) of Table 61.1, the term seems apropos for the broader group as well. It is clear that use of these signs in research studies requires more attention to such methodologic issues as appropriate control groups and inter- and intrarater reliability (16) than is customary with use of the traditional neurologic examination, but with proper attention to these matters, soft signs appear to be useful both in clinical diagnosis and clinical research (17).

SOFT SIGNS IN PSYCHIATRY

The use of specific batteries of soft signs has never become common in adult neurology, but has been widespread in pediatric neurology and in psychiatry. One possible explanation for this popularity of soft signs in psychiatry may be that standardized diagnostic systems exclude patients a priori from major psychiatric diagnoses (such as schizophrenia) if they have focal or demonstrable neurologic abnormalities that are considered responsible for their behavioral disturbance. It is only a slight exaggeration to say that by definition only soft signs, considered as nondiagnostic and/or nonlocalizing signs, are consistent with a formal psychiatric diagnosis of schizophrenia or bipolar affective disorder. Setting such considerations aside, however, it becomes clear from a review of almost four decades of work that soft signs have provided important clinical and research insights in the areas of psychiatry where they have been utilized.

Most of the reports of soft signs in psychiatric disorders can be grouped as follows: (1) soft signs in nonpsychotic behavioral disorders of children (primarily the attention deficit disorder spectrum); (2) soft signs in diagnostically mixed groups of early adolescents; (3) soft signs in diagnostically mixed adult and late-adolescent populations, particularly in adult schizophrenia and bipolar affective disorder patients; and (4) soft signs in childhood schizophrenia and in children of schizophrenic parents.

Children with Nonpsychotic Behavioral Disorders

As was noted in the introduction, the concept of MBD was an attempt to find an underlying connection between certain patterns of neurologic dysfunction and behavioral disturbances in children. The first ambitious attempts at delineation of syndromes of specific soft signs and specific behavioral problems, such as the choreiform syndrome of Prechtl (2), did not completely hold up because subsequent studies indicated that patterns of choreiform movements similar to those described in MBD can be seen in a rather large minority of normal schoolchildren and are only poorly predictive of behavioral difficulties in this group (3,4). Similar problems have occurred with use of hyperactivity as a single behavioral marker for a specific syndrome. An early study by Werry (18) examined 103 hyperactive children, aged 6 to 10 years, of whom 91% were males, and found that 39 (38%) had neurologic abnormalities. This work led to the development of a specific battery, the original Physical and Neurologic Examination of Soft Signs (PANESS) (10). However, an attempt to replicate the association between hyperactivity and abnormalities on the PANESS showed that the battery was unable to distinguish between hyperactive and normal children at different ages (19), even though the same study could demonstrate a significant relationship of these soft signs to age in both hyperactive and normal children.

Studies that included a variety of soft signs and/or a variety of abnormal behaviors tended to yield more positive results. Wender (20), whose definition of MBD includes five subtypes: classic hyperactive, neurotic, psychopathic, schizophrenic, and special learning disordered, reports a

prevalence of soft signs of approximately 50% in MBD referrals. One exception to this rule that one obtains a higher yield and greater patient-control discrimination by using a variety of signs comes from studies using mirror movements as a single sign of neurologic dysfunction: several such studies have found them usefully discriminatory in group studies. Woods and Eby (21) reported that in a group of psychiatrically hospitalized children and young adolescents, patients with a history of impulsive aggressive behavior had more mirror movements than patients without such a history. Szatmari and Taylor (22) looked at overflow movements in boys between 7 and 11 years old in four primary schools; 138 of 167 eligible children were actually examined. Eight (73%) of 11 children with the highest overflow scores had behavioral problems, compared with 2 (18%) of 11 with the lowest scores. Looked at from the other direction, 21% of the children with behavioral problems had excessive overflow scores, whereas only 3% of those without behavioral problems had similarly excessive scores.

In general, reported soft sign studies have been cross-sectional, but Shaffer et al (17) have reported a 10-year follow-up study of 162 subjects that correlated soft signs present at age 7 with psychiatric diagnoses at age 17. These results are as follows:

Psychiatric Diagnosis at Age 17	Signs at Age 7	
	No	Yes
No	54	42
Yes	25	41

In the 21 patients with a diagnosis of anxiety disorder at age 17, 6 of 6 girls and 12 of 15 boys had had soft signs at age 7. In general, the more soft signs present at age 7, the greater the risk of having a psychiatric disorder at age 17. These numbers illustrate one of the general principles about soft signs and psychiatric disorders: they have a greater than chance association, but often occur independently.

Early-Adolescent Mixed Psychiatric Disorders

Perhaps the first study of this category to rely more or less exclusively on soft signs or "equivocal signs" was that of Kennard in 1960 (23). This study looked at children hospitalized for psychiatric disorders who were between ages 13 and 16, and found that the average number of soft signs was greatest for those with an "organic" or "organic plus schizophrenia" diagnosis. Pure schizophrenic patients were next highest, and sociopathic and neurotic patients were lowest and appeared to be hardly different from the controls. Somewhat similar studies were carried out by Hertzig and Birch (24,25). These studies, which looked separately at adolescent girls and boys hospitalized for psychiatric illness, found an excess of neurologic abnormalities, primarily soft signs, in both groups. Approximately one-third of all patients had soft signs, whereas only a small percentage had hard (i.e., localizing) signs. In boys, the abnormalities cut across diagnostic categories, but in girls they were found to be concentrated among those diagnosed as psychotic. (It should be noted that in these earlier studies a large proportion of the patients were diagnosed as schizophrenic, consistent with American diagnostic practices prior to the third edition of the *Diagnostic and Statistical Manual of Mental Disorders* (DSM-III) (26), and it is unlikely that many of the patients would meet current criteria for that diagnosis.)

Soft Signs in Adult Psychiatric Disorders

There are several studies of soft signs that have either looked at consecutive admissions or compared patients from two or more diagnostic categories (with schizophrenia as one category). Rochford et al (27) used a broadly defined soft sign battery and looked at 65 patients (inpatients and outpatients), 26 (40%) of whom were diagnosed schizophrenic (once again, this proportion reflects pre–DSM-III diagnostic practice). Neurologic abnormalities (defined as one hard or two soft signs) were found in 24 (37%) of the 65 patients, including 17 (65%) of 26 schizophrenic patients. No affective patients met the preestablished criteria for neurologic abnormality, but 5 (42%) of 12 had one soft sign. Tucker et al (28) compared schizophrenic (pre–DSM-III criteria) and nonschizophrenic patients on four neurologic tests of cortical soft signs (type 4, Table 61.1). Twenty-two (58%) of the 38 schizophrenic patients had mild to moderate neurologic impairment, compared with 23 (32%) of 71 nonschizophrenic patients. Cox and Ludwig (8) also emphasized cortical soft signs but grouped their 76 patients diagnostically according to the Feighner criteria (29); in consequence, their 21 schizophrenic patients can be considered roughly comparable with DSM-III-diagnosed schizophrenic patients. They found that these 21 patients had more frontal signs than any other group, but overlapped with unipolar depressive patients in terms of having excessive parietal and total cortical impairment.

Nasrallah et al (30) compared DSM-III-diagnosed manic and schizophrenic inpatients with a hospital staff control group on a battery that also emphasized cortical soft signs, and concluded that the two patient groups both had significantly more soft signs than the control groups but did not differ significantly from one another. Two other studies that have compared schizophrenic patients with affective patients (31,32) found the schizophrenic patients to be more impaired, but both of those studies included unipolar depressed patients in the affective groups. However, in a prospective study that limited the affective patient group to DSM-III-diagnosed bipolar patients with a history of psychosis, Woods et al (33) found schizophrenic patients to have significantly more neurologic signs of potential etiologic significance than either manic-depressive patients or healthy controls (and replicated this finding on a different sample [34]), but did not find the schizophrenic group to differ significantly in terms of total scores or number of affected individuals from a group hospitalized for substance abuse. Their battery differed from that of Nasrallah et al (30) by emphasizing subtle hard signs and a limited number of classic motor soft signs.

In summary, these studies have all found that the psychiatric patients studied show more abnormalities on neurologic examination than nonpsychiatric control groups. Most studies have also found that schizophrenic patients have more neurologic abnormalities than other diagnostic groups, but one study (30) found a similar prevalence of abnormalities in manic patients, and another (33) did not show a statistically significant difference between schizophrenic and substance abuse inpatients. One study looked at both schizophrenic and bipolar patients with or without tardive dyskinesia (TD) and found that within both diagnostic groups the patients with TD had significantly more neurologic signs than those without TD (35).

Several groups have looked at the relationship of neurologic abnormalities to family history in schizophrenia. In a very influential early study, Mosher et al (36) reported that when identical twins, discordant for schizophrenia, were examined neurologically the schizophrenic probands had significantly more abnormalities than their nonschizophrenic twins. A more recent study of discordant twin pairs not only replicated this finding but also showed that the well twins from these pairs had significantly more signs than normal twin pairs (37). This study also looked at whether a history of obstetric complications was correlated with abnormal signs in discordant twin pairs and found that the correlation was significant for the well twins but fell short of significance for the schizophrenic twins. Similarly, Kinney et al looked at neurologic signs in the nonschizophrenic first-degree relatives of schizophrenic patients (38) and found an increase in subtle and soft signs in this group compared with normal controls, but no significant difference between relatives and probands.

Other variables that have been looked at in relation to neurologic abnormalities in schizophrenia include paranoid versus nonparanoid (no difference [39]), premorbid asociality versus emotionally unstable character disorder (different patterns of abnormality [40]), acute versus chronic (chronic showing more abnormalities [41]), good versus poor outcome (no difference in one study [42], but decreased signs after clinical improvement in another report [43]), lateral asymmetry of signs (none [44]), and institutionalized versus returned to the community (no difference [45]). One study that looked at the relationship of neurologic signs and cognitive measures to violence in schizophrenic patients reached the somewhat counterintuitive conclusion that there was an *inverse* relationship between a history of violent behavior and numbers of neurologic abnormalities and a *direct* relationship between higher levels of cognitive functioning and violent behavior (46).

A number of studies have looked at motor abnormalities, including primitive reflexes, and exposure to neuroleptic medications in schizophrenia. Owens and Johnstone (47),

Owens et al (48), Manschreck et al (49), Rogers (50), and Gupta et al (51) have all concluded that abnormalities of movement and tone seen in schizophrenia are not solely related to neuroleptic exposure, but were found prior to the introduction of neuroleptics and can still be found in never-exposed, more recently examined patients. Interestingly, when these neuroleptic-naive patients are compared with other patients exposed to neuroleptics, the naive patients show less overall signs but equal numbers of developmental signs (51).

It has also been suggested (49,52,53) that motor and cognitive deficits in these patients may be two facets of a common underlying defect, possibly localized to the prefrontal regions of the cerebral cortex. One somewhat conflicting conclusion has been postulated for bipolar disorder patients. Mukherjee et al (54) found soft sign abnormalities only in patients with long-term neuroleptic exposure. (This raises the interesting possibility that there are neurologic defects intrinsic to schizophrenia that can be induced by neuroleptics in patients with other psychiatric diagnoses [55].)

Most studies of soft signs in adult psychiatric disorders have been focused on schizophrenia or manic-depressive illness, but a recent study that looked at the diagnostic status of 22 of 300 psychiatric inpatients who had an abnormal palmomental reflex found that 6 (27.3%) were diagnosed schizoaffective, and 5 (18.2%) bipolar with psychosis, although those two diagnostic groups only constituted 5.9% and 4.1% respectively of the referral base population (56).

Soft Signs in Childhood Schizophrenia and in Children with a Schizophrenic Parent

Attempts have also been made to relate soft signs to schizophrenia in childhood schizophrenia. In a major early study, Gittelman and Birch (57) looked at 51 children for whom neurologic examination data and IQ scores were available. Thirty-eight (74.5%) of the 51 children evaluated had either moderate or severe neurologic dysfunction, and this impaired group had a mean full-scale IQ score 38 points lower than the neurologically unimpaired group. Fish (58) reviewed the whole issue of the nosology of childhood schizophrenia and concluded that it was "continuous with the most severe, chronic, adult schizophrenia" and that there was a "neurointegrative defect" already evident in infancy. Fish's work (58) in very young children estimated neurologic status based on constructs derived from the Gesell (59) developmental standards rather than from a specific neurologic battery.

Fish (60) is also one of the group of researchers who initiated a series of studies of soft signs in high-risk children, that is, children with one or two schizophrenic parents. The high-risk paradigm is an effort to delineate the antecedents of adult-onset schizophrenia by examining children known on statistical grounds to be at considerably greater risk than the general population for later developing the disorder.

Studies have looked at two periods in the life of these children: infancy/early childhood and later childhood/early adolescence. The infant neurologic data are to a considerable extent based on findings that are somewhat outside the soft sign spectrum and will not be reviewed, except to note that the available reports conflict as to whether these children have increased neurologic abnormalities or not (61). For older children the findings are less equivocal. Fish and Hagin (62) report perceptual disabilities, specific reading disabilities, and poor fine-motor coordination in 10-year-old high-risk subjects. Several different groups that participated in the Collaborative Perinatal Project (CPP) (63) found at least a trend for an excess of neurologic abnormalities, primarily motor, in older high-risk children (64–66).

In a separate high-risk study carried out in Israel, Marcus et al (67) found school-age offspring of schizophrenic parents had more neurologic soft signs, particularly poor motor coordination and perceptual dysfunctioning. Similar results were obtained in a Danish high-risk study (68), though that study found motor overflow as well as motor incoordination to be excessive. Interestingly, Marcus et al (69) have also provided some outcome data: 9 (18%) of 50 high-risk children in their study now have a schizophrenia spectrum diagnosis, and although only 24 (48%) of the 50 high-risk children had early neurobehavioral signs, 8 (89%) of the 9 with adult illness had such signs. Most recently, McNeil et al (70) reported results of neurological evaluations of a Swedish high-risk population at age 6 years. They found increased neuromotor abnormalities at age 6 in children of mothers diagnosed with schizophrenia or unspecified functional psychosis, but not children of mothers with schizoaffective disorder or bipolar disorder. These deficits did not correlate with a positive history of birth complications, and the children did not have an excess of cognitive or psychosocial deficits. Taken together, these studies suggest that high-risk children do show an excess of soft signs, especially before age 11 (61), and that the signs are predictive of later development of adult schizophrenic illness.

Utility and Limitations of Soft Signs in Psychiatry

The usefulness of soft signs can be considered from two perspectives: clinical practice and research. Clinically, examination for soft signs can be useful in all age ranges, but different signs are helpful in different age ranges. In children and younger adolescents the presence of the signs in group 1(a) (see Table 61.1), along with historical data and response to treatment, lends considerable weight to diagnosis of one or another form of the attention deficit/hyperactive disorder (ADHD) complex. Contrarily, the absence of such signs should lead to increased attention to the many environmental and psychosocial factors that can result in apparently similar patterns of disturbed childhood behavior. This distinction can be particularly important when one of the therapeutic alternatives in these children is use of amphetamines.

In young-adult psychiatric patients, the author has found that the motor soft signs of groups 1(a) and 1(b) are only infrequently present and that the more important abnormalities are the subtle lateralizing signs of group 2 (Table 61.1). Such signs may point to a mild "hemisyndrome," which in turn may correlate with other clinical data suggestive of unrecognized complex partial seizures. In older patients, soft signs of groups 1(b) and 4 are the most likely to provide early evidence for an underlying dementing process or other neurologic disorder responsible for the psychiatric symptoms. There are, however, several difficulties that arise in assessing soft signs in adult psychiatric patients, especially those who are psychotic. The first major problem is that tests that require the active cooperation of the patient are vulnerable to anything that interferes with that cooperation. Interference can come from preoccupation with internal stimuli, indifference, lack of arousal, cognitive misunderstanding, and even volitional resistance. It is extremely difficult to get reliable sensory examination data from acutely psychotic patients, but there are problems with other patients as well. For one thing, patients may not fully understand the task. For example, on testing of double simultaneous stimulation (either visual or tactile), patients often do not realize that the stimuli may be bilateral. If this is not fully explained, they may detect bilateral stimuli but not report what they believe is a "wrong" answer.

A second problem that also arises clinically is medication effects. Currently prescribed antipsychotic medications can interfere with both cognition and motor function. Neuroleptics can cause both choreiform movements and variations in motor tone. The author has on a number of occasions found acutely psychotic patients on large doses of neuroleptic medication to have both grasp reflexes and upgoing toes, only to have both findings disappear as the psychosis clears and the medication dosage is reduced.

From a research viewpoint, soft signs offer another potential avenue into understanding the etiology of a variety of disorders, but they pose considerable methodologic and interpretive difficulties as well. First, there is no agreed-on definition of just what the limits are of the soft sign concept, so every researcher tends to use a different group of signs. The result is that it is difficult to compare the results of such separate studies. Second, it is difficult to determine the degree of equivalency of different signs. One can argue that excess mirror movements and choreiform movements are more similar to one another than either is to astereognosis, but there are only limited data to support this assumption. Marcus et al (67) and Schroder (43) have used factor analysis to attack this problem and have come up with groupings of signs that appear consistent with what one might expect based on clinical grounds, but other investigators have not done this. Lacking such data, one cannot decide whether a given study that finds 10 signs that discriminate subjects and controls has found evidence for 10 separate defects or has simply assessed the same defect in 10 superficially different but fundamentally equivalent ways.

Still a third area of difficulty is that of reproducibility of results. One has to contend with variation between examiners, variation over time in the same examiner, and variation in the subject. The CPP study (63) is a good example. Examiners in the Boston area found many more neurologic abnormalities in all of their groups than examiners in other centers (65); the most probable explanation is that thresholds for accepting findings varied systematically between academic centers.

In spite of these caveats one cannot review the literature of soft signs without concluding that knowledge of the origins and mechanisms of soft signs will be a critical component for progress in understanding the whole complex of learning and behavioral disorders of children that are currently grouped under the ADHD umbrella. In the case of schizophrenia, the evidence that soft signs are the neurologic manifestation of a factor that is integral to the development of the illness is not so overwhelming as for ADHD, but the number of independent studies that have found a relationship is impressive and certainly points to the desirability of further investigation.

THE ORIGIN AND PATHOGENETIC SIGNIFICANCE OF SOFT SIGNS

The foregoing discussion of soft signs has suggested that there is both a broad and a narrow definition of soft signs and that many of the signs in the more broadly defined group might better be referred to as subtle signs. Clinically, such signs, which may be evidence for relatively mild or at least silent brain disorders, are important clues to etiology and may also be important guides to treatment. Scientifically, however, the signs that would seem to be of greatest interest are those either seen in childhood, or, if first seen in adult life, seen before the overt manifestations of psychiatric illness or even identifiable behavioral disturbances. There are a number of sources of such signs that should be considered.

Genetic Defects

The familial character of the ADHD syndrome suggests that its manifestations might have a genetic basis. Likely candidates might be genes that regulate the timing of development of certain nervous system structures. Such a defective gene might result, for example, in delays in the timetable of myelination, a process that is normally spread over at least three decades of life (71). If there were actually a temporal and spatial hierarchy of such regulatory genes, any one of which could be defective, then one might see a variety of sometimes independent, sometimes overlapping syndromes, as is the case in ADHD.

Another form of genetic defect that can lead to complex patterns of expression is a genetic susceptibility to some noxious environmental agent—infectious, toxic, or traumatic. The genetic predisposition to develop seizures after traumatic brain insults is an example of this kind of mechanism.

In recent years a great deal of attention has been given to the phenomenon of apoptosis, or programmed cell death. Apoptosis is a complex mechanism by which cells, including nerve cells, that are either damaged in a variety of ways or are simply functionally redundant initiate a cascade of reactions that leads to their own dissolution. Initial emphasis in studies of apoptosis in the nervous system focused on its role during normal development, in which it functions to eliminate redundant neurons. Subsequently, however, it has become evident that it can also be a response to cell damage arising from a variety of causes (72) and that the determinant of whether the result is necrosis (which does cause gliosis) or apoptosis may depend on the rapidity and severity of the damage rather than the special character of the causal agent (73).

Environmental Agents

Modern diagnostic tools, such as ultrasound, have greatly increased the ability of clinicians to detect cerebral insults occurring in the perinatal period. Many of these insults result in mild deficits that would have gone undetected in earlier years, only to manifest a few years later as learning or behavioral difficulties. The effects of (nonprogressive) brain insults during development not only vary with the nature of pathologic process, as would be true in adults, but with the exact point in development of the brain at which the insult occurs. Different neural systems are vulnerable at different times, so that the same process can have very different effects at different stages. The situation is still more complex in that the immature nervous system has a considerable capacity to reorganize functionally (and even structurally) after focal damage, and the result may be impairment that does not follow the localizing patterns expected from studies of adults (74–77).

In the case of schizophrenia, soft signs may be evidence of neurologic deficits that are another facet of the same process that causes the schizophrenia, which is suggested by the results of the high-risk studies, especially Marcus et al (67). Alternatively, the soft signs could bear witness to the residual effects of brain insults that have predisposed to schizophrenia by somehow intersecting with the effects of a primary hereditary factor, as could be inferred from the twin study of Mosher et al (36). Finally, schizophrenia could be a two-factor process, with both factors being familial/genetic, as is suggested by the findings of neurologic abnormalities dissociated from psychiatric abnormalities in the families of schizophrenic patients (38).

FUTURE DIRECTIONS FOR INVESTIGATION

One exciting new line of research is the beginning use of functional imaging, particularly functional magnetic resonance imaging (fMRI) to look for abnormalities in patterns of regional brain activation that correlate with soft signs. It has long been speculated that mirror movements can come about pathologically in hemiparetic patients because the intact hemisphere comes to control both hands, so that attempts to move the paretic hand overflow and result in the same movement in the intact hand (78). In a recent fMRI study that looked at cortical activation induced by unilateral hand movements by patients who were hemiparetic due to early unilateral brain lesions, the patients' intact hemispheres were equally activated by contralateral and ipsilateral hand movements (79).

CONCLUSIONS

The term "soft signs" has come to refer to two types of neurologic abnormalities: first, abnormalities primarily involving motor systems that are suggestive of disturbances in brain organization or developments that have occurred early in life; second, subtle and poorly localizing abnormalities suggestive of brain dysfunction that are seen in a context of adult-life behavioral disturbances. Both kinds of soft signs have been studied in psychiatric patients, and both would appear to be clinically useful in that patient population. In addition, the signs that suggest early-life brain injuries or disturbances of development may have important etiologic implications in a number of behavioral disorders, especially ADHD and schizophrenia. Continued study of soft signs in these disorders may shed further light on their underlying causes and mechanisms.

REFERENCES

1. Strauss A, Lehtinen L. Psychopathology and education of the brain-injured child. New York: Grune & Stratton, 1947.
2. Prechtl HFR, Stemmer CH. The choreiform syndrome in children. Dev Med Child Neurol 1962;4:119–127.
3. Wolff PH, Hurwitz J. The choreiform syndrome. Dev Med Child Neurol 1966;8:160–165.
4. Rutter M, Graham P, Birch HG. Interrelations between the choreiform syndrome, reading disability and psychiatric disorders in children of 8–11 years. Dev Med Child Neurol 1966;8:149–159.
5. Touwen BCH, Prechtl HFR. The neurological examination of the child with minor nervous system dysfunction. London: Heinemann Medical Books, 1970.
6. Peters JE, Romine JS, Dykman RA. A special neurological examination of children with learning disabilities. Dev Med Child Neurol 1975;17:63–78.
7. Luria AR. The working brain. New York: Basic Books, 1973.
8. Cox SM, Ludwig AM. Neurological soft signs and psychopathology. I. Findings in schizophrenia. J Nerv Ment Dis 1979;167:161–165.
9. Denckla MB. Revised neurological examination for subtle signs. Psychopharmacol Bull 1985;21:773–789.
10. Guy W. ECOEU assessment manual for psychopharmacology. Washington, DC: Department of Health, Education and Welfare, 1976.
11. Shaffer D, O'Connor PA, Shafer SQ, Prupis S. Neurological "soft signs": their origins and significance for behavior. In: Rutter M, ed. Developmental neuropsychiatry. New York: Guilford Press, 1983.
12. Kinsbourne M. Minimal brain dysfunction as a neurodevelopmental lag. Ann N Y Acad Sci 1973;205:268–273.
13. Denckla MB, Rudel RG. Anomalies of motor development in hyperactive boys. Ann Neurol 1978;3:231–233.
14. Ingram TTS. Paediatric aspects of cerebral palsy. Edinburgh: E & S Livingstone, 1961.
15. Noica M. Etude sur les mouvements associes. Encephale 1921;7:201–221.

16. Shafer S, Shaffer D, O'Connor PA, et al. Hard thoughts on neurologic "soft" signs. In: Rutter M, ed. Developmental neuropsychiatry. New York: Guilford Press, 1983.

17. Shaffer D, Schonfeld I, O'Connor PA, et al. Neurological soft signs: their relationship to psychiatric disorder and intelligence in childhood and adolescence. Arch Gen Psychiatry 1985;42:342–351.

18. Werry JS. Studies on the hyperactive child: an empirical analysis of the minimal brain dysfunction syndrome. Arch Gen Psychiatry 1968;19:9–16.

19. Camp JA, Bialer I, Sverd J, Winsberg BG. Clinical usefulness of the NIMH physical and neurological examination for soft signs. Am J Psychiatry 1978;135:362–364.

20. Wender PH. Minimal brain dysfunction in children. New York: Wiley-Interscience, 1974.

21. Woods BT, Eby M. Excessive mirror movements and aggression. Biol Psychiatry 1982;17:23–32.

22. Szatmari P, Taylor DC. Overflow movements and behavior problems: scoring and using a modification of Fog's test. Dev Med Child Neurol 1984;26;297–310.

23. Kennard MA. Value of equivocal signs in neurologic diagnosis. Neurology 1960;10:753–764.

24. Hertzig ME, Birch HG. Neurologic organization in psychiatrically disturbed adolescent girls. Arch Gen Psychiatry 1966;15:590–598.

25. Hertzig ME, Birch HG. Neurologic organization in psychiatrically disturbed adolescents. Arch Gen Psychiatry 1968;19:528–537.

26. American Psychiatric Association. Diagnostic and statistical manual of mental disorders. 3rd ed. Washington, DC: American Psychiatric Association, 1980.

27. Rochford JM, Detre T, Tucker GJ, Harrow M. Neuropsychological impairment in functional psychiatric disease. Arch Gen Psychiatry 1970;22:114–119.

28. Tucker GJ, Campion EW, Silberfarb PM. Sensorimotor functions and cognitive disturbance in psychiatric patients. Am J Psychiatry 1975;132:17–21.

29. Feighner JP, Robins E, Guze SB, et al. Diagnostic criteria for use in psychiatric research. Arch Gen Psychiatry 1972;26:57–63.

30. Nasrallah HJ, Tippin J, McCalley-Whitters M. Neurological soft signs in manic patients. J Affect Disord 1983;5:45–50.

31. Manschreck TC, Ames D. Neurologic features and psychopathology in schizophrenic disorders. Biol Psychiatry 1984;19:703–719.

32. Woods BT, Short MP. Neurological dimensions of psychiatry. Biol Psychiatry 1985;20:192–198.

33. Woods BT, Kinney DK, Yurgelun-Todd D. Neurologic abnormalities in schizophrenic patients and their families. Arch Gen Psychiatry 1986;43:657–663.

34. Kinney DK, Yurgelun-Todd D, Woods BT. Neurologic hard signs in schizophrenia and major mood disorders. J Nerv Ment Dis 1993;181:202–204.

35. Youssef HA, Waddington JL. Primitive (developmental) reflexes and diffuse cerebral dysfunction in schizophrenia and bipolar affective disorder: over-representation in patients with tardive dyskinesia. Biol Psychiatry 1988;23:791–796.

36. Mosher LR, Pollin W, Stabenau JR. Identical twins discordant for schizophrenia. Arch Gen Psychiatry 1971;24:422–430.

37. Cantor-Graae E, McNeil TF, Rickler KC, et al. Are neurological abnormalities in well discordant monozygotic co-twins of schizophrenic subjects the result of perinatal trauma? Am J Psychiatry 1994;151:1194–1199.

38. Kinney DK, Woods BT, Yurgelun-Todd D. Neurological abnormalities in schizophrenic patients and their families. II. Neurologic and psychiatric findings in relatives. Arch Gen Psychiatry 1985;43:665–668.

39. Nasrallah HA, McCalley-Whitters M, Kuperman S. Neurologic differences between paranoid and non-paranoid schizophrenia. I. Sensory-motor lateralization. J Clin Psychiatry 1982;42:303–305.

40. Quitkin F, Rifkin A, Klein DF. Neurologic soft signs in schizophrenia and character disorder. Arch Gen Psychiatry 1976;33:845–853.

41. Torrey EF. Neurological abnormalities in schizophrenic patients. Biol Psychiatry 1980;15:381–388.

42. Kolakowska T, Williams AO, Jambor E, et al. Schizophrenia with good and poor outcome. III. Neurological "soft signs," cognitive impairment, and their clinical significance. Br J Psychiatry 1985;146:348–357.

43. Schroder J, Niethammar R, Geider F-J, et al. Neurological soft signs in schizophrenia. Schizophr Res 1992;6:25–30.

44. Walker E, Green M. Soft signs of neurological dysfunction in schizophrenia: an investigation of lateral performance. Biol Psychiatry 1982;17:381–386.

45. Johnstone EC, Owens DGC, Gold A, et al. Institutionalization and the defects of schizophrenia. Br J Psychiatry 1981;139:195–203.

46. Lapierre D, Braun CMJ, Hodgins S, et al. Neuropsychological correlates of violence in schizophrenia. Schizophr Bull 1995;21:253–262.

47. Owens DGC, Johnstone EC. The disabilities of chronic schizophrenia—their nature and the factors contributing to their development. Br J Psychiatry 1980;136:384–395.

48. Owens DGC, Johnstone EC, Frith CD. Spontaneous involuntary disorders of movement. Arch Gen Psychiatry 1982;39:452–461.

49. Manschreck TC, Maher BA, Rucklos ME, et al. Disturbed voluntary motor activity in schizophrenic disorder. Psychol Med 1982;12:73–84.

50. Rogers D. The motor disorders of severe psychiatric illness: a conflict of paradigms. Br J Psychiatry 1985;147:221–232.

51. Gupta S, Andreasen NC, Arndt S, et al. Neurological soft signs in neuroleptic-naive and neuroleptic-treated schizophrenic patients and in normal control subjects. Am J Psychiatry 1995;152:191–196.

52. Liddle PF. Schizophrenic syndromes, cognitive performance and neurological dysfunction. Psychol Med 1985;17:49–57.

53. Flashman LA, Flaum M, Gupta S, Andreasen NC. Soft signs and neuropsychological performance in schizophrenia. Am J Psychiatry 1996;153:526–532.

54. Mukherjee S, Shukla S, Rosen A. Neurological abnormalities in patients with bipolar disorder. Biol Psychiatry 1984;19:334–345.

55. Holzman PS, Solomon CM, Levin S, Waternaux CS. Pursuit eye movement dysfunctions in schizophrenia. Arch Gen Psychiatry 1984;41:136–139.

56. Kostyk SK, Wheeler EL, Woods BT. The palmomental reflex in psychiatric patients: increased incidence in young patients with schizoaffective disorder and a subclass of bipolar disorder patients. Ann Neurol 1993;34:286. Abstract.

57. Gittelman M, Birch HG. Childhood schizophrenia: intellectual and neurological status, perinatal risk, prognosis and family pathology. Arch Gen Psychiatry 1967;17:16–25.

58. Fish B. Neurobiological antecedents of schizophrenia in children: evidence for an inherited congenital neurointegrative defect. Arch Gen Psychiatry 1977;34:1296–1313.

59. Gesell A. Developmental diagnosis. 2nd ed. New York: Paul B. Boeber, 1947.

60. Fish B. The detection of schizophrenia in infancy. J Nerv Ment Dis 1957;125:1–24.

61. Erlenmeyer-Kimling L, Cornblatt B, Friedman D, et al. Neurological, electrophysiological and attentional deviations in children at risk for schizophrenia. In: Nasrallah HA, Henn F, eds. Schizophrenia as a brain disease. New York: Oxford University Press, 1982.

62. Fish B, Hagin R. Visual-motor disorders in infants at risk for schizophrenia. Arch Gen Psychiatry 1973;28:900–904.

63. Nichols P, Chen T. Minimal brain dysfunction: a prospective study. Hillsdale: Erlbaum, 1981.

64. Hanson DR, Gottesman II, Heston LL. Some possible childhood indicators of adult schizophrenia inferred from children of schizophrenics. Br J Psychiatry 1976;129:142–154.

65. Reider RD, Nichols PL. Offspring of schizophrenics. III. Hyperactivity and neurological soft signs. Arch Gen Psychiatry 1979;36:665–674.

66. Marcuse Y, Cornblatt B. Children at high risk for schizophrenia: predictions from infancy to childhood functioning. In: Erlenmeyer-Kimling L, Miller NE, eds. Life-span research on the prediction of psychopathology. Hillsdale: Erlbaum, 1986.

67. Marcus J, Hans SL, Lewow E, et al. Neurological findings in high-risk children: childhood assessment and five-year followup. Schizophr Bull 1985;11:85–100.

68. Orvaschel H, Mednick S, Schulsinger F, Rock D. The children of psychiatrically disturbed parents: differences as a function of the sick parent. Arch Gen Psychiatry 1979;36:691–695.

69. Marcus J, Hans JF, Nagler S, et al. Review of the NIMH Israeli kibbutz-city study and the Jerusalem infant development study. Schizophr Bull 1987;13:425–427.

70. McNeil TF, Harty B, Blennow G, Cantor-Graae E. Neuromotor deviation in offspring of psychotic mothers: a selective developmental deficiency in two groups of children at heightened psychiatric risk? J Psychiatr Res 1993;27:39–54.

71. Yakovlev PI, Lecours AR. The myelogenetic cycles of regional development of the brain. In: Minkowski A, ed. Regional development of the brain in early life: symposium. Oxford: Balckwell Scientific Publications, 1967.

72. Carson DA, Ribeiro JM. Apoptosis and disease. Lancet 1993;341:1251–1254.

73. Bredenson DE. Neural apoptosis. Ann Neurol 1995;38:839–851.

74. Woods BT, Teuber H-L. Early onset of complementary specialization of cerebral hemisphere in man. Trans Am Neurol Assoc 1973;98:59–63.

75. Woods BT, Teuber H-L. Changing patterns of childhood aphasia. Ann Neurol 1978;3:273–280.

76. Woods BT. The restricted effects of right hemisphere lesions after age one: Wechsler test data. Neuropsychologia 1980;19:65–71.

77. Woods BT. The ontogenesis of hemispheric specialization: insights from acquired aphasia of childhood. In: Castro-Caldas A, Martins IP, Van Dorgen H, Van Hout A, eds. Acquired aphasia in children. Dordrecht, The Netherlands: Kluwer Academic, 1991:73–81.

78. Woods BT, Teuber H-L. Mirror movements after childhood hemiparesis. Neurology 1978;28:1152–1158.

79. Cao Y, Vikingstad EM, Huttenlocher PR, et al. Functional magnetic resonance studies of the reorganization of the human hand sensorimotor area after unilateral brain injury in the perinatal period. Proc Natl Acad Sci USA 1994;91:9612–9616.

Quantitative Assessment of Locomotor Activity in Psychiatry and Neurology

JANET M. LAWRENCE   MARTIN H. TEICHER   SETH P. FINKLESTEIN

INTRODUCTION

In recent years there has been a tremendous growth in the application of objective measures and sophisticated technology to the fields of psychiatry and neurology. Clinical practice in psychiatry has been directly influenced by the introduction of objective diagnostic criteria embodied in the research diagnostic criteria (RDC) and DSM-III criteria. Laboratory measurements using gas chromatography, high-performance liquid chromatography, and radioreceptor assays facilitate monitoring of neurotransmitter metabolites and psychotropic drug levels. Computerized tomographic scanning and magnetic resonance imaging have enabled researchers and clinicians to study quantitative neuroanatomy in living subjects. Positron emission tomography, brain electrical activity mapping, magnetoencephalography, and magnetic resonance spectroscopy promise to provide a quantum leap in the in vivo topographic analysis of brain function and activity. But despite these great strides in the application of contemporary technology to issues of brain anatomy and function, relatively little has occurred to enhance our ability to assess and quantify clinically relevant behaviors. One possible emerging contribution may be the development of reliable ambulatory activity monitors with solid-state memory.

Abnormalities in spontaneous locomotor activity have been observed in a variety of psychiatric and neurologic disorders. For some disorders they are the defining characteristics. In fact, several DSM-III-R psychiatric diagnostic criteria require clinicians to assess disruptions in psychomotor activity or rest–activity rhythms. Table 62.1 lists some psychiatric disorders in which motility disturbances are particularly prominent and often an important diagnostic criteria. The purpose of this chapter is to briefly review the

history of attempts to monitor psychomotor activity, to summarize what has been learned about disturbances in ambulatory activity in neuropsychiatric disorders, and to indicate the possible directions that these endeavors should take in the near future.

HISTORY OF ACTIVITY MONITORING IN HUMANS

Early reports in the psychiatric literature discussed the feasibility and potential utility of measurements of spontaneous activity in psychiatric inpatients (1,2). At first, techniques were devised for time sample ratings by human observers. Large devices were also designed to measure activity in patients confined to special beds, chairs, platforms, or rooms (3–6). More recently, a number of portable activity monitors have been devised that facilitate objective measurements.

Wrist-worn mechanical activity monitors were first described by Schulman and Reismann (7) and were based on modifications of the self-winding watch. Advances in technology soon made electronic sensors feasible. The most important of these early devices was the telemetered wrist activity monitor (8,9). Some four years later McPartland et al (10) described a very small self-contained unit employing a mercury switch to detect tilt from horizontal and a light emitting diode display. At about the same time Colburn et al (11) described a small monitor with solid-state memory. It differed from the McPartland model by use of a piezoelectric transducer to detect acceleration rather than position, and it stored activity counts at preselected intervals in a 256-byte solid-state memory that was read directly by computer. This proved to be the basis for nearly all contemporary motility monitors.

Table 62.1 Psychiatric Disorders and Related States in Which There Are Prominent Disturbances in Rest/Activity Rhythms or Activity Levels

Disorders characterized by excess motility or movements
ADHD
Major depression (psychomotor agitated subtype)
Bipolar disorder—manic phase
Generalized anxiety disorder
Tourette's disorder
Autistic disorders
Stereotypy/habit disorder
Amphetamine abuse
Cocaine intoxication
Caffeine intoxication
Neuroleptic-induced akathisia

Disorders characterized by psychomotor retardation, fatigue, or catatonia
Major depression (psychomotor retarded subtype)
Schizophrenia, catatonic type
Amphetamine withdrawal
Cocaine withdrawal
Inhalant intoxication
Neuroleptic-induced parkinsonism

Disorders characterized by disturbed sleep/wake or rest/activity cycles
Delirium
Insomnias
Daytime hypersomnias
Sleep/wake schedule disorders
Major depression
Bipolar disorder—manic or depressed phases

CONTEMPORARY STUDIES USING AMBULATORY MOTILITY MONITORING

Affective Illness: Disturbances in Overall Activity Levels

The focus of most research in this domain has been on activity and circadian rhythm disturbances in affective illness. A number of key findings about the nature of unipolar and bipolar depression have emerged from this work. Astute clinicians have recognized that patients with unipolar depression tend to be more agitated and angry than bipolar depressed patients, who are generally inactive and withdrawn (12). Quantitative measurements of locomotor activity have confirmed this observation. Kupfer et al (13,14) and Wehr et al (15) found that middle-aged adult bipolar depressed subjects were significantly less active than younger normal subjects (15) and were only half as active as unipolar depressed patients (13). Wehr et al (15) and Wolff et al (16) documented the clinical impression that bipolar patients are less active when depressed than when euthymic, and they are somewhat less active than younger normal controls even when they are no longer clinically depressed. However, as two of these activity monitor studies carried out at the National Institute of Mental Health (NIMH) appeared to be confounded by age differences [control subjects averaged

21 to 24 years, and the bipolar depressed patients averaged 40 to 42 years (15,16)], further clinical studies of this kind involving close matching by age and polarity would be desirable.

We have recently explored the effect of major unipolar depression on circadian activity rhythms of geriatric patients (17). We hypothesized that these subjects would be more agitated than their age-matched controls. As seen in Figure 62.1, the depressed patients (mean age 75, $n = 8$) as a group were significantly more active than their healthy controls (mean age 77, $n = 8$). This was true for both daytime and nighttime activity records. Furthermore, five of eight depressed patients were more active than any of the control subjects, suggesting that this degree of activity difference may be readily apparent clinically.

Kupfer et al (14) have found that lithium increased the activity of responsive bipolar depressed patients to the unipolar group level, and that amitriptyline increased (i.e., worsened) the activity of nonresponsive, but not responsive, unipolar depressed patients.

Joffe et al (18) examined levels and distribution of motor activity in a group of predominately bipolar depressed patients treated with carbamazepine and found that responders to the medication increased (i.e., normalized) their motor activity levels. The drug had no effect on motor activity levels in nonresponders.

Hypomania has been associated with an increase in daytime activity without an increase in nighttime activity. Clinically significant mania was associated with an increase in nighttime activity, and marked increases in this measure were associated with the development of severe, stage III (psychotic) mania (19).

Affective Illness: Disturbances in the Timing of Activity

In recent years, chronobiologic theories have emerged to explain several specific features of major affective illness, such as sleep disturbances, early morning awakening, and diurnal variations of symptom severity: long-term cyclic and seasonal recurrences, and responses to mood-altering drugs (20). These theories are based largely on observed disturbances in the phase of circadian rhythms in depressed patients. Foster and Kupfer (21) reported that middle-aged depressed patients showed blunting of the amplitude, or "desynchronization," of their 24-hour activity cycle, and emitted a greater than normal percentage of their daily activity during the night (8.5% versus approximately 5%). Young adult patients with primary depression (25 years old) emitted a significantly lower percentage of their total daily activity during the night (2.2%) than did age-matched controls (5.1%). As this group of depressed young adults suffered from prominent anergic and hypersomnolent symptoms, they may have been predominantly bipolar.

Using various models to analyze circadian rhythms, Wehr et al (15) found that the activity acrophase (peak time of

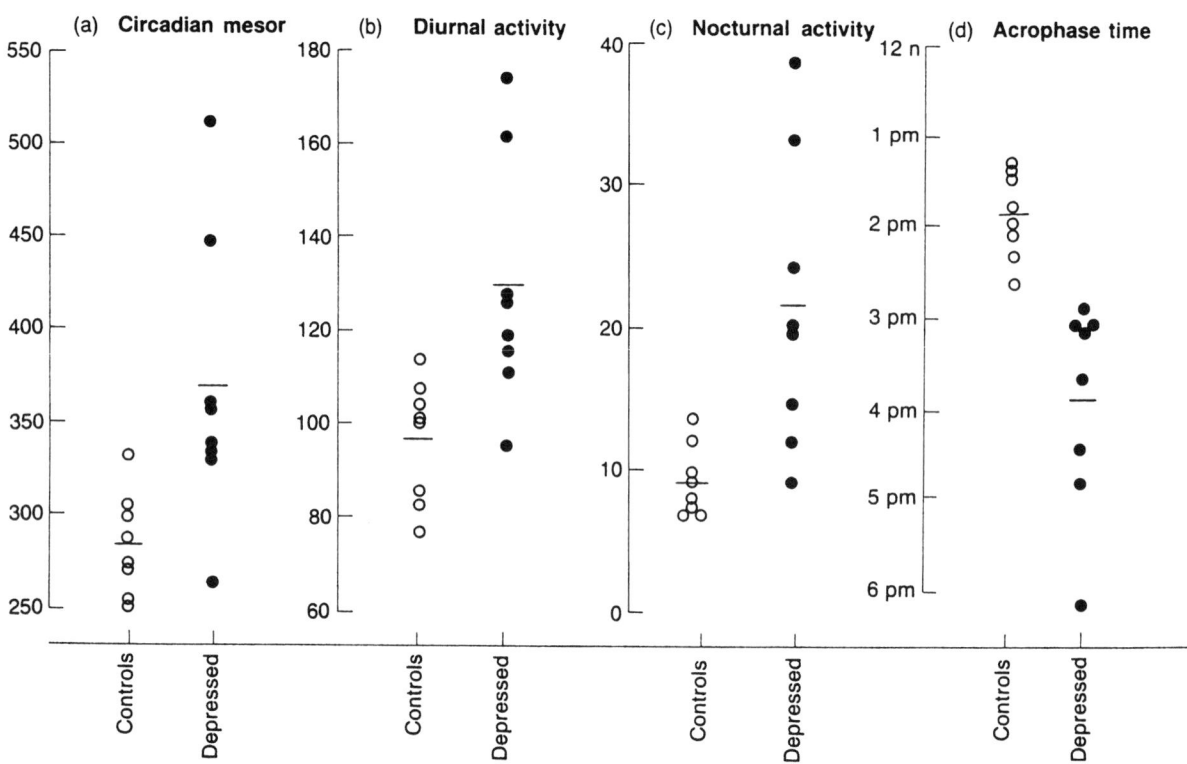

FIGURE 62.1 *Distribution of individual values of computed chronobiologic measures for elderly depressed and control subjects. (a) Mean hourly activity (1 cycle/day mesor); (b) diurnal activity levels (average total activity counts between 0730 and 2330 hours accumulated every 15 minutes during 48 hours of monitoring); (c) nocturnal activity levels (2330 to 0730 hours, as for b); (d) circadian acrophase by cosinor analysis (in hours); normal elderly controls (0) and depressed patients (0). Reproduced with permission from Teicher MH, Lawrence JM, Barber NI, et al. Increased activity and phase delay in circadian motility rhythms in geriatric depression. Arch Gen Psychiatry 1988;45:913–917.*

activity determined by a circadian cosinor analysis) of middle-aged bipolar depressed patients was 97 minutes earlier (phase advanced) than in younger controls. Body temperature and excretion of the norepinephrine metabolite 3-methoxy-4-hydroxy-phenethylene glycol showed a similar phase advance. Wolff et al (16) did not statistically replicate this result using a less sophisticated centroid analysis (time of day from 0700 hours on, when half of total daily activity was produced). Nevertheless, there was a trend for bipolar patients to show a 20-minute phase advance and for unipolar depressed patients to show an 8-minute phase delay compared with younger normal controls. These trends may have been more significant if phase differences had not been constricted by entraining both patients and controls to the same set ward environment with a fixed wake-up time (0700 hours), fixed mealtime, and a scheduled milieu (15,16).

We have found that geriatric patients with unipolar depression differ very strikingly from age-equivalent controls (17). Depressed patients were markedly phase delayed. The circadian activity acrophase occurred at 1300 hours in controls, and at 1554 hours in depressed patients (2.04-hour phase delay; Figs 62.1 and 62.2). More recently we have found that the primary disturbance in depressed children

and adolescents is a blunting of the circadian rhythm, which is a chronobiologic measure of diurnal variation.

Affective Illness: Summary

Locomotor activity is often altered in depression, and psychomotor activity change is the symptom factor most directly linked to endogenous depression (22). Motility levels can be either low or excessive when compared with normal subjects. Patients with bipolar disorder, when depressed, tend to be psychomotorically retarded and to have diminished mean activity levels and increased sleep time. Their circadian activity acrophase may occur earlier in the day than in nondepressed individuals and suggests the presence of a phase advance of their circadian rest/activity oscillator (internal clock). Unipolar depressed patients have elevated activity levels relative to most bipolar depressed patients, and they may be even more active than age-matched normal controls (17). Our findings in older, nonbipolar depressives suggest the intriguing possibility that peak activity may occur later in these patients and that their rest/activity oscillator may be phase delayed rather than phase advanced. These observations suggest the possibility that the measurement of spontaneous activity levels,

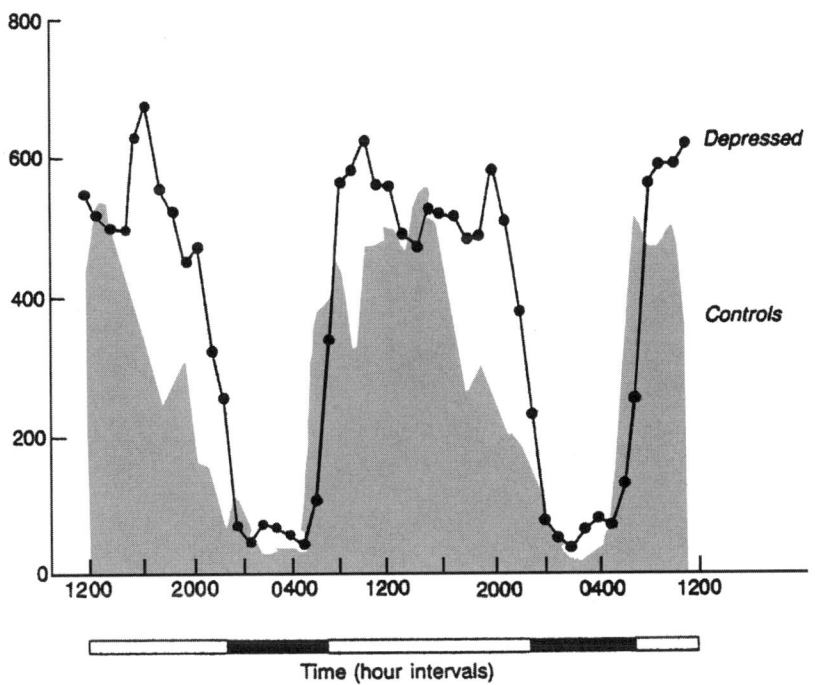

FIGURE 62.2 *Mean 48-hour activity profiles for elderly depressed and control subjects. The activity record commenced at 1200 hours, and the first point indicates the mean activity level for each subject accumulated between 1200 and 1300 hours. Overall, depressed patients were more active than controls during the period between 1700 and 2200 hours (all p < 0.05; Dunn multiple comparison test), but were less active than controls very early in the morning (0600 to 0700 hours; all p < 0.05). Reproduced with permission from Teicher MH, Lawrence JM, Barber NI, et al. Increased activity and phase delay in circadian motility rhythms in geriatric depression. Arch Gen Psychiatry 1988;45:913–917.*

and the determination of acrophase times, may help distinguish unipolar from bipolar depressive illness on initial assessment.

Relationship Between Nocturnal Motility and Sleep Electroencephalography

Researchers have found that the measurement of activity during just the first 2 hours of sleep time afforded an excellent correlation with sleep latency [0.85, $p < 0.01$ (23)] as determined by polysomnographic recording. Interestingly, this correlation with sleep latency held for depressed patients ($r = 0.88$, $n = 10$), and for those with personality disorders ($r = 0.87$, $n = 9$), but did not appear to hold in schizophrenic patients [$r = -0.07$, $n = 7$ (23)]. Kripke et al (24) have also explored the utility of wrist activity recording in sleep studies. They have described a fully automated system that can make on-line determinations of sleep/wake state from wrist activity data on a minute-to-minute basis that is in agreement 94% of the time with electroencephalography (EEG)-based determination. Unlike polysomnographic recordings, special rooms, expensive equipment, and the inconvenience of electrodes could be eliminated. More detailed sleep staging, however, has not yet been shown to be possible using activity measures alone.

Attention Deficit Hyperactivity Disorder

Using the NIMH-Colburn device, Porrino et al (25) have shown that children with attention deficit hyperactivity disorder (ADHD) are more active than age-matched controls at all times of day, including sleep. The greatest differences in activity levels, however, occurred during structured school tasks and disappeared during various playtime events. The effect of a single dose of dextroamphetamine lasted about 8 hours and resulted in a 28% decrease in activity, essentially normalizing the activity levels of the hyperactive children. The greatest inhibitory effects of dextroamphetamine were noted during classtime in reading and math, and play activity was not significantly attenuated (26).

We are currently examining whether motility monitoring can be used on an individual basis as an aid in the diagnosis of ADHD and as a means of documenting treatment response (27). Our emphasis has been on the individual subject, and we have used finer-resolution time series than reported by the NIMH group in an attempt to isolate features of the activity profile that might accomplish this goal. Figure 62.3 displays 64-hour activity profiles from two children: a 6-year-old with ADHD and a healthy 7-year-old control. Note that the ADHD child had virtually no daytime periods of quiet restfulness (activity scores of less than 50), while the seven-year-old did. So far this appears to be a reliable discriminative feature. Stimulant medication attenuated overall activity levels, and markedly increased the number of low-level diurnal activity periods (Fig 62.4). Overall, these data suggest that children with ADHD might have difficulty modulating their activity to conform to the demands of their environment and that this capacity might be enhanced by clinically effective doses of stimulant medications.

Activity Rhythm Disturbances in Psychosis

Schizophrenia and bipolar psychoses have often been characterized by profound disturbances in locomotor activity and movement. Catatonic patients can be profoundly

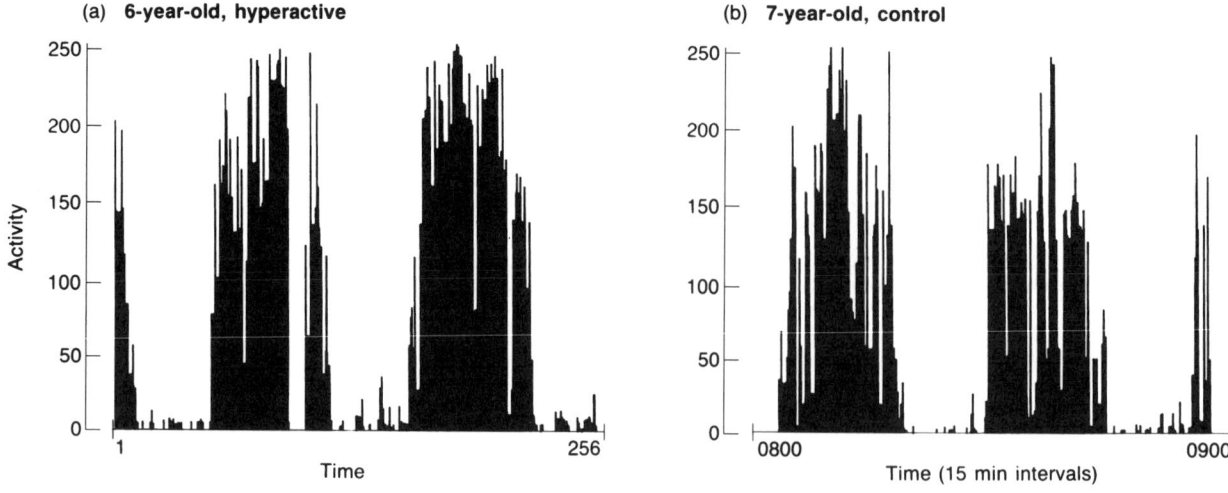

FIGURE 62.3   *(a) Sixty-four-hour activity profile of a hyperactive boy, and (b) 49-hour activity profile of a normal boy of similar age.*

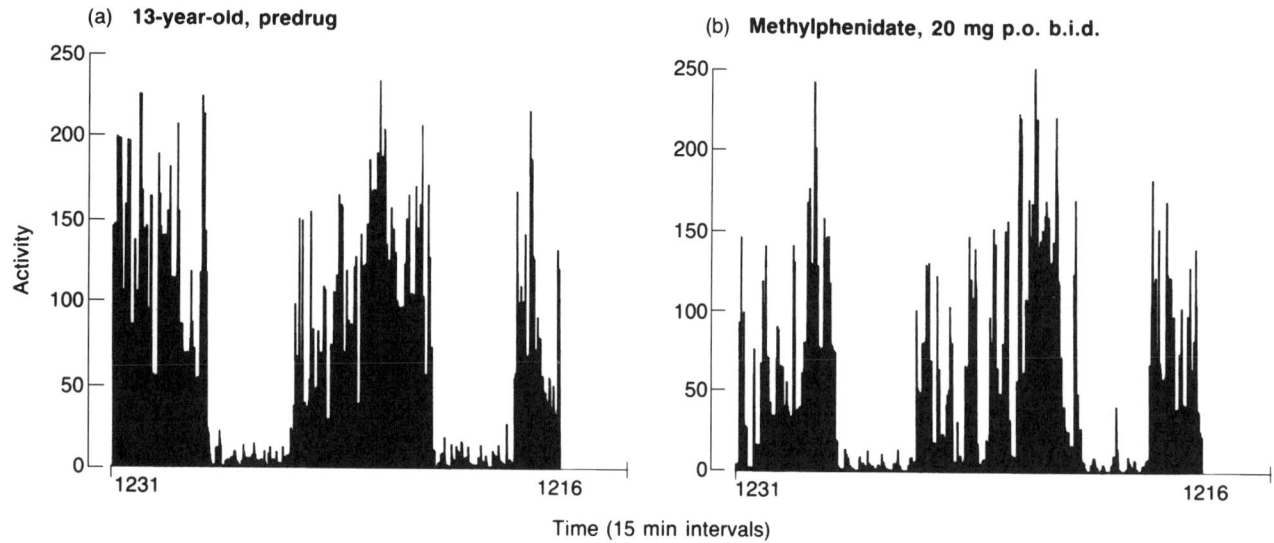

FIGURE 62.4   *(a) Forty-eight-hour activity profile of a 13-year-old hyperactive child prior to the initiation of treatment. (b) Forty-eight-hour activity profile of 13-year-old patient after the initiation of treatment with methylphenidate. Note that the patient displayed many more periods of quiet daytime restfulness after the initiation of treatment.*

psychomotorically retarded or wildly agitated. Patients with negative schizophrenic symptoms often show a paucity of purposeful movement, and patients in a manic frenzy can be both unmanageably active and incapable of sleeping. Very little is known about quantitative disturbances in rest/activity levels in these patients. In a preliminary study, we evaluated 20 psychotic inpatient (28). Altogether, five patients met strict DSM-III-R and RDC criteria for schizophrenia (mean age 28). Four patients were schizoaffective by DSM-III-R criteria (mean age 29), and 11 met criteria for bipolar disorder, manic phase, with psychotic features (mean age 28). The patients were monitored for 72 hours using a high-

resolution ambulatory activity monitor worn on the non-dominant wrist (see p. 417).

Patients in each of these groups were similar in mean age and on average they were treated with comparable medication regimens, although schizophrenic patients may have received slightly higher neuroleptic doses. As expected, mean activity levels (mesor) were greater in bipolar patients than in the other two groups (bipolar 7,399 $\pm$ 695; schizophrenic 5,376 $\pm$ 1,487; schizoaffective 4854 $\pm$ 664 ct/h). Schizoaffective and bipolar disorder patients, however, tended to display a shorter optimal (nonlinear least squares) circadian periodicity than schizophrenics (schizophrenic

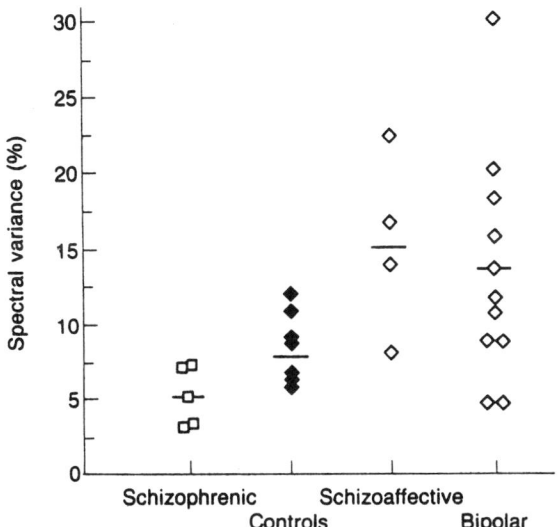

FIGURE 62.5   *Comparison of the magnitude of 2 cycles/day (12 hours) ultradian rest/activity rhythms in normal controls and patients with schizophrenia, schizoaffective disorder, and bipolar illness. Data are expressed as the percentage of variability in the subjects activity profile that can be accounted for by a 2 cycles/day oscillation. Thus a score of 10 means that 10% of the variance in the subjects 72-hour activity profile can be accounted for by a simple 2 cycles/day rhythm. By chance alone, we would only expect about 2% of a subjects variance to be accounted for by a rhythm of this frequency.*

24.27 ± 0.20; schizoaffective 23.78 ± 0.29; bipolar 23.69 ± 0.14 hour), and this was consistent with data from Goodwin et al (20) in which they postulated that a circadian oscillator may be running fast in some patients with bipolar illness.

Possibly the most interesting group difference was noted in a specific ultradian bandwidth; the 2 cycles/day (12-hour) rhythm. A significant 12-hour ultradian rhythm of plasma 4-methoxy-3-hydroxyphenylglycol excretion has been reported to occur in some patients with affective illness (29), and it appears to us that this ultradian parameter may be a specific chronobiologic index of "diurnal variation." As can be seen in Figure 62.5, there were very large differences in the magnitude of this rhythm between subjects. Schizophrenic patients had uniformly weak 2 cycles/day rhythms, whereas several of the patients with schizoaffective disorder and bipolar illness had extremely robust 2 cycles/day rhythms. Normal controls (*n* = 8) had 2 cycles/day rhythms of intermediate magnitude, and as a group their scores were clustered fairly tightly. These observations are intriguing, and raise the possibility that an ultradian rest–activity rhythm may be attenuated in schizophrenia and accentuated in some patients with psychotic affective illness. Further evaluation of this phenomenon is of course necessary, as these patients were medicated and the sample size was very limited. However, this pilot study does suggest that potentially important and novel information may be derived from undertaking a formal study of motility, rest–activity rhythms, and arousal processes in schizophrenia and other psychotic disorders.

Assessment of the Effects of Psychotrophic Medications on Daytime Activity

Motility monitoring has also been used to assess the carry-over effects of hypnotic medication. Flurazapam, administered to healthy volunteers at bedtime, was found to diminish 24-hour activity by 15% and to reduce the amplitude of the circadian motility rhythm by 19%, without affecting its phase (30). We have recently used ambulatory motility monitoring to help document a potential side effect of monoamine oxidase inhibitor treatment. Eight patients with hypersomnolent, anergic major depression benefited markedly from treatment with phenelzine or tranylcypromine, but experienced periods of intense afternoon somnolence often culminating in involuntary naps (31). This disruption in rest–activity rhythms was readily verified in five subjects using ambulatory motility monitoring (Fig 62.6). These observations suggest that activity monitoring could be valuable in determining drug effects on physical performance and may also be useful in assessing fatigue states.

Effects of Normal Aging

A commonly held assumption in our society is that elderly people are less vigorous and presumably less "active" than young adults. Animal studies have also suggested that circadian rhythms are disrupted with aging (32). We studied activity levels and rhythms in very healthy geriatric controls (mean age 73, *n* = 40) and healthy young adults (mean age 26, *n* = 29) at the MIT clinical research center. We found, contrary to our expectations, that the circadian rhythms of very healthy elderly subjects were not impaired, and that these subjects were at least as active and less sleepy than the younger controls (33). The amplitude and mesor of the circadian activity rhythm was greater in these healthy elderly subjects and, as expected, these elderly subjects arose earlier and were phase advanced by almost 2 hours (Fig 62.7). These findings suggest that levels and rhythms of daily activity in healthy elderly people are often well preserved and may not deteriorate as readily as has been assumed. It would be interesting to ascertain whether disrupted activity parameters in elderly individuals was an indicator of failing health.

Activity Level Disturbances in Neurologic Disorders

Very little research has been conducted on locomotor activity levels and circadian activity rhythms in patients with

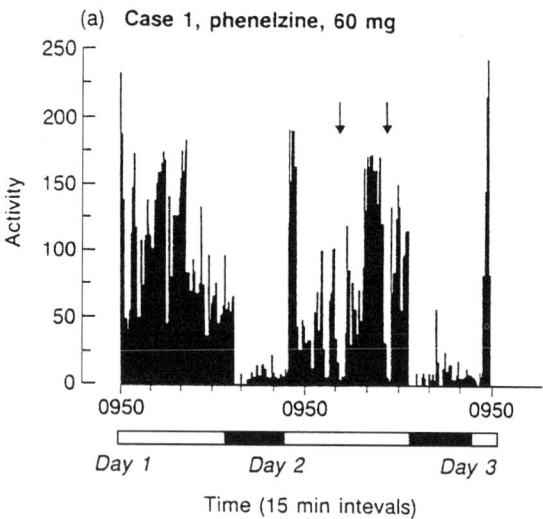

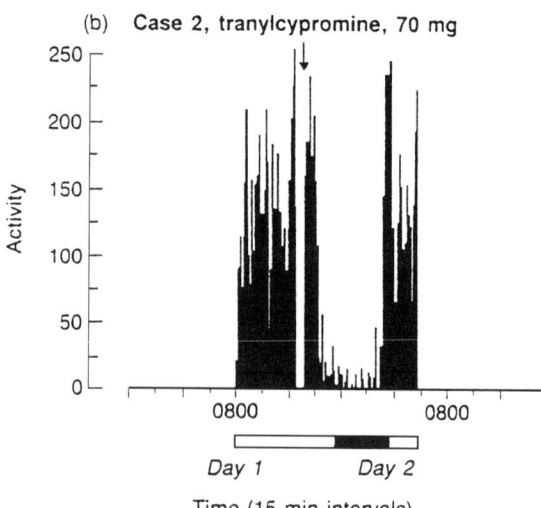

FIGURE 62.6   *Activity profiles of two patients receiving monoamine oxidase inhibitors as measured by electronic activity monitor. Data are displayed as activity counts versus time in 15-minute intervals over the course of days. The rectangular band below each half of the figure indicates successive days, and the white and black bands separate day from night. The start time for each profile is indicated by 24-hour time, and repeated at daily intervals. The arrows point to periods of intense fatigue culminating in naps. Reproduced with permission from Teicher MH, Cohen BM, Baldessarini RJ, Cole JO. Severe daytime somnolence in patients treated with an MAOI. Am J Psychiatry 1988;145:152–156.*

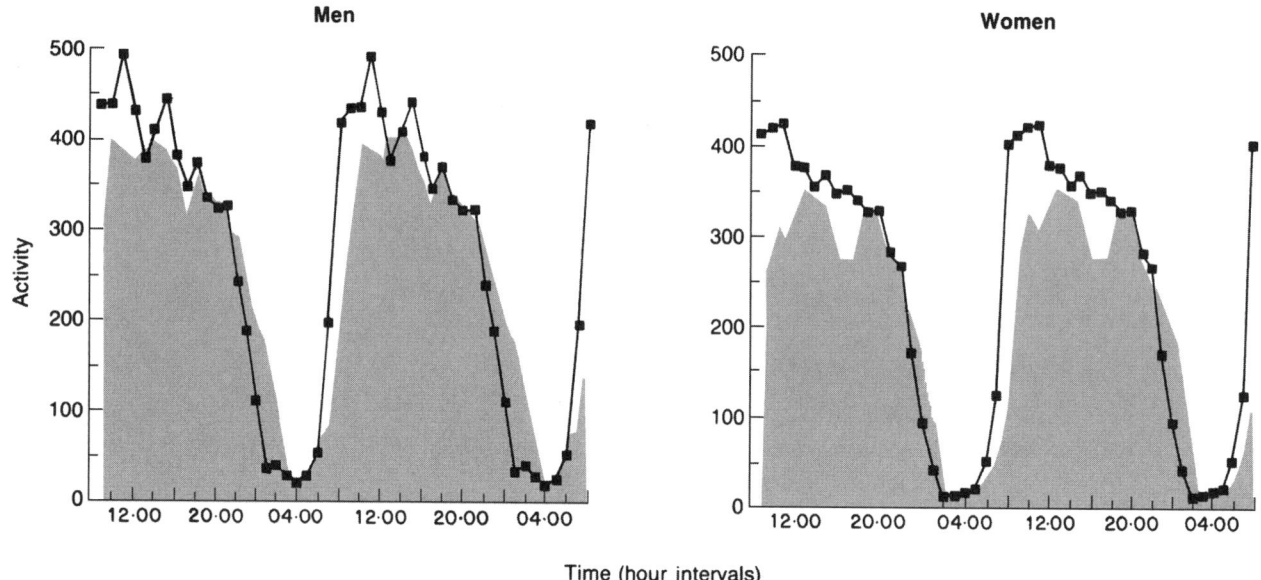

FIGURE 62.7   *Mean 48-hour activity double plots for healthy male and female young adult and elderly individuals. (Young men, n = 15, x = 24.3 years; elderly men, n = 17, x = 71.4 years; young women, n = 14, x = 28.1 years; elderly women, n = 23; x = 74.3 years.) Elderly normals arose earlier than the young adults and were more active during the morning hours. Young adults retired at a later hour and were more active during the late night. Reproduced with permission from Leiberman HR, Wurtman JJ, Teicher MH. Circadian rhythms of activity in healthy young and elderly humans. Neurobiol Aging 1989;10:259–265.*

neurologic illness. We thus sought to determine, in a preliminary study, whether activity rhythms were disrupted in patients with brain injury. Figure 62.8 displays activity profiles obtained with a modified Colburn–NIMH monitor of a representative 65-year-old normal control and patients with an idiopathic dementia, a right frontoparietal stroke,

and a 3-cm well-calcified parasagittal meningioma. Striking differences were observed in both circadian and more rapid ultradian rhythms between these patients and normal controls of similar age (34). We found a loss of circadian rhythmicity following stroke, and a marked 4-hour ultradian activity rhythm in patients with dementia and brain tumor

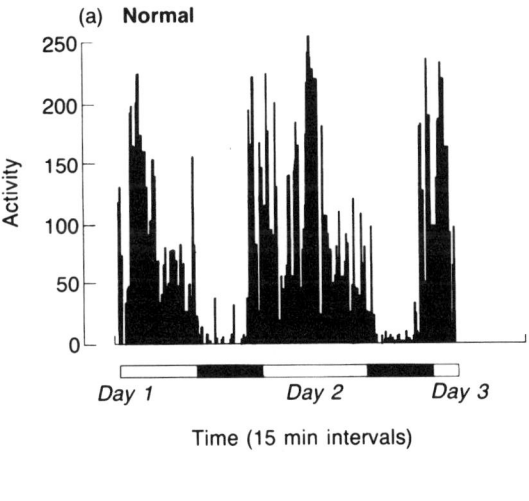

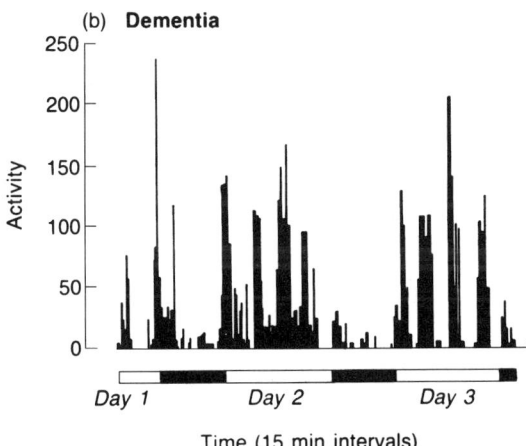

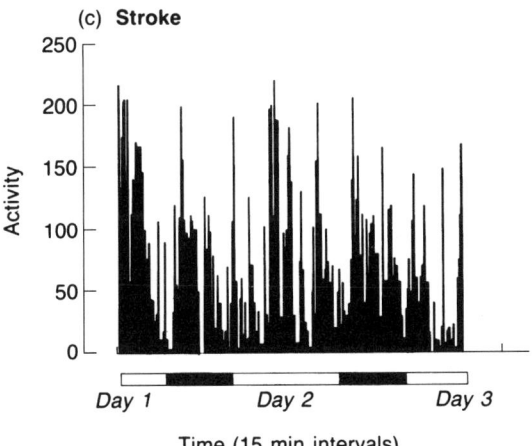

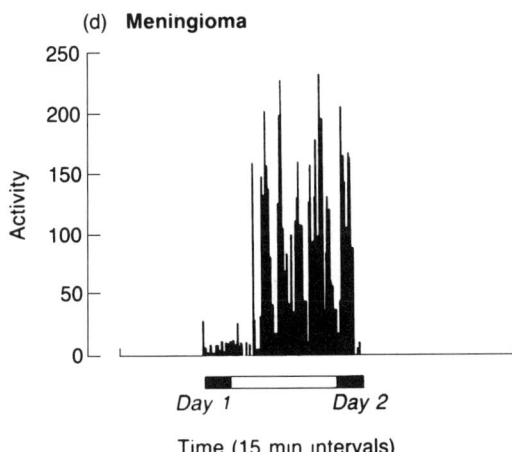

FIGURE 62.8 *Activity profiles of patients with neuropsychiatric disorders. Data are displayed as activity counts versus time in 15-minute intervals. (a) Shows the 48-hour activity profile of a healthy 65-year-old man; (b–d) displays the activity of individuals with dementia, stroke, and meningioma, respectively. Start times for the actigraph profiles are at 1130 hours, 1500 hours, 1600 hours, and 0245 hours, respectively. Reproduced with permission from Teicher MH, Lawrence JM, Barber NI. Altered locomotor activity in neuropsychiatric patients. Prog Neuropharmacol Biol Psychiatry 1986;10:755–761.*

(Fig 62.9). These initial studies dramatically demonstrated the potential utility of this tool for the study of brain function and suggested that activity monitoring might have some promise as a diagnostic tool.

In collaboration with Satlin (35), we obtained data on 17 elderly, severely demented patients with Alzheimer's disease and nine normal subjects of comparable age. Using an even more precise and flexible activity monitor, we substantiated some of the effects of this disorder on circadian rhythmicity. Patients with Alzheimer's disease showed increased levels of nocturnal activity and an increased proportion of percent nocturnal activity. In a subgroup of six patients characterized clinically by constant pacing, there were marked disturbances in daily activity levels (56% increase), nighttime activity levels (174% increase), and percent nocturnal activity (77% increase). These patients also had a smaller circadian amplitude (37% decrease), suggesting that the circadian

rest/activity oscillator may be weakened in this subgroup. Alzheimer patients also showed a consistent phase delay, with their acrophase (time of peak circadian activity) occurring about 1.75 hours later in the afternoon than in controls (35).

Piezoelectric determination of acceleration and tremor has also been applied to the study of movement disorders. For these purposes, a very sensitive detector is applied to a limb or digit (often at the end of a lever arm to further increase sensitivity), and data is recorded continuously and analyzed for time-dependent fluctuations in tremor amplitude. Using this approach, Tryon and Pologe (36) found that accelerometric measures from the right index finger could be used to correctly determine the presence of tardive dyskinesia following multiple discriminant analyses of movement amplitude, peak frequency, and the number of occurrences of large-amplitude movement spikes.

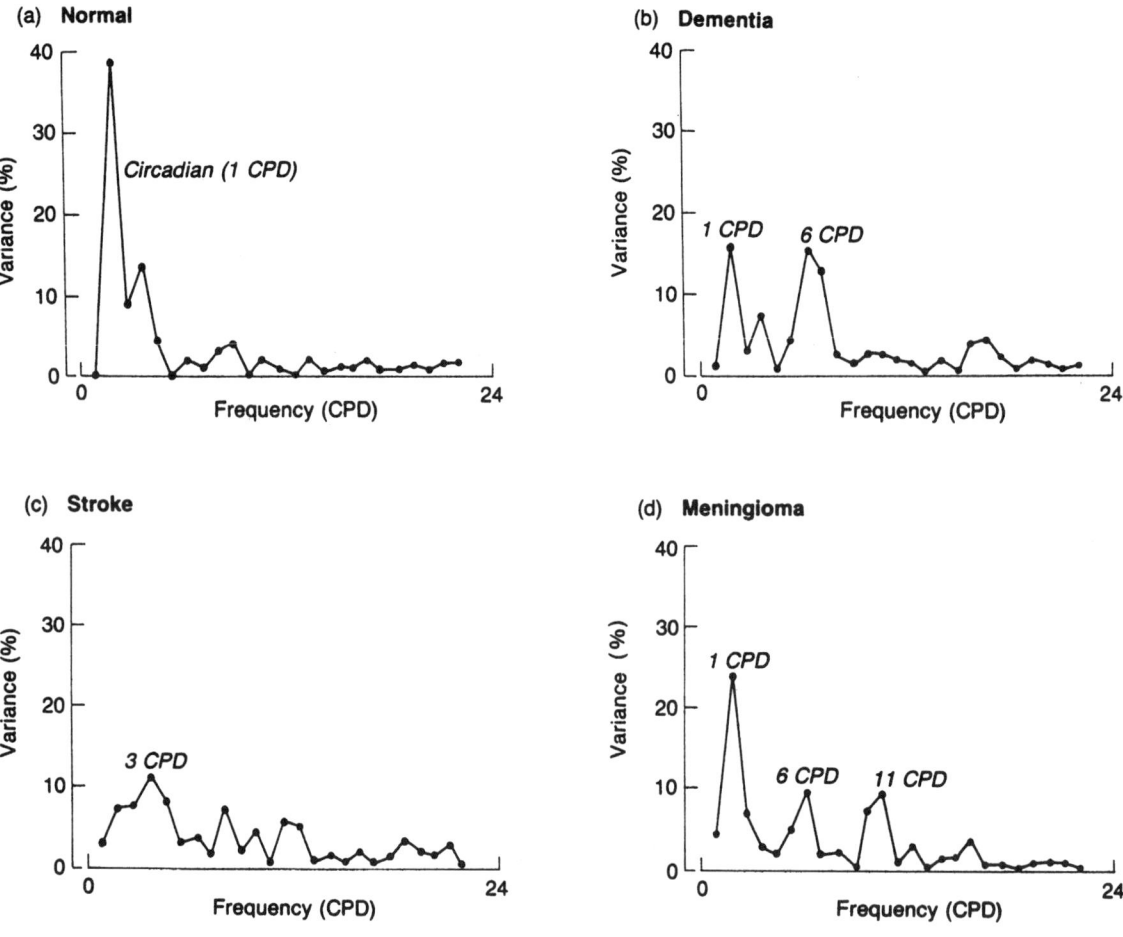

FIGURE 62.9   *Frequency distribution of activity rhythms in the healthy 65-year-old man and three neuropsychiatric patients shown in Figure 62.8. The graphs display individual variance spectra from 0 to 24 cycles/day (CPD) in 1 cycles/day increments, and are expressed as percent total variance. In each case, prominent peaks are indicated by arrows. Reproduced with permission from Teicher MH, Lawrence JM, Barber NI. Altered locomotor activity in neuropsychiatric patients. Prog Neuropharmacol Biol Psychiatry 1986;10:755–761.*

AMBULATORY MOTILITY MONITORING: TECHNICAL CONSIDERATIONS

Previous studies indicate that quantitative assessment of locomotor activity is feasible in patients with neuropsychiatric disorders and that such studies may in the future provide useful information regarding diagnosis and response to treatment. Nevertheless, it should be noted that most of these studies are limited by several factors. First, the sample size is often small. Second, this technology has until recently only been available to a limited number of researchers and there have been no agreed upon standards for the physical assessment of activity. The Colburn–NIMH device, which has been the *de facto* standard for solid-state monitors, is rather difficult to accurately crosscalibrate with other Colburn–NIMH monitors, and was limited in its flexibility. This might explain why these have been so few attempts to replicate or verify most of these reported findings. Third, no standards have been established regarding data analysis, and appropriate software has been very limited. Progress in this

field will be aided by the widespread introduction of a precisely calibrated, flexible, and reasonably affordable activity monitoring system and by the development of relevant software.

Instrument

Very reliable and accurately calibrated activity monitors are commercially available. For most of our work we have used an Actigraph (model AM-16) developed by Precision Control Design, Inc. (646 A Anchors Street, Ft. Walton Beach, FL 32548) and distributed by Ambulatory Monitoring, Inc. (731 Saw Mill River Road, Ardsley, NY 10502). This device has a programmable time base for studies of activity ranging from fractions of seconds to hours and has sufficient memory (16 kilobytes) to record activity in 5-minute epochs for 41 days. The device has dimensions of $15.2 \times 6.4 \times 4$ cm, and weighs about 88 g.

More recently, an even smaller version called the Mini-Motion Logger (AM-32) has become available from the same source. This device has physical dimensions of 3.8 × 3.3 × 1 cm and is only slightly larger than a man's wrist watch. Moreover, it is even more flexible in its programmable parameters and is capable of greater sensitivity, but the device can also accurately emulate the older monitor to produce comparable data and has greater storage capacity. The primary limitation of the new device is battery life, which is limited to about 14 days.

Data Analysis and Interpretation

Although it is now possible to obtain a reliable motility monitor and to measure activity levels, very little is known about the meaning of these levels. Activity profiles can contain an enormous amount of data, and powerful analytical techniques are needed to provide meaningful descriptive summary statistics. These activity profiles also display characteristic wave features (like electrocardiogram and EEG recordings), but little is known about their interpretation. There are also no standards available for determining how activity should be recorded.

Our approach to collecting activity data varies with clinical conditions. For most neuropsychiatric problems, we have recorded activity by having the subject wear the monitor on their nondominant wrist. In children we have had them wear the device on a belt, as a wrist-worn monitor was too distracting. For patients with advanced Alzheimer's disease, we have hidden the monitor in a secret pouch in a sweatshirt, which they then were able to wear. We are also using ankle activity monitoring for the study of neuroleptic-induced akathisia. Changing the location of the activity monitor affects the activity profile to a certain extent, although agreement between wrist, belt, chest, and leg monitors in normal individuals are very high ($r > 0.98$). In all cases, regardless of placement, we have recorded activity in 5-minute epochs over 3 to 4 days. These records provide a good basis for the quantification of activity levels and of circadian and ultradian activity rhythms.

Our approach to deciphering the data is as follows. First, the activity time series is analyzed for mean activity (ct/min), mean diurnal activity, mean nocturnal activity, percent diurnal activity, and estimated sleep duration. Then the data are plotted. The first analytical technique we used to examine the rhythmic structure of the data is a modified (nonlinear) form of cosinor analysis. Traditionally, this technique provides a linear least-squares fit of a cosine function to the raw time series data (37,38). The function is made linear by selecting a set frequency (1 cycle/day for circadian rhythms) and deriving least-squares estimators of mesor (mean daily activity level), amplitude, and acrophase (time of the activity peak). A nonlinear least-squares fit enables frequency to be fit as an additional variable and makes it possible to fit raw data simultaneously to oscillators operating at several frequencies (39). With the microcomputer program we have prepared (40), time-series for different groups can be analyzed simultaneously, parameters can be shared or constrained, and differences between parameters can be assessed by ANOVA methods.

In addition to analyzing circadian rhythm parameters, we have also been interested in higher frequency or ultradian (more than 1 cycle/day) rhythms in locomotor activity. The analysis of such rhythms is complex and unsettled, and most researchers in this area have adopted their own relatively unique statistical approach to the problem. We have chosen to follow the recommendation of Kripke (41) and use a harmonic technique known as "variance spectral analysis" (42,43). This approach represents one way of contending with the critical problem of the nonstationary character of the dominant ultradian rhythm. This problem occurs because ultradian rhythms are not entrained to any known regularly occurring external timing cue ("*zeitgeber*") and even under highly controlled conditions, they drift in and out of phase. Analysis of spectral variance allows use of a fairly narrow sampling (lag) window to scan the spectrum in smaller units and sacrifices some degree of frequency resolution to obtain a more accurate estimation of spectral magnitude. In addition to variance spectral analysis, the programming package written by Teicher and Barber (40) also yields autocorrelation function, periodograms, Fourier transforms, power spectra (at harmonic and nonharmonic intervals), and correlation spectra, if desired.

As indicated above, there is no actual consensus regarding the best time-series approach to use for the analysis of ultradian motility rhythms. It has been suggested that the computer is to the chronobiologist what the microscope is to the biologist. If this is true, then the various time-series strategies are analogous to the biologic stains used to highlight cellular structures. A time-series strategy is useful if it reveals the underlying rhythmic structure of interest, without the addition of significant artifacts or distortions. The analysis of spectral variance appears to readily meet this criteria.

The statistical significance of spectral changes are determined using the Kolmogorov–Smirnov test (44–46), and the significance of spectral peaks are determined using a technique described by Fisher (47). Group spectral differences are determined by calculation of deviation and probability spectra with correction for the number of multiple paired comparisons (48,49).

FUTURE DIRECTIONS

Now that activity monitoring devices are widely available it should be possible to build on the groundwork of previous studies. Further work is needed to make such techniques generally acceptable across a wide range of clinical conditions and settings. This will require the establishment of standardized testing procedures and data analysis. It will be important to ascertain whether there are characteristic patterns of activity in different disorders and whether these might have specificity, sensitivity, and predictive value of use as an aid to differential diagnosis. Activity patterns may also be useful as an aid to monitoring the effects of medication treatment and may facilitate prediction or early detection of treatment response.

SUMMARY

Disturbances in motor activity levels and patterns may occur in a variety of neuropsychiatric disorders. In the past, it was possible to assess these only by clinical observation. More recently, with the development of solid-state technology, ambulatory activity monitors have been devised that can record large amounts of data regarding activity. These data can then be transferred to a computer and analyzed for a variety of parameters.

At the present time, ambulatory activity monitors have been used in the study of conditions as diverse as depression, ADHD, Alzheimer's disease, and schizophrenia. Although such studies have many technical limitations, they suggest that characteristic abnormalities of motor activity level and pattern may occur in such illnesses.

Ambulatory activity monitoring has also been used in the study of sleep, and the effects of psychotropic medication. Activity monitoring has made it possible to corroborate clinical observed changes with medication in ADHD. Current availability of more technologically advanced activity monitors and increasing standardization of techniques may allow more widespread application of this technology. There is potential for ambulatory activity monitoring to be an important adjunct to clinical observation in the diagnosis and monitoring of treatment in a variety of neuropsychiatric illnesses.

ACKNOWLEDGMENTS

Supported in part by award MH-47370 and grant MH-43743 from the NIMH, by Biomedical Research Support Grant RR-05484 from the National Institutes of Health, by a grant from the Scottish Rite Schizophrenia Research Program, and by awards from the Hall Mercer Foundation, the Snider Family, the Marion Ireland Benton Trust Fund, and the William F. Milton Foundation. Cynthia McGreenery provided excellent secretarial assistance.

REFERENCES

1. Page J. An experimental study of the day and night motility records of normal and psychotic individuals. Arch Gen Psychol 1935;192:1–40.
2. Jones MR. Measurement of spontaneous movements in adult psychotic patients by time sample technique: methodological study. J Psychol 1941;11:285–295.
3. Wada T. An experimental study of hunger in its relation to activity. Arch Psychol 1922;8:1–65.
4. Foshee JG. Studies in activity level: 1. Simple and complex task performance in detectives. Am J Ment Defic 1958;62:882–896.
5. Griffiths E, Chapman N, Campbell D. An apparatus for directing and monitoring movement. Am J Psychol 1967;80:438–441.
6. Pfadt A, Tryon WW. Issues in the selection and use of mechanical transducers to directly measure motor activity in clinical settings. Appl Res Ment Retard 1983;4:251–270.
7. Schulman JL, Reisman JM. An objective measure of hyperactivity. Am J Ment Defic 1959;64:455–456.
8. Foster FG, Kupfer DJ, Weiss G, et al. Mobility recording and cycle research in neuropsychiatry. J Interdisc Cycle Res 1972;3:60–72.
9. Kupfer DJ, Foster FG. Sleep and activity in psychotic depression. J Nerv Ment Dis 1973;156:341–348.
10. McPartland RJ, Foster FG, Kupfer DR, Weiss BL. Activity sensors for use in psychiatric evaluation. IEEE Trans Biomed Eng 1976;23:175–178.
11. Colburn TR, Smith BM, Guarnini JJ, Simmons NN. An ambulatory activity monitor with solid state memory. Instrum Soc Am 1976;12:117–122.
12. Beigel A, Murphy DL. Unipolar and bipolar affective illness. Arch Gen Psychiatry 1971;24:215–220.
13. Kupfer DJ, Foster FG, Detre TP, Himmelhoch J. Sleep EEG and motor activity as indicators in affective states. Neuropsychobiology 1975;1:296–303.
14. Kupfer DJ, Weiss BL, Foster FG, et al. Psychomotor activity in affective states. Arch Gen Psychiatry 1974;30:765–768.
15. Wehr TA, Muscettola G, Goodwin FK. Urinary 3-methoxy-4-hydroxyphenylglycol circadian rhythm. Early timing (phase advance) in manic–depressive compared with normal subjects. Arch Gen Psychiatry 1980;37:257–263.
16. Wolff EA III, Putnam FW, Post RM. Motor activity in affective illness: The relationship of amplitude and temporal distribution to changes in affective state. Arch Gen Psychiatry 1985;42:288–294.
17. Teicher MH, Lawrence JM, Barber NI, et al. Increased activity and phase delay in circadian motility rhythms in geriatric depression. Arch Gen Psychiatry 1988;45:913–917.
18. Joffe RT, Uhde TW, Post RM, et al. Motor activity in depressed patients treated with carbamazepine. Biol Psychiatry 1987;22:941–946.
19. Weiss BL, Foster FG, Reynolds CF, Kupfer DJ. Psychomotor activity in mania. Arch Gen Psychiatry 1974;31:379–383.
20. Goodwin FK, Wirz-Justice A, Wehr TA. Evidence that the pathophysiology of depression and mechanism of action of antidepressant drugs both involve alterations in circadian rhythms. Adv Biochem Psychopharmacol 1982;32:1–11.
21. Foster FG, Kupfer DJ. Psychomotor activity as a correlate of depression and sleep in acutely disturbed psychiatric inpatients. Am J Psychiatry 1975;132:928–931.
22. Nelson JC, Charney DS. The symptoms of major depression. Am J Psychiatry 1981;138:1–13.
23. Reich LH, Kupter DJ, Weiss BL, et al. Psychomotor activity as a predictor of sleep efficiency. Biol Psychiatry 1974;8:253–256.
24. Kripke DF, Mullaney DJ, Messin S, Wyborney VG. Wrist actigraphic measures of sleep and rhythms. Electroencephalogr Clin Neurophysiol 1978;44:674–676.
25. Porrino LJ, Rapoport JL, Behar D, et al. A naturalistic assessment of the motor activity of hyperactive boys. Comparisons with normal controls. Arch Gen Psychiatry 1983;40:681–687.
26. Porrino LJ, Rapoport JL, Behar D, et al. A naturalistic assessment of the motor activity of hyperactive boys. II. Stimulant drug effects. Arch Gen Psychiatry 1983;40:688–693.
27. Wren FJ, Teicher MH, Baldessarini RJ, Lieberman H. Locomotor activity patterns and stimulant response in children with attention deficit hyperactivity disorder. Am Acad Child Adoles Psychiatry Abstr 1988;4:65.
28. Teicher MH, Sussman AJ, Baldessarini RJ, Lieberman HR. Motility rhythms in psychotic inpatients. Am Psychiatr Assoc Abstr 1988;141:104.
29. Halaris A. Normal and abnormal circadian patterns of noradrenergic transmission. In: Halaris A, ed. Chronobiology and Psychiatric Disorders. New York: Elsevier 1987;23–47.
30. Crowley TJ, Hydinger-MacDonald M. Bedtime flurazepam and the human circadian rhythm of spontaneous mobility. Psychopharmacology 1979;62:157–161.
31. Teicher MH, Cohen BM, Baldessarini RJ, Cole JO. Severe daytime somnolence in patients treated with an MAOI. Am J Psychiatry 1988;145:152–156.
32. Ingram D, London E, Reynolds M. Circadian rhythmicity and sleep: effects of aging in laboratory animals. Neurobiol Aging 1982;3:287–297.
33. Lieberman HR, Wurtman JJ, Teicher MH. Circadian rhythms of activity in healthy young and elderly humans. Neurobiol Aging 1989;10:259–265.
34. Teicher MH, Lawrence JM, Barber NI, et al. Altered locomotor activity in neuropsychiatric patients. Prog Neuropharmacol Biol Psychiatry 1986;10:755–761.
35. Satlin A, Teicher MH, Lieberman H, et al. Circadian locomotor activity rhythms in Alzheimer's disease. J Neuropsychopharmacol 1991;5:115–126.
36. Tryon WW, Pologe B. Accelerometric assessment of tardive dyskinesia. Am J Psychiatry 1987;144:1584–1587.
37. Halberg F, Johnson EA, Nelson W, et al. Autorhythmometry procedures for physiological self-measurements and their analysis. Physiol Teacher 1972;1:1.

38. Nelson W, Tong IL, Lee JK, Halberg F. Mehods for cosinor-rhythmometry. Chronobiologia 1979;6:305–323.

39. Rummel J, Lee JK, Halberg F. Combined linear–nonlinear chronobiologic windows by least squares resolve neighbouring components in a physiologic rhythms spectrum. In: Ferin M, et al., eds. Biorhythms and human reproduction New York: John Wiley, 1974:53–82.

40. Teicher MH, Barber NI. COSIFIT: An interactive program for simultaneous multi-oscillator cosinor analysis of time-series data. Computers Biomed Res 1990;23:283–295.

41. Kripke DF. Ultradian rhythms in sleep and wakefulness. In: Weitzman E, ed. Advances in sleep research. Vol. 1. New York: Spectrum, 1974:305–325.

42. Blackman RB, Tukey JW. The measurement of power spectra. New York: Dover, 1958.

43. Halberg F, Panofsky H. Thermovariance spectra: method and clinical illustration. Exp Med Surg 1961;19:284–309.

44. Siegel S. Nonparametric statistics for the behavioral sciences. New York: McGraw Hill, 1956:184–193.

45. Box GEP, Jenkins GM. Time series analysis: forecasting and control. San Francisco: Holden Day, 1970.

46. Wang DCC, Vangnucci AH. TSAN: A package for time series analysis. Computer Progr Biomed 1980;11:132–144.

47. Fisher RA. Tests of significance in harmonic analysis. Proc R Soc A 1929;125:54–59.

48. Teicher MH, Barber NI, Baldessarini RJ, Shaywitz BA. Amphetamine accelerates and attenuates ultradian activity rhythms in developing rats. Pharmacol Biochem Behav 1988;29:517–523.

49. Teicher MH, Barber NI, Lawrence JM, Baldessarini RJ. Motor activity and antidepressant drugs: a proposed approach to categorizing depression syndromes and their animal models. In: Koobs GF, Ehlers CL, Kupfers D, eds. Animal models of depression. Boston: Birkhauser, 1989:135–161.

Serotonin Syndrome

JERROLD G. BERNSTEIN

HISTORICAL INTRODUCTION

The serotonin syndrome (SS) is a movement disorder characterized by restlessness, myoclonus, hyperreflexia, tremor, and often incoordination. This syndrome, resulting from excess serotonin activity in the central nervous system, commonly includes a variety of autonomic signs such as shivering, diaphoresis, diarrhea, labile blood pressure, and tachycardia. Because of the prominent behavioral and mood effects of serotonin, it is not surprising that this syndrome is frequently associated with confusion and hypomania. Serotonin syndrome was first described in the clinical psychiatric literature in 1982 by Insel et al (1) in two patients previously treated with clorgyline, a selective inhibitor of monoamine oxidase (MAO) type A, who received the serotonergic tricyclic clomipramine one month after discontinuing clorgyline. Both patients—who were being treated for severe obsessive–compulsive disorder—experienced myoclonus, hyperreflexia, restlessness, and diaphoresis, which began within an hour of a single dose of clomipramine and abated within 24 hours. In retrospect, a similar syndrome with clonus, hyperreflexia, restlessness, diaphoresis, dizziness, and feelings of drunkenness had been reported in the neurology literature in 1960 by Oates and Sjoerdsma (2) following oral administration of L-tryptophan to seven patients being treated for hypertension with β-phenylisopropylhydrazine (Catron), a monoamine oxidase inhibitor (MAOI) that was marketed in the early 1960s as an antihypertensive drug. Those investigators attributed the symptoms, which abated within 24 hours, to excess brain levels of tryptamine and serotonin.

In the early days of neuropharmacologic investigation, many groups of investigators employed a variety of monoamine oxidase inhibitors to increase brain levels of serotonin and norepinephrine and subsequently administered neurotransmitter precursors, releasers, and other drugs to study effects on brain chemistry, behavior, and cardiovascular parameters. Tremor, increased muscle tone, myoclonus, and autonomic signs were noted in MAOI-treated animals following administration of tryptophan in studies of tissue levels and excretion patterns of serotonin metabolites in the 1959 publication of Hess et al (3). As a naive college freshman, conducting my first research in neuropharmacology in 1958, I observed diarrhea, increased salivation, shivering, increased muscle tone, and irritability following administration of reserpine to three dogs that had been pretreated with iproniazid, an MAO inhibitor. Because my mentors and I attributed these observations simply to reserpine administration, this finding was never published. In retrospect, it seems likely that reserpine, which releases serotonin and norepinephrine from binding sites in the brain, actually provoked the serotonin syndrome in these animals whose ability to catabolize serotonin was inhibited by pretreatment with iproniazid.

Symptoms consistent with SS have been found in all mammalian species studied, including mice, rats, rabbits, cats, dogs, and monkeys, most commonly provoked by the administration of the serotonin precursor L-tryptophan or a serotonin reuptake inhibitor such as clomipramine to animals who are simultaneously given or pretreated with a monoamine oxidase inhibitor (4). The earlier clinical literature generally focused on the occurrence of this syndrome in MAOI-treated patients who subsequently received L-tryptophan or a tricyclic antidepressant in an attempt to achieve a more robust antidepressant or antiobsessional effect (1,5–7). Serotonin syndrome has also been observed in patients receiving combined MAOI and tricyclic antidepressant regimens who have taken overdoses of either agent (5).

With the advent of a new class of serotonin selective reuptake inhibitors (SSRIs), the treatment of depression and obsessive–compulsive disorder was revolutionized and the incidence of SS was dramatically increased, since these drugs rapidly became the most widely prescribed antidepressant and antiobsessional agents (8–10). Serotonin syndrome was reported when tranylcypromine, an MAOI, was initiated two days following discontinuation of a two-week course of fluoxetine, the first SSRI to be marketed in the United States (9). In 1991, Sternbach (10), who had reported the first case of SS with an MAOI and fluoxetine, reviewed 12 clinical publications recounting a total of 38 patients who had developed SS during treatment with an MAOI and L-tryptophan or with clomipramine or fluoxetine and L-tryptophan or an MAOI. In each of the 38 SS patients reported in the literature prior to Sternbach's 1991 review, the preeminent symptoms were those of a movement disorder, including myoclonus, hyperreflexia, and restlessness. Some also experienced ataxia and many had a variety of autonomic symptoms including shivering, diaphoresis, diarrhea, and labile blood pressure; some patients were also noted to have mental status changes with agitation or hypomania. Prior to the finding of SS precipitation by fluoxetine and tranylcypromine, Steiner and Fountaine (8) noted a toxic reaction characterized by agitation, restlessness, and autonomic symptoms in a group of five fluoxetine-treated patients who were given L-tryptophan in an attempt to enhance therapeutic response. The assumption that a combination of two different serotonergic agents is required to produce SS would be comforting to the cautious clinician, who could avoid SS simply by avoiding such combinations. Unfortunately three elderly patients were reported to develop SS during treatment with a single agent—in one case with the SSRI citalopram and in two cases with moclobemide, a reversible inhibitor of MAO type A, following dosage increases (11).

As will be discussed subsequently in this chapter, the SS may occur in various degrees of severity. Indeed, some patients have only very mild reactions consisting of muscle tension or myalgia with or without abdominal cramping or diarrhea when given modest doses of SSRIs or MAOIs in the absence of other medications, while other patients have moderate to severe forms of SS when treated with an SSRI alone or in combination with other drugs (12). One patient was reported to develop mild signs of SS when treated with the heterocyclic antidepressant trazodone in combination with buspirone, a nonbenzodiazepine anxiolytic, presumably due to the combined serotonergic activity of both compounds (13). Serotonin syndrome has been noted when a nonprescription cough remedy containing dextromethorphan was combined with the SSRI paroxetine, underscoring the potential risk of over-the-counter products provoking serious interactions with prescription medications (14).

Although severe and life-threatening forms of SS appear to be very uncommon thus far, the similarities between SS and the potentially fatal complication of antipsychotic drugs known as "neuroleptic malignant syndrome" (NMS) is highlighted by the publication of a case of SS associated with

hyperthermia, rhabdomyolysis, disseminated intravascular coagulation, and myoglobinuric renal failure (15). This case report illustrates the importance of adhering to a lengthy period free of SSRI prior to initiating an MAOI and emphasizes the principle I have proposed that the long half-life of fluoxetine necessitates a longer drug-free interval, which must be longer still if higher doses are employed (12,15). Indeed, this patient, who developed the most severe SS documented in the literature, did so when tranylcypromine was initiated 24 days after discontinuing a 35-day course of treatment with fluoxetine at a dose of 40 mg daily (15).

DIAGNOSIS

The serotonin syndrome as encountered in clinical practice spans a wide range of severity from muscular discomfort and tremor through masseter spasm with painful tooth grinding, myoclonus, and hyperreflexia (12). These symptoms are often associated with a variety of autonomic symptoms including shivering, chills, diaphoresis, diarrhea, and labile blood pressure, as shown in Table 63.1. Most patients with SS experience motor restlessness. Although mental status changes including confusion and hypomania are commonly present, they are not necessary to make the diagnosis of SS, which results from excess central nervous system serotonergic activity (10,12). Indeed patients experiencing mental status changes without neuromuscular symptoms may be manifesting a side effect that is common to all antidepressants, including those that do not alter serotonergic activity (12). Patients who present with isolated neuromuscular symptoms such as myoclonus, hyperreflexia, myalgia, or bruxism, in the absence of autonomic or behavioral symptoms are likely to be suffering from a milder form of SS and should be managed accordingly (10,12).

Severe forms of serotonin syndrome may be difficult to differentiate from neuroleptic malignant syndrome (NMS) (12,15,16) as shown in Table 63.2. Generally SS as described in the literature falls into the category of moderate severity

Table 63.1 Serotonin Syndrome: Signs and Symptoms*

Mental status changes: confusion or hypomania
Restlessness or agitation
Myoclonus
Hyperreflexia
Diaphoresis
Shivering (or shaking chills)
Tremor
Diarrhea, abdominal cramps, nausea
Ataxia or incoordination
Headache

* Signs and symptoms tabulated from most to least frequent.

SOURCE: Adapted from Bernstein JG. Handbook of drug therapy in psychiatry. 3rd ed. St. Louis: Mosby, 1995.

Table 63.2   Comparison of Neuroleptic Malignant and Serotonin Syndromes

	Neuroleptic Malignant (NMS)	Serotonin Syndrome
Mental status	Dazed mutism	Confusion, Disorientation, Mania
Hyperthermia	Mild to marked	Mild to marked
Autonomic dysfunction	+	+
Tachycardia	+	+
Labile BP	+	+
Diaphoresis	+	+
Tremor	+	+
Incontinence	+	0
Sialorrhea	+	0
Dyspnea	+	0
Shivering	0	+
Restlessness	0	+
Extrapyramidal effects	+	0
Myoclonus	0	+
Hyperreflexia	0	+
Ataxia	0	+
Leukocytosis	+	0
CPK elevation	+	0
Muscular rigidity	+	0

SOURCE: Reproduced with permission from Bernstein JG. Handbook of drug therapy in psychiatry. 3rd ed. St. Louis: Mosby, 1995.

with mental status changes and autonomic symptoms accompanying signs of a movement disorder with irritability, hyperreflexia, and myoclonus (10,12). Very severe cases of SS have been reported that have included hyperthermia, rhabdomyolysis, disseminated intravascular coagulation, and myoglobinuric renal failure (15,17). There is one report of five patients who had a fatal outcome after taking overdoses of moclobemide in combination with either citalopram (an SSRI not marketed in the United States) or clomipramine, in spite of early recognition and intervention in two of the patients (17). Milder forms of what I would consider SS have been described in the literature as cases of bruxism or myoclonus during SSRI therapy without reference to serotonin syndrome (18–21).

In reviewing the literature and clinical experience with SS, it is apparent that clomipramine or any of the SSRIs in combination with L-tryptophan or with any MAOI, including the MAO type B selective agent selegiline, or moclobemide, the reversible inhibitor of MAO type A (RIMA), can provoke the syndrome if used simultaneously or in close time proximity of each other (12). Since 7 to 14 days may be required to regenerate MAO after its inhibition, at least two weeks must elapse after discontinuing an MAOI prior to initiating an SSRI, preferably three weeks if a higher dosage of MAOI has been employed (12). The time that

must elapse after discontinuing an SSRI before initiating an MAOI is dependent on the half-life of the SSRI that has been prescribed and on its dosage (12). Table 63.3 presents half-life data on currently available SSRIs.

Fluoxetine and its active metabolite have a half-life of approximately one week, and five half-lives must elapse to clear a drug from plasma and tissues, thus at least five weeks must elapse following discontinuation of this drug, prior to MAOI therapy, unless fluoxetine doses in excess of 20 mg per day have been employed, in which case, there may need to be a hiatus of 6 to 12 weeks between fluoxetine and MAOI therapy (12). Clomipramine and its active metabolite have a combined half-life of approximately four days, therefore, this agent should be discontinued approximately three weeks before starting an MAOI (12). As a rule of thumb, other currently marketed SSRIs have half-lives of approximately 24 hours and should generally be discontinued two weeks before an MAOI is initiated (12). Meperidine, a narcotic analgesic, has prominent central serotonergic activity and therefore may precipitate a syndrome resembling SS when given to MAOI-treated patients (12). There have been occasional reports suggesting that SS may be precipitated by either lithium or carbamazepine in conjunction with an MAOI or SSRI; however, generally these mood stabilizing agents can be used safely in MAOI- or SSRI-treated patients (12).

Serotonin syndrome is diagnosed clinically by history and physical examination, neither electroencephalogram (EEG) or brain imaging studies are likely to be useful in arriving at the diagnosis. Typically a patient who is currently receiving either an SSRI or MAOI will present with irritability and myalgia or bruxism and will show increased deep tendon reflexes and clonus on physical examination. Milder forms of SS may be seen in patients who are receiving monotherapy with a serotonergic drug who have not recently received another serotonergic agent. Individuals who have previously been treated with an MAOI or SSRI who receive the alternative serotonergic drug prior to dissipation of the pharmacologic effect of the first agent will present with moderate to severe SS, depending on the half-life of the first agent and the interval that has elapsed following its discontinuation prior to starting the second drug.

The most severe cases of SS are likely to be seen among patients who have received an MAOI and an SSRI, clomipramine, or L-tryptophan simultaneously or those who have taken an overdose of either or both agents. Most patients with SS will have tremors; many will experience shivering, diarrhea, abdominal cramps, nausea, headache, incoordination or ataxia. Although mild cases of SS generally do not have mental status changes, patients with moderate to severe SS most often will have mental status changes with confusion or hypomania.

Regardless of the severity of SS, in order to make the diagnosis clinically, neuromuscular symptoms including hyperreflexia and clonus must be present; generally there

T a b l e   6 3 . 3   Comparison of Serotonin-Selective Reuptake Inhibitors

	Half-Life[a] (mean)	Half-Life (metabolite)	Activity of Metabolite	Impairment of Drug Metabolism[a]
Fluoxetine (Prozac)	2–3 days	7–9 days	Equal to F	+ + + + +
Fluvoxamine (Luvox)	15 hr	Inactive	0	+ + +
Paroxetine (Paxil)	21 hr	Inactive	0	+ + +
Sertraline (Zoloft)	26 hr	2–4 days	Minimal	+
Venlafaxine (Effexor)	5 hr	11 hr	Equal to V	±
Clomipramine[b] (Anafranil)	32 hr	69 hr	CM/serotonin DCM/NEPI	+

[a] Impairment of drug metabolism parallels the potency of cytochrome P-450 inhibition and drug half-life (DeVane CL. J Clin Psychiatry 1992;53(2, suppl):13–20).
[b] Clomipramine-TCA (not SSRI) presented for comparison. The parent compound, clomipramine, is primarily serotonergic; the metabolite, desmethyl-clomipramine, is primarily noradrenergic. The half-life shown is for single-dose administration; it may be two to four times higher with continuous or high-dose regimens.
SOURCE: Adapted from Bernstein JG. Handbook of drug therapy in psychiatry. 3rd ed. St. Louis: Mosby, 1995.

will coexist myalgia and bruxism as well. Patients who develop bruxism during SSRI or MAOI monotherapy in the absence of other symptoms are likely to be suffering from a mild form of SS that may worsen with continued treatment at the same dosage level or with dosage increase and is likely to abate promptly with dosage reduction or discontinuation of the serotonergic drug.

The differential diagnosis of serotonin syndrome includes sleep myoclonus, essential myoclonus, epileptic myoclonus, SSRI-induced extrapyramidal reactions, carcinoid syndrome, and NMS (12,21–27). The nondrug-induced forms of myoclonus can generally be ruled out in patients who initially develop myoclonus during treatment with an MAOI or SSRI. Patients with a prior history of epilepsy or myoclonus may have worsening of seizure or myoclonic symptoms during MAOI or SSRI therapy (23). Infrequently dystonic, dyskinetic, or other extrapyramidal symptoms have been reported in SSRI-treated patients, many of whom have been receiving a neuroleptic previously or concurrently (24–26). In those patients who have had neuroleptics and SSRIs together, it is likely that the latter drug increased vulnerability to the neuroleptic. Indeed, in the "four neuron" model of the extrapyramidal system, serotonin may well function as a regulatory transmitter of motor function, and thus could be implicated in the causation of a movement disorder in the absence of other drugs (28).

SSRIs and MAOIs increase serotonin activity in the central nervous system as well as in other tissues. Carcinoid syndrome, caused by increased synthesis and release of serotonin and histamine by carcinoid tumors, produces a variety of symptoms including flushing, lacrimation, salivation, valvular heart disease, and diarrhea. Some SSRI-treated patients will have flushing, diaphoresis, salivation, and diarrhea without myoclonus or hyperreflexia and may well be manifesting symptoms of peripheral serotonin excess

without CNS manifestations. Neuroleptic malignant syndrome is generally more serious than SS and may indeed be life threatening (12) (see Table 63.3). In NMS the patient often presents as being dazed and mute with "lead pipe" rigidity, cogwheel signs, akinesia, and catatonia and often will become comatose. The NMS patient is usually febrile, often to 104°F to 106°F, and has pronounced sialorrhea and diaphoresis with marked tachycardia and labile blood pressure (12). Rigidity, cogwheeling, and catatonia are virtually never present in SS, and the autonomic signs of SS are generally much less intense than in NMS (12).

MANAGEMENT

The most effective approach to management of SS is to avoid simultaneous prescription of MAOIs with serotonergic drugs including SSRIs, clomipramine, tryptophan, and meperidine. Whenever any of these drugs is prescribed individually, the physician must remain vigilant and monitor the patient carefully since individual symptoms or mild cases of serotonin syndrome may occur in some patients receiving treatment with a single serotonergic drug. Myoclonus, which is a primary symptom of SS, was reported in patients receiving tricyclic and MAOI antidepressants individually prior to the use of SSRIs, with an incidence that paralleled serotonergic potency of the specific agent (29). Another important step to avoiding SS is to allow an adequate period of time to elapse between SSRI therapy and MAOI therapy when the medication change must be made in either direction. At least two weeks must elapse after an MAOI is discontinued before starting any SSRI. Two weeks must elapse after stopping fluvoxamine, paroxetine, sertraline, or venlafaxine before starting an MAOI. Three weeks should intervene between clomipramine and an MAOI. If the patient has been receiving fluoxetine at a dose of 20 mg per day or less, there must be at least five weeks between its discontinuation and initiation of an MAOI, while 6 to 12 weeks may need to elapse after higher doses of fluoxetine before starting an MAOI (12).

One area of controversy involves the safety of the simultaneous administration of two SSRIs or the simultaneous use of an SSRI with clomipramine. The major risk of combining two SSRIs arises if one of the drugs is fluoxetine, a potent inhibitor of cytochrome P 450 IID6, a drug metabolizing enzyme that is likely to increase the blood level of many coadministered drugs, including other SSRIs, thus potentially increasing the therapeutic as well as the toxic effect of coadministered drugs. Clomipramine, particularly at higher doses, may lower seizure-threshold and provoke convulsions; elevation of clomipramine serum concentration by fluoxetine could therefore produce the dangerous complication of seizures. Fluoxetine given along with another SSRI or clomipramine could provoke the serotonin syndrome. One study reported that administration of paroxetine to patients who had previously been treated with fluoxetine produced no greater adverse effects in patients who went directly to paroxetine from fluoxetine than in another group who had a two-week drug-free interval between fluoxetine and paroxetine (30). Reanalysis of those data by another investigator pointed out that those patients changing from fluoxetine to paroxetine without a washout period had higher incidences of headache, insomnia, nausea, and anxiety that were statistically significant (31). Patients switching from fluoxetine to sertraline without a washout period had similar complaints of adverse effects that were not seen when there was a three-week washout period after fluoxetine prior to initiating sertraline (31).

Another controversial aspect of SS and the issue of drug combinations is the risk entailed when MAO-A or MAO-B selective MAOIs are employed. Although there are but limited data on regimens combining SSRIs and moclobemide, the selective inhibitor of MAO type A, this combination has resulted in SS and thus should be avoided for optimally safe pharmacotherapy (17,31). Selegiline, a selective inhibitor of MAOI type B that is commonly used in the treatment of Parkinson's disease, does not require employment of a low-tyramine MAOI diet but has been reported to provoke SS in a very small number of patients simultaneously receiving an SSRI (31). It has been suggested that parkinsonian patients have reduced serotonergic function and may therefore be less likely to develop SS (31). A recently presented study surveying 63 Parkinson Study Group (PSG) investigators received data from 45 investigators indicating that 4,568 selegiline-treated patients had simultaneously received an antidepressant medication, with only 11 patients (0.24%) reporting some symptoms consistent with SS, which was judged to be serious in only two patients (0.04%) (32). Personal communication with one of the investigators (I.R.) suggested to me that only about six patients actually had indications of SS and that the complications in the two patients considered serious may well have

been independent of a serotonergic interaction (32). It is important to recognize that selegiline is selective for MAO-B at doses of 10 mg per day or less and becomes a nonselective inhibitor of MAO at daily doses of 20 mg or greater. Furthermore, when the range of antidepressant side effects are taken as a whole, SSRIs are generally more benign than tricyclic antidepressants or nonselective MAOIs. Therefore, SSRIs may be the safest antidepressants to employ in patients with Parkinson's disease. The previously mentioned study, in which a variety of antidepressants including TCAs and SSRIs were employed along with selegiline, suggests that if patients are carefully monitored and their physicians are vigilant for signs of impending SS, this combination therapy of conservative doses of SSRIs and selegiline may be safely utilized (32).

After prevention, which is practiced by avoiding potentially interacting drug regimens and allowing adequate washout periods between therapies, the next important step in management of SS requires the physician to discontinue SSRI, clomipramine, or MAOI in any patient appearing to develop SS. In general, physicians tend to prescribe doses of SSRIs that exceed the amount necessary to produce a therapeutic response; therefore, SS can be avoided in many instances by prescribing lower doses of any SSRI, particularly in patients who begin to show SS symptoms when treated with conventional or relatively higher doses of SSRIs or MAOIs.

Most cases of SS are uncomfortable but not serious or life threatening, and abate within one to three days of discontinuing the offending drug, although abatement may take more time following longer-acting drugs such as fluoxetine. Recurrence can generally be avoided by continuing treatment with a lower dose of serotonergic drug or an alternate nonserotonergic agent once symptoms have abated.

Pharmacologic intervention to treat SS is generally not necessary and there have been no controlled trials of alternative drug therapies for SS. Several published studies of SS have reported on small numbers of patients treated with a variety of pharmacologic interventions (10,12,31,33,34). Selective inhibitors of 5-HT$_1$ receptors are generally ineffective, although propranolol, a beta blocker that also blocks 5-HT$_{1A}$ sites may be useful (10,31). Nonselective serotonin receptor antagonists such as cyproheptadine (4 mg two to three times daily) or methysergide (2 mg two to three times daily) have both been helpful in rapidly alleviating symptoms of SS (10,31). Clonazepam has been very effective in eliminating myoclonus due to SSRIs and MAOIs, most often in doses of 0.5 mg two to three times daily, whether the myoclonus was a solitary symptom or appeared in the context of polysymptomatic SS (12,33). Since cyproheptadine and methysergide are nonselective serotonin antagonists, they will also inhibit the therapeutic effects of SSRIs or MAOIs and therefore should not be continuing components of SSRI or MAOI therapy (12). In patients who tolerate and respond therapeutically to SSRIs or MAOIs, myoclonus and neuromuscular irritability may be reduced or eliminated by coadministration of clonazepam (12). Although nausea is not uncommon when initiating SSRIs and may be a component of SS, it generally abates with continuing treatment, particularly following dosage reduction. Some patients who respond well to SSRIs but have continuing nausea at minimal effective dosages may benefit from simultaneous administration of cisapride, a 5-HT$_3$ antagonist, 5 mg twice daily (34).

BASIC SCIENCE

A variety of indole compounds, including 5-hydroxytryptamine (serotonin) were first isolated from enterochromaffin cells of the small intestine by Erspamer, who attributed to these compounds a role in regulating gastrointestinal motility. In 1948, Rapport, Green, and Page, who were trying to understand the physiology of hypertension, isolated and characterized serotonin from blood platelets where it was thought to function primarily as a vasoconstrictor substance controlling vasomotor tone (35). With the birth of the sciences of neuropharmacology and psychopharmacology in the early 1950s, the MAOI iproniazid was found to increase brain levels of norepinephrine and serotonin, and the neurotransmitter releaser, reserpine, was shown to deplete serotonin as well as norepinephrine from the brain (12).

Subsequently, with the recognition that MAOIs could provoke mania and that reserpine could produce depression, it was proposed that alteration of brain neurotransmitters could have a profound effect on mood giving rise to the monoamine theory of depression, popularized by Schildkraut, Klerman, and others (12).

Serotonin research is now only about 50 years old. The first 25 years were interesting but rather peaceful on the receptor front since it was clear that if serotonin were synthesized in the body there must be two or three different serotonin receptors, just as we knew that there were two or three acetylcholine receptors and two or three different adrenergic receptors (35). The most recent quarter-century of serotonin research has been filled with turmoil as new serotonin receptors and subtypes with different roles have become identified, studied, and characterized on a molecular level (36). There are, as of this writing, 14 separately identified serotonin receptors and subtypes, a number likely to expand with the extension of serotonin science and its clinical role (36). Table 63.4 outlines currently recognized serotonin receptors.

Serotonin is ubiquitous in all mammalian systems, with significant concentrations occurring in blood platelets, gastrointestinal tract, lungs, and the central nervous system. The numerous subtypes of serotonin receptors are present in different animal systems, not all of which have been identified

Table 63.4   Serotonin Receptors, Agonists, Antagonists, and Effects

Receptor	Subtype*	Agonist	Effect	Antagonist	Effect
5-HT$_1$	5-HT$_{1A}$	Buspirone	Anxiolytic	Pindolol Propranolol	Potentiate SSRIs ? treatment of SS
	5-HT$_{1B}$	Methysergide Sumatripan	5-HT$_{1B}$ not in humans	Pindolol Yohimbine	5-HT$_{1B}$ not in humans
	5-HT$_{1D}$	Sumatripan	Treatment of migraine	Buspirone	Anxiolytic
	5-HT$_{1E}$	None specific	Unknown	None specific	Unknown
	5-HT$_{1F}$	None specific	Unknown	None specific	Unknown
5-HT$_2$	5-HT$_{2A}$	None marketed	Platelet aggregation	Methysergide Risperidone Nefazodone, Trazodone	Treatment of migraine Antipsychotic Antidepressant
	5-HT$_{2B}$	None marketed	Gastric contraction	None marketed	Unknown
	5-HT$_{2C}$	Sumatripan (weak)	Treatment of migraine	Methysergide Cyproheptadine Risperidone Nefazodone, Trazodone	Treatment of SS & migraine Treatment of SS Antipsychotic Antidepressant
5-HT$_3$	5-HT$_3$	None marketed	Unknown	Odansetron	Antiemetic
5-HT$_4$	5-HT$_4$	Cisapride Metoclopramide	Gastric prokinetic Gastric prokinetic (used in GERD)	None marketed	Reduced GI motility
5-HT$_5$	5-HT$_{5A}$	None marketed	Unknown	None marketed	Unknown
	5-HT$_{5B}$	None marketed	Unknown	None marketed	Unknown
5-HT$_6$	5-HT$_6$	None marketed	Unknown	None marketed	Unknown
5-HT$_7$	5-HT$_7$	None marketed	Unknown	None marketed	Unknown

* Additional data on 5-HT receptor subtypes and ligands is to be found in Hoyer D, Clarke DE, Fozard JR, et al. VII International Union of Pharmacology classification of receptors for 5-hydroxytryptamine (Serotonin). Pharmacol Rev 1994; 46:157–203.
Data from references 12 and 36.

in humans (36). As can be seen in reviewing the variety of serotonin receptors, this rather simple molecule may have profound physiologic effects on platelet aggregation, gastrointestinal motility, vasomotor tone, headaches, cognition, mood, sexual function, extrapyramidal, and neuromuscular activity (36). The wide range of symptoms attributed to excess central and peripheral effects of serotonin as seen in SS and in some patients without SS who experience adverse effects of SSRIs and MAOIs is readily understandable (31). Likewise the symptoms of carcinoid syndrome can be readily associated with the peripheral effects of serotonin production by tumors that lie outside the central nervous system (27).

Since the movement disorder of SS is the focus of this chapter, it is important to review the interactions of the serotonin and dopamine neurotransmitter systems.

The serotonin antagonist, cyproheptadine, antagonizes neuroleptic-induced catalepsy and increases the anticataleptic effects of both L-dopa and amantadine (28). Indeed, comparably effective doses of respiridone, which blocks both D_2 dopamine sites and 5-HT$_2$ receptors, produce less extrapyramidal side effects than does haloperidol, which blocks D_2 but not 5-HT$_2$ receptor sites (12). Fluoxetine inhibits catecholamine synthesis in dopamine-rich areas of the forebrain, hippocampus, and striatum, suggesting that serotonin may inhibit dopamine neurons, which may thus explain extrapyramidal side effects such as akathisia, which is seen in some SSRI treated patients (28). In the "three neuron model" of extrapyramidal function, the first neuron entering the basal ganglia is the inhibitory nigrostriatal dopamine tract. Excitatory cholinergic interneurons are the second neuron, while the third neuron is represented by the inhibitory GABA-ergic tract that modulates voluntary motor activity (28). The "four neuron model" proposed by Hamilton and Opler adds a new first neuron that is serotonergic to the previously described "three neuron model" (24,28). In the "four neuron model," the serotonergic neuron of the raphe-striatal tract inhibits firing in the nigrostriatal tract, thus potentially inducing extrapyramidal symptoms that can parallel excessive serotonergic activity, which may be seen during SSRI treatment or in patients developing SS (28). The ability of the serotonin antagonist cyproheptadine to block cataleptic effects of neuroleptics lends further support to this model that includes serotonin in the cascade of transmitters involved in extrapyramidal motor control (24). This view of serotonergic tracts acting in opposition to dopaminergic transmission is challenged by other findings that suggest that effects mediated by 5-HT$_1$ and 5-HT$_3$ may enhance dopamine function. It is difficult, however, to extrapolate findings in one species to another, particularly since some subtypes of serotonin receptors are not present in all mammalian species and may subserve different functions in different organisms (36). 5-HT$_2$ receptors are generally viewed as having an inhibitory effect on dopaminergic activity, although some studies suggest heterogeneity of their physiologic actions on these

sites, and again species differences must be considered (36).

In addition to SS produced by SSRIs in combination with other drugs, a number of patients have been reported to develop akathisia, parkinsonian rigidity, and dystonic reactions when treated with ordinary doses of fluoxetine or other SSRIs (21,24–26,28). The most cogent explanation of these findings is that increased serotonin activity inhibits both nigrostriatal and tuberoinfundibular dopaminergic neurones, resulting in extrapyramidal symptoms and in many cases increased prolactin serum concentrations (24). Further support of the notion that serotonergic activity can suppress dopaminergic function comes from the finding that methysergide diminishes akinesia induced by section of nigrostriatal circuits in rats, suggesting that serotonergic fibers from the raphe dorsal nucleus can inhibit nigrostriatal dopaminergic fibers (24). Although extrapyramidal side effects of serotonergic drugs appear to be a separate entity from the serotonin syndrome, evaluation of patients with adverse neuromuscular consequences of SSRI therapy must also include consideration of these symptoms.

Another consequence of SSRI therapy that can cause considerable patient discomfort is suppression of libido and disturbance of erectile, ejaculatory, and orgasmic function. This constellation of sexual side effects is generally dose dependent and often responds favorably to dosage reduction, although some patients will require an alternate SSRI or nonserotonergic drug (12). Serotonin clearly functions as a central and likely peripheral mediator of sexual arousal and function, quite possibly in opposition to dopamine, which is generally viewed as enhancing sexual appetite and arousal (12). Patients who experience impairment of sexual function during serotonergic therapy should be evaluated for other clinical signs of serotonin excess as seen in SS, since clinically these sexual side effects of SSRIs are often significantly improved by serotonin antagonists such as cyproheptadine, although the latter will also inhibit therapeutic effects of SSRIs. Persistent sexual dysfunction in patients requiring long-term SSRI treatment may benefit from cautious coadministration of a dopaminergic drug such as amantadine or bromocriptine (12).

In summary, in spite of the dramatic therapeutic benefits of SSRI drugs in depression, obsessive–compulsive disorder, and phobic and panic disorders, these drugs may exert a variety of unwanted effects due to excessive central and peripheral effects of serotonin. These effects may arise when SSRIs are used alone but are more common when used improperly in conjunction with other serotonergic drugs. Combinations of two or more serotonergic agents simultaneously should be avoided, and patients should be closely monitored for adverse consequences of serotonin excess.

REFERENCES

1. Insel TR, Roy BF, Cohen RM, Murphy DL. Possible development of the serotonin syndrome in man. Am J Psych 1982;139:954–955.

2. Oates JA, Sjoerdsma A. Neurologic effects of tryptophan in patients receiving a monoamine oxidase inhibitor. Neurology 1960;10:1076–1078.

3. Hess SM, Redfield BG, Udenfriend S. The effect of monoamine oxidase inhibitors and tryptophan on the tryptamine content of animal tissues and urine. J Pharmacol Exp Ther 1959;127:178–181.

4. Squires RF. Monoamine oxidase inhibitors: animal pharmacology. In: Iversen L, Iversen S, Snyder S, eds. Handbook of psychopharmacology. Vol. 14. New York: Plenum, 1978:1–58.

5. White K, Simpson G. Combined MAOI-tricyclic antidepressant therapy: a reevaluation. J Clin Psychopharm 1981;1:264–282.

6. Lieberman JA, Kane JM, Reife R. Neuromuscular effects of monoamine oxidase inhibitors. J Clin Psychopharm 1985;5:221–228.

7. Pope HG, Jonas JM, Hudson JI, Kafka MP. Toxic reactions to a combination of monoamine oxidase inhibitors and tryptophan. Am J Psychiatry 1985;142:491–492.

8. Steiner W, Fontaine R. Toxic reaction following the combined administration of fluoxetine and 1-tryptophan: five case reports. Biol Psychiatry 1986;21:1067–1071.

9. Sternbach H. Danger of MAOI therapy after fluoxetine withdrawal (letter). Lancet 1988;2:850.

10. Sternbach H. The serotonin syndrome. Am J Psychiatry 1991;148:705–713.

11. Fischer P. Serotonin syndrome in the elderly after antidepressant monotherapy (letter). J Clin Psychopharmacol 1995;15:440–442.

12. Bernstein JG. Handbook of drug therapy in psychiatry. 3rd ed. St. Louis: Mosby, 1995.

13. Goldberg RJ, Huk M. Serotonin syndrome from trazodone and buspirone (letter). Psychosomatics 1992;33:235.

14. Skop BP, Finkelstein JA, Mareth TR, et al. The serotonin syndrome associated with paroxetine, an over-the-counter cold remedy, and vascular disease. Am J Emerg Med 1994;12:642–644.

15. Miller F, Friedman R, Tanenbaum J, Griffin A. Disseminated intravascular coagulation and acute myoglbinuric renal failure: a consequence of the serotonergic syndrome (letter). J Clin Psychopharmacol 1991;11:277–279.

16. Kline SS, Mauro LS, Scala-Barnett DM, Zick D. Serotonin syndrome versus neuroleptic malignant syndrome as a cause of death. Clin Pharmacy 1989;8:510–514.

17. Neuvonen PJ, Pohjola-Sintonen S, Tacke U, Vuori E. Five fatal cases of serotonin syndrome after moclobemide–citalopram or moclobemide–clomipramine overdoses. Lancet 1993;342:1419.

18. Ellison JM, Stanziani P. SSRI-associated nocturnal bruxism in four patients. J Clin Psychiatry 1993;54:432–434.

19. Garvey MJ, Tollefson GD. Occurrence of myoclonus in patients treated with cyclic antidepressants. Arch Gen Psychiatry 1987;44:269–272.

20. Bauer M. Severe myoclonus produced by fluvoxamine (letter). J Clin Psychiatry 1995;56:589–590.

21. Shihabuddin L, Rappaport D. Sertraline and extrapyramidal side effects (letter). Am J Psychiatry 1994;151:288.

22. Hopkins A. Clinical neurology: a modern approach. Oxford: Oxford University, 1993.

23. Deahl M, Trimble M. Serotonin reuptake inhibitors, epilepsy, and myoclonus. Brit J Psychiatry 1991;159:433–435.

24. Arya DK. Extrapyramidal symptoms with selective serotonin reuptake inhibitors. Brit J Psychiatry 1994;165:728–733.

25. Coulter DM, Pillans PI. Fluoxetine and extrapyramidal side effects. Am J Psychiatry 1995;152:122–125.

26. Fitzgerald K, Healy D. Dystonias and dyskinesias of the jaw associated with the use of SSRIs. Hum Psychopharmacol 1995;10:215–219.

27. Kaplan LM. Carcinoid tumors. In: Isselbacher KJ, Braunwald E, Wilson JD, Martin JB, et al., eds. Harrison's principles of internal medicine. 13th ed. New York: McGraw Hill, 1994:1537–1539.

28. Hamilton MS, Opler LA. Akathisia, suicidality, and fluoxetine. J Clin Psychiatry 1992;53:401–406.

29. Merikangas JR, Merikangas KR, Himmelhoch JM. Serotonergic activity and drug-induced myoclonus. Presented at the Annual Meeting of the American Psychiatric Association, Washington, DC, May 14, 1986. Abstract NR 157.

30. Kreider MS, Bushnell WD, Oakes R, Wheadon DE. A double-blind, randomized study to provide safety information on switching fluoxetine-treated patients to paroxetine without an intervening washout period. J Clin Psychiatry 1995;56:142–145.

31. Lane R, Fischler B. The serotonin syndrome: coadministration, discontinuation and washout periods for the selective serotonin reuptake inhibitors (SSRIs). J Serotonin Res 1995;3:171–180.

32. Richard I, Kurlan R, Tanner C. Serotonin syndrome and the combined use of deprenyl (selegiline) and an antidepressant in Parkinson's disease. Presented at the Annual Meeting of the American Academy of Neurology, San Francisco, March 28, 1996. Abstract P05.118.

33. Feighner JP, Boyer WF, Tyler DL, Neborsky RJ. Adverse consequences of fluoxetine-MAOI combination therapy. J Clin Psychiatry 1990;51:222–225.

34. Bergeron R, Blier P. Cisapride for the treatment of nausea produced by selective serotonin reuptake inhibitors. Am J Psychiatry 1994;151:1084–1086.

35. Cooper JR, Bloom FE, Roth RH. The biochemical basis of neuropharmacology. 7th ed. New York: Oxford University, 1996.

36. Sanders-Bush E, Mayer SE. 5-hydroxytryptamine (serotonin) receptor agonists and antagonists. In: Hardman JG, Limbird LE, Molinoff PB, et al., eds. Goodman and Gilman's the pharmacological basis of therapeutics. 9th ed. New York: McGraw-Hill, 1996:249–293.

Tics, Myoclonus, and Startle

Tic Disorders: An Overview

Roger Kurlan

HISTORICAL INTRODUCTION

Under the tutelage of Charcot, George Gilles de la Tourette undertook the task of clarifying conditions characterized by involuntary movements. After translating Beard's 1880 American journal article on "the Jumping Frenchmen of Maine," a condition characterized by excessive startle response, echolalia, and echopraxia, Tourette reasoned that if jumping Frenchmen existed in Maine they should be found in Paris as well. He searched the neurological institute of the Salpetriere for similar cases, but failed to identify any. Instead, he reported nine patients with motor and vocal tics some of whom had echo phenomena and coprolalia. In his now-famous publication of 1885 where he described the illness that bears his name, Gilles de la Tourette considered the disorder to be closely related to a group of startle disorders that included the jumpers. Although Tourette himself stated that the disorder was hereditary in nature, for many years the etiology of Tourette's syndrome (TS) was ascribed to psychogenic causes and the importance of genetic factors was neglected. The observations in the 1960s that neuroleptic drugs were successful in treating the condition refocused attention from a psychologic to an organic central nervous system etiology. It was not until the late 1970s that investigators demonstrated a familial concentration for TS and analysis of transmission patterns in families has suggested an autosomal dominant pattern of inheritance. Family studies indicate that the disorder may have variable clinical expression with milder variants including chronic motor or vocal tic disorder and transient tic disorder. Furthermore, recent evidence suggests that certain behavioral disturbances, including obsessive–compulsive disorder and attention deficit hyperactivity disorder, may be alternative expressions for the TS trait. Others have expressed a more extreme view that a wide range of psychopathologic conditions, such as

conduct disorder, panic disorder, bipolar affective disorder, and phobic disorder, may fall within the spectrum of TS symptoms. Notions concerning the clinical features and etiology of TS and related tic and behavioral disorders have undergone a dramatic evolution in recent years and will serve as a focus for this chapter (1).

DIAGNOSIS

Tics are brief movements (motor tics) or sounds produced by moving air through the nose, mouth, or throat (vocal tics) (2). In contrast to most other involuntary movements, tics are not constantly present (except when extremely severe) and occur out of a background of normal motor activity. Motor and vocal tics may take a variety of forms and can be divided conceptually into simple and complex types. Simple motor tics are abrupt, sudden, brief, isolated movements such as an eye blink, a shoulder shrug, or a head jerk. Although most simple motor tics are fast and abrupt, some may appear as slower, sustained, tonic movements (e.g., neck twisting, buttock tightening) that resemble dystonia and are therefore termed *dystonic tics* (3). Complex motor tics consist of more coordinated and complicated movements that may appear purposeful, as if performing a voluntary motor act. Examples include smelling, touching, copropraxia (obscene gestures), and echopraxia (mimicking movements performed by others). Motor tics usually recur in the same part of the body and multiple body regions can be involved. Over time, tics often recede from one body part and evolve elsewhere.

Simple vocal tics include a variety of inarticulate noises and single sounds, such as throat clearing, sniffing, and grunting. Complex vocal tics have linguistic meaning and consist of full or truncated words, such as echolalia (repeating the words of others), palilalia (repeating the individual's own words), and coprolalia (obscene words). Although coprolalia has been the symptom perhaps most responsible for the notoriety of TS, it is now clear this symptom may be mild and transient and occurs in only a minority of cases.

A recently emphasized symptom of TS is represented by "sensory tics," which are patterns of uncomfortable somatic sensations, such as pressure, tickle, or warmth, that are localized to specific body regions, such as face, shoulder, or neck (4). Patients attempt to relieve the uncomfortable sensations with movements often interpreted as voluntary, usually tonic tightening or stretching of muscles indicative of a dystonic tic. Relief is temporary, however, and the movements are repeated. Some patients produce vocalizations that are responses to a sensory stimulus in the larynx or throat. Such sensory tics are seen in approximately 40% of patients with TS.

A variety of primary tic disorders are now recognized and *Tourette's syndrome* can be considered to represent the most severe member of a family of tic disorders. Diagnostic criteria for TS include 1) the presence of multiple motor tics, 2) the presence of one or more vocal tics, 3) age at onset before 18 years, 4) duration of more than one year, and 5) the disturbance causes marked distress or significant impairment in daily functioning (5). The final criterion, that tics must be functionally impairing, is new to the latest edition of the Diagnostic and Statistical Manual of Psychiatry and is controversial since it runs contrary to recent genetic and epidemiologic information that indicates that the majority of individuals with TS have mild symptoms (6–8). Chronic tic disorder (CTD) differs from TS in that motor *or* vocal tics, but not both, are present. Transient tic disorder (TTD) differs from TS and CTD by a duration of less than one year. Both CTD and TTD are now generally viewed as milder variants of TS and possible expressions of the same genetic defect (see below) (9).

Although chronic multiple motor and vocal tics are usually the most prominent clinical features of TS and represent the signs upon which the diagnosis of the disorder is currently based, tics may also be accompanied by a variety of behavioral disturbances. Studies have demonstrated a high incidence of obsessive–compulsive disorder (OCD), generally about 50%, in TS patients (10). Common examples of such symptoms include compulsive checking, counting, and perfectionism and obsessive worries or fears. The notion that OCD may be an alternative expression of the TS genetic trait is supported by family studies showing an increased rate of OCD in first-degree relatives of TS probands (11) and by segregation analysis of TS families that indicates that OCD is etiologically related to TS and supports autosomal dominant inheritance with variable expression (TS, CTD, or OCD) and sex-specific penetrance (12). For males, penetrance is nearly complete when only tic disorders (TS or CTD) are considered. When OCD is included as an alternative expression of the putative TS gene, penetrance esti-

mates for females rise from 56% (when only TS or CTD is considered) to 70%.

About 50% of patients with TS will also show evidence of attention deficit hyperactivity disorder (ADHD), manifested by inattention, hyperactivity, and impulsivity. Following an inspection of many TS family pedigrees, Comings and Comings concluded that the TS genetic trait could also be expressed as ADHD without tics (13). Segregation analysis and family studies by Pauls and colleagues, however, do not indicate an etiologic relationship between ADHD and TS and suggest that the two traits segregate independently (14,15). These authors reason that the commonly observed association between ADHD and TS may be secondary to ascertainment bias, in that individuals with both problems may be more likely to be referred for medical evaluation. This difference in interpretation remains unsolved.

Comings and others have further suggested that TS is actually a very broadly based behavioral disorder and that the TS genetic trait can be expressed by tics or a variety of behavioral disorders alone, including ADHD, stuttering, dyslexia, conduct disorder, panic attacks, multiple phobias, OCD, depression, mania, and anxiety disorder (16,17). This view, however, has been subject to much debate (18). At present, the full spectrum of the TS behavioral disorder has not been accurately delineated.

It is now generally accepted that almost all cases of TS occur on a hereditary basis, although the mode of inheritance has not been fully established. Occasional cases of chronic tics may represent phenocopies of the genetic disorder, and examples include chronic neuroleptic exposure (tardive TS) (19), head trauma (20), viral encephalitis (21), and carbon monoxide intoxication (22). Tics may also be seen in a variety of neurologic disorders, including Huntington's disease, Parkinson's disease, progressive supranuclear palsy, Meige's syndrome, neuroacanthocytosis, and startle disorders (e.g., Lâtah, Myriachit, "Jumping" Frenchmen) (23). In contradistinction to primary tic disorders, for these conditions tics are usually combined with other disorders of movement (e.g., with chorea in Huntington's disease and neuroacanthocytosis).

Simple motor tics may be difficult to distinguish from the rapid muscle jerks of myoclonus (2). Even when most tics are simple jerks, however, more complex forms of motor tics or more sustained dystonic tics may also be present, allowing one to establish the diagnosis by association with these other forms of motor tics. Moreover, simple motor tics tend to have a less random, more predictable body distribution and a wider range of amplitude and forcefulness when compared to myoclonus. The characteristic voluntary suppressibility of tics and the tendency of myoclonus to increase with intentional acts may also help distinguish between the two. It should be emphasized, however, that voluntary suppressibility is a feature that is not specific for tics but can be seen to at least some degree for virtually the whole range of hyperkinetic movement disorders.

Repetitive eye blinking from tics and from blepharospasm, a form of focal dystonia, can usually be differentiated by the presence of other tics or dystonic movements at other sites. In addition, while tics typically begin in childhood, blepharospasm is predominantly a disorder with onset in later adult life. Dystonic tics may be differentiated from torsion dystonia in that the latter is a continual movement that can result in a sustained abnormal posture whereas dystonic tics usually cause an abnormal posture that is present for only a short duration (2). The presence of more typical clonic tics in other body regions would favor that the sustained contractions could be dystonic tics rather than torsion dystonia. In addition, dystonic tics are often preceded by localized uncomfortable sensations (sensory tics) that may be relieved by the movement. Such sensory phenomena are typically absent in torsion dystonia.

There are a variety of other movement disorders that present with complex movements but are generally considered distinct from tics (2). Hyperekplexia is an excessive startle syndrome that may be associated with echolalia, coprolalia, and echopraxia. It may be difficult to differentiate complex motor tics and compulsions. In contrast to tics, compulsions are closely associated with obsessions, performed in response to an obsession, and may be performed according to certain rules (rituals), such as a specified number of times or in a specified order. In addition, compulsive rituals may be performed with the thought of preventing discomfort or a future dreaded event. The repetitive complex motor acts, known as "stereotypies," of patients with mental retardation or psychosis may also be difficult to distinguish from motor tics. Repetitive "handwashing" or "hand caressing" movement may be seen in young girls with Rett's syndrome, characterized by autism, dementia, and motor dysfunction. The correct diagnosis of tics is usually made by the exclusion of these other conditions or by identifying associated simple motor or vocal tics. Response to drug therapy may be useful for differential diagnosis as well. For example, while tics usually respond predictably to dopamine antagonist medications, compulsions do not. Rather, antidepressant drugs that preferentially inhibit serotonin reuptake (e.g., fluoxetine, clomipramine) may be quite effective for compulsions (see below). Furthermore, as TS and related tic disorders occur on a hereditary basis, examination of affected family members may help clarify diagnosis.

MANAGEMENT

The diagnosis of TS or a related tic disorder will often be obvious to an experienced clinician after simple observation. Given the voluntary suppressibility of tics and the characteristic waxing and waning quality, however, tics may be absent at the time of an examination. It should be remembered that for most affected individuals with TS, tics are mild

and that severe symptoms are not required for diagnosis. Neuroimaging or other diagnostic studies are generally not required. The presence of a family history is particularly useful for establishing the diagnosis of TS. As current evidence indicates that the clinical manifestations of TS may be quite variable, including both motor and behavioral dysfunction, it is important to evaluate each patient carefully to determine which aspects of illness are most disabling (1). For most patients, one or two clinical problems (e.g., tics, ADHD) will predominate and can serve as specific target symptoms for therapy. Detailed assessments, including neurologic and psychiatric assessments and testing with standardized neuropsychological measures of attention and obsessive–compulsive behavior, are often required to sort out the relative contributions of motor and behavioral disturbances for an individual patient.

For patients with a duration of tics of less than one year or for an unknown time period, it is possible that transient tic disorder may be present and that the condition will spontaneously resolve. It is best to avoid drug therapy if possible during the initial one-year time period until the chronic nature of the disorder can be established. Even with chronic tics, most patients with mild symptoms who have made a good adaptation in their lives can avoid the use of any medications. Educating patients, family members, peers, and school personnel regarding the nature of TS, restructuring the educational environment, and supportive counseling are measures that may be sufficient to avoid drug therapy. Once it is determined that the symptoms of TS are functionally disabling and not remediable to psychosocial interventions, however, pharmacotherapy should be considered. A variety of medications are now available to treat the symptoms of TS (24), and these should be selected on the basis of specific target symptoms and potential side effects of therapy. For example, in one patient tic suppression may be the important goal, while treatment of obsessive–compulsive behavior may take precedence in another. Drug dosage is titrated slowly in order to achieve the lowest satisfactory dosage and the maximum dosage depends on achieving a tolerable suppression of symptoms.

Neuroleptic drugs, such as haloperidol (Haldol), pimozide (Orap), and fluphenazine (Prolixin), are the most predictably effective tic-suppressing agents. Risperidone (Risperidol) is a newer agent that may be efficacious (25). Clonidine (Catapres), clonazepam (Klonopin), reserpine, and tetrabenazine (currently available only experimentally) may also be useful for tic suppression. Recently introduced antidepressant drugs that inhibit serotonin reuptake, including fluoxetine (Prozac), clomipramine (Anafranil), and fluvoxamine (Luvox), may be effective for the treatment of OCD associated with TS. Children with impaired school performance due to associated ADHD may improve following treatment with tricyclic antidepressants, clonidine, or neuroleptics. Often these are ineffective, however, necessitating the use of stimulants such as methylphenidate (Ritalin) or pemoline (Cylert). Although treatment with stimulants remains somewhat controversial and may exacerbate tics in some patients, the occasional worsening of tics may be tolerable when these medications are effective in improving attentional abilities and alleviating hyperactivity. A combination of a neuroleptic and a stimulant drug can be used in selected problem patients. Clinicians should be cautious about combining clonidine and a psychostimulant since there have been recent concerns about sudden death in children receiving both drugs, although a true cause-and-effect relationship has not been established (26,27). Preliminary information suggests that the selective monoamine oxidase B inhibitor deprenyl may be useful in children with the combination of ADHD and chronic tics (28,29).

SCIENTIFIC CONTEXT

The confines of the clinical spectrum of TS remain incompletely delineated and open to debate. Recent genetic studies indicate that both chronic tic disorder (CTD) (motor or vocal) and TS are transmitted as hereditary traits in the same families and that CTD seems to represent a mild form of TS (12,30,31). Inspection of TS kindreds indicates that at least some family members with transient tic disorder (TTD) appear to be obligate carriers of the TS genetic trait, suggesting that TTD is also part of the clinical spectrum of TS and a possible expression of the same genetic defect (9). At present it remains unclear what percentage of the up to 16% of all children reported to experience tics at some time in the course of normal development carry the TS genetic trait (32,33). It has been suggested that TS resides at one end of a clinical spectrum that includes the normal childhood expression of tics (34).

The nature of the spectrum of the TS behavioral disorder remains controversial as well. In addition to the recognized association between TS and certain behavioral disturbances, current evidence suggests that the TS genetic trait can indeed be expressed by a behavioral disorder alone, even in the absence of tics. This notion appears to be well-supported for OCD, particularly in females (12). Recent data also supports ADHD as another possible behavioral variant of TS (15). However, it remains undetermined whether any other psychopathologic conditions represent alternative expressions of the disorder as well or rather are associated with TS on the basis of ascertainment bias or as a consequence of the illness.

The recognition of a specific inheritance pattern for TS and the identification of large kindreds affected by the illness suggest that the application of pedigree linkage analysis, using modern recombinant DNA technology, might be able to identify a genetic marker linked to the disease (7,8,35). The identification of such a linked marker would establish the hereditary pattern, facilitate diagnosis, improve genetic counseling, and hold promise for elucidating basic molecular genetic mechanisms and thereby fostering novel rational therapeutic strategies. The implications of clarifying the

pathogenesis of TS extend far beyond the population of TS sufferers as the study of TS pedigrees may represent the most promising approach for advancing scientific knowledge in such important and pervasive conditions as primary OCD and ADHD.

Studies investigating the mode of inheritance of TS in families have indicated major gene involvement, with the most widely held notion of hereditary transmission pattern being autosomal dominant (12). Recent information, however, suggests that the pattern of inheritance may be more complicated than previously thought. It has been observed, for example, that bilineal transmission, involving both the maternal and paternal sides, is common in TS families and may be related to the severity of symptoms (36,37). Thus, it is possible that polygenic influences are important, with clinical expression being determined by the number of "susceptibility loci" that are inherited from either mother or father. The best approaches to clarify the hereditary pattern of TS may therefore come from recent advances in the field of quantitative genetics (38). Such quantitative genetic approaches as sib-pair analysis (39), which does not require specification of exact transmission parameters and which can be applied to conditions with unknown or complex inheritance patterns, may be more productive in localizing the TS genetic defect than the traditional family linkage approach.

While genetic factors are now recognized as most important for the development of TS and related tic disorders, investigators continue to search for underlying neurobiologic disturbances that may be manifestations of the gene defect and involved in the pathogenesis of the disorder. Several lines of evidence support the notion that striatal dopamine receptor supersensitivity at least partly underlies the tic disorder. The observations of tic suppression by dopamine receptor antagonists, exacerbation of tics by dopaminergic medications such as amphetamines, reduced levels of the dopamine metabolite homovanillic acid in cerebrospinal fluid (4), and the phenomenon of tardive tics following chronic dopamine antagonist therapy (19) contribute to this hypothesis. The reported absence of staining for dynorphin in the globus pallidus of the postmortem brain from a patient with TS (41) and clinical observations that drugs affecting the endogenous opioid system may influence the symptoms of TS (42–44) have focused attention on the role of this neurochemical system in the pathophysiology of tic disorders. A possible dysfunction of secondary neurochemical messengers has been suggested by a recent study of postmortem TS brains that revealed reduced concentrations of adenosine 3,5-monophosphate (cyclic AMP) in cerebral cortex (45). A promising line of investigation regarding the pathogenesis of TS involves the role of sex hormones in brain developmental processes (46,47). Recent findings raise the possibility that sex hormones may mediate abnormal development of specific brain regions, particularly the basal ganglia and limbic system, resulting in TS. An interesting lead is the consistent finding from a variety of neuroimaging techniques—magnetic resonance imaging (MRI), single photon emission computed tomography (SPECT), positron emission tomography (PET)—that there is an abnormality in structural and functional relationships between the left and right sides of the brain, particularly in the region of the basal ganglia (48–51).

As both motor and mental disturbances are closely linked in this disorder, TS seems to be a particularly apt model for studying the relationship between brain biology and human behavior. It is anticipated that clarification of pathogenetic mechanisms for TS will contribute to our understanding of normal physiologic interactions between brain regions such as basal ganglia and limbic systems.

REFERENCES

1. Kurlan R. Tourette's syndrome: current concepts. Neurology 1989;39: 1625–1630.
2. Tourette Syndrome Classification Study Group. Definitions and classification of tic disorders. Arch Neurol 1993;50:1013–1016.
3. Jankovic J, Stone L. Dystonic tics in patients with Tourette's syndrome. Mov Disord 1991;6:248–252.
4. Kurlan R, Lichter D, Hewitt D. Sensory tics in Tourette's syndrome. Neurology 1989;39:731–734.
5. Diagnostic and Statistical Manual of Mental Disorders. 4th ed. Washington: American Psychiatric Association, 1994.
6. Kurlan R, Behr J, Medved L, et al. Severity of Tourette's syndrome in one large kindred: implication for determination of disease prevalence rate. Arch Neurol 1987;44:268–269.
7. Robertson M, Gourdie A. Familial Tourette's syndrome in a large British pedigree: associated psychopathology, severity and potential for linkage analysis. Brit J Psychiatry 1990;156:515–521.
8. McMahon WM, Leppert M, Filloux F, et al. Tourette syndrome in 161 related family members. Adv Neurol 1992;58:159–165.
9. Kurlan R, Behr J, Medved L, Como P. Transient tic disorder and the clinical spectrum of Tourette's syndrome. Arch Neurol 1988;45:1200–1201.
10. Frankel M, Cummings JL, Robertson MM, et al. Obsessions and compulsions in Gilles de la Tourette's syndrome. Neurology 1986;36:378–382.
11. Pauls DL, Towbin KE, Leckman JF, et al. Gilles de la Tourette's syndrome and obsessive-compulsive disorder: evidence supporting a genetic relationship. Arch Gen Psychiatry 1986;43:1180–1182.
12. Pauls DL, Leckman JF. The inheritance of Gilles de la Tourette's syndrome and associated behaviors: evidence for autosomal dominant transmission. N Engl J Med 1986;315:993–997.
13. Comings DE, Comings BG. Tourette's syndrome and attention deficit disorder with hyperactivity: are they genetically related? J Am Acad Child Psychiatry 1984;23:138–146.
14. Pauls DL, Hurst CR, Kruger SD, et al. Gilles de la Tourette's syndrome and attention deficit disorder with hyperactivity: evidence against a genetic relationship. Arch Gen Psychiatry 1986;43:1177–1179.
15. Pauls DL, Pakstis AJ, Kurlan R, et al. Segregation and linkage analysis of Tourette's syndrome and related disorders. J Am Acad Child Adolesc Psychiatry 1990;29:195–203.
16. Comings DE. A controlled study of Tourette syndrome. VII. Summary: a common genetic disorder causing disinhibition of the limbic system. Am J Hum Genet 1987;41:839–886.
17. Kerbeshian J, Burd L, Klug MG. Comorbid Tourette's disorder and bipolar disorders: an etiologic-perspective. Am J Psychiatry 1995;152:1646–1651.
18. Pauls DL, Cohen DJ, Kidd KK, Leckman JF. Tourette syndrome and neuropsychiatric disorders: is there a genetic relationship? (letter) Am J Hum Genet 1988;43:206–209.
19. Klawans HL, Falk DK, Nausieda PA, Weiner WJ. Gilles de la Tourette's syndrome after long-term chlorpromazine therapy. Neurology 1978;28:1064–1068.
20. Fahn S. A case of post-traumatic tic syndrome. In: Friedhoff AJ, Chase TN, eds. Gilles de la Tourette syndrome. New York: Raven, 1982:349–350.
21. Sacks OW. Acquired Tourettism in adult life. In: Friedhoff AJ, Chase TN, eds. Gilles de la Tourette Syndrome. New York: Raven, 1982:89–92.
22. Pulst SM, Walshe TM, Romero JA. Carbon monoxide poisoning with features of Gilles de la Tourette syndrome. Arch Neurol 1983;40:443–444.
23. Jankovic J. Tics in other neurologic disorders. In: Kurlan R, ed. The handbook of Tourette's syndrome and related tic and behavioral disorders. New York: Marcel Dekker, 1993:167–182.
24. Kurlan R, Trinidad KS. The treatment of tics. In: Kurlan R, ed. The treatment of movement disorders. Philadelphia: Lippincott, 1995:365–406.
25. Bruun RD, Budman CL. Risperidone as a treatment for Tourette's syndrome. J Clin Psychiatry 1996;57:29–31.
26. Fenichel RR. Combining methylphenidate and clonidine: The role of post-marketing surveillance. J Child Adolesc Psychopharm 1995;5:155–156.
27. Popper CW. Combining methylphenidate and clonidine: pharmacologic questions and news reports about sudden death. J Child Adolesc Psychopharm 1995;5:157–166.
28. Jankovic J. Deprenyl in attention deficit associated with Tourette's syndrome. Arch Neurol 1993;50:286–288.
29. Feigin A, Kurlan R, McDermott MP, et al. A controlled trial of deprenyl in children with Tourette's syndrome and attention deficit hyperactivity disorder. Neurology 1996;46:965–968.
30. Golden GS. Tics and Tourette's syndrome: a continuum of symptoms? Ann Neurol 1978;4:145–148.
31. Pauls DL, Cohen DJ, Heimburch R, et al. Familial pattern and transmission of Gilles de la Tourette syndrome and multiple tics. Arch Gen Psychiatry 1981;38:1091–1093.
32. Kellmer Pringle ML, Butler NR, Davie R. First report of national child development study. In: 11,000 seven-year-olds. London: National Bureau for Cooperation in Child Care, 1967:185.
33. Lapouse R, Monk M. Behavior deviations in a representative sample of children: variation by sex, age, race, social class and family size. Am J Orthopsychiatry 1964;34:436–446.
34. Kurlan R. Hypothesis II: Tourette's syndrome is part of a clinical spectrum that includes normal brain development. Arch Neurol 1994;51:1145–1150.
35. Kurlan R, Behr J, Medved L, et al. Familial Tourette's syndrome: report of a large pedigree and potential for linkage analysis. Neurology 1986;36:772–776.
36. Kurlan R, Eapen V, Stern J, Robertson MM. Bilineal transmission in Tourette's syndrome families. Neurology 1994;44:2336–2342.
37. McMahon WM, van de Wetering BJM, Filloux F, et al. Bilineal transmission and phenotypic variation of Tourette's disorder in a large pedigree. J Am Acad Child Adolesc Psychiatry 1996;35:672–680.
38. Plomin R, Owen MJ, McGuffin P. The genetic basis of complex human behaviors. Science 1994;264:1733–1739.
39. Risch N, Zhang H. Extreme discordant sib pairs for mapping quantitative trait loci in humans. Science 1995;268:1584–1589.
40. Singer HS, Butler IJ, Tune LE, et al. Dopaminergic dysfunction in Tourette's syndrome. Ann Neurol 1982;12:361–366.
41. Haber SN, Kowell NW, Vonsattel JP, et al. Gilles de la Tourette's syndrome: a postmortem neuropathological and immunohistochemical study. J Neurol Sci 1986;75:225–241.
42. Gilman MA, Sandyk R. The endogenous opioid system in Gilles de la Tourette syndrome: a postmortem neuropathological and immunohistochemical study. Med Hypotheses 1986;19:371–378.
43. Lichter D, Majumdar L, Kurlan R. Opiate withdrawal unmasks Tourette's syndrome. Clin Neuropharmacol 1988;11:559–564.
44. Kurlan R, Majumdar L, Deeley C, et al. A controlled trial of propoxyphene and naltrexone in Tourette's syndrome. Ann Neurol 1991;30:19–23.
45. Singer HS, Hahn I-H, Krowiak E, et al. Tourette's syndrome: a neurochemical analysis of postmortem cortical brain tissue. Ann Neurol 1990;27:443–446.
46. Kurlan R. The pathogenesis of Tourette's syndrome: a possible role for hormonal and excitatory neurotransmitter influences in brain development. Arch Neurol 1992;49:874–876.
47. Peterson BS, Leckman JF, Scahill L, et al. Steroid hormones and sexual dismorphisms modulate symptom expression in Tourette's syndrome. Psychoneuroendocrinology 1992;17:553–563.
48. Braun AR, Stoetter B, Randolph C, et al. The functional neuroanatomy of Tourette's syndrome. An FDG-PET study. Neuropsychopharmacology 1993;9:277–291.
49. Peterson B, Riddle MA, Cohen DJ, et al. Reduced basal ganglia volume in Tourette's syndrome using three-dimensional reconstruction techniques from magnetic resonance images. Neurology 1993;43:941–949.
50. Singer HS, Reiss AL, Brown JE, et al. Volumetric MRI changes in basal ganglia of children with Tourette's syndrome. Neurology 1993;43:950–956.
51. Dimitsopulos T, Fett K, Klieger P, et al. Asymmetry of cerebral perfusion in Tourette's syndrome as shown by single photon emission computed tomography (SPECT). Mov Disord 1993;8:415–416. Abstract.

Gilles de la Tourette's Syndrome

ORRIN DEVINSKY   BRUCE D. GELLER

INTRODUCTION

The biographical accounts of Samuel Johnson (1709–1874), the prominent English author, provide one of the earliest descriptions of Gilles de la Tourette's syndrome. He suffered from akathisia, unusual complex compulsions, and a variety of motor and vocal tics. Itard (1), the French physician who is best remembered for his work on the education of deaf mutes and the study of feral children, reported the first definite case of Tourette's syndrome. He described a French noblewoman who began to have multiple tics at 7 years of age and later uttered explosive shrieks, senseless words, and curses. He regarded this behavior not as a new disorder, but "as one of the most extraordinary forms that clonic convulsions can assume" (1). This woman, who had a vocal tic disorder until her death at the age of 85, was presented incorrectly by Charcot, at his famous Tuesday lectures, as having psychogenic illness.

In 1885, George Albert Edouard Brutus Gilles de la Tourette (2) presented nine cases of the syndrome that now bears his name. As a 28-year-old student of Charcot at the Salpetriere, he gave an account of the onset and progression of the symptoms and introduced the term *coprolalia* to describe the use of obscenities. He personally examined six of the nine patients. Tics, present in all patients, were associated with one or more disturbances involving involuntary vocalizations, coprolalia, echolalia, and echopraxia. Because two patients had family members with tics, Tourette suggested that hereditary factors are important.

Later, psychosis was reported to be a frequent development in patients with Tourette's syndrome (3,4). During the first 60 years of this century, medical research in Tourette's syndrome was done principally by psychoanalytic physicians. The cursing, uncontrolled sexual impulses, and aggressive behavior led some psychiatrists to postulate that Tourette's syndrome resulted from a primary disturbance in the psyche's capacity to repress the forbidden. Neither the theory nor practice of psychoanalysis, however, advanced the understanding and treatment of the syndrome. The modern era of research on Tourette's syndrome began with the successful use of haloperidol by Seignot (5) in 1961, which led to the pharmacologic and neurochemical investigation of the disorder.

EPIDEMIOLOGY AND GENETICS

There is a 3:1 male predominance among sufferers of Tourette's syndrome. The lifetime risk of the syndrome is approximately 0.3 to 0.5 per 1,000 people. The annual incidence of new cases in the United States is about 4.6 per 1 million people. Tourette's syndrome has been found in all races and appears to be uniformly distributed among members of different socioeconomic classes. The clinical picture is quite uniform between different cultural groups with the exception that coprolalia is uncommon in Japanese patients.

The role of hereditary factors was originally suggested by Gilles de la Tourette and has been supported by further research. The concordance rate for monozygotic twins is 77% (6). In first-degree family members, the incidence of tics varies from 14% to 85%, and the incidence of Tourette's syndrome varies from 4% to 7.4% (7). The specific patterns of inheritance within families have not been established. Some investigators speculate that in certain family members transient tic of childhood, chronic motor tic, obsessive–compulsive personality disorder (8), and sleep disorder may be formes frustes of Tourette's syndrome. Nevertheless, the relatives of a patient with Tourette's syndrome should be informed that their risk of contracting the disease is low, and patients and relatives of childbearing age should be counseled that they have an excellent chance of having an unaffected child. However, they should be informed that there is a high incidence of tics among relatives of an affected person, and if both parents have tic disorders, the risk of having an affected child is probably greater.

CLINICAL FEATURES AND DIAGNOSIS

Phenomenology of Tics

A motor tic is an involuntary, rapid, nonrhythmic movement. Vocal tics consist of a variety of noises and sounds. Although tics are usually sudden and brief muscle contractions (clonic tics), they are occasionally sustained movements (dystonic or tonic tics). The patient often experiences an irresistible "itch to tic" (9). This urge can usually be suppressed for some time, but at the expense of increased psychic tension, which can only be allayed by the production of the tic.

Motor and vocal tics are classified as either simple or complex, although the distinction is often arbitrary. Simple motor tics include eye blinking, forced staring, facial grimace, head or neck jerk, shoulder shrug, and contraction of abdominal muscles. Blepharospasm occasionally occurs as a dystonic tic. Simple vocal tics, consisting of laryngeal, lingual, labial, and nasal tics, include throat clearing, coughing, grunting, clicking, snorting, shrieking, and animal sounds (e.g., barking, hooting, hissing, growling, quacking). Complex motor tics, which are often on a continuum with compulsive acts, may be stereotyped and include facial expressions, grooming behaviors, touching, smelling an object or body part, and aggressive actions against self or others. Complex vocal tics include words and phrases, often emitted in a loud gushing stream with an unusual pitch or cadence. These tics are often repeated. Obscenities describing sexual behavior or body elimination functions are used more commonly than religious profanities (e.g., God damn). The obscenities are often slurred or mispronounced to conceal their content. Coprolalia may occur at the most socially inappropriate times. For example, a patient shouting "F—ing nigger" or "F—ing oink-oink" when passing a black man or policeman.

Tics are usually exacerbated by stress, anxiety, or fatigue and are diminished during absorbing activities, such as reading an interesting novel, and in sleep. However, tics may occur during both rapid eye movement (REM) and non-REM sleep (10).

Associated Disorders

In addition to motor and vocal tics, patients with Tourette's syndrome have a variety of other symptoms. More than half of the patients under age 20 have attentional deficit disorder with hyperactivity. Other common concomitants of the syndrome are obsessions and compulsions, including obtrusive sexual and aggressive thoughts and actions in about 50% of patients. Sleep disorders, compulsive touching, palilalia (compulsively repeating one's own sounds or words, most often the first or last syllable with increasing speed and decreasing clarity), echolalia (repeating the sounds or words from an external source, often the last heard sound), echopraxia (repeating movements made by another person), and copropraxia (obscene gestures such as simulating masturbation) also occur in roughly decreasing order of frequency.

Diagnostic Criteria and Course of the Illness

According to the Diagnostic and Statistical Manual of Mental Disorders (p. 103) (11) the criteria for the diagnosis of Tourette's syndrome are as follows:

1. Both multiple motor and one or more vocal tics have been present at some time during the illness, although not necessarily concurrently.
2. The tics occur many times a day (usually in bouts) nearly every day or intermittently throughout a period of more than one year, and during this period there is never a tic-free period of more than three consecutive months.
3. The disturbance causes marked distress or significant impairment in social, occupational, or other important areas of functioning.
4. Onset before age 18 years.
5. The disturbance is not due to the direct physiologic effects of a substance (e.g., stimulants) or a general medical condition (e.g., Huntington's disease or postviral encephalitis).

The onset of symptoms occurs between 2 and 15 years of age (mean age 7 years) in more than 90% of patients. However, symptoms may begin as early as age 1 or younger or as late as the fourth decade of life. The initial symptom is most often a tic in the upper body, commonly around the eyes, some other part of the face, or the neck. Vocal tics constitute the original manifestation in 15% to 30% of patients and begin within three years of the onset in most others (7,12). The vocal tics typically begin as inarticulate sounds but progress in complexity in about 60% of patients. Coprolalia, previously thought to be common, is actually relatively uncommon. Tourette's syndrome is usually a lifelong illness, but the intensity of symptoms varies. The symptoms may remit after adolescence, especially coprolalia, which is often the most socially disabling manifestation of the disorder.

Patients with Tourette's syndrome usually have normal intelligence. Their IQ distribution parallels that of the general population (12). Patients may have difficulties with reading, writing, and arithmetic (10). Although Tourette's syndrome has been described as "psychosis with multiple tics," thought disorder only rarely occurs. Their emotional response to external stimuli, their experience of affect, and their perception of other people's affect appear entirely normal. Instead, the syndrome may represent a disorder of the expression of affect. Thus, the absence of inhibition of sexual and aggressive impulses has been described as emotional incontinence (13).

Complications

Profound social stigma is the most important complication of moderate and severe Tourette's syndrome. Many patients are considered "crazy" and their involuntary tics attributed to sociopathic behavior. Social and employment opportunities are often limited by vocal tics; secondary depression is not uncommon and is often overlooked.

Physical sequelae may also occur in these patients. The violent and repeated contractions associated with the tics may cause a compressive neuropathy, radiculopathy (14), or myelopathy (10). Other injuries include joint disorders, especially affecting the neck and knee, blindness due to retinal detachment, dermatologic disorders from compulsive picking, and in rare instances, self-mutilation from biting or head banging.

Classification and Differential Diagnosis of Tic Disorders

The tic disorders form a continuum along a spectrum from physiologic tics in normal persons (i.e., mannerisms or habits) to Tourette's syndrome. Transient tic disorder, which occurs in up to 15% of children and adolescents, is characterized by simple motor or vocal tics that last from 2 weeks to 1 year. The tics may briefly recur during adulthood, especially during periods of stress. In chronic tic disorder, the tics last longer than 1 year and occur almost every day, and usually many times a day. They typically begin before the age of 21. Chronic motor tic disorder occurs more commonly among family members of patients with Tourette's syndrome. Patients with chronic motor tic disorder do not have vocal tics.

In addition to the primary tic disorders, tics may also be present in a variety of neuropsychiatric disorders. They are also seen in hereditary neurologic disorders, such as Huntington's disease, dystonia musculorum deformans, and neuroacanthocytosis. Tics are frequently sequelae of central nervous system infectious and postinfectious diseases, including encephalitis, especially von Economo's encephalitis lethargica, and Sydenham's chorea. Tics may be secondary to medications, including amphetamines, methylphenidate, cocaine, L-dopa, carbamazepine, phenytoin, phenobarbital, and antipsychotics (tardive tics). Other causes of secondary tics are strokes, head trauma, carbon monoxide poisoning, static perinatal encephalopathy, neurocutaneous syndromes, and degenerative disorders.

Tics must be differentiated from other hyperkinetic movement disorders, such as chorea, tremor, athetosis, hemiballismus, and tardive dyskinesia. According to Jankovic (10), tics are distinguished by three features: 1) the occurrence of an unusual sensation and an irresistible urge to move prior to the tic, 2) the ability to voluntarily suppress the tic for variable periods, and 3) occurrence during all stages of sleep. When taken together, these features are quite useful for differentiating tics from other hyperkinesias.

TREATMENT

There is no cure for Tourette's syndrome. For the majority of patients, however, medical therapy successfully controls the tics so that they play only a minor part in the patients' lives. Some patients, especially children with mild symptoms, may not require therapy. The therapeutic approach must be individualized and include, in addition to medical factors, consideration of the patient's social and behavioral function.

Psychotherapy and Behavioral Therapy

Structured psychotherapy is of no proven benefit in the treatment of tics. However, consultation with a psychiatrist, psychologist, or social worker may be helpful for some patients as they learn to cope with the emotional and behavioral problems of Tourette's syndrome (7). Individual or group therapy may be of benefit in the patient's social and educational development. The difficulties encountered by some patients following successful control of their tics, with resultant loss of their source of secondary gain, may be managed effectively with supportive psychotherapy.

The role of behavioral therapy for tics is uncertain. Massed (negative) practice (trying to inhibit the tic by voluntarily repeating the movement) and operant conditioning (contingency management using aversion shock and time out periods) have been tried with no evidence of long-term benefit. Relaxation techniques may temporarily reduce the severity of tics.

Pharmacotherapy

Pharmacotherapy is the mainstay of treatment in Tourette's syndrome (Table 65.1). It is critical to tailor the treatment to the patient and to try different medications in refractory cases. The drug of first choice is usually an antidopaminergic agent, such as haloperidol, pimozide, or trifluoperazine. These agents are highly efficacious but also moderately toxic. If a specific neuroleptic does not work or cannot be tolerated, the chances of successful therapy with another drug of this class are still good. Because of the potent side effects of neuroleptics, some physicians advocate an initial trial of clonidine.

The systematic approach to pharmacotherapy of Tourette's syndrome is more important than which drug is

Table 65.1 Drugs Used in the Treatment of Tourette's Syndrome

Drugs	Efficacy	Daily Dose	Side Effects Sedative	Extrapyramidal	Anticholinergic
Neuroleptic					
Haloperidol	+++	1–100 mg	+	+++	+
Trifluoperazine	+++	1–40 mg	+	+++	+
Thioridazine	+++	40–500 mg	+++	+	++
Fluphenazine	++	0.5–20 mg	+	+++	+
Thiothixene	+++	1–40 mg	+	+++	+
Pimozide	+++	0.5–20 mg	+	+++	+
Tetrabenazine	+ to ++	50–150 mg	+	+[a]	0
Alpha₂ agonist					
Clonidine	+ to ++[b]	0.1–1 mg	++	0	0

[a] Tardive dyskinesia has not been reported.
[b] More effective in obsessive–compulsive behavior than in tics.

tried first and which ones follow in refractory cases. The lowest effective dose should be prescribed initially and increased gradually to avoid excessive side effects. However, each drug should be increased to maximally tolerated dosages before it is considered inefficacious.

Neuroleptics

Haloperidol is the drug most frequently used in the treatment of moderate to severe Tourette's syndrome. It is initially effective in two-thirds of patients, but may have to be discontinued in 30% to 50% of them because of serious side effects or the development of tolerance to the drug (i.e., symptoms recur despite dosage increases). In some of these patients, a later trial of haloperidol may prove beneficial (15).

The starting dose of haloperidol is 0.25–0.5 mg/day, with a gradual increase of 0.25–0.5 mg/week, depending on the clinical response and signs of toxicity. The usual daily dose is 8 mg or less, but some patients may require 20–40 mg. Side effects include mental dullness, sedation, drowsiness, depression, hypersensitivity, extrapyramidal symptoms (parkinsonism, dystonic reactions, neuroleptic malignant syndrome, akathisia, tardive dyskinesia), weight gain, hepatotoxicity, and agranulocytosis. Haloperidol has fewer anticholinergic side effects than other neuroleptics.

Pimozide, fluphenazine, trifluoperazine, thioridazine, and perphenazine are other dopamine receptor blocking agents that are as effective as haloperidol in reducing tics. Of the neuroleptics, pimozide and fluphenazine cause the least sedation and therefore are important alternatives to haloperidol. Pimozide, which has a serum half-life of approximately 55 hours, may be given once daily. However, the therapeutic effects of pimozide and fluphenazine may not be as long-lasting as that of trifluoperazine and thioridazine (15).

Other Drugs

Tetrabenazine, a benzoquinoline derivative, depletes monoamines and blocks presynaptic and postsynaptic dopamine receptors. Preliminary studies (10) suggest that it is moderately efficacious in Tourette's syndrome, with children responding better than adults. The drug's side effects are sedation, depression, mild tremor, acute dystonic reactions, and parkinsonism. Unlike other neuroleptics, tetrabenazine has not been reported to cause tardive dyskinesia.

Clonidine, an alpha₂ receptor agonist, is reported to provide significant relief of tics and especially obsessive–compulsive behaviors. The drug is less efficacious than the neuroleptics in improving tics, particularly in adults (15). Sedation, dry mouth, and orthostatic hypotension are the most common side effects, but extrapyramidal symptoms do not occur. Therefore, clonidine may be an important alternative to neuroleptic treatment of Tourette's syndrome, especially in children.

The role of benzodiazepines in the management of Tourette's syndrome is controversial. Diazepam, alprazolam, and clonazepam may be used to treat anxiety, which may exacerbate tics. The development of tolerance to these drugs limits their efficacy, however, and they are useful primarily in mild cases or as an adjunct to other medications. There have been anecdotal reports of reduced tic symptoms with reserpine, carbamazepine, calcium channel blockers, corticosteroids, and clomiphene.

Botulinum toxin injected into local muscles has been used to successfully treat painful dystonic tics characterized by more sustained muscle tightening or twisting. Obsessive-compulsive symptoms often respond to selective serotonin reuptake inhibitors. Attention deficit hyperactivity disorder can be treated with clonidine or stimulants. Unfortunately, stimulants can exacerbate tics and clonidine can worsen the sedation produced by dopamine receptor blockade.

RESEARCH STUDIES

Neurochemical and Pharmacologic Studies

The role of the central dopaminergic system in Tourette's syndrome has been the focus of attention in neurochemical and pharmacologic studies. It is now well accepted that drugs that block postsynaptic dopamine (D_2) receptors tend to relieve symptoms, whereas drugs that increase dopaminergic activity (e.g., amphetamines, L-dopa, methylphenidate) acutely exacerbate tics.

The accumulation of homovanillic acid (HVA), one of the principal metabolites of dopamine in the cerebrospinal fluid, is often used as an index of dopaminergic activity in the brain. In patients with Tourette's syndrome, some but not all studies have shown low baseline and accumulated levels of HVA, but positron emission tomography (PET) studies (10) of dopaminergic binding activity have not demonstrated any consistent abnormality. The decreased dopaminergic activity in Tourette's syndrome is consistent with a primary loss of dopaminergic cells, resulting in hypersensitive postsynaptic receptors, or a primary hypersensitivity, causing feedback inhibition of the dopaminergic cell.

Abnormalities of serotonin metabolism in Tourette's syndrome have been reported. In addition, abnormal regulation of brain serotonergic activity is the most widely accepted pathophysiologic mechanism for obsessive–compulsive disorder. After probenecid loading, cerebrospinal fluid levels of 5-hydroxyindolacetic acid (5-HIAA), the major metabolite of serotonin, are decreased in some patients with Tourette's syndrome (16,17). This finding suggests hypersensitivity of serotonin receptors, leading to feedback inhibition, loss of serotonergic neurons, or both. PET studies (10) show that serotonergic receptor activity in patients with Tourette's syndrome is normal.

Alterations in norepinephrine and acetylcholine metabolism in Tourette's syndrome also have been reported, but there is less direct evidence for these changes (18). The neurotransmitter studies are complicated by the poorly understood interactions between the dopaminergic, serotonergic, noradrenergic, and cholinergic systems. It is clear, however, that abnormalities of the central nervous system biogenic amines do occur in Tourette's syndrome, and any hypothesis concerning the etiology of the disorder must address the neurochemical and neuropharmacologic findings.

Electrophysiologic Studies

The electroencephalogram (EEG) of patients with Tourette's syndrome is often nonspecifically abnormal, showing background disorganization and mild slowing in 20% to 80%. The incidence of these abnormalities is increased in patients with abnormal neurologic signs and in those taking neuroleptics. Infrequently, the EEG shows spikes and sharp waves (7). Studies of evoked potentials in patients with Tourette's syndrome have not revealed significant abnormalities (19). One of the most interesting EEG findings in Tourette's syndrome is the absence of the premovement negative wave (20). In back-averaged EEG recordings, this potential normally occurs 500–800 ms before a voluntary movement. This observation supports the belief that tics are involuntary and suggests that they probably originate in subcortical structures or utilize pathways other than those subserving the control of voluntary movement.

Neuroradiologic and Neuropathologic Studies

Computerized tomography and magnetic resonance imaging have not revealed definite abnormalities in patients with Tourette's syndrome (7,21). Preliminary PET studies (21) demonstrated decreased glucose utilization in the frontal, cingulate, and possibly insular cortex and inferior corpus striatum. Furthermore, there was a significant inverse correlation between tic severity and glucose utilization rates in these areas.

There have been few neuropathologic studies in patients with Tourette's syndrome. Dewulf and van Bogaert (22) examined the brain of a 30-year-old man in whom Tourette's syndrome developed at 18 years of age. They found no evidence of central nervous system abnormalities despite "minutely detailed histologic study" of the motor cortices, basal ganglia, cerebellum, red and olivary nuclei, and the anterior horns of the cervical cord. Balthasar (23) reported an increased number and packing density of small neurons in the striatum of a 42-year-old man who first had tics at age 3. There were deposits of mononuclear cells in the subarachnoid and perivascular spaces, mild neuronal loss in the third and fifth cortical layers, without gliosis, and a very small unilateral lesion in the medial thalamus, with cell loss and gliosis. The only important abnormality was thought to be in the striatum; it was considered to be a developmental anomaly and responsible for Tourette's syndrome in this patient.

Using the usual histopathologic methods, Haber et al (24) found no abnormalities in the brain of a 57-year-old man who had Tourette's syndrome since age 5. However, immunochemical studies showed a reduction in dynorphin-like staining of the external segment of the globus pallidus, and less so in the substantia nigra. Striatal neurons give rise to the dynorphin-immunoreactive fibers in the pallidum. The relevance of this finding remains uncertain, as it is from a single case report, and the behavioral effects of dynorphin in humans is unknown.

Encephalitis Lethargica: A Model Illness

In encephalitis lethargica, the periaqueductal gray and midbrain tegmentum are the principal sites of involvement (25).

One might speculate that loss of ascending dopamine fibers, which arise in the ventral tegmental area, to the frontal cortex and limbic system might result in failure to suppress forbidden thoughts and emotions. Indeed, encephalitis lethargica is one of the few illnesses in which specific lesions of the nervous system are correlated with the development of motor and vocal tics and obsessive–compulsive behavior. These symptoms are especially frequent among postencephalitic patients who experience oculogyric crises (18,26). In fact, in many of these patients, the symptoms only occur as a prodrome to or during the oculogyric crisis. Emotional factors often precipitate oculogyric crises. During the attacks, the patient might be overwhelmed with anxiety and "forbidden thoughts." For example, at the onset of an oculogyric crisis, one patient repeated the words, "rape my sister, rape my mother, kill my brother, kill my father" (26). Forbidden and emotionally charged thoughts may trigger abnormal movements in both encephalitis lethargica and Tourette's syndrome.

Several observations suggest a relationship between tics, oculogyric crises, and dopamine receptor activity. Alterations of the dopaminergic system may explain why oculogyric crises develop only in postencephalitic patients who have parkinsonism and why tics and obsessive–compulsive behavior are observed in patients with Tourette's syndrome and oculogyric crises. Sacks (27) described a series of patients with postencephalitic parkinsonism in whom L-dopa therapy was initiated; many of them returned from an immobile, aphonic, and apathetic state to one of activity. Unfortunately, their "awakening" often left them on a tightrope, balanced between various symptoms. Shortly after the initiation of L-dopa therapy, oculogyric crises ceased and tics often developed. When the L-dopa dosage was reduced, oculogyric crises recurred and the tics would usually remit.

The oculogyric crises and parkinsonism in encephalitis lethargica may be considered to develop in two stages. First, loss of dopaminergic neurons leads to diminished levels of dopamine at the postsynaptic receptor. This change is initially compensated for by increased activity of remaining dopamine-synthesizing neurons and the development of hypersensitive receptors. Second, the number and sensitivity of the receptors eventually plateau, while the level of dopamine present at the postsynaptic receptor continues to fall because of progressive loss of dopaminergic neurons.

From these observations in patients with encephalitis lethargica and other studies (18), it appears that oculogyric crises occur when supersensitive dopamine receptors are exposed to decreased dopaminergic activity and that tics result from stimulation of these supersensitive receptors. Interestingly, true tics occur as side effects of L-dopa therapy in patients with postencephalitic parkinsonism but not in patients with idiopathic Parkinson's disease, although L-dopa-induced hyperkinesia could be mistaken for tics. If oculomotor tics of lateral or vertical gaze are seen in Parkinson's disease, it indicates that the patient had a pre-existing tic disorder. Tics of gaze are not seen as a side effect of L-dopa in idiopathic Parkinson's disease (28).

Anatomy of Vocalization

Vocal tics are the single most characteristic feature of Tourette's syndrome, and the anatomy of vocalization is therefore especially relevant. The forms of vocalization observed in the syndrome have not been produced by neocortical stimulation in either humans or monkeys (29,30). The cingulate gyrus is of particular interest in Tourette's syndrome, although stimulation of the human cingulate gyrus produces neither vocalization nor interruption of speech (31). In monkeys, however, stimulation of the cingulate gyrus results in gutteral sounds and clear calls, but only a small fraction of the animal's normal vocal repertoire has been reproduced (30). The cingulate gyrus connects to cortical and limbic structures known to be involved in vocalization. It also receives a dopaminergic projection from the ventral tegmental area, and lesions of the anterior cingulate or its connections are sometimes successful in relieving obsessive and compulsive symptoms.

Stimulation of the midbrain periaqueductal gray in cats and monkeys (30,32) produces a wide range of species-specific vocalizations. Transection of the midbrain–diencephalic junction does not eliminate vocalization after midbrain stimulation or noxious stimuli, demonstrating that the midbrain can medicate these responses without the participation of more rostral brain areas. Although many limbic structures are involved in emotional vocalization, circuitry sufficient to elicit a diverse group of affective vocalizations may therefore exist in the brainstem. More rostral areas, such as the anterior cingulate gyri, amygdalae, and hypothalamus may be important in learning certain responses and initiating and modifying vocalization in response to complex sensory associations and affective states.

CONCLUSIONS

The pathophysiology of Tourette's syndrome remains a mystery. The role of dopamine and the involvement of specific brain areas such as the midbrain, pallidum, and cingulate gyrus are speculative. Application of modern techniques, including electron microscopy, tests for the presence of foreign antigens or abnormal genetic material, and assays for neurotransmitters, enzymes, and receptors, may provide new insights into the etiology of Tourette's syndrome.

ACKNOWLEDGMENT

The editorial assistance of B. J. Hessie is greatly appreciated.

REFERENCES

1. Itard JMG. Memoire sur quelques fonctions involontaires des appareils de la locomotion de la prehension et de la voix. Arch Gen Med 1825;8:385–407.

2. Gilles de la Tourette G. Etude sur une affection nerveuse caracterisee par de l'incoordination motrice accompagnee d'echolalie et de copralalie. Arch Neurol 1885;9:19–42.

3. Guinon G. Tics convulsifs et hysterie. Rev Med 1887;7:509–519.

4. Meige H, Feindel E. Tics and their treatment. Wilson SAK (trans.). London: Appleton, 1907.

5. Seignot MJN. Un cas de maladie des tics de Gilles de la Tourette syndrome gueri par le R-1625. Ann Med Psychol 1961;119:578–579.

6. Price RA, Kidd KK, Cohen DJ, et al. A twin study of Tourette syndrome. Arch Gen Psychiatry 1986;42:815–820.

7. Lees AJ. Tics and related disorders. New York: Churchill Livingstone, 1985.

8. Pauls DL, Leckman JF. The inheritance of Gilles de la Tourette's syndrome and associated behaviors. N Engl J Med 1986;315:993–997.

9. Bliss J. Sensory experiences of Gilles de la Tourette's syndrome. Arch Gen Psychiatry 1980;37:1343–1347.

10. Jankovic J. The neurology of tics. In: Marsden CD, Fahn S, eds. Movement disorders 2. London: Butterworth, 1987.

11. American Psychiatric Association, Diagnostic and statistical manual of mental disorders. 4th ed. Washington: American Psychiatric Association, 1994.

12. Shapiro AK, Shapiro ED, Brunn RD, et al. Gilles de la Tourette's Syndrome. New York: Raven, 1978.

13. Mahler MS, Rangell L. A psychosomatic study of maladie des tics (Gilles de la Tourette's disease). Psychiatr Q 1943;17:579–603.

14. Goetz CG, Klawans HL. Gilles de la Tourette's syndrome and compressive neuropathies. Ann Neurol 1980;8:453.

15. Mesulam MM, Petersen RC. Treatment of Gilles de la Tourette's syndrome: Eight-year, practice-based experience in a predominantly adult population. Neurology 1987;37:1828–1833.

16. Cohen DJ, Shaywitz BA, Caparulo B, et al. Chronic multiple tics of Gilles de la Tourette's disease: CSF acid monoamine metabolites after probenecid administration. Arch Gen Psychiatry 1978;35:245.

17. Butler IJ, Doslow SH, Seifert WE, et al. Biogenic amine metabolism in Tourette's syndrome. Ann Neurol 1979;6:37–39.

18. Devinsky O. Neuroanatomy of Gilles de la Tourette's syndrome: possible midbrain involvement. Arch Neurol 1983;40:508–514.

19. Krumholz A, Singer HS, Niedermeyer E, et al. Electrophysiologic studies in Tourette's syndrome. Ann Neurol 1983;14:638–641.

20. Obeso JA, Rothwell JC, Marsden CD. Simple tics in Gilles de la Tourette's syndrome are not prefaced by a normal premovement potential. J Neurol Neurosurg Psychiatry 1981;44:735–738.

21. Chase TN, Geoffrey V, Gillespie M, Burrows GH. Structural and functional studies in Gilles de la Tourette's syndrome. Rev Neurol 1986;142:851–855.

22. Dewulf A, van Bogaert L. Etudes anatomo-clinique de syndromes hypercinetiques complexes. III. Une observation anatomo-clinique de maladie des tics (Gilles de la Tourette). Monatsschr Psychiatr Neurol 1941;104:53–61.

23. Balthasar K. Ubes das anatomische substrat der generalisierten tic-krankheit (maladie des tics, Gilles de la Tourette): entwicklung-shemmung des corpus striatum. Arch Psychiatr Nervenkr 1957;195:531–549.

24. Haber SN, Kowall NW, Vonsattel JP, et al. Gilles de la Tourette's syndrome: A postmortem neuropathological and immunohistochemical study. J Neurol Sci 1986;75:225–241.

25. Von Economo C. Encephalitis lethargica. Newman KO (trans.). Oxford: Oxford University Press, 1931.

26. Jelliffe SE. Psychological components in postencephalitic oculogyric crises: contribution to a genetic interpretation of compulsive phenomena. Arch Neurol 1929;21:491–532.

27. Sacks O. Awakenings. New York: Random House, 1976.

28. Shale H, Fahn S, Mayeaux R. Tics in a patient with Parkinson's disease. Mov Disord 1986;1:79–83.

29. Penfield W, Jasper H. Epilepsy and the functional anatomy of the human brain. Boston: Little, Brown, 1954.

30. Jurgens U, Ploog D. Cerebral representation of vocalization in the squirrel monkey. Exp Brain Res 1970;10:532–554.

31. Lewin W, Whitty CWM. Effects of anterior cingulate stimulation in conscious human objects. J Neurophysiol 1960;23:445–447.

32. Magoun HW, Atlas D, Ingersoll EH, et al. Associated facial, vocal, and respiratory components of emotional expression: an experimental study. J Neurol Psychopathol 1937;17:241–255.

Myoclonus and Asterixis

MICHAEL RONTHAL   PENNY GREENSTEIN

MYOCLONUS

Definition

Myoclonus is best defined as a "sudden shock-like contraction of a muscle." The modern use of the term would add that the contraction be triggered by an event within the central nervous system (1). The contraction or "jerk" may be minimal or severe enough to produce movement of the adjacent joint. It may be localized or diffuse, and irregular or regular and rhythmic.

While bedside diagnosis is often easy, the differentiation from other movement disorders can at times be problematic. Tremor, chorea, and tic syndromes may be confused with myoclonus. A brief pause or so-called silent period between jerks distinguishes myoclonus from tremor, which is more continuous and rhythmic. Choreiform movements are usually more irregular or random and flowing; they often appear to be fragments of normal movements. Tics can be voluntarily inhibited, at least for a brief period.

A firm diagnosis may require video taping, combined with electroencephalogram (EEG) and electromyogram (EMG) monitoring.

History

"Myoclonus" as a descriptive term was first used by Friedreich in 1881 (2). He reported a 50-year-old man with a five-year history of muscle jerking as an isolated neurologic sign and called the syndrome "paramyoclonus multiplex," believing that the movements arose in the spinal cord. Various case reports followed and were reviewed by Unverricht in 1891 (3). Although he rejected about three-quarters of the patients, Unverricht agreed that the syndrome as described by Friedreich existed. It fell to Lundborg (4), who

included Unverricht's cases with his own, to recognize an epileptic component and name the condition "progressive myoclonic epilepsy" as distinct from "paramyoclonus multiplex" or "essential myoclonus." He included a third group called "symptomatic myoclonus."

Myoclonic jerks as part of the symptomatology of epilepsy, although not so named, were described during the nineteenth century by various authors. West (1861) (5) reported what would now be called infantile spasms, and Reynolds (1861) (6) discussed interictal "clonic spasms". Myoclonus was thought to be a fragment of epilepsy by Muskens (1928) (7) and Hodskins and Yakovlev in 1930 remarked on the presence of interictal myoclonus in patients with epilepsy (8). In 1945, Lennox (9) included myoclonus as part of petit mal.

Myoclonus, cerebellar ataxia, and epilepsy as a clinical syndrome was named "dyssynergia cerebellaris myoclonica" by Hunt in 1921 (10), and in 1963, Lance and Adams (11) described intention or action myoclonus as a similar clinical symptom complex, but as a posthypoxic phenomenon.

Myoclonus attributed to an infectious process was described by Walsh (1920), (12) Reimold (1925) (13), and Von Economo (1929) (14) in encephalitis, and myoclonus in what we now know to be a slow virus encephalitis was described by Creutzfeldt (1920) (15) and Jakob (1921) (16). Subacute sclerosing pan encephalitis, now known to be part of measles infection was described by Dawson in 1934 (17).

Palatal myoclonus, the prototype of segmental myoclonus, was first described by Kupper in 1873 (18) and the classical papers including clinical descriptions together with pathology were written by Guillaine and Mollaret in 1931 (19) and 1932 (20). The essential features are rhythmic jerking of the palate and sometimes face, pharynx, and diaphragm usually at a rate of 120/min, persisting during sleep.

Physiologic myoclonus, that is, a diffuse jerk as one falls asleep, so-called hypnic jerks, are common but the first written description was that of DeLisi in 1932 (21). Symonds reviewed the subject in 1953 (22).

Clinical Correlations of Myoclonus

Myoclonus should be regarded as a relatively nonspecific sign of central nervous system dysfunction and should prompt further investigation as to the cause. Although there is an extremely wide differential diagnosis, broad clinical categories can be defined. The commonest of these include myoclonus as part of a confusional state or delirium, myoclonus as part of a dementia, and myoclonus in association with epilepsy.

Myoclonus in the Setting of a Confusional State

The presence of myoclonus or asterixis (see below) in a confused or delirious patient should alert the physician to the possibility of a toxic or metabolic encephalopathy and should trigger an extensive search for its cause. The myoclonic jerks may be of large amplitude or present as low-amplitude twitches. They may be regular or irregular, and synchronous or asynchronous and chaotic. Occasionally multiple scattered and irregular low-amplitude jerks are associated with chaotic and irregular but conjugate eye movements—polymyoclonia with opsoclonus. At times, the myoclonus is partly or wholly stimulus sensitive—reflex myoclonus.

The etiology may be obscure at the bedside, but laboratory studies will usually define the cause. Organ failure or drug intoxication is a frequent source and a careful search for sepsis may be required. Occasionally other exogenous toxins such as heavy metal poisoning may be the cause.

Myoclonus in the Setting of Dementia

Almost all patients with Creutzfeldt-Jakob disease, whatever the mode of onset, will at some point develop myoclonic jerks (23). Initially the myoclonus may be unilateral, but it soon progresses to become bilateral, widespread, and synchronous. Periodic EEG activity, while not pathognomonic, helps with the diagnosis and is seen in over 95% of patients (24).

Some patients with Alzheimer's dementia will, after years, develop myoclonus clinically reminiscent of that seen in the spongiform encephalopathy of Creutzfeldt–Jakob dementia; electrophysiologic studies, however, suggest a different mechanism (24). Myoclonus may be an accompaniment of the AIDS-dementia complex (25).

Myoclonus in the Setting of Epilepsy

Myoclonic seizures are almost always associated with other forms of seizure.

Generalized Idiopathic Epilepsy

In older children and adolescents, myoclonus may be part of photomyoclonic epilepsy, with spontaneous and photic reflex myoclonic jerks and an EEG that shows generalized polyspike or spike–wave bursts, or it may be part of classical petit mal epilepsy when myoclonus accompanies an absence attack. Early morning myoclonic jerks in adolescents with idiopathic generalized epilepsy are usually limited to the arms. Juvenile myoclonic epilepsy in some families is inherited as an autosomal dominant trait. The gene has been mapped to 6p21.1–p11 (26).

Almost continual localized myoclonic jerking, occurring for a minimum of one hour and recurring at intervals of no more than 10 seconds without loss of consciousness, suggests the diagnosis of epilepsia partialis continua with a focal cortical discharging lesion; the pathology varies from case to case, and often no definite pathology can be identified (27). Chronic, prolonged focal myoclonic jerking in children suggests the possibility of a focal chronic progressive encephalitis (Rasmussen) (28).

Progressive Myoclonic Epilepsy

The triad of myoclonic seizures, tonic–clonic seizures, and progressive neurologic deficit, particularly dementia and ataxia, suggests the diagnosis of progressive myoclonic epilepsy (PME) (29). The clinical syndrome is nonspecific and its presence should prompt a search for the underlying pathology. The triad may be initially incomplete and years may elapse before the neurologic deficit becomes apparent, thus excluding more benign forms of epilepsy with myoclonus. The diagnosis of PME is therefore usually made after a period of observation with documented neurologic deterioration despite optimal treatment.

Definitive diagnosis of the pathology frequently requires tissue study. Modern molecular methods have elucidated the genetic basis for the clinical phenotype in many cases.

Neuronal Ceroid Lipofuscinosis

The accumulation of abnormal amounts of lipopigment in lysosomes in brain, eccrine secretory cells, muscle, appendix, or rectal mucosa is characteristic (30). Usually a skin or rectal biopsy with electron microscopy is definitive. The inclusions take various forms that correlate with the clinical subtypes (31). Curvilinear bodies are characteristic of the late infantile form (Bielschowsky–Jansky disease), and fingerprint profiles are seen in the juvenile (Spielmeyer–Vogt disease) and the adult syndrome (Kufs' disease).

The infantile form (Batten's disease) does not present as a PME syndrome. The late-infantile form is an autosomal recessive disease with onset between age of $2^{1}/_{2}$ and 4 with epilepsy and, within a few months, stimulus-sensitive myoclonic seizures. Dementia and ataxia follow. Late blindness with macular degeneration may occur. The EEG shows marked photic sensitivity and the electroretinogram (ERG) shows absent B waves, while the visual evoked response (VER) is amplified. Onset of the juvenile type occurs between age 4 and 10, usually with visual failure as the first symptom. Dementia, seizures, and dysarthria follow in about two years. Extrapyramidal rigidity is late. Sometimes seizures are the presenting symptom. Optic atrophy and macular degeneration are seen. The ERG shows absent B waves but a diminished VER. The adult form is inherited as an autosomal recessive, but a dominant pattern has been described. While the PME triad is usually present, psychiatric and extrapyramidal signs may be prominent and the optic fundi are normal.

Urinary screening for dolichol in the sediment is positive in 92% of late-infantile cases and in 85% of the juvenile type of neuronal ceroid lipofuscinosis. False positives are seen in 15% of healthy controls (32), and in adults the test is probably too sensitive and nonspecific to be of value. The gene for Batten's disease has been cloned and mutational analysis will replace dolichol screening. The gene for the late-infantile form has been mapped to 13q21.1 (33).

Mitochondrial Encephalomyopathy

Two clinical syndromes are described–MELAS (mitochondrial myopathy, encephalopathy, lactic acidosis, and stroke-like episodes) (34) and MERRF (myoclonus epilepsy, and ragged red fibres) (35). Although MELAS does not present as PME, overlapping forms occur. Because of heteroplasmy (mixing of normal and mutant mtDNA), there is wide phenotypic heterogeneity within families. Patients with MERRF usualy present in the second decade, and the diagnosis may be suggested by the presence of short stature, hearing loss, optic atrophy, neuropathy, or hypoventilation. The diagnosis is usually suggested by the finding of "ragged red fibers" in the muscle biopsy stained with Gomori's trichrome, but not all cases have this abnormality. Sophisticated studies of mitochondrial metabolism by way of magnetic resonance spectroscopy, positron emission tomography, and from in vitro studies of mitochondrial respiration may help. Mitochondrial enzyme defects have been established in some patients (36). In MERRF, two-point mutations in the tRNA^{Lys} gene have been described (37). Molecular genetic analysis of some of the more common mitochondrial DNA mutations is now a commercially available laboratory test.

Sialidosis

Visual failure with cherry red spots at the maculae, myoclonus, and normal intelligence are the diagnostic clues. The sialidoses are a group of lysosomal storage diseases associated with a deficiency of alpha-N-acetylneuraminidase (sialidase) and, in some, with additional deficiency of beta-galactosidase (38). Urinary excretion of sialyloligosaccharides is markedly increased, and the enzyme deficiency can

be demonstrated in leukocytes or cultured fibroblasts (39,40).

A simple classification is that of a normosomatic or type 1 sialidosis and a dysmorphic or type 2 sialidosis. In sialidosis type 1 (41), myoclonus begins in adolescence and grand mal seizures, peripheral neuropathy, ataxia, and lens opacities may be associated; other somatic and bony abnormalities are absent. These patients may have a primary defect of neuraminidase. Sialidosis type 2 includes a number of subcategories, and dysostosis multiplex and Hurler-like features are common (40). Some have, in addition, a defect of galactosidase—galactosialidosis (42). The gene for galactosialidosis has been mapped to 20q13.1 (43). There are multiple point mutations in the cathepsin A gene resulting in absent or defective protective protein cathepsin A, which lacks catalytic activity and results in combined beta-galactosidase and neuraminidase deficiency (43).

Lafora Body Disease

This is an autosomal recessive storage disease characterized by the presence of polyglucosan acid-Schiff positive inclusions (Lafora bodies) in cells of brain, liver, muscle, and skin in sweat gland ducts (44,45). An axillary skin biopsy is usually diagnostic (46). Onset occurs at a mean age of 14 years, and dementia is always present, with variable myoclonus and occipital seizures. Behavioral change or school failure may be the first sign. Death occurs within 2 to 10 years of onset. Rarely, a more benign course is seen (44,45). Using linkage studies in three Italian families with Lafora disease, Pennacchio et al (47) demonstrated that the gene is located at a locus other than that for the Unverricht-Lundborg type (see below) on chromosome 21q22.3 and Serratosa et al (48) assigned the gene to 6q23-q25.

Unverricht-Lundborg Disease: "Baltic Myoclonus"

Great confusion has surrounded the classification of this entity. The most recent clinical reviews (49–51) differentiate the syndrome from other causes of PME and describe the presentation and course in 93 cases in Finland. Onset is at a mean age of 10.8 years, and the condition is inherited as an autosomal recessive trait. There has been no specific test for the syndrome, but the recent demonstration (47) in these patients of a defect in the gene encoding Cystatin B (21q22.3), which inactivates proteases that leak out of lysosomes, is likely to provide a laboratory-based test for diagnostic purposes. Myoclonus is constant and typically provoked by external stimuli including sound, light, or touch. It may be triggered by movement or stress and repetitive morning myoclonus may culminate in a clonic–tonic–clonic seizure. Autopsy studies show widespread degeneration in the brain, the most prominent of which is loss of Purkinje cells in the cerebellum without storage material. The clinical counterpart is the inevitable development of ataxia of gait, dysarthria, and intention tremor. Dementia is mild and intellectual decline is said to occur at the rate of 10 IQ points per decade. The EEG shows generalized spike–wave patterns and photosensitivity.

Miscellaneous Causes of PME

These include Gaucher's disease (52), GM2 gangliosidosis (53), biotin responsive encephalopathy (54), neuraxonal dystrophy (55), action myoclonus–renal failure syndrome (56), dentatorubral-pallidoluysian atrophy (DRPLA) (57), PME and deafness (May–White syndrome) (58), and PME and lipomas (59). Hallervorden–Spatz disease and globoid-cell leukodystrophy are other rare causes (60). The gene defects underlying many of these syndromes are summarized in Table 66.1.

Action Myoclonus

The term *action myoclonus* is applied to "arrythmic muscular jerking induced by voluntary movement. It is made worse by attempts at precise or coordinated movement (intention myoclonus) and may also be provoked by certain sensory stimuli" (61). The nosology of this syndrome continues to be controversial. Intention tremor and dysarthria occur in the first or second decade, myoclonus—frequently of the action type—develops late, and cerebellar ataxia progresses. Dementia, if it occurs, is mild and late, and seizures are rare.

The syndrome has usually been regarded as one of the "system degenerations" but should probably be regarded simply as a syndrome of cerebellar ataxia with myoclonus of multifactorial causes. It is distinct from Baltic myoclonus in that epilepsy is rare. Mitochondrial myopathy is frequent, and a primary mitochondrial dysfunction may be the underlying pathology in most patients (31).

Posthypoxic Myoclonus

Chronic action myoclonus in association with cerebellar ataxia following an episode of cerebral anoxia is often called the Lance–Adams syndrome (11). Autopsy studies have shown no consistent pathology, but the underlying defect may relate to a deficiency of serotonin. A rather dramatic response to therapy with 5-hydroxytryptophan has been reported (62).

Focal Myoclonus

The syndromes of focal myoclonic jerking includes palatal myoclonus, epilepsy partialis continua, and segmental myoclonus.

Palatal Myoclonus

Following a lesion of the central tegmental tract (red nucleus to inferior olive), or occasionally of the dentate nucleus, regular and rhythmic movements of the palate, sometimes spreading to the pharynx, larynx, external ocular muscles, and diaphragm may be seen (63). The lesion itself is often

an infarction, but the syndrome has been seen in neoplastic, inflammatory, degenerative processes, and in dialysis encephalopathy. At autopsy, an enlarged inferior olive is seen, an example of transsynaptic degeneration of sorts. The movements are permanent and persist during sleep. They may represent release of primitive gill movements.

Epilepsy Partialis Continua

Repeating, regular myoclonic jerking of an extremity or part thereof, without loss of consciousness, represents partial motor seizure activity arising in cortex.

Segmental Myoclonus

Spinal cord trauma, neoplasm, or, occasionally, inflammatory lesions may cause repetitive myoclonic jerking in an arm or leg (64). Affected muscles show co-contraction of agonists and antagonists, and activity in flexor muscles predominates.

Pathophysiology of Myoclonus

In 1967, Halliday (65) divided myoclonus into three major categories on the grounds of their electrophysiologic correlates: pyramidal, extrapyramidal, and segmental myoclonus. In pyramidal myoclonus, a very short interval between the cortical discharge and the EMG activity in the jerking muscle is seen. Because of the short latency (15 to 40 ms), he proposed that the discharge was propagated via the pyramidal pathways. In extrapyramidal myoclonus, the cortical event was often less obvious but the EMG discharge was prolonged. The cortical event was often not strictly time-locked to the muscle event, and Halliday considered that the myoclonus might be arising in some extrapyramidal site.

Subsequent authors have preferred to classify myoclonus as being of cortical or subcortical origin.

Cortical Myoclonus

The basis for an epileptic myoclonic jerk is a prominent spontaneous cortical spike discharge. In cortical reflex myoclonus (66,67), that is, a myoclonic jerk in response to an external trigger, the cortical event is not obvious and the technique of back averaging the EEG using the EMG activity as the trigger will demonstrate transient, relatively subtle time-locked cortical events preceding the myoclonic jerk.

In most patients with cortical reflex myoclonus, giant sensory evoked potentials are seen. It may be that this type of myoclonus results from cerebellar pathology with loss of inhibitory cerebellar influences on motor cortical function, leading to pathologic facilitation of long-loop transcortical stretch and/or cutaneous reflexes (1,68).

Subcortical Myoclonus

Subcortical myoclonus may be spontaneous or reflex in origin. Hallett et al (69) described the characteristics of

T a b l e   6 6 . 1   Genetic Basis of Myoclonus

Name of Disease	Frequency	Mode of Inheritance	Mutant Gene Product	Chromosomal Location	Altered DNA Structure	Disturbed Protein Function	Disrupted Cell and Organ Function
DRPLA (87–90)	$1:1 \times 10^6$; in Japan	Autosomal dominant	Unknown	12p13.31	Expansion of $(CAG)_n$ repeats: copy number >49–75 in DRPLA patients	Unknown, gain of function postulated invoking polyglutamine tracts	Neuronal cell degeneration in the dentate, red nucleus, pallidum, and subthalamic nucleus
Prion disease (91)	$1:1 \times 10^6$; worldwide for all forms	Autosomal dominant	Prion protein gene (PRNP)	20pter		PrP^{sc} accumulation	CNS spongiform degeneration
Sialidosis (92)	50–100 cases	Autosomal recessive	Lysosomal α-neuraminidase	10pter-q23	Unknown	Deficient enzyme activity	Accumulation of oligosaccharides causes tissue damage
Galactosialidosis (93)	Uncommon, but not rare in Japan	Autosomal recessive	Lysosomal protective protein/cathepsin A	20q13.1	Multiple alleles, point mutations	Absent or defective lysosomal protective protein/ cathepsin A, lacking catalytic activity and causing combined β-galactosidase and neuraminidase deficiency	Lysosomal accumulation of primarily sialylated oligosaccharides, producing dysostosis multiplex, Hurler-like features and neurologic abnormalities
Unverricht–Lundborg (94)	1:20,000 in Finland; rare elsewhere	Autosomal recessive	Cystatin B protease inhibitor	21q22.3	3-splice site mutation and a translation stop codon mutation	Reduced amounts of Cystatin B	Despite ubiquitous expression of this protein, it is not understood why mutations in this gene cause such a tissue-specific phenotype
Lafora body disease (95)	Few cases described	Autosomal recessive	Unknown	6q23-q25	Unknnown	Unknown	Intracellular Lafora bodies suggesting amyloid are found in the brain, heart, liver, and retina
GM$_2$ gangliosidosis hexosaminidase α-subunit deficiency (variant B, Tay–Sachs disease) (96)	1:300,000; 100 × higher in Ashkenazi Jews	Autosomal recessive	α subunit of β-hexosaminidase (HEXA)	15q23-q24	Multiple alleles, deletion (French-Canadian) and nondeletion	Absent or defective hexosaminidase A ($\alpha\beta$) activity	Accumulation of ganglioside GM$_2$ in lysosomes causes neuronal dysfunction
GM$_2$ gangliosidosis hexosaminidase 3-subunit deficiency (Sandhoff disease) (96)	1:300,000	Autosomal recessive	β-subunit of β-hexosaminidase (HEXB)	5q13	Multiple alleles, both deletion and nondeletion	Absent or defective hexosaminidase A ($\alpha\beta$) and B ($\beta\beta$) activity	Accumulation of ganglioside GM$_2$ and water-soluble substrates causes neuronal dysfunction and organomegaly
Myoclonic epilepsy and ragged-red fiber disease (MERRF) (97)	Unknown	Maternal inheritance	IRNA	mtDNA	Two-point mutations in the $tRNA^{lys}$ gene	Abnormal mitochondrial protein synthesis producing abnormal oxidative phosphorylation	Variable combinations of myoclonic epilepsy, mitochondrial myopathy, and cardiac, neurologic, endocrine, and renal manifestations
Gaucher disease type 3: juvenile neuronopathic (98)	Rare, genetic isolate in Norbotten, Sweden	Autosomal recessive	Glucocerebrosidase	1q21	1448T-C	Small decrease in catalytic activity and unstable enzyme protein results in significantly decreased lysosomal glucocerebrosidase	Accumulation of glucosylceramide in lysosomes of macrophages, which leads to injury of them and surrounding neurons
Globoid cell leukodystrophy (Krabbe's disease) (99)	1:50,000 in Sweden; much lower in other places	Autosomal recessive	Lysosomal galactosylceramidase (galactocerebroside β-galactosidase)	14q24.3-q32.1	Unknown	Absent enzyme activity	Accumulation of a toxic natural substance (galactosysphingosinepsychosine) lead to disappearance of oligodendroglia and no subsequent myelination with destruction of CNS white matter

Table 66.1 *Continued*

Name of Disease	Frequency	Mode of Inheritance	Mutant Gene Product	Chromosomal Location	Altered DNA Structure	Disturbed Protein Function	Disrupted Cell and Organ Function
Neuronal ceroid lipofuscinosis (CLN5) late-infantile (100)	Few families in Finland	Autosomal recessive	Unknown	13q21.1-q32	Unknown	Unknown	Accumulation of autofluorescent lipopigment in neurons and retinal ganglion cells
Juvenile myoclonic epilepsy (101)	Unknown	Autosomal dominant	Unknown	6p21.1-p11	Unknown	Unknown	Unknown
Hallervorden–Spatz disease (102)	Rate	Autosomal recessive	Unknown	Unknown	Unknown	Unknown	Spheroid bodies (axonal swellings) widely distributed in globus pallidus, substantia nigra and caudate nucleus, medulla, and spinal cord
Neuroaxonal dystrophy (103)	Very rare, few case reports	Autosomal recessive	Unknown	Unknown	Unknown	Unknown	Spheroid bodies (axonal swellings) widely distributed in hypothalamus, infundibulum neurohypophysis, and colonic myenteric plexus
Striatonigral degeneration (infantile)	Rare	Autosomal recessive	Unknown	Unknown	Unknown	Unknown	Symmetrical degeneration of caudate, putamen, and globus pallidus
Benign adult familial myoclonus epilepsy (104)	5 Japanese kindreds	Autosomal dominant	Unknown	Not linked to DRPLA; gene locus, unknown	Unknown	Unknown	Unknown

reticular reflex myoclonus, which they believed to be generated in the reticular formation of the brain. Using the back averaging technique, the cortical event is not time-locked to the muscle event in muscles innervated by brain stem nuclei, nor is it prefaced by their activity. The syndrome has been described in posthypoxic myoclonus, uremia, and other metabolic dysfunctions (70).

Treatment of Myoclonus

The most potent agents curently available for suppressing myoclonic activity act to enhance gamma-aminobutyric acid (GABA)-mediated inhibition and/or to diminish amino acid induced excitation (71). Clonazepam facilitates GABA-ergic transmission by a direct effect on bezodiazepine receptors (72). GABA receptors lie on the cell bodies of dorsal raphe neurons and GABA inhibits raphe cell firing (73). Clonazepam decreases 5-hydroxytryptophan (5-HTP) utilization in brain and blocks the egress of 5-hydroxyindoleacetic acid (HIAA) from brain, but its precise mode of action in blocking myoclonus is unknown (74,75).

Valproate inhibits GABA catabolism (76). GABA metabolism may be abnormal in certain myoclonic syndromes, and low levels have been described in the cerebrospinal fluid of patients with postanoxic intention myoclonus, progressive myoclonus epilepsy (77). Valproate produces an increase in the concentration of tryptophan and HIAA but only minimal changes in the functional pool of 5HT were seen in experimental animals (78). The changes seen do not explain its antimyoclonic activity. Valproate has been shown

to decrease the levels of the excitatory amino acids aspartate and glycine, but the role of aspartate in myoclonus has not been investigated (79).

Myoclonus, in contrast to most forms of epilepsy, may respond to treatment with drugs that enhance serotonin activity. The serotonin precursor 5-hydroxytryptophan (HTP) with carbidopa has been useful (80).

ASTERIXIS

Adams and Foley first used the term *asterixis* to denote an almost rhythmical, recurrent abrupt lapse in postural tone of the outstretched arms (81). The movement or "flap" is characterized by a cessation or pause in muscle activity that can be demonstrated on the EMG (82). Bilateral asterixis is a sign used to support the bedside diagnosis of a toxic or metabolic cause of a confusional state or encephalopathy and may be accompanied by an irregular tremulousness also due to short, often incomplete pauses in EMG activity (82).

Shahani and Young used the term *negative myoclonus* to emphasise the EMG silent periods, even though the movements may look superficially myoclonic (83). They suggested that asterixis is a disorder of those central nervous system (CNS) programs or mechanisms responsible for the maintenance of posture or of slow unidirectional movements as distinct from those concerned with movement itself (84).

Whereas bilateral asterixis invariably suggests the diagnosis of a diffuse metabolic or toxic encephalopathy, unilateral asterixis may be seen with focal lesions within the CNS, sometimes triggered by anticonvulsants such as phenytoin. Such focal lesions are often poorly defined in case reports but are frequently correlated with lesions in posterior parietal cortex, ventrolateral thalamus, rostral midbrain, or supplementary motor area (85).

Marsden et al (1,86) have demonstrated that transcutaneous electrical stimulation of the human cortex produces either twitches of the appropriate body part or, if stimulus parameters are changed, brief silent periods in voluntarily contracting muscles that are associated with postural lapses. They concluded that activity in the motor cortex may cause either muscle contraction or asterixis. At any CNS level, bursts of inhibitory activity, an active phenomenon, may be the basic pathogenesis of asterixis.

REFERENCES

1. Marsden C. The physiology of myoclonus and its relation to epilepsy. Res Clin Forums 1980;2:31–45.
2. Friedreich N. Neuropathologische beobachtung beim paramyoklonus multiplex. Virchows Arch Pathol Anat Physiol Klin Med 1881;86:421–434.
3. Unverricht H. Die myoklonie. Leipzig: Franz Deutike, 1881.
4. Lundborgh H. Die progressive myoklonus-epilepsie. Uppsala: Almqvist and Wiksell, 1903.
5. West W. On a peculiar form of infantile convulsions. Lancet 1861;1:724–725.
6. Reynolds J. Epilepsy: its symptoms, treatment and relation to other convulsive diseases. London: John Churchill, 1861.
7. Muskens L. Epilepsy: comparative pathogenesis, symptoms, treatment. New York: William Wood, 1928.
8. Hodskins M, Yakolev P. Anatomico-clinical observation on myoclonus in epileptics and on related symptom complexes. Am J Psychiatry 1930;9:827–848.
9. Lennox W. The petit mal epilepsies. JAMA 1945;129:1069–1074.
10. Hunt J. Dyssynergia cerebellaris myoclonia—primary atrophy of the dentate system: a contribution to the pathology and symptomatology of the cerebellum. Brain 1921;44:490–538.
11. Lance J, Adams R. The syndrome of intention or action myoclonus as a sequel to hypoxic encephalopathy. Brain 1963;86:111–136.
12. Walsh F. On the symptom complexes of lethargic encephalitis with special reference to the involuntary muscular contractions. Brain 1920;43:197–219.
13. Reimold W. Uber die myoklonische form der encephalitis. Z Gesampte Neurol Psychiatr 1925;95:21–36.
14. Von Economo C. Die encephalitis lethargica, ihre nachkrantheiten und ihre behandlung. Berlin: Urban and Schwarzenberg, 1929.
15. Creutzfeldt H. Uber eine eigenartige herdfomige erkrankung des zentral nervensystems. Z Gesamte Neurol Psychiatr 1920;57:1–18.
16. Jakob A. Uber eigenartige erkrakungen des zentralnervensystems mit bemerkenswerten anatomischen befunden (spastische pseudosklerose, encephalomyelopathie mit disseminierten degenerationsherden). Z Gesamte Neurol Psychiatr 1921;64:147–228.
17. Dawson J. Cellular inclusions in cerebral lesions of epidemic encephalitis. (Second Report). Arch Neurol Psychiatry 1934;31:685–700.
18. Kupper A. Uber klonische krampfe der schingmuskulatur. Archiv Ohrenheilkunde 1873;1:296–297.
19. Gullain G, Mollaret P. Deux cas de myoclonies synchrones et rhythmees velopharyngo-laryngo-oculo-diaphragmatiques. Le probleme anatomique et physio-pathologique de ce syndrom. Rev Neurol (Paris) 1931;2:545–566.
20. Gullain G, Mollaret P. Nouvelle contribution a l'etude des myoclonies velopharyngo-laryngo-oculo-diaphragmatiques. Rev Neurol (Paris) 1932;2:249–264.
21. DeLisi LD. Sudi un fenomeno motorio constante del sonno normale: le mioclonie ipniche fisiologiche. Rev Pathol Nerv Ment 1932;39:481–496.
22. Symonds C. Nocturnal myoclonus. J Neurol Neurosurg Psychiatry 1953;16:166–171.
23. Brown P, Cathala F, Castaigne P, Gajdusek D. Creutzfeldt–Jakob disease: clinical analysis of a consecutive series of 230 neuropathologically verified cases. Ann Neurol 1986;20:597–602.
24. Wilkins D, Hallet M, Berardelli A, et al. Physiologic analysis of the myoclonus of Alzheimer's disease. Neurology 1984;34:898–903.
25. Navin B, Jordan B, Price R. The AIDs–dementia complex I. Clinical features. Ann Neurol 1986;19:517–524.
26. Liu A, Delgado-Escueta A, Serratosa J, et al. Juvenile myoclonic epilepsy locus in chromosome 6p21.2-p11: linkage to convulsions and electroencephalography trait. Am J Hum Genet 1995;57(2):368–381.
27. Thomas J, Reggan R, Klass D. Epilepsia partialis continua. A review of 32 cases. Arch Neurol 1977;34:266–275.
28. Rasmussen T. Further observations on the syndrome of chronic encephalitis and epilepsy. Appl Neurophysiol 1978;41(1–4):1–12.
29. Berkovic S, Andermann F, Carpenter S, Wolfe L. Progressive myoclonus epilepsies: specific causes and diagnosis. N Engl J Med 1986;315:296–305.
30. Siakotos A. Neuronal ceroid lipofuscinosis. In: Vinken P, Bruyn G, eds. Handbook of clinical neurology. Vol. 42. Amsterdam: North Holland, 1981.
31. Lake B. Lysosomal enzyme deficiencies. In: Adams J, Corsellis J, Duchen L, eds. Greenfield's neuropathology. 4th ed. New York: John Wiley, 1984.
32. Wolfe L, Palo J, Santavuori P, et al. Urinary sediment dolichols in the diagnosis of neuronal ceroid-lipofuscinosis. Ann Neurol 1986;19:270–274.
33. Savukoski M, Kestila M, Williams R, et al. Defined chromosomal assignment of CLN5 demonstrates that at least four loci are involved in the pathogenesis of human ceroid lipofuscinoses. Am J Human Genet 1994;55:695–701.
34. Pavlakis S, Phillips P, DiMauro S, et al. Mitochondrial myopathy, encephalopathy, lactic acidosis and stroke-like episodes: a distinctive clinical syndrome. Ann Neurol 1984;16:481–488.
35. Fukuhara N, Tokiguchi S, Shirakawa K, Tsubaki T. Myoclonus epilepsy associated with ragged-red fibers (mitochondrial abnormalities): disease entity or syndrome? Light- and electron-microscopic studies of two cases and a review of the literature. J Neurol Sci 1980;47:117–133.
36. Dimauro S, Bonilla E, Zeviani M, et al. Mitochondrial myopathies. Ann Neurol 1985;17:521–538.
37. Hammans S, Sweeney M, Brockington M, et al. The mitochondrial DNA transfer RNA^{Lys} A-G$^{(8334)}$ mutation and the syndrome of myoclonic epilepsy with ragged red fibres (MERRF). Brain 1993;116:617–632.
38. Tsuji S, Yamada T, Tsutsumi A, Miyatake T. Neuraminidase deficiency and accumulation of sialic acid in lymphocytes in adult type sialidosis with partial B-galactosidase deficiency. Ann Neurol 1982;11:541–543.
39. Lowden J, O'Brien J. Sialidosis: A review of human neuraminidase deficiency. Am J Hum Genet 1979;31:1–18.
40. Warner T, O'Brien J. Genetic defects in glycoprotein metabolism. Annu Rev Genet 1983;17:395–441.
41. Thomas P, Abrams J, Swallow D, Stewart G. Sialidosis type 1: cherry red spot–myoclonus syndrome with sialidase deficiency and altered electrophoretic mobility of some enzymes known to be glycoproteins. 1. Clinical findings. J Neurol Neurosurg Psychiatry 1979;42:873–880.
42. Matsuo T, Egawa I, Okada S, et al. Sialidosis type 2 in Japan: clinical study in 2 siblings, cases and review of literature. J Neurol Sci 1983;58:45–55.
43. d'Azzo A, Andria G, Strisciuglio P, Galjaard H. Galactosialidosis. In: Scriver C, Beaudet A, Sly W, Valle D, eds. The metabolic and molecular bases of inherited disease. 7th ed.; Vol. 2. New York: McGraw Hill, 1995:2825–2837.
44. Ham MVH, Jager H. Progressive myoclonus epilepsy with Lafora bodies: clinical-pathological features. 1963;4:95–119.
45. Ham MVH. Lafora disease: a form of progressive myoclonus epilepsy. In: Vinken P, Bruyn G, eds. Handbook of clinical neurology. Vol. 15. Amsterdam: North Holland, 1974:382–422.
46. Carpenter S, Karpati G. Sweat gland duct cells in Lafora disease: diagnosis by skin biopsy. Neurology 1981;31:1564–1568.
47. Pennacchio L, Lehesjoki A, Stone N, et al. Mutations in the gene encoding Cystatin B in progressive myoclonus epilepsy (EPM1). Science 1996;271:1731–1734.
48. Serratosa J, Delgado-Escueta A, Posada I, et al. The gene for progressive myoclonus epilepsy of the Lafora type maps to chromosome 6q. Hum Molec Genet 1995;4:1657–1663.
49. Koskiniemi M, Donner M, Majuri H, et al. Progressive myoclonus epilepsy: a clinical histopathological study. Acta Neurol Scand 1974;50:307–332.
50. Koskiniemi M. Psychological findings in progressive myoclonus epilepsy without Lafora bodies. Epilepsia 1974;15:537–545.
51. Koskiniemi M, Toivakka E, Donner M. Progressive myoclonus epilepsy: electroencephalographical findings. Acta Neurol Scand 1974;50:333–359.
52. King J. Progressive myoclonus epilepsy due to Gaucher's disease in an adult. J Neurol Neurosurg Psychiatry 1977;40:470–478.
53. Brett E, Ellis R, Haas L, et al. Late onset GM2 gangliosidosis: clinical, pathological and biochemical studies on 8 patients. Arch Dis Child 1973;48:775–785.

54. Bressman S, Fahn S, Eisenberg M, Brin M, Maltese W. Biotin responsive encephalopathy with myoclonus, ataxia and seizures. Adv Neurol 1986;43:119–125.

55. Dorfman I, Pedley T, Tharp B, Scheithaver B. Juvenile neuraxonal dystrophy: clinical, electrophysiological and neuropathological features. Ann Neurol 1978;3:419–428.

56. Andermann E, Andermann F, Carpenter S, et al. Action myoclonus–renal failure syndrome. Adv Neurol 1986;43:87–103.

57. Lizuka R, Hirayama K, Machara K. Dentato-rubro-pallido-Luysian atrophy: a clinico-pathological study. J Neurol Neurosurg Psychiatry 1984;47:1288–1298.

58. May D, White H. Familial myoclonus, cerebellar ataxia and deafness: specific genetically determined disease. Arch Neurol 1968;19:331–338.

59. Ekbom K. Hereditary ataxia, photomyoclonus, skeletal deformities and lipoma. Acta Neurol Scand 1975;51:393–404.

60. Rozdilsky B, Cumings J, Huston A. Hallervorden-Spatz disease—late infantile and adult types; report of two cases. Acta Neuropathol (Berl) 1968;10:1–16.

61. Lance J. Action myoclonus, Ramsay Hunt syndrome, and other cerebellar myoclonic syndromes. Adv Neurol 1986;43:33–35.

62. Thal I, Sharpless N, Wolfson L, Katzman R. Treatment of myoclonus with L 5 hydroxytryptophan and carbidopa: clinical, electrophysiological and biochemical observations. Ann Neurol 1980;7:570–576.

63. Lapresle J. Palatal myoclonus. In: Fahn S, Marsden C, Woert MV, eds. Advances in neurology. Vol. 43. New York: Raven, 1986;265–273.

64. Frenken C, Notermans S, Korten J, Horstink M. Myoclonic disorders of spinal origin. Clin Neurol Neurosurg 1978;79:107–118.

65. Halliday A. The electrophysiological study of myoclonus in man. Brain 1967;90:241–284.

66. Shibasaki H, Motomura S, Ymashita Y, et al. Periodic synchronous discharge and myoclonus in Creutzfeldt-Jakob disease: diagnostic application of jerk-locked averaging methods. Ann Neurol 1981;9:150–156.

67. Hallett M, Chadwick D, Marsden C. Cortical reflex myoclonus. Neurology 1979;29:1107–1125.

68. Marsden C, Merton P, Morton H. Is the human stretch reflex cortical rather than spinal? Lancet 1973;1:759–761.

69. Hallett M, Chadwick D, Adam J, Marsden C. Reticular reflex myoclonus: a physiological type of human post-anoxic myoclonus. J Neurol Neurosurg Psychiatry 1977;40:253–264.

70. Chadwick D, French A. Uraemic myoclonus: an example of reticular reflex myoclonus? J Neurol Neurosurg Psychiatry 1979;42:52–55.

71. Meldrum B. Drugs acting on amino acid neurotransmitters. In: Fahn S, Marsden C, Woert MV, eds. Advances in neurology. Vol. 43. New York: Raven, 1986;687–706.

72. Meldrum B. Epilepsy and GABA-mediated inhibition. Int Rev Neurobiol 1975;17:1036.

73. Gallager D. Benzodiazepines: potentiation of a GABA inhibitory response in the dorsal raphe nucleus. Eur J Pharmacol 1978;39:357–364.

74. Wiener W, Goetz C, Nausieda P, Klawans H. Clonazepam and 5-hydroxytryptophan induced myoclonic stereotypy. Eur J Pharmacol 1977;46:21–24.

75. Hwang E, Woert MV. Antimyoclonic action of clonazepam: the role of serotonin. Eur J Pharmacol 1979;60:31–40.

76. Chapman A, Keane P, Meldrum B, et al. Mechanism of anticonvulsant of valproate. Prog Neurobiol 1982;19:315–359.

77. Airaksinen E, Leino E. Decrease of GABA in the cerebrospinal fluid of patients with progressive myoclonus epilepsy and its correlation with the decrease of 5 HIAA and HVA. Acta Neurol Scand 1982;66:666–672.

78. Hwang EC, Woert MV. Effect of valproic acid on serotonin metabolism. Neuropharmacology 1979;18:391–397.

79. Kukino K, Deguchi T. Effects of sodium dipropylacetate on gamma aminobutyric acid and biogenic amines in rat brain. Chem Pharm Bull (Tokyo) 1977;25:2257–2262.

80. Woert M, Hwang EC. Biochemistry and pharmacology of myoclonus. Clin Neuropharmacol 1978;3:167–184.

81. Adams R, Foley J. The neurological changes in the more common types of severe liver disease. Trans Am Neurol Assoc 1949;74:217–219.

82. Leavitt S, Tyler H. Studies in asterixis. Arch Neurol 1964;10:360–368.

83. Shahani B, Young R. Physiological and pharmacological aids in the differential diagnosis of tremor. J Neurol Neurosurg Psychiatry 1976;39:772–783.

84. Shahani B, Young R. Asterixis—a disorder of the neurological mechanisms underlying sustained muscle contraction. In: Shahani M, ed. The motor system—neurophysiology and muscle mechanisms. Amsterdam: Elsevier, 1976:301–316.

85. Young R, Shahani B. Asterixis: one type of negative myoclonus. In: Fahn S, Marsden C, Woert MV, eds. Advances in neurology. Vol. 43. New York: Raven, 1986:137–156.

86. Marsden C, Hallett M, Fahn S. The nosology and pathophysiology of myoclonus. In: Marsden C, Fahn S, eds. Movement disorders. London: Butterworth Scientific, 1982:196–248.

87. Burke J, Enghild J, Martin M, et al. Huntingtin and DRPLA proteins selectively interact with the enzyme GAPDH. Nat Med 1996;2:347–350.

88. Hirayami K, Takayanagi T, Nakamura R, et al. Spinocerebellar degenerations in Japan: a nationwide epidemiological and clinical study. Acta Neurol Scand 1994;89:1–22.

89. Ikeuchi T, Koide R, Tanaka H, et al. Dentatorubral-pallidoluysian atrophy: clinical features are closely related to unstable expansions of trinucleotide (CAG) repeat. Ann Neurol 1995;37:769–775.

90. Nagafuchi S, Yanagisawa H, Sato K, et al. Detatorubral and pallidoluysian atrophy: expansion of an unstable CAG trinucleotide on chromosome 12p. Nat Genet 1994;6:14–18.

91. Prusiner S. Prior diseases. In: Scriver C, Beaudet A, Shy W, Valle D, eds. The metabolic and molecular bases of inherited disease. Vol. 3. St. Louis: McGraw-Hill, 1995:4511–4546.

92. Thomas G, Beaudet A. Disorders of glycoprotein degradation and structure: α-mannosidosis, β-mannosidosis, fucosidosis, sialidosis, aspartylglucosaminuria, and carbohydrate-deficient glycoprotein syndrome. In: Scriver C, Beaudet A, Shy W, Valle D, eds. The metabolic and molecular bases of inherited disease. Vol. 2. St. Louis: McGraw-Hill, 1995:2542–2545.

93. d'Azzo, Andria G, Strisciuglio P, Galjaard H. Galactosialidosis. In: Scriver C, Beaudet A, Shy W, Valle D, eds. The metabolic and molecular bases of inherited disease. Vol. 2. St. Louis: McGraw-Hill, 1995:2825–2837.

94. Pennacchio L, Lehesjoki A, Stone N, et al. Mutations in the gene encoding Cystatin B in progressive myoclonus epilepsy (EPM1). Science 1996;271:1731–1734.

95. Serratosa J, Delgado-Escueta A, Posada I, et al. The gene for progressive myoclonus epilepsy of the Lafora type maps to chromosome 6q. Human Molec Genet 1995;4:1657–1663.

96. Gravel R, Clarke JT, Kaback M, et al. The G_{M2} gangliosidoses. In: Scriver C, Beaudet A, Shy W, Valle D, eds. The metabolic and molecular bases of inherited disease. Vol. 2. St. Louis: McGraw-Hill, 1995:2839–2863.

97. Hammans S, Sweeney M, Brockington M, et al. The mitochondrial DNA transfer RNA^{Lys}A-G$^{(8334)}$ mutation and the syndrome of myoclonic epilepsy with ragged red fibres (MERRF). Brain 1993;116:617–632.

98. Beutler E, Grabowski G. Gaucher disease. In: Scriver C, Beaudet A, Shy W, Valle D, eds. The metabolic and molecular bases of inherited disease. Vol. 2. St. Louis: McGraw-Hill, 1995:2641–2670.

99. Suzuki K, Suzuki Y, Suzuki K. Galactosylceramide lipidosis: globoid-cell leukodystrophy (Krabbe disease). In: Scriver C, Beaudet A, Shy W, Valle D, eds. The metabolic and molecular bases of inherited disease. Vol. 2. St. Louis: McGraw-Hill, 1995:2671–2692.

100. Savukoski M, Kestila M, Williams R, et al. Defined chromosomal assignment of CLN5 demonstrates that at least four loci are involved in the pathogenesis of human ceroid lipofuscinoses. Am J Human Genet 1994;55:695–701.

101. Liu A, Delgado-Escueta A, Serratosa J, et al. Juvenile myoclonic epilepsy locus in chromosome 6p21.2-p11: linkage to convulsions and electroencephalography trait. Am J Hum Genet 1995;57:368–381.

102. Rozdilsky B, Cumings J, Huston A. Hallervorden-Spatz disease—late infantile and adult types; report of two cases. Acta Neuropath (Berl) 1968;10:1–16.

103. Dorfman I, Pedley T, Tharp B, Scheithaver B. Juvenile neuraxonal dystrophy: clinical, electrophysiological, and neuropathological features. Ann Neurol 1978;3:419–428.

104. Kuwano A, Takakubo F, Morimoto Y, et al. Benign adult familial myoclonus epilepsy (BAFME): an autosomal dominant form not linked to the dentatorubral pallidoluysian atrophy (DRPLA) gene. J Med Genet 1996;33:80–81.

Startle Syndromes

Anthony B. Joseph   Marie-Helene Saint-Hilaire

INTRODUCTION

Startle is a universal mammalian behavior. The basic startle response in humans and other species may be part of a constellation of orienting behaviors that allow an animal to assess and respond to sudden discontinuous stimuli. These signal discrete and abrupt changes in the environment that might portend danger and threaten the individual. The ability to orient toward and then analyze these environmental stimuli may well optimize survival.

In humans, startle is a nonsuppressible reflex with a usual latency of less than 100 ms and a usual duration of less than 1,000 ms (1,2). Although audiogenic startle has been the most studied model, startle can be induced by sudden discontinuous input from other sensory modalities and can also be modified by cognitive and neurophysiologic processes such as learning and habituation (3,4).

The pattern of startle reaction induced by a loud, unexpected sound starts proximally with an eyeblink response and progresses distally with a generalized flexion of the head, trunk, and limbs, sometimes followed after more than a second by a secondary response (5). Although the flexor response predominates, there is also a significant occurrence of startle in the extensor muscles. The secondary stage of the response varies greatly among individuals and has voluntary and autonomic components.

The acoustic startle response can still be elicited in decerebrate animals, indicating that the neural circuit mediating the reflex is located at the level of the midbrain or below (6). In humans, the noise-induced startle reflex originates in the caudal brainstem and uses relatively slowly conducting spinal efferent pathways to recruit trunk and limb muscles (7).

Most evidence suggests that the pathway of the acoustic startle response consists of the cochlear nucleus, the inferior colliculus, the reticular formation, the reticulospinal tract, and the lower motor neurons. It is probably elaborated through the nucleus reticularis and pontis caudalis (8). Rats with lesions of this area show a significant decrement in responsiveness to startle-eliciting stimuli of two different sensory modalities, and electrical stimulation of this specific area elicits a response that looks very much like acoustic startle (9). The anatomic organization of the reticular formation probably explains its role in the organization of the startle response. It receives input from many sensory modalities and gives rise to long descending projections to the spinal cord.

Startle modulation is mediated by polysynaptic brainstem mechanisms with further modulation by cortically mediated attention toward or away from eliciting stimuli (10,11). Startle amplitude can be altered by changes in the parameters of the eliciting stimuli, surrounding environment, general state of the subject, and by a variety of drugs. For example, in rats, dopaminergic stimulation enhances startle response amplitude (12), and serotonin infused into the lateral ventricle reduces it (13). Adrenergic agonists and antagonists also play a role (14). In addition, the startle reflex shows habituation or sensitization depending on the parameters used. In animals, the habituation response is impaired by lesions of the inferior colliculus and midbrain reticular formulation (15).

In humans, the startle reflex seems to be present in the fetus after 30 weeks of gestation (16), but the brainstem mechanisms that mediate startle response modulation undergo development during childhood and do not mature until about 8 years of age (17). In adults, the intensity of the startle reaction varies from subject to subject, increasing with fatigue and anxiety.

There is probably a genetic predisposition to startle in the normal population (18). In American recruits, at least

1 in 2,000 had an excessive startle response (19). This becomes pathologic when the frequency or intensity are such that startling interferes with daily functioning, causes falls or other injuries, or leads patients to perceive themselves as dysfunctional.

In this chapter, we will give an overview of the main startle syndromes. Startle disease is described in more detail in Chapter 68.

CLASSIFICATION OF STARTLE SYNDROMES

Evidence for the existence of a number of startle syndromes exists in the literature. Several schemes for the classification of startle have been proposed (20–22). We do not suggest that the one that follows is either fully correct or definitively complete; we merely hope that it is useful.

We have divided startle into three main categories. The first consists of conditions in which startle is the primary symptom: startle disease and startle epilepsy. The second category includes startle caused by specific central nervous system conditions such as brainstem lesions and startle associated with increased adrenergic states. Startle can be a relatively minor component of some of these disorders. The third category consists of the so-called culture-bound syndromes, of which "lâtah" and the "jumping Frenchmen of Maine" are the best known. These disorders have been described worldwide and their pathophysiology is still a subject of controversy. This classification is outlined in Table 67.1.

STARTLE DISEASE: HYPEREKPLEXIA

Hyperekplexia was first described in 1966 by Suhren et al (23) as a hereditary disorder characterized by hypertonia in infancy, with poor feeding, apneic spells, and motor delay. An exaggerated startle response appears between infancy and early adulthood and can lead to falling and injuries, without loss of consciousness. More than 50% of the patients have nocturnal myoclonus (24), and a small number has generalized seizures (23). A minor form of hyperekplexia has been described in families with major hyperekplexia (22,25,26) and in sporadic cases (27). This form is also characterized by an excessive startle reaction appearing in childhood but without stiffness (23).

Hyperekplexia can be sporadic or inherited in autosomal dominant or recessive form (28). The dominant form is caused by mutations in the alpha 1 subunit of the inhibitory glycine receptor resulting in the substitution of an uncharged amino acid for Arg 271 in the mature protein (28,29). A mutation resulting in the substitution of asparagine for isoleucine at another location has been associated with a recessive form of the disease (25). These mutations were not found in sporadic cases (29) or in the minor form of hyperekplexia (30).

Physiologic studies suggest that the exaggerated startle response in hyperekplexia originates from the same brain-

Table 67.1 Clinical Classification of Startle

Startle reflex
  Benign hyperstartle
Psychogenic startle
Primary pathologic startle syndromes
  Startle epilepsy syndrome
    Startle-induced epilepsy
    Startle synkinesis
  Startle disease; hyperekplexia
    Major of minor
    Hereditary (dominant or recessive) or sporadic
Secondary pathologic startle syndromes
  Associated with increased adrenergic states
    Posttraumatic stress disorder
    Anxiety states
    Drug or alcohol withdrawal
    Hyperthyroidism
    Physical or sexual abuse
  Associated with disorders of the central nervous system
    Gilles de la Tourette
    Cerebral palsy
    Stiff-man syndrome
    Arnold Chiari and other lesions of the cervicomedullary junction
    Brainstem lesions: stroke, encephalitis, demyelination
    Occlusion of posterior thalamic arteries
    Postanoxic encephalopathy
    Hexosaminidase A deficiency (Tay Sachs)
Culturally linked startle syndromes
  Lâtah (Malaysia and Indonesia)
  Yaun (Burma)
  Bah-tsche (Thailand)
  Mali-mali and silok (Philippines)
  Myriachit, ikota, and amurakh (Siberia)
  Lapp panic (Lapland)
  Imu (Japan)
  Belin (Manchuria)
  Belenci (Inner Mongolia)
  Jumping Frenchmen of Maine (Canada; northeastern United States)
  Goosey (United States)
  Hyperstartlers (United States)
  Raging Cajuns (Louisiana)
  Unnamed varieties (Africa)

stem efferent system as the normal auditory startle reflex (22). However, the physiology of major hyperekplexia might differ from minor hyperekplexia, even in the same family (31).

Clonazepam appears to be the treatment of choice (21). Sodium valproate, 5-hydroxytryptophan, and piracetam have also been reported as useful (24).

STARTLE EPILEPSY

Startle epilepsy does not refer to a specific entity but to a type of phenomenon that can occur in several different clinical contexts. It was first described in 1901 by Gowers (32) and further characterized in 1955 by Alajouanine and Gastaut (33). In this rare form of epilepsy, which usually starts in the first two decades of life, seizures are triggered by unexpected stimuli of the kind likely to induce startle. It has been described mainly in patients with infantile hemiparesis or quadriparesis and diffuse cerebral dysfunction secondary to perinatal anoxia. It has also been reported in Down syndrome (34), Sturge-Weber disease (35), and Lennox–Gastaut syndrome (36).

Two types of patients can be distinguished. In patients with hemiparesis, the seizures consist of an abrupt startle response followed by a tonic phase involving the paretic hemibody (33). Loss of consciousness can be observed during long-lasting attacks. Atonic, hemiclonic seizures and automatisms have also been described accompanying the attacks. In patients with epileptic manifestations during an attack, there is little doubt about their ultimate epileptogenic nature (21). In others it can be difficult to decide whether the abnormal startle reaction itself is an epileptic phenomenon, and such attacks have been referred to as "startle synkinesis" by Alajouanine and Gastaut. This distinction may be artificial, however, as some patients may not present epileptic discharges on the surface electroencephalogram (EEG) (37,38).

In the second group, patients have widespread cerebral dysfunction and severe intellectual impairment. Unexpected stimuli induce a generalized tonic contraction, followed by a generalized clonic or atonic seizure (36).

In addition, startle-induced seizures are a recognized phenomenon in partial epilepsy, especially with involvement of the postcentral area, and in cases of secondary generalized epilepsy (27). The surface EEG pattern has been described as showing vertex polyspikes followed by desynchronization of the background and focal or generalized epileptic activity, or a vertex spike followed by a generalized or unilateral 10 cycles/sec rhythmic activity and postictal slow waves (39). Depth electrode studies in two patients revealed that the origin of the seizures was in the supplementary motor area, in the interhemispheric fissure in one patient and, in the other, in the mesiofrontal structures in the vicinity of the paracentral lobule (37,38). It was hypothesized that the startle epilepsy was secondary to the activation of an epileptogenic focus by the proprioceptive input of the startle reaction. On the other hand, there may have been focal or diffuse cortical excitability to the startling stimuli, as several of the patients had an excessive startle response (36). As suggested by Andermann, diffuse encephalopathies may affect the same neuronal systems as the genetically determined startle disease (21).

Clonazepam has been reported to be the most effective medication in the treatment of startle epilepsy (40) but may be more effective in children than in adults (21). Valproic acid and carbamazepine have also been found to be effective in certain patients. Carbamazepine seems to be most effective in patients with predominantly unilateral hemispheric lesions and hemiparesis (36).

A reasonable summary of startle epilepsy at this time is that epileptic startle can occur in a wide variety of patients with focal or generalized cerebral dysfunction of either a primary or secondary nature. It can occur as part of a distinct syndrome, as a secondary epileptic phenomenon, or startling itself can act as an activator of focal or generalized seizures.

SECONDARY STARTLE DISORDERS

Pathologically exaggerated startle can occur as a component of many disorders such as cervicomedullary compression or posterior thalamic artery occlusion (41,42), or general anxiety disorders and alcohol and benzodiazepine withdrawal (43). The pathophysiology of the exaggerated startle response is not fully understood in all these conditions. In some, like postanoxic encephalopathy, startle is a form of brainstem reticular reflex myoclonus (44), while in others, like brainstem encephalitis, it probably represents a pathologic exaggeration of the normal startle reflex (22).

PSYCHOGENIC STARTLE

One report has described the clinical presentation of five patients who presented with stimulus sensitive jerks and had been diagnosed as having either reflex myoclonus or pathologic startle (45). Two patients had generalized body jerks in response to sudden stimulation, one patient had prolonged repetitive limb jerking triggered by loud noise, one patient had jerking of the head and left arm triggered by noise and touch, and one patient had leg jerks triggered by tapping the patella. Electrophysiologic studies showed that the latencies between the stimuli and the jerks were long, and greater than that seen in cortical or brainstem reflex myoclonus. In addition, the pattern of muscle recruitment varied with each jerk. One patient's jerks resolved completely when the possibility that symptoms were voluntary was discussed with her.

THE LÂTAH GROUP AND AMERICAN HYPERSTARTLERS

There is quite an extensive literature on a group of disorders that exists worldwide, transculturally, and may overlap with sporadic and familial forms of benign hyperstartle. The two best studied forms of this disorder are "lâtah" and the "jumping Frenchmen of Maine." These disorders are characterized by an excessive startle response associated with any or all of the following phenomena: echolalia, echopraxia, coprolalia, and automatic obedience. They occur in sporadic and familial forms.

These syndromes first attracted attention in the medical literature in 1878 and 1880, when George Beard reported his observations of "jumpers" in the Moosehead lake region of Maine (46). His subjects displayed a startle reaction consisting of jumping, raising the arms, yelling, hitting, obeying sudden commands, or repeating sentences. The intensity of the response was proportional to the frequency of stimulation, and sometimes entailed risk of injury. Most "jumpers" were considered shy, retiring, and excessively ticklish. Lâtah on the other hand, has been known in Malaysia since at least the fifteenth century (47). The characteristics of this startle reaction are practically identical to "jumping" and the subjects are also described as timid and passive.

Similar syndromes occur throughout the world in different cultures and are known by a variety of names (21,48,49); these are shown in Table 67.1.

There is a controversy as to whether or not all these disorders are in fact the same. This is difficult to resolve. Certainly, the specific combination of hyperstartle, coprolalia, automatic obedience, echolalia, and echopraxia occurs in the conditions so far described. Descriptions of many of these disorders, however, were often not neurologically oriented, and those that were often omitted significant data on patterns of inheritance, partial penetrance, and other factors that would allow phenotypically similar syndromes to be differentiated. Similarly, the majority of these reports preceded the availability of modern neurological laboratory evaluation and thus salient data from modalities such as EEG, computerized tomography, and magnetic resonance imaging are also missing.

These caveats aside, the striking similarity of clinical histories from all over the world does tend to suggest that this group of disorders in fact represents a list of local names for cultural variations of the same basic entity.

Another controversial point is whether lâtah is a "true" neuropsychiatric disorder or a "psychologic state." The resolution of this point is confounded by reliable observations that people with lâtah may exaggerate or falsify aspects of their dysfunction to achieve other goals (48). In some communities and cultures, lâtah is perceived as an acceptable excuse for indulging in swearing and erotic or sexually overt acts under the pretext of startle-induced coprolalia, automatic obedience, and echopraxia.

Lâtah was first thought to be related to Gilles de la Tourette's disease (50), then to represent a specific hereditary tic syndrome (21). Although descriptions of lâtah and "jumping" describe a familial incidence of these conditions, they can develop in the absence of other afflicted relatives (51). In a study of eight patients with "jumping," three reported a positive family history. The eight subjects had in all 46 children, none of whom was affected. The patterns of heritability in the two families in which there was more than one affected individual were not consistent with any mendelian pattern (51). A specific genetic disorder also cannot explain why "jumping" appears predominantly in young, adolescent males, and lâtah almost exclusively in females (52).

"Jumping" is a behavior that has been related to a specific situation, in which young men who had started working as lumberjacks were teased by their companions as a form of distraction during the long winter nights. This was a fairly common occurrence in lumber camps and was not restricted to subjects of French-Canadian descent. Some subjects may also have been exposed to this kind of game as children in their villages (53). Despite the fact that Beard described "jumping" in young men, this specific phenomenon is not found in young people in these same cultural contexts any more, probably because of the modification of the way of life in lumber camps (51–53). In conclusion, "jumping" is a behavior that is related to a specific situation and is explainable as an operant conditioned response. Subjects always described themselves as ticklish and reacted to sudden stimuli more intensely than usual. Their enhanced startle reaction when teased by their companions was reinforced by the positive attention it attracted. This conditioned response became less intense and less complex when the subjects left the environment that was characterized by frequent stimuli and positive reinforcement.

Lâtah is basically similar to jumping, as it is associated with an excessive startle response and occurs in ticklish subjects who are teased for the entertainment of others. It occurs characteristically in women, who can often be startled with impunity because of their lower social status than men. In addition to the startle response, echopraxia, echolalia, and automatic obedience, the subjects can perform "role lâtah," which consists of an elaborated, prolonged response to amuse onlookers that sometimes mimics suggestive sexual behaviors.

Bartholomew reviewed 37 cases of lâtah from within his own family (52) and divided them into two categories. In the first, which included most of the patients, startle was associated with coprolalia. The second category consisted of a few subjects with severe lâtah, with automatic obedience and performances lasting up to 10 minutes occurring in large social gatherings. The author concluded that the first form was a culturally conditioned habit used as a coping strategy, permitting the exhibition of verbal obscenity with impunity, and the second form was a conscious ritual exhibited for social gain.

These observations support the concept that at least some cases of the lâtah phenomenon are due to culturally specific exploitation of a universal neurophysiologic response, the startle reflex. The themes illustrated by the startle phenomenon and the groups in which it appears are often culture specific (48). What remains unanswered is whether some of the cases are also due to cultural influences affecting the behavior of individuals already prone to develop the lâtah syndrome because of a neurophysiologically or psychopathologically determined vulnerability.

A final point of interest is the existence of American hyperstartlers. These individuals were found by Simons in response to an advertising campaign searching for American equivalents of lâtah (48). Their histories were very similar to those gathered in other forms of lâtah, and the data obtained from this investigation were consistent with the hypothesis that sporadic lâtah occurs in America but often goes unnamed and unremarked upon in the medical literature.

SUMMARY

Startle is a universal mammalian behavior that serves as an orienting reflex to allow the assessment of abrupt discontinuous stimuli in the external environment. The ability has obvious survival value. This response is stereotyped and is mediated at the level of the reticular formation, with modulation by cortical mechanisms.

It has also been suggested that afferent information processing in the dorsal cord, amygdala, and hippocampus are important in the startle response, and that pathologic startle occurs when these processes go away (48,49).

In humans, the intensity of the startle response varies among individuals and also depends on the subject's emotional state. Exaggerated forms of startle may be benign, but others may shade into true pathologic states, especially when the response becomes embarrassing or interferes with normal functioning. Pathologic startle can be primary or secondary. Secondary startle can be caused by a large number of diseases and events, including neurologic diseases, psychiatric diseases, toxic and metabolic states. The primary startle disorders are fewer in number and divide into those with a neurologic presentation—the startle diseases and startle epilepsies—and those in which the excessive startle response is modulated by the cultural environment and presents psychiatrically, if at all.

REFERENCES

1. Ekman P, Friesen WV, Simons RC. Is the startle reaction an emotion? J Pers Soc Psychol 1985;49:1416–1426.
2. Bernston GG, Boysen ST. Cardiac startle and orienting responses in the great apes. Behav Neurosci 1984;98:914–918.
3. Davis M. Pharmacological and anatomical analysis of fear conditioning using the fear-potentiated startle paradigm. Behav Neurosci 1986;100:814–824.
4. Ison JR, Hoffman HS. Reflex modification in the domain of startle: II. The anomalous history of a robust and ubiquitous phenomenon. Psychol Bull 1983;94:3–17.
5. Landis C, Hunt WA. The startle pattern. New York: Farrar and Rinehart, 1939.
6. Forbes A, Sherrington CS. Acoustic reflexes in the decerebrate rat. Am J Psychol 1914;35:367–376.
7. Brown P, Rothwell JC, Thompson PD, et al. New observations on the normal auditory startle reflex in man. Brain 1991;114:1891–1902.
8. Leitner DS, Powers AS, Hoffman HS. The neural substrate of the startle response. Physiol Behav 1980;25:291–297.
9. Gendelman DS, Davis M. The primary acoustic startle circuit. Soc Neurosci Abstr 1979;5:494.
10. Hackley SA, Graham FK. Early selective attention effects on cutaneous and acoustic blink reflexes. Physiol Psychol 1984;11:235–242.
11. Silverstein LD, Graham FK, Bohlin G. Selective attention effects on the reflex blink. Psychophysiology 1981;18:240–247.
12. Davis M. Cocaine: excitatory effects on sensorimotor reactivity measured with acoustic startle. Psychopharmacology 1985;86:31–36.
13. Davis M, Astrachan DI, Kass E. Excitatory and inhibitory effects of serotonin on sensori-motor reactivity measured with acoustic startle. Science 1980;209:521–523.
14. Davis M, Kehne JH, Commissaris RL. Antagonism of apomorphine-enhanced startle by alpha-1-adrenergic antagonists. Eur J Pharmacol 1985;108:233–241.
15. Jordan WP, Leaton RN. Habituation of the acoustic startle response in rats after lesions in the mesencephalic reticular formation or the inferior colliculus. Behav Neurosci 1983;97:710–724.
16. Divon MY, Platt LD, Cantrell CJ, et al. Evoked fetal startle response: a possible intrauterine neurological examination. Am J Obstet Gynecol 1985;153:454–456.
17. Ornitz EM, Guthrie D, Kaplan AR, et al. Maturation of startle modulation. Psychophysiology 1986;23:624–634.
18. Andermann F, Keene DL, Andermann E, Quesney LF. Startle disease or hyperekplexia. Further delineation of the syndrome. Brain 1980;103:985–997.
19. Thorne FC. Startle neurosis. Am J Psychiatry 1944;101:105–109.
20. Wilkins DE, Hallett M, Wess MM. Audiogenic startle reflex of man and its relationship to startle syndromes. Brain 1986;109:561–573.
21. Andermann F, Andermann E. Excessive startle syndromes: startle disease, jumping, and startle epilepsy. Adv Neurol 1986;43:321–333.
22. Brown P, Rothwell JC, Thompson PD, et al. The hyperekplexias and their relationship to the normal startle reflex. Brain 1991;114:1903–1928.
23. Suhren O, Bruyn GW, Tuynman JA. Hyperekplexia. A hereditary startle syndrome. J Neurol Sci 1966;3:577–605.
24. Saenz-Lope E, Herranz-Tanarro FJ, Masdeu JC, Chacon Pena JR. Hyperekplexia: a syndrome of pathological startle responses. Ann Neurol 1984;15:36–41.
25. Dooley JM, Andermann F. Startle disease or hyperekplexia: adolescent onset and response to valproate. Pediatr Neurol 1989;5:126–127.
26. Pascotto A, Coppola G. Neonatal hyperekplexia: A case report. Epilepsia 1992;33:817–820.
27. Gastaut H, Villeneuve A. The startle disease or hyperekplexia, pathological surprise reaction. J Neurol Sci 1967;5:523–542.
28. Rees MI, Andrew M, Jawad S, Owen MJ. Evidence for recessive as well as dominant forms of startle disease (hyperekplexia) caused by mutations in the alpha-1-subunit of the inhibitory glycine receptor. Hum Mol Genet 1994;3:2175–2179.
29. Shiang R, Ryan SG, Zhu YZ, et al. Mutational analysis of familial and sporadic hyperekplexia. Ann Neurol 1995;38:85–91.
30. Tijsen MAJ, Shiang R, Van Deutekom J, et al. Molecular genetic reevaluation of the Dutch hyperekplexia family. Arch Neurol 1995;52:578–582.
31. Tijssen MA, Padberg GW, Gert van Dijk J. The startle pattern in the minor form of hyperekplexia. Arch Neurol 1996;53:608–613.
32. Gowers WR. Epilepsy and other chronic convulsions. London: Churchill Livingstone, 1901.
33. Alajouanine A, Gastaut H. La syncinésie—sursaut et l'épilepsie—sursaut à déclenchement sensoriel ou sensitif inopiné. Rev Neurol (Paris) 1955;93:29–41.
34. Gimenez-Roldan S, Martin M. Startle epilepsy complicating Down syndrome during adulthood. Ann Neurol 1980;7:78–80.
35. Nakamura M, Kanai H, Miyamoto Y, et al. A case of Sturge-Weber syndrome with startle epilepsy. No To Shinkei 1975;27:324–331.
36. Saenz-Lope E, Herranz FJ, Masdeu JC. Startle epilepsy: a clinical study. Ann Neurol 1984;16:78–81.
37. Bancaud J, Talairach J, Bonis A. Physiopathogénie des épilepsies—sursaut (à propos d'une épilepsie de l'aire motrice supplémentaire). Rev Neurol (Paris) 1967;117:441–453.
38. Bancaud J, Talairach J, Lamarche M, et al. Hypothèses neurophysiopathologiques sur l'épilepsie—sursaut chez l'homme. Rev Neurol (Paris) 1975;131:559–571.
39. Aguglia U, Tinuper P, Gastaut H. Startle-induced epileptic seizures. Epilepsia 1984;25:712–720.
40. Gimenez-Roldan S, Martin M. Effectiveness of clonazepam in startle-induced seizures. Epilepsia 1979;20:255–261.
41. Fariello RG, Schwartzman RJ, Beall SS. Hyperekplexia exacerbated by occlusion of posterior thalamic arteries. Arch Neurol 1983;40:244–246.
42. Winston K. Hyperekplexia relieved by surgical decompression of the cervicomedullary region. Neurosurgery 1983;13:708–710.
43. Howard R, Ford R. From the jumping Frenchmen of Maine to post-traumatic stress disorder: the startle response in neuropsychiatry. Psychol Med 1992;22:695–707.
44. Hallett M, Chadwick D, Adam J, Marsden CD. Reticular reflex myoclonus: a physiological type of human post-hypoxic myoclonus. J Neurol Neurosurg Psychiatry 1977;40:253–264.
45. Thompson PD, Colebatch JG, Brown P, et al. Voluntary stimulus sensitive jerks and jumps mimicking myoclonus or pathological startle syndromes. Mov Disord 1992;7:257–262.
46. Beard G. Experiments with the jumpers of Maine. Pop Sci Monthly 1880;18:170–178.

47. Chapel JL. Lâtah, Myriachit and jumpers revisited. NY State J Med 1970;70:2201–2204.

48. Simons RC. The resolution of the Lâtah paradox. J Nerv Ment Dis 1980;168:195–206.

49. Joseph AB. Startle disease. Neurosurgery 1984;14:786–787.

50. Gilles de la Tourette G. Etude sur une affection nerveuse caractérisée par de l'incoordination motrice accompagnée d'écholalie et de coprolalie (jumping, lâtah, myriachit). Arch Neurologique 1885;9:19–42, 158–200.

51. Saint-Hilaire M-H, Saint-Hilaire J-M, Granger L. Jumping Frenchmen of Maine. Neurology 1986;36:1269–1271.

52. Bartholomew RE. Disease, disorder, or deception? Lâtah as habit in a Malay extended family. J Nerv Ment Dis 1994;182:331–338.

53. Rabinovitch R. An exaggerated startle reflex resembling a kicking horse. Can Med Assoc J 1965;93:130.

Startle Disease

ANDREA BERNASCONI   FREDERICK ANDERMANN   EVA ANDERMANN

Startle is a basic alerting reaction to unexpected, particularly audiogenic stimuli; it is common to all mammals. A rapid reflex not amenable to voluntary control, startle was studied extensively in 1929 by Strauss (1) and is the subject of a monograph by Landis and Hunt (2) and a more recent study by Gogan (3). In the human adult, except for minor interpersonal variations, a stereotyped motor pattern is seen, consisting of eye blinking, facial grimacing, flexion of the head, elevation of the shoulders, and flexion of the elbows, trunk, and knees. With repeated stimulation, the intensity of the surprise reaction decreases, but never completely disappears. Tension, fatigue, and heightened expectation of the stimulus enhance it. The intensity is greater in infancy where it appears at the same time as the Moro reflex (an extensor response to sudden stimuli). However, startle becomes more noticeable in time, while the Moro reflex disappears (4).

Animal studies, mostly in rats, demonstrated that the origin of the efferents of the audiogenic startle reflex, which involves several structures in the brainstem, is mediated by the bulbopontine median reticular formation (5–7). Habituation of the audiogenic startle reflex most likely results from synaptic depression of brainstem interneurons (8). The motor response in the normal auditory startle reflex in humans is also organized in the medial reticular formation, which may be activated by subcortical or cortically relayed afferent inputs (9). The specific motor response may result from a caudally and rostrally spreading single volley (9) or from a polysynaptically generated muscle activation organized by a reticular generator capable of spatiotemporal sequencing (8,10).

The pathophysiology of audiogenic startle in man was reviewed by Wilkins et al (11). This basic reflex can be present in a pathologically exaggerated form that is always embarrassing, sometimes interferes with normal activities,

and occasionally may be dangerous. The electromyogram (EMG) changes in subjects with abnormal startle response were well described by Gastaut and Villeneuve (12): isolated or grouped volleys of 10 to 12 elements with a latency of 10 to 40 ms (starting from the frontal muscles and going to those of the leg). According to the number of motor units recruited, the amplitude varied from 1 to 10 mV while the duration was of 20 to 60 ms. Activity of interferential type followed, sometimes after an interval of about 20 ms, and lasted from a fraction of a second to several seconds, thus lengthening the initial jerk. These muscle potentials were generalized to the agonist and antagonist muscular system without reciprocal innervation. Their amplitude decreased from the head and neck to the trunk, from the root of the limbs to their extremities, and from the upper to the lower limbs. More recent electrophysiologic studies by Brown et al (13) and by Matsumoto et al (14) have shown rostrocaudal propagation of the EMG motor responses from the orbicularis oculi, to the sternocleidomastoid, the masseter, and the musculature of the trunk and of the limbs. Brown et al (13) suggested that the physiologic and the pathologic audiogenic startle reflexes utilize the same bulbospinal efferents. Chokroverty et al (8) found that in a patient with clinically exaggerated startle the masseter response preceded that of the sternocleidomastoid response 90% of the time. They suggested the following electrophysiologic criteria, as measured by EMG, to define the abnormal startle reflex: 1) excessive duration of the myogenic response, 2) persistence of extracranial muscular contractions after two bursts of consecutive stimuli, and 3) reduced habituation.

Abnormal, excessive startle is a feature of three distinct conditions: startle disease or hyperekplexia, "jumping" (the "jumping Frenchmen of Maine"), and startle epilepsy (Table 68.1). The first of these three disorders is described in this chapter.

Table 68.1   Startle Disorders of Humans

	Startle Disease or Hyperekplexia	Jumping	Startle Epilepsy
Onset	Birth, rarely later	Variable	Variable
Excessive startle	+	+	+
Stiffness	+	−	−
Generalized hyperreflexia	+	−	−
Attacks of spontaneous clonus	+	−	−
Falling	+	Rarely	With some attack patterns
Insecure gait	+	−	±
Echolalia	−	+	−
Echopraxia	−	+	−
Forced obedience	−	+	−
Crying out, swearing	−	+	−
Fighting stance	−	+	−
Epileptic seizures, nonstartle related	Rarely	−	Sometimes
Epileptogenic EEG abnormality	Rarely	−	Usually
Inheritance	Autosomal dominant; autosomal recessive; or sporadic	Autosomal dominant with variable penetrance	Acquired
Treatment	Valproic acid, clonazepam	Clonazepam?	Antiepileptic drugs, clonazepam?

Case Study

Twenty years ago a mother brought her two girls, who had been diagnosed and treated for epilepsy, complaining that the older girl was falling when startled. Both girls had a mechanical, broad-based gait that suggested cerebellar dysfunction, but they were not ataxic. They were hyperreflexic. Since extensive questioning did not solve the problem, a kidney basin was dropped to the stone floor and the older girl fell forward like a log, hit her head on the foot of the metal examining table, and began to cry. This response was far greater than anticipated. The patient, the family, and the examiner were quite mortified, and the girl has always been wary in her neurologist's presence since.

Kirstein and Silfverskiold first described startle disease in 1958 (15). Two sisters, their father, and the daughter of one of the sisters suffered from sudden violent falls precipitated by stress, fright, or surprise. Three of these family members also had nocturnal myoclonus. The authors cautiously considered the disorder to represent an unusual, genetically determined form of drop seizures.

In a letter to Lancet in 1962, Kok and Bruyn (16) drew attention to a hereditary disease affecting 29 individuals in six generations of a German-Dutch family with 127 members. In 1966, Suhren (née Kok) et al (17) described this family in much greater detail. The affected individuals had a strikingly excessive response to startle elicited by visual, auditory, and proprioceptive stimuli that failed to produce a response in most normal individuals. These authors coined the term *hyperexplexia* (excessive jerking or jumping) to describe the condition. The disorder occurred in two forms: a minor form in which the response

was quantitatively different from normal (i.e., the startle response was more violent), and a major form in which there were also additional clinical symptoms. In the major form, patients when startled experienced momentary generalized muscular stiffness with loss of voluntary postural control causing them to fall, as if frozen, with their arms at their sides, unable to carry out protective movements. As soon as they hit the ground, muscle tone and control of voluntary movements returned, and there was never evidence of loss of consciousness. Kirstein and Silfverskiold (15) described brief loss of consciousness in association with these falls, but this was probably related to concussion. Urinary incontinence may occur and is probably due to increased intra-abdominal pressure associated with the extensor spasm. This abnormal response was almost always present from the time the affected child first attempted to walk. It was increased by emotional tension, nervousness, fatigue, and the expectation of being frightened, while alcohol, phenobarbital, and chlordiazepoxide lessened its intensity to some degree.

In the major form of hyperekplexia, there was also transient generalized hypertonia during infancy. As babies, when awakened or handled, affected individuals had an immediate increase in muscle tone in flexion that disappeared during sleep. This abnormality diminished as spontaneous activity increased during the first year of life. About the time of its disappearance, frequent, violent, and often repetitive jerks of the limbs were described as the child fell asleep. The jerks could lift the child off the bed.

The neonatal form of this condition was redescribed by Klein et al (18) as a "familial congenital disorder resembling stiff-man syndrome" occurring in 10 individuals from three generations of a family. The family stressed the onset of stiffness within 4 or 5 hours after birth, the absence of crawling (with the children scooting about in a seated position propelling themselves with their arms), and some delay in walking. Stiffness disappeared during sleep. Difficulty in swallowing and frequent choking were also described. The infants had hard, tense shoulder girdle muscles and faces set in a somewhat unhappy and inappropriate expression. Lingam et al (19), in a second report on the hereditary stiff-baby syndrome, suggested the identity of this condition with startle disease. The infants have a high incidence of umbilical and other hernias, previously noted by Suhren et al (17) and probably related to their hypertonicity. A boy with a convincing history of hyperekplexia also had a thoracic meningomyelocele, Arnold–Chiari malformation, and hydrocephalus (20). The disorders could be fortuitously associated but intrauterine hypertonicity could perhaps be a factor in the development of the closure defect. Interestingly, the symptoms of hyperekplexia were relieved by surgical decompression of the cervicomedullary region. Exceptionally the symptoms of startle disease will arise later in life. Dooley and Andermann (21) studied an adolescent boy with normal neonatal history who developed generalized stiffness, which made it impossible for him to take part in sports, as well as falling attacks. Rare members of the family described by Suhren et al (17) also had onset of symptoms later than in the neonatal period. Apnea due to spasm of respiratory muscles may also occur and has sometimes led to the children's death (17,22–24).

A positive family history may be difficult to elicit in this condition because of this phenotypic variation. In the first family we described, the disorder was obvious in the proband and her sister. Only the minor form was present in the probands, children, and only when they were ill. For years, it was impossible to obtain a history of abnormal startle from either of the proband's parents. Eventually it became clear that, in the years leading up to the mother's divorce from her alcoholic husband, she startled excessively and literally jumped off her chair when the telephone rang. Thus autosomal dominant inheritance with variable expressivity was again confirmed. In the second family reported by us, however, no other member was found to be affected by either the major or the minor form, even on intensive questioning. This may be explained by a new mutation in the proband or by lack of penetrance of the gene in other family members. One sporadic patient with this disease was also described by Boudouresques et al in 1964 (25) and Saenz-Lope et al (26) described three additional sporadic patients and five affected siblings.

Gastaut and Villeneuve (12) in 1967 reported in detail 12 patients with sporadic startle disease. The authors stressed the psychogenic precipitation of startle and falling. Eleven of their patients had falling attacks and in at least one these were, according to their description, identical to those occurring in familial cases. The incidence of mild retardation or low intelligence was higher than expected and

similar to that noticed by Andermann et al (27) and by Suhren et al (17). Nine had nocturnal jerking of the legs. The authors felt that their patients were different from those described by Suhren et al, although it seems likely that at least some of them had the same disorder but without an obvious family history. They corrected the Greek spelling to *hyperekplexia* rather than *hyperexplexia* and this spelling has been generally used since.

There is no good evidence that the patients with sporadic startle disease differ from the familial cases described by Suhren et al (17), as Gastaut and Villeneuve (12) have suggested. Our own cases, familial or sporadic, appeared to have the same syndrome. These two forms would thus appear to represent a single genetically determined disorder.

Using systematic linkage analyses in several unrelated families with the major form of hyperekplexia, Ryan et al (22,28) identified the locus of the major form of hyperekplexia on the distal portion of the long arm of chromosome 5 (5q33–q35), an area that contains the genes for several neurotransmitter receptors, including glycine receptors. Subsequent sequence analysis of the gene encoding for the alpha$_1$ subunit of the inhibitory glycine receptor (GLRA1) revealed two different missense mutations occurring in the same base pair of exon 6 of GLRA1. These mutations replace arginine at position 271 with either leucine or glutamine (G1192A and G1192T) (29–31). GLRA1 is a constituent of the inhibitory glycine receptor in the mammalian central nervous system and is antagonized by strychnine, which in sublethal doses in the mouse causes hypertonia and an exaggerated startle response comparable to the symptoms in hyperekplexia (32,33). Agonist binding to GLRA1 initiates the opening of a chloride-selective channel that modulates the neuronal membrane potential (34). These mutations reduce the glycine sensitivity of GLRA1 (35,36) and result in the redistribution of GLRA1 single-channel conductances to lower conductance levels (37). We analyzed this gene in a family of Swiss-Italian origin and found a G1192A mutation changing an ARG to a LEU codon in three affected females with major startle disease (30,38).

The major and minor forms of startle disease can occur in the same family, as illustrated in the large family reported by Suhren et al (17) and those reported by Andermann et al (27,39,40) and by Dooley and Andermann (21). The minor form of the disease, which must be distinguished from psychogenic startle (41), consists only of excessive startle (17,23,24,27). A parent with the minor form can have children with the major form and vice versa, but siblings tend to be affected to the same degree. Therefore it is likely, as Suhren et al have suggested, that these two forms represent different phenotypic expressions of the same (autosomal dominant) gene. Recent reports, however, showed that only clinically typical or major hyperekplexia is consistently associated with GLRA1 (G1192A) mutations (42). Tijssen et al (31) reanalyzed the family described in 1966 by Suhren et al (17) and observed that patients with the minor form never transmitted the major form and found the mutation of the GLRA1 receptor only in patients with a major form of the disorder. They postulated that the minor form could represent a variant of the physiologic startle reaction.

Based on clinical observations, Hayashi et al (43,44) suggested the possibility of recessive transmission of the disorder in some families. Rees et al (45) recently reported a different mutation in the same exon of GLRA1 also causing a recessive form of the disease in a 22-year-old girl with major startle disease.

We recently examined four individuals from four families with the major form of hyperekplexia in whom all the described GLRA1 mutations were not found. A recent report in another family (46) confirmed our observation. It is therefore evident that the clinical phenotypes of hyperekplexia, both the major and the minor form, can result from more than one genetic abnormality, providing evidence for genetic heterogeneity. The three strains of mutant mouse that bear a striking resemblance to the startle disease phenotype are *spastic* (33,47), *spasmodic* (48), and *oscillator* (49). These animals have a genetic defect involving glycine receptors (32,33). In the case of *spasmodic*, a missense mutation in the alpha$_1$ subunit gene has been identified (32,50). A defect in the glycine receptor beta-subunit has been found in *spastic* (33). In humans, mutations in other subunits of the glycine receptor that are defective remain to be discovered (51).

Suhren et al (17) and Gastaut and Villeneuve (12) suggested that, as jerking of the legs occurred only at night, it presumably represented an exaggerated form of hypnagogic myoclonus. Two of our patients had such attacks in the daytime as well, and all limbs were involved, although the legs always more than the arms. When the attacks occurred at night, the patients woke with a feeling described as unsteadiness, similar to their diurnal state when unexpected stimuli would be particularly likely to provoke a fall. The jerking would begin later, lasting for several minutes. There were no electrographic features to suggest an epileptic etiology. Clinically, these attacks strongly resembled spontaneous generalized clonus, most marked in the lower extremities and usually triggered by emotion. De Groen and Kamphuisen (52) studied the periodic nocturnal myoclonic jerks of one of Suhren and Bruyn's patients. They concluded that these were due to spontaneous arousal reactions caused mainly by increase in excitability of motor neurons, hyperexcitability of the brainstem arousal system, and markedly increased influence of respiratory variables on reticular hyperexcitability.

The electroencephalographic (EEG) correlates of startle were similar in the patients reported by Suhren et al (17), Andermann et al (27), and Gastaut and Villeneuve (12). The EEG response consisted of an initial spike recorded from the centroparietal vertex followed by a short-lasting train of slow waves, and then by desynchronization of background activity lasting 2 to 3 seconds. The response was abolished by intravenous diazepam. This complex discharge, the most consistent electrographic correlate of excessive startle, may represent an evoked response to various sensory stimuli. Averaged somatosensory, visual, and brainstem auditory evoked responses, however, have shown no significant abnormality in patients with the major form of startle disease, according to Rosenblatt and Majnemer (personal communication).

Other polygraphic features were sudden lowering of skin resistance, variable but often persistent tachycardia, rise of arterial blood pressure (mainly systolic), and a fall in systolic peripheral blood flow. Frequently the most intense stimuli induced, after the early muscular potential, an interferential muscular activity sufficient to engender a tonic spasm lasting several seconds. The spasm was accompanied by a vegetative discharge bringing on an apnea lasting several seconds and a heart rate accelerated by 100% (52).

In their review, Wilkins et al (11) suggested that hyperekplexia could represent the known combination of reticular reflex myoclonus and cortical reflex myoclonus as described by Hallet et al (53). They tentatively concluded that hyperekplexia should be considered as an independent phenomenon within the spectrum of stimulus-sensitive myoclonic disorders. Spasticity, hyperreflexia, and muscle stiffness in patients with hyperekplexia are probably not related to spinal hyperexcitability. Testing spinal inhibitory pathways in five patients with hereditary hyperekplexia, Floeter et al (54) found definite abnormalities only in one of the two forms of inhibition mediated by glycinergic interneurons. Fariello et al (55) reported the case of a patient in whom a posterior infarction involving the subthalamic nucleus and the dentatorubroventrolateral thalamic pathway led to the reappearance of a preexisting hyperekplexia. They postulated that interruption of the thalamic pathways can eliminate the descending inhibition of the startle reflex. Hochman et al (56) reported a patient with hyperekplexia with decreased cerebral blood flow in the frontal lobe using single photon emission computed tomography (SPECT), and assumed that this abnormality could represent a functional cortical abnormality involving a descending pathway that normally inhibits the startle reflex. The widespread nature of hyperexcitability in hyperekplexia is corroborated by the EEG abnormalities (57) and the enlarged somatosensory evoked potentials (13,55,58) found in some of the patients. Our results of proton magnetic resonance spectroscopy imaging studies in four patients with familial hyperekplexia show a variable degree of neuronal dysfunction (i.e., reduction of the relative NAA resonance intensity) in both frontocentral regions. This finding agrees with the hypothesis of a facilitatory role of cortical dysfunction in sensorimotor pathways leading to the generation of the pathologic startle reaction seen in some patients with familial hyperekplexia.

Suhren et al (17) considered the disorder to be nonepileptic. They believed that the abnormality in these patients probably resulted from retarded maturation of control of brainstem centers by higher inhibitory mechanisms, particularly by the rhombomesencephalic reticular formation. However, epileptogenic EEG abnormalities were found in several of their patients who fell, and many had excessive slow activity that they attributed to the repeated head injuries. Some patients, though, display evidence of more widespread cerebral dysfunction not explainable by a maturational defect in a specific system alone, and unlikely to be due merely to the repeated falls. One of the patients of Andermann et al (27) had an active generalized spike–wave discharge and another had a parietal sharp wave focus; neither had epileptic seizures or episodes other than the specific clinical phenomena just described. Indeed, the spike–wave discharge was blocked by startle. Several of the patients reported by Gastaut and Villeneuve (12) had a low convulsive threshold, and one had seizures as well. Four of their patients had, or were suspected to have, mild mental retardation. Low average intelligence was also encountered in two of the three patients of Andermann et al (27) with the major form, suggesting diffuse cerebral dysfunction. The hypertonicity and hyperreflexia implies an abnormality of the pyramidal system. No pathologic studies of individuals with these conditions are available.

The diagnosis of startle disease should not be difficult if one is aware of this syndrome. The condition is probably rare, and one would suspect that it is commonly misdiagnosed as epilepsy, as it was at first in most patients. Hypertonia in infancy is easily misinterpreted as spastic quadriplegia, as it was in the cases of Andermann et al (27), where its disappearance was quite baffling. The most puzzling symptom is the unsteady gait that the physician may attribute to a cerebellar disorder instead of the uncertainty and fear of falling, which actually causes it.

The course of the condition is variable (59). Some patients with early onset eventually improve, whereas in others the symptoms only arise or increase later in life. In our patients there has been little change over the years, although on the whole the manifestations were more severe in childhood, when the hypertonicity was striking and the falls very frequent. The disorder is not entirely benign considering the risk of sudden death in infancy attributable to spasm of respiratory muscles and also the possible complication of hernias. Later, patients may suffer multiple fractures including skull fractures as well as repeated lacerations and cerebral concussions.

At the present time clonazepam (22,38), a benzodiazepine and potent serotonin agonist, and valproic acid appear to be the drugs of choice in the treatment of this condition. In small doses (0.1 mg/kg), clonazepam abolishes the falling attacks and greatly reduces the episodic jerking. There is a remarkable disappearance of the uncertainty of the gait and patients walk more freely, no longer holding hands or continuously touching the wall. Although clonazepam does not cause the startle response to return to normal, its effect is greater than that of diazepam, and appears to be sustained. Excessive backward jerking of the

head elicited by tapping the forehead or nose (60) persists and appears to represent residual reticular reflex myoclonus. Under conditions of exceptional emotional stress, falling or nocturnal leg jerking occasionally recur. The effect of clonazepam suggests that a serotoninergic mechanism may be involved. Valproic acid abolished the clinical manifestations in a patient studied by Dooley and Andermann (21). Alcohol, phenobarbital, phenytoin, primidone, and chlordiazepoxide, although they have some effect on the falling attacks, startle, and repetitive jerks, are not the drugs of choice for treatment of this disorder. According to Saenz-Lope et al (61) 5-hydroxytryiptophan and piracetam may also be helpful. When intelligence is normal and the symptoms are successfully treated, people affected with this disorder lead normal lives. Genetic counseling and close supervision during delivery of babies at risk and during infancy are indicated.

REFERENCES

1. Strauss H. Das Zusammenschrecken. Experimentell kinematographische Studie zur Physiologie und Pathophysiologie der Reaktivbewegungen. J Psychol Neurol 1929;39:111–231.
2. Landis C, Hunt WA. The startle pattern. New York: Ferrar and Rinehart, 1939.
3. Gogan P. The startle and orienting reactions in man. A study of their characteristics and habituation. Brain Res 1970;18:117–135.
4. Goldstein K, Landis C, Hunt WA, Clarke FM. Moro reflex and startle pattern. Arch Neurol Psychiatry 1938;40:322–377.
5. Davis M. The mammalian startle response. In: Neuronal mechanisms of startle behavior. New York: Plenum, 1984:287–351.
6. Davis M, Gendelman DS, Tischler MD, Gendelman DM. A primary acoustic startle circuit: lesion and stimulation studies. J Neurosci 1982;2:791–805.
7. Leitner DS, Powers AS, Hoffman HS. The neural substrate of the startle response. Physiol Behav 1980;25:291–297.
8. Chokroverty S, Walczak T, Hening W. Human startle reflex: technique and criteria for abnormal response. Electroencephal Clin Neurophysiol 1992;85:236–242.
9. Brown P, Rothwell JC, Thompson PD, et al. New observations on the normal auditory startle reflex in man. Brain 1991;114:1891–1902.
10. Bisdorff AR, Bronstein AM, Gresty MA. Responses in neck and facial muscles to sudden free fall and a startling auditory stimulus. Electroencephal Clin Neurophysiol 1994;93:409–416.
11. Wilkins DE, Hallett M, Wess MM. Audiogenic startle reflex of man and its relationship to startle syndromes. A review. Brain 1986;109:561–573.
12. Gastaut H, Villeneuve A. The startle disease or hyperekplexia. Pathological surprise reaction. J Neurol Sci 1967;5:523–542.
13. Brown P, Rothwell JC, Thompson PD, et al. The hyperekplexias and their relationship to the normal startle reflex. Brain 1991;114:1903–1928.
14. Matsumoto J, Fuhr P, Nigro M, Hallett M. Physiological abnormalities in hereditary hyperekplexia. Ann Neurol 1992;32:41–50.
15. Kirstein L, Silfverskiold B. A family with emotionally precipitated drop seizures. Lancet 1958;33:471–476.
16. Kok O, Bruyn GW. An unidentified hereditary disease (letter). Lancet 1962;1:1359.
17. Suhren AL, Bruyn GW, Tuyman JA. Hyperekplexia: a hereditary startle syndrome. J Neurolog Sci 1966;3:577–586.
18. Klein R, Haddow JE, DeLuca C. Familial congenital disorder resembling stiff-man syndrome. Am J Dis Child 1972;124:730–731.
19. Lingam S, Wilson J, Hart EW. Hereditary stiff-baby syndrome. Am J Dis Child 1981;135:909–911.
20. Winston K, Hyperekplexia relieved by surgical decompression of the cervicomedullary region. Neurosurgery 1983;13:708–710.
21. Dooley JM, Andermann F. Startle disease or hyperekplexia: adolescent onset and response to valproate. Pediatr Neurol 1989;5:126–127.
22. Ryan SG, Sherman SL, Terry JC, et al. Startle disease, or hyperekplexia: response to clonazepam and assignment of the gene (STHE) to chromosome 5q by linkage analysis. Ann Neurol 1992;31:663–668.

23. Vigevano F, Di Capua M, Dalla-Bernardina B. Startle disease: an avoidable cause of sudden infant death (letter). Lancet 1989;1:216.
24. Kurczynski TW. Hyperexplexia. Arch Neurol 1983;40:246–248.
25. Boudouresques J, Roger J, Tassinari CA, et al. Réflexions à propos d'un sursaut pathologique. Rev Neurol (Paris) 1964;111:561–570.
26. Saenz-Lope E, Herranz FJ, Masdeu JC. Startle epilepsy: a clinical study. Ann Neurol 1984;16:78–81.
27. Andermann F, Keene DL, Andermann E, Quesney LF. Startle disease or hyperekplexia: further delineation of the syndrome. Brain 1980;103:985–997.
28. Ryan SG, Dixon MJ, Nigro MA, et al. Genetic and radiation hybrid mapping of the hyperekplexia region on chromosome 5q. Am J Hum Genet 1992;51:1334–1343.
29. Shiang R, Ryan SG, Zhu YZ, et al. Mutations in the alpha 1 subunit of the inhibitory glycine receptor cause the dominant neurologic disorder, hyperekplexia. Nat Genet 1993;5:351–358.
30. Schorderet DF, Pescia G, Bernasconi A, Regli F. An additional family with startle disease and a G1192A mutation at the alpha 1 subunit of the inhibitory glycine receptor gene. Hum Mol Genet 1994;3:1201.
31. Tijssen MA, Shiang R, van Deutekom J, et al. Molecular genetic reevaluation of the Dutch hyperekplexia family. Arch Neurol 1995;52:578–582.
32. Ryan SG, Buckwalter MS, Lynch JW, et al. A missense mutation in the gene encoding the alpha 1 subunit of the inhibitory glycine receptor in the spasmodic mouse. Nat Genet 1994;7:131–135.
33. Kingsmore SF, Giros B, Suh D, et al. Glycine receptor beta-subunit gene mutation in spastic mouse associated with LINE-1 element insertion. Nat Genet 1994;7:136–141.
34. Grenningloh G, Rienitz A, Schmitt B, et al. The strychnine-binding subunit of the glycine receptor shows homology with nicotinin acetylcholine receptors. Nature 1987;328:215–220.
35. Rajendra S, Lynch JW, Pierce KD, et al. Startle disease mutations reduce the agonist sensitivity of the human inhibitory glycine receptor. J Biol Chem 1994;269:18739–18742.
36. Langosch D, Laube B, Rundstrom N, et al. Decreased agonist affinity and chloride conductance of mutant glycine receptors associated with human hereditary hyperekplexia. EMBO J 1994;13:4223–4228.
37. Rajendra S, Lynch JW, Pierce KD, et al. Mutation of an arginine residue in the human glycine receptor transforms B-alanine and taurine from agonist into competitive antagonists. Neuron 1995;14:169–175.
38. Bernasconi A, Regli F, Schorderet DF, Pescia G. Familial hyperekplexia—a startle disease. Rev Neurol (Paris) 1996;152:447–450.
39. Andermann F, Andermann E. Startle disease, or hyperekplexia (letter). Ann Neurol 1984;16:367–368.
40. Andermann F, Andermann E. Excessive startle syndromes: startle disease, jumping, and startle epilepsy. Adv Neurol 1986;43:321–338.
41. Thompson PD, Colebatch JG, Brown P, et al. Voluntary stimulus-sensitive jerks and jumps mimicking myoclonus or pathological startle syndromes. Mov Disord 1992;7:257–262.
42. Shiang R, Ryan SG, Zhu YZ, et al. Mutational analysis of familial and sporadic hyperekplexia. Ann Neurol 1995;38:85–91.
43. Hayashi T, Tachibana H, Kajii T. Hyperekplexia: pedigree studies in two families. Am J Med Genet 1991;40:138–143.
44. Hayashi T, Kajii T. Autosomal recessive startle disorder (letter; comment). Acta Pediatr 1993;82:124.
45. Rees MI, Andrew M, Jawad S, Owen MJ. Evidence for recessive as well as dominant forms of startle disease (hyperekplexia) caused by mutations in the alpha 1 subunit of the inhibitory glycine receptor. Hum Mol Genet 1994;3:2175–2179.
46. Turecki G, Grandmaison F, Lemieux B, Rouleau G. Hyperexplexia and the alpha-1 subunit glycine receptors gene (GLRA1). Arch Neurol 1996;53:836–837.
47. Heller AH, Hallett M. Electrophysiological studies with the *spastic* mutant mouse. Brain Res 1982;234:299–308.
48. Buckwalter MS, Testa CM, Noebels JL, Camper SA. Genetic mapping and evaluation of candidate genes for *spasmodic*, a neurological mouse mutation with abnormal startle response. Genomics 1993;17:279–286.
49. Buckwalter MS, Cook SA, Davisson MT, White WF, Camper SA. A frameshift mutation in the mouse alpha 1 glycine receptor gene (Glra1) results in progressive neurological symptoms and juvenile death. Hum Mol Genet 1994;3:2025–2030.
50. Saul B, Schmieden V, Kling C, et al. Point mutation of glycine receptor alpha 1 subunit in the *spasmodic* mouse affects agonist responses. FEBS Lett 1994;350:71–76.
51. Rajendra S, Schofield PR. Molecular mechanisms of inherited startle syndromes. Trends Neurosci 1995;18:80–82.
52. de Groen JH, Kamphuisen HA. Periodic nocturnal myoclonus in a patient with hyperexplexia (startle disease). J Neurol Sci 1978;38:207–213.
53. Hallett M, Chadwick D, Marsden CD. Cortical reflex myoclonus. Neurology 1979;29:1107–1125.
54. Floeter MK, Andermann F, Andermann E, et al. Physiological studies of spinal inhibitory pathways in patients with hereditary hyperekplexia. Neurology 1996;46:766–772.
55. Fariello RG, Schwartzman RJ, Beall SS. Hyperekplexia exacerbated by occlusion of posterior thalamic arteries. Arch Neurol 1983;40:244–246.
56. Hochman MS, Chediak AD, Ziffer JA. Hyperekplexia: report of a nonfamilial adult onset case associated with obstructive sleep apnea and abnormal brain nuclear tomography. Sleep 1994;17:280–283.
57. Uesaka Y, Terao Y, Ugawa Y, et al. Magnetoencephalographic analysis of cortical myoclonic jerks. Electroencephal Clin Neurophysiol 1996;99:141–148.
58. Markand ON, Garg BP, Weaver DD. Familial startle disease (hyperexplexia). Electrophysiologic studies. Arch Neurol 1984;41:71–74.
59. Bruyn GW. Hyperekplexia (startle disease). In: Handbook of clinical neurology. Vol. 42. Amsterdam: North-Holland, 1981:228–229.
60. Shahar E, Brand N, Uziel Y, Barak Y. Nose tapping test inducing a generalized flexor spasm: a hallmark of hyperexplexia. Acta Paediatr 1991;80:1073–1077.
61. Saenz-Lope E, Herranz-Tanarro FJ, Masdeu JC, Chacon-Pena JR. Hyperekplexia: a syndrome of pathological startle responses. Ann Neurol 1984;15:36–41.

Startle Epilepsy

Frederick Andermann   Eva Andermann

The startle reflex is common to all mammals and its stereo-typed motor pattern leads to a posture that prepares them for flight. In humans this pattern consists of blinking, grimacing, and flexion of the head, elbows, trunk, and knees with elevation of the shoulders. The response is reduced with repeated stimulation and increased with tension, fatigue, and heightened expectation. It is increased in children and is distinct from the Moro reflex, which disappears in time.

The physiologic mechanism of the startle reflex has been reviewed by Gogan (1) and the pathophysiology by Wilkins et al (2). The physiologic response to startle may be enhanced and may usher in or trigger an epileptic seizure. This represents a form of reflex epilepsy where the startle reflex contributes the stimulus that activates the epileptic discharge and clinical manifestations.

Alajouanine and Gastaut (3) first described two types of abnormal startle associated with seizures occurring in individuals with infantile hemiparesis or quadriparesis and diffuse cerebral dysfunction: 1) startle synkinesis, consisting of a 5- to 10-sec tonic contraction of the affected side without other clinical or electrographic evidence of epileptic discharge, and 2) startle epilepsy where, in addition to this excessive response and tonic contraction, there are other clinical or electrographic epileptic manifestations. These patients also had clear evidence of lateralized or diffuse cerebral abnormality. The distinction between these two types of abnormal startle, however, was somewhat artificial, since surface epileptic discharges may not be striking or obvious in some patients, as subsequently shown by Bancaud et al (4,5).

Cases of startle-induced epileptic manifestations in patients with secondary generalized corticoreticular epilepsy have been described by Gastaut and Villeneuve (6), Bancaud et al (4), and by Ohtahara et al (7). Startle epilepsy has been also described in association with Sturge–Weber syndrome (8) and Down syndrome (9), and cases of startle epilepsy with impressive clinical histories but without good electrographic correlation continue to be presented in the literature (10–12). Activation by startle is relatively common in patients with partial epilepsy, particularly those whose symptoms and signs suggest involvement of the precentral and postcentral areas. Exceptionally, startle epilepsy may occur in patients with no neurologic abnormality and who have normal intelligence (13).

Imaging studies frequently show atrophic lesions, with a preponderance of mesial frontal areas of atrophy in 6 of 16 patients in the series reported by Aguglia et al (13). Inter-ictal frontal and/or central spikes were noted on electro-encephalographic (EEG) recording in over 50% of patients and could be brought out in over one-third (13). During sleep, frontal spike foci were found in all patients who had sleep recordings. In over 50%, startle seizures were the only seizure pattern and spontaneous attacks also occurred in the remainder. The clinical pattern of the attacks consisted of a bilateral startle reaction followed by a generalized tonic spasm (37.5%) or by a global atonic attack (6.25%), whereas a unilateral startle reaction was followed by hemitonic spasm (50%) or a hemiatonic attack (6.25%). The severity of this syndrome is probably overestimated as published series describe cases that are resistant to treatment. The neurologic examination is often abnormal and often shows hemiatrophy or spastic hemiparesis associated with hemisensory disturbance and hemiatrophy. Mental retardation is present in half of cases.

Implanted electrode studies were carried out by Bancaud et al (4) in a patient with hemiplegia and startle epilepsy. They demonstrated the origin of the seizures to be in the supplementary motor area, in the interhemispheric fissure. A second patient studied by Bancaud and his group (5) had excessive startle, at times without clear additional epileptic manifestations; at other times, startle was clearly associated with other epileptic features. The area of epileptogenic abnormality involved mesial frontal structures in the vicinity of the paracentral lobule. The authors concluded that the startle reflex may be responsible through a feedback mechanism for triggering the epileptic focus. Surgical treatment and removal of epileptogenic area in their first patient led to complete cessation of seizures and startle phenomena during a three-year follow-up.

A third study from this group by Chauvel et al (14) reviewed a group of 20 patients with a perinatal lesion, usually a porencephalic cyst. High-frequency ictal discharges occurred in the abnormal motor and premotor cortex including the supplementary motor area. They spread rapidly toward the mesial frontal area including the cingulate gyrus, the parietal lobe (the anterior portion of which was always included in the initial extent of the discharge), and especially to the contralateral frontal lobe. The ictal discharge was preceded by a high amplitude evoked response localized to the motor cortex and/or the supplementary motor area.

Attacks began as an intense startle reaction, followed by a complex partial motor seizure. Polygraphic studies showed that this startle pattern was asymmetric, predominant, or limited to the hemiplegic side, focused on one muscle, and subject to habituation. The seizure itself, either tonic or tonic–clonic, started in the limb (or muscle) first involved by the startle reflex and propagated to the corresponding contralateral limb as well as to the ipsilateral side. After the initial localized startle response, motor signs appeared. These were almost always tonic with flexion and abduction of the paretic arm, extension of the ipsilateral leg, and flexion of the head and trunk. The tonic motor signs then rapidly spread to the other side. Thus, a unilateral tonic seizure became bilateral, or a bilateral tonic seizure developed that predominated over the paretic side. The seizure then continued with tonic, tonic–clonic, or clonic manifestations. If the patient was standing, he would fall. There was often tonic adversion of the head away from the side of origin. Speech arrest occurred. Consciousness may be altered but loss of memory for the attack was rare. There were intense autonomic manifestations with flushing and mydriasis. Seizures usually lasted from 10 to 30 seconds and only rarely more than one minute. Patients could use their nonparetic hand to hold on to the affected arm and said this may arrest the seizure. Initial sensory manifestations were rare.

Spontaneous seizures also occur in patients with startle seizures but may be rare. These are more often tonic attacks, and rarely clonic or other seizures.

Activation of a diffusely abnormal cortex by the startle reflex can lead to the generalized spike and wave discharges accompanied by a massive myoclonic jerk described by Gastaut and Villeneuve (6), Gastaut and Tassinari (15), and in some of their patients by Gimenez-Roldan and Martin (16). This illustrates that startle-induced epileptic events can occasionally be a feature of secondary generalized epilepsy, just as startle can activate partial cortical epileptic discharge.

According to Gastaut and Broughton (17), conventional anticonvulsant drug therapy is of little value in the treatment of startle epilepsy, although some patients with partial epilepsy respond to carbamazepine (18). Booker et al (19) suggested that extinction techniques may be useful in the treatment of this condition, but this approach has met with little acceptance. Chlordiazepoxide was found effective in the treatment of a patient with startle epilepsy as early as 1961 (20). Recently, Gimenez-Roldan and Martin (16) have shown the effectiveness of clonazepam in treating startle-induced seizures in children. Two patients with hemiparesis who had startle seizures as the only epileptic manifestation remained permanently controlled after a mean of 34 months of continuous therapy. Startle-induced seizures reoccurred after one and four years, respectively, in two patients with the Lennox–Gastaut syndrome. The authors postulated that clonazepam inhibits abnormal brainstem mechanisms mediating pathologically enhanced startle reactions in these patients, thus avoiding activation of a discharging focus in the vicinity of the supplementary motor area. The reported effect of clonazepam further supports the concept of a common pathway in the pathophysiology of startle disorders. In our experience, however, clonazepam was ineffective in controlling startle epilepsy in three young adults with this disorder. Aguglia et al (13) found clobazam effective in arresting startle attacks in 61% of their patients and it reduced the frequency of these attacks by two-thirds in another 23%, whereas 15% were unresponsive to the drug. In 75% of those initially controlled, the effect was maintained for a mean of two years.

Reduction in startle seizures or startle myoclonus was also found following anterior callosal section in one patient (21). The operation initially led to a reduction of nonstartle-related epileptic events. The addition of clonazepam proved to be more effective than it has been prior to callosotomy in reducing the startle-dependent attacks.

In summary, in patients with cerebral dysfunction startle may activate either focal or generalized epileptic discharges, although the former have been much better studied than the latter. The startle response itself may be abnormal or excessive in these patients, and on the other hand, there may be focal or diffuse cortical hyperexcitability in response to the startle reflex. Finally, in some patients diffuse encephalopathies may affect the same neuronal systems and lead to similar clinical manifestation as are found in genetically determined startle disease. Occurrence of such nonepileptic abnormal startle in patients with diffuse encephalopathy has been suggested by Gastaut and Villeneuve (6).

Clinical, genetic, electrographic, and imaging studies enable a definite diagnosis to be made in most people with abnormal startle with or without associated epileptic seizures.

REFERENCES

1. Gogan P. The startle and orienting reactions in man: a study of their characteristics and habituation. Brain Res 1970;18:117–135.
2. Wilkins DE, Hallett M, Wess MM. Audiogenic startle reflex of man and its relationship to startle syndromes. Brain 1986;109:561–573.
3. Alajouanine T, Gastaut H. La syncinésie-sursaut et l'épilepsie-sursaut à déclanchement sensoriel ou sensitif inopiné. Rev Neurol (Paris) 1955;93:29–41.
4. Bancaud J, Talairach J, Bonis A. Physiopathogénie des épilepsies-sursaut: a propos d'une épilepsie de l'aire motrice supplémentaire. Rev Neurol (Paris) 1967;117:441–453.
5. Bancaud J, Talairach J, Lamarche M, et al. Hypothèses neurophysiopathologiques sur l'épilepsie-sursaut chez l'homme. Rev Neurol (Paris) 1975;131:559–571.
6. Gastaut H, Villeneuve A. The startle disease or hyperekplexia: pathological surprise reaction. J Neurol Sci 1967;5:523–542.
7. Ohtahara S, Oka E, Ban T, et al. Startle epilepsy with the Lennox syndrome. Rinsho Shinkeigaku 1971;11:201–207.
8. Nakamura M, Kanai H, Miyamoto Y, et al. A case of Sturge–Weber syndrome with startle epilepsy. No To Shinkei 1975;27:325–331.
9. Gimenez-Roldan S, Martin M. Startle epilepsy complicating Down syndrome during adulthood. Ann Neurol 1980;7:78–80.
10. Baier WK. The startle disease in brain-damaged patients: report of a case. Neuropaediatrie 1980;11:72–75.
11. Bermejo PF, Peralta AMR, Picornell DI. Epilepsia sobresalto. A proposito de un caso. Arch Neurobiol 1975;38:247–259.
12. Bhandari B, Gupta BM, Garg AR. Touch epilepsy. Indian J Pediatr 1973;40:111–113.
13. Aguglia U, Tinuper P, Gastaut H. Startle induced epileptic seizures. Epilepsia 1984;25:712–720.
14. Chauvel P, Liegeois C, Chodkiewicz JP, et al. Startle epilepsy with infantile hemiplegia: the physiopathological data leading to surgical therapy. Abstracts of the 15th Epilepsy International Symposium 1983:180.
15. Gastaut H, Tassinari CA. Triggering mechanisms in epilepsy: the electroclinical point of view. Epilepsia 1966;7:85–135.
16. Gimenez-Roldan S, Martin M. Effectiveness of clonazepam in startle-induced seizures. Epilepsia 1979;20:555–561.
17. Gastaut H, Broughton R. Epileptic seizures. Clinical and electrographic features. Diagnosis and treatment. Springfield: Charles C Thomas, 1972:153–155.
18. Saenz-Lope E, Herranz FJ, Masdeu JC. Startle epilepsy; a clinical study. Ann Neurol 1984;16:78–81.
19. Booker HE, Forster FM, Klove H. Extinction factors in startle (acousticomotor) seizures. Neurology 1965;15:1095–1103.
20. Cohen NH, McAuliffe M, Aird R. Startle epilepsy treated with chlordiazepoxide (Librium). Dis Nerv Syst 1961;22:20–27.
21. Avila JO, Radvany J, Huck FR, et al. Anterior callosotomy as a substitute for hemispherectomy. Acta Neurochir 1980;30(suppl):137–143.

Ballismus, Chorea, and Athetosis

Ballism

Jeremy M. Shefner

Ballism is a movement disorder of particular interest because of its precise relationship to lesions in a very localized area of the brain. While exceptions have been reported, the vast majority of cases of ballism occur in association with damage to the subthalamic nucleus or its outflow tracts. With the possible exception of Parkinson's disease, this specificity is unmatched by any other movement disorder. The invariance of the relationship between clinical findings and pathology is probably the reason that appropriate anatomic localization for this disorder was made as early as 1897 (1).

CLINICAL DESCRIPTION

According to the Ad hoc Committee Classification of Extrapyramidal Disorders (2), ballism is defined as involuntary limb movements that are violent and flinging in nature; when unilateral, they are called "hemiballism." Whittier (3), in his extensive review, attributed the term *hemiballism* to Kussmaul in 1895; others at approximately the same time described similar patients but viewed the movements as a form of chorea (4).

Early case reports provide quite complete descriptions of the clinical syndrome. Typically, abnormal movements begin suddenly, often without warning (5). The arm is usually affected first, and rarely may be the only limb involved. More often, both arm and leg participate in wild, rapid flinging movements that occur at irregular intervals. Movements originate proximally within a limb and are often most extreme in shoulder and hip girdle musculature. These is usually a clear rotatory component to the movement, which is more clear in the arms than the legs. In a study reviewing the world's literature on hemiballism prior to 1950, all patients reported had abnormal upper extremity movements, and all but one had lower extremity movements (6).

Two-thirds of the patients in this series had abnormal facial movements as well, with a smaller percentage exhibiting glossal and palatal movements. Despite this, however, most patients are able to eat. With great effort on the part of the patient, movements can usually be controlled for periods of seconds. Generalized arousal increases the frequency and amplitude of movements, which are often violent enough to cause lacerations and bruises because of the limb banging against bedrails and other furniture. Movements are strikingly reduced when the patient is relaxed, and entirely absent during sleep.

Limbs involved in hemiballistic movements usually have normal strength. Tone may be normal, increased, or decreased, but most often is slightly reduced. Deep tendon reflexes are either unchanged or mildly reduced. While gross sensation is usually normal, some patients will report an initial, transient hyperalgesia of limbs affected by the movement disorder. In a series of 14 patients with hemiballism, four reported initial hyperalgesia (7). Other signs sometimes associated with hemiballism include confusion and agitation (8,9), speech difficulties, and hemianopia (6).

Ballism occurs considerably less frequently than hemiballism, usually as a result of bilaterally symmetric or diffuse processes. Hoogstraten et al (10) found 12 cases reported in the literature. They described a patient in which bilateral ballistic movements began six weeks postpartum and involved flinging movements of both arms, abnormal facial movements, and continuous movements of both legs. As in cases of hemiballism, movements were violent enough to cause multiple ecchymoses and lacerations, but disappeared during sleep. CT scan showed a single right frontotemporal lesion.

As will be discussed later, the most common etiology for hemiballism is infarction/hemorrhage in the deep gray matter; it is not surprising, then, that the age of onset of hemiballism coincides well with the average age of onset of symptomatic cerebral vascular disease in general. Average age of the patients reported before 1950 was 64 years, with a slight female predominance (3,6). Age of onset in more recent series was 75 years (11), 67 years (12), and 48 years (13), with the younger age reported in the latter series due to the fact that stroke was thought to be the etiology in less than half of the patients.

In most early reports, hemiballism, once established, persisted relatively unchanged until the patient's death, usually within six weeks, although occasional long-term survival was noted. Death was often attributed to exhaustion. However, although the natural history of more recent cases has been complicated by the effects of treatment, most recent reports do not confirm the grave prognosis initially suggested. Of the 14 patients discussed by Hyland and Forman (7), 10 recovered spontaneously over the course of five days to three months. In two additional patients, recovery was associated with drug therapy. Most of the 21 patients studied by Dewy and Jankovic (13) were treated with a variety of drugs; however, approximately 25% of their patients showed spontaneous recovery without drugs; 75% showed good recovery with or without medication. The severity of hemiballism can wax and wane; Bedwell (14) reported a patient in whom episodic hemiballism was noted in association with increased blood sugar, and Martin (15) discussed a patient with chronic hemiballism whose movements normalized with febrile illnesses.

ANATOMY AND PATHOPHYSIOLOGY

The clinical syndrome of hemiballism has been associated with lesions of the subthalamus since approximately 1900. Martin, in 1927, reviewed the world's literature on hemiballism and found 12 reports with associated pathology (8). Eleven of the twelve patients had lesions in the area of the contralateral subthalamus, but in most patients lesions were either multiple or so large that multiple white and grey matter structures were affected. Pathology in two patients (16,17), however, showed lesions that were restricted to the subthalamus. Martin himself reported a case of hemiballism in which a small hemorrhage was seen nearly limited to the contralateral subthalamus, although minimal involvement of the zona incerta and the H2 field of Forel also was noted (Fig 70.1). He proposed that damage to the contralateral subthalamus produced a specific syndrome involving hemiballism most prominently of the contralateral shoulder and hip girdle but also including facial and palatal muscles.

Subsequent case reports have mostly confirmed the localization of hemiballism to damage to the subthalamus. Whittier (3) reviewed literature prior to 1947 and found 30 cases in which hemiballism could be attributed to subthalamic lesions. More recently, using computed tomography (CT) imaging rather than pathology, subthalamic lesions have

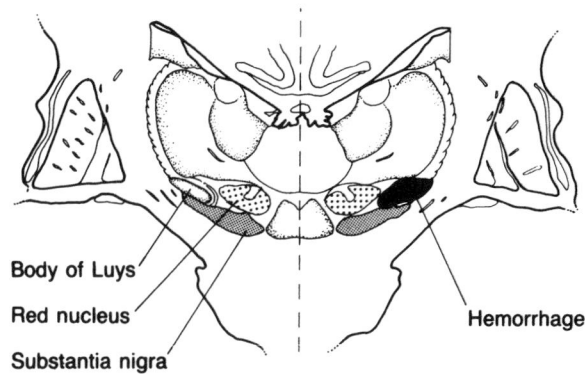

FIGURE 70.1   *Diagram showing a small hemorrhage in the left subthalamic nucleus in a patient with right body hemiballism. (Modified from Martin JP. Hemichorea resulting from a local lesion in the brain (the syndrome of the body of Luys). Brain 1927;50: 637–651.)*

been frequently identified in patients with hemiballism (13,18,19).

In six additional cases described by Whittier (3), the subthalamus was spared but damage to outflow tracts was noted; in three reports describing typical hemiballism, lesions were remote to the subthalamus or its outflow. Martin (15) also described two cases where pathologically confirmed lesions were in subthalamic outflow tracts. Other locations where local damage has been attributed to cause hemiballism include the striatum (20–24), the thalamus (13,25), neocortex (3), and cerebellum (26).

Studies on experimental animals have added significantly to the current understanding of hemiballism and the connections of the subthalamus with other brain structures. Whittier and colleagues (27–29) produced stereotactic lesions of variable size in and around the subthalamic nucleus in 80 rhesus monkeys. By tracing subsequent degeneration, they demonstrated the existence of profuse connections from subthalamus to globus pallidus, as well as from globus pallidus to subthalamus. No clear descending connections from subthalamus were noted, implying that the function of the subthalamus might be to modulate the output of the pallidum.

After lesions were placed, the behavior of the monkeys was monitored both acutely and chronically. In 24 of 50 animals in which the lesions were later proved to involve subthalamic damage, a movement disorder closely resembling hemiballism was seen. Movements were more severe in the leg than arm and persisted relatively unchanged until the death of the animal. Subsequent pathologic analysis showed that animals were likely to display the movement disorder when more than 20% of the subthalamic nucleus was damaged or if the outflow tract from subthalamus to globus pallidus was destroyed. If just the globus pallidus was damaged, no hemiballism-like movements were seen; in addition, if animals displaying the movement disorder were given a second lesion in the ipsilateral globus pallidus, the movements ceased or were significantly alleviated. Thus, these studies suggest that the subthalamus provides an inhibitory influence upon globus pallidus and that damage to subthalamus or its outflow causes abnormal movements by releasing this inhibition.

More recent anatomic studies have provided more details regarding the connections of the subthalamic nucleus. That the subthalamus lesion itself and not interruption of fibers of passage is crucial for producing hemiballism was demonstrated by the production of hemiballism using an injection of a neurotoxin into the subthalamic region (30). The strong efferent connections with both lateral and medial globus pallidus have been confirmed with degeneration studies (31), autoradiography (32), and retrograde transport (33,34). In addition, an efferent connection to the pars reticulata of the substantia nigra has been documented (35,36); it seems that the same neurons that project to the medial globus pallidus send branches that descend to the substantia nigra (37). Cerebral cortex also receives a projection from the lateral portion of the subthalamus (38), as well as, to a small extent, do the ventral anterior and ventral lateral nuclei of the thalamus, and the putamen (32,39).

Afferent projections to the subthalamic nucleus are most numerous from the lateral globus pallidus, with inputs arranged in a somatotopic fashion (33,34,40). Broad areas of frontal cortex also project to the subthalamus, including primary motor cortex as well as the premotor areas (41,42).

Both physiologic and radioactive tracer studies have added insight into the nature of the afferent and efferent connections of the subthalamus. Whittier's hypothesis that the subthalamus exerted inhibitory control over the globus pallidus has been confirmed by studies showing that subthalamopallidal fibers going to both medial and lateral segments utilize the inhibitory neurotransmitter gamma aminobutyric acid (GABA) (43–45). Very localized injections of antagonists of GABA (such as picrotoxin or bicuculline) in monkey brains produced hemiballistic movements if the injections were made in the subthalamus, but not in the globus pallidus or related structures (46,47). This finding suggests that at least some interneurons within the subthalamus also use GABA as their transmitter. The fact that injection of GABA antagonists into the globus pallidus did not produce ballistic movements was an unexpected finding but may reflect the fact that the inhibitory projections of the subthalamopallidal pathway are rather diffuse, and localized injections do not result in significant blockade of the pathway.

Other connections of the subthalamus are less well described. The efferent connections of subthalamonigral fibers are most likely excitatory (48) with L-glutamate as the putative neurotransmitter (49); since these fibers bifurcate and send branches to the medial globus pallidus, this is most likely an excitatory pathway as well. Subthalamic afferents

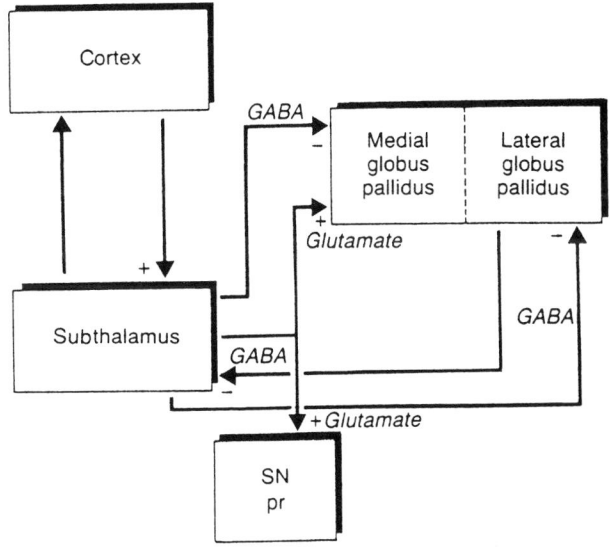

FIGURE 70.2 *Afferent and efferent connections of the subthalamus. Plus and minus signs represent excitatory and inhibitory synapses when known. SN pr refers to the pars reticulata of the substantia nigra. Pathways thought to use the neurotransmitter GABA and glutamate are shown.*

from the lateral globus pallidus are thought to be inhibitory, probably also utilizing GABA as the neurotransmitter (50,51). Cortical-subthalamic fibers are probably excitatory (52), while it is unclear whether subthalamocortical fibers are inhibitory or excitatory. Figure 70.2 summarizes the afferent and efferent connections of the subthalamus.

The recently developed technique of 2-deoxyglucose autoradiography provides further evidence for the importance of inhibition of the subthalamopallidal pathway in the production of hemiballism. This technique assesses local brain metabolic activity by measuring the uptake of radioactively labeled glucose. In monkeys in which hemiballism was induced by microinjection of GABA antagonist drugs into the subthalamus, both the subthalamic nucleus and its projection to the globus pallidus showed significantly reduced glucose uptake (53,54). If, as seems likely, decreased glucose utilization reflects a reduction of synaptic activity, these data suggest that hemiballism results from a reduction in activity of the inhibitory subthalamopallidal pathway.

Although the subthalamus is best known for its hypoactivity syndrome, hemiballism, it has recently been suggested that another pathologic movement disorder results from overactivation. In a 77-year-old woman with Parkinson's disease, hemiballism developed contralateral to an acute lacunar infarct localized radiographically in the region of the putamen. Interestingly, the signs of Parkinson's disease were abolished on the side of the hemiballism (55). This suggested that the putamen was exerting a tonic excitatory effect on the subthalamic nucleus and that a putamenal lesion reduced the level of activity of the subthalamus causing the hemiballism and reducing the signs of parkinsonism. Further support for the idea that parkinsonism may be related to subthalamic overactivity comes from a study in which monkeys made parkinsonian by the drug methyl phenyl tetrahydropyridine (MPTP) showed significantly increased activity of subthalamic nucleus neurons as compared to normal monkeys (56). When an ablative lesion was made in the subthalamus, contralateral extrapyramidal symptoms were markedly reduced.

CAUSES OF HEMIBALLISM AND BALLISM

By far the most common reported etiology of hemiballism is cerebral vascular disease, with localization of lesions as discussed in the previous section. In Whittier's (3) review of the early literature, 11 of 13 patients with subthalamic lesions and hemiballism showed pathology related to vascular disease, with three cases of infarction and eight hemorrhages. Similarly, the cases of Martin (8), Martin and Alcock (9), and Melamed et al (19) all showed small hemorrhages in the subthalamic areas on autopsy or CT scan. In contrast, of the 21 patients reported by Dewey and Jankovic (13), 9 of 10 patients with hemiballism who were over 55 years of age showed evidence of infarction on CT scan, but hemorrhage was not noted in any patient. Eleven patients were under 55 years of age, and stroke was thought to be the etiology of their movement disorder in only one of these patients.

Multiple other diseases that result in focal brain lesions have been reported to produce hemiballism. Infections have been implicated, including tuberculous mass lesions (14) and tuberculous meningitis (57), as well as toxoplasmosis associated with AIDS (58,59). AIDS without an associated mass lesion has also been reported to cause hemiballism (60). Nonketotic hyperglycemia has also been associated with hemiballismus; if recognized, appropriate treatment results in prompt resolution of symptoms (61,62). Other rare causes include encephalitis, neonatal anoxia, central nervous system (CNS) lupus (13), perhaps associated specifically with antiphospholipid antibodies (63), Behçet's disease (64), and neurosurgery, particularly for the amelioration of Parkinson's disease (65). In diseases such as lupus and Behçet's disease, small vascular lesions due to vasculitis may be the underlying mechanism.

Metastatic tumors have also been reported to produce hemiballism (18,66–68). Not surprisingly given the relatively slow growth of neoplastic lesions, the development of the movement disorder has been reported as being gradual and intermittent, rather than occurring with a sudden onset as is characteristic of vascular lesions. In a review of the literature conducted by Glass et al (18), five of nine reported cases and lung cancer as the primary lesion, with three cases of breast cancer and one patient with biliary cancer.

In contrast to hemiballism, bilateral ballism generally results from processes that produce diffuse pathology or multiple lesions. In the literature surveyed by Hoogstraten et al (10), 6 of the 12 cases were thought to be vascular in origin, with bilateral atrophy, bilateral infarction of deep grey matter structures, or bilateral hemorrhages being noted. Two cases were reported of bilateral ballism during postictal states, with one case following a toxic ingestion of diphenylhydantoin (DPH), and one case associated with a heredodegenerative disorder. In the case of drug toxicity, ballistic movements waned in close association with declining drug levels and other more common manifestations of DPH toxicity (69). In one unusual case, bilateral ballistic movements were reported to repeatedly follow reduction of ventricular size by ventricular peritoneal shunting (70). Multiple sclerosis has been reported as a cause of both hemiballism (71) and bilateral ballism (72); in the bilateral case, demyelinating plaques were noted in both subthalamic nuclei.

TREATMENT

Assessing the efficacy of treatment for hemiballism is difficult because many patients recover spontaneously over variable time intervals. However, sufficient numbers of patients show static disease that the effects of treatment can be documented. Initial attempts to alleviate hemiballism were surgical in nature. Lesions at all levels of the neuraxis have been studied, from cortical ablation (73,74), which reduced the movements but caused hemiplegia, to partial cordotomy (75), which also produced unacceptable negative effects. Good relief of involuntary movements without significant weakness was produced both by lesions of the ventrolateral thalamus (76) and the globus pallidus (77). No significant differences were noted between the results produced by lesions in the two sites, although there was a suggestion that lesions in the ventrolateral thalamus, which receives afferents from the globus pallidus, produced more immediate relief.

The use of surgical ablation to reduce symptoms of hemiballism has waned with the discovery that pharmacologic management can be quite effective. Neuroleptic drugs were probably the first to show significant effect; two of the three patients given chlorpromazine by Hyland and Forman (7) showed improvement. Phenothiazines and butyrophenones continue to be the most widely used drugs for hemiballism, including haloperidol (78–80), perphenazine (11), chlorpromazine (12), and thiopropazate hydrochloride (Rowlands, 1972). The presumed mechanism of action of these drugs is to block dopaminergic synapses in the striatum. Tetrabenazine and reserpine, which reduce dopaminergic activity by depleting intracellular stores, have also been reported to improve hemiballism (81,82).

The fact that inhibition of dopaminergic transmission or central dopamine depletion improves symptoms of hemiballism suggests that increased activity of dopaminergic systems might be present. Increased dopamine turnover is also suggested by studies showing increased levels of the dopamine metabolite homovanillic acid in cerebrospinal fluid (12,83). Thus, hemiballism may in part be due to a release of inhibition of dopaminergic pathways, mediated either directly or indirectly by reduced activity of the inhibitory subthalamopallidal pathways.

As the major outflow tract of the subthalamic nucleus to the basal ganglia is GABA mediated, drugs that enhance GABA transmission might be expected to be useful in the treatment of hemiballism. Progabide, a GABA-mimetic agent, has been used successfully (84), as has sodium valproate (85,86). Lang (22) used sodium valproate to no effect in his patients; however, these patients had lesions outside the subthalamic nucleus, suggesting that enhancement of GABA-ergic transmission may be more important when the subthalamopallidal pathway is damaged.

Occasionally, hemiballismus after stroke may be quite persistent and resistant to pharmacotherapy. Chronic thalamic stimulation can be quite effective in reducing symptoms in such situations. Tsubokawa et al (87) treated two patients with resistant hemiballism from stroke with continuous high-frequency stimulation to the VL and nucleus ventralis intermedius of the thalamus. Near complete reduction in symptoms was noted within several weeks, and symptoms returned when stimulation was stopped. Good release was obtained for up to 16 months.

Making inferences about pathophysiology from the therapeutic effects of different drugs can be a treacherous undertaking. However, when the results of drug studies are combined with the anatomic studies discussed previously, a fairly consistent picture emerges. Lesions in the subthalamic nucleus or its outflow tracts produce hemiballismus primarily because of a loss of inhibitory influences on the globus pallidus. This can occur because of interruption of subthalamopallidal, subthalamonigral, or subthalamoputamenal connections. The fact that dopaminergic blocking drugs are effective in reducing hemiballism suggests that the nigrostriatal dopaminergic system is modulated in part by any of the three subthalamic outflow systems mentioned above. This hypothesis is also consistent with the experimental finding that parkinsonian monkeys show increased activity in subthalamic neurons (56), perhaps via a negative feedback loop. Pharmacologic enhancement of GABA-ergic transmission likely ameliorates hemiballism by mimicking activity in the inhibitory subthalamopallidal pathway.

REFERENCES

1. Bonhoeffer K. Ein beitrag zur localisation der choreatischen bewegungen. Monatschr Psychiatr Neurol 1897;1:6–41.
2. Ad hoc Committee. Classification of extrapyramidal disorders. J Neurol Sci 1981;51:311–327.
3. Whittier JR. Ballism and subthalamic nucleus (nucleus hypothalamicus; corpus Luysi). Review of the literature and study of thirty cases. Arch Neurol Psychiatry 1947;58:672–692.
4. von Economo CJ. Beitrag zur kasuistik und zur erklarung der posthemiplegischen chorea. Wien Klin Wochenschr 1910;23:429–431.
5. Buruma OJS, Lakke JPWF. Ballism. In: Vinken P, Bruyn G, Klawans H, ed. Handbook of clinical neurology. vol. 5. New York: Elsevier, 1986:369–380.
6. Carpenter MB, Carpenter CS. Analysis of somatotopic relations of the corpus Luysi in man and monkey. J Comp Neurol 1951;95:349–370.
7. Hyland HH, Forman DM. Prognosis in hemiballismus. Neurology 1957;7:381–391.
8. Martin JP. Hemichorea resulting from a local lesion of the brain (the syndrome of the body of Luys). Brain 1927;50:637–651.
9. Martin JP, Alcock NS. Hemichorea associated with lesion of corpus Luysii. Brain 1934;57:504–516.
10. Hoogstraten MC, Lakke JPWF, Zwarts MJ. Bilateral ballism: a rare syndrome. Review of the literature and presentation of a case. J Neurol 1986;233:25–29.
11. Johnson WG, Fahn S. Treatment of vascular hemiballism and hemichorea. Neurology 1977;27:634–636.
12. Klawans HL, Moses H, Nausieda PA, et al. Treatment and prognosis of hemiballismus. N Engl J Med 1976;295:1348–1350.
13. Dewey RB, Jankovic J. Hemiballism-hemichorea. Clinical and pharmacologic findings in 21 patients. Arch Neurol 1989;46:862–867.
14. Bedwell SF. Some observations on hemiballismus. Neurology 1960;10:619–622.
15. Martin JP. Hemichorea (hemiballismus) without lesions in the corpus Luysi. Brain 1957;80:1–11.
16. Fischer O. Zur frage der anatomischen grundlage der athetose double und der posthemiplegischen bewegungsstorung uberhaupt. Z Neurol Psychiatr 1911;7:463–486.
17. Pette H. Zur localization hemichoreatischer bewegungsstorungen7-408. Zentralbl Neurol Psychiatr 1922;30:40.
18. Glass JP, Jankovic J, Borit A. Hemiballism and metastatic brain tumor. Neurology 1984;34:204–207.
19. Melamed E, Korn-Lubetzk I, Reches A, Siew F. Hemiballismus: detection of focal hemorrhage in subthalamic nucleus by CT scan. Ann Neurol 1978;4:582.
20. Dubinsky RM, Greenberg M, Di Chiro G, et al. Hemiballismus: study of a case using positron emission tomography with 18-fluoro-2-deoxyglucose. Mov Disord 1989;4:310–319.
21. Kase CS, Maulsby GO, deJuan E, Mohr JP. Hemichorea-hemiballism and lacunar infarction in the basal ganglia. Neurology 1981;31:452–454.
22. Lang AE. Persistent hemiballismus with lesions outside the subthalamic nucleus. Can J Neurol Sci 1985;12:125–128.
23. Lodder J, Baard WC. Paraballism caused by bilateral hemorrhagic infarction in basal ganglia. Neurology 1981;31:484–486.
24. Srinivas K, Rao VM, Subbulakshmi N, Bhaskaran J. Hemiballism after striatal hemorrhage. Neurology 1987;37:1428–1429.
25. Antin SP, Prockop LD, Cohen SM. Transient hemiballism. Neurology 1967;17:1068–1072.
26. Tognetti F, Donati R. Hemiballism of ischemic origin. Report of a case with unusual anatomical location. Acta Neurol (Napoli) 1986;8:150–152.
27. Whittier JR, Mettler FA. Studies on the subthalamus of the rhesus monkey. I. Anatomy and fiber connections of the subthalamic nucleus of Luys. J Comp Neurol 1949;90:281–314.
28. Whittier JR, Mettler FA. Studies on the subthalamus of the rhesus monkey. II. Hyperkinesia and other physiologic effects of subthalamic lesions, with special reference to the subthalamic nucleus of Luys. J Comp Neurol 1949;90:319–372.
29. Carpenter MB, Whittier JP, Mettler FA. Analysis of choreoid hyperkinesia in the rhesus monkey. J Comp Neurol 1950;92:293–331.
30. Hammond C, Feger J, Bioulac B, Souteyrand JP. Experimental hemiballism in the monkey produced by unilateral kainic acid lesion in corpus Luysii. Brain Res 1979;171:577–580.
31. Carpenter MB, Strominger N. Efferent fiber projections of the subthalamic nucleus in the rhesus monkey. A comparison of the efferent projections of the subthalamic nucleus, substantia nigra and globus pallidus. Am J Anat 1967;121:41–72.
32. Nauta HJW, Cole M. Efferent projections of the subthalamic nucleus: an autoradiographic study in monkey and cat. J Comp Neurol 1978;180:1–16.
33. Carpenter MB, Batton RR, Carleton SC, Keller JT. Interconnections and organization of pallidal and subthalamic nucleus neurons in the monkey. J Comp Neurol 1981;197:579–603.
34. Carpenter MB, Carleton SC, Keller JT, Conte P. Connections of the subthalamic nucleus in the monkey. Brain Res 1981;224:1–29.
35. Deniau JM, Hammond C, Chevalier G, Feger J. Evidence for branched subthalamic nucleus projections to substantia nigra, entopeduncular nucleus and globus pallidus. Neurosci Lett 1978;9:117–121.
36. Kanazawa I, Marshall GR, Kelly JS. Afferents to the rat substantia nigra studied with horseradish peroxidase, with special reference to fibres from the subthalamic nucleus. Brain Res 1976;115:485–491.

37. Van Der Kooy D, Hattori T. Single subthalamic nucleus neurons project to both the globus pallidus and substantia nigra in rat. J Comp Neurol 1980;192:751.

38. Jackson A, Crossman AR. Subthalamic nucleus efferent projection to the cerebral cortex. Neuroscience 1981;6:2367–2377.

39. Smith Y, Hazrati LN, Parent A. Efferent projections of the subthalamic nucleus in the squirrel monkey as studied by the PHA-L anterograde tracing method. J Comp Neurol 1990;294:306–323.

40. Kim R, Nakano K, Jayaraman A, Carpenter MB. Projections of the globus pallidus and adjacent structures: an autoradiographic study in the monkey. J Comp Neurol 1976;169:263–289.

41. Hartmann-von Monakow K, Akert K, Kunzle H. Projections of the precentral motor cortex and other cortical areas of the frontal lobe to the subthalamic nucleus of the monkey. Exp Brain Res 1978;33:395–403.

42. Kunzle H. An autoradiographic analysis of the efferent connections from premotor and adjacent prefrontal regions (areas 6 and 9) in Macaca fascicularis. Brain Behav Evol 1978;15:135–234.

43. Larsen KD, Sutin J. Output organization of the feline entopeduncular and subthalamic nuclei. Brain Res 1978;157:21–31.

44. Nauta HJW, Cuenod M. Perikaryal cell labeling in the subthalamic nucleus following the injection of 3H-gamma-aminobutyric acid into the pallidal complex: an autoradiographic study in cat. Neuroscience 1982;7:2725–2734.

45. Rouzaire-Dubois B, Scarnati E, Hammond C, et al. Microiontophoretic studies on the nature of the neurotransmitter in the subthalamo-entopeduncular pathway of the rat. Brain Res 1983;271:11–20.

46. Crossman AR, Sambrook MA, Jackson A. Experimental hemiballismus in the baboon produced by injection of a gamma aminobutyric acid antagonist into the basal ganglia. Neurosci Lett 1980;20:369–372.

47. Crossman AR, Sambrook MA, Jackson A. Experimental hemichorea/ hemiballismus in the monkey. Brain 1984;107:579–596.

48. Hammond C, Deniau JM, Riszk A, Feger J. Electrophysiological demonstration of an excitatory subthalamo nigral pathway in the cat. Brain Res 1978;151:235–244.

49. Smith Y, Parent A. Neurons of the subthalamic nucleus in primates display glutamate but not GABA immunoreactivity. Brain Res 1988;453:353–356.

50. Tsubokawa T, Sutin J. Pallidal and tegmental inhibition of oscillatory slow waves and unit activity in the subthalamic nucleus. Brain Res 1972;2:101–118.

51. Van Der Kooy D, Hattori T, Shannak K, Hornykiewicz O. The pallidosubthalamic projection in rat: anatomical and biochemical studies. Brain Res 1981;204:253–216.

52. Kitai ST, Deniau JM. Cortical inputs to the subthalamus: intracellular analysis. Brain Res 1981;214:411–415.

53. Mitchell IJ, Sambrook MA, Crossman AR. Subcortical changes in the regional uptake of 3H-2-deoxyglucose in the brain of the monkey during experimental choreiform dyskinesia elicited by injection of a gamma-aminobutyric acid antagonist into the subthalamic nucleus. Brain 1985;108:405–422.

54. Mitchell IJ, Jackson A, Sambrook MA, Crossman AR. Common neural mechanisms in experimental chorea and hemiballismus in the monkey. Evidence from 2-deoxyglucose autoradiography. Brain Res 1985;339:346–350.

55. Scoditti U, Rustichelli P, Calzetti S. Spontaneous hemiballism and disappearance of parkinsonism following contralateral lenticular lacunar infarct. Ital J Neurol Sci 1989;10:575–577.

56. Bergman H, Wichmann T, DeLong MR. Reversal of experimental parkinsonism by lesions of the subthalamic nucleus. Science 1990;249:1436–1438.

57. Udani PM, Parekh UC, Dastur DK. Neurological and related syndromes in CNS tuberculosis. J Neurol Sci 1971;14:341–357.

58. Sanchez-Ramos JR, Facor SA, Weiner WJ, Marquez J. Hemichorea-hemiballismus associated with acquired immune deficiency syndrome and cerebral toxoplasmosis. Mov Disord 1989;4:266–273.

59. Nath A, Jankovic J, Pettigrew LC. Movement disorders and AIDS. Neurology 1987;37:37–41.

60. Reyes-Iglesias Y, Grant TH. Hemiballism-chemichorea: unusual neurologic presentation in acquired immunodeficiency syndrome. Bol Assoc Med PR 1991;83:17–18.

61. Lin JJ, Chang MK. Hemiballism-hemichorea and non-ketotic hyperglycemia. J Neurol Neurosurg Psychiatry 1994;57:748–750.

62. Lietz TE, Huff JS. Hemiballismus as a presenting sign of hyperglycemia. Am J Emerg Med 1995;13:647–648.

63. Tam LS, Cohen MG, Li EK. Hemiballismus in systemic lupus erythematosus: possible association with antiphospholipid antibodies. Lupus 1995;4:67–69.

64. Salomez J, Francois M, Petit H. Hemiballisme au corps d'une maladie de Behçet. LARC Med 1982;10:869–870.

65. Modesti LM, Van Buren JM. Hemiballismus complicating stereotactic thalamotomy. Appl Neurophysiol 1979;42:267–283.

66. Bronster DJ, Yahr MD. Hemiballism secondary to a metastatic neoplasm of the subthalamic nucleus as demonstrated by CT scan. Mt Sinai J Med 1983;50:351–355.

67. Manorama Devi TK, Kumar D, Rajasekharan Nair K. Hemiballismus and intracranial metastases. Acta Neurol (Napoli) 1986;8:491–494.

68. Taylor RL. Metastatic hemiballism again. Neurology 1984;34:1126.

69. Opida CL, Korthals JK, Somasundaram M. Bilateral ballismus in phenytoin intoxication. Ann Neurol 1978;3:186.

70. Walker FO, Hunt VP. Ballism: an association with ventriculoperitoneal shunting. Neurology 1990;40:1004.

71. Riley D, Lang AE. Hemiballism in multiple sclerosis. Mov Disord 1988;3:88–94.

72. Masucci EF, Saini N, Kurtzke JF. Bilateral ballism in multiple sclerosis. Neurology 1989;39:1641–1642.

73. Alpers BJ, Jaeger R. Hemiballism and its control by ablation of the motor cortex. Arch Neurol 1950;64:285–287.

74. Juba A, Dobi A. Der hemiballismus. Monatschr Psychiatr Neurol 1956;132:48–61.

75. Brown MH, Walsh MN. The effect of ventral quadrant section of the spinal cord on hemiballism. J Neurosurg 1954;11:409–412.

76. Martin JP, McCaul IR. Acute hemiballismus treated by ventrolateral thalamolysis. Brain 1959;82:104–108.

77. Gioino GG, Dierssen G, Cooper IS. The effect of subcortical lesions on production and alleviation of hemiballic or hemichoreic movements. J Neurol Sci 1966;3:10–36.

78. Davis JM. Response of hemiballismus to haloperidol. JAMA 1976;235:2812.

79. Gilbert GJ. Response of hemiballismus to haloperidol. JAMA 1975;233:535–536.

80. Gilbert GJ. Response of hemiballismus to haloperidol. JAMA 1976;236:1576.

81. Obeso JA, Marti-Masso JF, Astudillo W, et al. Treatment of hemiballism with reserpine. Ann Neurol 1978;4:581.

82. Pearce J. Reversal of hemiballismus by tetrabenazine. JAMA 1972;219:1345.

83. Kostic V, Djuricic B, Paschen W. Hemiballismus: changes in cerebrospinal fluid. Acta Neurol Scand 1988;78:115–117.

84. Gonce M, Schoenen J, Charlier M, Delwaide PJ. Successful treatment of hemiballismus with progabide, a new GABA-mimetic agent. J Neurol 1983;229:121–124.

85. Chandra V, Wharton S, Spunt AL. Amelioration of hemiballismus with sodium valproate. Ann Neurol 1982;12:407.

86. Lenton RJ, Cofti M, Smith RG. Hemiballismus treated with sodium valproate. Br Med J 1981;283:17–18.

87. Tsubokawa T, Katayama Y, Yamamoto T. Control of persistent hemiballismus by chronic thalamic stimulation. J Neurosurg 1995;82:501–505.

Chorea: A Clinical and Scientific Overview

STEPHEN A. BERMAN   RICHARD M. ZWEIG   NEIL W. KOWALL

To urgent unknown music she danced . . .
—*Maureen Howard,*
Facts of Life *(1978)*

THE CLINICAL PHENOMENON OF CHOREA

Chorea refers to involuntary forceful rapid jerks without a specific rhythmic pattern. These movements can involve the upper extremities, lower extremities, neck, trunk, and face. They can even include grimacing and abnormal movements of the respiratory muscles, producing grunts and other sounds, which may interrupt normal speech and cause an associated dysarthria (1). When the patient walks, such movements frequently intensify, and the sudden jerking, thrusting, and twitching produce a gait resembling a dance (2,3), as reflected in the Greek meaning of the word "chorea."

Chorea resembles several other types of involuntary movements. It is similar to myoclonus, except that the myoclonic jerks are faster and may involve single muscles, and even parts of muscles, rather than whole muscle groups. It also resembles ballismus, except that ballistic movements are generally larger, characteristically rotatory, and involved more with proximal muscle groups, usually the arm, shoulder, and leg of one side (hemiballismus). Ballismus is well described in Chapter 70. Finally, choreic movements often overlap with athetotic movements, which are more sinuous and writhing, as well as slower and more distal. Thus, some authorities use "choreoathetosis" as a general reference to movement disorders in which one can usually find some more specifically choreic movements, other more clearly athetotic movements, and still other movements that have features of both. The reader should refer to Chapter 72, "Athetosis and the Common Athetoid Syndromes," for an excellent discussion of the differences between these terms placed in an historical perspective.

Numerous diseases produce chorea as a part of their clinical spectrum. In some, chorea can aid the physician in making a differential diagnosis. In addition, treatment with antiparkinson medicines frequently induces choreiform movements, and many antipsychotics produce tardive dyskinesia that resembles chorea.

Apart from drug-induced choreas, the most clear-cut information about a patient with chorea may be that another family member has similar symptoms. Thus, we will first divide the choreiform disorders into two large groups: hereditary and sporadic. Of course, the reader must be aware that frequently the family history is inaccurate. Information about hereditary conditions may be forgotten, lost, or even hidden. After reviewing the specific choreiform disorders, we will present a current model of basal ganglia pathophysiology that helps to rationalize this interesting phenomenon. Finally, we will explore present and proposed approaches to treatment.

HEREDITARY CHOREIFORM DISORDERS

The three most common hereditary choreiform disorders are Huntington's disease, hereditary chorea-acanthocytosis, and benign hereditary chorea. In addition, the physician should consider hereditary essential myoclonus and the large category of hereditary spinocerebellar degenerations when assessing the patient and family presumably afflicted with a hereditary choreiform illness. Of course, hereditary essential myoclonus does not involve chorea at all, but, as noted above, myoclonus can resemble chorea. On the other hand, true chorea can be present in patients with certain hereditary spinocerebellar degenerations, as we shall describe later. Finally, there are a number of rare hereditary diseases that have chorea or choreoathetosis as one component of their complex multifaceted problems.

Huntington's Disease

Patients with Huntington's disease (HD) usually present between the ages of 35 and 50 with one or both of two types of problems: a movement disorder (of which chorea is the most characteristic feature, though it might not be noticeable as such initially) and a disorder of thinking (of which dementia is characteristic, though—like the chorea—a frank dementia may not be apparent right away and, instead, the complaint may be depression, difficulty concentrating, psychotic episodes, or other types of unusual behavior). There is also a childhood form, the Westphal variant, which frequently displays rigidity and hypokinesia with little or no chorea or choreoathetosis. Such children present at ages 3 to 12 and follow a rapidly worsening course with severe loss of mental milestones and steadily worsening rigidity and/or chorea. Epileptic seizures are also common in this variant (4).

Because the genetic pedigree pattern of the juvenile form is the same as that of the adult, the basis for the distinction had not been clear. It was long realized that most children so afflicted inherited the illness from the father, but the juvenile cases still constituted a small subset of those who inherit HD from their father. We now know that an unstable site in the HD gene causes HD when the gene expands beyond a certain length. This gene is more likely to expand when inherited from the father, and the larger (more expanded) the gene, the earlier the onset of symptoms (and generally the worse the overall biological severity of the disease). Thus, in the juvenile cases, the gene has expanded enough beyond the extent of the parent's (usually the father's) gene to make the disease severe enough to manifest very early.

In the initial stages, without a family history as a guide, choreiform movements may be interpreted as clumsiness, unsteadiness, minor tics, or just fidgety movements. As HD progresses, the chorea becomes more manifest. Although no specific sign can prove that chorea is due to HD, certain classic descriptions of the chorea in HD are worthwhile to remember. For example, many patients exhibit a "stereotyped extension/flexion of one particular finger, or abduction of one leg or shrugging of one shoulder" (4). Other common patterns include "opening of the hand to a fully extended pronated posture with pronation of the wrist to closure with a trapped thumb and supinated wrist" (5), "a downward sweep of the chin with pursing of the lips followed by extension of the head with labial retraction" (5), "swaying to and fro of the head with inappropriate hyperflexion," "stereotyped opening and closing of the mouth, associated with tongue protrusion," "alternately [flexing or extending] one or two fingers," or inappropriate pouting or brow raising (4). Compared with Sydenham's chorea, which we will describe later, the movements of HD are slower and involve a wider range of associated muscle groups. Thus the chorea of Huntington's disease more easily blends into normal movement patterns, at least at the outset, and,

indeed, some patients can incorporate the abnormal movements into normal actions. The facio-lingual-buccal movements of HD differ somewhat from those of tardive dyskinesia. For example, it is rare for patients with HD to be able to keep the tongue protruded for more than 15 seconds, whereas those with tardive dyskinesia can do so easily. As the patient worsens, more muscle groups become involved. Involvement of the tongue, throat, and facial muscles produces dysarthria. The patient's difficulty in speaking may falsely increase the appearance of dementia (4).

Genetic Factors in Huntington's Disease

It had long been known that HD follows an autosomal dominant hereditary pattern, with an extremely high penetrance (i.e., if an individual with a gene for HD lives long enough, he or she will almost inevitably show the effect of the disease) (6–8). But the modern approach to the study of HD really began in the early 1980s when Houseman and Gusella (9) suggested the possibility of cloning the gene for HD using molecular biological methods. They proposed taking DNA from affected and nonaffected members of families with Huntington's disease, digesting the DNA with enzymes (restriction endonucleases), separating the DNA fragments by size via gel electrophoresis, and visualizing certain fragments using a battery of DNA probes (in a manner that we will describe below) in the hope of finding specific fragments that correlated with the existence of the disease. This might have seemed like a hopeless task at the time, but they argued that 150 to 600 nonoverlapping (and essentially uniformly spaced) DNA segments or probes should span the genome adequately, making it likely that at least one such probe would lie close enough to the gene to detect, in a given family, a characteristically sized DNA fragment (a restriction fragment length polymorphism, or RFLP) in a very high percentage (say 90%) of patients with the disease.

While today we may assume that scientists can clone the gene for most any hereditary disease, in the early 1980s many believed that Houseman and Gusella had undertaken an almost impossible task. In those days cloning genes still largely depended on specific assays for or antibodies to known proteins. For a disease such as HD, no specific biochemical marker was available. Gene discovery schemes such as that outlined by Houseman and Gusella (9) were termed reverse genetics because they reversed the usual order of first finding a defective protein and then cloning the gene. Today we use a more informative term, positional cloning, to describe such strategies to emphasize the fact that one uses a combination of knowledge concerning 1) the positions of specific sequences in the DNA itself (the physical map), 2) the position of markers and bands on the layout of the chromosomes that can be examined microscopically (the cytogenetic map), and 3) the relative positions of genetic markers derived from pedigree (family tree) information, often using combinations of clinical observations, biochemical tests, and, today, specific genetic tests produced by other cloning projects to progressively refine the locale of a gene (the genetic map).

Eleven years after their exciting proposal, the same authors, as part of a phalanx of investigators known as the Huntington's Disease Collaborative Research Group, with Gusella the corresponding member, reported cloning the HD gene, culminating an inspired and inspiring team effort (10). They found a 210-kb gene, IT15, that encoded a 348-kd protein, now called huntingtin. Its reading frame contains a polymorphic CAG repeat (10,11). In healthy individuals there are a limited number of repeats, usually 11 to 34, whereas HD patients have 42 or more repeats. In the original paper reporting the discovery of the HD gene, 66 was the highest repeat number seen in any HD patient, but now patients with higher numbers of repeats have been reported. Those with the highest repeat numbers (especially 100 or more) are often patients with juvenile onset of HD. Indeed, there is a good inverse correlation between age of onset and length, though the confidence interval is too broad to allow this fact to help much in counseling individual patients (12).

Now that the gene has been cloned, the major question has shifted to what the gene does and how the increased number of CAG repeats causes the disease. Antibodies raised to huntingtin show that it is present in most cells, including neurons, without significant changes in the localization pattern between normal and HD cells. The CAG repeats do become transcribed into complementary mRNA (13) and are then expressed on the protein level as increased stretches of polyglutamine near the N-terminus of the protein (14). Total lack of huntingtin in mice nullizygous for Hdh (the mouse version of huntingtin) produces severe developmental abnormalities, including significant programmed cell death in the ectoderm (15). On the neuropathologic level, the abnormalities in such mice appear different from the HD pathology, leading to the thought that HD huntingtin probably produces the disease by a gain in function, that is, the HD huntingtin probably possesses a new and different property than the normal huntingtin (or, perhaps, an exaggeration of a normal property) (16).

The levels of huntingtin produced in the brains of HD patients are not significantly different from those produced in healthy individuals after adjustment is made for neuronal loss. Because most HD patients are heterozygous, it is reasonable to expect expression of both the normal and the abnormal version of the protein. Indeed, both are found in amounts not very different from each other in relatively spared brain areas such as the hippocampus and cerebellum (17). In the caudate itself and in the neocortex, the expression level of the mutant protein is actually lower than that of the normal protein, and a blurring of the mutant protein's pattern on protein electrophoresis suggests that some degradation or abnormality in conformation has occurred (17). Thus, though researchers can now approach the pathophysiology of HD from the basis of having the gene in hand, as described above, the possession of the huntingtin gene has not yet yielded an understanding of the disease. The methods to be described below, therefore, continue to have great importance in HD and the other choreiform disorders.

Two laboratories now have evidence of a possible pathogenic mechanism, based on altered binding to a specific protein or proteins. One group has discovered a huntingtin-associated protein (HAP-1) to which huntingtin binds more tightly in the mutant than in the normal form. This protein is also enriched in brain (18). In a different bur somewhat similar approach, other investigators immobilized 20-glutamine peptides and 60-glutamine peptides to a matrix and investigated which brain proteins bound to either peptide. Interestingly, few proteins bound to either in significant amounts. But the important metabolic enzyme glyceraldehyde 3-phosphate dehydrogenase (GAPDH) bound significantly to the 60-glutamine peptide but not the shorter one. Conversely, immobilized GAPDH binds the polyglutamine-containing protein associated with dentatorubropallidoluysian atrophy (DRPLA) as well as fragments of the huntingtin protein. Such work suggests that perhaps proteins such as the DRPLA protein and huntingtin may share common protein binding mechanisms through their expanded polyglutamine tracts (19).

Pathogenesis and Pathophysiology

It is the tissue pathology of Huntington's disease, both gross and microscopic, that has given us many of the clues on which the current limited understanding of HD has been built. The most obvious pathology involves the neostriatum, with atrophy, accompanied by neuronal loss and gliosis, in both the caudate and putamen. Indeed, caudate atrophy on pneumoencephalogram, computed tomography (CT), and now magnetic resonance imaging (MRI) scans has long served as a hallmark of the disease that is readily apparent to the clinician. However, there are subpopulations of neurons within those regions that are more specifically at risk and whose loss may explain many features of the disease (20,21). This correlates broadly with the often stated fact that total destruction of the caudate, such as by an infarct, does not cause chorea. Within the striatum the medium-sized spiny striatal neurons show the earliest and most severe alterations. Large and medium-sized aspiny neurons are largely unaffected (20,22–26). Early in the disease dendrites show proliferative alterations in their branching patterns and an increase in the number and size of their dendritic spines. Much later they show degenerative changes, including spine loss (25,27,28). There is also differential involvement of the regional striatal compartments, with the matrix elements being affected most significantly, whereas the patch or striasomal compartments are relatively spared (22–24,29–33).

Less striking loss is found in other subcortical regions, including the globus pallidus, thalamus (mainly ventral lateral nucleus), subthalamic nucleus, substantia nigra (quite mild), cerebellum (more so in juvenile form), and brainstem. Changes, mainly variable degrees of gliosis, hyperchromasia of anterior horn cells, and lipofuscin deposition, have even been noted in the spinal cord. In the cortex, loss is noted in the third, fifth, and sixth cortical layers. Considerable gliosis is associated with the neuronal loss (34,35). Pharmacologically, a generalization upon which several therapeutic trials have been based is that there is a GABAergic and cholinergic decrease coexisting with an absolute or relative dopaminergic increase. More recent studies of early cases indicate that the neurons primarily destroyed are the GABAergic neurons that project from the striatum (20,21).

While exact correlations between the pathology and the symptoms are not known, there are some helpful generalizations. In assessing the dementia of Huntington's disease, neuropsychological studies show that HD patients display frontal-system cognitive deficits as well as difficulties with sequential motor programming that are not attributable to the movement disorder alone. Such findings are indicative of a subcortical dementia in which there is a frontal syndrome (36).

The chorea appears to be related to the basal ganglia pathology. More specifically, neuropathologic findings (20,37) and data from primate models (38,39) suggest that chorea results from loss of inhibitory striatal input to the external pallidum. This allows the external pallidum to excessively inhibit the subthalamic nucleus, which, in turn, decreases the activation of the internal segment of the pallidum and reduces inhibition of the thalamus, allowing the thalamus to overexcite the cortex, causing chorea. Later in this chapter we will more fully discuss the current state of knowledge of the alterations in neural pathways underlying choreiform movements and related movement disorders (see the section entitled "Model of Basal Ganglia Function").

What actually damages the neurons in HD? A current idea is that certain excitatory neurotransmitters, or closely related substances, may do the damage. Injection of kainic acid, an analogue of the excitatory neurotransmitter glutamic acid, into the neostriatum of rats causes loss of striatal neurons with (relative) sparing of incoming axons, their afferent terminals, and fibers transversing the striatum; a decrease in both GABAergic and cholinergic function; and decreases in both GABA and glutamic acid decarboxylase. All these changes mimic the pathology seen in HD, but the rats do not develop choreiform movements (40–43). Bilateral injections of another excitotoxin, ibotenic acid, produce similar lesions in rats as well as motor hyperactivity and disturbances in maze learning that are considered to be analogous to the deficits seen in humans with Huntington's chorea (44). In addition, when kainic acid lesions are made in the striatum of macaque monkeys, one can produce chorea via systemic administration of L-dopa (but not with the kainic acid or the L-dopa alone) (45).

Beal et al (46,47) improved on the kainic acid model using N-methyl D-aspartate (NMDA) excitotoxins, including quinolinic acid, to produce lesions that show selective neuronal sparing. Application of an excitotoxin, quinolinic acid, in mice appears to raise huntingtin expression; this method may ultimately help explain the locale and even the mechanism of damage (48). In the monkey model such lesioning produces a close correspondence to the neuropathologic, neurochemical, and clinical features of Huntington's disease (49). However, no known excitotoxins such as quinolinic acid are actually increased in HD. A recent hypothesis of interest is that normal glutamate levels may cause excitotoxicity in HD via impaired energy metabolism (50,51). Normally a voltage-dependent magnesium block restrains the activity of the calcium channel linked to the NMDA receptor. Partial membrane depolarization, which occurs with energy depletion, can remove or diminish this block, leading to increased calcium movements through the channel, causing excitotoxic lesions in model systems (52–56). In HD, alteration of certain electron transport chain enzymes may give rise to energy depletion (57–60).

Based on this reasoning 3-nitropropionic acid (3-NP), an irreversible inhibitor of succinate dehydrogenase, has been used to create new model systems that show excitotoxic damage based on decreased cellular energy levels (61,62). Striatal injection of 3-NP in rats produces age-dependent striatal lesions with many neuropathologic and neurochemical features of HD (63,64). A recently developed chronic primate model, based on 3-NP administration, shows significant similarity to many pathologic and clinical features of HD (27,46,47,49,65–67).

It is also possible that huntingtin may affect mitochondrial function through involvement with transport of intracellular molecules. Evidence has accumulated that huntingtin is found in synaptosomes and other vesicles; thus it may have a role in movement of intracellular molecules (so-called trafficking) (68). In one recent study, huntingtin showed no enrichment in the striatum. It was present in the cell bodies of neurons, reduced in nuclei and mitochondria, and concentrated at nerve terminals (69). Another study found it present in the cytoplasm and dendrites, particularly around vesicles, but not enriched at terminals (68). Still other investigators have found huntingtin to be enriched in the striatum in a patchy distribution (70). The vesicular association appears to be a consistent finding at the subcellular level. Involvement with transport could affect mitochondrial function regardless of lack of mitochondrial concentration of the protein itself (70,71).

Hereditary Chorea-Acanthocytosis

Hereditary chorea-acanthocytosis (72) originally was more commonly reported in Japan, but it is now increasingly recognized all over the world. It can be either autosomal dominant or recessive. There are less severe choreiform movements in this condition than are seen in HD. There are also other abnormal movements, including myoclonic jerks and various tics and uncontrollable vocalizations such as humming and tongue clicking. A marked dystonia of the bulbar musculature causes dysphagia and can even result in mutilation of the lips.

Neuropathologically, there is atrophy and gliosis of the caudate and putamen with no cortical neuronal loss (73). The name derives from the hematologic finding of acanthocytes (erythrocytes with spiky protrusions) even in freshly drawn peripheral blood. Areflexia is one sign of the axonal neuropathy that is part of the condition. An increased creatinine phosphokinase is suggestive of a concomitant muscle disorder. Although muscle biopsies show centralization of nuclei and fiber splitting to some degree, it has been argued that the myopathic features are secondary to denervation (72,74).

Benign Hereditary Chorea

Benign hereditary chorea (also known as chronic juvenile hereditary chorea or hereditary chorea of early onset) is a generalized familial (usually dominant) chorea that begins in early childhood (often at younger than 2 years, almost always younger than 11) and continues into adulthood but does not progress to a profound physical disability, nor, usually, is it accompanied by any mental disability. The chorea typically involves the limbs, face, and trunk with a distal predominance (75).

Positron emission tomography (PET) scanning shows decreased glucose utilization in the caudate similar to the results seen in HD (76). The chorea may look similar to myoclonus, and thus the disease may look similar to benign hereditary myoclonus (72). Of course, by chance one or more individuals in a family with benign hereditary chorea could have a separate dementing condition, and thus confusion with HD could be created.

There had been a controversy regarding whether at least one subset of these patients might represent a distinct subtype of HD. More typical Huntington's patients do *not* appear in the pedigrees (75). Recently, use of the G8 probe to determine the rate of recombination or crossing over between the G8 locus and benign hereditary chorea indicated no significant linkage. Thus, benign hereditary chorea is not due to a defect in the same gene as that of HD (77).

Paroxysmal Choreoathetosis

The term paroxysmal choreoathetosis covers several different hereditary disorders, predominantly autosomal dominant, that have appeared in various case reports since the initial description (78) of what is now often called paroxysmal dystonic choreoathetosis (PDC). In PDC, attacks of unilateral or bilateral dystonia and superimposed choreo-

athetosis may be provoked by "alcohol, other beverages, chocolate (occasionally), fatigue, (rest after) physical exertion, hunger, cold, stress, excitement, concentration, urge, menses" (79). Attacks are of variable length (from at least 5 minutes to hours).

In a second disorder, paroxysmal kinesigenic choreoathetosis (PKC), unilateral dystonia and choreoathetosis are provoked by a physical trigger such as a quick movement or effort. Often there is an aura. Attacks are brief—always less than 5 minutes, and frequently a small fraction of that. Therapeutic response to many anticonvulsants (phenytoin, phenobarbital, carbamazepine) is good. There are also recessive and sporadic cases of this variety (79).

Finally, there is an overlap syndrome, intermediate paroxysmal choreoathetosis, that has a physical trigger like PKC but has attacks that are as long in duration as PDC (79). Fink et al (80) have studied a Polish American kindred that shows tight linkage between certain markers on the q region of chromosome 2. The location is near a cluster of sodium channel genes. In Chapter 73, Bakdash and Goetz present an improved classification in which the duration of attack is the key. Thus, there are two familial groups: prolonged familial paroxysmal dyskinesias (PFPD), which includes the old PDC and the intermediate form, and brief familial paroxysmal dyskinesias (BFPD), which includes the familial PKC cases. The class of sporadic cases is termed brief sporadic paroxysmal dyskinesia (BSPD). These are usually similar clinically to the BFPD cases.

Benign Hereditary Myoclonus

As implied above, this could also enter the differential diagnosis of a hereditary chorea.

Hereditary Sydenham's Chorea

Although Sydenham's chorea is usually sporadic (a presumed reaction to streptococcal or pneumococcal infection), there are many reports of familial cases. The hereditary pattern is not clear (8). Perhaps there is a hereditary predisposition to react to certain strains of streptococcal infections in such a way as to produce the condition.

Wilson's Disease

Wilson's disease, or hepatolenticular degeneration, is a recessive hereditary disorder that produces mental changes, including dementia, and a movement disorder, which can include choreiform movements (see Chapter 40, but it is not likely to cause major confusion with HD.

Spinocerebellar Degenerations

Spinocerebellar degenerations can be either autosomal dominant or recessive; as implied by their name, the major neurologic damage is in either the spinal cord or the cerebellum, though some also have associated peripheral neuropathies. At present the genes responsible for many of these syndromes have been either partially localized or entirely cloned (81–88). Although chorea is sometimes seen as part of the overall constellation of signs, the problem is generally one of diagnostic confusion because spinal, cerebellar, and neuropathic movement problems can produce various degrees of clumsiness and incoordination that may be hard to distinguish from true chorea in the early stages. Combining the movement problems with a family history of similar disturbances and the fact that some spinocerebellar degenerations, such as olivopontocerebellar atrophy, can include a dementia, explains how these conditions could be confused with HD. In addition to the diagnostic confusion, true chorea, athetosis, and/or choreoathetosis are seen in a small percentage (perhaps 2%) of spinocerebellar patients (89). However, even in these cases, chorea is usually not the major movement abnormality, nor is it a distinguishing diagnostic sign. In addition, genetic tests available for HD as well as those for some of the spinocerebellar degenerations can now cut through any potential confusion. The one spinocerebellar degeneration that does frequently manifest considerable chorea is the rare dentatorubropallidoluysian atrophy (DRPLA) (89). In fact, the autosomal dominant pattern and the clinical findings, which include both dementia and chorea, previously made it very difficult to distinguish DRPLA from HD (90). Interestingly, now that the genes for both have been cloned, we know that both are triplet expansion syndromes; that is, there is an increase in the number of times that a three-base sequence (in both cases, CAG) is repeated in the midst of the affected gene (91). The neuropathology of DRPLA typically involves the subthalamic nuclei, pallidum, dentate nuclei of the cerebellum, and red nuclei with striatal sparing (92).

Lesch–Nyhan Syndrome

This X-linked recessive disease is caused by a defect in the hypoxanthine-guanine phosphoribosyltransferase (HPRT) gene. The enzymatic defect leads to accumulation of uric acid in all major bodily fluids, as well as urate crystal deposition in the joints (causing gout) and the kidney (causing nephropathy) (93,94).

With respect to symptoms and signs referable to the central nervous system, spasticity, choreoathetosis, and loss of intellectual milestones begin in the first year of life. By the second year, the patient displays the self-mutilating behavior (severely biting his or her own lips and fingers) that is highly characteristic of the disease. Patients typically die of kidney failure before the age of 40. Despite the fact that the gene for this condition has been cloned, there is presently no good understanding of the link between the gene product (i.e., HPRT) and the neurologic deterioration. Uric acid does not appear to be the immediate cause of the neurologic problems. The basal ganglia of patients with Lesch-Nyhan syndrome have abnormally low levels of dopamine metabolites, but it is not clear why this occurs or whether this is a significant factor (93,94).

Hallervorden–Spatz Disease

Hallervorden-Spatz disease, an autosomal recessive condition starting in childhood, can show manifestations of chorea and/or choreoathetosis amidst a plethora of other motor problems consisting of stiffness, spasticity, and dystonia that frequently involve the face (causing clenched teeth and dysphagia), dysarthria, and bizarre facial expressions (see Chapter 41). Children with this condition may live for several decades or may die before age 10, usually from infection (95).

There is iron deposition in the basal ganglia, which show nonspecific changes on CT and MRI (the caudate is often atrophic). Cortical atrophy of variable degree may be seen as well (95).

Pelizaeus–Merzbacher Disease

Pelizaeus-Merzbacher disease is an X-linked recessive disorder either present at birth (connatal form) or beginning during infancy (classic variety). It can be caused by any one of several mutations in the proteolipid protein gene (96–98). Patients display nystagmus and a head-rolling tremor from the outset of the disease. Choreoathetosis occurs several years later amidst a constellation of motor signs, including spasticity and ataxia, as the children are slowly acquiring limited developmental milestones such as crawling and rudimentary speech. Individuals with the connatal form usually die in the first year before even achieving this level, and, thus, they rarely show chorea at all. The others can live to adolescence or even somewhat later. Dementia is not necessarily profound, though the children are usually mute due to motor problems (95).

There is a severe decrease in the amount of myelin in most central structures, though peripheral myelin is spared. Ventricular dilatation is evident on MRI and CT, along with marked cerebellar atrophy and decreased differentiation between gray and white matter (95).

SPORADIC CHOREAS

Sydenham's Chorea

Just as HD is the archetype for the hereditary choreas, Sydenham's chorea (variously called St. Vitus' dance and chorea minor) is probably the most commonly thought of sporadic chorea.

Sydenham's chorea is seen in cases of streptococcal infection, often as a part of the constellation of rheumatic fever, a condition now less common than in the past due to early antibiotic treatment. One presumption is that it is an autoimmune disorder. Anticaudate and antisubthalamic nucleus antibodies (99) have been described in the condition, but a specific antigen has not been identified. In general, the movements are swifter and smaller than those seen in Huntington's disease. They often have a darting quality, do not involve as many muscles, and are less likely to blend into ordinary movements. Nonetheless, in individual cases there could be great difficulty distinguishing the two from the movements alone. In fact, we think that the most significant differentiating point is that the chorea of Sydenham's almost always occurs in children whereas the chorea of HD almost always occurs in adults. Generally, the former chorea goes away completely in weeks to months. There is usually no severe neurologic residua (however, a rheumatic heart condition could be a severe residua of the whole episode). Some individuals will have one or more relapses of the chorea, presumably due to a new infection.

The literature contains conflicting statements about how often there is significant neurologic residua. Very careful long-term studies show that over half of the patients do have some choreiform movements as a residua (100). Often the chorea goes completely away and then gradually comes back, to a more minor degree, years later. Typically, patients and families do not even recognize it as such. Sometimes an action tremor is noted, or the minor movements are ascribed to nervousness. Also, post-Sydenham patients appear more likely to manifest choreiform movements if they are later treated with "amphetamines, phenylethylamines, thyroid hormone [or] phenytoin" (100). They also appear more likely to manifest chorea with birth control pills or pregnancy (100).

Pathology of Sydenham's Chorea

There has not been as much study of pathologic material in this condition as in HD. In examined cases, there has been "swelling, chromatolysis and atrophy" of neurons and "perivascular infiltrates, evidence of overt arteritis or the presence of focal petechial hemorrhage" (100). Much of the change has been concentrated in the caudate and putamen, but the cortex, thalamus, and other basal ganglia structures are not spared. It is interesting to note that autopsies of patients who died of rheumatic fever but who never manifested chorea have showed similar findings (100).

It is reasonable to assume that some of the same neuroanatomic structures and neurochemical pathways involved in HD may be under attack in Sydenham's chorea. Thus, it is also reasonable to try the same medications. However, there do appear to be differences in the pharmacotherapy. Essentially, the chorea of Sydenham's responds better than that of HD and also responds to more medications. The dopamine antagonists offer some relief, as they do in Huntington's disease. Sodium valproate may also help, however, in Sydenham's chorea (101). Other treatments are discussed in the section on therapy.

Chorea Gravidarum and Oral Contraceptive Chorea

Chorea gravidarum is the occurrence of chorea during pregnancy. A large fraction (about one-third) of such patients have previously experienced Sydenham's chorea (100,102). Thus, one hypothesis has been that chorea gravidarum is a reactivation of Sydenham's chorea in these cases, due to a new infection. But more recently a possible hormonal link has been emphasized because there is usually no good evidence of a new streptococcal infection. Also, there is experimental evidence that oophorectomy reduces sensitivity to dopamine agonists in experimental animals (103,104).

The pathology in chorea gravidarum is similar to Sydenham's chorea. Work-up should include a screen for collagen diseases. There is usually no reason to terminate the pregnancy (105).

Appearance of chorea with the use of birth control pills strengthens the suspicion of some hormonal link with this particular movement disorder. A large number (41%) of such patients have also had a prior history of Sydenham's chorea (104). Some workers feel that oral contraceptive chorea, as well as chorea induced by other pharmacologic agents, reflects an increased susceptibility of the relevant basal ganglia structures due to prior (detected or undetected) injuries (105). Regardless of the theories, stopping the birth control pills stops the contraceptive-induced chorea.

Other Causes of Chorea

Hyperthyroidism may sometimes cause chorea, in which case cure of the hyperthyroidism usually produces a cure of the chorea, or at least an amelioration of the condition. Polycythemia vera is an unusual cause of chorea that may affect the basal ganglial structures via its effects on blood flow. Arteritis, for example, lupus, is another rare cause of choreiform or choreoathetoid movements. Again, the presumption is that at least some of the same neurologic circuity affected in HD is also affected by the arteritis (35,72,106).

Consistent with the pharmacologic/pathophysiologic model presented later, L-dopa administration can sometimes induce chorea. Typically this occurs in the context of treatment of a parkinsonian patient. Many parkinsonian patients treated with L-dopa for several years will not get relief from bradykinesia without being given some degree of choreoathetosis from L-dopa. Most patients prefer mobility even with some choreoathetoid movements.

Neuroleptics (phenothiazines, butyrephenones, and related compounds) cause tardive dyskinesias that resemble chorea but which are usually more stereotyped and repetitive and tend to emphasize facial movements (oral-lingual-buccal dyskinesias) (35). Nevertheless, in some cases it is fair to apply the term chorea to these movements (106).

Finally, there is a sporadic form of brief paroxysmal choreoathetosis, which was mentioned above and is covered in Chapter 73.

Although this discussion has covered the usual causes and many of the rare ones, it is not exhaustive. There are rare cases reported of chorea caused by head trauma, brain tumors, and cerebrovascular disorders (106). In addition, there are a host of infections, presumed autoimmune disorders, drugs and other chemical agents, and hereditary diseases (other than the ones we have described above) that have produced occasional cases of chorea. The review by Padberg and Bruyn (106) provides the most exhaustive list that we have seen.

LABORATORY STUDIES IN THE CHOREAS

CT and MRI scans are usually quite characteristic in HD, particularly in the later stages, when enlarged ventricles and a markedly atrophied caudate nucleus are seen. PET scans using radiolabeled 2-deoxyglucose reveal decreased glucose metabolism in both the caudate and the putamen in HD (107). As mentioned above, similar PET findings can be seen in benign hereditary chorea (76).

The electroencephalogram (EEG) provides no specific information valuable to the diagnosis, though there are generally some diffuse findings, such as slowing, particularly when the other signs and symptoms have become manifest. A more sophisticated technique, which time-locks EEG activity to preceding motor activity, has revealed a cortical negativity that precedes the choreiform movements in hereditary chorea-acanthocytosis and is not seen in HD. In the past this may have offered occasional utility in separating the two disorders, though it would be much easier to look at the peripheral blood for acanthocytes (108). Of course, genetic testing for the specific gene involved is the method of choice in applicable cases.

MODEL OF BASAL GANGLIA FUNCTION

We now present a more detailed model of chorea that attempts to rationalize the phenomenon in the context of current physiologic and pharmacologic models of basal ganglia function. Basal ganglia output from the traditionally recognized output nuclei, that is, the globus pallidus interna (GPi) and substantia nigra pars reticulata (SNr), is inhibitory and directed primarily toward regions of motor thalamus. This tonic inhibitory output influences the firing pattern of thalamic neurons. Excessive inhibition of thalamocortical activity by the GPi (and the SNr) is thought to underlie the hypokinetic features of Parkinson's disease (PD) (109). Increased GPi (and SNr) activity in PD is thought to be due to a shift in balance between so-called direct and indirect basal ganglia pathways (39,110). This results from loss of dopaminergic input to the striatum from the substantia nigra pars compacta (SNc) (Fig 71.1).

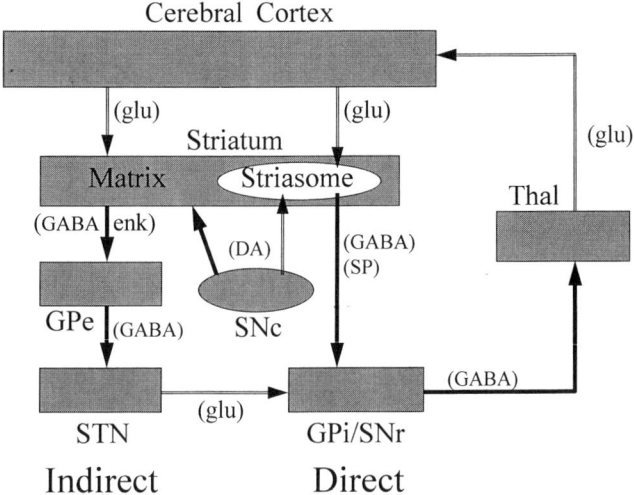

FIGURE 71.1   *The direct/indirect model of basal ganglia function (39,110). Only pathways contributing to the model are included in this figure. Additional pathways that may contribute significantly to basal ganglia function (111) are discussed in the text. Abbreviations: DA = dopamine, enk = enkephalin, GABA = γ-aminobutyric acid, glu = glutamate, GPe = globus pallidus externa, GPi/SNr = globus pallidus interna and substantia nigra pars reticulata, SP = substance P, STN = subthalamic nucleus, Thal = thalamus. Open arrow = excitatory pathway; closed arrow = inhibitory pathway.*

Dopaminergic innervation has a differential effect on spiny projection neurons within the striatum (for a detailed review, see reference 111). In summary, an excitatory action, via D_1 receptors on GABA/substance P–containing neurons most densely concentrated within the striasomal compartment, results in inhibition of GPi (and SNr). This direct inhibition of GPi (and SNr) is complemented by inhibition of an indirect pathway by dopamine via D_2 receptors on GABA/enkephalin-containing neurons most densely concentrated within the striatal matrix. The output of these neurons inhibits GABAergic neurons within the globus pallidus externa (GPe), thereby disinhibiting glutaminergic neurons within the subthalamic nucleus (STN). Output from the STN has an excitatory action on GPi (and SNr). Thus, through an excitatory action on the direct pathway and an inhibitory action on the indirect pathway, dopaminergic innervation of the striatum leads to GPi (and SNr) inhibition. Therefore, *loss* of dopaminergic innervation in PD results in decreased direct and increased indirect pathway function and excessive inhibition of the thalamus from the GPi (and SNr). A shift in balance in the opposite direction (i.e., increased direct and decreased indirect pathway activity) would be expected to result in increased thalamocortical activity. In theory, this could account for or contribute to the expression of certain dyskinesias, including ballism, athetosis, and chorea (112).

This model is fully consistent with hemiballismus resulting from acute lesions of the contralateral subthalamic nucleus, thereby inactivating the indirect pathway. Similarly, peak-dose dyskinesia, seen in some patients with PD on levodopa therapy and which typically has a choreiform or choreoathetotic appearance, has been attributed to excessive excitation of the direct pathway and excessive inhibition of the indirect pathway by dopamine (112,113). In HD, pathologic studies suggest selective vulnerability of striatal projection neurons, with most studies indicating earlier and greater involvement of enkephalin-containing neurons that project to the GPe (indirect pathway) than substance P–containing neurons that project to the GPi (direct pathway) (114,115).

The direct/indirect model of basal ganglia function is elegant in its relative simplicity and in its ability to account for certain clinical observations. This model has also provided a rationale for the surgical procedure of posterior (sensorimotor) GPi pallidotomy in patients with PD (116). As is predicted by this model, experimental hemiparkinsonism in primates induced by intracarotid injection of the dopamine-depleting toxoid 1-methyl-4-phenyl-1,2,3,6-tetrahydropyridine (MPTP) is associated with increased activity within the STN and the GPi (109,117). Lesioning of the STN in this model attenuates the parkinsonism (118). However, the clinical experience with pallidotomy in patients with PD raises fundamental questions concerning the accuracy of the direct/indirect model and the pathophysiology of hyperkinetic states such as chorea. Specifically, although lesioning of the posterior GPi predictably attenuates the major motor signs associated with parkinsonism (tremor, rigidity, akinesia, bradykinesia, and the gait disorder), levodopa-induced dyskinesia (including chorea) is also greatly attenuated (116,119). Rather than increasing hyperkinetic signs, which would be an expected consequence of disinhibition of thalamus, pallidotomy appears to *normalize* extrapyramidal motor function in patients with PD. Thus, pallidotomy is actually an effective treatment for one of the most prevalent causes of chorea, levodopa-induced chorea associated with the treatment of PD. Moreover, GPi pallidotomy also attenuates hemiballismus from experimental subthalamic nucleus lesions, as was first demonstrated in 1950 (120).

What could account for the apparent paradox of improvement in both hypokinetic signs (e.g., bradykinesia) and hyperkinetic signs (e.g., chorea) by a single lesion within the posterior GPi, that is, in the sensorimotor region of the principal basal ganglia outflow nucleus? The answer to this question is, as of this writing, still unknown (121). However, the direct/indirect model leaves out numerous additional connections among basal ganglia structures and between these nuclei and other brain regions that might contribute to extrapyramidal motor function (111). Some of these pathways support the model. For example, a direct inhibitory output from the GPe to GPi parallels GPe inhibition of

STN excitation of the GPi (122). Although the GPe is not traditionally considered a basal ganglia outflow nucleus, an inhibitory output from the GPe to the reticularis nucleus of the thalamus (123) appears to result in disinhibition of both pallidal and cerebellar receiving areas within the thalamus (124). When this pathway is inhibited, as occurs in patients with PD, reticularis nucleus inhibition of the thalamus results in a shift in thalamic neuronal activity from a so-called transfer to a bursting mode. This shift in thalamic activity, resulting from hyperpolarization of thalamic neurons, may be related to tremor and rigidity in patients with PD (125–127). Of note, this cerebellar receiving area appears to be the optimal localization for therapeutic thalamotomy for the treatment of parkinsonian tremor (128,129).

Other basal ganglia pathways counter the direct/indirect model. For example, in addition to projecting to GPi and SNr (direct pathway), GABAergic striosomal compartment (striatal) neurons that receive an excitatory dopaminergic input provide an inhibitory feedback to the SNc. In fact, Hedreen and Folstein have provided pathologic evidence of earliest striatal neuronal loss in HD within striosomes (130), arguing that the resultant lack of inhibition of SNc and increased dopaminergic activity in the striatum may contribute to chorea (i.e., inhibition of indirect and excitation of remaining direct pathways). Inhibition of the STN by the GPe is balanced by an excitatory feedback from the STN to the GPe (as reviewed in reference 111). The cerebral cortex projects directly to the STN. Although this pathway could possibly augment subthalamic excitation of GPi inhibition of the thalamus (indirect pathway), subthalamic excitation of GPe could result in thalamic disinhibition via the inhibitory pathways noted above involving the reticularis nucleus of thalamus.

Probably the least well understood structures involved with extrapyramidal motor function are the thalamus and supplementary motor cortex (and other motor-related cortical regions) that receive excitatory projections from the thalamus. These projections are reciprocal. However, the role of excitatory corticothalamic projections to motor thalamus is unknown. Connectivity within the thalamus, for example, between pallidal and cerebellar receiving areas, is also poorly understood. Beyond recognizing a role of input in modulating between bursting and transfer firing patterns (noted above), regulation of thalamic activity is poorly understood. Corticothalamic activity arising in somatosensory cortical areas has been demonstrated to modulate responsiveness to tactile stimuli by facilitating activity of certain ventroposterolateral (sensory) thalamic neurons (131). Other studies have demonstrated both direct excitatory responses and inhibitory responses (e.g., via inhibitory interneurons) of corticothalamic activity on cortically projecting thalamic neurons (132). Whether corticothalamic projections modulate responsiveness to input from the GPi (or SNr) has not yet been established. However, it is possible that corticothalamic and cortico-striatal-pallidal-thalamic pathways interface in the thalamus, with the resultant corticothalamic activity determined by a logical operation at this site. If cortico-striatal-pallidal-thalamic activity is aberrant (as reflected in abnormal pallidal outflow, whether increased or decreased), then elimination of this input, that is, therapeutic pallidotomy, might allow normalization of corticothalamic activity (133).

In addition to the motor thalamus, basal ganglia outflow nuclei project to several other sites. Some of these include the center-median parafascicular (CM-PF) nucleus of the thalamus, the pedunculopontine nucleus (PPN) in the midbrain, the lateral habenular nucleus, and from the SNr, the superior colliculus (111). The CM-PF thalamus provides a large input back to the striatum. The PPN provides an excitatory projection back to the GPi and SNr. This nucleus also projects to the SNc and connects bidirectionally with the STN. Numerous nonextrapyramidal connections of the PPN include additional brainstem sites, the spinal cord, cerebellum, basal forebrain, and thalamus (for review of PPN connectivity and possible functions, see reference 134).

As with the thalamus and other sites receiving basal ganglia output, disinhibition of the PPN by levodopa or surgical pallidotomy (in patients with PD) may have specific clinical consequences. However, the PPN cannot be released from inhibition by treatment if there is significant neuronal loss within the nucleus by the disease process. Studies have, in fact, demonstrated variably severe neuronal loss within this structure in patients with PD (135–137). In contrast to PD, neuronal loss within the PPN in patients with progressive supranuclear palsy (PSP) appears to be uniformly severe (136–138). Moreover, the brainstem pathology in PSP is much more widespread than in PD, including within the midbrain tegmentum (and tectum). Patients with PSP have minimal or no response to treatment with levodopa (139). Moreover, they do not develop levodopa-induced dyskinesias. Finally, they do not respond to pallidotomy (and, in fact, have severe neuronal loss within the pallidum as part of the disease process). It is possible that the positive phenomenology of PD, including response to levodopa (both therapeutic and dyskinetic) or pallidotomy, requires certain intact brainstem systems. Of note, the PPN is unaffected in HD (R. Zweig, unpublished observation).

TREATMENT OF CHOREA (EMPHASIS ON HUNTINGTON'S DISEASE AND SYDENHAM'S CHOREA)

Generations of physicians have employed therapies for the choreas, and such treatments have often provided a degree of amelioration. A much earlier discussion in a highly regarded neurology textbook held that

From among the large number of drugs which have been introduced in the therapy of Sydenham's chorea, only three appear to me to have a specific effect:

arsenic, antipyrin and cannabis indica. Arsenic is incontestably the most efficient of the pharmacological agents, and should hence be preferred . . . Besides these drugs, it may be necessary to prescribe hypnotics for a longer or shorter time, as it is of great importance that the patients sleep long and deeply (140).

With respect to HD, the same author was less optimistic: "The therapy is purely symptomatic, and, as such, gives little prospect of results. Only in very early stages arsenic and scopolamin (0.5–2.0 mg per dose once a day) appear to be able to procure alleviation" (140).

Today, there are rational therapies based on the previously discussed neuropharmacology of the movement disorder as well as attempts at chemoprotection from the effects of the putative excitotoxins. In most cases it is not obvious, however, that our better rationalized therapies are much more effective than the older nostrums.

For therapeutic purposes, the neuropharmacologic relationships previously described can be simplified further to the concept that the GABAergic and cholinergic systems of the basal ganglia have been weakened in comparison with the dopaminergic ones. Thus, rational candidates for therapy would be 1) drugs that enhance the GABA systems, 2) drugs that enhance cholinergic systems, and 3) drugs that block dopaminergic systems.

In the first group, diazepam and other benzodiazepines, which bind near the GABA receptor and increase GABA binding (GABA also increases benzodiazepine binding), may thus enhance GABAergic transmission and, indeed, have been found to be somewhat useful in controlling the choreiform movements of HD. Sodium valproate inhibits GABA transaminase and, thus, may raise GABA levels. It also increases GABA binding. However, it does not appear to give significant benefit in this condition. It may help, however, in Sydenham's chorea (101). Finally, baclofen, a $GABA_B$ agonist that is useful in treating spasticity, does not appear to be useful in treating HD chorea (141).

In general, anticholinergics worsen the chorea, whereas cholinergic drugs often confer some benefits. For example, physostigmine improves chorea (142). Not all patients benefit, but those who do may also respond to choline administration. Not every cholinergic drug works. For example, arecoline provides no benefit (143). Scopolamine, used by the earlier neurologists (140), ameliorates the chorea but worsens coordination (144). Indeed, there is evidence that the efficacy of the cholinergic drugs may depend on their sedative effect more than on a specific cholinergic action (145). This possibility should be considered in all the drugs that appear to ameliorate chorea. However, drugs whose antichoreic action is due to a sedative effect can still be useful in providing symptomatic relief.

Probably the most useful drugs are those which influence the dopamine system. These include

1. Dopamine receptor blockers such as the phenothiazines and butyrophenones (e.g., haloperidol). In particular, haloperidol has been shown to ameliorate choreiform movements in a manner dependent on the serum haloperidol concentration (146).

2. Dopamine depleters such as reserpine and tetrabenazine (147). Tetrabenazine, in particular, has the advantage that it is not only quite effective but also has no tendency to produce tardive dyskinesias (147). Reserpine, a much older drug, has a long history of producing depression in patients who have used it for hypertension. While it is listed for completeness, we do not recommend it.

As was true in an earlier era (140), Sydenham's chorea appears more amenable to treatment than does HD. Of course it also resolves spontaneously. We have already mentioned the response to sodium valproate. Carbamazepine, which may also act through the GABA system, has been reported to be effective as well, as have dopamine antagonists (e.g., haloperidol). Sedative/hypnotics (e.g., chloral hydrate) are also useful, though their action may not be specific. We believe that enthusiasm for specific pharmacologic treatment should be tempered by the fact that most cases resolve spontaneously with little or no severe neurologic residua. We therefore recommend caution in the treatment of these children and believe that medication such as haloperidol, which can itself produce permanent dyskinesias, should be used only as a last resort.

Differences in the Treatment Approach to Choreas Caused by Other Conditions

Familial paroxysmal chorea (see Chapter 73) is especially responsive to the anticonvulsants, including phenytoin, carbamazepine, and phenobarbital, but not to sodium valproate or diazepam. Generally, the pharmacologic literature on this and the other choreic syndromes, aside from HD and Sydenham's chorea, consists of scattered reports involving small numbers of cases. The best counsel we can offer is that all the drugs that work in any one case of chorea may work in any other, but that one should carefully consider the severity of the chorea, the likely length of the condition, the age of the patient, and the possible side effects of treatment. For example, it usually would be unwise to treat birth control pill–induced chorea in any other way than by discontinuing the birth control pills. If the pills were extremely important to the patient, different formulations could be tried. Continuing the offending medication and adding haloperidol, for example, in an attempt to suppress the chorea should be considered only as a last resort.

Chemoprotection

If, as some investigators suspect, the neuronal damage in HD is caused by excitatory neurotransmitters, why not try to prevent or slow the progression of the disease by blocking them? Baclofen has been considered a possible candidate for a chemoprotective role because in addition to (or perhaps as a consequence of) its GABAergic action it can decrease glutaminergic transmission (72). Indeed, there is evidence that baclofen can retard the corticostriatal release of both glutamate and aspartate, another excitatory amino acid that could also have a role in the neuronal death found in HD (141). However, in a recent randomized controlled trial (141), baclofen provided no benefit. Dextromethorphan has also been tested in an attempt to block the subset of glutamate receptors sensitive to *N*-methyl D-aspartate. No beneficial effect was found in a recent open-label trial (148). However, the trials of chemoprotective agents are still in their infancy, and we believe that this is a promising approach. The work of Albin et al (21), showing reduction of NMDA glutamate receptors on the inhibitory GABAergic striatal neurons in HD, suggests that NMDA receptor blockade may be beneficial. It is possible that the specific blocking agent and/or the dose has not been optimal in early trials. Thus, despite negative trial results (148), we still think that the excitotoxin blocking approach holds promise.

Neurotransplantation

An additional therapeutic possibility is transplantation of fetal neuronal material to replace the neurons that have been destroyed. In the previously mentioned ibotenic acid–induced rat model, transplantation of fetal striatal neurons produced amelioration of the condition (44,149). A combined approach using transplantation of fetal cells plus other cells engineered to secrete trophic factors may be of value (150). Further studies are needed.

REFERENCES

1. Adams RD, Victor M. Principles of neurology. 4th ed. New York, McGraw-Hill, 1989:391.
2. Koller WC, Trimble J. The gait abnormality of Huntington's disease. Neurology 1985;35:1450–1454.
3. Gilman S. Gait disorders. In: Rowland LP, ed. Merritt's textbook of neurology. 8th ed. Philadelphia: Lea and Febiger, 1989:57.
4. Bruyn GW, Went LN. Huntington's chorea. In: Vinken PJ, Bruyn GW, Klawans HL, eds. Handbook of clinical neurology. Vol. 5 (49), Extrapyramidal disorders. Amsterdam: Elsevier, 1986:267–313.
5. Bruyn GW. Huntington's chorea. Historical, clinical and laboratory synopsis. In: Vinken PJ, Bruyn GW, eds. Handbook of clinical neurology. Vol. 6, Diseases of the basal ganglia. Amsterdam: North-Holland: 1968:298–378.
6. Huntington G. On chorea. Med Surg Reporter 1872;26:317–321.
7. Vessie PR. On the transmission of Huntington's chorea for 300 years: the Bures family group. J Nerv Ment Dis 1932;76:553–573.
8. Ionasescu V, Zellweger H. Genetics in neurology. New York: Raven Press, 1983.
9. Houseman D, Gusella J. Molecular genetic approaches to neural disorders. In: Schmitt FO, Bird SJ, Bloom FE, eds. Molecular genetic neuroscience. New York: Raven Press, 1982.
10. Huntington's Disease Collaborative Research Group. A novel gene containing a trinucleotide repeat that is expanded and unstable on Huntington's disease chromosomes. Cell 1993;72:971–983.

11. Hoogeveen AT, Willemsen R, Meyer N, et al. Characterization and localization of the Huntington disease gene product. Hum Mol Genet 1993;2:2069–2073.

12. Andrew SE, Goldberg YP, Kremer B, et al. The relationship between trinucleotide (CAG) repeat length and clinical features of Huntington's disease. Nat Genet 1993;4:398–403.

13. Stine OC, Li SH, Pleasant N, et al. Expression of the mutant allele of IT-15 (the HD gene) in striatum and cortex of Huntington's disease patients. Hum Mol Genet 1995;4:15–18.

14. Persichetti F, Ambrose CM, Ge P, et al. Normal and expanded Huntington's disease gene alleles produce distinguishable proteins due to translation across the CAG repeat. Mol Med 1995;1:374–383.

15. Zeitlin S, Liu JP, Chapman DL, et al. Increased apoptosis and early embryonic lethality in mice nullizygous for the Huntington's disease gene homologue. Nat Genet 1995;11:155–163.

16. Duyao MP, Auerbach AB, Ryan A, et al. Inactivation of the mouse Huntington's disease gene homolog Hdh. Science 1995;269:407–410.

17. Schilling G, Sharp AH, Loev SJ, et al. Expression of the Huntington's disease (IT15) protein product in HD patients. Hum Mol Genet 1995;4:1365–1371.

18. Li XJ, Li SH, Sharp AH, et al. A huntingtin-associated protein enriched in brain with implications for pathology. Nature 1995;378:398–402.

19. Burke JR, Enghild JJ, Martin ME, et al. Huntingtin and DRPLA proteins selectively interact with the enzyme GAPDH. Nat Med 1996;2:347–350.

20. Albin RL, Reiner A, Anderson KD, et al. Striatal and nigral neuron subpopulations in rigid Huntington's disease: implications for the functional anatomy of chorea and rigidity-akinesia. Ann Neurol 1990;27:357–365.

21. Albin RL, Young AB, Penney JB, et al. Abnormalities of striatal projection neurons and N-methyl-D-aspartate receptors in presymptomatic Huntington's disease. N Engl J Med 1990;322:1293–1298.

22. Ferrante RJ, Kowall NW, Beal MF, et al. Selective sparing of a class of striatal neurons in Huntington's disease. Science 1985;30:561–563.

23. Ferrante RJ, Beal MF, Kowall NW, et al. Sparing of acetylcholinesterase-containing striatal neurons in Huntington's disease. Brain Res 1987;411:162–166.

24. Ferrante RJ, Kowall NW, Beal MF, et al. Morphologic and histochemical characteristics of a spared subset of striatal neurons in Huntington's disease. J Neuropathol Exp Neurol 1987;46:12–27.

25. Ferrante RJ, Kowall NW, Richardson EP Jr. Proliferative and degenerative changes in striatal spiny neurons in Huntington's disease: a combined study using the section Golgi method and calbindin D28k immunocytochemistry. J Neurosci 1991;11:3877–3887.

26. Dawbarn D, DeQuidt ME, Emson PC. Survival of basal ganglia neuropeptide Y-somatostatin neurones in Huntington's disease. Brain Res 1985;340:251–260.

27. Ferrante RJ. Huntington's disease: morphometric and immunocytochemical alterations. In Bignami A, ed., New issues in neuroscience, basal ganglia and movement disorders. New York: Thieme, 1991:191–201.

28. Graveland GA, Williams RS, DiFiglia MA. Evidence for degenerative and regenerative changes in neostriatal spiny neurons in Huntington's disease. Science 1985;227:770–773.

29. Ferrante RJ, Kowall NW, Beal MF, et al. Topography of enkephalin, substance P, and acetylcholinesterase staining in Huntington's disease striatum. Neurosci Lett 1986;71:283–288.

30. Seto-Ohshima A, Emson PC, Lawson E, et al. Loss of matrix calcium-binding protein-containing neurons in Huntington's disease. Lancet 1988;1:1252–1255.

31. Faull RL, Waldvogel HJ, Nicholson LF, Synek BJ. The distribution of GABAA-benzodiazepine receptors in the basal ganglia in Huntington's disease and in the quinolinic acid-lesioned rat. Prog Brain Res 1993;99:105–123.

32. Glass M, Faull RL, Dragunow M. Loss of cannabinoid receptors in the substantia nigra in Huntington's disease. Neuroscience 1993;56:523–527.

33. Morton AJ, Nicholson LF, Faull RL. Compartmental loss of NADPH diaphorase in the neuropil of the human striatum in Huntington's disease. Neuroscience 1993;53:159–168.

34. Roos RAC. Neuropathology of Huntington's chorea. In: Vinken PJ, Bruyn GW, Klawans HL, eds. Handbook of clinical neurology. Vol. 5 (49), Extrapyramidal disorders. Amsterdam: Elsevier, 1986:315–326.

35. Fahn S. Huntington disease and other forms of chorea. In: Rowland LP, ed. Merritt's textbook of neurology. 8th ed. Philadelphia: Lea and Febiger, 1989:647–652.

36. Cummings JL, Benson DF. Dementia: a clinical approach. 2nd ed. Boston: Butterworth, 1992:96–98.

37. Reiner A, Albin RL, Anderson KD, et al. Differential loss of striatal projection neurons in Huntington's disease. Proc Natl Acad Sci U S A 1988;85:5733–5737.

38. Crossman AR. Primate models of dyskinesia: the experimental approach to the study of basal ganglia-related involuntary movement disorders. Neuroscience 1987;21:1–40.

39. DeLong MR. Primate models of movement disorders of basal ganglia origin. Trends Neurosci 1990;13:281–285.

40. Coyle JT, Schwarcz R. Model for Huntington's chorea: lesion of striatal neurons with kainic acid. Nature 1976;263:244–246.

41. Coyle JT, McGeer EG, McGeer PL, Schwarcz R. Neostriatal injections: a model for Huntington's chorea. In: McGeer EG, Olney JW, McGeer PL, eds. Kainic acid as a tool in neurobiology. New York: Raven Press, 1978:139–160.

42. McGeer GE, McGeer PL. Duplication of biochemical changes of Huntington's disease by intrastriatal injections of glutamic and kainic acids. Nature 1976;263:517–519.

43. McGeer EG, McGeer PL, Hattori T, Vincent SR. Kainic acid neurotoxicity and Huntington's disease. In: Chase TN, Wexler NS, Barbeau A, eds. Advances in neurology. Vol. 23, Huntington's disease. New York: Raven Press, 1979:577–591.

44. Isacson O, Dunnett SB, Bjorklund A. Graft-induced behavioral recovery in an animal model of Huntington disease. Proc Natl Acad Sci U S A 1986;83:2728–2732.

45. Kanazaw I, Kimura M, Murata M, et al. Choreic movements in the macaque monkey induced by kainic acid lesions of the striatum combined with L-dopa. Pharmacological, biochemical and physiological studies on neural mechanisms. Brain 1990;113:509–535.

46. Beal MF, Kowall NW, Ellison DW, et al. Replication of the neurochemical characteristics of Huntington's disease with quinolinic acid. Nature 1986;321:168–171.

47. Beal MF, Kowall NW, Swartz KJ, et al. Differential sparing of somatostatin-neuropeptide Y and cholinergic neurons following striatal excitotoxin lesions. Synapse 1989;3:38–47.

48. Tatter SB, Galpern WR, Hoogeveen AT, Isacson O. Effects of striatal excitotoxicity on huntingtin-like immunoreactivity. Neuroreport 1995;6:1125–1129.

49. Ferrante RJ, Kowall NW, Cipolloni PB, et al. Excitotoxin lesions in primates as a model for Huntington's disease: histopathologic and neurochemical characterization. Exp Neurol 1993;119:46–71.

50. Albin R, Greenamyre JT. Alternative excitotoxic hypotheses. Neurology 1992;42:733–738.

51. Beal MF. Does impairment of energy metabolism result in excitotoxic neuronal death in neurodegenerative illnesses? Ann Neurol 1992;31:119–130.

52. Olney JW. Neurotoxicity of excitatory amino acids. In: Olney JW, McGeer RL, eds. Kainic acid as a tool in neurobiology. New York: Raven Press, 1978:95–122.

53. Novelli AJ, Reilly A, Lysko PG, Henneberry RC. Glutamate becomes neurotoxic via the N-methyl-D-aspartate receptor when intracellular energy levels are reduced. Brain Res 1988;451:205–212.

54. Zeevalk GD, Nicklas WJ. Mechanisms underlying initiation of excitotoxicity associated with metabolic inhibition. J Pharmacol Exp Ther 1991;257:870–878.

55. Mariani AP, Neff NH, Hadjiconstantinou M. MPTP treatment decreases dopamine and increases lipofuscin in mouse retina. Neurosci Lett 1986;72:221–226.

56. Ramsay RR, Krueger MJ, Youngster SK, Singer TP. Interaction of 1-methyl-4-phenylpyridium ion (MPP+) and its analogs with the rotenone/piericidin binding site of NADH dehydrogenase. J Neurochem 1991;56:1184–1190.

57. Brennan WAJ, Bird ED, Aprille JR. Regional mitochondrial respiratory activity in Huntington's disease brain. J Neurochem 1985;44:1948–1950.

58. Parker WJR, Boyson SJ, Luder AS, Parks JK. Evidence for a defect in NADH ubiquinone oxidoreductase (complex I) in Huntington's disease. Neurology 1990;40:1231–1234.

59. Mann VM, Cooper JM, Javoy-Agid F, et al. Mitochondrial function and parental sex effect in Huntington's disease. Lancet 1990;336:749.

60. Browne SE, Beal MF. Oxidative damage and mitochondrial dysfunction in neurodegenerative diseases. Biochem Soc Trans 1994;22:1002–1006.

61. Hamilton BF, Gould DH. Nature and distribution of brain lesions in rats intoxicated with 3-nitropropionic acid: a type of hypoxic (energy deficient) brain damage. Acta Neuropathol 1987;72:286–297.

62. Ludolph AC, He F, Spencer PS, et al. 3-Nitropropionic acid—exogenous animal neurotoxin and possible human striatal toxin. Can J Neurol Sci 1991;18:492–498.

63. Brouillet E, Jenkins BG, Hyman BT, et al. Age-dependent vulnerability of the striatum to the mitochondrial toxin 3-nitropropionic acid. J Neurochem 1993;60:356–359.

64. Beal MF, Brouillet E, Jenkins B, et al. Age-dependent striatal excitotoxic lesions produced by the endogenous mitochondrial inhibitor malonate. J Neurochem 1993;61:1147–1150.

65. Brouillet E, Hantraye P, Ferrante RJ, et al. Chronic mitochondrial energy impairment produces selective striatal degeneration and abnormal choreiform movements in primates. Proc Natl Acad Sci U S A 1995;92:7105–7109.

66. Beal MF, Ferrante RJ, Swartz KJ, Kowall NW. Chronic quinolinic acid lesions in rats closely resemble Huntington's disease. J Neurosci 1991;11:1649–1659.

67. Bossi SR, Simpson JR, Isacson O. Age dependence of striatal neuronal death caused by mitochondrial dysfunction. Neuroreport 1993;4:73–76.

68. DiFiglia M, Sapp E, Chase K, et al. Huntingtin is a cytoplasmic protein associated with vesicles in human and rat brain neurons. Neuron 1995;14:1075–1081.

69. Sharp AH, Loev SJ, Schilling G, et al. Widespread expression of Huntington's disease gene (IT15) protein product. Neuron 1995;14:1065–1074.

70. Gutekunst CA, Levey AI, Heilman CJ, et al. Identification and localization of huntingtin in brain and human lymphoblastoid cell lines with anti-fusion protein antibodies. Proc Natl Acad Sci U S A 1995;92:8710–8714.

71. Gu MM, Gash T, Mann VM, et al. Mitochondrial defect in Huntington's disease caudate nucleus. Ann Neurol 1996;39:385–389.

72. Marsden CD, Fahn S. Problems in the dyskinesias. In: Marsden CD, Fahn S, eds. Movement disorders 2. London: Butterworth and Co, 1987:305–308.

73. Adams RD, Victor M. Principles of neurology. 4th ed. New York: McGraw-Hill, 1989:935.

74. Limos LC, Ohnishi A, Sakai T, et al. "Myopathic" changes in chorea-acanthocytosis. Clinical and histopathological studies. J Neurol Sci 1982;55:49–58.

75. Bruyn GW, Myrianthopoulous NC. Chronic juvenile hereditary chorea (benign hereditary chorea of early onset). In: Vinken PJ, Bruyn GW, Klawans HL, eds. Handbook of clinical neurology. Vol. 5 (49), Extrapyramidal disorders. Amsterdam: Elsevier, 1986:335–348.

76. Suchowersky O, Hayden MR, Martin WRW, et al. Cerebral metabolism of glucose in benign hereditary chorea. Mov Disord 1986;1:33–44.

77. Quarrell OW, Youngman S, Sarfarazi M, Harper PS. Absence of close linkage between benign hereditary chorea and the locus D4S10 (probe G8). J Med Genet 1988;25:191–194.

78. Mount LA, Reback S. Familial paroxysmal choreoathetosis: preliminary report on a hitherto undescribed clinical syndrome. Arch Neurol Psych 1940;44:841–846.

79. Buruma OJS, Roos RAC. Paroxysmal choreoathetosis. In: Vinken PJ, Bruyn GW, Klawans HL, eds. Handbook of clinical neurology. Vol. 5 (49), Extrapyramidal disorders. Amsterdam: Elsevier, 1986:349–358.

80. Fink JK, Rainer S, Wilkowski J, et al. Paroxysmal dystonic choreoathetosis: tight linkage to chromosome 2q. Am J Hum Genet 1996;59:140–145.

81. Matilla T, Volpini V, Genis D, et al. Presymptomatic analysis of spinocerebellar ataxia type 1 (SCA1) via the expansion of the SCA1 CAG-repeat in a large pedigree displaying anticipation and parental male bias. Hum Mol Genet 1993;2:2123–2128.

82. Banfi S, Zoghbi HY. Molecular genetics of hereditary ataxias. Baillieres Clin Neurol 1994;3:281–295.

83. Banfi S, Servadio A, Chung MY, et al. Identification and characterization of the gene causing type 1 spinocerebellar ataxia. Nat Genet 1994;7:513–520.

84. Ranum LP, Schut LJ, Lundgren JK, et al. Spinocerebellar ataxia type 5 in a family descended from the grandparents of President Lincoln maps to chromosome 11. Nat Genet 1994;8:280–284.

85. Subramony SH. Degenerative ataxias. Curr Opin Neurol 1994;7:316–322.

86. Kameya T, Abe K, Aoki M, et al. Analysis of spinocerebellar ataxia type 1 (SCA1)-related CAG trinucleotide expansion in Japan. Neurology 1995;45:1587–1594.

87. Teh BT, Silburn P, Lindblad K, et al. Familial periodic cerebellar ataxia without myokymia maps to a 19-cM region on 19p13. Am J Hum Genet 1995;56:1443–1449.

88. Twist EC, Casaubon LK, Ruttledge MH, et al. Machado Joseph disease maps to the same region of chromosome 14 as the spinocerebellar ataxia type 3 locus. J Med Genet 1995;32:25–31.

89. Brown JR. Diseases of the cerebellum. In: Baker AB, Baker LH, eds. Clinical neurology. Hagerstown, MD: Harper and Row, 1981:21–29.

90. Kondo I, Ohta H, Yazaki M, et al. Exclusion mapping of the hereditary dentatorubropallidoluysian atrophy gene from the Huntington's disease locus. J Med Genet 1990;27:105–108.

91. Nagafuchi S, Yanagisawa H, Ohsaki E, et al. Structure and expression of the gene responsible for the triplet repeat disorder, dentatorubral and pallidoluysian atrophy (DRPLA). Nat Genet 1994;8:177–182.

92. Goto I, Tobimatsu S, Ohta M, et al. Dentatorubropallidoluysian degeneration: clinical, neuroophthalmologic, biochemical, and pathologic studies on autosomal dominant form. Neurology 1982;32:1395–1399.

93. White HH, Rowland LP. Disorders of purine metabolism. In: Rowland LP, ed. Merritt's textbook of neurology. 8th ed. Philadelphia: Lea and Febiger, 1989:499–500.

94. Gibbs RA, Patel PI, Strout JT, Caskey CT. Lesch-Nyhan syndrome: Human hypoxanthine phosphoribosyltransferase deficiency. In: Rowland LP, Wood DS, Schon EA, DiMauro S, eds. Molecular genetics in diseases of brain, nerve, and muscle. New York: Oxford University Press, 1989:211–220.

95. Rapin I. Hallervorden-Spatz disease. In: Rowland LP, ed. Merritt's textbook of neurology. 8th ed. Philadelphia: Lea and Febiger, 1989:556–557.

96. Pratt VM, Naidu S, Dlouhy SR, et al. A novel mutation in exon 3 of the proteolipid protein gene in Pelizaeus-Merzbacher disease. Neurology 1995;45:394–395.

97. Kawanishi C, Sugiyama N, Osaka H, et al. Pelizaeus-Merzbacher disease: a novel mutation in the 5′-untranslated region of the proteolipid protein gene. Hum Mutat 1996;7:355–357.

98. Boespflug-Tanguy O, Mimault C, Melki J, et al. Genetic homogeneity of Pelizaeus-Merzbacher disease: tight linkage to the proteoliprotein locus in 16 affected families. Am J Hum Genet 1994;55:461–467.

99. Husby C, Van de Rijn I, Zabriske JB. Antibodies reacting with cytoplasm of subthalamic and caudate nuclei neurons in chorea and acute rheumatic chorea. J Exp Med 1976;144:1094–1110.

100. Nausieda PA. Sydenham's chorea, chorea gravidarum and contraceptive induced chorea. In: Vinken PJ, Bruyn GW, Klawans HL, eds. Handbook of clinical neurology. Vol. 5 (49), Extrapyramidal disorders. Amsterdam: Elsevier, 1986:359–367.

101. Daoud AS, Zaki M, Shakir R, al-Saleh Q. Effectiveness of sodium valproate in the treatment of Sydenham's chorea. Neurology 1990;40:1140–1141.

102. Nausieda PA, Bieliauskas LA, Bacon L, et al. Chronic dopaminergic sensitivity after Sydenham's chorea. Neurology 1983;31:750–754.

103. Nausieda PA, Koller WC, Weiner WJ. Modification of post synaptic dopaminergic sensitivity by female sex hormones. Life Sci 1979;25:521–526.

104. Nausieda PA, Koller WC, Weiner WJ. Chorea induced by oral contraceptives. Neurology 1979;29:1605–1609.

105. Carter S. Sydenham chorea. In: Rowland LP, ed. Merritt's textbook of neurology. 8th ed. Philadelphia: Lea and Febiger, 1989:645–647.

106. Padberg GW, Bruyn GW. Chorea: differential diagnosis. In: Vinken PJ, Bruyn GW, Klawans HL, eds. Handbook of clinical neurology. Vol. 5 (49), Extrapyramidal disorders. Amsterdam: Elsevier, 1986:549–564.

107. Kuhl DE, Phelps ME, Markhau CH, et al. Cerebral metabolism and atrophy in Huntington's disease determined by 18FDG and computed tomographic scans. Ann Neurol 1982;12:425–434.

108. Shibaski H, Sakai T, Nishimura H, et al. Involuntary movements in chorea-acanthocytosis: a comparison with Huntington's chorea. Ann Neurol 1982;12:311–314.

109. Filion M, Tremblay L. Abnormal spontaneous activity of globus pallidus neurons in monkeys with MPTP-induced parkinsonism. Brain Res 1991;547:142–151.

110. Albin RL, Young AB, Penney JB. The functional anatomy of basal ganglia disorders. Trends Neurosci 1989;12:366–375.

111. Flaherty AW, Graybiel AM. Anatomy of the basal ganglia. In: Marsden CD, Fahn S, eds. Movement disorders 3. London: Butterworth-Heinemann Ltd, 1994:3–27.

112. Boyce S, Clarke CE, Luquin R, et al. Induction of chorea and dystonia in parkinsonian primates. Mov Disord 1990;5:3–7.

113. Clarke CE, Sambrook MA, Mitchell IJ, Crossman AR. Levodopa-induced dyskinesia and response fluctuations in primates rendered parkinsonian with 1-methyl-4-phenyl-1,2,3,6-tetrahydropyridine (MPTP). J Neurol Sci 1987;78:273–280.

114. Richfield EK, Maguire-Zeiss KA, Vonkeman HE, Voorn P. Preferential loss of preproenkephalin versus proprotachykinin neurons from the striatum of Huntington's disease patients. Ann Neurol 1995;38:852–861.

115. Albin RL. Selective neurodegeneration in Huntington's disease. Ann Neurol 1995;38:835–836. Editorial.

116. Baron MS, Vitek JL, Bakay RAE, et al. Treatment of advanced Parkinson's disease by posterior GPi pallidotomy: 1-year results of a pilot study. Ann Neurol 1996;40:355–366.

117. Miller WC, DeLong MR. Altered tonic activity of neurons in the globus pallidus and subthalamic nucleus in the primate MPTP model of parkinsonism. In: Carpenter MB, Jayaraman A, eds. The basal ganglia II. New York: Plenum Press, 1987:415–429.

118. Bergman H, Wichmann T, DeLong MR. Reversal of experimental parkinsonism by lesions of the subthalamic nucleus. Science 1990;249:436–438.

119. Dogali M, Fazzini E, Kolodny E, et al. Sterotactic ventral pallidotomy for Parkinson's disease. Neurology 1995;45:753–761.

120. Carpenter MB, Whittier JR, Mettler FA. Analysis of choreoid hyperkinesia in the rhesus monkey. Surgical and pharmacological analysis of hyperkinesia resulting from lesions in the subthalamic nucleus of Luys. J Comp Neurol 1950;92:293–332.

121. Marsden CD, Obeso JA. The functions of the basal ganglia and the paradox of stereotaxic surgery in Parkinson's disease. Brain 1994;117:877–897.

122. Hazrati LN, Parent A, Mitchell S, Haber SN. Evidence for interconnections between the two segments of the globus pallidus in primates: a PHA-L anterograde tracing study. Brain Res 1990;533:171–175.

123. Hazrati LN, Parent A. Projection from the external pallidum to the reticular thalamic nucleus in the squirrel monkey. Brain 1991;550:142–146.

124. Ilinksy IA, Kultas-Ilinsky K. Reticular thalamic nucleus input to the nuclei of the monkey thalamus: light and electron-microscopic study. Soc Neurosci 1993;19:1436. Abstract.

125. Ohye C, Shibazaki T, Hirai T, et al. Further physiologic observations on the ventralis intermedius neurons in the human thalamus. J Neurophysiol 1989;61:488–500.

126. Llinas RR. The intrinsic electrophysiological properties of mammalian neurons: insights into central nervous system function. Science 1988;242:1654–1664.

127. Buzsaki G, Smith A, Berger S, et al. Petit mal epilepsy and parkinsonian tremor: hypothesis of a common pacemaker. Neuroscience 1990;36:1–14.

128. Narabayashi H. Stereotaxic vim thalamotomy for treatment of tremor. Eur Neurol 1989;29(suppl 1):29–32.

129. Tasker RR, Lenz F, Yamashiro K, et al. Microelectrode techniques in localization of stereotactic targets. Neurosci Res 1987;9:105–112.

130. Hedreen JC, Folstein SE. Early loss of neostriatal striosome neurons in Huntington's disease. J Neuropathol Exp Neurol 1995;54:105–120.

131. Ghosh S, Murray GM, Turman AB, Rowe MJ. Corticothalamic influences on transmission of tactile information in the ventroposterolateral thalamus of the cat: effect of reversible inactivation of somatosensory cortical areas I and II. Exp Brain Res 1994;100:276–286.

132. Jones EG, Powell TPS. An electron microscopic study of the mode of termination of cortico-thalamic fibers within the sensory relay nuclei of the thalamus. Proc R Soc Lond Biol 1969;172:173–185.

133. Zweig RM. Functions of the basal ganglia. Brain 1995;118:882.

134. Inglis WL, Winn P. The pedunculopontine tegmental nucleus: where the striatum meets the reticular formation. Prog Neurobiol 1995;47:1–29.

135. Zweig RM, Jankel WR, Hedreen JC, et al. The pedunculopontine nucleus in Parkinson's disease. Ann Neurol 1989;26:41–46.

136. Hirsch EC, Graybiel AM, Duyckaert C, Javoy-Agid F. Neuronal loss in the pedunculopontine tegmental nucleus in Parkinson disease and progressive supranuclear palsy. Proc Natl Acad Sci U S A 1987;84:5976–5980.

137. Jellinger K. The pedunculopontine nucleus in Parkinson's disease, progressive supranuclear palsy and Alzheimer's disease. J Neurol Neurosurg Psychiatry 1988;51:540–543.

138. Zweig RM, Whitehouse PJ, Casanova MF, et al. Loss of pedunculopontine neurons in progressive supranuclear palsy. Ann Neurol 1987;22:18–25.

139. Litvan L, Agid Y, Calne D, et al. Clinical research criteria for the diagnosis of progressive supranuclear palsy (Steele-Richardson-Olszewski syndrome): report of the NINDS-SPSP international workshop. Neurology 1996;47:1–9.

140. Bing RA. Textbook of nervous diseases. New York: Rebman Company, 1921:85.

141. Shoulson I, Odoroff C, Oakes D, et al. A controlled clinical trial of baclofen as protective therapy in early Huntington's disease. Ann Neurol 1989;25:252–259.

142. Klawans HL, Goetz CH, Perlik S. Presymptomatic and early detection in Huntington's disease. Ann Neurol 1980;8:343–347.

143. Nutt JG, Rosin A, Chase TN. Treatment of Huntington disease with a cholinergic agonist. Neurology 1978;28:1061–1064.

144. Nutt JG, Morgan NT. Acute effects of scopolamine in Huntington's disease. In: Fahn S, Calne DB, Shoulson I, eds. Experimental therapeutics of movement disorders. Advances in neurology, Vol. 37. New York: Raven Press, 1983:291–297.

145. Nutt JG. Effect of cholinergic agents in Huntington's disease: a reappraisal. Neurology 1983;33:932–935.

146. Barr AN, Fischer JH, Koller WC, et al. Serum haloperidol concentration and choreiform movements in Huntington's disease. Neurology 1988;38:84–88.

147. Jankovic J, Orman J. Tetrabenazine therapy of dystonia, chorea, tics and other dyskinesias. Neurology 1988;38:91–94.

148. Walker FO, Hunt VP. An open label trial of dextromethorphan in Huntington's disease. Clin Neuropharmacol 1989;12:322–330.

149. Freeman TB, Sanberg PR, Isacson O. Development of the human striatum: implications for fetal striatal transplantation in the treatment of Huntington's disease. Cell Transplant 1995;4:539–545.

150. Shannon KM, Kordower JH. Neural transplantation for Huntington's disease: experimental rationale and recommendations for clinical trials. Cell Transplant 1996;5:339–352.

Athetosis and the Common Athetoid Syndromes

RAYMOND D. ADAMS   MARIA SALAM-ADAMS

INTRODUCTION

Athetosis, a term introduced into the medical lexicon in 1871 by Hammond to specify an "inability to retain the fingers and toes in any position in which they might be placed and by their continual movement," is the dominant feature of a number of basal ganglionic diseases. For this reason alone it deserves a chapter in this volume. It must be conceded, however, that from the beginning the term has been surrounded by controversy and was the focus of a polemic among some of the great figures in nineteenth-century neurology, such as Charcot (1), Gowers (2), and Bonhoeffer (3).

Disputed was the relation of athetosis to chorea and dystonia. The term chorea was already in use to designate a type of wide-ranging, arrhythmic involuntary movement such as is displayed by patients with Sydenham's chorea. Was it necessary, Charcot asked, to employ another term merely because the movements were of slower, sinuous quality and of predominantly distal appendicular localization? Gowers, who earlier had described the movement disorder of what was later called hepatolenticular degeneration as "tetanoid chorea," accepted the term and used it in his textbook.

The term dystonia had a somewhat different origin and meaning, being first used by Oppenheim (4) in 1911 to refer to a movement disorder peculiar to childhood in which the large proximal limb and trunk muscles were implicated in involuntary movements and in grotesque posturing. True, the movements were slow and involuntary and associated with distal athetosis. In these respects and in the cocontraction of agonist, antagonist, and fixator muscles, dystonia was like athetosis, yet the clinical setting and the topography of the movements were different. Other writers, who referred to any fixed posture as dystonia, preferred to group choreo-athetosis and dystonia under a single heading as expressions of extrapyramidal diseases.

The authors of this chapter plead for the separation of chorea, athetosis, and dystonia, believing that each has its own unique pathophysiology and morbid clinical linkages. The term athetosis is used in the following pages to specify involuntary slow sinuous movements of any muscle group, including the tongue and face, but presenting most prominently in the hand and foot. Chorea will refer here to wide-ranging quick involuntary movements, but slower than myoclonus, on a background of reduced muscular tone. Dystonia refers to a fixed attitude or abnormal postural set of any part of the body. It may accompany athetotic movements of proximal and trunk muscles or of distal muscles and provide the postural background of corticospinal paralysis (hemiplegic dystonia) or some other extrapyramidal disorder (the flexion dystonia of Parkinson's disease). The slightest degree of athetosis of the hand or foot may present as a dystonic posture, and the most advanced stage of dystonia musculorum deformans may end in a fixed deformity of the neck, trunk, or proximal parts of limbs.

PATHOPHYSIOLOGY AND PATHOGENESIS OF ATHETOSIS

The foundations of all phenomena classed as extrapyramidal motor manifestations were originally established by the anatomic study of the nervous system of diseased patients. These victims of a variety of pathologic states were known to have manifested tremor, rigidity, bradykinesia, chorea, dystonia, and athetosis, even when the major motor pathways, that is, the corticospinal systems, were essentially intact.

This is not the place to review the detailed anatomy and pathophysiology of these clinical phenomena. It need only be pointed out that most of our knowledge is recent and is even now incomplete. With reference to athetosis, the corpus striatum and parts of the thalamus were found to figure importantly in the highly intricate motor system. Recently it has become popular to delineate motor circuits emanating from the prefrontal, premotor, and parietal cortices and traversing the caudate and putamenal nuclei to reach the globus pallidus and then the intralaminar thalamic nuclei before reverting to the cortex. These circuits are believed to be essential in the planning of voluntary movement and in encoding information about the amplitude, velocity, and organization of movement. Such preparation for movement takes place before the motor cortex and corticospinal system are activated for the performance of willed movement. Interruption of these striatal circuits results in the abnormalities of movement that are under consideration. Our only objection to this physiologic formulation is that it surely represents an oversimplification. Actually, each nuclear structure in these loops is under feedback and feed-forward control of adjacent structures. By analogy it is more like a vast computer network. The most up-to-date review of this subject will be found in the article of DeLong and Alexander (5).

From pathologic studies of diseases with athetosis as a dominant clinical finding, certain principles can be deduced.

1. *The diseases in question selectively involve specific neuronal systems.* Only if certain striatal and thalamic structures are injured is it possible for athetosis and athetoid dystonia to become manifest. Of equal importance is the integrity of other structures. Most anatomic pathologists agree that the corticospinal and probably other systems of neurons must remain relatively functional in order for these disorders to express themselves. One must therefore think of the lesion in terms both of parts impaired and of parts preserved, constituting a kind of anatomic constellation.

2. *Only certain diseases have the potential for producing athetosis.* A respected principle in anatomic pathology, applicable here, is that certain diseases have a predilection for certain parts of the brain, and certain parts of the brain are especially vulnerable to certain diseases. Vogt (6) denoted these relationships by the term pathoclisis. More explicitly, hypoxia, hyperammonemia, hyperbilirubinemia, hypocalcemia, and Hallervorden-Spatz disease with iron deposit regularly and severely involve these parts of the nervous system. In contrast, lesions such as the common ischemic and hemorrhagic vascular lesions, tumors, trauma, etc., if they include these parts, are so destructive or widespread in their effects on all structures in the region that athetosis is relatively infrequent.

3. *A variable temporal relation exists between lesion and onset of athetosis.* Unlike most of the deficits or negative effects of lesions on nervous function, which are immediate, with respect to the athetotic syndromes there may be a long interval of months or years after the receipt of the lesion before the appearance of the involuntary movements. There

are several explanations of this delay. In the infant affected at birth, the athetosis will be delayed because of the nonfunctional state of parts of the immature nervous system, for example, the corticospinal system. At a later age, the initial involvement of the corticospinal system and associated parts of the nervous system may cause an initial paralysis; only after partial recovery of the paralysis, which may take months or years, can the athetosis from the basal ganglionic lesion show itself. When the delay is in terms of many years, and particularly in late life, one suspects always the addition of some other disease or of the aging process unmasking an older athetotic lesion. Some neuropathologists have also postulated the occurrence of chain degenerations in connected neuronal systems, but this idea is difficult to affirm or negate.

4. *Athetosis may be based on either a physiologic or pathologic block of function, or both.* It is obvious that athetosis may result from a diversity of pathologic processes. In some conditions a well-defined structural change of a certain type can be discerned; in others, such as tardive dyskinesia, it seems doubtful if there is any lesion at the light microscopic level. In some diseases that cause definite cellular changes, the pathogenetic mechanism also has an important physiologic effect, and the visible lesion is only the most advanced and irreversible aspect of it. The functional or physiologic block for each disease of this type has its own time course and may advance progressively or intermittently or regress. These possibilities require that each pathologic process be considered in all its physiologic and anatomic possibilities. For these several reasons correlations between visible lesion and athetotic syndrome are often imprecise. Most obscure of all the causative diseases are the ones that cause the intermittent athetoses, which may depend in part on fluctuations in pathogenetic mechanism but also on the status of the nervous system from time to time, for example, during sleep, fatigue, or excitement.

CLINICAL ATTRIBUTES OF ATHETOTIC MOVEMENTS

The instability of posture and involuntary movements are most characteristically displayed in the hand. The fingers slowly flex and extend, as does the wrist; the thumb is opposed and flexed; and there are variable degrees of pronation and supination of the forearm. Seldom are the swings of movement complete, and small flexions and extensions of one or two fingers are frequent. The speed of movement is variable, sometimes fairly rapid, often seemingly slowed in proportion to the degree of rigidity or spasticity. However, the slower athetotic movement, in contrast to chorea, does not exactly parallel the rigidity. When at rest the habitual position of the hand tends to be one of hyperextension at metacarpophalangeal joints and flexion and pronation of the wrist. Lengthening and shortening reactions to passive movement are gradually abolished. In this pattern of athetotic movement and posture, Denny-Brown (7,8) discerned an uninhibited and unstable alteration of grasp and avoidance reactions. We feel uncertain about this interpretation because the patterns have been so variable in our cases.

The affected foot often adopts a position of inversion with flexion of the toes but at times is also seen to extend (dorsiflex) with abduction of the smaller toes. As a rule the involuntary movements of the foot are less prominent than those of the hand.

Affection of the neck takes the form of extension with side-to-side tipping or turning of the head. Conspicuous hypertrophy of cervical muscles attends protracted involuntary head movements. Slow grimace, pursing and parting of the lips, and drawling dysarthria represent involuntary contractions of the facial and tongue muscles.

In all these involuntary movements one observes fluctuations of posture, which as the disease progresses may terminate in relatively fixed attitudes. In milder degree, when the patient is quiet and relaxed, however, the limb may be quite flaccid. Any relative fixation of posture may have either a plastic or spastic quality, depending on the associated findings.

A spread or overflow of innervation to muscles not required in an intended movement is another common feature of athetosis. Indeed this is one of the most effective stimuli for the induction of the involuntary movements. For example, a command to "make a fist" results in visible contraction of the muscles of the upper arm and shoulders, with spread at times even to the other arm, trunk, and legs.

Careful analysis of volitional movement by surface electromyograms has revealed a loss of natural reciprocation of agonist and antagonist muscles. The antagonist muscles are not suppressed as the agonist contracts (9). Sometimes this results in a movement in a direction opposite to the patient's wish. Denny-Brown remarks on the modification by concurrent mass movements of the neck and of the labyrinthine reflex movements.

COMMON DISEASES PRESENTING WITH ATHETOSIS

Diseases known to present with athetosis and dystonia are classified in Table 72.1.

Posthemiplegic Athetosis

The original observations of Hammond (10) in posthemiplegic athetosis have been regularly duplicated in individuals who have suffered a cerebrovascular stroke. Carpenter (11) has reviewed all published writings on this subject up to 1950, and Dooling and Adams (12) up to 1975. The usual sequence has been a hemiplegic stroke that improves over a period of weeks, months, or years. Once it has reached a stable state, motility in the arm and leg becomes progressively impaired by the emergence of athetosis. The hand

Table 72.1   Classification of Diseases Known to Dispose to Athetosis and Dystonia

Generalized Persistent Athetotic Syndromes
Double athetosis, birth trauma, Little's disease
Kernicterus
Hallervorden-Spatz disease
Fahr's disease
Acquired and familial hepatocerebral degeneration
Other hereditary metabolic diseases
Dystonia musculorum deformans

Persistent Hemiathetotic Syndromes
Ischemic
    Embolic, thrombolic
Hemorrhagic
    Arteriovenous malformations
    Hypertensive

Persistent Segmental Athetoses
Blepharospasm
Spasmodic torticollis
Writer's cramp
Orofacial oromandibular dyskinesia
Lumbar athetosis

Intermittent Athetoses
Paroxysmal generalized athetosis
Dopamine athetosis

becomes engaged in constant slow involuntary movements and adopts some of the previously described postures. The plantar response, which earlier had been extensor with the foot in equinovarus position, now begins to flex on plantar stimulation, in conjunction with a tonic downward contraction of all five toes. However, in some instances any stimulus applied to the sole of the foot may produce extension and fanning of the toes. But this reaction differs in time and duration from the classic Babinski sign. The side of the face may be pulled into a contracture with deepening of the nasolabial fold, retraction of the corner of the mouth, and narrowing of the palpebral fissure. Some of the patients have had a hemisensory syndrome. Abnormalities of movement other than athetosis may be conjoined—such as tremor, myoclonus, hemichorea, hemiballismus, hemirigidity, and akinesia or hemiataxia, depending presumably on the anatomy of the lesion.

As to the pathologic anatomy of posthemiplegic athetosis, our cases, which were without sensory deficit, had ischemic necrosis or hemorrhage of the putamen and to a variable extent the globus pallidus. When sensory loss was prominent the lesion lay in the ventromedian and ventroanterior thalamus and intralaminar nuclei. Secondary degeneration of these thalamic zones in the patients with the striopallidal lesions was reflected in gliosis. The corticospinal tract from the level of the internal capsule was relatively intact.

Generalized Athetosis (Double Athetosis)

This bilateral lesion is usually caused by hypoxia, hyper-bilirubinemia at birth, or a genetic abnormality. The syndrome usually appears an interval of time after birth, at 1 to 2 or more years of age, when the corticospinal tract fully matures. The hyperbilirubinemic cases are featured by deafness, vertical gaze palsy, and relatively normal intelligence. The hypoxic cases are more variable in their clinical expression, merging with cerebral diplegia (Little's disease) and accompanied not infrequently by some degree of mental retardation. The typical lesion, found only in consequence of hypoxic-ischemic injury at birth, has been neuronal loss, gliosis, and a peculiar condensation of myelinated fibers, imparting a marble-like appearance (état marbré) to the striatum and thalamus. The initial observation of this pathologic change was made by Anton (13) in 1896 but the precise definition is forever associated with the Vogts (14). In addition they described a condition called status dysmyelinatus, which many neuropathologists believe to be the lesion of kernicterus.

The hereditary form of generalized athetosis, known as idiopathic torsion dystonia and usually expressed as a mendelian dominant trait, tends to leave intelligence and other cerebral functions intact.

Hereditary Metabolic Diseases with Athetosis

Choreoathetosis has been the principal clinical manifestation of several metabolic diseases of the nervous system. It is a feature of three of the known disturbances of organic acid metabolism: glutaric acidemia, D-glyceric acidemia, and sulfite oxidase deficiency. We have observed rare instances of choreoathetosis in such infants when only 8 or 9 months old. Dislocated lenses are a feature of sulfite oxidase deficiency. In older children, athetosis and rigidity may be the dominant symptoms in Lesch-Nyhan disease, hepatocerebral degeneration (Wilson's disease), acquired forms of chronic cirrhosis of the liver, adolescent Niemann-Pick disease, familial calcification of the basal ganglia and hypoparathyroidism, Huntington's chorea, and Hallervorden-Spatz disease. Space does not permit a description of each of these relatively rare conditions. In almost all instances of these diseases there are other neurologic abnormalities, some in the sphere of cognitive functioning, that set each of them apart. The definitive diagnostic criterion is the biochemical or cellular abnormality.

Paroxysmal Generalized Athetosis

Mount and Reback (15) were the first to report examples of this condition. As later pointed out by Lance (16), some are familial. The movements take the form of either episodic dystonic spasms or a diffuse choreoathetosis. The onset is abrupt, the duration of an episode a matter of minutes to

an hour, and all parts of the body are affected. The age of onset has ranged from 1 to 22 years. The frequency of attacks varies from one or two per month to several per day. Possible predisposing factors are excitement, fatigue, alcohol, and coffee, but usually none is recognizable. The state of consciousness remains clear and the electroencephalogram (EEG) normal. Many of the patients have had no family history of a similar disorder, and the neurologic examination discloses no abnormalities between attacks. In a small subgroup the paroxysmal athetosis occurs on a background of multiple sclerosis, basal ganglionic scarring, or cerebral palsy. No microscopic pathology was found in one of Lance's cases that came to autopsy. It is the only fatal case of several hundred that have been reported.

The nature of the disease remains controversial. Claims that it represents epilepsy due to a focus in the basal ganglia are contradicted by the normal EEG and the clear mentation of the patient. Yet response to carbamazepine, in a few cases, is a point in favor of this hypothesis. A more likely possibility is the presence of some subtle structural abnormality, possibly genetic, whose presence is exposed by a change in body metabolism or in the level of a neurotransmitter. In some of the cases, called kinesiogenic, a sudden movement after a period of rest has regularly evoked an attack. Startle has been another initiating event in a few cases.

Dopa-Responsive Athetosis and Dystonia

In recent years this autosomal dominant hereditary disease of children has emerged as an important clinical entity (17). Individuals with this disorder are at first normal (for 2 to 5 years after birth), then athetotic movements and dystonic postures of feet and hands appear. About three-quarters of these cases exhibit diurnal variation. As the condition worsens, postural instability tremor, rigidity, and bradykinesia become prominent, giving the clinical syndrome a parkinsonian aspect. In adolescence and adult life the parkinsonian features dominate. The fluctuating form is sometimes called Segawa's disease. A distinguishing feature has been the remarkable response to small doses of L-dopa.

A more common type of episodic choreoathetosis and dystonia occurs in the Parkinson patient in relation to L-dopa therapy. L-Dopa itself has no central nervous system activity but is a precursor of the neurotransmitter dopamine. The usual situation is for the patient, after continuous use of L-dopa for a number of years, to have periods of athetotic dyskinesia when slightly overdosed. The movement disorder usually coincides with the time of maximal therapeutic effect and lasts for 30 to 45 minutes. The types of abnormal movement are similar to those seen in tardive dyskinesia and include shrugging of the shoulders, head turning, grimacing, blepharospasm, and mandibular movements. When severe they may extend to all the musculature and even assume a ballistic or myoclonic range and velocity. The mechanism is believed to be excitation of a striatum rendered excessively sensitive because of denervation (loss of activating nigral cells).

Special Types of Focal Athetosis

In recent years a number of types of involuntary movement, restricted to certain segments of the body, have been reclassified as segmental athetosis or dystonia. Formerly they were mistakenly called tics, meaning habitual movements of quasivoluntary nature, and were known to be more frequent in childhood and old age. Included in this group of focal or segmental athetoses are blepharospasm, spasmodic torticollis, oromandibular and orofacial dyskinesia, writer's and other occupational cramps, and axial athetosis (dystonia).

In blepharospasm there are intermittent contractions of the orbicularis oculi muscles that forcefully close the eyes at irregular intervals for periods of 15 to 20 seconds or longer. Persistent spasms may be counteracted by patients pulling their eyes open with their fingers or by resorting to some trick such as opening the mouth and yawning. The spasms continue even when the patient is placed in complete darkness or when the corneas are anesthetized. This indicates that it is not an exaggerated blink reaction to tactile or visual stimuli. Nevertheless, the spasms may be increased by bright light and wind. Most of the subjects are elderly and have no family history of athetotic or familial extrapyramidal disease. In some patients the spasms spread to perioral and mandibular muscles, causing grimacing and jaw opening. This was noted in half of Marsden's 26 collected cases (18). We have also observed blepharospasm as the initial event in an adolescent who later manifested typical dystonia musculorum deformans. Usually the condition in the elderly is confined to the eyes and is mainly a source of annoyance in all visual activities.

In spasmodic torticollis, the most frequent of the segmental athetoses, the patient, usually a middle-aged adult, begins to have an irregular tipping or turning of the head to one side. With continual contraction the sternomastoid and trapezius and other muscles are seen to contract and become hypertrophied. The condition for a long time was thought in some medical circles to be psychogenic, even though the patient disavowed the movements' voluntary nature and the ability to suppress them. For a time they are present only when the patient maintains an upright posture and cease upon lying down. Later they may persist even in recumbency. Once started they continue unabated throughout life. In a personal experience with more than 100 such cases, only 2 have eventually remitted. Equally rare is the spread to other muscles. Various attempts to subdivide torticollis into arthritic (painful), vestibular, reflex, and ocular types (19) have proven to be relatively useless.

In oromandibular and orofacial or lingual dyskinesias, the affected muscles are thrown continually in irregular, slow spasms. The result is an unattractive grimace, a pursing of the lips, grinding of the teeth (bruxism), or protrusion of the tongue; all these may occur singly or in some combination. The grotesque expression of the face is reminiscent of some of the characters in a Brueghel painting, hence the name Brueghel syndrome. Like spasmodic torticollis, these conditions tend to occur in middle or late adult life and to merge with spastic dysphonia and other localized spasms. They may also be the solitary manifestation of tardive dyskinesia.

In writer's cramp the muscles of the hand or forearm tend to engage in involuntary spasms, either persistent or irregular during cursive movements. To overcome them the patient adopts new ways of holding the pen, but even then the natural fluidity of movement of the fingers is impaired. The spasms are irregular, rarely rhythmic, and present only in writing. If the patient substitutes the nondominant hand, it too eventually may be involved. Other activities to which the hand is put remain facile. Nonetheless other highly complex, practiced skills, such as instrument playing or typing, may be affected in a similar manner. Two of our younger patients with athetotic writer's cramp later developed spasmodic torticollis.

In axial athetosis an adult patient develops intermittent contractions of the lumbar and lower thoracic paravertebral muscles. The back arches and the abdomen is thrust forward when standing and walking. Later the contractions persist even while lying in bed. Another of our patients with an initial torticollis later began to hunch his shoulders and intort the arms. In childhood and adolescence, segmental athetosis of a shoulder or hip not infrequently is a forerunner of dystonia musculorum deformans.

The above types do not exhaust the repertoire of involuntary athetotic movements seen in a neurologic clinic. There is an endless array of so-called vocal tics, bleatings, sniffing, head tossing, etc., most of which occur without identifiable cause. They are nosologically listed in books as tics, spasms, dyskinesias, dystonias, restricted choreas or athetoses, and tremors, but their physiology is so poorly understood that they are difficult to classify. None has an identifiable pathology. They have become more frequent since the introduction of neuroleptic drugs for the treatment of psychiatric diseases. For the most part they are readily distinguishable from myotonia, facial spasm, nerve irritation and aberrant regeneration, fasciculation, and myokymia and cramp.

THERAPEUTIC STRATEGIES

Largely on the basis of observed dopamine effects in patients with Parkinson's disease and a lack of a definable pathology of tardive dyskinesia, it has been assumed that chorea, athetosis, and dystonia may be due to depletion of a neurotransmitter or a hypersensitivity of the extrapyramidal structures that it naturally activates. This has led to a search for drugs that might enhance the release of the neurotransmitter or a replacement for it.

With respect to athetosis as well as chorea, drug therapy (tetrabenazine, haloperidol, trihexyphenidyl, amantadine, baclofen) has had relatively little beneficial effect. The only exception to this statement is the L-dopa-responsive athetosis and Parkinson's disease of children. Several neuropharmacologists have acclaimed carbamazepine or clonidine as means of controlling paroxysmal choreoathetosis. Bromocriptine is said to have alleviated a generalized athetosis (dystonic) in one case (20).

Taking advantage of the fact that progressive relaxation tends to reduce all extrapyramidal movement disorders, physiotherapists have employed this method systematically with claims of benefit. Biofeedback techniques are sometimes used to warn the patient of oncoming muscle contraction. In mild cases the patient may seem to keep the athetosis under better control, but we have not been impressed with it as a long-term therapy. We have had no experience with cervical cord stimulation by implanted intraspinal electrodes, as proposed by Waltz and Davis (21) for torticollis. Cerebellar stimulation by implanted surface electrodes, introduced by Cooper (22) for generalized athetosis and dystonia, has not been used in our hospital. McClellan et al (23), after employing it in a series of cases, concluded that less than half of them were improved, and the long-term results are unknown.

Stereotaxic surgery on the basal ganglia was advanced as a therapy after the demonstration of lasting improvement in the Parkinson patient. But the results in athetosis have been distressingly inconsistent, and the procedure is not without risk. Andrew et al (24) published one of the most objective reports on stereotaxic thalamotomy for athetosis and dystonia. They have described their results in cases of focal, segmental, hemi-, and generalized athetosis. They compared them with those of Cooper (22), Marsden and Fahn (25), and Bertrand (26). A radiofrequency lesion was made in the ventromedial nucleus of the thalamus, on both sides of the cerebrum in both the generalized and segmental cases, and on one (contralateral) side in hemiathetosis. The location of the lesion was checked by stimulation and recording techniques. Of their 45 patients, 16 had generalized athetosis, mostly of dystonia musculorum deformans type, 27 had segmental or focal athetosis (22 with spasmodic torticollis), and 12 had hemiathetosis. Of the 16 patients with generalized dystonia, 6 experienced lasting improvement (1-year follow-up). By the end of 1 year, 4 unimproved patients had died, 2 improved temporarily, and 2 were left unchanged. There was one postoperative death. Of the 12 with hemiathetosis, all except one had a lasting reduction of the movement disorder. Of the 22 cases of spasmodic torticollis, 12 were at least partly relieved; 16 of this group had had bilateral thalamotomies and 10 of them obtained a good result. Two of the 6 with unilateral thalamotomies improved. The operations carried some liability to further neurologic deficit. Hemiparesis of mild degree (and usually transitory) occurred

in 16 of the 55 cases. Dysarthria developed in 9; the latter symptom and other pseudobulbar effects were complications of bilateral thalamotomies.

Our own neurosurgical results conform to those of Andrew et al (24). We have been most apprehensive about the effect of bilateral thalamotomies. Nevertheless, in some cases of generalized dystonia musculorum deformans, when a favorable outcome is obtained in a patient whose disease has resisted all pharmacologic agents, one is encouraged to resort to thalamotomy and assume the risk of the procedure.

With focal and segmental athetosis it is always debatable as to whether a thalamotomy should be undertaken. Sometimes a myotomy or peripheral denervation of the few affected muscles or a cervical radiculotomy, as in spasmodic torticollis, seem to be procedures of less risk. For very restricted dystonias intramuscular injections of botulinus toxin are being used with considerable success. With a single injection the muscle spasm can be relieved for weeks to months. This treatment has virtually replaced surgical intervention.

REFERENCES

1. Charcot JM. Lectures on diseases of the nervous system. Sigerson G, trans. Philadelphia: Henry C Lea, 1897:390.
2. Gowers WR. Diseases of the nervous system. Philadelphia: Blakiston and Co., 1888.
3. Bonhoeffer K. Ein Beitrag zur Localisation des Choreoatischen Bewegungen. Monatsschr Psychiatr Neurol 1897;1:6–41.
4. Oppenheim H. Über eine eigenartige Krampfkrankheit des Kindlichen und jugendlichen Alters (dysbasia lordotica progressiva, dystonia musculorem deformans). Neurol Zentralbl 1911;30:1090–1107.
5. DeLong MR, Alexander GE. Organization of basal ganglia. In: Asbury AK, McKhann GM, McDonald WI, eds. Diseases of the nervous system. Philadelphia: WB Saunders, 1986:394–401.
6. Vogt C. Nature et localisation de la paralysie pseudobulbaire congenitale et infantile. J Psychol Neurol 1911;18(suppl):293–308.
7. Benny-Brown D. The cerebral control of movement. Liverpool: Liverpool University Press, 1966.
8. Denny-Brown D. The basal ganglia and their relation to disorders of movement. London: Oxford University Press, 1962.
9. Hallett HM, Shahani BT, Young RR. EMG analysis of patients with cerebellar deficits. J Neurol Neurosurg Psychiatry 1975;38:1163–1169.
10. Hammond WA. A treatise on diseases of the nervous system. New York: D. Appleton, 1871.
11. Carpenter MR. Athetosis and the basal ganglia. Arch Neurol 1950;63:895–901.
12. Dooling EC, Adams RD. Pathologic anatomy of posthemiplegic athetosis. Brain 1975;98:29–48.
13. Anton G. Ueber die Beteiligung der basalien Gehirnganglien bei Bewegungsstorungen unbesondere bei Chorea. Jahrb Psychiatrie 1896;14:141–182.
14. Vogt C, Vogt O. Zur Lehre der Erkrankungen des striaten Systems. J Psychol Neurol 1920;25:627–846.
15. Mount LA, Reback S. Familial paroxysmal choreoathetosis. Arch Neurol Psychiatry 1940;44:841–847.
16. Lance JW. Familial paroxysmal dystonic choreoathetosis and its differentiation from related syndromes. Ann Neurol 1977;2:285–293.
17. Segawa M, Nomura Y. Hereditary progressive dystonia with marked diurnal fluctuations. Adv Neurol 1993;60:568.
18. Marsden CW. The problem of adult onset idiopathic torsion dystonia. In: Eldridge MR, Fahn S, eds. Advances in neurology. vol. 14. New York: Raven Press, 1976:259–276.
19. Wilson SAK. Diseases of mobility and muscle tone with special reference to the corpus striatum (Croonien lectures). Lancet 1925;i:215–291.

20. Gautier JC, Awada A. Dystonia musculorum deformans: effet favorable de la bromocriptine. Rev Neurol 1983;139:449–551.
21. Waltz JM, Davis JA. Cervical cord stimulation in the treatment of athetosis and tremor. Adv Neurol 1983;37:225–237.
22. Cooper IS. Involuntary movement disorders. New York: Paul Hoeber, 1969.
23. McClellan DL, Selwyn M, Cooper IS. Time course of clinical and physiological effects of stimulating the cerebellar surface. J Neurol Neurosurg Psychiatry 1978;41:150–158.
24. Andrew J, Fowler CJ, Harrison MJG. Stereotaxic thalamotomy in fifty-five cases of dystonia. Brain 1983;106:981–1001.
25. Marsden CD, Fahn S. Surgical approaches to the dyskinesias. In: Marsden CD, Fahn S, eds. Movement disorders. London: Butterworths, 1974.
26. Bertrand D. Evolution and indications for surgery of involuntary movement. Union Med Can 1982;109:20–25.

Familial and Primary Sporadic Paroxysmal Dyskinesias

Tarif Bakdash   Christopher G. Goetz

INTRODUCTION

The paroxysmal dyskinesias (PDs) are a heterogenous group of disorders with significant clinical differences. As the pathophysiology is unknown, a phenomenologic rather than etiologic definition will be used here. We define a PD as an abnormal dystonic and/or choreoathetotic movement that is only intermittently present. The attacks are stereotyped and usually are preceded by an aura, raising the possibility of seizures. And, as in the reflex epilepsies, they have characteristic precipitants. Furthermore, because the movements may involve the orobuccolingual musculature, occasionally there may be tongue biting; when the movements involve the lower extremities, patients may fall and injure themselves. However, the movement is unaccompanied by altered consciousness or incontinence, the patient is not amnestic for the episode, and there is no accompanying or residual confusion (1).

In 1940, Mount and Reback described a syndrome of paroxysmal dystonia and choreoathetosis, lasting up to 2 hours, in a 23-year-old male textile worker (2). Twenty-seven family members through five generations were likewise affected. Mount and Reback named the syndrome familial paroxysmal choreoathetosis. To date there are over 200 cases of PD reported in the literature, published under at least 16 different appellations. These include l'epilepsie extrapyramidale (3), subcortical epilepsy (4), striatal epilepsy (5), tonic seizures (6), epilepsie reflexe (7), periodic dystonia (8), paroxysmal kinesigenic choreoathetosis (9), paroxysmal dystonic choreoathetosis (10), seizures induced by movement (11), hypnogenic paroxysmal dystonia (12), and familial dystonic choreoathetosis with myokymia, a sleep-responsive disorder (13).

In his attempt to establish nosographic categories, Lance reviewed the literature on "tonic seizures" and differentiated between sporadic and familial varieties (14). Kertesz followed, coining the adjective "kinesigenic" to distinguish the more common and often movement-induced short dyskinesias (9) from the less common prolonged type described by Mount and Reback (2). The predominantly dystonic character of the movements was later appropriately emphasized by Richards and Barnett (10). Lugaresi and Cirignotta underscored the resemblance between sleep-related hypnogenic dystonia and the other paroxysmal dyskinesias (12). In 1994, Fahn (15) suggested a broader classification that included six categories: 1) kinesigenic paroxysmal choreoathetosis, 2) nonkinesigenic paroxysmal dystonic choreoathetosis, 3) intermediate paroxysmal dystonic choreoathetosis, 4) hypnogenic paroxysmal dyskinesia, 5) benign paroxysmal dystonia/torticollis in infancy, and 6) miscellaneous. More recently, Demirkiran and Jankovic (16) proposed a classification based chiefly on precipitating events but also on duration and etiology.

Lance's classification is the most widely used (17). He divided the PDs into two basic groups: prolonged (paroxysmal dystonic choreoathetosis) and brief (paroxysmal kinesigenic choreoathetosis). He had a third intermediate form with a single family that may easily be incorporated into his prolonged group. The brief group was further divided into familial and sporadic, with the latter split into primary and secondary. Goodenough et al divided the PDs into familial and acquired, with primary sporadic being included in the former group (18). We have recently incorporated Lugaresi and Cirignotta's observations into Lance's classification (Table 73.1) (1,19).

The important descriptive classification categories are daytime versus nocturnal, brief versus prolonged, familial versus nonfamilial, and primary or sporadic disorders without other neurologic abnormalities versus acquired or secondary disorders in which the movement disorder is one

Table 73.1   Classification of Paroxysmal Dyskinesias

Daytime		Nocturnal	
Prolonged (more than 5 min)	**Brief (less than 5 min)**	**Prolonged**	**Brief**
Familial	Familial	Familial	Familial
Sporadic	Sporadic	Sporadic	Sporadic
Primary?	Primary?	Primary?	Primary?
Secondary?	Secondary?	Secondary?	Secondary?

feature of a larger syndrome. Among these divisions, the most pivotal distinction for prognosis and natural history is the issue of primary versus secondary forms, as both familial and primary sporadic cases are usually benign, nonprogressive, and readily responsive to pharmacotherapy. In contrast, those cases secondary to or associated with other neurologic abnormalities follow the course of the underlying illness and are often difficult to treat. As a group, secondary paroxysmal dyskinesias have a later age of onset. For this reason, the PDs are treated in two chapters. The first discusses familial and primary sporadic cases, and the next chapter focuses on the acquired forms. Some authors have stressed the distinction between action-induced (kinesigenic) and nonkinesigenic dyskinesias (16), but these occur in all groups and action is one of many precipitants in such spells.

PROLONGED FAMILIAL PAROXYSMAL DYSKINESIAS

Following Mount and Reback's (2) initial description, there are now about 35 published cases of prolonged familial paroxysmal dyskinesias (PFPD). The age of onset has ranged from birth to age 22, with two in three cases beginning prior to age 5. Two-thirds of reported patients were male. Most authors agree that the disorder is autosomal dominant with variable penetrance.

Alcohol, caffeine, fatigue, nervousness, and exposure to cold are the most frequent inciting factors. The patient of Mount and Reback "was certain to have one [an attack] if he drank a cocktail after dinner," and on three occasions, typical attacks were provoked in the hospital by $90\,cm^3$ of whisky orally (2). Patient V:II of Forssman "had to draw the line at one glass of schnapps" (20). Caffeine in the form of cola, tea, chocolate, coffee, and analgesics is also an effective precipitant. Patient IV:II of Forssman "got an attack of almost unprecedented length and severity: following consumption of his wife's headache powder which contained caffeine" (20). Startle, sudden fright, swimming, overexertion, excitement, walking, and menstruation have all been described to precipitate the attacks (10,12,17,21,22). Sudden movement can induce paroxysms, but is not a regular precipitant.

A variety of stereotypic sensory phenomena may herald an attack. The auras generally last several seconds, but occasionally continue for up to 5 minutes. Mount and Reback's patient described "a feeling as if the collar and belt are too tight" (2). Others related a "tugging" feeling, "pins and needles," and "stiffness" (10,12,20). Some are unable to describe the sensation but "could feel when [it was] coming on" (20). Usually, the sensations are located in the limb in which the attack begins.

Following a typical aura, the attack commences with dystonic posturing of a single extremity. For instance, flexion or extension of the hand, abduction or adduction of the shoulder, or equinovarus posturing of the foot. In most patients, the posture progresses to involve all four extremities and axial muscles, with varying amounts of facial grimacing and opisthotonos. The oromandibular dystonia often leads to dysarthria and sometimes anarthria. But the attack is never associated with aphasia, altered mental status, or loss of consciousness. The spasms of case III:4 of Lance "may affect one side of the body for half an hour then ease, or it may progress to involve the other side" (17). When bilateral, ambulation is often impaired and the patient may fall. Choreoathetosis is superimposed on the dystonia in differing amounts. This may be distal and mild, or proximal and ballistic. In rare instances, chorea may be the predominant dyskinesia. Other movements described as part of the syndrome include clonus and twitching (12,20).

Many patients are able to partly or completely suppress their attacks. The most common method employed is rest. Often, lying quietly is sufficient, although some patients may actually need to go to sleep. An occasional patient may require the opposite effort. Case 5 of Richards said that "activity seems to help. Lying down is the worst thing in the world for me" (10). Some patients obtain relief from engaging in alternate activities, either mental or physical, or by rubbing the affected limb (12,21,22). One patient claimed that she was able to abort an attack by "grasping [the] Bible tightly in [her] hand" (20).

The frequency varies from five episodes a day to five a year, but averages about one a week. Most attacks last between 20 minutes and 2 hours, and the longest reported attack was 2 days (22). In terms of natural history, after beginning in childhood, the spells tend to increase in both frequency and severity through the teens and young adulthood; thereafter, most patients improve.

In contrast to the high prevalence of secondary dyskinesias or other neurologic signs in the nonfamilial PDs, familial patients rarely had associated neurologic abnormalities, although there may be an association with epilepsy. Two patients had a seizure disorder, one with primary generalized simple absence with a typical 3-Hz spike and wave electroencephalogram (EEG) abnormality, the other with generalized tonic-clonic spells (10). It is unclear whether the latter was primary, with concomitant epilepsy, or secondary, whereby the movement is the behavioral manifestation of the ictal discharge (17). Both of the above cases demonstrated abnormalities on their neurologic examinations: facial diplegia in the former; mental retardation from birth, atrophy on computed tomography (CT) brain scan, and diffuse slowing on EEG in the latter. A third patient had febrile seizures during infancy (12).

In two cases, EEGs have been normal during an attack, including one case in which the patient was paralyzed with a neuromuscular blocker during an episode while her EEG was being recorded (12,20). Jacome and Risko reported a case of an 82-year-old woman with rare attacks of strictly right-sided PFPD who had photic stimulation-induced lateralized epileptiform discharges (PLED) emanating from her contralateral hemisphere (23).

The original patient of Mount and Reback displayed an atypical Kayser-Fleischer ring. There has not been a second report of a Kayser-Fleischer ring, but Weber described a family in which case 2 had a minimally elevated serum copper level (21). However, cases 3 and 4 had progressive dysarthria and disdiadochokinesia, and cases 2 to 4 had continual dystonia at rest. Therefore, these cases are not typical PFPD, and it is unclear whether these cases should be considered as a secondary form of PFPD or whether they represent another disease entity.

Numerous agents have been used for the treatment of these dyskinesias. Few, however, have demonstrated efficacy. The most successful have been benzodiazepines, especially clonazepam. Recently, Kurlan and Shoulson reported a patient who, following transient improvement with daily oxazepam, derived further benefit from alternate-day oxazepam therapy (24). Based on studies that demonstrated a reduced number of receptors (downregulation) in response to chronic benzodiazepine administration, they suggested that the alternate-day therapy would maximally stimulate the benzodiazepine receptors while allowing for functional recovery of receptors. Phenytoin, tetrabenazine, and trihexyphenidyl have been used in small numbers of patients with kinesigenic dyskinesias (16).

Lance described the only postmortem study of PFPD in an unfortunate 21-month-old boy who died a "crib death" after suffering from PFPD since the age of 2 months (17). Study of sections from the cortex, hippocampus, basal ganglia, cerebellum, midbrain, pons, medulla, and cord failed to reveal any macroscopic or microscopic abnormality, other than congestion and edema consistent with sudden death.

BRIEF FAMILIAL PAROXYSMAL DYSKINESIAS

This group largely constitutes the kinesigenic group described by Kertesz (9). While these cases are usually kinesigenic, some are not, yet are otherwise phenomenologically indistinguishable and respond to similar pharmacologic agents. Therefore, we use the term brief, rather than kinesigenic. There are over 30 reported cases of brief familial paroxysmal dyskinesias (BFPD). The age of onset ranged from age 2 to 18, with more than half of the cases beginning between 8 and 12 years of age. Three-quarters of the patients were male. As with the PFPD, most authors agree that the disorder is autosomal dominant with variable penetrance.

Most attacks are precipitated by activity, usually a quick movement with a change of posture after a period of rest, for example, arising from a chair and taking rapid steps. In addition, excitement and emotional upset often evoke a paroxysm. Furthermore, hyperventilation, startle, embarrassment, self-consciousness, and running have all been implicated in inducing attacks (25–27).

Auras last from one to several seconds. Tingling, numbness, and pins and needles are typical. These are usually localized to a single extremity. Some patients describe a sensation of movement, formication or a "vacant feeling" (26,28). Other patients describe a "sensation of muscle contraction" or stiffness (17,29).

The majority of attacks are dystonic and begin with unilateral posturing of an upper or lower extremity: leg extension with equinovarus foot posturing or arm abduction, elbow flexion, and wrist extension. In addition, there may also be torso torsion and facial grimacing. Half of all cases have only unilateral spasms, although they may alternate sides. The remaining cases have spasms that begin unilaterally and extend to involve both sides or begin bilaterally. In other cases, the attacks are characteristically choreatic or ballistic. When attempting to walk, case 1 of Pryles et al was interrupted by "swaying, prancing movements . . . in the lower limbs throwing him off balance and to the floor" (28). The attacks of case 1 of Hudgins and Corbin "were characterized by a series of involuntary truncal distortions, facial grimaces, and writhing and flinging motions of his four extremities" (30).

Although the movements are involuntary, many patients are able to suppress or abort their spasms. Usually, resting, cessation of ongoing activity, or tightly holding the affected limb will be effective.

The episodes last from 5 seconds to 3 minutes, with the majority between 10 and 30 seconds. Nearly all patients experience daily attacks. Half of the patients suffered several a day, and as many as 100 attacks a day have been reported (31).

Seizures have been the most frequently reported associated disease of BFPD. Additionally, numerous patients had abnormal EEGs. These abnormalities include 3-Hz spike and wave with and without hyperventilation, diffuse θ waves with and without hyperventilation, diffuse slowing, and focal slowing (26,28,31,32). Despite the associations of BFPD with seizures and abnormal EEG, such changes are not prerequisite to the movement disorder since there have also been several reports of normal EEGs both interictally and during attacks (25,29,33,34).

Of the various agents and combinations of agents used to treat BFPD, the anticonvulsants are the most cost effective. Phenytoin, phenobarbital, the combination of phenytoin and phenobarbital, and carbamazepine all have demonstrated efficacy. Phenytoin is probably the drug of choice considering dosing schedule and expense. Homan et al attempted to correlate plasma phenytoin concentration with response (35). However, their sample was too small (five cases) to draw significant conclusions.

Only one case to date has been autopsied. This patient (whose diagnosis was made posthumously) died at age 56 from pneumonia. There was only slight asymmetry of the zona compacta of the substantia nigra (26).

PRIMARY BRIEF SPORADIC PAROXYSMAL DYSKINESIAS

About one-third of the 150 reported cases of brief paroxysmal dyskinesias are primary, without associated disease or focal cerebral dysfunction that could be implicated in its pathophysiology. As in BFPD, many cases of primary brief sporadic paroxysmal dyskinesias (BSPD) are associated with nonspecific but abnormal EEG. Over two-thirds of patients are male. Their ages range from 1 to 33, with 80% between 8 and 17. Only a few cases began after the age of 20, and they were young adults (26,36).

As in BFPD, where all are kinesigenic, nearly all of these cases are also kinesigenic (35,37). The case described by Homan et al, like some of the prolonged PD cases, was induced by alcohol (35). In a patient with brief, nonfamilial episodes that are not kinesigenic, an aggressive search for secondary causes is recommended.

The most frequently described precipitant is a quick movement, usually with a change in posture, following a period of rest. This pattern resembles that seen with BFPD. Arising from a chair, turning in bed, dancing, running, swimming, and hopping, as well as startle, fright, nervousness, embarrassment, and tension are well-known inciting factors. In some cases, passive movement of a limb was enough to precipitate an attack (4). Finally, hyperventilation has also been reported to induce attacks (26,38,39). Case 2 of Kinast et al even reported that "anticipation of movement" could induce an attack (37). Likewise, one patient claimed that "reading about running" could bring on an episode (7).

Most patients described their prodrome as numbness, tingling, pins and needles, and an odd or funny feeling. The sensation usually begins in a distal extremity and passes through the body. Also described is a "current-like sensation" and a feeling like being "high on drugs" (40,41). Both primary and secondary patients had similar auras, although only one patient with primary disease complained of pain (11). By contrast, several patients with secondary BSPD complained of painful, burning, and horrid prodromes (5,9,38,42,43).

Most attacks are bilateral and predominantly dystonic in character, and are indistinguishable from the BFPD. In contrast to the primary cases, most patients with secondary dyskinesias are unable to suppress or abort their attacks (see Chapter 74).

Many patients have nonspecific but abnormal EEG. These abnormalities include diffuse slowing, focal slowing, 3-Hz activity with hyperventilation, and a focal photoconvulsive response (26,27,44–46). In addition, one patient had a history of early childhood seizures. A patient with right arm dyskinesias also manifested an action dystonia of his right arm (38). Other abnormalities have included brainstem atrophy on a CT brain scan, right leg atrophy from childhood polio, migraine, capillary hemangioma of the forehead, psychiatric problems, and obesity (9,40,44,46,47).

As in the familial variety, the treatment of choice for primary BSPD is anticonvulsant therapy. The most effective anticonvulsants are dilantin, phenobarbital, the combination of dilantin and phenobarbital, and carbamazepine. In contrast to the prolonged dyskinesias, benzodiazepines are not regularly useful, although some patients have complete resolution of attacks with clonazepam (16). Demirkiran and Jankovic (16) found that kinesigenic spells, whether short or long-acting, were associated with a better response to medication than were nonkinesigenic dyskinesias. Of interest is the single case report of primary BSPD responsive to L-dopa (30). Also of interest is the single case of a morbidly obese woman whose dyskinesias ceased following weight reduction (9).

These is only one reported pathologic study, case 4 of Kertesz (9). After developing BSPD at the age of 10, the patient apparently hanged himself at age 13. An autopsy revealed diffuse vascular congestion. Slides of the cortex, cerebellum, striatum, and pons revealed normal cytoarchitecture and myelination. There was a suggestion of a slight loss of neurons in the area of the locus ceruleus because of the presence of some melanin-pigmented macrophages in this area.

NOCTURNAL PAROXYSMAL DYSKINESIAS

Lugaresi and Cirignotta defined a syndrome of nocturnal paroxysmal dystonia that is phenomenologically similar to daytime dyskinesias (12). The attacks may be either prolonged or brief, and the brief attacks, in this case less than 1 minute, have a strong association with seizures. Lee et al

(48) have also described a familial variety of nocturnal dyskinesias; primary and secondary sporadic cases have also been described (43,49). Horner and Jackson reported a family with paroxysmal dyskinesias, with either or both nocturnal and daytime dyskinesias occurring in multiple family members (50,51).

In two families, with a total of 13 patients, their age of onset ranged from 2 to 23 years, with all but one beginning prior to age 13 (48,50). The familial cases were predominantly male, and the genetic pattern appeared to be autosomal dominant with variable penetrance. Bryne et al (13) reported a family with paroxysmal dystonic choreoathetosis transmitted as a dominant trait over five generations, with marked responsiveness of the episodes to short periods of sleep in several family members and associated with prominent myokymia in some cases.

Over 14 sporadic cases have been reported. The age of onset was slightly older than the familial, ranging from 3 to 47 years, with only 5 cases beginning before age 13 (43,49,51).

In patients who experienced both daytime and nocturnal attacks, the daytime attacks were initiated by sudden changes in posture as in typical daytime PD (50). The majority of patients with nocturnal PD, however, do not have daytime attacks, and the contorsions are isolated to sleep or to awakening in the morning. Some patients were able to induce their episodes by hyperventilation. In addition, antecedent heavy work and stress were also reported to be aggravating factors (48).

When the attacks awakened patients from sleep they were unable to relate an aura. Patients with daytime attacks typically experienced pins and needles prodromes.

The familial attacks of Horner and Jackson consisted of "violent episodes of nocturnal paroxysmal choreoathetosis" lasting 2 to 5 minutes (50). The nocturnal episodes were never observed by these authors; however, a daytime episode was induced by hyperventilation. The patient "developed trismus and rigidity of facial and neck muscles, rapid flexion and extension movements of the fingers, wrists, and elbows, and violent flailing, twisting movements of the arms and legs" (48). The dyskinesias were bilateral, primarily dystonic, with opisthotonus and were accompanied by occasional clonic movements. The duration was less than a minute. Unlike in the previous family, these attacks were described as being painful.

The sporadic cases, both long and short, also demonstrated bilateral dystonic, choreoathetotic movements. The brief episodes lasted less than 1 minute, often only 15 seconds. The prolonged episodes often continued for 30 minutes or more. Although the two types of attacks appeared similar, the duration is important therapeutically (see below). Secondary cases may be either long or short.

The attacks occur at least weekly, and almost nightly. Most patients experience more than one episode a night, some up to 20 a night.

The familial patients with nocturnal PD described by Horner and Jackson had no associated diseases, and their neurologic examinations and EEGs were normal. However, several other family members, without nocturnal dyskinesias but with daytime dyskinesias, had choreoathetosis at rest. The familial cases of Lee et al (48) had no associated abnormality, except patient 3, who had febrile convulsions at age 1.

By contrast, the sporadic cases have a high incidence of abnormal EEGs and associated epilepsy. Of the 12 cases studied by Lugaresi et al, 4 suffered from primary generalized epilepsy and 4 others had episodes suggestive of partial seizures (51). In patients studied with polysomnography, most of the EEGs demonstrated an arousal pattern preceding the attacks (51). Cases have also occurred secondary to multiple sclerosis (43,49). In addition, a patient with a family history of Huntington's disease also had nocturnal paroxysms. Twenty years later this patient manifested cognitive decline and chorea at rest, resulting in a diagnosis of Huntington's disease.

The brief attacks, including those secondary to multiple sclerosis, have been sensitive to phenytoin and phenobarbital, and, more recently, to carbamazepine (50,51). Patient 1 of Lee et al (48) responded to carbamazepine and amitriptyline, and Demirkiran and Jankovic's patient responded well to lorazepam (16). By contrast, the prolonged attacks have been particularly resistant to pharmacotherapy, including benzodiazepines, anticonvulsants, and phenothiazines.

There have been no postmortem studies to date.

LABORATORY INVESTIGATIONS

The extent of the investigation should be based on the clinical suspicion of an associated abnormality. However, certain screening tests are particularly useful, including magnetic resonance imaging (MRI) brain scan (CT brain scan with infusion if an MRI is unavailable), EEG awake and sleep deprived, serum glucose, sodium, calcium, phosphorus, thyroid functions, copper, and ceruloplasmin. There are some guidelines that may help the clinician in the evaluation of a patient with paroxysmal movements. First, kinesigenic episodes can occur in all of the categories discussed. However, they have been described in all cases of BFPD and nearly all cases of primary BSPD. Second, painful attacks are uncommon in the familial and primary sporadic cases. Third, seizures are associated with all categories. However, they are most commonly associated with brief episodes, both daytime and nocturnal. Finally, the movements may be extremely bizarre, and because there is no alteration in consciousness, these patients have been labeled hysterical. This disease should be entertained when a diagnosis of conversion reaction is based on abnormal movements.

NATURAL HISTORY AND PROGNOSIS

In cases of primary PD, the patients often present soon after their movements begin, and there is a good response to medication. Infrequently, patients will be controlled on one medication for a period of months to years and then the medication will lose efficacy. A second medication is then introduced, often successfully. Some patients give a long history of abnormal movements. For instance, they may begin with occasional facial grimacing at age 1, followed by dyskinesias of one or more extremities in the ensuing years. In some cases the movements cease on their own, whereas in others they fluctuate. While there may be some progression of the movements, the course of the primary PD is generally benign. Should a patient develop an abnormal neurologic examination between attacks, this should be taken as a sign that the patient has secondary PD or another illness, and further diagnostic evaluations should be instituted. The natural history of the secondary PD is closely tied to the underlying disease (see Chapter 74).

PATHOPHYSIOLOGY

The pathophysiology of these intriguing movements remains elusive. There is evidence that the disorder may relate to cortical or subcorticobasal ganglionic dysfunction. The phenomenologic resemblance of the dystonic-choreoathetotic movements to those of Huntington's chorea, Wilson's disease, and primary torsion dystonia suggests that the disorder relates directly to basal ganglionic dysfunction. In addition, several other types of action-induced (kinesigenic) involuntary movements are well accepted as being of basal origin, especially the focal dystonias, for example, blepharospasm, oromandibular dystonia, and writer's cramp, and possibly generalized intention myoclonus (52–54). On the other hand, some authors have favored a cortical epileptic genesis of the disorder, based on the high incidence of associated seizures, abnormal EEG, the short duration of the paroxysms, the stereotypy of the movements, and the few reports of EEG paroxysms related to the movements. These data suggest that the same or similar paroxysmal movements may be generated by abnormalities in either the cortex or basal ganglionic nuclei. Although the response of the PDs to anticonvulsants has also been offered as evidence of an epileptic origin of the movements, phenytoin has known behavioral and pharmacologic effects on the striatum, and carbamazepine has been used successfully to treat dystonias (55,56).

An animal model has been developed that may clarify elements of the pathopharmacology of the disorder. In the mutant hamster dt^{sz}, episodic dystonic spasms develop with handling or environmental stimuli. Drugs that augment γ-aminobutyric acid (GABA) function decrease the abnormal movements, and *N*-methyl D-aspartate (NMDA) antagonists delayed the disorder's progression in a dose-dependent fashion (57,58). Further studies suggest that the GABA-gated chloride ion channel may be directly involved in this disorder, specifically in the connections among basal ganglia, frontal association cortex, and thalamus (59).

Based on available anatomic and physiologic evidence demonstrating the intimate relationship between the basal ganglia, thalamus, and the premotor cortex, Penney and Young have suggested a corticostriatopallidothalamocortical feedback circuit as the mechanism whereby the basal ganglia influence motor behavior (60,61). The backbone of this circuit is a positive-feedback corticothalamocortical loop that the cortex utilizes to maintain motor output. Inhibitory efferents from the medial globus pallidus modulate this activity. The various PDs could result from imbalances within this circuit, either from excessive cortical output or deficient pallidal inhibition. Because this circuit receives direct input from the motor cortex and input from the reticular activating system via the intralaminar thalamic nuclei, arousal, alerting, sudden movement, and exercise could all be expected to activate this system. In this way, PD movements could be precipitated by diseases of many different etiologies affecting any part of this pathway.

REFERENCES

1. Bennett DA, Goetz CG. Paroxysmal dyskinesias. In: Chokroverty S, ed. Movement disorders. Costa Mesa: PMA Publishing, 1990:287–307.
2. Mount LA, Reback S. Familial paroxysmal choreoathetosis: preliminary report on a hitherto undescribed clinical syndrome. Arch Neurol 1940;44:841–847.
3. Sterling W. Le type spasmodique tetanoide et tetaniforme de l'encephalite epidemique: remarques sur l'epilepsie "extrapyramidale." Rev Neurol 1924;2:484–492.
4. Spiller WG. Subcortical epilepsy. Brain 1927;50:171–187.
5. Wilson SAK. Nervous semeiology, with special references to epilepsy. Lecture III—symptoms indicating increase of neural function. Br Med J 1930;2:90.
6. Cooper MJ. Tonic epileptic attacks precipitated by fright or surprise. Arch Neurol Psychiatry 1933;30:462–464.
7. Pitha V. Epilepsie reflexe. Rev Neurol 1938;70:178–181.
8. Smith LA, Heersema PH. Periodic dystonia. Proc Mayo Clin 1941;16:842–846.
9. Kertesz A. Paroxysmal kinesigenic choreoathetosis: an entity within the paroxysmal choreoathetosis syndrome. Description of 10 cases, including 1 autopsied. Neurology 1967;17:680–690.
10. Richards RN, Barnett HJM. Paroxysmal dystonic choreoathetosis. A family study and review of the literature. Neurology 1968;18:461–469.
11. Lishman WA, Symonds CP, Whitty CWM, Willison RG. Seizures induced by movement. Brain 1962;85:93–108.
12. Lugaresi E, Cirignotta F. Hypnogenic paroxysmal dystonia: epileptic seizures or a new syndrome? Sleep 1981;4:129–138.
13. Bryne E, White O, Cook M. Familial dystonic choreoathetosis with myokymia: a sleep responsive disorder. J Neurol Neurosurg Psychiatry 1991;54:1090–1092.
14. Lance JW. Sporadic and familial varieties of tonic seizures. J Neurol Neurosurg Psychiatry 1963;26:51–59.
15. Fahn S. The paroxysmal dyskinesias. In: Marsden CD, Fahn S, eds. Movement disorders 3. Oxford: Butterworth-Heinemann, 1994:310–345.
16. Demirkiran M, Jankovic J. Paroxysmal dyskinesias: clinical features and classification. Ann Neurol 1995;38:571–579.
17. Lance JW. Familial paroxysmal dystonic choreoathetosis and its differentiation from related syndromes. Ann Neurol 1977;2:285–293.
18. Goodenough DJ, Fariello RG, Annis BL. Chun RWM. Familial and acquired paroxysmal dyskinesias: a proposed classification with delineation of clinical features. Arch Neurol 1978;35:827–831.
19. Bennett DA, Goetz CG, Ristanovic RK, Morrell F. Paroxysmal dyskinesias: clinical and laboratory features in nine cases. Neurology 1978;37(suppl 1):262.
20. Forssman H. Hereditary disorder characterized by attacks of muscular contractions, induced by alcohol amongst other factors. Acta Med Scand 1961;170:517–533.
21. Weber MB. Familial paroxysmal dystonia. J Nerv Ment Dis 1967;145:221–226.
22. Walker ES. Familial paroxysmal dystonic choreothetosis: a neurologic disorder simulating psychiatric illness. Johns Hopkins Med J 1981;148:108–113.
23. Jacome DE, Risko M. Photicinduced-driven PLEDs in paroxysmal dystonic choreoathetosis. Clin Electroencephalogr 1984;15:151–154.
24. Kurlan R, Shoulson I. Familial paroxysmal dystonic choreoathetosis and response to alternate-day oxazepam therapy. Ann Neurol 1983;13:456–457.
25. Soffer D, Licht A, Yaar I, Abramsky O. Paroxysmal choreoathetosis as a presenting symptom in idiopathic hypoparathyroidism. J Neurol Neurosurg Psychiatry 1977;40:692–694.

26. Stevens H. Paroxysmal choreoathetosis—a form of reflex epilepsy. Arch Neurol 1966;14:415–420.

27. Hishikawa E, Furuya E, Yamamoto J, Nan'No H. Dystonic seizures induced by movement. Arch Psychiatr Nervenkr 1973;217:113–138.

28. Pryles CV, Livingston S, Ford FR. Familial paroxysmal choreoathetosis of Mount and Reback. Pediatrics 1952;9:44–47.

29. Jung S, Chen KM, Brody JA. Paroxysmal choreoathetosis. Neurology 1973;23:749–755.

30. Hudgins RL, Corbin KB. An uncommon seizure disorder: familial paroxysmal choreoathetosis. Brain 1966;89:199–205.

31. Kato M, Araki S. Paroxysmal kinesigenic choreoathetosis: report of a case relieved by carbamazepine. Arch Neurol 1969;20:508–513.

32. Garello L, Ottonello GA, Regesta G, Tanganelli P. Familial paroxysmal kinesigenic choreoathetosis: report of a pharmacological trial in two cases. Eur Neurol 1983;22:217–221.

33. Suber DA, Riley TL. Valproic acid and normal computerized tomographic scan in kinesigenic familial paroxysmal choreoathetosis. Arch Neurol 1980;37:327.

34. Smith LA, Heersema PH. Periodic dystonia. Proc Mayo Clin 1941;16:842–846.

35. Homan RW, Vasko MR, Blaw M. Phenytoin plasma concentrations in paroxysmal kinesigenic choreoathetosis. Neurology 1980;30:673–676.

36. Lang AE. Focal paroxysmal kinesigenic choreoathetosis. J Neurol Neurosurg Psychiatry 1984;47:1057–1058.

37. Kinast GE, Erenberg G, Rothner AD. Paroxysmal choreoathetosis: report of five cases and review of the literature. Pediatrics 1980;65:74–77.

38. Matthews WB. Tonic seizures in disseminated sclerosis. Brain 1958;81:193–206.

39. Williams J, Stevens H. Familial paroxysmal choreoathetosis. Pediatrics 1963;3:656–659.

40. Juson RMD. Idiopathic paroxysmal choreoathetosis—report of two cases and review of literature. Med J Malaysia 1983;38:224–227.

41. Plant GT. Focal paroxysmal kinesigenic choreoathetosis. J Neurol Neurosurg Psychiatry 1983;46:345–348.

42. Drake ME Jr, Jackson RD, Miller CA. Paroxysmal choreoathetosis after head injury. J Neurol Neurosurg Psychiatry 1986;49:837–338.

43. Berger JR, Sheremata WA, Melamed E. Paroxysmal dystonia as the initial manifestation of multiple sclerosis. Arch Neurol 1984;41:747–750.

44. Lishman WA, Symonds CP, Whitty CWM, Willison RG. Seizures induced by movement. Brian 1962;85:93–108.

45. Whitty CWM, Lishman WA, Fitzgibbon JP. Seizures induced by movement: a form of reflex epilepsy. Lancet 1964;i:1403–1406.

46. Goodenough DJ, Fariello RG, Annis BL, Chun RWM. Familial and acquired paroxysmal dyskinesias: a proposed classification with delineation of clinical features. Arch Neurol 1978;35:827–831.

47. Watson RT, Scott WR. Paroxysmal kinesigenic choreoathetosis and brainstem atrophy. Arch Neurol 1978;36:522.

48. Lee BI, Lesser RP, Pippenger CE, et al. Familial paroxysmal hypnogenic dystonia. Neurology 1985;35:1357–1360.

49. Joynt RJ, Green D. Tonic seizures as a manifestation of multiple sclerosis. Arch Neurol 1962;6:293–299.

50. Horner FH, Jackson LC. Familial paroxysmal choreoathetosis. Prog Neurogenet Excerpta Med 1969;745–751.

51. Lugaresi E, Cirignotta EF, Montagna P. Nocturnal paroxysmal dystonia. J Neurol Neurosurg Psychiatry 1986;49:375–380.

52. Lance JW. Action myoclonus, Ramsey Hunt syndrome, and other cerebellar myoclonic syndromes. In: Fahn S, et al, eds. Advances in neurology. Vol. 32, Myoclonus. New York: Raven Press, 1986.

53. Lees AJ, Hardie RJ, Stern GM. Kinesigenic foot dystonia as a presenting feature of Parkinson's disease. J Neurol Neurosurg Psychiatry 1984;47:885.

54. Marsden CD. The problem of adult-onset idiopathic torsion dystonia and other isolated dyskinesias in adult life (including blepharospasm, oromandibular dystonia, dystonic writer's cramp, and torticollis or axial dystonia). In: Eldridge R, Fahn S, eds. Advances in neurology. Vol. 14. New York: Raven Press, 1976.

55. Geller M, Kaplan B, Nicholas C. Treatment of dystonic symptoms with carbamazepines. In: Eldridge R, Fahn S, eds. Advances in neurology. Vol. 14. New York: Raven Press, 1976.

56. Elliott PNC, Jenner P, Chadwick D, et al. The effects of diphenylhydantoin on central catecholamine containing neuronal systems. J Pharm Pharmacol 1977;27:41.

57. Richter A, Fredow G, Löscher W. Antidystonic effects of the NMDA receptor antagonists memantine, MK-801 and CGP 37849 in a mutant hamster model of paroxysmal dystonia. Neurosci Lett 1991;133:57–60.

58. Fredow G, Löscher W. Effects of pharmacological manipulation of GABAergic neurotransmission in a new mutant hamster model of paroxysmal dystonia. Eur J Pharmacol 1991;192:207–219.

59. Nobrega JN, Richter A, Burnhamn WM, Löscher W. Alterations in the brain GABA A/benzodiazepine receptor complex in a genetic model of paroxysmal dystonia. Neuroscience 1994;64:229–239.

60. Goldberg G. Supplementary motor area structure and function: review and hypotheses. Behav Brain Sci 1985;8:567–616.

61. Penney JB Jr, Young AB. Speculations on the functional anatomy of basal ganglia disorders. Ann Rev Neurosci 1983;6:73–94.

Acquired Paroxysmal Dyskinesias

CHRISTOPHER G. GOETZ   TARIF BAKDASH

INTRODUCTION

In the previous chapter, we defined a paroxysmal dyskinesia as an abnormal dystonic and/or choreoathetotic movement that is only intermittently present. The movement is unaccompanied by altered consciousness or incontinence, the patient is not amnestic for the episode, and there is no accompanying or residual confusion (1). The movements may be diurnal or nocturnal, short (less than 5 minutes) or prolonged (more than 5 minutes), familial or sporadic. The latter may be primary or secondary (acquired). Because the primary sporadic dyskinesias are phenomenologically indistinguishable and follow the same natural history as the familial, they were covered in the preceding chapter. This chapter will address the acquired dyskinesias. Table 74.1 lists various disorders known to present with or be complicated by paroxysmal dyskinesias.

MULTIPLE SCLEROSIS

Spiller was probably the first to report paroxysmal dyskinesias in a patient with multiple sclerosis (MS) (2), but Matthews coined the term "tonic seizures" and first systematically studied them (3). Over 80 cases of paroxysmal dyskinesias secondary to MS have now been reported (2–19). In addition to tonic seizures, some of these cases are referred to as spinal seizures (10,11,13). The age of onset ranges from 16 to 62, with the average age being about 40. There is a slight female preponderance. The majority of paroxysms occur after the diagnosis of MS has been established. However, at least 18 patients, including 2 personally observed cases, presented with their paroxysmal dyskinesia as the first manifestation of their demyelinating disease (5,6,14, and unpublished observations). All of the cases but two were diurnal. Case 4 of Joynt and Green had a single diurnal attack, the remainder awakening him from sleep (8), and case 7 of Berger et al only had nocturnal attacks (6).

Diagnosis

The majority of attacks are kinesigenic and brief. When the patient begins to move following a period of rest, a paroxysm is induced. A classic occurrence is for an attack to be brought on when turning over in bed or suddenly arising from a chair. Sometimes a purposeful movement is necessary to provoke a spasm, such as reaching out to grab something (7). Hyperventilation may be a potent stimulus for an episode. On occasion, passive manipulation of a limb may also cause the dyskinesia.

Most MS patients with paroxysmal dyskinesias describe sensory auras preceding the paroxysm. Often these are vague paresthesias, such as a feeling of trembling, an odd undescribable feeling, or tingling. In contrast to the familial dyskinesias, burning or pain may be the aura. These sensory complaints often begin in a distal extremity and spread throughout the body. Within seconds they are followed by the tonic attack, which usually begins distally with dystonic posturing. The hand is flexed and the arm oronated and extended. The toes are plantar flexed and the foot held in an equinovarus posture. Only rarely is there superimposed choreoathetosis. The axial musculature is not spared and the patient is often twisted. In over half of the cases the spasm is distinctly painful. The whole episode rarely lasts longer than 1 minute, and may recur up to 50 times a day. About 80% of cases are unilateral, the remainder being bilateral, with some alternating sides. Nearly 20% include the face, most on the same side as the body, but some contralateral to the body (16), a fact that has obvious implications regarding anatomic substrate and pathophysiology.

Table 74.1   Diseases Associated with Acquired Paroxysmal Dyskinesias

Multiple sclerosis
Myelopathy
Vascular or developmental anomalies
Drug-induced paroxysmal dyskinesias
Cerebral ischemia
Head trauma
Cerebral palsy
Hemiparesis
Focal seizures
Encephalitis
Radiculopathy
Hypoparathyroidism
Thyrotoxicosis
Hypoglycemia
Psychogenic
Reflex sympathetic dystrophy

A subgroup of MS patients with paroxysmal dyskinesias has been described who have a "reverse" Brown-Séquard syndrome (6,10,11,14). These patients have a unilateral sensation of heat followed by pain, then the spasm on the contralateral side. Similar episodes have also been described as a result of disseminated encephalomyelitis (10) and idiopathic transverse myelitis (20).

In about 80% of cases the dyskinesia occurs in the setting of an established diagnosis of MS. When the dyskinesia is the presenting feature, the history and physical examination will often suggest the diagnosis of MS and be supported by analysis of the cerebrospinal fluid. One would suspect that magnetic resonance imaging (MRI) would also suggest the diagnosis of MS. In a case of acute transverse myelitis presenting with a paroxysmal dyskinesia, the MRI of the brain was normal, but the cord showed a lesion at C2 (20). The authors claimed that this patient probably had MS in view of her typical paroxysmal dyskinesia. Two other cases of "idiopathic" transverse myelitis also eventually developed MS (21). Although MS is the most widely described cause of secondary paroxysmal dyskinesias, the differential diagnosis is wide, and other causes must be investigated.

Treatment

First reported by Kuroiwa and Shibasaki in 1967 (9), carbamazepine is the drug of choice for paroxysmal dyskinesias and other paroxysmal symptoms in MS (5,12, 14,15,22–24). Phenytoin is the second drug (5,12). Acetazolamide has also been reported to be successful in seven patients with various paroxysmal disturbances with MS including paroxysmal dyskinesias (16,25). However, the success has not been universal (21). Phenobarbitone is also useful, if necessary (5), and Clorazepate was beneficial in one patient (6). Of interest, prednisone and lioresol were reported to be ineffective (6,21). Finally, case 4 of Shibasaki and Kuroiwa, whose dyskinesias always started in the left

hand, responded to a left axillary nerve block with 1% procaine hydrochloride (12). Her dyskinesias were also successfully treated with phenytoin and carbamazepine.

Pathophysiology

Spiller initially thought the disorder was a form of epilepsy (2). He was reluctant to restrict himself to the striatum, and therefore called it subcortical epilepsy. For Wilson, the fact that "the muscular contractions themselves were dolorous and (in particular) that they arose in consequence of active, voluntary movement, in my opinion render their ascription to any of the epilepsies, as ordinarily understood, more than a little dubious" (26, p. 91). Matthews originally thought of them as a form of tetany of central origin (3). Ekbom et al assumed that an irritative lesion that did not interrupt sensory and motor pathways could, at a specific spinal level, transversely activate axons, leading to both the tonic spasm and the sensory disturbance (10). Osterman and Westerberg also considered the paroxysmal phenomenon a result of transverse ephaptic excitation of axons within an area of partial demyelination "somewhere in the central nervous system" (14, p. 196). Alternatively, when the corticospinal tract is activated by voluntary movement, it could spread ephaptically when it reaches an area of demyelination (20). The location of the ephaptic spread would determine the clinical symptomatology of a particular paroxysm, that is, ipsilateral face, arm and leg; ipsilateral face with contralateral arm and leg; or ipsilateral motor arm and leg and contralateral sensory arm and leg, without face, corresponding to cerebrum, brainstem, and spinal cord, respectively. A case of MRI-documented thalamic demyelination was associated with contralateral paroxysmal hemidystonia in one case of MS (27), and bilateral basal gangliar lesions have been associated with alternating-side paroxysmal dyskinesias (28).

MYELOPATHY

These cases include several reports of transverse myelitis (11,20,21,29), some of which turned out to be MS (13,20), a case of spinal cord meningioma (26), and a case of acute disseminated encephalomyelitis (10). Isolated high cervical lesions without added evidence of multiple sclerosis lesions can also cause paroxysmal dyskinesias (30). We group these cases together because they all have a myelopathy by neurologic examination, and phenomenologically similar movements. All of these cases are diurnal and brief. Because of its unusual character, we will present only spinal cord meningioma here, as the others were dealt with in the section on MS.

Diagnosis

This patient was a 75-year-old woman who presented with attacks of a burning pain in the left lower limb followed by stiffening of the leg. These were very painful, lasted about

30 seconds and occurred up to 10 times a day. Her examination suggested a midthoracic myelopathy, and a myelogram showed a complete block at the first thoracic vertebra. This eventually turned out to be a meningioma.

Treatment

She had a prompt, albeit short-lived, response to dilantin. Eventually she consented to surgical decompression, resulting in cessation of her movements.

Pathophysiology

Nathanson believed that this case supported "observations that the spinal cord . . . may initiate their own seizure discharge" (26). However, pathologic studies of the spinal cord at the area of compression demonstrate areas of demyelination, presumably secondary to ischemia (31). It is conceivable that these areas can give rise to an abnormal spread of ephaptic transmission similar to demyelinated areas from MS.

VASCULAR AND DEVELOPMENTAL ANOMALIES

Several isolated cases of unusual structural aberrations have been associated with paroxysmal dyskinesias, including porencephalic cysts (32) and arteriovenous malformations (33). These spells are phenomenologically typical in character, being brief, dystonic, and kinesigenic.

DRUG-INDUCED PAROXYSMAL DYSKINESIAS

There are isolated cases of drugs inducing paroxysmal dystonic movements. A case of methylphenidate usage in a boy with attention deficit disorder was complicated by induction of new kinesigenic dystonia, which persisted after drug cessation (34). Carbamazepine controlled the movements, but they recurred if he stopped the anticonvulsant. Another stimulant, cocaine, has been associated with paroxysmal movements, although whether these related to vascular, epileptic, or acute intoxication is not clear from the report (35).

CEREBRAL ISCHEMIA

Gastaut and Fischer-Williams performed the classic study to differentiate the convulsive movements of syncope from those of seizures (36). Using ocular pressure, they induced at least 10 seconds of cardiac arrest in 20 patients. They demonstrated that there was no epileptic electroencephalographic (EEG) correlate to the clonic movements of convulsive syncope. By carotid compression, they were also able to induce isolated contralateral clonic movements without an epileptic EEG correlate (37). Despite these elegant studies, transient abnormal movements as a manifestation of intermittent cerebral ischemia are rarely reported. Fisher was probably the first to mention transient cerebral ischemia presenting a "shaking" movement (38). There are now more than 35 such cases in the literature (38–49). These cases are distinct from postinfarction movement disorders.

Diagnosis

The movements are usually precipitated by a change in posture, usually standing, walking, or neck extension (40,49), though this is not always necessary (46). Even when induced by standing, the patients rarely show significant orthostatic hypotension. However, there have been similar cases observed in patients with autonomic insufficiency (42). The movements are described as "shaking," "jerking," "trembling," or "flapping" (40,46,47). The spells typically involve the hand and arm, but sometimes extend to the leg. The face is usually spared. A few cases have reported affection of both upper extremities simultaneously. The spells last between several seconds and an hour, but most often only a few minutes. Transient ischemic attacks in the same cerebral territory may be interspersed between movement spells.

The age of onset is between 44 and 88, with the vast majority of patients presenting in their sixth and seventh decade. Almost without exception, there is a history of cerebrovascular risk factors. About 70% have a history of a prior cerebrovascular accident (CVA) in the hemisphere contralateral to the dyskinesia.

Computed tomography (CT) scanning may or may not reveal a CVA in the hemisphere contralateral to the dyskinesia. EEG fails to reveal any epileptic activity; however, there may be focal slowing in the hemisphere contralateral to the movements. Finally, arteriography nearly always demonstrates either severe stenosis or occlusion of the contralateral carotid. One patient's work-up only revealed a cardiac source of emboli (43).

Treatment

Therapy has usually been surgical: patients with a carotid occlusion receiving an extracranial-intracranial bypass, those with severe stenosis receiving endarterectomy. The results have been good to excellent in 14 of 18 patients to whom follow-up was given (46,48,49). Baquis et al treated two patients with antiplatelet agents (46). In one patient, the movements ceased; the other continued to have episodes, but did not suffer a subsequent CVA. Bennett and Fox reported one patient whose movements were terminated by aspirin (40). Phenytoin was without benefit in four patients (40,46).

Pathophysiology

The angiographically demonstrated vascular disease in the appropriate vascular distribution and the results of vascular surgery suggest some type of ischemic irritability as the etiology of the movements.

HEAD TRAUMA

Several cases of paroxysmal dyskinesias have been reported following head trauma with loss of consciousness (50–53). Case 5 of Lishman et al (50), cases 4 and 5 of Hishikawa et al (51), and Robin's case (52) are all typical idiopathic brief sporadic paroxysmal dyskinesias, except for the history of head trauma with loss of consciousness lasting for several minutes (54). Their posttraumatic neurologic examinations were normal. Because these cases are so typical of the idiopathic dyskinesias, it is hard to definitely implicate the head trauma in their pathogenesis and we will not discuss them. Other cases, however, are phenomenologically distinct (53,55).

Diagnosis

Several young men sustained severe closed head injuries resulting in coma for 2 weeks and residual motor deficits. The movements began within months after regaining consciousness. Some patients complained of a prodrome of pain and fatigue and paresthesias in the involved extremity. In one patient, movements were induced by passive manipulation of the limb, and in another, attempts at volitional movement and stress precipitated the attacks. The attacks were described as "clonic jerking, writhing, spasmodic flexion, and ballistic flailing" lasting a few to several minutes. In two cases they could be aborted by grasping or squeezing the involved limbs. EEGs were unremarkable, evoked potentials were not helpful, and brain scans were not reported. In cases described by Demirkiran and Jankovic (56), peripheral trauma could be associated with later development of paroxysmal dystonia.

Treatment

Two patients were controlled with phenobarbital, and one with lorazepam. Carbamazepine was helpful in one patient but had to be discontinued because of nausea. Phenytoin and diazepam were ineffective.

Pathophysiology

The pathophysiology of paroxysmal dyskinesia is controversial, and investigators are not certain whether this condition is an unusual form of epilepsy or a primary movement disorder related to putative aberrant ephaptic transmission involving basal gangliar structures. The putamen has been the site of primary anatomic interest. The case of Biarry et al (55) involved a 15-year-old boy with severe head injury, coma, and hemiplegia who developed nocturnal hemidystonia during non–rapid eye movement sleep. He responded to acetazolamide, and the authors suggested that trauma-induced putamenal abnormalities seen on MRI accounted for the paroxysmal events that never occurred during wakefulness.

CEREBRAL PALSY AND HEMIPARESIS

Several cases have been reported in which hemiatrophy is evident by examination, or a history of perinatal injury is obtained (4,7,57,58). Specifically, the syndrome of alternating hemiplegia with accompanying paroxysmal dystonia has been described (60,61). These cases probably represent a heterogenous population of patients rather than a specific nosologic group (58).

Diagnosis

These patients are usually younger, between 5 and 14, and they present specifically for evaluation of their movements. The movements are usually precipitated by startle or movement, and often are not preceded by a sensory aura. They may be unilateral, in which case they are all on the same side (18,62), or bilateral (57). When bilateral they consist of tonic extension of the extremities followed by marked athetosis. In one case the movements were painful (4). One patient had rare intermittent dystonic posturing of the hand in addition to his hemiatrophy (58). An abnormal ictal EEG was obtained in one patient (see "Seizures") (7). In the case of alternating hemiplegia with dystonia, attacks were longer and not precipitated by activity, although startle could induce paroxysmal events (60,63).

Treatment

Phenytoin was effective in two patients (57,58); tincture of belladonna and diphenhydramine were ineffective (57), as was "intensive psychotherapy" (58). In one case of alternating hemiparesis with dystonia, flunarizine abolished the spasms (60).

SEIZURES

Several patients phenomenologically had paroxysmal dyskinesias associated with seizures. In one, painful spasms were associated with clearly established focal epileptic activity of cortical origin in the frontal-sagittal area (63). In two cases the movements themselves were thought to be epileptic (62,64), and in two others, typical paroxysmal dyskinesias blended imperceptibly with generalized seizures (65). Kotagal et al reported a large series of patients with complex partial seizures of temporal lobe origin who presented with unilateral dystonic posturing with superimposed choreoathetosis (66). We have seen a similar case from a mesial frontal focus (62).

Diagnosis

A 29-year-old man experienced episodes characterized by a "feeling of tension in the right quadriceps," followed by a stiffening of the right leg, arching of the trunk to the right, and abduction of the right shoulder with extension of the elbow (64). Episodes lasted 10 to 20 seconds and occurred up to 40 times a day. They could be precipitated by movement, especially when awakening from sleep, or by stress or attack. Numerous EEGs recorded during his spells failed to reveal epileptic activity. Eventually, an EEG following injection of 5% Metrazol provoked a spell, which developed into a generalized convulsion. The EEG demonstrated a prominent 20 cps left central rhythm, which rapidly slowed to 9 cps. This was interpreted as a probable seizure focus. Skull radiographs, pneumoencephalogram, and cerebral angiogram were all negative.

A 7-year-old boy had a history of cerebral palsy, experiencing episodes of choreoathetotic movements of the right hand, followed by abduction of the shoulder and head dropping (62). The episodes lasted several seconds and occurred up to 100 times daily. They could be suppressed by tightly holding the extremity. Routine EEGs were negative; however, an EEG with double-density electrodes over the vertex showed bursts of 20 to 40 μV 3-Hz epileptiform activity maximal at Cz. Blood chemistries, evoked potentials, CT, and MRI brain were all negative

Two additional cases had typical brief sporadic paroxysmal dyskinesias culminating in generalized seizures (65). One of these patient's EEG demonstrated medium voltage spikes in the contralateral frontotemporal region.

Treatment

The first patient failed trials of primidone, Epanutin, phenobarbitone, and sodium amytal (64). A craniotomy was eventually performed, and a 1.5 × 0.5 cm cortical scar was removed from 2 cm anterior to the Rolandic fissure.

Case 2 had some response to phenytoin, but was better controlled with carbamazepine (62). The last two patients were successfully treated with primidone and phenytoin.

Pathophysiology

In these cases there was good evidence of the attack being epileptic in nature. Penfield and Jasper were able to produce similar tonic posturing of one or both extremities and the trunk by stimulation of the mesial frontal lobes (67). Kennedy described the case of a young woman whose seizures began with a "horrible indescribable feeling in her left foot or a stabbing feeling in her left hip" followed by tonic posturing (68). The EEG demonstrated a spike focus at the vertex. Pneumoencephalogram was consistent with an atrophic lesion of the right hemisphere. Vague sensory complaints and speech arrest can also be elicited, in addition to the posturing, by stimulation of the supplementary motor areas (69). Similar responses may also be obtained by stimulation of the cingulate gyrus (69,70). This evidence suggests that the seizures may arise in the supplementary motor area, or possibly in the cingulate gyrus (63).

ENCEPHALITIS

Three cases of prolonged (71,72), and one case of brief (7) paroxysmal dyskinesias were described complicating the course of encephalitis. The attacks began during the acute illness.

Diagnosis

Sterling's patients were both male, aged 12 and 56 (72). The attacks consisted of painful dystonic posturing lasting minutes to hours. They occurred several times daily. They eventually stopped without therapy.

A third patient developed normally until a "febrile illness" at 6 months of age, when he exhibited "running movements of the legs and jerking of the arms" (71). At age 9 this boy developed severe athetoid and dystonic posturing brought on by sudden movement, stress, or startle; they occurred four to five times daily, lasting 5 to 30 minutes.

The last patient had biopsy-proven enteroviral encephalitis (7). She was a 50-year-old woman with an immune deficiency syndrome. She experienced up to 100 daily episodes of painful left arm dystonic posturing with superimposed choreoathetosis. The movements were often precipitated by movement and lasted less than a minute. Numerous EEGs obtained during her episodes failed to reveal epileptic activity. An MRI demonstrated multiple intercranial lesions.

Treatment

Sterling's patients followed a self-limited course without treatment (72). The boy responded to benztropine mesylate. The woman had a reasonable response to carbamazepine and intrathecal infusion of immunoglobulins via an Ommaya reservoir.

Pathophysiology

The spasms are thought to relate to spread of ephaptic impulses, as seen in the painful episodes in MS (7).

RADICULOPATHY

A single case of a paroxysmal dyskinesia was reported secondary to an L4-5 disk (26). This case resembles some of the dyskinesias associated with reflex sympathetic dystrophy (73).

Diagnosis

A 62-year-old man experienced episodes of knife-life pain in the low back that radiated down the posterior right leg. Each episode was accompanied by "twitching and jumping of [the] leg and foot" (26). Episodes could be precipitated by leaning on his right side. Occasionally the examiner could induce one by applying pressure over the sciatic notch. They lasted several seconds and occurred up to 30 times a day.

Treatment

Phenytoin was initially helpful, but the episodes soon returned. He had several attacks the first week following operation and none since.

Pathophysiology

This case is intriguing because of its resemblance to the painful leg moving toes syndrome, trigeminal neuralgia, and hemifacial spasm.

HYPOPARATHYROIDISM

There are few documented cases of hypoparathyroidism presenting with paroxysmal dyskinesias. The movements were present from months (74) to years (75) prior to diagnosis. Two patients experienced brief episodes; the third had spells that lasted minutes to hours (76). A fourth case of possible hypoparathyroidism is suggested by the patient's response to therapy (77).

Diagnosis

The patients with brief spells had their attacks induced by either sustained movement (74,75) or sudden movement (74). The first patient's hands "felt tight" and he had a peculiar feeling in his legs (74). This was followed by his hands and face becoming stiff. Episodes lasted seconds and he had up to 20 a day. His examination revealed brisk reflexes and Chvostek's sign. Laboratory analysis demonstrated a low calcium level. The second patient also had a Chvostek's sign and low calcium level (75). His skull laminagram demonstrated calcification of the basal ganglia.

The patient with prolonged episodes had spells characterized by choreoathetotic movements with facial grimacing (77). Of note, because of her bizarre behavior, she was initially placed on a psychiatric ward. She had several cutaneous stigmata of hypocalcemia, including thick and cracked nails, thin and scanty hair, and hypoplastic teeth with enamel hypoplasia, in addition to areflexia. Her electrocardiogram demonstrated a prolonged QT interval. Skull radiographs and EEG were not helpful. Her serum calcium level was markedly reduced.

Treatment

Patient 1 failed to respond to phenobarbital prior to the diagnosis. All patients drastically improved with calciferol or vitamin D, and calcium. As mentioned above, a fourth patient responded to a combination of dihydrotachysterol, calciferol, and phenytoin. His serum calcium level was not given, but Chvostek's sign was absent.

Pathophysiology

Arden viewed his case as a form of tetany (74). Tabaee-Zadeh et al thought that the basal ganglionic calcifications suggested an extrapyramidal origin (75). This is further supported by another reported case of paroxysmal dyskinesias associated with basal ganglionic calcifications (78). This patient did not suffer from hypoparathyroidism. However, an epileptic etiology should not be discounted, as hypoparathyroidism is also an unusual cause of both focal (79) and generalized (77) seizures.

THYROTOXICOSIS

Tremor, chorea, and periodic paralysis are known movement and paroxysmal disorders associated with hyperthyroidism (80). Muscle spasms, exacerbated by movement and stress, were reported as a complication of hyperthyroidism (81). However, only a single case of paroxysmal choreoathetosis has been reported with hyperthyroidism (82).

Diagnosis

A 35-year-old woman had a history of generalized seizures since age 13. An episode of status epilepticus at age 26 left her with residual memory impairment. She developed myasthenia gravis at age 34. At the same time she began to have episodes of generalized tonic spasms. They were precipitated by raising her arms above her head, fatigue, and stress. They lasted 1 to 2 minutes, and occurred up to four times daily. The movement consisted of a progressive flexion of the left side with shaking of the hand, which would rapidly spread to the right side. The legs were tonically extended, and the face contorted.

Her examination revealed a low-grade fever, tachycardia, and diaphoresis. She had bilateral otosis, decreased eye movement, nasal speech, slight choreiform movements of the hands and feet; the vital capacity was reduced; CT and EEG were negative; and thyroid function tests revealed moderate hyperthyroidism.

Treatment

She did not respond to phenytoin, diphenhydramine, or benztropine. However, she improved with propranolol, propylthiouracil, and potassium iodide.

HYPOGLYCEMIA

A single case of paroxysmal choreoathetosis during hypoglycemia has been reported (83).

Diagnosis

Two episodes of generalized choreoathetosis were reported in a 45-year-old diabetic woman. Both episodes occurred while the patient was hypoglycemic with a serum glucose of 20 and 38 mg/dl. On both occasions, the movements lasted several minutes, being relieved by therapy; CT scans and other blood work were negative.

Treatment

Intravenous dextrose promptly terminated the choreoathetosis.

PSYCHOGENIC

Abnormal bizarre movements can be a perplexing diagnostic dilemma to the most experienced clinician. One patient mentioned above was admitted to a psychiatric unit despite obvious stigmata of hypoparathyroidism (77). Another patient with prolonged familial paroxysmal dyskinesias received 24 electroshock treatments during five psychiatric hospitalizations over 2 years (84). However, abnormal movements are a common expression of conversion disorders. Recently, a patient who abruptly developed twitching of his left foot and both hands was suspected of having a functional disorder because of his clinical course (85). Back-averaging EEG was used to identify the *Bereitschaftspotential*, or readiness potential, which correlates with normal willed movements. His abnormal movements were associated with the same electrophysiologic correlate as normal willed motion. The authors used this information to support a diagnosis of conversion disorder. To date, back-averaging has not been performed on patients with "organic" paroxysmal dyskinesias.

Lang (86) reported on 18 cases of psychogenic dystonia; 10 experienced paroxysmal worsening, often with a specific trigger point. The importance of recognition of psychogenic paroxysmal dyskinesia is underscored by Demirkiran and Jankovic (56), who reported that among 23 patients with established etiologies, psychogenic paroxysmal dyskinesia was the most frequent diagnosis. This diagnosis accounted for 9 cases, compared with only 2 with multiple sclerosis and 4 with cerebral vascular disease.

REFERENCES

1. Bennett DA, Goetz CG. Paroxysmal dyskinesias. In: Chokroverty S, ed. Movement disorders. Costa Mesa: PMA Publishing, 1990:287–307.
2. Spiller WG. Subcortical epilepsy. Brain 1927;50:171–187.
3. Matthews WB. Tonic seizures in disseminated sclerosis. Brain 1958;81:193–206.
4. Lance JW. Sporadic and familial varieties of tonic seizures. J Neurol Neurosurg Psychiatry 1963;26:51–59.
5. Twomey JA, Espir MLE. Paroxysmal symptoms as the first manifestations of multiple sclerosis. J Neurol Neurosurg Psychiatry 1980;43:296–304.
6. Berger JR, Sheremata WA, Melamed E. Paroxysmal dystonia as the initial manifestation of multiple sclerosis. Arch Neurol 1984;41:747–750.
7. Bennett DA, Goetz CG, Ristanovic RK, Morrell F. Paroxysmal dyskinesias: clinical and laboratory features in nine cases. Neurology 1987;37(suppl 1):262.
8. Joynt RJ, Green D. Tonic seizures as a manifestation of multiple sclerosis. Arch Neurol 1962;6:293–299.
9. Kuroiwa Y, Shibasaki H. Carbamazepine for tonic seizure in multiple sclerosis. Lancet 1967;i:116.
10. Ekbom KA, Westerberg CE, Osterman PO. Focal sensory-motor seizures of spinal origin. Lancet 1968;i:67.
11. Castaigne P, Cambier J, Brunet P. Spinal sensory-motor seizures. Lancet 1968;i:357.
12. Shibasaki H, Kuroiwa Y. Painful tonic seizure in multiple sclerosis. Arch Neurol 1974;30:47–51.
13. Castaigne P, Cambier J, Barbizet J, et al. Crisis sensitivomotrices d'origine spinale au cours d'une sclerose in plaques a poussee aigue terminale. Rev Neurol 1974;130:261–271.
14. Osterman PO, Westerberg CE. Paroxysmal attacks in multiple sclerosis. Brain 1975;98:189–202.
15. Matthews WB. Paroxysmal symptoms in multiple sclerosis. J Neurol Neurosurg Psychiatry 1975;38:617–623.
16. Voiculescu V, Apostol BP, Alecu C. Treatment with acetazolamide of brain-stem and spinal paroxysmal disturbances in multiple sclerosis. J Neurol Neurosurg Psychiatry 1975;38:191–193.
17. Toyokura Y, Sakuta M, Nakanishi T. Painful tonic seizures in multiple sclerosis. Neurology 1976;26:18–19.
18. Heath PD, Nightingale S. Clusters of tonic spasms as an initial manifestation of multiple sclerosis. Ann Neurol 1982;5:494–495.
19. Tranchant C, Bhatia KP, Marsden CD. Movement disorders in multiple sclerosis. Mov Disord 1995;4:418–423.
20. Sozzi G, Marotta P, Piatti L, et al. Paroxysmal sensor motor attacks due to a spinal cord lesion identified by MRI. J Neurol Neurosurg Psychiatry 1987;50:490–492.
21. Cherrick AA, Ellenberg M. Spinal cord seizures in transverse myelopathy: report of two cases. Arch Phys Med Rehabil 1986;67:129–131.
22. Espir MLE, Millac P. Treatment of paroxysmal disorder in multiple sclerosis with carbamazpine (Tegretol). J Neurol Neurosurg Psychiatry 1970;33:528–531.
23. Miley CE, Forster FM. Paroxysmal signs and symptoms in multiple sclerosis. Neurology 1974;24:458–461.
24. Perks WH, Lascelles RG. Paroxysmal brain stem dysfunctions presenting features of multiple sclerosis. Br Med J 1976;2:1176–1177.
25. Sethi KD, Hess DC, Huffnagle VH, Adams RJ. Acetazolamide treatment of paroxysmal dystonia in central demyelinating disease. Neurology 1992;42:919–921.
26. Nathanson M. Paroxysmal phenomena resembling seizures related to spinal cord and root pathology. J Mt Sinai Hosp 1962;29:147–151.
27. Burguera JA, Catalá J, Casanova B. Thalamic demyelination and paroxysmal dystonia in multiple sclerosis. Mov Disord 1991;4:379–383.
28. Lugaresi A, Uncini A, Gambi D. Basal ganglia involvement in multiple sclerosis with alternating side paroxysmal dystonia. J Neurol 1993;240:257–261.
29. Previdi P, Buzzi P. Carbamazepine for paroxysmal dystonia due to spinal cord lesions. Ital J Neurol Sci 1993;14:337.
30. Previdi P, Buzzi P. Paroxysmal dystonia due to a lesion of the cervical cord: case report. Ital J Neurol Sci 1992;13:521–523.
31. Adams RD, Victor M. Principles of neurology. New York: McGraw-Hill, 1985:665–698.
32. Hamano S-I, Tanaka Y, Nara T, et al. Paroxysmal kinesigenic choreoathetosis associated with prenatal brain damage. Acta Paediatr Jpn 1995;37:401–404.
33. Shintani S, Shiozawa Z, Tsunoda S, Shiigai T. Paroxysmal choreoathetosis precipitated by movement, sound and photic stimulation in a case of arteriovenous malformation in the parietal lobe. Clin Neurol Neurosurg 1991;93:237–239.
34. Gay CT, Ryan SG. Paroxysmal kinesigenic dystonia after methylphenidate administration. J Child Neurol 1994;9:45–46.
35. Parera IC, Gatto E, Fernández Pardal MM, et al. Complicaciones neurologicas por abuso de cocaina. Medicina (B Aires) 1994;54:35–41.
36. Gastaut H, Fischer-Williams M. Electro-encephalographic study of syncope. Its differentiation from epilepsy. Lancet 1957;ii:1018–1025.
37. Rogert J, Naquet R, Gastaut H, et al. Electroencephalographic and electrocardiographic manifestations provoked by carotid compression in cerebral circulatory insufficiencies. In: Meyer JS, Gastaut H, eds. Cerebral anoxia and the electroencephalogram. Springfield: Charles C Thomas, 1961:439–451.
38. Fisher CM. Concerning recurrent transient cerebral ischemic attacks. Can Med J 1962;87:1091–1099.

39. Caplan LR, Sergay S. Positional cerebral ischemia. J Neurol Neurosurg Psychiatry 1976;39:383–391.

40. Bennett DA, Fox JH. Paroxysmal dyskinesias secondary to cerebral vascular disease—reversal with aspirin. Clin Neuropharmacol 1989;12:215–216.

41. Riley TL, Friedman JM. Stroke, orthostatic hypotension and focal seizures. JAMA 1981;245:1243–1244.

42. Yanagihara T, Klass DW. Rhythmic involuntary movement as a manifestation of transient ischemic attacks. Trans Am Neurol Assoc 1981;106:46–48.

43. Margolin DI, Marsden CD. Episodic dyskinesias and transient cerebral ischemia. Neurology 1982;32:1379–1380.

44. Landi G, Perrone P, Guidotti M. Bilateral TIAs and unilateral seizures due to orthostatic hypotension. A case report. Ital J Neurol Sci 1983;2:239–241.

45. Ross Russell RW, Page NGR. Critical perfusion of brain and retina. Brain 1983;106:419–434.

46. Baquis GD, Pessin MS, Scott RM. Limb shaking—a carotid TIA. Stroke 1985;106:444–448.

47. Margolin DI. Transient dyskinesia and cerebral ischemia. Neurology 1985;35:445. Letter.

48. Stark SR. Transient dyskinesia and cerebral ischemia. Neurology 1985;35:445. Letter.

49. Yanagihara T, Piepgras DG, Klass DW. Repetitive involuntary movement associated with episodic cerebral ischemia. Ann Neurol 1985;18:244–250.

50. Lishman WA, Symonds CP, Whitty CWM, Willison RG. Seizures induced by movement. Brain 1962;85:93–108.

51. Hishikawa Y, Furuya E, Yamamoto J, Nan'no H. Dystonic seizures induced by movement. Arch Psychiatr Nervenkr 1973;217:113–138.

52. Robin JJ. Paroxysmal choreoathetosis following head injury. Ann Neurol 1977;2:447–448.

53. Drake ME, Jackson RD, Miller CA. Paroxysmal choreoathetosis after head injury. J Neurol Neurosurg Psychiatry 1986;49:837–843.

54. Richardson JC, Homes JC, Alimski MJ, et al. Kinesigenic choreoathetosis due to brain injury. Can J Neurol Sci 1987;14:626–628.

55. Biarry N, Singh B, Bahou Y, et al. Posttraumatic paroxysmal nocturnal hemidystonia. Mov Disord 1994;1:98–99.

56. Demirkiran M, Jankovic J. Paroxysmal dyskinesias: clinical features and classification. Ann Neurol 1995;38:571–579.

57. Rosen JA. Paroxysmal choreoathetosis. Associated with perinatal hypoxic encephalopathy. Arch Neurol 1965;11:385–387.

58. Kinast M, Erenberg G, Rothner AD. Paroxysmal choreoathetosis: report of five cases and review of the literature. Pediatrics 1980;65:74–77.

59. Donat JF, Wright FS. Episodic symptoms mistaken for seizures in the neurologically impaired child. Neurology 1990;40:156–157.

60. Andermann F, Ohtahara S, Andermann E, et al. Infantile hypotonia and paroxysmal dystonia: a variant of alternating hemiplegia of childhood? Mov Disord 1994;2:227–229.

61. Hart YM, Tampieri D, Andermann E, Andermann F. Alternating paroxysmal dystonia and hemiplegia in childhood as a symptom of basal ganglia disease. J Neurol Neurosurg Psychiatry 1995;59:453–454.

62. Bennett DA, Ristanovic RK, Morrell F, Goetz CG. Dystonic posturing in seizures. Neurology 1989;39:1270–1271.

63. Bokstein F, Neufeld MY, Nisipeanu P, Korczyn AD. Painful paroxysmal dystonia associated with focal epileptic activity. J Neurol Neurosurg Psychiatry 1995;58:257–258.

64. Falconer MA, Driver MV, Serafetinides EA. Seizures induced by movement: report of a case relieved by operation. J Neurol Neurosurg Psychiatry 1963;26:300–307.

65. Whitty CWM, Lishman WA, Fitzgibbon JP. Seizures induced by movement: a form of reflex epilepsy. Lancet 1964;i:1403–1406.

66. Kotagal P, Luders H, Morris HH, et al. Dystonic posturing in complex partial seizures of temporal lobe onset: a new lateralizing sign. Neurology 1989;39:196–201.

67. Penfield W, Jasper H. Epilepsy and the functional anatomy of the human brain. Boston: Little Brown, 1954:93–99.

68. Kennedy WA. Clinical and electroencephalographic aspects of epileptogenic lesions of the medial surface and superior border of the cerebral hemisphere. Brain 1959;82:147–161.

69. Van Buren JM, Fedio P. Functional representation on the medial aspect of the frontal lobes in man. J Neurosurg 1976;44:275–289.

70. Talairach J, Bancaud J, Geier S, et al. The cingulate gyrus and human behavior. Electroencephalogr Clin Neurophysiol 1973;34:45–52.

71. Mushet GR, Dreifues FE. Paroxysmal dyskinesia: a case responsive to benztropine mesylate. Arch Dis Child 1967;42:654–656.

72. Sterling W. Le type spasmodique tetanoide et tetaniforme de l'encephalite epidemique remarque sur l'epilepsie "extrapyramidale." Rev Neurol 1924;2:484–492.

73. Schwartzman RJ, Kerrigan J. The movement disorder of reflex sympathetic dystrophy. Neurology 1990;40:57–61.

74. Arden F. Idiopathic hypoparathyroidism. Med J Aust 1953;2:217–219.

75. Tabaee-Zadeh MJ, Frame B, Kapphahn K. Kinesigenic choreoathetosis and idiopathic hypoparathyroidism. N Engl J Med 1972;286:762–763.

76. Soffer D, Licht A, Yaar I, Abramsky O. Paroxysmal choreoathetosis as a presenting symptom in idiopathic hypoparathyroidism. J Neurol Neurosurg Psychiatry 1977;40:692–694.

77. Cox RE. Hypoparathyroidism: an unusual cause of seizures. Ann Emerg Med 1983;12:314–315.

78. Micheli F, Pardal MMF, Parera IC, Giannaula R. Sporadic paroxysmal dystonic choreoathetosis associated with basal ganglia calcification. Ann Neurol 1986;20:750.

79. Willison RG, Whitty CWM. Parathyroid deficiency presenting as epilepsy. Br Med J 1957;1:802–803.

80. Swanson JW, Kelly JJ, McConahey WM. Neurologic aspects of thyroid dysfunction. Mayo Clin Proc 1981;56:504–512.

81. Van Geusau RBA, Howeler DH. Reversible muscle spasms in hyperthyroidism. J Neurol Neurosurg Psychiatry 1986;49:1322–1323.

82. Fishbeck KH, Layzer RB. Paroxysmal choreoathetosis associated with thyrotoxicosis. Ann Neurol 1979;6:453–454.

83. Newman RP, Kinekel WR. Paroxysmal choreoathetosis due to hypoglycemia. Arch Neurol 1984;41:341–342.

84. Walker ES. Familial paroxysmal dystonic choreoathetosis: a neurologic disorder simulating psychiatric illness. Johns Hopkins Med J 1981;148:108–113.

85. Toro C, Torres F. Electrophysiologic correlates of a paroxysmal movement disorder. Ann Neurol 1986;20:731–734.

86. Lang AE. Psychogenic dystonia: a review of 18 cases. Can J Neurol Sci 1995;22:136–143.

Painful Legs and Moving Toes

Christopher G. Goetz   Aron S. Buchman

INTRODUCTION

"Painful legs and moving toes" (PLMT) is a clinical syndrome first described in detail by Spillane et al in 1971 (1). It has since been described by multiple authors and is usually associated with lesions of the peripheral nervous system. Occasionally, no etiologic factor has been identified, and cases have been presented that vaguely suggested central system abnormalities. Electrophysiologic examinations have shown a wide variety of patterns, and treatment has generally been ineffective.

CLINICAL DESCRIPTION

The syndrome includes sensory and motor phenomena, and may involve one or both lower extremities (Table 75.1). The sensory problem is a discomfort or pain that may range from being mildly irritating to excrutiatingly severe. In most cases, it has the character of a constant, deep, boring pain. Occasionally, patients will describe it as fiery or crushing, but it does not have the electric or shooting sensation of a radicular syndrome. The pain is not confined to specific dermatomes, myotomes, or peripheral nerve distributions, nor is it predominant in either flexor or extensor muscle groups. In patients who have had previous sciatic pain, the sensation of PLMT is usually described as quite unlike the former. Furthermore, the pain is distinctive in that it is not affected by coughing, Valsalva maneuvers, or bending (1). In some cases the description of the pain is similar to the pain described with causalgia.

No patients have been reported with PLMT with vasomotor, sudomotor, subcutaneous, or cutaneous features suggestive of reflex sympathetic dystrophy (RSD). Four of 20 patients in a recent series had radiological evidence of Sudeck's osteoporosis (2). Various abnormal movements have been reported to be associated with reflex sympathetic dystrophy (3). It is not known why following similar trauma one person develops abnormal movements and reflex sympathetic dystrophy and another develops PLMT. It is not clear whether patients with "painless moving toes" represent variants of PLMT (4).

The movements seen in this syndrome show less variety than the sensory complaints and are usually highly characteristic. They are generally isolated to the toes but occasionally extend into the foot. Rarely, they can be more proximal and involve the thigh muscles (5). However, in all reported cases reviewed, toes are the predominant area of involvement, and if movements are seen elsewhere in the lower extremities, they are not marked in severity. The movements themselves consist of flexion and extension and adduction and abduction of the phalanges. They cause a continual "sinuous clawing and restraightening, fanning and circular movements of the toes" (1). In almost all cases, the movements are continuous while the patient is awake, although there may be lapses of seconds or minutes when the foot is quiet. Unlike chorea, these movements are rather stereotypic in appearance and continue to repeat themselves incessantly. In cases where the movements quietly abate for periods of time, an attempt to imitate the movement voluntarily cannot even approximate the involuntary movement. While there may be mild control of the movements with effort, once the patient is distracted, the movements quickly recur. Only rarely do the movements persist during sleep (6). Unlike akathisia, the patient feels no relief from the moving and instead fruitlessly longs to have the toes quiet. Although it is described as a lower extremity syndrome, extension to the upper extremities can occur (6). In one case of a brachial plexus lesion associated with breast carcinoma and radiotherapy, a similar syndrome of painful arm and moving fingers developed (7). Recently there have

Table 75.1   Clinical Features of PLMT*

Male/female ratio: 16 : 34	
Average age of onset: 58.8 years (range, 28–80)	
Associated findings in PLMT (number of cases)	
Radiculopathy	16
Peripheral neuropathy	11
Entrapment neuropathy (tarsal tunnel syndrome)	1
Trauma	
Peripheral	11
Cauda equina	2
Herpes zoster	2
Sacral cyst	1
Unknown	6

* Features of the 50 patients reported in references (5,6,12–16).

been reports of patients with abnormal movements that were similar to those described in PLMT, but pain was lacking (2,4).

In the original description of these movements, an attempt was made to distinguish whether the pain and involuntary movements coincided temporally with one another both in their original development and their daily manifestations. In almost all cases, pain is remembered by patients to have originally preceded the involuntary movements. Furthermore, in cases where sympathetic blockade was associated with temporary abatement of symptoms, pain could often be blocked prior to the cessation of movements. Such observations have led some investigators to suggest that the origin of the disorder involves sensory systems primarily, with the movements as a consequence of distorted sensory inputs. Nathan (5) suggested that the syndrome's origin could be in the posterior roots, as large coordinated movements of the limbs similar to the movements of moving toes can occur when the posterior lumbar or cervical roots are surgically stimulated. The fact that patients can develop this syndrome after herpes zoster further supported his notion. Curiously, however, after sympathetic blockade, movements often recur prior to the resumption of any pain.

Peripheral nerve injury and stimulation have been shown to change the patterns of central neuronal activity. After peripheral nerve trauma, changes have been observed in the dorsal horn of the spinal cord, dorsal column nuclei, and ventral thalamus, as well as the sensory cortex. Persistent patterns of peripheral stimulation can also alter the neuronal activity of the cortex (8–11). Since many PLMT cases occur following various injuries or trauma to various components of the peripheral nervous system, it has been suggested that PLMT develops following peripheral nerve injury with the concomitant change in central sensory and motor pathways. Further studies are necessary to determine whether PLMT, movement disorders associated with peripheral trauma, and

reflex sympathetic dystrophy share common underlying pathophysiologic mechanisms.

The development of the syndrome is slow and indolent. Factors that aggravate the pain are typically motor activities involving the lower limbs, specifically walking. Factors that may relieve the pain include immersion of the lower body into hot or cold water and rest, although often there is nothing but sleep that provides the patient with respite.

ASSOCIATED NEUROLOGIC FINDINGS AND PAST HISTORY

In many cases, the objective neurologic examination is normal, except for the obvious abnormal involuntary movements. There is no evidence of sympathetic dysfunction in the form of altered temperature, skin turgor, or vasodilatation. A past history of lumbago or sciatic nerve irritation has been present in approximately half the reported cases. In such cases, low back or sciatic notch tenderness can sometimes be found with hypothesia along the posterior thigh and lateral leg. Polyradiculopathies have also accompanied some cases of the syndrome (5,6), and in these instances, the neurologic examination shows the expected sensory, motor, and tendon reflex changes of such syndromes as they occur in any other context. In cases of polyradiculopathy, altered sensation in specific dermatomes with associated weakness in muscles supplied by the roots involved will occur along with depressed knee or ankle jerks if L2-4 or S1 are involved, respectively. When PLMT occurs in the context of polyneuropathy, bilateral distal hypothesia is detected along with mild weakness of distal muscles and depressed ankle jerks.

The role of trauma in the genesis of this disorder has been commented on by several authors and studied by Schott (12). The trauma is minor and usually involves seemingly inconsequential injury to the lower leg, foot, or back. Examples would include bruising with tenderness, sprains, and soft tissue injuries. Other forms of trauma have been compressive root lesions by cysts, cauda equina lesions, local surgery, and herpes zoster infection involving the lower extremities. The role of surgery per se in patients who have had chronic lumbar back disease or preexisting bony deformity is arguable. The time course between trauma and the first development of the syndrome of PLMT has been months, so that direct relationships to acute trauma are difficult to establish.

DIAGNOSTIC EVALUATION

In an attempt to define the anatomic level of dysfunction in the PLMT syndrome, investigators have performed a variety of diagnostic tests with a wide gamut of reported findings (13,14). The disparity in results from electrophysiologic studies performed in published studies may in part stem from the different neurologic problems that can result in PLMT.

A study of six patients by Schoenen et al (15) reported two distinct electromyographic (EMG) patterns. The first pattern was simple and erratic, consisting of spontaneous repetitive single-unit discharges that occurred in an unpredictable fashion, most often synchronously in antagonistic muscles with an irregular frequency. The second pattern was more complex and consisted of arrhythmic bursts of longer duration and higher amplitude (1–3 versus 0.1 mV and 160–500 versus 10–80 ms). These bursts showed alternating antagonistic muscle involvement and were of a slower frequency compared with the simple bursts (1.5–3 Hz versus 4–6 Hz).

Posterior tibial nerve blockade was used to localize the origin of involuntary movements. The successful blockade of movement with this anesthetic maneuver implied that the site of origin was proximal to the site of blockade. Conversely, persistence of movements following nerve block suggested that the site of movement generation was distal to the point of nerve anesthesia.

In two patients with the complex alternating pattern, posterior tibial nerve blockade abolished the abnormal discharges. Observing that such patients also had evidence of dyskinesias in other body parts besides the legs (orofacial, truncal, or diaphragmatic), the authors concluded that this pattern "favored a central disorder . . . implying a more general disturbance of sensorimotor control" (15, p. 1112). The authors, however, did not perform additional tests to define the proposed central lesion.

In spite of this convenient classification, however, careful reading of this study reveals that there did not seem to be a clear correlation between the types of EMG patterns recorded (simple erratic versus complex alternating) and the patients' clinical features. One patient with chronic back pain had the simple erratic pattern and was felt to represent a peripheral lesion, but his movements were ameliorated with a peripheral nerve block and he had facial dyskinesias. These features were used in two other patients to suggest a more central lesion.

In this study, however, the response to nerve blockade did seem to correlate with the associated clinical complaints. Patients with radicular complaints (numbers 1, 4, and 5) exhibited prompt blockade of their involuntary movements with posterior tibial nerve block, whereas those with clinical signs of peripheral neuropathy (numbers 2 and 3) did not. The study demonstrates the potential utility of sequential motor unit blockade to delineate the site of origin of the abnormal involuntary movements in this heterogenous syndrome; with further refinement, this technique could help delineate more subgroups than proposed so far.

Barnett et al (13) performed detailed EMG studies on two patients with PLMT syndrome in association with radicular lesions at L5-S1. Absent H reflex was seen in both patients, and F wave prolongation occurred in one. Dener-

vation in the distribution of the S1-innervated muscles and of the paraspinal muscles at L5-S1 levels was seen in both. These findings suggested a proximal root origin of the problem in these patients. The investigators further studied the muscular genesis of the involuntary movements and, through samplings of different foot muscles, determined that the movements in their patients originated in the abductor digiti quinti. They attempted to block movements and pain by a number of injection maneuvers: lower lumbar sympathetic ganglia blockade did not change the symptoms; S1 radicular block produced transient motor and sensory improvement; and posterior, but not anterior, tibial nerve block provided temporary relief. Although these studies suggest that a proximal root lesion can cause the syndrome of PLMT, it did not determine whether sensory or motor abnormalities are of primary pathogenic significance.

The evolution of the motor disorder detected on EMG relative to the symptom of pain was studied in one patient by Nathan (5). He examined the subject when he presented with unexplained deep pain in the leg only; the EMG examination was normal. Over months, however, spontaneous motor unit firing increased and at 3 years, when involuntary movements were visible, clear spontaneous motor units of short and long flexors and extensors, adductors and abductors of the toes fired synchronously with the movements.

Review of the literature suggests that electrophysiologic testing in patients with PLMT has not definitively clarified the site(s) of origin of these involuntary movements or shed direct light on their pathophysiology. We propose the following testing scheme that would allow for comparison between individual reports and facilitate an understanding of the unifying and distinguishing features of the various forms of this syndrome (Table 75.2).

Table 75.2 Electrophysiologic Evaluation of PLMT

Evaluate for associated neurologic findings
    Motor nerve conduction studies
    Sensory nerve conduction studies
    Paraspinal EMG
    Appropriate peripheral extremity muscles
    H reflexes
    F responses
    Dermatomal somatosensory evoked potentials
    Somatosensory evoked responses
EMG pattern of involuntary movements using surface or needle electrodes
    Duration
    Frequency
    Amplitude
    Sequence of muscle activation
Sequential blockade of the motor unit
    Nerve blockade
    Neuromuscular junction blockade
    Spinal or general anesthesia

We suggest that there are three steps necessary for adequate evaluation of patients with PLMT. First, the patient must be screened for the most common causes of these involuntary movements (see Table 75.1). A careful neurologic history and examination will be pivotal to this step. Second, an electrophysiologic description of the pattern of movements should be established by the use of surface or needle electrodes. Finally, sequential blockade of the motor unit should be utilized to allow for more accurate localization of the site or origin of the movements.

As with all electrophysiologic evaluations, testing must be individualized, based on the patient's complaint and clinical examination. Testing should evaluate for the presence of radiculopathy and neuropathy, as these are the two common abnormalities associated with this syndrome. Peripheral motor and sensory conduction studies should be performed in all patients. In patients with a history of peripheral trauma, more extensive nerve conduction studies will be necessary for evaluation of possible mononeuropathy. Screening for radiculopathy includes evaluation of paraspinal and appropriate extremity muscles as well as H reflexes and F responses as indicators of proximal nerve or root dysfunction. Somatosensory potentials and/or dermatomal somatosensory evoked potentials should be considered when the putative lesion is radicular or within the central nervous system. Following these studies, surface or needle recordings should focus on the sequence of muscle activation in the involuntary movements. The duration, frequency, amplitude, and relationship of agonist to antagonist muscles should be clarified.

Sequential blockade of different levels of the motor unit can then be performed to localize the level of origin or organization of the involuntary movements. The first and simplest blockade is the peripheral innervating nerve. Persistence of movements would imply that the site of generation is distal to the site of the block. Neuromuscular blockade with curare can then be performed to allow further localization to the distal nerve segment or muscle cells below the site of the block. If the initial nerve block abolishes the movements, then more proximal blockade is required to define the site of origin of the movements. Proximal nerve block, spinal block, and general anesthesia would be the logical sequence of progressive blockade.

Although PLMT is probably a heterogenous disorder, standardization of testing will allow a more accurate estimation of its various causes, localization of its site(s) of origin, and comparison between individual studies. Only after the above described minimal testing can one begin to design studies to elucidate the more fundamental question of the pathophysiology of the syndrome in its different forms.

TREATMENT

Sympathetic block by local anesthesia has been associated with temporary abolition of pain and movements. The improvement can occur within minutes or can persist for days after the injections. The procedure described by Spillane et al (1) involved 40 mg of bupivacaine hydrochloride 0.25% to block the lumbar sympathetic chain. The relief afforded by such injections is temporary. Sympathectomies or phenol injections, however, have not been consistently associated with long-term improvement. Although improvement can occur for weeks, a slow return is usually seen in the reported cases. Treatment with anticonvulsants, specifically, phenytoin and carbamazepine; baclofen; and antidepressants has not met with consistent success. In isolated cases where a putative structural etiology can be defined, as in Nathan's case of a sacral cyst compressing the posterior spinal roots, improvement can follow decompression.

REFERENCES

1. Spillane JD, Nathan PW, Kelly RE, Marsden CD. Painful legs and moving toes. Brain 1971;94:541–556.
2. Dressler D, Thompson PD, Gledhill RF, Marsden CD. The syndrome of painful legs and moving toes. Mov Disord 1994;9:13–21.
3. Schwartzman RJ, Kerrigan J. The movement disorder of reflex sympathetic dystrophy. Neurology 1990;40:57–61.
4. Walters AS, Hening WA, Shah SK, Chokroberty S. Painless legs and moving toes: a syndrome related to painful legs and moving toes? Mov Disord 1993;8:377–379.
5. Nathan PW. "Painful legs and moving toes": evidence on the site of lesion. J Neurol Neurosurg Psychiatry 1978;41:934–939.
6. Montagna P, Cirignotta F, Sacquegna T, et al. "Painful legs and moving toes" associated with polyneuropathy. J Neurol Neurosurg Psychiatry 1983;46:399–403.
7. Verhagen WIM, Horstink MWIM, Notermans SLH. Painful arm and moving fingers. J Neurol Neurosurg Psychiatry 1985;48:384–389.
8. Wall PD, Devor M. Consequences of peripheral nerve damage in the spinal cord and in neighbouring intact peripheral nerves. In: Culp WJ, Ochoa J, eds. Abnormal nerves and muscles as impulse generators. Oxford: Oxford University Press, 1982:588–603.
9. DeCaballos ML, Baker M, Rose J, et al. Do enkephalins in basal ganglia mediate a physiological rest mechanism? Mov Disord 1986;1:223–233.
10. Kass JH, Merzenich MM, Killackey HP. The reorganization of sensory cortex following peripheral nerve damage in adult and developing mammals. Ann Rev Neurosci 1983;6:325–356.
11. Wang X, Merzenich MM, Sameshima K, Jenkins WM. Remodeling of hand representation in adult cortex determined by timing of tactile stimulation. Science 1995;378:71–75.
12. Schott GD. "Painful legs and moving toes": the role of trauma. J Neurol Neurosurg Psychiatry 1981;44:344–346.
13. Barnett RE, Singh N, Fahn S. The syndrome of painful legs and moving toes. Neurology 1981;31:79.
14. Wulff CH. Painful legs and moving toes. Acta Neurol Scand 1982;66:283–287.
15. Schoenen J, Gonce M, Delwaide PJ. Painful legs and moving toes: a syndrome with different pysiopathologic mechanisms. Neurology 1984;34:1108–1112.
16. Pla MER, Dillingham TR, Spellman NT, et al. Painful legs and moving toes associated with tarsal tunnel syndrome and accessory soleus muscle. Mov Disord 1996;11:82–86.

Tremor and Dystonia

Tremor: An Overview

Robert R. Young

INTRODUCTION

Tremors, among the simpler and most common movement disorders, may involve the face, voice, neck, upper or lower extremities. They are rhythmic, involuntary, and wax and wane in amplitude from second to second but, in any one patient, the frequency does not change. The term tremor, like weakness, is a symptom or sign, not a specific illness; tremors have a number of different causes and are parts of unrelated syndromes. Some tremors are the only symptom of a disorder; others are part of multisymptom disorders. Therapies for tremor therefore vary depending on the type of tremor and the underlying causative or associated disorder. Simple quantitative techniques are available to measure tremor and are essential for clinical studies of its progress or to monitor its response to therapy (1).

ENHANCED PHYSIOLOGIC TREMORS

Any contraction of muscle, voluntary or otherwise, is accompanied by a tremor due to unfused contractions of muscle fibers whose motor units are being recruited at subtetanic rates and to consequent vibrations of muscle. These mechanical perturbations of a second-order (spring-mass) system, consisting of the muscle and body parts to which it is attached, cause the system to oscillate at its natural frequency (2). That frequency is proportional to the stiffness of the muscle and to the inverse of the mass of the system: fingers extended by strong cocontraction of their extensors and flexors oscillate at a much higher frequency than the whole leg lifted off the bed by weak contraction of the hip flexors. These tremors are ubiquitous but are usually very small; an accelerometer or similar mechanical amplifier is needed to demonstrate them. They are called physiologic tremor.

When such muscle contractions are maintained for a few moments or, for a variety of other reasons listed below, the amplitude of this tremor increases, it becomes visible to the naked eye. Such symptomatic tremors are called enhanced physiologic tremors (3) and are experienced from time to time by all normal subjects and by most patients with neurologic or other conditions. Only persons without stretch reflexes (see below) because of neuropathies or myelopathies cannot develop enhanced physiologic tremor.

Most often, enhanced physiologic tremors are caused by a hyperadrenergic state. Anxiety, fear, stage fright, and serious competition in sports or battle are the usual precipitants. Sometimes getting "psyched up" or getting "the adrenalin flowing" is useful for a successful outcome, even though enhanced physiologic tremor is an unwanted accompaniment. At other times that appears not to be the case. For example, it has been demonstrated that concert musicians play better after taking a single dose of propranolol to block the tremor associated with stage fright, a practice that has become widespread (4). A number of widely used medications such as bronchodilators and lithium also produce enhanced physiologic tremor (1). The pathophysiology of these tremors is complex and only partially understood; adrenergically mediated changes in mechanical properties of skeletal muscle (contraction and half-relaxation times, for example) alter the timing of muscle spindle afferent input from the contracting muscle to already active spinal motor neurons. This tends to synchronize their discharges, which produces bursts of electromyographic (EMG) activity and rhythmic contractions of muscle (i.e., tremor). Because these mechanisms operate via the stretch reflex arc, patients with neuropathies that interfere with operation of the stretch reflex (absent tendon jerks) cannot develop enhanced physiologic tremor. In addition to emotional/affective/psychic causes for hyperadrenergic states (mediated presumably through increased activity of the locus coeruleus) that produce enhanced physiologic tremor, the following are a few other causes: thyroid hormone excess, amphetamines, β_2 agonists (terbutaline, isoproterenol, etc.), fatigue, hypoglycemia, withdrawal syndromes, L-dopa, and xanthines such as caffeine in coffee and soft drinks. In some circumstances, tremors such as these can be alleviated by treatment of the underlying disorder, reduction of the causative medication, or addition of β adrenergic blocking agents; in other circumstances, none of the above are appropriate and the patient learns to live with the tremor.

Because tremors are additive, enhanced physiologic tremor is often more troublesome in patients who are prone to some other tremor than in the general population. For example, patients with mild essential-familial tremor or Parkinson's disease (PD) may have little tremor except when anxious or when being treated for asthma. A patient with PD whose tremor is only bothersome when he or she gives a lecture or speaks on television should be treated for enhanced physiologic tremor (e.g., 40 mg propranolol by mouth 45 minutes before going on stage) and should not have his or her L-dopa increased.

ESSENTIAL-FAMILIAL TREMOR

Like enhanced physiologic tremor, this is an action tremor. That is, patients with essential-familial tremor are completely tremor free when muscles or limbs are at rest. When the arms are held outstretched against gravity, however, or when the patient tries to drink from a cup, write, and so on, the tremor is bothersome. Essential-familial tremor and enhanced physiologic tremor look much alike, but a careful history will differentiate them. The latter occurs, usually for short periods of time, under the circumstances outlined above, whereas the former is present at all times, however relaxed the person feels. Essential-familial tremor, the most common of the movement disorders, is inherited more than 50% of the time. It can occur at any age but is rare in children; there are peaks of occurrence in the second and sixth decades. Naturally it becomes more prevalent in later life. The same tremor is sometimes called senile if it develops after age 65; if it is not obviously familial, it is called essential. Apart from these historical features, there is no difference between essential, familial, and senile tremor. It appears to be worsened temporarily by anxiety or other causes of enhanced physiologic tremor, which then becomes added to it; it is temporarily improved by small amounts of oral alcohol and can be treated by primidone (25 or 50 mg two or three times a day) or propranolol (40 mg three or four times a day) with success about three-quarters of the time. Propranolol and other peripheral β adrenergic blockers produce an acute and short-lived reduction in enhanced physiologic tremor by action on β_2 adrenergic structures within the limb itself, but it is propranolol's central nervous system (CNS) action (not shared with all β blockers) that produces a chronic, long-lived reduction in essential-

familial tremor (5). Stereotaxic neurosurgery (vim thalamotomy) results in permanent cure of this tremor (as well as that seen with PD) in the limbs contralateral to the surgical lesion (6). Deep brain stimulation (DBS) with electrodes chronically implanted in the vim thalamus also reduces or eliminates these tremors (7). Patients with essential-familial tremor have an increased incidence of dystonia and PD. For an excellent review of clinical aspects of essential-familial tremor, see Lou and Jankovic (8).

TREMORS SEEN WITH PD

Most characteristic of PD is a slow, distal pill-rolling tremor seen when the patient is sitting still. It is attenuated, sometimes only briefly, when the patient uses the limb. Although termed tremor at rest, it is absent when the patient is truly at rest, for example, lying without postural contraction in axial and limb girdle muscles. It is not clinically obvious in all patients with PD, is primarily an embarrassment rather than a handicap, and is difficult to treat medically. Any of the medications for PD—L-dopa, dopamine agonists, or the older centrally acting anticholinergics—may reduce tremor at rest but are not as effective at that as at treating bradykinesia (1).

The pathophysiology of tremor at rest or of essential-familial tremor is not understood. Both arise from malfunctions within the CNS, are cured by ventrolateral thalamotomy, and do not require stretch reflex arcs to be operative. Both can occur in the same patient. In fact, evidence exists to support the clinical observation that essential-familial tremor is more common in PD than one would expect by chance. Enhanced physiologic tremor also occurs in patients with PD. There are one or two other tremors seen with PD, including a tremor only when the patient tries to write. It is obvious, therefore, that not all the tremors seen in patients with PD are Parkinson tremors if, by that term, one means the tremor at rest. Furthermore, each of these tremors responds to a mode of therapy different from the other.

MISCELLANEOUS TREMORS

Anxious patients sometimes describe an internal feeling of tremulousness that is not associated with visible or measurable tremor of the types noted above. Whether this is related somehow to enhanced physiologic tremor is unclear but, clinically, one should reserve judgment as well as antitremor (as opposed to anxiolytic) therapy unless a tremor can be seen. For a discussion of factitious or psychogenic tremors, see Chapter 100.

Certain patients produce tremors for reasons of secondary gain, and others produce tremors for reasons that are not clear. Whether these should be termed factitious, voluntary, or psychogenic tremors is continually debated. Such tremors may be difficult to categorize and to differentiate from tremors mentioned above, but often they can be seen, with long-term observation of the patient, to be erratic in nature (for example, they may disappear when the patient thinks no one is looking). The clinical setting also differs from that seen with classic tremors.

Myoclonus (see Chapter 66), defined as quick, lightning-like jerky movements of parts of muscles, parts of limbs, or the whole body, may appear tremulous at times. Myoclonus may be due to brief contractions of muscles (positive myoclonus) or to equally brief relaxation of tonically contracting muscles (negative myoclonus, also termed asterixis). Asterixis is most often the result of a wide variety of metabolic encephalopathies, including reactions to general anesthesia and to almost every anticonvulsant. In addition to the gross lapses of posture reflected in the flaps of a dorsiflexed hand or brief, lightning-like relaxations of any tonically contracting muscle, asterixis often has a tremulous quality due to recurrent, brief, partial relaxations of active muscles. These relaxations, large or small, are associated with brief periods of silence in the ongoing EMG, which can be used to differentiate asterixis from true tremors. The EMG silent periods recur irregularly, and asterixis is visibly less rhythmic or regular than true tremor. However, because it occurs very frequently in a general hospital, asterixis accounts for most of the so-called tremors seen on an inpatient movement disorder consultation service (9).

Patients with disorders of the cerebellar system—whether they are due to lesions of the spinocerebellar inflow pathways, of the cerebellum itself, or of cerebellar efferent tracts—demonstrate a number of motor abnormalities (see Chapter 39), including a slow, rhythmic ataxia or dysmetria. It is usually demonstrated by increasing side-to-side oscillations of the arm near the end points of finger-nose-finger testing, but it may also occur with postural contractions of axial musculature. The latter rhythmic oscillations of neck and head posture and proximal arms are particularly prominent with lesions of cerebellar outflow pathways in the midbrain and have been called rubral tremor. The oscillations on finger-nose-finger testing, writing, drinking, and so on are most often seen with spinocerebellar degenerations of the Friedreich type in which there is usually little visible derangement of the cerebellum itself. They have been called intention tremor. Although these rhythmic cerebellar dysmetrias are often classified with tremors, they deserve a separate categorization because of their peculiar neuropathology, their predominantly proximal nature, and the fact that they are slower and less regular than the action tremors or tremor at rest mentioned above.

Patients with Wilson's disease and with other rare basal ganglia degenerations may, in addition to various movement disorders, have tremor or ataxic dysmetria. In the elderly, a tremor of the jaw may appear that looks like that seen with PD but which is unresponsive to L-dopa. It is difficult to categorize this and other unusual tremors. Rather than review long lists of tremors seen with uncommon neurologic conditions, attention is more profitably focused on

these movement disorders as syndromes which themselves sometimes include movements that resemble tremor. This chapter emphasizes common situations in which tremor is the major (or sometimes the only) movement disorder.

Patients with neuropathies can, on rare occasion, have a superimposed tremor. Most often this is simply due to the simultaneous inheritance of essential-familial tremor and a familial neuropathy of the Charcot-Marie-Tooth type (1). In other patients with neuropathic sensory loss (particularly proprioception), an irregular, slow sensory ataxia of the fingers may be seen with arms outstretched and eyes closed. These movements look more like choreoathetosis than tremor, but use of the limbs even with eyes open is clumsy, awkward, and occasionally ataxic. Very rarely, patients with chronic relapsing, steroid-sensitive dys-γ-globulinemic polyneuropathies have a true action tremor, the amplitude of which waxes and wanes in direct proportion to the severity of the neuropathy (1).

In muscles with considerable weakness due to denervation, action fasciculations may be seen. These are visible twitches during contraction of the few remaining, often enlarged, motor units. Clonus, seen with hyperreflexia, is rhythmic and involuntary, fulfilling the definition of tremor, but its clinical context differentiates it from tremor. The same is true for shivering that is tremulous.

SUMMARY

Several types of tremor are common, easily recognizable, and responsive to an etiology-specific therapy. Others are uncommon, difficult to diagnose, and impossible to treat. One must not be satisfied simply to recognize that a tremor is present or to assume a patient must have PD because a tremor is present. In neuropsychiatric practice, tremors are often seen, and although not all require therapy, attempts should be made to account for the presence of the tremor.

REFERENCES

1. Young RR. Tremor. In: Asbury AK, McKhann GM, McDonald WI, eds. Diseases of the nervous system. 2nd ed. Philadelphia: WB Saunders, 1992:353–367.
2. Young RR, Wiegner AW. Tremor. In: Swash M, Kennard C, eds. Scientific basis of clinical neurology. Edinburgh: Churchill Livingstone, 1985:116–132.
3. Young RR, Hagbarth KE. Physiological tremor enhanced by manoeuvres affecting the segmental stretch reflex. J Neurol Neurosurg Psychiatry 1980;43:248–256.
4. Brantigan CO, Brantigan TA, Joseph N. Effect of beta blockade and beta stimulation on stage fright. Am J Med 1982;72:88–94.
5. Young RR. Essential-familial tremor. In: Johnson RT, Griffin JW, eds. Current therapy in neurologic disease. 5th ed. St. Louis: Mosby, 1997:294–296.
6. Mohadjer M, Goerke H, Milios E, et al. Long-term results of stereotaxy in the treatment of essential tremor. Stereotact Funct Neurosurg 1990;54:125–129.
7. Benabid AL, Pollak P, Gao D, et al. Chronic electrical stimulation of the ventralis intermedius nucleus of the thalamus as a treatment of movement disorders. J Neurosurg 1996;84:203–214.
8. Lou JS, Jankovic J. Essential tremor: clinical correlates in 350 patients. Neurology 1991;41:234–238.
9. Young RR, Shahani BT. Asterixis—one type of negative myoclonus. In: Fahn S, Marsden CD, van Woert M, eds. Myoclonus. New York: Raven, 1986:137–156.

Primary Torsion Dystonia

Stanley Fahn

INTRODUCTION

Dystonia is a syndrome of sustained muscle contractions, frequently causing twisting and repetitive movements or abnormal postures (1–3). It is classified by etiology (primary, dystonia-plus, secondary, or heredodegenerative), by age at onset (childhood, adolescent, or adult onset), and by distribution of involvement of body parts (focal, segmental, generalized, hemidystonia). This chapter will review briefly the clinical features of idiopathic torsion dystonia. The reader is referred to the reviews by Fahn et al (2), Jankovic and Fahn (3), and Calne and Lang (4) for details of symptomatic dystonias.

The term dystonia was coined in 1911 by Oppenheim (5) to emphasize the variability of muscle tone and the ultimate postural deformities that develop with time. Flatau and Sterling (6), later in 1911, emphasized torsion spasms as the major clinical feature and suggested that the name for the disorder should be progressive torsion spasm. They also pointed out that it is likely an inherited disease. Although the term dystonia has been widely accepted as the name of the disorder, the views of Flatau and Sterling are part of the current concepts of the disease.

PHENOMENOLOGY OF DYSTONIC MOVEMENTS

The abnormal movements making up dystonia are diverse, with a wide range in speed, amplitude, repetitiveness, torsion, forcefulness, distribution in the body, and relationship to rest or voluntary activity.

The first step toward diagnosis of dystonia is to recognize the presence of dystonic movements. Once this recognition is made, the etiology is then determined, specifically,

whether the disorder is 1) primary (pure dystonia); 2) with features of parkinsonism or myoclonus (dystonia-plus); 3) secondary; or 4) heredodegenerative (1).

The pattern of abnormal dystonic movements is so highly variable (7) that it is important to recognize the most cardinal features of the contractions, namely, that they are sustained at the height of the movement, that the movements tend to be twisting and repetitive, and that they involve the same muscle groups continually. The speed of dystonic movements varies from slow to rapid. The speed can be so fast that they have the appearance of repetitive myoclonic jerking. The term myoclonic dystonia has been applied to such types of dystonia (8–11).

Dystonic movements typically worsen during voluntary movement. If dystonia appears only during a voluntary movement, it is referred to as action dystonia. Idiopathic torsion dystonia commonly begins with a specific action and then often progresses to be present with other actions, then with actions in other parts of the body, and finally is present with the body part at rest (7,12). A quantitative scale for measuring severity of dystonia takes into account this feature of inducing factors (13). An example of such progression is a child who develops idiopathic dystonia in one leg. It often first appears only when walking forward, and is usually absent when running or when walking backward. As the disease progresses, other actions of the affected leg may activate the dystonia, then voluntary actions of other parts of the body can induce dystonic movements of the involved leg, so-called overflow. With still further worsening, the affected limb develops dystonic movements while it is at rest. Eventually sustained posturing of the leg can develop. Thus, dystonia at rest is usually a more severe form than pure action dystonia. One of the most common forms of action dystonia is writer's cramp, a dystonia of the arm when used for this task-specific activity. Playing a musical instrument is another fairly common task that is associated with action dystonia (musician's cramp).

With time, primary dystonia often spreads to involve other parts of the body, usually in a contiguous fashion. Age at onset is important as to whether dystonia will spread to involve other parts of the body. As a general rule, the younger the age at onset, the more likely for dystonia to spread; childhood onset usually leads to eventual generalized dystonia (14,15). Adult-onset dystonia tends to remain as a focal dystonia, such as blepharospasm, torticollis, spastic dysphonia, writer's cramp, and oromandibular dystonia (16).

A characteristic feature of dystonic movements is that they are often diminished by sensory tricks that are frequently tactile or proprioceptive. Thus, touching the involved body part can reduce the muscle contractions. This is frequently seen in patients with torticollis; they will often place a hand on the chin or side of the face to reduce nuchal contractions.

Dystonia usually is present continually throughout the day whenever the affected body part is in use, or in more severe cases at rest, and disappears with deep sleep. Dystonic movements tend to increase with fatigue, stress, and emotional states; they tend to be suppressed with relaxation, hypnosis, and sleep.

A form of torsion dystonia with diurnal fluctuations needs to be recognized because it is exquisitively sensitive to L-dopa. This curious clinical feature of diurnal fluctuation was emphasized by Segawa et al (17). The patient is relatively free of dystonic movements and postures in the morning and is afflicted severely in the late afternoon, evening, and night. More recently it has been recognized that dopa-responsive dystonia may not always have such diurnal fluctuation (18). Other important clinical features are the presence of elements of parkinsonism (19), with patients having slowness of movement (bradykinesia) and loss of postural reflexes (positive pull test). The age of onset of dopa-responsive dystonia is in childhood before the age of 16, often with a gait disorder. When it begins in adult life, it can present as a focal dystonia or as parkinsonism.

EXAMINATION OF THE PATIENT

In primary dystonia, the only neurologic abnormality is the presence of dystonic postures and movements, and occasionally the presence of tremor. There is no associated weakness, spasticity, ataxia, reflex change, amyotrophy, abnormality of eye movements, disorder of retina, dementia, or seizures except where they may be the result of a concomitant problem such as a complication from a neurosurgical procedure undertaken to correct the dystonia, or the presence of some other incidental neurologic disease. As many of the symptomatic dystonias have these neurologic findings, the presence of any of these findings in a patient with dystonia immediately suggests that one is dealing with symptomatic

dystonia. However, the absence of such neurologic findings does not necessarily exclude the possibility of a symptomatic dystonia, which may rarely present as a pure dystonia. Table 77.1 lists clinical features that help distinguish between primary and symptomatic dystonias.

Clinical clues suggesting that a patient may have symptomatic dystonia come from both the history and the physical findings. Exposure to drugs known to cause dystonia is obviously relevant. Dopamine receptor blocking agents, most commonly antipsychotic drugs, are the most common drugs causing acute dystonic reactions and tardive dystonia (20); tardive dystonia is reviewed in Chapter 15. Previous head trauma, encephalitis, birth injury, stroke, or toxin exposure can all cause dystonia, often with a delay before manifestation of the dystonic symptoms.

Special mention should be made of psychogenic dystonia. At one time the diagnosis of dystonia due to hysteria was overly carried out, with as many as 40% of dystonic patients being so labeled at one time or another in the course of their illness, including patients with focal dystonia such as torticollis or writer's cramp (21). It is now firmly recognized, however, that psychogenic dystonia does occur but is not common (22). Table 77.2 lists clues to help the clinician be suspicious of psychogenic dystonia. Findings that are suggestive of psychogenic dystonia are the presence of any of the following: false weakness, false sensory

T a b l e 77.1 Clues to the Diagnosis of Primary versus Symptomatic Dystonia

Feature	Primary Dystonia	Symptomatic Dystonia
Action dystonia	Typical onset	Uncommon, usually postural change
Dystonia at rest	As disorder progresses	Typical onset
Other neurologic findings on exam	None	Commonplace
Hemidystonia	Uncommon	Very common
Generalized dystonia	Childhood onset after disease progresses	Common with metabolic diseases early in course in children, e.g., Wilson's disease, Leigh's disease
Focal dystonia	Common with adult onset	Common after trauma
History of drugs, i.e., dopamine receptor blockers	No history of exposure, or no temporal relation to exposure	Tardive dystonia develops during administration of these drugs or within 3 days after discontinuing drugs
Birth history	Normal	Abnormal birth history can lead to dystonia with delayed onset
Brain imaging	CT and MRI are normal	CT and MRI may be abnormal

Table 77.2   Clues Suggesting the Diagnosis of Psychogenic Dystonia

Abrupt onset
Presence of additional types of movements
Decrease of movements with distraction
False weakness
False sensory complaints
Multiple somatizations
Self-inflicted injuries
Obvious psychiatric disturbances
Inconsistent and incongruous movements and postures
Dystonia usually presents as a fixed dystonia or as paroxysmal dystonia

complaints, multiple somatizations, obvious psychiatric disturbances (e.g., self-inflicted injuries), and incongruous and inconsistent dystonic movements and postures (e.g., exacerbation when the child does not get his or her way and disappearing when the parents give in to the child). Care is required to avoid misinterpreting normal variations of dystonia as psychiatric phenomena. Relief with sensory tricks or variations with change of posture or voluntary motor activity are common in primary dystonia. Psychogenic dystonia can be severe enough to lead to fixed permanent contractures (22) and to surgical procedures (22,23).

GENETICS OF PRIMARY TORSION DYSTONIA

Primary torsion dystonia consists of familial and non-familial (sporadic) types. Although most patients with torsion dystonia have a negative family history for this disorder, when dystonia is mild, it is often not recognized. Moreover, patients usually do not distinguish between the form of dystonia they may have with the form appearing in a family member. For example, a child with generalized dystonia may have a relative with writer's cramp or with torticollis, and no family member considered there to be a connection between them. It is critical that personal examination of family members be conducted to be absolutely certain about the presence or absence of dystonia.

Zeman and Dyken (24) had established that a pattern of autosomal dominant transmission exists in many families. For a long time it was considered that primary dystonia in the Ashkenazi Jewish population, the ethnic group with the highest frequency of the disorder, is due to the expression of an autosomal recessive gene (25). It has now been established beyond any doubt that this ethnic group also transmits dystonia in an autosomal dominant pattern, with a penetrance rate of 0.3 (26).

In the general population, the frequency of familial generalized dystonia has been estimated at 1/160,000 (24). In the Ashkenazi Jewish population, prevalence is much higher, estimated to range from 1/15,000 to 1/23,000 (25,27).

Using restriction fragment length polymorphism analysis of a large, non-Jewish kindred in which the mode of inher-

itance is consistent with autosomal dominant transmission and with a penetrance rate of 0.75, Ozelius et al (28) found the locus of the dystonia gene to reside on chromosome 9q32–34 and then (29) showed the mutation to be a deletion of one of a pair of guanosine-adenosine-guanosine triplets that codes for glutamic acid in the ATP binding protein, torsion A. This discovery is a major advance in the biology of torsion dystonia and may lead to understanding the pathophysiology and to new therapy of the disorder.

A form of X-linked recessive heredodegenerative dystonia occurs on Panay Island in the Philippines (30). This disorder was shown to be associated with parkinsonism (31) and due to striatal degeneration with a mosaic pattern of gliosis (32).

Dopa-responsive dystonia is due to a variety of mutations in the gene that codes for the enzyme, GTP cyclohydrolase 1 (33). This enzyme catalyzes the first step in the biosynthesis of tetrahydrohipterin, the co-factor for tyrosine hydroxylase and other similar enzymes.

PATHOPHYSIOLOGY AND ANATOMY

The classic pathophysiologic characteristic of dystonia is sustained simultaneous contractions of agonists and antagonists that can be detected by electromyography (34,35). Rothwell et al (35) described three types of contractions: 1) continuous activity lasting 30 seconds and terminated by short periods of silence; 2) repetitive, often rhythmic, contractions lasting 1 to 2 seconds each and separated by equal periods of relative electromyographic silence; and 3) rapid, irregular, brief jerks lasting only 100 milliseconds resembling myoclonus. They also found 6 to 10 Hz tremor of the outstretched arms resembling essential tremor in 6 of 35 patients. Four of the patients had brief jerks lasting 100 to 500 milliseconds in the affected limbs during voluntary activity.

Primary torsion dystonia is not associated with any known pathologic lesion. On the other hand, symptomatic dystonia is most often associated with a lesion of the basal ganglia, particularly the putamen (36). Lesions producing dystonia can also involve connections to and from these nuclei, such as the thalamus and the cortex (37).

BIOCHEMISTRY

Neurochemical analysis of primary torsion dystonia is very limited. Hornykiewicz et al (38) examined the biochemistry of the brain in two patients with childhood-onset generalized idiopathic dystonia. Dopamine was decreased in the accumbens and striatum, but homovanillic acid was normal. Norepinephrine was reduced in some regions (hypothalamus, mammillary bodies, subthalamic nucleus, locus ceruleus) and increased in others (septum, thalamus, colliculi, red nucleus, dorsal raphe). Serotonin was decreased in the dorsal raphe and increased in the globus pallidus, subthalamic nucleus, and locus ceruleus. Jankovic et al (39) found similar biochemical changes, with the red nucleus and substantia nigra showing large increases in norepinephrine, and the substantia nigra a large increase in dopamine in a single case of adult-onset idiopathic cranial segmental dystonia. In a patient with symptomatic dystonia due to neuroacanthocytosis, de Yebenes et al (40) found large increases in norepinephrine in the caudate, putamen, globus pallidus, and dentate nucleus. Many more biochemical studies need to be carried out in order to be certain what neurotransmitter change predominates consistently in this disorder.

TREATMENT OF DYSTONIA

Treatment strategy depends on the type of dystonia encountered. The first step usually is to evaluate L-dopa. As dopa-responsive dystonia is so easy to treat, it is important not to miss this special form of dystonia. A trial of L-dopa/carbidopa up to 25/250 mg four times a day is adequate to make this evaluation. Next, one should consider injections of botulinum toxin if the dystonia is focal or if the major serious part of the dystonia is focal. The best responses for these injections are the dystonias involving the vocal cords (spastic dysphonia), the eyelids (blepharospasm), the neck (torticollis), the jaw (oromandibular dystonia), and the fingers (varieties of writer's and musician's cramps). The smaller the muscle involved, the smaller the dose of the injection. A summary of doses and results has been presented by Brin et al (41).

If the dystonia involves multiple sites, such as in segmental and generalized dystonia, then systemic pharmacotherapy is indicated. In terms of percentage of patients responding to drugs, the most efficacious agents are the anticholinergics, given in high doses, usually greater than 40 mg/day of trihexyphenidyl, and often greater than 80 mg/day. Our group has reached up to 160 mg/day in some patients. One starts with a low dose and gradually increases it until benefit or central adverse effects are encountered. Peripheral adverse effects, such as dry mouth, blurred vision, and difficulty with micturition are treated with peripheral anticholinesterases, such as pyridostigmine, and with pilocarpine eye drops. Central adverse effects may sometimes be overcome by switching to a sustained-release preparation of trihexyphenidyl or to some other anticholinergic, hoping that less side effects will occur. Greene et al (42) found that about 60% of children and 40% of adults will respond favorably to anticholinergics. Adults are more intolerable to adverse effects and cannot tolerate as high a dosage as children (42,43).

Often anticholinergics fail to provide sufficient benefit, and other drugs must be used in addition. Baclofen and clonazepam have been found to show benefit in about 15% of patients (42). Carbamazepine shows a smaller percentage of successful response. When these agents fail, a trial of dopamine depleters (reserpine, tetrabenazine), sometimes

with lithium (44) or dopamine receptor blockers (45), may be effective.

Hemidystonia often fails to respond to pharmacotherapy, but can be benefited by contralateral thalamotomy (46) or pallidotomy (47). Bilateral operations may be indicated in patients with severe, disabling dystonia that fails to respond to pharmacotherapy.

REFERENCES

1. Fahn S, Bressman S, Marsden CD. Classification of dystonia. Mov Disord 1997;12(suppl 3):1–5.
2. Fahn S, Marsden CD, Calne DB. Classification and investigation of dystonia. In: Marsden CD, Fahn S, eds. Movement disorders 2. London: Butterworths, 1987:332–358.
3. Jankovic J, Fahn S. Dystonic disorders. In: Jankovic J, Tolosa E, eds. Parkinson's disease and movement disorders, 3rd ed. Baltimore: Williams and Wilkins, 1998:513–551.
4. Calne DB, Lang AE. Secondary dystonia. Adv Neurol 1988;50:9–33.
5. Oppenheim H. Uber eine eigenartige Krampfkrankheit des kindlichen und jugendlichen Alters (Dysbasia lordotica progressiva, Dystonia musculorum deformans). Neurol Centrabl 1911;30:1090–1107.
6. Flatau E, Sterling W. Progressiver Torsionspasms bie Kindern. Z Gesamte Neurol Psychiatr 1911;7:586–612.
7. Fahn S. The varied clinical expressions of dystonia. Neurol Clin 1984;2:541–554.
8. Davidenkow S. Auf hereditar-abiotrophischer Grundlage akut auftretende, regressierende und episodische Erkrankungen des Nervensystems und Bemerkungen uber die familiare subakute, myoklonische Dystonie. Z Gesamte Neurol Psychiatr 1926;104:596–622.
9. Obeso JA, Rothwell JC, Lang AE, Marsden CD. Myoclonic dystonia. Neurology 1983;33:825–830.
10. Kurlan R, Behr J, Medved L, Shoulson I. Myoclonus and dystonia: a family study. Adv Neurol 1988;50:385–389.
11. Quinn NP, Rothwell JC, Thompson PD, Marsden CD. Hereditary myoclonic dystonia, hereditary torsion dystonia and hereditary essential myoclonus: an area of confusion. Adv Neurol 1988;50:391–401.
12. Cooper IS, Cullinan T, Riklan M. The natural history of dystonia. Adv Neurol 1976;14:157–169.
13. Burke RE, Fahn S, Marsden CD, et al. Validity and reliability of a rating scale for the primary torsion dystonias. Neurology 1985;35:73–77.
14. Marsden CD, Harrison MJG, Bundey S. Natural history of idiopathic torsion dystonia. Adv Neurol 1976;14:177–187.
15. Fahn S. Generalized dystonia: concept and treatment. Clin Neuropharmacol 1986;9(suppl 2):S37–S48.
16. Marsden CD. The focal dystonias. Clin Neuropharmacol 1986;9(suppl 2):S49–S60.
17. Segawa M, Hosaka A, Miyagawa F, et al. Hereditary progressive dystonia with marked diurnal fluctuation. Adv Neurol 1976;14:215–233.
18. Nygaard TG, Marsden CD, Duvoisin RC. Dopa-responsive dystonia. Adv Neurol 1988;50:377–384.
19. Nygaard TG, Trugman JM, de Yebenes JG, Fahn S. Dopa-responsive dystonia: the spectrum of clinical manifestations in a large North American family. Neurology 1990;40:66–69.
20. Burke RE, Fahn S, Jankovic J, et al. Tardive dystonia: late-onset and persistent dystonia caused by antipsychotic drugs. Neurology 1982;32:1335–1346.
21. Lesser RP, Fahn S. Dystonia: a disorder often misdiagnosed as a conversion reaction. Am J Psychiatry 1978;153:349–452.
22. Fahn S, Williams DT. Psychogenic dystonia. Adv Neurol 1988;50:431–455.
23. Batshaw ML, Wachtel RC, Deckel AW, et al. Munchausen's syndrome simulating torsion dystonia. N Engl J Med 1985;312:1437–1439.
24. Zeman W, Dyken P. Dystonia musculorum deformans. Handbook of clinical neurology. Amsterdam: North-Holland, 1968;6:517–543.
25. Eldridge R. The torsion dystonias: literature review and genetic and clinical studies. Neurology 1970;20:1–78.
26. Bressman SB, de Leon D, Brin MF, et al. Idiopathic torsion dystonia among Ashkenazi Jews: evidence for autosomal dominant inheritance. Ann Neurol 1989;26:612–620.
27. Zilber N, Korczyn AD, Kahana E, et al. Inheritance of idiopathic torsion dystonia among Jews. J Med Genet 1984;21:13–20.

28. Ozelius L, Kramer PL, Moskowitz CB, et al. Torsion dystonia gene located on chromosome 9q32–34. Neuron 1989;2:1427–1434.

29. Ozelius LJ, Hewett JW, Page CE, et al. The early-onset torsion dystonia gene (DYT1) encodes an ATP binding protein. Nat Genet 1997;17:40–48.

30. Lee LV, Pascasio FM, Fuentes FD, Viterbo GH. Torsion dystonia in Panay, Philippines. Adv Neurol 1976;14:137–151.

31. Fahn S, Moskowitz C. X-linked recessive dystonia and parkinsonism in Filipino males. Ann Neurol 1988;24:179.

32. Waters CH, Faust PL, Powers J, et al. Neuropathology of Lubag (X-linked dystonia-parkinsonism). Mov Disord 1993;8:387–390.

33. Ichinose H, Ohye T, Takahashi E, et al. Hereditary progressive dystonia with marked diurnal fluctuation caused by mutations in the GTP cyclohydrolase 1 gene. Nat Genet 1994;8:236–242.

34. Yanagisawa N, Goto A. Dystonia musculorum deformans: analysis with electromyography. J Neurol Sci 1971;13:39–65.

35. Rothwell JC, Obeso JA, Day BL, Marsden CD. The pathophysiology of dystonias. Adv Neurol 1983;39:851–863.

36. Burton K, Farrell K, Li D, Calne DB. Lesions of the putamen and dystonia: CT and magnetic resonance imaging. Neurology 1984;34:962–965.

37. Marsden CD, Obeso JA, Zarranz JJ, Lang AE. The anatomical basis of symptomatic hemidystonia. Brain 1985;108:463–483.

38. Hornykiewicz O, Kish SJ, Becker LE, et al. Brain neurotransmitters in dystonia musculorum deformans. N Engl J Med 1986;315:347–353.

39. Jankovic J, Svendsen CN, Bird ED. Brain neurotransmitters in dystonia. N Engl J Med 1987;316:278–279.

40. de Yebenes JG, Vazquez A, Martinez A, et al. Biochemical findings in symptomatic dystonias. Adv Neurol 1988;50:167–175.

41. Brin MF, Fahn S, Moskowitz C, et al. Localized injections of botulinum toxin for the treatment of focal dystonia and hemifacial spasm. Mov Disord 1987;2:237–254.

42. Greene P, Shale H, Fahn S. Analysis of open-label trials in torsion dystonia using high dosages of anticholinergics and other drugs. Mov Disord 1988;3:46–60.

43. Fahn S. High dosage anticholinergic therapy in dystonia. Neurology 1983;33:1255–1261.

44. Jankovic J, Orman J. Tetrabenazine therapy of dystonia, chorea, tics, and other dyskinesias. Neurology 1988;38:391–394.

45. Marsden CD, Marion M-H, Quinn N. The treatment of severe dystonia in children and adults. J Neurol Neurosurg Psychiatry 1984;47:1166–1173.

46. Andrew J, Fowler CJ, Harrison MJG. Stereotaxic thalamotomy in 55 cases of dystonia. Brain 1983;106:981–1000.

47. Iacono RP, Kuniyoshi SM, Lorsen DR, et al. Simultaneous bilateral pallidoansotomy for idiopathic dystonia musculorum deformans. Pediat Neurol 1996;14:145–148.

Hereditary Progressive Dystonia/ Dopa-Responsive Dystonia

TORBJOERN G. NYGAARD   ROGER C. DUVOISIN

INTRODUCTION

Dystonia is the term for sustained muscle contractions that frequently cause twisting and repetitive movements (1). Hereditary progressive dystonia/dopa-responsive dystonia (HPD/DRD), also known as Segawa syndrome, is a syndrome of selective nigrostriatal dopamine deficiency caused by genetic defects in the dopamine synthetic pathway without nigral cell loss (2, 2a), the key clinical features of which include

1. onset with "dystonia," usually affecting gait, in childhood;
2. the concurrent or subsequent development of parkinsonian signs; and
3. a dramatic therapeutic response to L-dopa, which is sustained without long-term L-dopa–induced complications such as motor fluctuations and dyskinesia.

The mode of presentation may suggest a variety of other diagnoses, including diplegic cerebral palsy, spastic paraplegia, childhood-onset parkinsonism (3), and ataxic syndromes. Often reported are a diurnal fluctuation of symptoms, worsening of dystonia with exercise, and improvement following sleep. These fluctuations vary widely in degree and do not occur in a quarter of cases. There is frequently a family history, and autosomal dominant inheritance with reduced penetrance is most common. Recent observations suggest that benign adult-onset parkinsonism may be the expression of the disease in at-risk individuals who do not manifest dystonia in childhood (4,5).

This review focuses on the clinical features of HPD/DRD based on data from 132 treated cases appearing in the literature (2,4–51); 63 were personally examined by one of the authors (T.G.N.).

The nosologic designations used in originally reporting these cases appear in Table 78.1. The designation HPD/DRD minimizes confusion with other disorders causing childhood-onset parkinsonism that do not have the good long-term prognosis of HPD/DRD, with the realization that a quarter of the cases do not report diurnal fluctuation (2). The key features linking all cases are dystonia and its dopa responsiveness.

HISTORICAL BACKGROUND

The first apparent report of affected individuals was by Beck (52), who described a girl and her paternal uncle affected with "dystonia musculorum deformans." The girl, at age $8\frac{1}{2}$, began to "kick up her left heel" on walking. The other leg became similarly affected and within 6 months she could walk only with support. Rest tremor appeared in the hands. She stood and walked with hips and knees flexed, her legs adducted and internally rotated, and her feet in equinovarus. Corner (53) drew attention to diurnal fluctuation of symptoms in this patient and in her then-affected brother. A dramatic response to low doses of trihexyphenidyl (Artane) occurred in this pair. Substitution with L-dopa therapy in the early 1970s resulted in maintenance or improvement in prior symptomatic response. After the introduction of L-dopa for the treatment of Parkinson's disease in 1967 (54), it was tried in a variety of patients with dystonia with little positive effect (55–57), but there were a few exceptions (56–60).

In 1971, Castaigne et al (6) reported two brothers with a "progressive extrapyramidal disorder," and Segawa et al (7) reported two cousins with "hereditary basal ganglia disease with marked diurnal fluctuation," who had a remarkable response to L-dopa therapy. Cooper tempered the general

Table 78.1   Designation of Previously Reported Cases of HPD/DRD

Hereditary basal ganglia disease with marked diurnal fluctuation (7)
Hereditary dystonia-parkinsonism (15)
Hereditary progressive dystonia with marked diurnal variation (16)
Segawa's syndrome (34)
Dopa-sensitive progressive dystonia (35)
Hereditary dystonia-parkinsonism syndrome of juvenile onset (37)
Fluctuating dystonia (42)
Biopterin-deficient progressive dystonia with diurnal variation (47)

use of L-dopa for dystonia in the United States by warning that L-dopa rendered patients less responsive to thalamotomy (59), a major treatment modality for dystonia at the time. Eldridge et al (60) also urged caution in L-dopa use, but added that about 5% of patients with dystonia reported greatest therapeutic benefit from this treatment. Isolated reports of L-dopa-responsive dystonia continued to appear (8–11,13,14).

At the First International Symposium on Torsion Dystonia in 1975, Allen and Knopp (15) reported a family afflicted with a disorder characterized by onset of dystonia in childhood with later development of parkinsonian features. These patients were responsive to L-dopa and anticholinergic medication in low doses. At the same symposium Segawa et al (16) presented further L-dopa-responsive patients. They stressed the progressive nature of the dystonia and the diurnal fluctuation of symptoms. They also described features of parkinsonism, including cogwheel-like rigidity and rest tremor in the older patients, frozen gait, pulsion, and a mask-like face.

THE TYPICAL CASE

The onset is between 14 months and 12 years of age with a curious abnormality of gait, including toe-walking, equinovarus, or other abnormal postures of the leg. Standing or walking often induces an accentuated lumbar lordosis or a crouched posture. The gait often has a long stride and wide base. Postural instability and a tendency to fall are common. Additional features are brisk reflexes in the legs, with varying degrees of clonus, and dystonic extension of the big toe spontaneously or on plantar stimulation— "the striatal toe" (61), which may be misinterpreted as a Babinski response.

The dystonia is progressive and more pronounced in the legs than the arms, but also affects the axial musculature with increased lumbar lordosis, scoliosis, and occasionally retrocollis or torticollis. In some earlier-onset cases, generalization of the dystonia with severe disability did not occur and disability remained mild until more overt parkinsonism appeared in the fifth or sixth decade. No individual with onset in the teenage years progressed to severe generalized dystonia.

The elements of parkinsonism in most patients with HPD/DRD are what separate this disorder clinically from

idiopathic torsion dystonia (ITD) (2). Although muscle tone may vary moment to moment in an affected limb in ITD, rigidity is not a feature. Similarly, decrementing amplitude, inability to sustain movement, or arrests on repetitive motor tasks (i.e., finger tapping or foot tapping) are not part of the motor impairment in ITD. Postural instability very rarely occurs in ITD even in severely affected generalized cases. Our prospective evaluation of new patients with dystonia has revealed that these features are invariably present in the early course of HPD/DRD.

In HPD/DRD, the earliest symptomatic parkinsonism is often postural instability and is frequently coincident with appearance of overt dystonia. There is a variable degree of rigidity, sometimes with cogwheeling, and a marked effect of activation (contralateral motor activity during passive limb testing). These features are often apparent in limbs unaffected by dystonia. Rapid fatiguing of effort with repetitive or sustained motor tasks is often prominent and a characteristic feature. Tremor appearing early in the disease is usually postural, resembling that of essential tremor, but typical parkinsonian rest tremor may occur later in the course.

Although early development is usually normal in affected children, there has been recent awareness of delayed motor milestones (late independent sitting and walking) in several children (49). In many other cases, pigeon-toed gait and poor balance from the onset of walking (at a normal age) (51) were observed. The disorder remained static in these children for several years before the appearance of more overt symptomatic involvement.

There is no history of birth abnormality, no precipitating illness or drug exposure, no evidence of retinal, sensory, cerebellar, or intellectual disturbance, and no obvious etiology (e.g., abnormal copper metabolism).

SUMMARY OF CLINICAL FEATURES OF 132 CASES

There was a 2.9:1 predominance of affected females. Although average age of onset was slightly earlier for females than males (5.6 versus 6.2 years) and occurred earlier in patients with diurnal fluctuation (5.7 versus 6.1 years), there was broad overlap among these groups.

Among the 132 cases, the most frequent presenting features (Table 78.2) were gait abnormality and dystonia in the leg, typically equinovarus posture of a foot. Although presentation with one of these two features occurred in 126 cases (95%), it is significant to note that 2 patients presented with difficulty in an arm (16,44), 2 with torticollis (2,44), and another with retrocollis and arm involvement (48). Slowness dressing was the mode of presentation in the remaining patient (7).

Some element of parkinsonism was present in 20% of cases at onset, and appreciated in at least 67% before initiation of treatment. This low frequency of parkinsonism at onset is undoubtedly an underestimate due to the retrospective nature of our analysis. Oculogyria (periodic invol-

Table 78.2   Clinical Features in the 132 Patients Reviewed
(98 female, 34 male)

	At Onset[a]	At Full Expression
Gait disorder	108	132
Dystonia	110	132
Leg	106	131
Arm	8	98
Neck[b]	5	35
Lumbar lordosis or scoliosis	4	56
Postural tremor	5	28
Parkinsonism	27	96
Rest tremor	0	16
Bradykinesia	16	59
Hypomimia	3	34
Postural instability	22	60
Cogwheel rigidity	?	65
Oculogyria	0	4
Diurnal fluctuation[c]	102	102

[a] Age at onset (in months) between 14 months and 12 years (average 5.8 years).
[b] Three patients with torticollis at onset. Seventeen patients with torticollis at full expression; the remainder had retrocollis or anterocollis.
[c] One patient had fluctuations only with her early symptoms, with subsequent disappearance of variation. Another patient developed fluctuations after several years of illness.

untary upward gaze) occurred in four cases with advanced symptoms (9,35,37), but did not recur following L-dopa therapy. Early treatment may have masked the appearance of these features in some patients.

DIURNAL FLUCTUATION AND SLEEP BENEFIT

Segawa et al have stressed diurnal fluctuation and sleep benefit as distinguishing characteristics of this disorder (16). However, among the 132 cases included here, diurnal fluctuation was absent in 29 (22%). Women reported fluctuations slightly more often than men (79% versus 74%). The degree of fluctuation was variable, with some cases "normal" in the morning, the others merely "better" in the morning though still obviously affected. The degree of fluctuation diminished with the progression of the disorder in some, and fluctuations disappeared after a few years in at least one individual. One case only experienced fluctuation after several years of illness (24). In four families there were affected members with and others without diurnal fluctuation (35,44,51). In another family, the degree of fluctuation among affected members varied markedly (35).

Sleep benefit has been said to require rapid eye movement (REM) sleep (16), but others have noted the effectiveness of non-REM sleep (32). Several personally examined cases showed significant benefit from a period of rest without sleep.

A survey of 51 patients with leg-onset ITD beginning before age 18 years and not responsive to L-dopa assessed

the nosologic value of these phenomena (48). Thirty-five percent of this group reported sleep benefit, 37% reported exercise-induced exacerbation of their symptoms, and 12% felt clearly more affected in the afternoon. Thus, diurnal fluctuation, at least to some degree, sleep benefit, and worsening with exercise do not reliably discriminate patients with HPD/DRD from others with early-onset dystonia and cannot be counted on to predict responsiveness to L-dopa.

INHERITANCE

In 39 families, representing 75 treated cases, there was more than one affected member. Autosomal dominant inheritance was evident (male-to-male transmission) in 12 kindreds (2,4,16,35,37,41,44,48,49). The pattern of inheritance in the remaining families was unclear, possibly due to the extremely variable degree of symptomatology in affected individuals. There were 57 cases with apparently "sporadic disease." Autosomal dominant inheritance with incomplete penetrance and variable expressivity appears likely.

A high proportion of cases have Japanese or Anglo-Saxon heritage, though cases have come from a variety of other ethnic backgrounds. ITD is 5- to 10-fold more prevalent among individuals of Ashkenazi Jewish origin. However, to date there are only five known sporadic cases of HPD/DRD recognized with Ashkenazic origin.

The study of one large North American family with autosomal dominant HPD/DRD found the penetrance of dystonia to be 30% (5). The frequency of dystonia in either sex was similar, though severity was greater in women. A review of 61 personally examined cases made a similar observation, that as a group, women demonstrated greater severity (51), suggesting that the female predominance observed in various series may reflect ascertainment bias related to gender differences in disease severity.

DIFFERENTIAL DIAGNOSES

The most common presentation was with insidious development of an inturning foot, often only on walking, with or without diurnal fluctuation. This generally progressed to a frankly dystonic gait, sometimes with unsteadiness and frequent falls. This clinical picture may be indistinguishable from that of childhood-onset ITD. However, impairment of balance and falls are not features of the early stages of ITD. As a group, children with ITD have a somewhat later mean age of onset (9 years) and may have a slight male predominance of disease (62). Two studies found no sex difference in severity of ITD (63,64). These latter observations do not aid the distinction in an individual case.

About 20% of this group presented with severe dystonia of the legs simulating paraplegia. Abnormalities found on examination included slight to moderate increases of muscle tone in the legs, unsustained or sustained ankle clonus, brisk knee jerks, and variable extensor plantar responses. The gait appeared spastic with flexed knees, scissoring, and scuffing of the plantigrade feet. Initial impressions included diplegic cerebral palsy or sporadic (hereditary) spastic paraplegia. The absence of abnormal birth history and normal intellectual development, and, most important, the progressive nature of disease should allow distinction from cerebral palsy. The recent observation in a few children of delayed motor milestones and a static illness for several years before more overt signs and symptoms develop can add to the confusion in some cases (49). Lack of serial examinations to show progression may be a factor in some cases. The presence of extrapyramidal features in the upper limbs would be unexpected in spastic diplegia.

Recognition of rigidity, bradykinesia, hypomimia, and tremor led to considerations of childhood-onset parkinsonism in 5% of these cases. In HPD/DRD, the dystonic elements tend to predominate with early progression, but a significant degree of parkinsonism may be apparent. One series identified several cases with similar onset to HPD/DRD in whom wearing-off and dose-related dyskinesias (complications of therapy similar to those encountered in Parkinson's disease) developed a few years after initiation of treatment (51). These children had onset of their illness somewhat later than the mean age of onset in HPD/DRD (no case had onset before age 8) but individually had little to distinguish them from other cases with HPD/DRD. None of these cases came from a family with autosomal dominant disease. The observation of a long-term response to therapy without complications may be necessary to allow this differentiation (51).

A few patients had diagnoses of odd ataxic syndromes when they presented with bizarre, unsteady gait, not typically dystonic, with unexpected and unexplained falls.

Thus, HPD/DRD needs to be considered in the differential diagnosis of a variety of clinical syndromes presenting with gait disorder in childhood or adolescence.

FREQUENCY OF HPD/DRD

There has been no epidemiologic study of HPD/DRD. ITD has an estimated population frequency of 1/160,000 in the general population (65). Data from the London Dystonia Research Centre and Dystonia Clinical Research Center (New York) suggest that 5% to 10% of children or young adolescents presenting with primary dystonia may have HPD/DRD (48). Crude estimates of the population frequency of HPD/DRD in Japan and the United Kingdom, based on reported cases, are similar at 0.5 per million and fit well with estimates based on the figures above.

LABORATORY INVESTIGATIONS

Blood counts, routine blood chemistries, studies of copper metabolism, computed axial tomography (CT) and magnetic resonance imaging (MRI) have been normal. Electromyography (EMG) showed typical cocontraction in agonist-antagonist muscles (16,29). Sleep studies showed decreased movement during sleep and decreased time in REM sleep that reversed with L-dopa therapy (16).

Cerebrospinal fluid homovanillic acid levels (CSF HVA) were low in most patients studied (2,15,18,25,32,35, 36,39,43,45,47). Seven patients had diurnal HVA level determinations that showed a mild rise, still below the normal range, or a fall in most patients (18,32,35,45). Various patients had elevated (18), normal (2,25,26,36,39,43,45,48), or decreased (2,45,48) levels of CSF 5-hydroxyindoleacetic acid (5-HIAA).

Nine patients had decreased CSF tetrahydrobiopterin [BH$_4$, a tyrosine hydroxylase (TH) cofactor] and neopterin (a BH$_4$ precursor) levels (36,45,48). We have found this to be a consistent finding in several other patients with HPD/DRD. We are not aware of any patient with HPD/DRD with normal CSF biopterin. CSF biopterin has been normal in ITD but has been low in several cases of childhood-onset parkinsonism (R.A. Levine, personal communication, 1989).

The dramatic response to low doses of L-dopa suggests intact dopa-decarboxylase activity and dopamine turnover. In Parkinson's disease, wearing off may reflect the loss of dopaminergic neurons (66,67), which results in impaired fluorodopa retention in positron emission tomography (PET) (68). The long-term stability observed in most HPD/DRD patients suggests preservation of dopaminergic neurons. Labeled fluorodopa PET scanning was normal (69,70), or "near-normal" (71), in eight cases studied as adults. The subtle abnormalities detected in this latter report do not represent fluorodopa uptake values outside of the control range but a difference detected in the mean uptake values comparing HPD/DRD and controls. Examination of the data suggests that there is very little decline in fluorodopa uptake with longer duration of disease. Another case, a 12-year-old girl, had a decreased putamenal signal similar to the finding in early Parkinson's disease (69). This study was limited, however, by being restricted to the analysis of only a single tomographic slice. Two cases of childhood-onset parkinsonism (72,73) had markedly abnormal studies consistent with findings in PD (74). A similarly abnormal scan was present in one young man (24) originally thought to have HPD/DRD, but reclassified to childhood-onset parkinsonism after the appearance of prominent wearing off (51,71).

These findings with PET differ from a recent analysis of the kinetics of labeled tyrosine metabolism in HPD/DRD (50). These authors concluded that HPD/DRD is the result of a reduced biologic half-life of dopamine, possibly because of impaired storage. A major limitation of this study would appear to be the lack of a parallel analysis of labeled L-dopa metabolism.

MOLECULAR PATHOGENESIS

Tetrahydrobiopterin (BH$_4$) is the essential natural cofactor for tyrosine hydroxylase (TH), which converts L-tyrosine to L-dopa, the rate limiting step in the synthesis of dopamine (DA) (Fig 78.1). In the production of BH$_4$ from guanosine triphosphate (GTP), GTP cyclohydrolase I (GCH-I) cat-

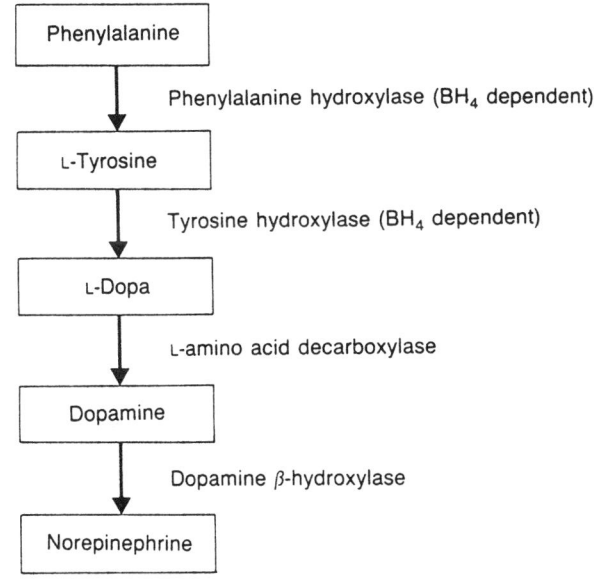

FIGURE 78.1   *Catecholamine biosynthetic pathway.*

alyzes the rate limiting step. If, as in most patients with HPD/DRD, GCH-I is defective because of one of several mutations in the gene responsible for it, BH_4 will be deficient and DA deficiency will result (75–78). Production of DA will also be deficient with mutations in the gene for TH (79). Mutations in both of these genes have been reported in patients with HPD/DRD.

Replacement of L-dopa, normally the product of TH, reverses the metabolic deficit accounting for this disorder. Over the long run, the nigrostriatal system then functions normally because in patients with HPD/DRD there are enzymatic defects in the synthesis of DA but there is no loss of nigral dopaminergic neurons (2a). Loss of the latter underlies Parkinson's disease (PD), where it also accounts for deficient dopamine transporter (DAT) in dopaminergic axon terminals in the striatum (2a).

Because multiple mutations have been found in the GCH-I gene and more are likely to be found, it is often impossible to confirm or reject a clinical diagnosis of HPD/DRD by mutation studies. However, with defects in the GCH-I gene, but not with those in the TH gene, one finds a deficit in CSF neopterin, a degradation product in the synthesis of BH_4 from GTP (2a). Single-photon emission computed tomography (SPECT) shows DAT is normal in the striatum of patients with HPD/DRD but is reduced in patients with PD, juvenile PD being a major diagnostic alternative to HPD/DRD (2a,80).

In most instances, HPD/DRD is due to autosomal dominant inheritance with incomplete penetrance, but there are also patients with autosomal recessive inheritance. Mutations in the GCH-I gene were not found in all patients with HPD/DRD and a mutation was found in the TH gene in

a family with autosomal recessive HPD/DRD (75,78,81). There appears to be a relatively high spontaneous mutation rate for defects in the GCH-I gene. Although heterozygous GCH-I mutations cause HPD/DRD, homozygous defects in GCH-I are associated with mental retardation and seizures in addition to dystonia (82).

RESPONSE TO TREATMENT

L-Dopa

The dramatic response to L-dopa sets this group apart from ITD and the other disorders with which it may be confused (83). Patients with HPD/DRD have an immediate benefit from small doses of L-dopa. Full benefit has occurred within several days to a few months after initiation of therapy, with patients returning to normal or near normal. Hyperreflexia and apparent spasticity have resolved (2,8,18,20,24,42,45,46,49). The Babinski response disappeared (perhaps the response of the striatal toe to therapy) in several patients (2,18,24,42,46,49). Full functional capacity is generally achieved, although minor abnormalities of gait may persist. Daily doses as small as 100 mg and not exceeding 3 g (average 500–1,000 mg) have yielded maximum benefit. No dose greater than 400 mg/day has been necessary with L-dopa given in combination with carbidopa (Sinemet). L-Dopa-induced dyskinesias occurred in at least 15% of cases at the initiation of therapy (2,6,13,15–18,24,33,37,40,42,45,46,49), but these subsided with dose reduction and have not reappeared with long-term therapy.

The duration of response following discontinuation of chronic L-dopa therapy has been variable: 12 hours to several days (in one patient several months) may pass before symptom reemergence. At least one patient remains symptom free on a single dose of medication on alternate days. L-Dopa in combination with a dopa-decarboxylase inhibitor (benserazide or carbidopa) appears to give a smoother long-term response and is preferable to treatment with L-dopa alone (53).

Twenty-four individuals in whom the illness had remained untreated for 20 to 60 years still had an impressive response at initiation of therapy (2,4,5,13,15,16,35, 37,44,45,51). A stable response continues in all 39 for whom we have follow-up after more than 10 years of L-dopa therapy (2,9,18,38,44,46,49,51). A few patients taking plain L-dopa required modest dose increases over time. Fluctuations, on–off phenomena, and freezing episodes have not appeared. This latter point is an important, but retrospective, difference from childhood-onset Parkinson's disease. Several authors have reported the early appearance of L-dopa-induced dyskinesias in juvenile parkinsonism (84–86). One case of torsion dystonia responding to L-dopa developed freezing after 2½ years of L-dopa therapy (87). These cases may have a clinical presentation that is virtually indistinguishable from HPD/DRD, including prominent diurnal fluctuation. Five cases reported in an earlier series have developed wearing-off or peak-dose dyskinesias during the first 5 years of L-dopa treatment and represent misclassified cases (51). Thus, the definition of HPD/DRD must be modified to include at least 5 years of stable response to L-dopa, if a family history of stable response is not available (51).

Other Drugs

There was prior treatment with trihexyphenidyl and other anticholinergics in at least 27 of these patients. A dramatic response occurred in 10 cases (38,51,53), a moderate response in 12 others (48), and no response in the remaining 5 patients (32,37,51). Doses were 10 mg of tri-hexyphenidyl a day or less in these latter cases, and it is uncertain whether the higher doses currently used in typical ITD would have yielded greater benefit in those patients with poor response (88). Because of decreasing efficacy through their teenage years, a few cases required increasing doses of trihexyphenidyl, to as high as 100 mg/day. Bradykinesia, rigidity, and postural instability tended to become more obvious during this period. All patients judged L-dopa to be superior to trihexyphenidyl, except two (who already felt normal on trihexyphenidyl) in whom the response was equal.

Carbamazepine was initially effective in one patient (12) but was inconsistent over time, with prolonged periods seemingly without response (51). One patient had a moderate response to this drug, and another reported only improvement in speech; other patients noted no significant effect (51).

Bromocriptine had an effect equivalent to that of L-dopa in two patients (32,43). BH$_4$, given intravenously, had a short effect in two patients (36), but did not improve three others (47). Amytriptyline had a moderate symptomatic effect in two sisters (45). Exposure to a dopamine receptor blocking drug has provoked worsening of dystonia during the period of exposure in a few patients with HPD/DRD (39,51). No other medication has had significant effect.

SUMMARY

HPD/DRD is a distinctive clinical entity and an unexpectedly common subgroup of torsion dystonia. Selective nigrostriatal dopamine deficiency underlies this disorder. It is caused by mutations affecting enzymes (especially GCH-I) in the dopamine synthetic pathway without nigral cell loss. Diminished CSF biopterin levels may serve as a marker of disease and serve to distinguish cases from ITD. SPECT scanning allows differentiation from childhood-onset parkinsonism. Clinically, diurnal fluctuation is often, but not always, present and does not reliably distinguish the disorder from idiopathic torsion dystonia.

HPD/DRD must be considered in the differential diagnosis of the child or adolescent presenting with a dystonic gait disorder, diplegic cerebral palsy, sporadic spastic paraplegia, and ataxic syndromes. The response to L-dopa is so dramatic and occurs so quickly that a diagnostic therapeutic trial should be considered in all patients presenting with these syndromes. The distinction from childhood-onset parkinsonism in cases without autosomal dominant disease may be difficult and may require a period of follow-up.

REFERENCES

1. Fahn S. Concept and classification of dystonia. Adv Neurol 1988;50:1–8.
2. Nygaard TG, Marsden CD, Duvoisin RC. Dopa-responsive dystonia. Adv Neurol 1988;50:377–384.
2a. Jeon BS, Jeon J-M, Park S-S, et al. Dopamine transporter density measured by [^{123}I]β-CIT single-photon emission computed tomography is normal in dopa-responsive dystonia. Ann Neurol 1998;43:792–800.
3. Gershanik OS, Nygaard TG. Parkinson's disease beginning before age 40. Adv Neurol 1990;53:251–258.
4. Nygaard TG, Gardner-Medwin D, Marsden CD. Dopa-responsive dystonia: the spectrum of clinical manifestations in a family. In: Crossman AR, Sambrook MA, eds. Neural mechanisms in disorders of movement. London: John Libbey, 1989;367–370.
5. Nygaard TG, Trugman JM, de Yebenes JG, Fahn S. Dopa-responsive dystonia: the spectrum of clinical manifestations in a large North American family. Neurology 1990;40:66–69.
6. Castaigne P, Rondot P, Ribadeau-Dumas JL, Said G. Affection extrapyramidale evoluant chez deux jeunes freres: effects remarquables du traitement par la L-dopa. Rev Neurol 1971;124:162–166.
7. Segawa M, Ohmi K, Itoh S, et al. Childhood basal ganglia disease with remarkable response to L-dopa, "hereditary basal ganglia disease with marked diurnal fluctuation." Shinryo 1971;24:667–672.
8. Maekawa K, Kitani N, Satake Y. Remarkable effect of L-dopa on idiopathic dystonia. A case report. No To Hattatsu 1972;4:274–281.
9. Rajput AH. Levodopa in dystonia musculorum deformans. Lancet 1973;i:432.
10. Hongladarom T. Levodopa in dystonia musculorum deformans. Lancet 1973;i:1114.
11. Mel'nichuk PV, Sosnovskai LS. Lechenie deformiruiushchei myshechnoi dystonii u detei preparatom L-DOP. Zh Neuropatol Psikhiatr 1973;73:1495–1498.
12. Geller M, Kaplan B, Christoff N. Dystonic symptoms in children: treatment with carbamazepine. JAMA 1974;229:1755–1757.
13. Winkelmann W. L-Dopa Langzeitbehandlung einer Torsionsdystonie. J Neurol 1975;208:319–323.
14. Schenck E, Kruschke U. Familiare progressive Dystonie mit Tagesschwankungen. Fallbeschreibung. Erfolgreiche Behanlung mit L-dopa. Klin Wochenschr 1975;53:779–780.
15. Allen N, Knopp W. Hereditary Parkinsonism-dystonia with sustained control by L-dopa and anticholinergic medication. Adv Neurol 1976;14:201–214.
16. Segawa M, Hosaka A, Miyagawa F, et al. Hereditary progressive dystonia with marked diurnal variation. Adv Neurol 1976;14:215–233.
17. Haidvogl M, Stogmann W. Hereditare progressive Dystonie mit Tagesschwankungen (Abstract). Jahrestag Ost Ges Kinderheilkd Millstatt 1976;24:9.
18. Ouvrier RA. Progressive dystonia with marked diurnal fluctuation. Ann Neurol 1978;4:412–417.
19. Montanini R, Basso PF, Gasco P. Trattamento con levodopa di un caso di spasmo di torsione con atetosi. Minerva Med 1979;70:1551–1553.
20. Bugiani O, Gatti R. L-Dopa in children with progressive neurological disorders. Ann Neurol 1980;7:93.
21. Segawa M. Hereditary progressive dystonia (HPD) with marked diurnal fluctuation. Adv Neurol Sci 1981;25:73–81.
22. Balottin U, Lanzi G, Zambrino CA. Illustrazione di un caso di dystonia musculorum deformans trattato con L-dopa. Riv Neurobiol 1981;27:584–590.
23. Garg BP. Dystonia musculorum deformans: implications of therapeutic response to levodopa and carbamazepine. Arch Neurol 1982;39:376–377.
24. Gordon N. Fluctuating dystonia and allied syndromes. Neuropediatrics 1982;13:152–154.
25. Hakamada S, Watanabe K, Hara K, Miyazaki S. A case of "hereditary progressive dystonia with marked diurnal fluctuation." No To Hattatsu 1982;14:44–48.
26. Rolando S, Cremonte M. Dystonia progressive con marcata fluttuazione mattine-sera. Instituto Gaslini 1982;14:176–179.

27. LeWitt PA, Newman RP, MIller LP, et al. Treatment of dystonia with tetrahydrobiopterin. N Engl J Med 1983;308:157–158.

28. Martinius J, Neuhauser G. Segawa-syndrom: Torsiondystonie mit Beginn im Kindersalter und deutlicher Fluktuation der Symptomatik im Tagesverlauf. Kasuistischer Beitrag. Padiatr Prax 1983;28:45–49.

29. Richards CL, Bedard PJ, Fortin G, Malouin F. Quantitative evaluation of the effects of L-dopa in torsion dystonia: a case report. Neurology 1983;33:1083–1087.

30. Chan-Lui WY, Low LCK. Progressive dystonia with marked diurnal fluctuation in a Chinese family. Aust Paediatr J 1984;20:143–146.

31. Chan-Lui WY, Low LCK. A patient with myasthenia gravis and progressive dystonia with marked diurnal fluctuation. Dev Med Child Neurol 1984;26:665–668.

32. Kumamoto I, Nomoto M, Yoshidome H, et al. Five cases of dystonia with marked diurnal fluctuation and special reference to homovanillic acid in CSF. Clin Neurol 1984;24:697–702.

33. Bertelsmann FW, Smith LME. Progressive dystonia with marked diurnal fluctuation. Clin Neurol Neurosurg 1985;87:123–126.

34. Deonna T, Ferreira A. Idiopathic fluctuating dystonia: a case of foot dystonia and writer's cramp responsive to L-dopa. Dev Med Child Neurol 1985;27:819–821.

35. Deonna T. Dopa-sensitive progressive dystonia of childhood with fluctuations of symptoms—Segawa's syndrome and possible variants. Neuropediatrics 1986;17:81–85.

36. LeWitt PA, Miller LP, Levine RA, et al. Tetrahydro-biopterin in dystonia: identification of abnormal metabolism and therapeutic trials. Neurology 1986;36:760–764.

37. Nygaard TG, Duvoisin RC. Hereditary dystonia-parkinsonism syndrome of juvenile onset. Neurology 1986;36:1424–1428.

38. Segawa M, Nomura Y, Kase M. Hereditary progressive dystonia with marked diurnal fluctuation: clinico-pathophysiological identification in reference to juvenile Parkinson's disease. Adv Neurol 1987;45:227–234.

39. Shimoyamada Y, Yoshikawa A, Kashii H, et al. Hereditary progressive dystonia—an observation of the catecholamine metabolism during L-dopa therapy in a 9-year-old girl. No Ho Hattatsu 1986;18:505–509.

40. Torelli D, Lamontanara G, Bracciolini M, Ciaravolo GA. Hereditary progressive dystonia with marked diurnal fluctuation in a family with pigmentary retinopathy. Acta Neurol 1986;8:626–632.

41. Vogel HP. Zum Problem der L-dopa-sensiblen Dystonie. Akt Neurol 1986;13:102–105.

42. Costeff H, Gadoth N, Mendelson L, et al. Fluctuating dystonia responsive to levodopa. Arch Dis Child 1987;62:801–804.

43. Nomura K, Yamamoto N, Takahashi I, et al. Bromocriptine and L-dopa therapy: comparison in a case of hereditary progressive dystonia with marked diurnal fluctuation. No To Hattatsu 1987;19:244–248.

44. de Yebenes JG, Moskowitz C, Fahn S, Saint-Hilaire MH. Long-term treatment with levodopa in a family with autosomal dominant torsion dystonia. Adv Neurol 1988;50:101–111.

45. Fink JK, Barton N, Cohen W, et al. Dystonia with marked diurnal variation associated with biopterin deficiency. Neurology 1988;38:707–711.

46. Boyd K, Patterson V. Dopa-responsive dystonia: a treatable condition misdiagnosed as cerebral palsy. Br Med J 1989;298:1019–1020.

47. Fink JK, Ravin P, Argoff CE, et al. Tetrahydrobiopterin administration in biopterin-deficient progressive dystonia with diurnal variation. Neurology 1989;39:1393–1395.

48. Nygaard TG. Dopa-responsive dystonia: 20 years into the levodopa era. In: Quinn NP, Jenner PG, eds. Disorders of movement—clinical, pharmacological and physiological aspects. London: Academic Press, 1989:323–337.

49. Nygaard TG, Waran SP, Chutorian AM. Unexplained cerebral palsy: dopa-responsive dystonia? Ann Neurol 1989;26:485.

50. de Jong APJM, Haan EA, Manson JI, et al. Kinetic study of catecholamine metabolism in hereditary progressive dystonia. Neuropediatrics 1989;20:3–11.

51. Nygaard TG, Marsden CD, Fahn S. Dopa-responsive dystonia: long-term treatment response and prognosis. Neurology 1991;41:174–181.

52. Beck DK. Dystonia musculorum deformans with another case in the same family. Proc R Soc Med 1947;40:551.

53. Corner BD. Dystonia musculorum deformans in siblings. Treated with Artane (trihexyphenidyl). Proc R Soc Med 1952;45:451–452.

54. Cotzias GC, Van Woert MH, Schiffer LM. Aromatic amino acids and modification of parkinsonism. N Engl J Med 1967;276:374–379.

55. Barrett RE, Yahr MD, Duvoisin RC. Torsion dystonia and spasmodic torticollis. Results of treatment with L-dopa. Neurology 1970;20:107–113.

56. Chase TN. Biochemical and pharmacologic studies of dystonia. Neurology 1970;20:122–130.

57. Mandell S. The treatment of dystonia with L-dopa and haloperidol. Neurology 1970;20:103–106.

58. Coleman M, Barnet A. L-Dopa reversal of muscular spasm, vomiting and insomnia in a patient with an atypical form of familial dystonia. Trans Am Neurol Assoc 1969;94:91–95.

59. Cooper IS. Levodopa-induced dystonia. Lancet 1972;ii:1317–1318.

60. Eldridge R, Kanter W, Koerber T. Levodopa in dystonia. Lancet 1973;ii:1027–1028.

61. Duvoisin RC, Yahr MD, Lieberman J, et al. The striatal foot. Trans Am Neurol Assoc 1972;97:267.

62. Zeman W, Dyken P. Dystonia musculoram deformans; clinical genetic and pathoanatomical studies. Psychiatr Neurol Neurochir 1967;70:77–121.

63. Burke RE, Brin MF, Fahn S, et al. Analysis of the clinical course of non-Jewish, autosomal dominant torsion dystonia. Mov Disord 1986;1:163–178.

64. Bressman SB, deLeon D, Brin MF, et al. Inheritance of idiopathic torsion dystonia among Ashkenazi Jews. Ann Neurol 1988;50:45–56.

65. Eldridge R. The torsion dystonias: literature review: genetic and clinical studies. Neurology 1970;20(suppl 2):1–78.

66. Marsden CD, Jenner P. L-Dopa action in Parkinson's disease. Trends Neurosci 1981;4:148–150.

67. Fabbrini G, Mouradian MM, Juncos JL, et al. Motor fluctuations in Parkinson's disease: central pathophysiological mechanisms, part 1. Ann Neurol 1988;24:366–371.

68. Leenders KL, Palmer AJ, Quinn N, et al. Brain dopamine metabolism in patients with Parkinson's disease measured with positron emission tomography. J Neurol Neurosurg Psychiatry 1986;49:853–860.

69. Lang AE, Garnett ES, Firnau G, et al. Positron tomography in dystonia. Adv Neurol 1988;50:249–253.

70. Martin WRW, Stoessl AJ, Palmer M, et al. PET scanning in dystonia. Adv Neurol 1988;50:223–229.

71. Sawle GV, Leenders KL, Brooks DJ, et al. Dopa-responsive dystonia: [18-F] dopa positron emission tomography. Ann Neurol 1991;30:24–30.

72. Horowitz G, Greenberg J. Pallido-pyramidal syndrome treated with levodopa. J Neurol Neurosurg Psychiatry 1975;38:238–240.

73. Naidu S, Wolfson LI, Sharpless NS. Juvenile parkinsonism: a patient with possible primary striatal dysfunction. Ann Neurol 1978;3:453–455.

74. Eidelberg D, Moeller JR, Dhawan V, et al. The metabolic anatomy of Parkinson's disease: complementary ^{18}F-fluorodeoxyglucose and ^{18}F-fluorodopa positron emission tomographic studies. Mov Disord 1990;5:203–213.

75. Ichinose H, Ohye T, Takahashi E, et al. Hereditary progressive dystonia with marked diurnal fluctuation caused by mutations in the GTP cyclohyrolase I gene. Nat Genet 1994;8:236–242.

76. Rajput AH, Gibb WRG, Zhong XH, et al. Dopa-responsive dystonia: pathological and biochemical observations in a case. Ann Neurol 1994;35:396–402.

77. Furukawa Y, Shimadzu M, Rajput AH, et al. GTP-cyclohydrolase I gene mutations in hereditary progressive and dopa-responsive dystonia. Ann Neurol 1996;39:609–617.

78. Furukawa Y, Lang AE, Trugman JM, et al. Gender-related penetrance and de novo GTP-cyclohydrolase I gene mutations in dopa-responsive dystonia. Neurology 1998;50:1015–1020.

79. Ludecke B, Dworniczak B, Bartholome K. A point mutation in the tyrosine hydroxylase gene associated with Segawa's syndrome. Hum Genet 1995;95:123–125.

80. Naumann M, Pirker W, Reiners K, et al. [^{123}I]β-CIT single-photon emission tomography in DOPA-responsive dystonia. Mov Disord 1997;12:448–451.

81. Bandmann O, Daniel S, Marsden CD, et al. The GTP-cyclohydrolase I gene in atypical parkinsonian patients: a clinico-genetic study. J Neurol Sci 1996;5:27–32.

82. Hyland K. Other biopterin deficient diseases. Mov Disord 1997;12:35–36 (abstract).

83. Fahn S. Clinical variants of idiopathic torsion dystonia. J Neurol Neurosurg Psychiatry 1989;52(suppl):96–100.

84. Martin WE, Resch JA, Baker AB. Juvenile parkinsonism. Arch Neurol 1971;25:494–500.

85. Gershanik OS, Leist A. Juvenile onset Parkinson's disease. Adv Neurol 1987;45:213–216.

86. Quinn N, Critchley P, Marsden CD. Young onset Parkinson's disease. Mov Disord 1987;2:73–91.

87. Still CN, Herberg K-P. Long-term levodopa therapy for torsion dystonia. South Med J 1976;69:564–566.

88. Burke RE, Fahn S, Marsden CD. Torsion dystonia: a double-blind, prospective trial of high-dosage trihexyphenidyl. Neurology 1986;36:160–164.

Spasmodic Torticollis

Edward Tarlov

INTRODUCTION

It is most satisfying for a physician to write on a clinical disorder when the cause is well known, the natural history understood, and effective therapy available. At present none of these situations applies to spasmodic torticollis. Patients suffering from this disorder, and their physicians, still have to make do with less than satisfactory treatment in most cases. If this chapter makes the point that really satisfactory and effective therapy does not exist for most patients with spasmodic torticollis, its goal will have been met. In treating this disorder physicians must rely heavily on their bedside manner, on encouragement, reassurance, and moral support, making every effort to avoid surgery except in the most severely affected patients.

CLINICAL FEATURES

In most cases spasmodic torticollis is an organic disorder, not a purely psychogenic one. Certainly there are exceptions, and astute clinicians will have to rely on their own careful history, examination, and, most of all, judgment to come to a correct diagnosis.

Stress makes any symptoms worse. Depression may have the same effect. Nevertheless, the stereotyped clinical features of typical spasmodic torticollis are so characteristic that anything other than an organic basis seems most unlikely. It typically affects patients in early to middle adulthood. It usually slowly worsens over a period of years—or is felt to be worsening by a discouraged and embarrassed patient. It is characteristically reduced by light contactual stimulus, such as by the placing of the patient's own finger on the chin lightly forcing the head back to a normal position—or even the same gesture without actually touching the chin. Variations, including retrocollis, where the head is

markedly extended, or antecollis, where the head is flexed forward, are rare but do occur. The sternomastoid and trapezius are typically affected asymmetrically. The most usual pattern is for the head to be rotated with the chin to one side and the neck extended with the occiput approximated to the shoulder on the side opposite that to which the chin is rotated. Spasmodic intermittent muscular contractions are present, although in the late stages, after years, the abnormal posture may take a tonic form.

The congenital wryneck occurring in early life, most probably relating to injury at birth in the majority of cases, is not likely to be clinically confused with typical spasmodic torticollis as described above. It is not spasmodic. In most instances, it arises from muscular injury with a histology of affected neck muscles resembling Volkmann's contracture. In rare instances such as that recently reported by Larkins and Halin, "a congenital anomaly at the craniocervical junction may present with a fixed irregular deformity" (1).

CAUSES OF TORTICOLLIS

Before turning attention to torticollis of the so-called idiopathic variety, it may be useful briefly to comment on the differential diagnosis of torticollis, as the diagnosis of idiopathic torticollis is made by excluding any identifiable cause.

1. Birth injury. Fixed abnormalities of cervical posture can arise from birth injury, as mentioned earlier.
2. Trauma. Trauma in adults as well can lead to torticollis, often with intense pain. Pain may be due to muscular injury or to nerve root compression. The former is common in trauma, whereas the latter is unusual.

The weight of the head on the neck causes it to act like a pendulum in acceleration-deceleration injuries. "Whiplash," a term invented by attorneys to capture the imagination of jurors and increase the financial benefits of otherwise minor injuries, is usually used to describe the painful stretching of the neck muscles that can be caused by trauma. This is common, and almost never serious unless excessive medical treatment is given.

Occasionally a severe rotatory injury results in unilateral dislocation of a pair of cervical facet joints. There may be an associated fracture, but not uncommonly the injury can be ligamentous. The condition is intensely painful and may cause nerve root compression because of the decreased diameter of the intervertebral foramen at the level of facet dislocation. Diagnosis is made by X-ray examination and can be documented in a most elegant fashion by computed tomography (CT). Closed reduction by traction may be attempted, but operative reduction is usually necessary.

3. Inflammatory. Inflamed lymph nodes in the pediatric age group can cause torticollis. Intra- or extraspinal abscess and cellulitis of the soft tissues of the neck can be a cause. Meningitis is an unusual cause of torticollis.

4. Neoplasms. Destructive neoplasms involving the cervical vertebrae can produce torticollis by causing pain.

5. Tonsillar herniation. In children with raised intracranial pressure and tonsillar herniation, a twisted neck posture may be present as a compensatory mechanism to reduce pain.

6. Trochlear nerve palsy. A voluntary compensatory torticollis to reduce diplopia may be a sign of unilateral fourth nerve palsy.

7. Labyrinthitis. Associated with severe vertigo and labyrinthitis, it is an unusual cause of torticollis.

8. Cervical disc herniation. A few words about this are worthwhile as this diagnosis is often offered, usually incorrectly, to explain spasmodic torticollis. True cervical disc herniation is an unusual cause of neck pain. Degenerative changes in the facet joints and in the cervical discs are very common. It is important to distinguish these because true cervical disc herniation, if radicular pain is intense, may require surgical treatment, whereas the ubiquitous degenerative changes in the facet joints and cervical discs that cause most cervical symptoms are not benefited by surgical intervention. Intense radicular pain right down the arm to the hand with sensory disturbance in the thumb and index finger (C6), the middle finger (C7), or the ring and little finger (C8) are prominent symptoms in cervical disc herniation, which most often occurs at C5-6 compressing the C6 root and rarely occurs above C5. Biceps weakness (C6) or triceps weakness (C7 or C8) with accompanying reflex diminution or intrinsic hand-muscle weakness (C8 or T1) may be present. The most important clinical feature of cervical disc herniation is intense pain, and although there may be accompanying torticollis, torticollis itself has in my experience never been the sole presenting symptom of cervical disc rupture.

Cervical spondylosis is widespread in the adult population and is never the cause of torticollis. In spite of this, we still occasionally see patients who have undergone decom-

pressive laminectomy operations in the hope of helping spasmodic torticollis. They are always disappointed to say the least.

SPASMODIC TORTICOLLIS

The spasmodic, intermittent, apparently involuntary movements of the neck described in the opening paragraphs of this chapter are the hallmark of spasmodic torticollis. Their occurrence is highly variable, but usually more pronounced under stress. The cause of isolated spasmodic torticollis in humans is unknown at present. It can be a part of a more generalized dystonia such as dystonia muscular deformans or choreoathetosis, but when the abnormal movements are confined to the neck itself, the cause has not been identified.

Histologic examination of the brain in a well-documented case has revealed no abnormality (2).

We can only speculate at this stage that an underlying disorder of neurotransmitters may be present.

Certainly in some cases the disorder is psychogenic, but I am convinced that in the majority of the many cases I have observed the disorder has an organic basis.

It is of theoretic interest that experimental unilateral vestibular nerve section in lower animals and experimental unilateral brainstem lesions including the vestibular nuclei in lower animals cause a postural abnormality closely resembling spasmodic torticollis. The same lesions, however, in the higher apes and in humans do not cause torticollis (3). Clearly an understanding of the pathophysiology of idiopathic spasmodic torticollis in humans must await further research. This literature has been reviewed elsewhere (2).

Differential Diagnosis

It is obvious from the list of causes of torticollis in Table 79.1 that a careful history and general physical and neurologic examination should lead to the correct diagnosis and should avoid confusing these various entities with one another, thereby avoiding inappropriate tests and therapies.

THERAPIES

Discussion here will be confined to the therapy of spasmodic torticollis, summarized in Table 79.2. Treatment of the other entities listed in Table 79.1 are outside the scope of this chapter.

It is most important to keep in mind when discussing this condition that no therapy has been predictably highly effective over the long run. Claims for short-term relief in small series have been made. Enthusiastic reports have been given. It has been my experience that lasting relief has not been shown by objective criteria with any of these methods. In fact the most effective approach for a physician faced

Table 79.1   Causes of Torticollis

Fixed, Nonspasmodic
Congenital wryneck secondary to birth injury
Cervical trauma
Muscular pain and spasm
Cervical fracture
Unilateral facet dislocation, "locked" facets
Inflammatory
Intra- or extraspinal
Abscess or cellulitis, soft tissues
Cerebellar tonsillar herniation
IV nerve palsy
Labyrinthitis
Cervical disc herniation—be careful in this diagnosis—likely to be wrong unless there are associated definite radicular symptoms and signs in C6, C7, or C8 nerve roots
"Idiopathic"
Spasmodic Torticollis
Psychogenic (unusual)
As part of a more generalized dystonia
"Idiopathic"

Table 79.2   Therapies of Spasmodic Torticollis

Medical	Sedatives—not effective
	Muscle relaxants—no predictable effect
	Antiparkinsonian drugs—no predictable effect
Biofeedback	Occasionally felt to be effective, harmless
Injection	Botulinum toxin, reportedly safe, can give months of relief
Surgery	See indications in text
	1. Peripheral division of XI branches to sternomastoid, trapezius. Safe. Can be somewhat helpful in some cases.
	2. Selective peripheral denervation of neck muscles. Safe. Can be helpful. Probably will prove more effective than procedure 1.
	3. Cervical laminectomy. Anterior cervical rhizotomy C2-4 with or without intradural division of XI nerve. Carries definite serious hazard to life; long-term effectiveness ±.
	4. Thalamotomy. Reportedly helpful, but risks probably outweigh benefits.

with a patient with spasmodic torticollis is a sympathetic examination and an explanation of the alternative therapies and their risks. If this is done, many or most patients given reassurance may elect to live with their symptoms—a decision I strongly support in the present state of our knowledge of this disorder.

It is important in planning therapy to tailor this to the patient's symptoms. For example, pain is a common symptom. This may not be always helped by steps to reduce the power of the cervical musculature.

Medical Therapy

If properly supervised, most of the commonly used medical regimens—sedatives, muscle relaxants, antiparkinsonian medications—are harmless enough.

The usual approaches have included anticholinergics, antidopaminergics, dopaminominetics, and drugs that modify serotonin or aminobutyric acid. Few if any have any obvious beneficial effect.

Pain is often a prominent symptom. Medication for a chronic disorder such as this is not likely to be effective and over the long term is likely to cause dependency or other unwanted side effects.

Biofeedback

This has been effective in some cases. I believe it to be a safe therapy. The physician should not be surprised if it is not effective.

Injections

Botulinum A toxin, which has been successfully used in several ophthalarologic disorders, can reduce the force of unwanted muscle contraction without producing weakness. Its action can last 6 to 8 weeks. For injection, 40 mg of botulinum A toxin was diluted to 1 ml and injections of 0.25 mL were injected into two sites in the two most active of the sternomastoid, splenius capitis, and trapezius for 21 patients reported in one study (4); the results were felt to demonstrate benefit in a significant number. This reviewer doubts the significance of the findings and can only conclude that this form of therapy is in its preliminary stages.

SURGICAL THERAPIES

Peripheral division of the XI nerve branches to the sternomastoid and trapezius. A clinical decision as to which muscles are predominantly effective is necessary in making a judgment about which muscles to denervate. Although in theory such a statement seems logical, I find it very difficult to be sure which muscles are most active, particularly as all the cervical muscles act together in any neck movement. Nevertheless, being superficial the sternomastoid and trapezius are easy enough to examine. The XI nerve branch to the sternomastoid can be divided at the posterior border of the midportion of this muscle, and the proximal end doubled back on itself to discourage regeneration. The XI branches to the upper part of the trapezius on the affected side are similarly divided, avoiding denervating the lower part of this muscle, to avert shoulder drooping. This operation has safety to recommend it, but it has been only marginally effective in the long run in most cases.

In an effort to safely provide more widespread denervation, Bertrand et al (5) have advocated selective peripheral denervation not only of cervical muscles innervated by XI but also of cervical muscles innervated by C1 to C4 or C5. Preoperative electromyography to identify the most active muscles has been carried out, and the suspected muscles are then infiltrated with xylocaine to test the effect of their denervation. The denervation is performed under light anesthesia. He has reported carrying out the procedure in 20 patients, 2 of whom experienced transient difficulties in swallowing. The procedure is claimed to be effective, but reports of long-term follow-up are needed, particularly as some degree of regeneration would be expected and would not have to progress far to reinnervate the cervical musculature.

Cervical laminectomy for intradural section of C1 to C4 anterior roots on the side more severely affected, C1 to C3 anterior roots on the less severely affected side, and bilateral intradural section of the spinal accessory nerves at the level of C1 has been in use for many years, since the original descriptions of McKenzie (6) and Dandy (7). The operation is often quite effective (8,9), but there have been occasionally devastating complications (10,11), including cerebral infarction, vascular catastrophe, and paralysis of both arms, due perhaps to spinal cord ischemia. The occasional occurrence of such serious complications has made surgeons consider even more carefully the indications for surgery in such a benign condition as this.

Thalamotomy has been occasionally used for spasmodic torticollis (12). The lesions in the ventral thalamus (VO1) somewhat anterior to the target for standard thalamotomy in another movement disorder may have to be bilateral to be effective. The incidence of speech and swallowing disturbances and impairment in intellect has been unacceptably high in most series of bilateral lesions. In general, thalamotomy does not appear to be the best answer for spasmodic torticollis.

SUMMARY

We are faced here with a disorder that is at present very difficult to treat effectively. Once correct diagnosis is established, it is my feeling that the patient should be made well aware of the very serious limitations and risks of the major surgical approaches. Until we reach a better understanding of the cause of this disorder—and perhaps with this will come safer, more effective therapy—I would advise a course of biofeedback therapy and sympathetic reassurance that the condition is a benign one that is unlikely to cause any significant functional impairment. In patients who are most severely affected, peripheral intraspinal denervation procedures may be worth considering, providing the patient understands their limitations. More effective therapy will no doubt come when we better understand the cause of this annoying disorder.

REFERENCES

1. Larkins MV, Halin J. Unusual presentation of torticollis. 5th Annual Meeting of Joint Section on Disorders of the Spine and Peripheral Nerves. American Association of Neurological Surgeons/Congress of Neurological Surgeons, February 11–15, 1989. Abstract 21.
2. Tarlov E. On the problem of the pathology of spasmodic torticollis in man. J Neurol Neurosurg Psychiatry 1970;33:457–463.
3. Tarlov E. The postural effect of lesions of the vestibular nuclei: a note on species differences among primates. J Neurosurg 1969;31:187–195.
4. Tsui K, Eisen A, Stoessl DB. Double-blind study of botulinum toxin in spasmodic torticollis. Lancet, 1986:245–246.
5. Bertrand C, Molina-Negro P, Martinez SN. Technical aspects of selective peripheral denervation for spasmodic torticollis. Appl Neurophysiol 1982;45:326–330.
6. McKenzie KG. The surgical treatment of spasmodic torticollis. Clin Neurosurg 1955;12:37–42.
7. Dandy WE. An operation for the treatment of spasmodic torticollis. Arch Surg 1930;20:1021–1033.
8. Sorenson BF, Hamby WB. Spasmodic torticollis: results in 71 surgically treated patients. Neurology 1966;16:867–878.
9. Hamby WB, Schiffer S. Spasmodic torticollis: results after cervical rhizotomy in 50 cases. J Neurosurg 1969;31:323–326.
10. Adams CBT. Vascular catastrophe following the Dandy-McKenzie operation for spasmodic torticollis. J Neurol Neurosurg Psychiatry 1984;47:990–994.
11. Sweet WH. What should the neurosurgeon do when faced with a malpractice suit? Clin Neurosurg 1975;23:112–124.
12. Bertrand C, Molina-Negro P, Martinez SN. Combined stereotactic and peripheral surgical approach for spasmodic torticollis. Appl Neurophysiol 1978;41:122–133.

Disorders of Movement Associated with Sleep

Cataplexy

J. GILA LINDSLEY

The term *cataplexy* is derived from the Greek *kataplexis* and literally means to be struck down, as from amazement or terror. In that sense well-named, cataplexy refers to a complete or partial flaccid paralysis generally precipitated by an emotional event. The attacks are brief. Their usual duration is between 5 and 30 seconds, although a 2-minute duration is not uncommon. There are rare reports of cataplectic attacks enduring for 30 minutes (1).

HISTORY AND OVERVIEW

Historically, the consideration of cataplexy is almost completely embedded in the narcolepsy literature because cataplexy occurs most commonly as a feature of that syndrome. Especially because until recently the effort has been to seek a common mechanism for the precipitous sleep attacks of narcolepsy and the associated auxiliary symptoms including cataplexy, only on occasion has cataplexy been singled out for independent scholarly treatment. Although an idiopathic form of cataplexy is described in this chapter, it is by virtue of its historical association to narcolepsy that a chapter devoted to the movement disorder cataplexy is placed with other sleep-related movement disorders.

Gelineau (2), credited with the first identification of narcolepsy as a differentiated syndrome, was likely also the first to describe what we now know as cataplexy in relation to the syndrome narcolepsy. His expressed sentiment at the time was that it was a type of neurosis. Henneberg (3), in the early twentieth century, also described cataplexy with narcolepsy. Adie (4), in 1926, provided further characterization of a cataplectic episode. His objective examination of patients showed that tendon reflexes had completely disappeared during a cataplectic attack. It was, however, Wilson (5) in 1928 who is generally credited with having provided the first personal description of a cataplectic attack. Accord-

ing to Wilson, during attacks not only the tendon reflexes but also the H-reflex are abolished. Wilson noted also that during a cataplectic attack plantar responses are extensor, and he later characterized cataplectic attacks as inhibitory epileptic attacks (6).

In 1957, Yoss and Daly (7), in their characterization of the narcolepsy tetrad, included cataplexy as one of the four major components of the syndrome. The notion of a narcoleptic tetrad persists to this day.

Description

A cataplectic attack can vary with respect to muscle groups affected and the degree to which they are affected. Guilleminault et al (8) described the spectrum of involvement as ranging from the "entire voluntary musculature" through "limited involvement of specific muscle groups" to a "generalized fleeting sense of weakness." The extraocular muscles generally are not involved. The most common manifestation, according to Guilleminault and colleagues, are a sagging jaw and inclined head and a slight buckling of the knees. Flexor and extensor muscles are involved. Consciousness is maintained.

Cataplexy as a feature of narcolepsy rarely is the first of the syndrome to develop but rather generally begins a period of time after the onset of severe daytime sleepiness. Once present, the rate at which attacks occur varies. Some individuals have attacks only on occasion. At the other extreme are some few reported cases of virtually continuous cataplectic attacks. Roth (1) and more recently Aldrich (9), for instance, reported cases of status catiplecticus.

From the vantage point of the patient, complete cataplectic attacks can be overwhelming experiences. They have a very rapid onset and are for that reason generally unavoidable. Moreover, they may involve dropping to the floor, which, even if the episode endures for only a matter of seconds, can be extremely disruptive and embarrassing. Perceptual distortions associated with a cataplectic attack can be equally unnerving. The following description was made by a patient at our sleep disorders center. Not incidentally, before being treated for cataplexy he reported an average of about 20 cataplectic attacks daily. We were witness to a number of these. Central nervous system (CNS) lesion was ruled out for this patient.

Case Study
The trigger is always emotional. Conflictual laughing. Horsing around such as when I am dancing. Never when I am crying. When I feel angry but am restraining it. The attack develops from head to foot. Head and neck muscles are affected before the rest of my body. If I have a partial attack, just my eyes [rolling back] or my jaw are affected. I can abort the attack by tightening major muscle groups or by sliding down a wall and squatting—if I catch it in time. There are some anticipatory cues. I feel extremely sleepy just beforehand, yet very alert. I do not experience the confusion, disorientation, and automatic behavior that I experience in the wake of a sleep attack. [During a cataplectic attack] my eyes close. It feels like a cone fitting on my face, as if my eyes were pulling together, [as if the] skin were pulling together. It is as if my eye muscles had moved. This is different from the unfocusing of each eye—that is each eye moving independently—which happens with a sleep attack. This experience of a change in my eyes is hard to describe, but is an important part of the experience. I feel as if my eyebrows were below my nose. The feeling of sleepiness abates when the loss of muscle tone is complete. At times I feel some disorientation, at times it is extreme. The paralysis is very different from the paralysis I experience with an episode of sleep paralysis [see Chapter 81]. For instance [in the case of cataplexy] even the stimulation from a burning cigarette does not release it. I am fully paralyzed. Once I have fallen down, nothing will break it until it breaks spontaneously. [With sleep paralysis, generally a light touch or the calling of the patient's name will break the episode.] I do not have cataplectic attacks if I am lying down. When I come out of a sleep paralysis attack, I am not sure where I am. When I come out of a cataplectic attack, I am very oriented.

Objective Studies

There are a few objective studies of patients during a cataplectic attack (8,10,11).

Electroencephalographic Findings
Data from all three studies provide strong objective evidence that the patient is awake during the cataplectic attack; that the attack variously does or does not lead to drowsiness and eventually sleep; and that if sleep does ensue, it generally is a sleep onset rapid eye movement (REM) period

(SOREMP). Guilleminault et al (8) found in all of their subjects that at least for short periods the recording was indistinguishable from REM sleep. Data from the Rechtschaffen and Dement study (11) would also suggest that all sensory systems are intact during the attack.

Electromyographic Findings
During the attacks, either hypotonia or complete atonia is recorded. Electromyography (EMG) shows decrease in tone of both agonists and antagonists. In addition, short bursts of muscle discharges are observed. Rechtschaffen and Dement's 1967 study (11) also documented inhibition of tendon reflexes but persistence of voluntary eye movements. The 1974 study by Guilleminault and co-workers (8) indicated that during an attack the eyelids might drop and eye movements might be uncoordinated. If the atonia affected upper and lower limbs, the pertinent jerk reflexes were also absent. The H-reflex, as well, was abolished. With attacks that affected only the jaw and neck muscles, abolition of the H-reflex was limited to the beginning of the attack, at the same time as transient decrease of tone was recorded in the legs. If the stimulation associated with elicitation of the H-reflex led to pain, the H-reflex would return with transient bursts of muscle activity.

Precipitants

Since it was first characterized, cataplexy has been understood generally to have strong emotion as its precipitant (12). There has not, however, been a systematic study of the kinds of emotional precipitants likely to trigger a cataplectic attack. Based largely upon anecdotal data, Roth (1) suggested that laughter is the highest probability trigger for cataplexy. Sudden joy, sudden excitement, surprise, anger, fatigue, and heavy meals are also described as common triggers (13). This is consistent with the findings from an unpublished study conducted with members of the Narcolepsy Network, a national self-help group.

The affect that triggers cataplexy does not have to be intense. One of our own patients reported that simply chuckling at a newspaper cartoon was sufficient to elicit an attack. Roth also describes rage—if associated with violent movements—and "any abrupt movement, even unaccompanied by emotion" as triggers for an attack. Reports are cited indicating that sneezing, coughing, and nose blowing might be effective stimuli. Less commonly cataplexy also occurs spontaneously, that is in the absence of any obvious trigger (1,8).

Incidence

Cataplexy is variously reported to develop in 67% to 95% (13) and in 60% to 70% (1) of all cases of narcolepsy. It has the highest probability of occurrence in an individual if SOREMPs are demonstrated with objective recording.

Independent Cataplexy

Cataplexy also can occur in an independent form, that is, not as a component of a narcoleptic syndrome. The incidence rate of independent cataplexy is unknown. There are very few descriptions of it. Roth (1) documented that 3 of 360 patients he studied had "monosymptomatic" cataplexy. He cautioned, however, that on occasion cataplexy can be the first symptom of narcolepsy and that the characteristic sleep attacks of narcolepsy may not develop for several years.

Gelardi and Brown (14) first documented the transmission of independent cataplexy as an isolated dominant trait. They reviewed four generations of a family with a high incidence rate of apparently independent cataplexy. The transmission of laughter-induced drop attacks—that is, idiopathic cataplexy—is described as an unmixed autosomal dominant trait of high penetrance. In virtually all of the cases, laughter was the precipitant. Tickling led to virtual paralysis in one family member. Onset was early, as many family members had their first episode at 4 to 5 years of age. Attacks seemed to decrease in frequency after age 30. Attacks were described as sudden limpness of the arms and legs, drooping of the mouth, eyelids, and head, buckling of the knees, and collapse to the ground. Episodes lasted from a few moments up to 30 seconds.

Hartse et al (15) also studied several generations of one family with laughter or tickle-induced drop attacks. Onset in this family was very early—3 to 8 months of age. Based primarily upon symptom history, the authors estimated that 30% of the 89 family members considered were affected. In all but one case, transmission appears to have been through the maternal line. The impression was of an autosomal dominant mode of transmission with incomplete penetrance. Three affected family members were studied objectively. Common signs of narcolepsy—SOREMP during sleep and pathologic sleepiness during the daytime—were not present.

DIAGNOSTIC CONSIDERATIONS

Diagnosis of cataplexy when it is part of the narcoleptic syndrome generally is indirect. The diagnosis is based upon findings consistent with narcolepsy–cataplexy.

1. History. The patient complains either of generalized daytime sleepiness or precipitous sleep attacks; and of sudden muscle weakness generally in response to an affective stimulus, exercise, or eating.
2. Objective establishment of a diagnosis of narcolepsy. This entails nighttime polysomnographic monitoring and a multiple sleep latency test (MSLT) during the following day.

The polysomnographic study permits other causes of excessive daytime sleepiness—such as obstructive sleep apnea and periodic limb movement disorder (previously referred to as "nocturnal myoclonus")—to be ruled out. Frequently, a SOREMP (in which REM, or dreaming, sleep occurs very close to the beginning of the sleep period instead of 90 minutes or so after sleep is initiated) is found for narcoleptics.

The MSLT consists of four to six 20-minute opportunities to sleep, spaced at 2-hour intervals. The expected result for a narcoleptic patient would be sleep latencies of about 5 minutes and the rapid development of REM sleep in at least two of the naps. If the findings of the objective studies are positive, it is unlikely that further diagnostic efforts of the cataplectic symptoms are necessary.

In the absence of complaints of complete drop attacks, it is possible that the clinician might miss the diagnosis of cataplexy. In this regard, the clinician should be cognizant that complete cataplectic attacks, during which the patient falls to the ground, are less common. More common are cataplectic attacks of very brief duration that affect only a portion of the musculature, for example, a sagging jaw and inclined head and slight buckling of the knees (13). Especially if the patient reports these episodes to occur in association with emotional events and/or if there is a concurrent complaint either of generalized daytime sleepiness or precipitous sleep attacks, cataplexy should be suspected.

When cataplectic-like symptoms occur in isolation from complaints of daytime sleepiness or in the apparent absence of emotional precipitants, establishment of the diagnosis is more difficult. Independent cataplexy, a true cataplexy, must be differentiated from other disorders that can affect muscle tonus, for example, transient ischemic attacks (TIA) and multiple sclerosis. We have seen one case in which the patient's description of what ultimately was diagnosed as a TIA so strongly suggested cataplectic attacks that the patient was referred for sleep evaluation. In differentiating cataplexy from other disorders, the completely reversible, highly transient character of cataplexy and maintenance of consciousness should be kept in mind.

Under certain circumstances, the possibility of CNS lesion should also be taken into consideration. Such circumstances include the case of isolated cataplectic symptoms with no related family history and late-onset cataplexy with or without associated daytime sleepiness. The usual age of onset for narcolepsy is in the second decade of life. Rarely, cataplexy is the first symptom. More commonly, cataplexy develops up to several years after the onset of the characteristic sleepiness. In some cases, there may be no cue to consider a CNS lesion. Unfortunately it is possible for CNS insult to mimic idiopathic narcolepsy with cataplexy (see below). As a rule of thumb, if age of onset, additional symptomatology, family history, and so forth are atypical, the possibility that the presenting symptoms of narcolepsy–cataplexy are secondary to CNS insult should be considered.

CATAPLEXY SECONDARY TO CNS INSULT

Anderson and Salmon (16) described a patient who developed, in succession over several years, excessive daytime sleepiness with nap attacks, postdormital sleep paralysis, and finally full cataplectic attacks. The cataplexy was spontaneous or secondary to startle and was not elicited either by laughter or anger. Despite an unremarkable developmental sequence for narcolepsy, necropsy (cause of death unrelated) suggested the cataplexy at least was secondary to damage to the rostral brainstem reticular nuclei. Major abnormalities in the area of the third ventricle, pituitary stalk, septum pellucidum, internal capsule, lenticular nuclei, and in the upper brainstem also were demonstrated.

D'Cruz et al (17) described two patients with isolated cataplexy with concurrent multiple sclerosis. Magnetic resonance imaging (MRI) studies demonstrated pontomedullary lesions in both the patients.

Virtually continuous cataplexy in association with sleep attacks and sleep paralysis was observed in a patient with a midbrain tumor (18). Similarly, severe cataplexy, over 100 cataplectic attacks per day, was found in a patient with a posterior fossa tumor that impinged upon the anterolateral aspects of the left cerebellar hemisphere (19). The cataplexy had been preceded 20 years earlier by the development of excessive daytime sleepiness. The development of transient cataplexy after removal of a craniopharyngioma (20) and chronic cataplectic-like episodes in association with cortical meningiomas (21) also have been documented. Ethelberg (22) presented two case studies describing cataplectic-like symptoms in association with a depressed fracture over the lateral surface of the frontal lobes. Both were resolved with corrective surgery of the skull defect.

CATAPLEXY WITH OTHER MEDICAL ILLNESSES

Cataplectic symptoms in association with excessive daytime sleepiness and hypnagogic hallucinations have also been observed as part of other medical illnesses. It has been documented as part of a cataplexy–muscle weakness–McCardle's syndrome (23) in association with systemic lupus erythematosus (24). Weakness attacks were lateralized to the right side and were triggered by laughter. Speech was also impaired during the attacks although, as with cataplexy in general, consciousness persisted. In none of the foregoing cases of cataplexy in the context of another medical illness was it possible to determine whether the cataplexy was independent or causally related to the concurrent disorder. Cataplexy was also recently reported in a patient with Norrie disease (25), which is an X-linked recessive disorder causing ocular atrophy, mental retardation, deafness, and dysmorphic features, and in multiple sclerosis, as above (17).

Pseudocataplexy, apparently indistinguishable from true cataplexy, was documented in an 11-year-old girl with Niemann–Pick disease (26). Behaviorally the events presented as stereotypic giggling followed immediately by loss of muscle tone; they occurred numerous times daily. Electroencephalography (EEG) demonstrated these to be gelastic–atonic seizures. Twelve attacks were captured by EEG studies. The stereotypic giggling was shown to be part of the developing seizure, not a precipitant of the "cataplectic" attack.

A rule of thumb regarding diagnosis of cataplexy is first to determine, on the basis of history and objective study, if it is part of a narcoleptic syndrome. If positive and mitigating factors are absent, there is no need for further diagnostic procedures. In the presence of isolated symptoms of cataplexy, in the presence of unusual presentation or absence of family history, and certainly in the presence of additional pathologic symptoms, further diagnostic procedures should be undertaken. The type of additional diagnostic procedure (e.g., computerized tomography scan or MRI EEG, and so forth) would depend upon the nature of the symptomatology.

TREATMENT

Treatment of cataplexy, both independent cataplexy and cataplexy as part of the narcoleptic syndrome, is pharmacologic. Tricyclic antidepressants with anticholinergic side effects have become the most commonly used anticataplectic drugs. Akimoto et al (27) introduced this form of treatment for cataplexy after they studied the effects of numerous classes of drugs on the various symptoms of narcolepsy in 80 cases. They found that stimulants mitigated daytime sleepiness but had no effect on cataplexy. Imipramine 50 mg produced complete control of cataplexy in 9 of 10 of their cases. The effect began an hour after ingestion of the imipramine and persisted for several days. The Japanese group questioned whether the effect of imipramine on cataplexy was direct or mediated by its effect on emotion. Perhaps as a partial answer to how this class of drugs might treat cataplexy, Nishino et al (28) and Mignot et al (29), using a canine model of cataplexy, concluded that the affinity of these medications for the alpha-1 central noradrenergic postsynaptic receptors is the effective site of action.

Since Schmidt et al (30) demonstrated protriptyline to be an effective anticataplectic agent in 1977, protriptyline at a dosage level of approximately 20 mg/day has in the United States become widely used. Clomipramine, studied as a treatment for cataplexy by Parkes and Schachter in 1979 (31), is widely used in Europe. Desipramine, another tricyclic antidepressant with anticholinergic side effects, is also used in the treatment of cataplexy, with a usual dosage of approximately 200 mg/day (32). The atropine-like properties of these more anticholinergic tricyclic antidepressants are assumed by many to be central to their effectiveness. This impression is supported by the recent work of Reid et al (33) on the neurochemistry of canine cataplexy.

However, there is some indication that fluoxetine (34,35) and viloxazine (36), tricyclic antidepressants without atropine-like and cholinergic side effects, might also be effective.

Freemon (37) found that anticholinergic antiparkinsonian medications were more effective than the tricyclic antidepressants with anticholinergic side effects. He favored trihexyphenidyl (Artane), 2 mg three times a day, but also suggested alternatives such as benztropin (Cogentin) 1 mg three times a day; biperiden (Akineton) 2 mg three times a day; ethopropazine (Parsidol) 10 mg three times a day; and procyclidine (Kemadrin) 5 mg three times daily. His experience is that with these drugs the patient does not develop a tolerance to the anticataplectic side effects and therefore that drug holidays are unnecessary. We have had success treating severe cataplexy in one patient with trihexiphenidyl in the slow-release formulation. When used in the nonslow-release form, however, the patient continuously cycled between relief from cataplexy and what appeared to be rebound episodes of strikingly severe cataplectic attacks.

Because of some of the undesirable side effects of tricyclic antidepressants, especially impotence, there has been an effort to develop alternative pharmacologic approaches. Anticataplectic effectiveness has been claimed for clonidine, an alpha-adrenergic blocker with significant REM effects (38); zimelidine, a serotonin reuptake inhibitor (39); clonazepam (31), a benzodiazepine that acts on the gamma-aminobutyric acid (GABA) system; and L-tyrosine (40), a dietary precursor of the catecholamines. The effective starting dose for the latter was eight 400 mg capsules for women and ten 400 mg capsules for men, divided into A.M. and midday doses. Concurrent treatment with vitamin B6 compromised the effectiveness.

Gamma-hydroxybutyrate (GHB), one of the more promising treatments for cataplexy, is in the final stages of FDA clinical testing (recommended dose will likely be 4.5–9.0 g) (41–42b). There are some data suggesting that GHB, a normal metabolite of GABA in the nervous system, may itself be either a neurotransmitter or neuromodulator in the brain. It is a dopamine release blocker and potentiates the central release of acetylcholine in the striatum. Its effect in normals when administered at night is to decrease REM latency and to increase percent of total sleep time in delta (deep non-REM) sleep. In narcoleptics, GHB addresses a number of the auxiliary symptoms of narcolepsy, especially including cataplexy. The deduction regarding its mechanism of action for narcoleptics is that it induces the symptoms of narcolepsy (? a natural narcoleptogenic compound) and when taken at night, contains these to the sleep period. One of the main disadvantages of GHB, at this point, is that it must be administered at intervals during the night, generally about 2.25–3 g taken two to three times per night.

For the patient with cataplexy, especially if it is severe, it is likely that there will also be beneficial effects from some form of psychotherapy or a therapeutic support group. A primary issue is the handling of emotions. It is not unusual for patients affected with severe cataplexy to present with an apparent absence of emotional expression and indeed to expend significant effort avoiding situations that might induce emotional responses and secondarily a cataplectic attack. Information regarding support groups, where strategies for dealing with emotion are shared among participants, can be obtained from the national office of the Narcolepsy Network, a national self-help group.

SCIENTIFIC ISSUES

A canine model of narcolepsy has been developed in recent years (43) through selective breeding for cataplexy. While there continues to be controversy in the field regarding whether the canine model is a useful human analogue (44), development of the model has resulted in the identification of genetic loci common to narcoleptic dogs and humans. These may only be genetic markers for narcolepsy (or at least cataplexy), but it is equally possible that they actually code for narcolepsy–cataplexy. Whichever of these possibilities is true, at least in dogs it is unambiguously clear that cataplexy can be genetically transmitted. The suggestion is strong that narcolepsy is genetically transmitted in humans as well. Unraveling of the genetics of the disorder is still very much in process. However, even once the genes that code for narcolepsy are identified, there will still remain a related question: What are the factors for which these genes code that result in sudden, transient atonia during wakefulness?

Cataplexy as a Dissociated Fragment of REM Sleep

One possibility is that the involved genes code for the dissociation of components of REM sleep. A prevailing assumption is that narcolepsy is a disorder of REM sleep and that cataplexy, as well as sleep paralysis, reflect the inappropriate timing of the motor inhibition aspect of REM sleep (8,10,45,47,48). The argument is that REM sleep is the only state during which there is the spontaneous development of complete muscle atonia (see Chapter 81 on sleep paralysis and Chapter 82 on REM sleep behavior disorder for more detail regarding the substrates of motor inhibition during REM sleep).

Conceptualized therefore as a fractional or dissociated manifestation of REM sleep occurring during wakefulness, the atonia of cataplexy (and sleep paralysis) is correspondingly assumed to share the same physiologic substrates as motor inhibition during normal REM sleep (46). According to this formulation, it is possible that the loci that code for narcolepsy in some way code for this dissociation of the elements of REM sleep, and therefore for a vulnerability to cataplectic attacks.

Cholinergic Mediation?

The assumption that REM atonia and the atonia of cataplexy share common mechanisms has generated a significant amount of research, primarily pharmacologic. The cholinergic system has been a main focus as a significant body of basic research data suggests that the timing of REM sleep depends upon cholinergic systems (see Chapters 81 and 82). The demonstrated effectiveness of powerfully anticholinergic tricyclic antidepressants and the apparent anticataplectic effectiveness of antiparkinsonian anticholinergic medications suggest a dependence of cataplexy upon a cholinergic chemical pathway. Also consistent, cataplectic-like behavior has been induced in cats after microinjection of carbachol (an acetylcholine agonist) into the pontine reticular formation (49).

The canine model of cataplexy offers more direct assessment of possible cholinergic mediation. Reid et al (33) concluded that the cholinergic aspect of cataplexy in canine narcolepsy is mediated by M2 muscarinic receptors in the pontine reticular formation.

Involvement of Other Neurochemical Systems?

The neurochemistry of cataplexy may involve more that one system. Analogizing the neurochemical mediation of cataplexy to the neurochemical mediation of REM sleep, Hishikawa and Shimizu (12) postulated an error in the balance between cholinergic and cholinoceptive REM sleep-on neuronal population and the monoaminergic REM sleep-off neuronal population. They speculated that there may be either hypersensitivity or hyperactivity of the cholinergic system, or hypoactivity of the monoaminergic system in the brainstem areas involved with REM sleep.

There is now ample documentation that drugs that do not act directly on cholinergic systems are also effective in attenuating cataplexy (see above). The primary question these data raise is whether they contradict the acetylcholine theory of cataplexy. The putative effectiveness of zimelidine and fluoxetine, both serotonin reuptake inhibitors, might suggest that the atonia of cataplexy depends upon hypoactivity of the central serotonin system. Unquestionably the anticataplectic effects of zimelidine depend neither upon the suppression of REM sleep nor directly upon antagonism of cholinergic systems: zimelidine is a serotonin reuptake inhibitor, and neither REM sleep during naps nor SOREMPs during nighttime sleep were eliminated with zimelidine treatment despite the suppression of cataplexy.

These findings do not necessarily contradict either the acetylcholine hypothesis or the (generally associated) hypothesis that cataplexy and REM sleep share common substrates. Zimelidine may act on a different aspect of the emotion–atonia circuitry. Montplaisir and Godbout (50) interpreted their data to suggest that zimelidine's anticata-

plectic effects depend upon interference with the neural processes by which emotions lead to cataplexy.

Klonopin, a benzodiazepine that therefore affects GABA receptors, also reportedly attenuates cataplexy when given at bedtime. Similar to zimelidine, its effectiveness in mitigating cataplexy does not necessarily contradict a cholinergic substrate for cataplexy's muscle atonia. Foutz et al (47) argued that its effect on cataplexy may be indirect, mediated by attenuation of disruptive myoclonic activity during nighttime sleep rather than by directly correcting inappropriately timed alpha motor neuron suppression. When administered in the daytime, it can produce sleepiness and muscle weakness.

In the absence of further follow-up, however, it is equally possible that these data can be interpreted to mean that the mechanisms giving rise to the atonia of cataplexy are different from those producing the atonia of normal REM sleep. That is, the catecholamines and indoleamines may also be involved. In that regard, the L-tyrosine data described earlier, if replicated, would suggest hypoactivity of catecholamines, possibly dopamine, may be involved in the development of cataplexy. The fact that it is possible to affect cataplexy without affecting the characteristic SOREMP periods of narcolepsy and without suppressing REM sleep during daytime naps would suggest that the contributions of chemical pathways other than the acetylcholine pathway must still be seriously evaluated.

The Affect–Cataplexy Link

An aspect of cataplexy that is extremely salient—elicitation of cataplectic attacks by affectively charged stimuli—has generated a surprisingly small body of research. This potential clue to the substrates of cataplexy was pursued vigorously in 1964 by Vizzioli (51), who proposed that cataplexy might be the prolongation of the normal version of knee buckling with emotion. The similar positions of Wilder (52) and van Bogaert (53), who considered cataplexy to be the pathologic exaggeration of normal tonic inhibition in association with any emotion, were cited in this context. Vizzioli proposed that abnormal activation of inhibitory systems among pontine structures, hippocampus, and the amygdala occur secondary to emotion and that the limbic system might be initiating the cataplectic attack. This idea has not been well pursued since then, although Nan'no et al (54) did hypothesize several years later that neural systems commonly active during anger, surprise, and so forth might facilitate the descending inhibition of motor output during cataplectic attacks.

More recently, the possible causal relationship between emotional reactivity and cataplexy has led to a focus on the autonomic nervous system. The possible roles of cardioacceleration, aberrant baroreceptor responsivity, and emotion as they might relate to cataplexy are under current consideration (55–59). Findings are not consistent and the body of literature is as yet too small to permit conclusions. This approach, however, may prove fruitful.

In conclusion, the scientific issues regarding cataplexy that are most intensively being pursued are several: 1) How is cataplexy transmitted? 2) What is the complete set of elements in the neural circuit necessary to account for all aspects of the cataplectic attack, from elicitation through atonia to spontaneous resolution? What are the associated chemistries? 3) More specifically, is cataplexy in fact a dissociated fragment of REM sleep and does the atonia of cataplexy rely upon the same biologic substrate as the atonia of REM sleep? 4) By what mechanism does emotion trigger cataplexy? For instance, does it rely upon a hyperresponsive limbic system component? Does the association rely upon aberrant autonomic control affecting a motor inhibition pathway?

REFERENCES

1. Roth B. Cataplexy. In: Roth B, ed. Narcolepsy and Hypersomnia. Schlierlová M (trans.) Basel: Karger, 1980:68–73.
2. Gelineau J. De la narcolepsi. Gaz Hop Paris 1880;53:626–628.
3. Henneberg R. Uber Genuine Narcolepsie. Neurol Zentralbl 1916;35:282–290.
4. Adie WJ. Idiopathic narcolepsy: a disease sui generic. Brain 1926;49:257–306.
5. Wilson SAK. The narcolepsies. Brain 1928;51:63–109.
6. Wilson SAK. Neurology. Vol. II. London: Edward Arnold, 1940.
7. Yoss RE, Daly DD. Criteria for the diagnosis of the narcoleptic syndrome. Proc Mayo Clin 1957;32:320–328.
8. Guilleminault C, Wilson RA, Dement WC. A study on cataplexy. Arch Neurol 1974;31:255–261.
9. Aldrich MS. The neurobiology of narcolepsy-cataplexy. Prog Neurobiol 1993;41(5):533–541.
10. Hishikawa Y, Kancho Z. Electroencephalographic study on narcolepsy. Electroencephalogr Clin Neurophysiol 1965;18:249–259.
11. Rechtschaffen A, Dement WC. Studies on the relationship of narcolepsy, cataplexy and sleep with low voltage high frequency EEG activity. In: Kety S, ed. Sleep and altered state of consciousness. Baltimore: Williams & Wilkins, 1967:488–505.
12. Hishikawa Y, Shimuzu T. Physiology of REM sleep, cataplexy and sleep paralysis. Adv Neurol 1995;67:245–271. Review.
13. Guilleminault C. Cataplexy. In: Guilleminault C, Dement W, Passouant P, eds. Narcolepsy. New York: Spectrum, 1976:125–144.
14. Gelardi JM, Brown JW. Hereditary cataplexy. J Neurol Neurosurg Psychiatry 1967;30:455–457.
15. Hartse KM, Zorick FJ, Roth T, Sicklesteel JM. Isolated cataplexy: a familial study. Sleep Res 1980;9:205.
16. Anderson M, Salmon MV. Symptomatic cataplexy. J Neurol Neurosurg Psychiatry 1977;40:186–191.
17. D'Cruz OF, Vaughn BV, Gold SH, Greenwood RS. Symptomatic cataplexy in pontomedullary lesions. Neurology 1994;44(11):2189–2191.
18. Stahl SM, Layzer RB, Aminoff MJ, et al. Continuous cataplexy in a patient with a midbrain tumor: the limp man syndrome. Neurology 1980;30:1115–1118.
19. Gozukirmizi E, Hartse KM, Karacan I, et al. Narcolepsy–cataplexy associated with posterior fossa tumors: a case report. Sleep Res 1981;10:249.
20. Schwartz W, Stakes JW, Hobson JA. Transient cataplexy after removal of a craniopharyngioma. Neurology 1984;34:1372–1375.
21. Smith T. Cataplexy in association with meningiomas. Acta Neurol Scand 1983;94(suppl):46–47.
22. Ethelberg S. Symptomatic "cataplexy" or chalastic fits in cortical lesions of the frontal lobe. Brain 1950;73:499–512.
23. Kramer M, McGinnis W. Cataplexy–muscle weakness–McCardle's syndrome: a case report. Sleep Res 1986;15:193.
24. Lascelles RG, Mohr PD, Peart I. Unilateral cataplexy associated with systemic lupus erythematosus. J Neurol Neurosurg Psychiatry 1976;39:1023–1026.
25. Vossler DG, Wyler AR, Wilkus RJ, et al. Cataplexy and monoamine oxidase deficiency in Norrie disease. Neurology 1996;46(5):1258–1261.
26. Jacome D, Risko M. Pseudocataplexy: gelastic-atonic seizures. Neurology 1984;34:1381–1383.
27. Akimoto H, Honda Y, Takahashi Y. Pharmacotherapy in narcolepsy. Dis Nerv Syst 1960;21:704–706.
28. Nishino S, Fruhstorfer B, Arrigoni J, et al. Further characterization of the alpha-1 receptor subtype involved in the control of cataplexy in canine narcolepsy. J Pharmacol Exp Ther 1993;264(3):1079–1084.
29. Mignot E, Renaud A, Nishino S, et al. Canine cataplexy is preferentially controlled by adrenergic mechanisms: evidence using monoamine selective uptake inhibitors and release enhancers. Psychopharmacology 1993;113(1):76–82.
30. Schmidt HS, Clark RW, Human PR. Protriptyline: an effective agent in the treatment of the narcolepsy-cataplexy syndrome and hypersomnia. Am J Psychiatry 1977;134:183–185.
31. Parkes JD, Schachter M. Clomipramine and clonazepam in cataplexy. Lancet 1979;ii:1085–1086.
32. Guilleminault C. Narcolepsy syndrome. In: Kryger MH, Roth T, Dement WC, eds. Principles and practice of sleep medicine. Philadelphia: WB Saunders, 1989:338–346.
33. Reid MS, Tafti M, Nishino S, et al. Cholinergic regulation of cataplexy in canine narcolepsy in the pontine reticular formation is mediated by M2 muscarinic receptors. Sleep 1994;17(5):424–435.
34. Langdon N, Bandak S, Shindler J, Parkes JD. Fluoxetine in the treatment of cataplexy. Sleep 1986;9:371–372.
35. Frey J, Darbonne C. Fluoxetine suppresses human cataplexy: a pilot study. Neurology 1994;44(4):707–709.
36. Guilleminault C, Mancuso J, Quera Salva MA, et al. Viloxazine hydrochloride in narcolepsy: a preliminary report. Sleep 1986;9:275–279.
37. Freemon FR. The treatment of narcolepsy and cataplexy. Compr Ther 1985;11:44–47.
38. Putkonen P, Bergstrom L. Clonidine alleviates cataplectic symptoms in narcolepsy. In: Koella WP, ed. Sleep 1980 (Fifth European Congress of Sleep Research). Basel: Karger, 1980:414–416.
39. Godbout R, Montplaisir J. The effects of zimelidine, a serotonin reuptake blocker, on cataplexy and daytime sleepiness of narcoleptic patients. Clin Neuropharmacol 1986;9:46–51.
40. Mouret J, Sanchez P, Taillard J, et al. Treatment of narcolepsy with L-tyrosine. Lancet 1988;2:1458–1459.
41. Mamelak M, Scharf MB, Woods M. Treatment of narcolepsy with gamma-hydroxybutyrate. A review of clinical and sleep laboratory findings. Sleep 1986;9:285–289.
42. Lammers GJ, Arends J, Declerck AD, et al. Gammahydroxybutyrate and narcolepsy: a double-blind placebo-controlled study. Sleep 1993;16(3):216–220.
42a. Scharf MB, Brown D, Woods M, et al. The effects and effectiveness of gamma-hydroxybutyrate in patients with narcolepsy. J Clin Psychiatry 1985;46:222–225.
42b. Scrima L, Hartman PG, Johnson FH, Hiller F. Efficacy of gamma hydroxybutyrate versus placebo in treating narcolepsy-cataplexy; double blind subjective measurements. Biol Psychiatry 1989;26:331–343.
43. Boehme RE, Baker TL, Mefford IN, et al. Narcolepsy: cholinergic receptor changes in an animal model. Life Sci 1984;34:1825–1828.
44. Thompson C, Schachter M, Parkes JD. Drugs for cataplexy. Ann Neurol 1982;12:62–63.
45. Rechtschaffen A, Dement W. Narcolepsy and hypersomnia. In: Kales A, ed. Sleep physiology and pathology: a symposium. Philadelphia: JB Lippincott, 1969:119–130.
46. Siegel JM, Nienhuis R, Fahringer HM, et al. Activity of medial mesopontine units during cataplexy and sleep-waking states in the narcoleptic dog. J Neuroscience 1992;12(5):1640–1646.
47. Foutz A, Delashaw J, Guilleminault C, Dement WC. Monoaminergic mechanisms and experimental cataplexy. Ann Neurol 1981;10:360–376.
48. Bixler EO, Kales A, Vela-Bueno A, et al. Narcolepsy/cataplexy III: Nocturnal sleep and wakefulness patterns. Int J Neurosci 1986;29:306–316.
49. Mitler M, Dement W. Cataplectic-like behavior in cats after micro-injection of carbachol in the pontine reticular formation. Brain Res 1974;68:335–343.
50. Montplaisir J, Godbout R. Serotonergic reuptake mechanisms in the control of cataplexy. Sleep 1986;9:280–284.
51. Vizzioli R. Les bases neurophysiologiques de la cataplexie. Electroencephalogr Clin Neurophysiol 1964;16:191–193.
52. Wilder J. Narkolepsie. In: Bumke O, Foerster O, eds. Handbuch der neurologie. Berlin: Springer, 1935:XVII:87–141.

53. Van Bogaert L. Les aspects familiaux dex paroxysmes reflexes du tonus. Contribution a l'etude des faits de cataplexie et d'hypertonie dites affectives et de leurs relations avec la pathologie constitutionnelle. Ann Med Psychol 1936;94:1–27.

54. Nan'no H, Hishikawa Y, Koida H, et al. A neurophysiological study of sleep paralysis in narcoleptic patients. Electroencephalogr Clin Neurophysiol 1970;28:282–390.

55. Scrima L. An etiology of narcolepsy–cataplexy and a proposed cataplexy neuromechanism. Int J Neurosci 1981;15:69–86.

56. Siegel JM, Fahringer H, Tomaszewski KS, et al. Heart rate and blood pressure changes associated with cataplexy in canine narcolepsy. Sleep 1986;9:216–221.

57. Guilleminault C, Salva MAQ, Mancuso J, Hayes B. Narcolepsy, cataplexy, heart rate and blood pressure. Sleep 1986;9:222–226.

58. Lai YY, Siegel JM. Determinants of cataplexy induced by stimulation of the medial medulla. Sleep Res 1986;15:8.

59. Banruch HL, Kelwala S, Kapen S. The cardioacceleratory response to arecoline infusion during sleep in narcoleptic subjects and controls. Sleep 1987;10:272–278.

Sleep Paralysis

J. Gila Lindsley

BACKGROUND

As a movement disorder, sleep paralysis is a rather intriguing one. The defining characteristic of sleep paralysis is state specific: it occurs during the sleep-onset period or during awakening(s) from sleep, but does not occur outside the sleep-related period (unless there is a concomitant disorder). The pathophysiology of the disorder, therefore, would appear to be intimately enmeshed with the physiology of sleep.

Sleep paralysis is defined as complete or near complete atonia of the neck and antigravity muscles, occurring in association with falling asleep or waking up (1–3). Variably, during a sleep paralysis episode the individual may also lose the ability to communicate (4–11) but may retain the ability to move or open the eyes (7). There is some suggestion in the literature (4,5,8,9,12) that in a given individual sleep paralysis tends either to occur during the sleep-onset period (predormital) or in association with awakening from sleep (postdormital), but rarely under both circumstances. The inability to move generally endures for only a brief period of time (i.e., several minutes). Most reports indicate that a light touch (4,6,7,9), gentle shaking (12), or hearing one's name called (9) can lead to prompt termination of the episode. Motor control then returns precipitously and completely. There are, however, a number of reports of patients who have had up to eight sequential episodes of sleep paralysis before they were able to fall fully asleep or become fully awake (unpublished data) (4,8,12). In at least one of these cases, the only way to prevent repetitive episodes during a given night was for the patient to get fully out of bed for at least an hour before resuming efforts to fall asleep.

HISTORY

The central focus of this historical review and the remainder of this chapter will be on idiopathic—generally referred to as either isolated or independent—sleep paralysis. As a symptom, sleep paralysis has had a modicum of attention in the narcolepsy literature (2) because it has been considered an auxiliary symptom of this disorder. However, this movement disorder appears to be independent of narcolepsy, or at least able to occur independent of it. Chodoff, in 1944 (13), made the point quite clearly that sleep paralysis is not diagnostic of narcolepsy. In fact, the earliest identified reference to this disorder described a case of sleep paralysis isolated from a narcoleptic syndrome. Furthermore, although sleep paralysis is—among many medical practitioners—thought of as part of the so-called narcoleptic tetrad, the majority of literature addressing sleep paralysis specifically focuses on the isolated form of the disorder. Finally, it is unclear whether or not the sleep paralysis that occurs in some narcoleptics is an integral part of the narcolepsy syndrome, or even if it has the same pathophysiology as idiopathic/isolated sleep paralysis.

The history of the recognition of sleep paralysis as a sleep-related phenomenon and its characterization thereof is delightfully colorful. Schneck (14) feels that it likely was known in the eighteenth century. His interpretation of Henry Fuseli's famous 1781 painting *The Nightmare* is that it actually depicts sleep paralysis. The painting is of a demoniacal creature, the nightmare, squatting upon the abdomen and chest of a supine woman. The woman's body is partly off the bed, as might be the case for affected persons amid an episode who are trying to break out of the paralytic attack. Consistent with this image of sleep paralysis, Ness (9) later described that according to folklore in Newfoundland, the cause of the symptom of sleep paralysis is "being hagged"—being attacked by an old woman who squats upon one's chest, and by so doing crushes away one's breath and causes paralysis. Liddon (15) also recognizes as probably sleep paralysis Macnish's 1834 (16) similar description of a nightmare:

> At one moment he [the victim] may have the consciousness of a malignant demon at his side; then to shun the sight of so appalling an object, he will close his eyes, but still the fearful being makes its presence known; ... if he looks up, he beholds horrid eyes glaring upon him, and an aspect of hell grinning at him with even more hellish malice. . . . Or, he may have the idea of a monstrous *hag squatted upon his breast—mute, motionless* and malignant (italics have been added here for emphasis).

Binns (17) (1842), however, is generally credited with the first definite case report of sleep paralysis. Binns's term for it was "daymare," since in the case reported it occurred in association with a daytime nap. It likely is a description of isolated or idiopathic sleep paralysis, as a concurrent narcoleptic syndrome is not noted. The patient is described as having utter incapacity for motion or speech, difficult respirations, and extreme dread. His experience was of being completely awake during the "daymare" episode. Mitchell's published report of "night palsy" then followed in 1876 (18). He described the problem also as "nocturnal paralysis" and contributed his finding that it occurred in people who were emotionally and physically healthy. Pfister described it in the German literature in 1903 (19) as "protracted psychomotor awakening," and Trömner (20) in 1911 used the term "dissociated awakening." Rosenthal (21), also in Europe, characterized it in 1927 as an "awakening phenomenon," and Lhermitte and Dupont (22), a year later in France referred to it as "awakening cataplexy."

It was Wilson (23), in 1928, who is credited with the first use of the term currently used, "sleep paralysis." He also noted that attacks were precipitated by terrifying dreams.

The first published association of sleep paralysis to narcolepsy was in 1933 by Levin (24), who noted in his patients as Wilson had done earlier that attacks were precipitated by terrifying dreams. In 1934, Daniels (25) (in the context of a lengthy treatise on narcolepsy) mirrored Lhermitte and Dupont in describing sleep paralysis as cataplexy of awakening (see Chapter 80 for an independent treatment of cataplexy). Krabbe and Magnussen's equaly lengthy treatise on narcolepsy several years later (26) promised this author further description of sleep paralysis in the context of narcolepsy (the term used by them simply as a label for a disorder of severe, intractable daytime sleepiness). However, much to the chagrin and disappointment of this author, their fascinating and extremely well-documented piece likely was, instead, one of the first published works on the familial incidence of obstructive sleep apnea! They describe

perfectly the characteristics and natural history of sleep apnea.

Although there was an increase in the rate of reporting individual sleep paralysis case studies beginning at about the time of World War II, there were still only a handful of reports. Lichtenstein and Rosenblum (27) published in 1942 a description of a 69-year-old diabetic woman who had had sleep paralysis since childhood. The episodes occurred exclusively when she awakened from sleep. Symptoms were inability to move, inability to speak, some residual capacity to open the eyes partially, and fear at times. Light touch reportedly broke the episode. However, this might then be followed by another episode. The authors ruled out diabetes as etiologic to the patient's sleep paralysis.

Through the end of the war and postwar period, the primary information available in the literature about sleep paralysis continued to be in the form of individual cases or case study series (13,28,29). Van der Heide and Weinberg (29) in 1945 presented three case studies for which they believed the sleep paralysis was an outcome of combat fatigue. This report was the forerunner of many suggesting that stress and exhaustion might be contributory to the disorder. It likely was also one of the first reports of what we now refer to as "posttraumatic stress syndrome." As an interesting aside, in our own sleep disorders center we have seen many patients with a diagnosis of posttraumatic stress disorder (PTSD) who also complain of night terrors. Hudson et al (30) reported sleep paralysis in association with hypnopompic hallucinations and REM sleep in a 36-year-old woman diagnosed with PTSD. As will be developed in a later section, night terrors may be intimately related to sleep paralysis.

Van der Heide and Weinberg in their paper introduced the theme, picked up later by Schneck (5,31,32), that psychiatric conflict underlies the symptom of sleep paralysis.

CONTEMPORARY TREATMENT

Sleep paralysis, at least in the literature of the United States, seemed until the 1960s to be treated largely as a curiosity. The rule was intensive individual case studies with, for the most part, the assumption that sleep paralysis was relatively rare. Some of the early authors indicated that they felt the incidence of sleep paralysis might be more prevalent than believed, but it was not until 1962 that the first systematic large-scale studies were carried out to assess this directly. Larger scale studies and more frequent case reports, in turn, afford us now with the possibility of making general statements about the incidence, antecedent conditions, comprehensive symptom picture, and possible etiology of sleep paralysis.

Incidence and Epidemiology of Sleep Paralysis

Estimates of the incidence of sleep paralysis in narcoleptics vary considerably. In 1933, Levin (24) accumulated reports of sleep paralysis from the narcolepsy literature and identified 16 cases in the 200 cases of narcolepsy reported up to that point (i.e., 8% of the cases studied). Yoss and Daly (33) saw sleep paralysis in 24% of the narcoleptics they studied. Roth (34,35) found it in 36 of 104 narcoleptics (i.e., in 34.4% of their cases). Hishikawa (36) reported sleep paralysis in 57% of 102 narcoleptics studied. The method of diagnosing narcolepsy and cultural distinctions (see below) may account for the discrepancy between the American and Japanese reports in estimates of probability of sleep paralysis co-occurring with narcolepsy.

The broader question, however, is what is the incidence rate of sleep paralysis, and the association of sleep paralysis to narcolepsy, in the general population? That information, among its other uses, will bear upon what has been assumed to be a necessary, intrinsic association of sleep paralysis to narcolepsy.

Estimates of incidence rates of isolated sleep paralysis also vary extensively. It is unclear whether the wide range of estimates reflect the populations studied, and therefore true differences among study samples, or if they more reflect artifacts of methodology.

The 1982 report by Coleman et al (37) of statistics from a national cooperative study among 11 sleep–wake disorders clinics showed that idiopathic sleep paralysis represented only 0.2% of the over 5,000 patients (i.e., about 10 patients) who had presented to the sleep centers and whose records formed the database for the study. It should be kept in mind that because of the self-selected sample, this is not an effective estimate of the prevalence of idiopathic (isolated) sleep paralysis in the general population. It would certainly suggest, however, that idiopathic sleep paralysis severe enough that the person seeks medical help occurs only infrequently.

In 1962, Goode (38) undertook the first extensive, systematic study, by questionnaire survey, of a general population—that is, neither specifically narcoleptics nor specifically patients who had presented to a specialized sleep–wake disorders clinic for help. Subjects were medical students, nursing students, and hospital patients. Three hundred and fifty-nine responded to the questionnaire surveys. Seventeen positive cases (4.7% of the study sample) were identified, with the rate of sleep paralysis cases four times greater for males than females. None of these cases had additional symptoms consistent with narcolepsy. Conversely, the single narcoleptic identified denied sleep paralysis. That is, in the sample studied, the correlation between narcolepsy and sleep paralysis was zero.

A year later, Everett's sequel (6) to Goode's study was published. Everett also questioned whether the past impression of sleep paralysis as unusual in the isolated form (versus as in association with narcolepsy) was accurate. He felt that isolated sleep paralysis was considerably more prevalent than had been believed and therefore also chose to survey a more random population rather than a population of narcoleptics. Subjects were healthy medical students. The database was

from survey questionnaires and follow-up interviews. Fifty-two students responded. An incidence rate of 15.4% for at least one episode of sleep paralysis was found.* Seven of the 47 male students (14.9%) and one of the five female students (20%) endorsed the experience. Although the ratio of male to female differs from Goode (38), the total number of females studied between the two studies is too small to permit extraction of population estimates by gender for this disorder. Age of onset for the group varied. The number of lifetime attacks varied between three and 50. All eight cases identified appeared to be of independent sleep paralysis. As in Goode's study, one narcoleptic was in addition identified. That person denied sleep paralysis. Again, the correlation between sleep paralysis and narcolepsy was zero.

Penn et al (10), also studying a sample of medical school students, found an incidence rate exceeding Everett's. Respondents with at least one episode of sleep paralysis accounted for 20% of the 80 students studied. The study made an important distinction in the type of sleep paralysis. Fourteen percent of the respondents reported sleep paralysis with awakening from sleep (postdormital) and 6% reported sleep paralysis during the sleep-onset period (predormital). Of these, 4% reported sleep paralysis under both circumstances. As in the foregoing cases, there was no obvious association of sleep paralysis to narcolepsy. The incidence rate was approximately the same in a group of 164 Nigerian medical students who were studied (39), 26.2% of whom reported the experience. There was s slight preponderance of female over male reports (31% and 21%, respectively, of the study sample).

In a more recent study of sleep paralysis in normal subjects (40), no sex differences in incidence of sleep paralysis were found among the 1,822 male and 876 female subjects who completed the questionnaire used to collect data. Overall, 6.7% of the study sample reported at least one episode of sleep paralysis.

In their 1984 study, Bell et al (41) introduced ethnicity as a variable possibly bearing upon incidence rate. They studied 108 black subjects, consisting of generally healthy subjects and psychiatric patients. Estimates of incidence rate of isolated sleep paralysis were considerably higher than in the previous studies: 41% of the sample had had at least one episode of sleep paralysis. This is at least twice the incidence rate described by the earlier American epidemiologic studies. Also in contrast to the foregoing studies, the male/female ratio slightly favored females. Eighteen (40.9%) of the identified cases were male, and 26 (59.1%) were female.

---

* It is possible that the true versus reported rate may have been higher. Questionnaires were distributed in a psychiatry class after a description had been offered of sleep paralysis and other symptoms generally associated with the narcolepsy syndrome. Everett later found out that presenting the questionnaire in this context may have decreased the number of people willing to acknowledge sleep paralysis. At least one student noted that he was hesitant because he feared being seen as in need of psychiatric help.

Sleep paralysis is apparently known also in the West Indies (42), in Newfoundland (9), and in Japan (11). Data are not currently available for the incidence of what is known as *Kokma* in the West Indies. De Jong provided an excellent review of cases of sleep paralysis in Portuguese, Guinean, Dutch, Moroccan, and Surinamese patients in the context of their respective cultures (43).

Ness's 1978 study of the old hag phenomenon in Newfoundland showed that 62% of 69 extensively interviewed adults reported one or more attacks. The male-female ratio was 70% male to 30% female, among the positive cases. The 1987 study by Fukuda et al (11) of *Kanashibari* in Japan, based on data collected from 635 college students, also suggests a high prevalence rate, with a gender ratio favoring females. Forty-three percent of the students studied had had at least one attack; 39.8% clearly had isolated sleep paralysis. With respect to the male-female ratio, 51.5% of the females, but only 37.7% of the males, had had the experience. The majority of those interviewed had had only a few episodes. However, two of the female respondents had virtually daily attacks. Of direct pertinence to the association of sleep paralysis to narcolepsy, the symptom cataplexy had a higher probability of being found in subjects who did not report sleep paralysis than in those who did. This would, again, suggest a negligible association of sleep paralysis to narcolepsy. Cataplexy is more generally assumed to be an intrinsic component of the narcolepsy syndrome.

The difference between the American studies on the one hand and the Newfoundland and Japanese studies on the other, with respect to prevalence rate, is striking. Fukuda et al (11) and Ness (9) both make cogent arguments that the discrepancy between their prevalence estimates and those of Goode (38), Everett (6), and Penn et al (10) may reflect the rate of reporting rather than the true incidence. *Kanashibari* and the old hag syndrome are well-embedded in their respective nations' folklores. They are seen as deriving from external influences and therefore as not reflecting upon an individual. In contrast, for the American medical students and nurses studied, endorsing this experience carried with it the perceived threat of stigmatization. These differences may have led to a higher rate of reporting in the Fukuda et al and Ness studies than in the American studies. It remains to be determined, however, if the differences are real or reflect only rate of reporting.

Antecedent Conditions of Isolated Sleep Paralysis

A number of investigators have attempted to cull out factors that might predispose to episodes of sleep paralysis. The majority of information is derived from persons who have had only a few episodes of sleep paralysis in their lives. The paucity of large sample studies, and absence in the literature of concentrated focus on those who have frequent sleep paralysis, prevent any generalizations regarding predisposing factors.

Psychologic stress is a frequently mentioned contributing factor. Van der Heide and Weinberg (29) described sleep paralysis in the context of combat fatigue in three army air force fliers. The medical school students poled by Everett (6) identified as contributory the sleep deprivation and overtiredness they experienced as medical students. Similarly, Luck (12) associated at least sleep-onset sleep paralysis with mental stress. Bell et al (41) also saw sleep paralysis as a stress-related phenomenon. As the reader will recall, their estimate of the incidence of isolated sleep paralysis in a black population far exceeded earlier estimates of prevalence in other (predominantly Caucasian) American populations. They attributed the difference to the stress in the daily life of American blacks, in fact likening their situation to that of Van der Heide and Weinberg's subjects with combat fatigue. Finally, Fukuda et al (11) identified tiredness, psychologic stress, irregular life patterns, and sleep loss with the development of *Kanashibara*. In a later paper, Fukuda et al (44) used the MMPI and Maudsley Personality Inventory to evaluate the personality structure of persons reporting *Kanashibara*. They found a slight tendency for elevated scores on the paranoia scale of the MMPI for this group compared to controls. More recently, Suarez (45) found in a hispanic population an increased incidence rate of sleep paralysis among adults diagnosed with "anguish crisis."

Snyder (42) reported two cases of isolated sleep paralysis following immediately upon rapid time-zone changes (i.e., in association with jet lag). It is possible that jet lag might represent a variant of stress. Alternatively, alterations in the sleep–wake cycle may represent the mediating variable between stress and sleep paralysis episodes. (See below, under "Physiology of sleep paralysis.")

Curiously, sleeping in the supine position is a recurrent theme in the description of antecedent conditions. In Newfoundland (the old hag syndrome), respondents identified falling asleep on the back as a factor that increased the probability of their "being hagged" (being attacked during the sleep period by the old hag, which results in paralysis) (9). This was almost universally identified as an antecedent condition in the Newfoundland sample studied. In fact, many guesses by the respondents regarding etiology of the disorder began with the empirical observation that the supine position predisposed them to sleep paralysis. This would appear not to be culture specific. Everett's medical school respondents (6) also identified sleeping on the back as a predisposing factor. Possibly related, there is some evidence that one of the aspects of sleep architecture in narcoleptics (sleep onset rapid eye movement (REM) periods (SOREMP)) depends upon the patient being in the supine position when falling asleep. Also possibly related, in our own experience (unpublished data) a number of patients with a primary complaint of disruptive nightmares (presumably also a disturbance of REM sleep) identify sleeping in the supine position as a predisposing factor.

Familial Incidence of Isolated Sleep Paralysis

There is some indication in the literature that heredity, or at least familial history, might predispose to sleep paralysis. The case study series available focus upon patients and their families for whom sleep paralysis occurs recurrently rather than only on rare occasion.

Rushton (28) published one of the first descriptions of a familial occurrence of sleep paralysis. He described a nephew and an aunt.

Roth et al (8) studied two families with isolated sleep paralysis. In family 1, 14 people across four generations were studied. The index case in this family and affected family members had the same clinical pictures. Sleep paralysis occurred only in association with midcycle awakenings from sleep, generally at 0400 hours. It did not occur with sleep onset or with the final awakening of the day. The paralysis inevitably occurred in association with wild, terrifying dreams. All affected family members reported that they were fully aware during these episodes, but they were unable to communicate until the episode was terminated. The experiences were generally associated with anxiety but apparently not initiated by anxiety. Within a given night, there was a high probability of recurrence if the person did not awaken fully for about an hour before attempting to return to sleep. Repetition frequency was between once and twice a month to two to three times per week. Stress at bedtime appeared to increase its probability of occurrence. Additional symptoms included nervousness, lassitude, pressure in the head, and increased irritability. Onset was quite early, between 5 and 8 years old. The index case had an additional medical disorder: unilateral cryptorchidism, hypotrophic genital organs, and feminine hair growth. His electroencephalogram (EEG) was normal, but drowsy. Narcolepsy, nonetheless, was ruled out. In retrospect, the patient may have had Prokoler–Will syndrome, known to be associated with abnormalities of REM sleep. The gonadal abnormality likely was not causally related to the disorder. It was not present in the other affected family members.

The second case study series reported by Roth and coworkers was of four family members across three generations. The index member of family 2 was 22 years old. He complained of humming in the ears while falling asleep and an associated inability to move. He also experienced some respiratory difficulties. He experienced himself to be fully conscious, and felt that if he made a considerable effort to move, that he could snap himself out of it. Sleep-onset sleep paralysis might repeat itself up to eight times in succession during efforts to establish sleep. In contrast to the first index case, sleep paralysis in association with midcycle awakenings from sleep was the exception rather than the rule. The sleep paralysis did not occur in association with dreams and was not associated with anxiety as in the first case. It did occur in association with daytime naps and also at sleep onset. Cataplexy and difficulty falling asleep were denied. Narcolepsy

was ruled out. The same clinical features applied to the other three family members interviewed.

In both families, the incidence of sleep paralysis was greater among men than women. The family genogram indicated, in both families, that transmission was exclusively through the maternal line. The authors hypothesized that heredity is X-linked and questioned whether the mode of genetic transmission for isolated sleep paralysis is different from that of transmission for narcolepsy.

Ness (9) did not collect systematic information on familial occurrences of independent sleep paralysis in his Newfoundland sample. It was his impression, however, that two families had "more frequent attacks distributed among more family members than did the other 73 families in the community" (p. 29).

One of our own patients, whose vivid description of sleep paralysis appears in a later section (p. 559) provides the following family history. We have not had the opportunity to speak directly with family members.

Case Study
The patient's paternal uncle has been told that he has narcolepsy, although this was never objectively confirmed. The uncle's primary symptom is excessive daytime sleepiness, which could have arisen from other sources. That uncle does not have sleep paralysis. The patient's paternal grandmother had difficulty sleeping at night, but no other sleep-related complaints. This patient's sister has had moderate difficulties with sleep paralysis and also with hypnogogic hallucinations. Especially in association with daytime naps, she awakens disoriented secondary to hallucinated disorientation of the room. For instance, she has tried to lay back down on a bed that was not there. A second sister had sleep paralysis until age 12, which then resolved. It never happened unless she was in the prone (versus supine!) position. It actually disappeared when she began sleeping in the supine position. Our patient's sleep paralysis, in contrast, was not position dependent. Interestingly, imipramine 30 mg at h.s. led to an increased rate of recurrent sleep paralysis episodes on a given night. This patient has more recently reported that his 4-year-old son has begun to describe similar episodes, not prompted by him or his wife.

There is some suggestion, in our own case records, that different components of a sleep paralysis syndrome (see below, under "Auxiliary symptoms of sleep paralysis") may be represented within a family. For instance, one patient, who has had sleep paralysis for virtually her entire life, has a daughter and granddaughter with both sleep paralysis and frequent sleepwalking. Another patient, who presented with a primary complaint of night terrors (i.e., nocturnal panic attacks), reports that his mother has severe sleep paralysis. Night terrors resemble the affective component of sleep paralysis described below. Possibly related, Bell et al (46) found for patients with panic attacks that were not associated with sleep a high incidence in first-degree through third-degree relatives of the isolated form of sleep paralysis. Suggesting possibly that sleep paralysis is part of the narcolepsy spectrum, but that it can be inherited in its isolated form, is the report of another of our patients. This 27-year-old woman just recently diagnosed with isolated narcolepsy (i.e., narcolepsy in the absence of cataplexy) reported that her brother has severe sleep paralysis.

Another of our patients polled her immediate family and found that both her siblings—a brother and a sister—have very frequent sleep paralysis. The three had never discussed this until she did the family poll. Her brother reportedly is able to induce sleep paralysis by altering his sleep–wake rhythm on preceding days.

Auxiliary Symptoms of Sleep Paralysis

Sleep paralysis most frequently is thought of as one of the auxiliary symptoms of narcolepsy. When sleep paralysis is not part of a narcoleptic picture, however, it of itself tends to have auxiliary symptoms.

Some of the auxiliary symptoms present as an intrinsic component of the sleep paralysis attack. Sleep paralysis occurring with the beginning of the sleep period tends to occur in association with visual hallucinations (5–7, 9,12,13,15,47). The content is either mundane (i.e., the hallucination of a bed where none was actually present), bizarre (gargoyles hanging out of the curtains), or idiosyncratic. The sense (often previsual) of a presence (as of a person) in the room is common, as is the visual experience of actually seeing someone in the room (4). Auditory hallucinations are also reported (1), at times described as a loud buzzing sound or as the sound of wind or waves.

One of our own patients, whose sleep paralysis occurred in association with cocaine use, had repeated hallucinations of a "man cartwheeling in the air" in association with the sleep paralysis. Parenthetically, the sleep paralysis and hallucinations disappeared with cocaine discontinuation.

At times, the experience of someone being in the room has a somatic component. Schneck (5) reported that his patient felt, during the course of her sleep paralysis, that the mattress moved as if someone had just gotten up from the mattress. Possibly related, our patient with cocaine-associated sleep paralysis also described feelings as if the mattress had moved. This experience, however, persisted at least through the first 3 weeks following cocaine discontinuation. In another of our patients whose sleep paralysis was associated with a narcoleptic syndrome, the somatic hallucination of the bed itself moving through the air during an episode is common.

Sleep paralysis can occur in association with more complex perceptual hallucinatory events. Liddon (48) reports two cases admitted for inpatient psychiatric treatment carrying a diagnosis of formal thought disorder. One had hallucinations, associated with sleep paralysis, of his grandmother telling him to kill himself. These began 6 years

prior to hospitalization. A second hallucinated a witch coming toward him and climbing on his stomach. There was at times an auditory component. During these episodes, the patient was fearful of dying.

Distinct from, but likely related to, associated hallucinatory experiences are dream reports.

Sleep paralysis has not routinely been classified in the literature as predormital (occurring during the beginning of the sleep period) or postdormital (occurring once the sleep phase of the circadian sleep–wake cycle already has been established, in association with an awakening from sleep). The dream-related descriptions, however, would indicate that the following relate to postdormital sleep paralysis.

There are numerous reports of sleep paralysis occurring with awakenings from wild, terrifying dreams (4,6–8,10,15). Weitzner (4) described this in detail. His patient reported that the early parts of the associated dreams were typically dream-like, with the expected bizarre material. The latter half of the dream, however, which was most directly associated with the sleep paralysis, was of a different quality. These latter dream events were vividly real, without the kinds of distortions expected in dreams.

Reports of respiratory disturbance in association with the sleep paralysis—often a sense of suffocation, heaviness of the chest, choking—are frequent (6–8,10,15). Sometimes this somatic experience is anthropomorphized. One of Payn's patients hallucinated a fat person holding her down (7). At times, the images reflect the popular folklore. The report of Ness (9) for his Newfoundland population that an old hag sitting on one's chest is a frequent component of the hallucination (perhaps not unlike Liddon's patient hallucinating a witch climbing onto his stomach) is consistent with this. Similarly, Fukuda et al (11) note that 30% of the sample they interviewed in Japan reported the image of a Buddha sitting on the chest.

Distortions of perception also can occur in the auditory modality. Weitzner (4) reported that extreme amplification of sound was a component part of his patient's sleep paralysis episodes. Schneck (5) described for his patient a shrill sound of constant pitch, a hissing in the ear, a roaring in the head. Liddon (15), as described earlier, reported humming in the ears at sleep onset in association with sleep paralysis. The patient described by Luck (12) complained of associated loud buzzing noise. Possibly related, Roth et al (8) described a pressure in the head.

Other auxiliary symptoms of isolated sleep paralysis seem more a reaction to the experience. In the majority of cases, there is an affective component as well, concurrent with the sleep paralysis episode. The way in which affect is associated with sleep paralysis should be underscored. Sleep paralysis has been called, by some, a variant of cataplexy (treated in detail in Chapter 80). It is important to recognize that the affect associated with sleep paralysis appears to be triggered by the paralysis. This is in contrast to the case of cataplexy, wherein the cataplectic attacks appear to be triggered *by*, rather than being the trigger for, the affective event. Anxiety, fear, tension, and even terror have been reported (4–8,10,15,27). The anxiety, terror, and so forth apparently are in response to not being able to move despite extensive effort.

The following previously unpublished description by one of our own patients poignantly emphasizes how frightening an attack of sleep paralysis can be, especially when accompanied by some of the auxiliary symptoms. At the time he provided the description, this patient had suffered with sleep paralysis for several years, often with episodes on multiple successive nights. Within a night, sleep paralysis episodes occurred repeatedly, in succession. He describes four distinct variants of postdormital sleep paralysis:

I wake up and my body is totally paralyzed. However, I am aware of my surroundings. I can see if someone enters or leaves the room. Sometimes I can hear. I have verified things with my wife [about what I experienced when I was paralyzed]. When muscle tone returns first [on the] left [side and] then [on the] right and then muscle tone is fully returned, but I feel exhausted.

I wake up and my body is totally paralyzed. However, with much effort I can move my body but it feels as if chains and lead are all over me. When moving across the room I lose my balance easily and it is difficult to get up. Often I will fall back asleep regardless of how I fight it and wake up seemingly minutes afterwards [with] full motor function except the normal waking up grogginess [No hallucinations].

Same as above, but in association with hallucinations. The patient has had the experience of waking up, dressing, leaving his room, only then to "awaken" and find himself in bed; then again dressing, leaving his room, to find himself in bed—repetitive hallucinations of having awakened that were sufficiently compelling that when he actually did awaken, get dressed and leave his room he was unsure if it were reality or hallucination until he was able to leave the house.

I wake up and my body is totally paralyzed. However, with much effort I can move my body but it feels as if chains and lead are all over me. But when I move/push hard to move even inches to grasp something, I discover it [the movement] was an illusion; that I had not moved at all.

Other affective components, likely reactions to the experience, are also described for the sleep paralysis attack. Ness (9) describes for his Newfoundland population that anxiety tends not to be a frequent component. However, the majority of those he interviewed reported feelings of exhaustion at the end of an experience, similar to that described by our patient. In like fashion, Luck (12) described exhaustion at the end of an episode. Possibly related, profuse sweating at the end of an episode (9) and heart pounding at the end of an episode (4) are also reported.

Efforts to break out of the paralytic episode (but possibly fear as well) may account for these symptoms. Many patients with recurrent sleep paralysis have found that if they have been able to accomplish even a minor movement (as of an appendage) that the sleep paralysis episode will suddenly break and full motor control return. Many therefore try violently during an episode to move. The female patient with sleep paralysis described by Luck (12) underwent testing for epilepsy, due to the twitching observed. EEG findings were negative. Schneck (49) believes the twitching may have reflected the woman's efforts to break out of the episode. We have had a similar case. This 22-year-old woman has recurrent episodes of sleep paralysis, during which she reports making frantic attempts to break the paralysis. Similar to Luck's patient, her husband observed that during these episodes she twitched as if she were having a convulsion. Sleep EEG, during natural nighttime sleep, was however, negative for epileptic waveforms.

Physiology of Sleep Paralysis

All of the thinking regarding sleep paralysis focuses upon its dissociation from—but also contiguity with—sleep, and particularly upon the psychomotor dissociation that it represents. Prior to the technologic developments of the past several decades, efforts to understand sleep paralysis were solely at the functional level of analysis. Levin (24) approached it from a Pavlovian perspective. He considered it to be a form of localized sleep, resulting from a dissociation of the motor and consciousness components of cerebral function during wakefulness and/or during the sleep-onset period.

The superficial similarity of sleep paralysis to cataplexy (see Chapter 80) was central to many other conceptualizations of sleep paralysis. Wilson (23), who first used the term *sleep paralysis*, considered it to be a transient physiologic disorder, that is a physiologic cataplexy. Brain (50) also noted its similarity to cataplexy and considered it to be a dissociative event, with motor and postural centers of the brain asleep and the mind awake. He contrasted sleep paralysis with somnambulism, characterizing the latter in exactly the opposite terms: motor and postural centers alert and mind asleep. Chodoff (13) also considered that sleep paralysis and cataplexy might be related. A similarity between the two was suggested by the common characteristic of temporary paralysis, but also because of the association of hypnogogic hallucinations to both.★ With some significant caveats discussed in a separate chapter (see Chapter 80), Chodoff sees both cataplexy and sleep paralysis as general disturbances in sleep and motility mechanisms, similar to the overall disturbance in narcolepsy.

★ Note that there are few reports in the literature of hypnagogic hallucinations accompanying cataplexy, while such reports for sleep paralysis are common.

Weitzner (4) postulated a possible role for aberrant carbohydrate metabolism in the development of narcolepsy and therefore of sleep paralysis (the assumption at that time was the sleep paralysis was a reflection of the primary "lesion" giving rise to the narcoleptic syndrome). Weitzner had previously noted that insulin-induced hypoglycemia was helpful to a narcoleptic, and subsequently published a paper in 1952 indicating that insulin-induced hypoglycemia had also corrected a sleep paralysis problem. He therefore posited pathophysiologic control by the hypothalamus of glucose metabolism as one etiology of sleep paralysis. Possible diencephalic (hypothalamic or thalamic) involvement has not been mentioned since that time. However, recent work linking the reticular nuclei of the thalamus to spindle generation during sleep, and spindle generation to inhibition of external sensory stimuli processing, may be related (50a).

The thrust of contemporary understanding of the pathophysiology of sleep paralysis (and cataplexy as well) still remains largely at the functional level, but considerably more direct observations of physiologic function during paralytic episodes are now available. The general formulation is that it represents a dissociation and displacement of a subset of the physiologic events that generally occur as a unit during a fully developed REM period (8,15,51–53).

Before proceeding, therefore, a description of the full complement of physiologic events that seem to be unique to REM sleep is in order. Not obviously related to the overall symptom picture of sleep paralysis are the following events that are specific to REM sleep. REM sleep is named for the characteristic rapid eye movements that occur during this unique stage of sleep. These phasic movements, which can occur singly or in bursts of varying density, are associated with volleys of spike activity in the pons, lateral geniculate nerve of the thalamus, and in the occipital cortex (pontogeniculo-occipital spikes). Other phasic neuromuscular events also occur during this sleep state. Phasic leg twitches, movement of digits especially the great toe, facial twitches, and so forth are common. During this sleep stage one also sees phasic autonomic changes reflected in brief changes in respiratory rate and heart rate, often in association with bursts of rapid eye movements. Blood pressure and core temperature also change in syndromic ways. To date, these events of REM sleep have not been related directly to the overall symptom picture of sleep paralysis (although one author has related blood pressure changes to cataplexy, see Chapter 80).

The two events of REM sleep most directly related to events observed with sleep paralysis are muscle atonia and dreaming. During REM sleep in normal subjects, complete atonia of neck and antigravity muscles occurs. The knee jerk reflex is generally depressed in sleep but is completely absent during REM sleep. Hodes and Dement (54), Kubota et al (55), and Shimizu et al (56) have demonstrated the virtual complete absence of the H reflex (an electrically stimulated tibial reflex) during REM sleep, but only a diminution of

this reflex during non-REM (NREM) sleep. Hodes and Dement noted further that the dramatic depression precedes REM sleep onset by a few minutes and also flows over into the beginning of the following NREM (stage 2) sleep period. Both they and Shimizu and co-workers observed far greater H-reflex suppression during intense rapid eye movement activity within this sleep period. Hodes and Dement also documented that as a given REM period progressed, H-reflex suppression, relatively speaking, diminished. Possibly related to the inability during a sleep paralysis attack to call out (and possibly related also to the experience of associated respiratory distress), suppression of the H reflex was preceded by a decrease in tone of the laryngeal muscles. Of particular interest to sleep paralysis occurring with the final awakening of the day, a depressed H reflex occurred also with the final arousal of the night.

The atonia during REM sleep has long been assumed to arise from pontine activation of a bulbar inhibitory region whose output results in hyperpolarization of alpha motor neurons in the spinal cord. Holmes et al (57) report that in the cat, at least, the source of the inhibitory efferents is the ventromedial medullary reticular formation, originally identified in the classic neurophysiologic studies of Magoun and Rhines (58). Selective lesions to this area with quisqualic acid in cats were associated with an absence of atonia specific to REM sleep. Neuromuscular activity during wakefulness and NREM sleep was unaffected. Yet during REM sleep, the cats showed increased tonus of the neck musculature and vigorous movements of the limbs.

Dreaming as an event specific to REM sleep is supported by a higher frequency of dream recall (versus more linear cognitive activity) when a subject is awakened from REM versus from NREM sleep.*

The assumption, with respect to sleep paralysis, is that the muscle atonia and cognitive dream events of REM sleep translate into sleep paralysis and hypnogogic hallucinations if the processes underlying them occur when the person is awake. The implied assumption is that these events of REM sleep and those that occur in the context of sleep paralysis have a common neurophysiologic substrate. This necessarily implies that the mediators of REM-related atonia and internally generated perceptual events are dissociable from sleep and therefore from REM sleep.

There is some precedent in the experimental literature with normal humans and cats that sleep and the foregoing events of REM are dissociable. Speaking to this point are Hodes and Dement's (54) findings that a suppression of the H reflex, consistent with what is found during REM sleep, occurs with the final awakening of the night (even if the person was not in REM sleep just before the final awakening of the day). Hodes and Dement, in fact, designated NREM as "sleep" and REM as "dreaming" to underscore their sense that the two are distinctly different states.

---

* There now exists, however, a considerable body of literature with contrary findings.

Broughton (59) also distinguished between a REM substrate potential and expression of REM sleep. He described a REM-tendency curve, with the REM substrate tendency greatest at the end of the usual sleep period and during the following several hours in the morning. Broughton related this to the finding that memory tasks requiring significant memory load are best carried out in the early part of the day, that is, that the cortical activation associated either with REM sleep or with REM substrate potential is contributory to this effect.

The sleep paralysis literature also is consistent with the assumption that sleep paralysis and auxiliary symptoms represent a displacement of a subset of REM sleep "symptoms" into periods of wakefulness bracketing the sleep period.

In association with daytime EEG studies of narcoleptics and normal controls, Hishikawa et al (60) found that in 16 of 20 induced awakenings from REM sleep, episodes of sleep paralysis and hypnogogic hallucinations occurred. This was not so with awakenings from NREM sleep stages. Their research also corroborated that the patient is subjectively awake when these events occur spontaneously. Yet, further complicating our understanding of REM events versus sleep, their data showed that subjectively awake patients when experiencing sleep paralysis were, according to objective (i.e., polysomnographic) criteria, in REM sleep! That is, even the EEG waveforms consistent with REM sleep, including sawtooth waves, were present for these patients during episodes of sleep paralysis. The overwhelming majority of the spontaneous episodes occurred when narcoleptic patients developed REM sleep immediately upon entering sleep (i.e., SOREMP).* Hishikawa and co-workers established through a behavioral testing paradigm that during SOREMP many of their subjects were at about the same or even at a slightly higher level of awareness than they had been during the just preceding drowsy state.

Based on these data, Hishikawa's group—along the same lines as investigators working with normal adults and cats described earlier—made a most provocative distinction between REM and sleep. They characterized sleep paralysis as falling into REM while still in the awake state. They propose, as a corollary, that one can be in REM-awake, REM-drowsy, and REM-asleep! In other words, the REM process and state of arousal are seen as orthogonal variables.

The work of Roth et al (8) also carried out sleep recordings during episodes of sleep paralysis, and like Hishikawa's group also identified the typical polysomnographic findings of REM sleep: sawtooth waves in the EEG, atonicity of the neck muscles, and rapid eye movements. They, too, made the point that sleep paralysis appears to be a dissociated form of paradoxical sleep and pointed for support to the association of sleep paralysis with hypnogogic events and wild dreams.

There are other objectively verifiable points of similarity between normal REM sleep and sleep paralysis. Hishikawa et al (60) applied the H-reflex paradigm of Hodes and Dement (54) and Shimizu et al (56) to a group of narcoleptics and normal controls further to determine if the muscle atonia of sleep paralysis is the same as (or an intimately related phenomenon to) the muscle atonia of REM sleep. The alternative hypothesis assessed was that sleep paralysis might represent somatokinesthetic hallucinations. They observed, as had been observed previously, that during REM sleep in general the tonic electromyographic (EMG) activity disappeared. They also observed transient phasic discharges at irregular intervals at a frequency greater than in stage 2 or delta sleep. During SOREMP, tonic EMG discharge and the H reflex almost completely disappeared, as was the case in the earlier study (with a normal population). A low-voltage H reflex was present on occasion. Two subjects were awakened at this point, and they provided reports of paralysis but neither hallucinations nor dreams. The SOREMP EMG and H-reflex phenomena disappeared with induced (objective) wakefulness. We emphasize that the induced wakefulness is in reference to objective measures of wakefulness (versus sleep), as these subjects reported that they had been awake prior to their "awakening" by the experimenter. Two other subjects, however, when awakened reported that they had been dreaming. These subjects did not report that they had been paralyzed. Importantly, for the narcoleptic and normal subjects, awakenings by the experimenter from later episodes of REM sleep did not produce these findings, that is, the experience of sleep paralysis and hypnogogic hallucinations seemed specific to SOREMP. This finding is curious, since Hodes and Dement's data (54) clearly indicated that in normal subjects H-reflex suppression was present with the final awakening during the night. One would therefore expect reports of sleep paralysis in at least some subjects with induced awakenings later in the night.

The distinction between early and late REM periods in other ways currently is elusive. In the study by Hishikawa et al (60), SOREMP and late REM periods seemed indistinguishable with respect to EEG pattern, changes in respiratory and heart rates, and to the somatic muscle and reflex activities described above. They did reach the conclusion that during a SOREMP in narcoleptics, consciousness seems to remain high and that, if this is correct, sleep paralysis in narcolepsy likely is not a part of a hypnogogic hallucination but an experience of true paralysis.

Nan'no et al (52) pursued the work of Hishikawa et al (60), testing further the hypothesis that sleep paralysis represents psychomotor dissociation that occurs in the early part of a SOREMP in narcoleptics. They stimulated narcoleptics and normal controls during REM sleep by repeatedly playing a tape of their names. Normal controls showed a behavioral response whereas the narcoleptics did not. However, both groups were equivalent in their correct reporting of the stimulations as having occurred. The

---

* This is in contrast to the expectation in normals that the first REM period of the night will not occur until about an hour and a half of sleep time has elapsed.

investigators take their data as supporting the hypothesis of Hishikawa's group of a sensory–motor dissociation specific to SOREMP for narcoleptics. This dissociation was not demonstrated for any of the subjects with stimulation during other stages of sleep. Nan'no and co-workers postulated further that in narcoleptics, motor suppression associated with REM sleep is unusually persistent, that is, narcoleptics failed to respond behaviorally because of a motor incapacity to do so. They also noted that for narcoleptics there was during REM sleep an increase in excitability and spontaneous activity leading to phasic activity, but there was an equally vigorous, active suppression of more tonic motor output. They noted that the excitability and phasic activity with sleep onset is prominent in narcoleptics. They posited that the primary problem for narcoleptics is an equally powerful centrifugal suppression, and postulated also that the ascending (centripetal) reticular formation is less responsive to modifying influences by sensory stimuli during SOREMP than during other conditions.

The thrust of the available research, therefore, suggests that physiologically sleep paralysis and associated hypnogogic hallucinations (for narcoleptics and nonnarcoleptics alike) are the waking equivalents of muscular atonia and dream events during REM sleep.

Summary

The following points, derived from the foregoing review of the sleep paralysis literature, need be underscored:

1. The true prevalence rate of isolated sleep paralysis is unknown. With respect to gender, it is unclear whether isolated sleep paralysis is more prevalent in one gender than another. The data presented so far do not demonstrate a consistent finding with respect to gender ratios.

2. Sleep paralysis and narcolepsy/cataplexy may be independent disorders. Apropos of this position, sleep paralysis in narcoleptics tends to occur during the sleep-onset period (predormitally), while in patients with independent sleep paralysis, episodes have the highest probability of occurrence postdormitally (i.e., in association with awakenings from sleep, once the sleep period has been firmly established). There are not yet sufficient empirical data to determine whether sleep paralysis in the context of narcolepsy has a significantly higher probability of occurrence than in the general population. Certainly these data do demonstrate that one can have sleep paralysis in the absence of narcolepsy.

3. Sleep paralysis occurs, by definition, only during the periods of wakefulness bracketing the sleep period. However, sleep-onset (predormital) sleep paralysis and sleep paralysis occurring in association with awakenings from sleep (postdormital sleep paralysis) may represent distinct phenomena, even for patients with isolated sleep paralysis. The small database available in this regard indicates that there is a considerably higher probability for an individual

to have experienced only one or the other, than to have experienced both. The small number of studies assessing transfamilial occurrence of independent sleep paralysis would indicate a homogeneity of sleep paralysis type within a multigenerational family.

4. The individual descriptions of symptoms associated with sleep paralysis lead to the impression that sleep paralysis, at least in its recurrent form, may be a component of a more comprehensive syndrome (one distinct from narcolepsy). This latter needs to be pursued. The literature implies that a distinction needs be made between a syndrome, to be called "isolated (idiopathic) sleep paralysis," and the single symptom of sleep paralysis. Isolated sleep paralysis disorder would be characterized by frequent, recurrent, sleep paralysis episodes and would also include the auxiliary symptoms described.

DIAGNOSIS

If a patient presents with a complaint of feeling paralyzed in association with the sleep period, it is necessary to inquire of the patient whether this happens repeatedly or if it was an isolated event. If the former, the patient can simply be reassured with an explanation of the phenomenon and advised that in vulnerable individuals this tends to occur with excessive fatigue, with abrupt changes of the sleep–wake cycle (as with jet lag), and with assumption of the supine position.

If the sleep paralysis happens recurrently, the remainder of the considerations in this section obtain.

The symptom of sleep paralysis requires no further diagnostic procedure than elicitation of the patient's report. It is necessary, however, to determine from that report if she or he is actually describing sleep paralysis. During sleep paralysis, the patient is truly paralyzed. She or he is wholly unable to move★ for up to many minutes. This complaint should be differentiated from complaints of tremendous heaviness of the limbs or such severe exhaustion upon awakening that movement or thought requires great effort but is possible. This latter set of symptoms would more suggest sleep disorders associated with excessive somnolence, such as obstructive sleep apnea.

A narcolepsy/isolated sleep paralysis differential should be carried out. If the patient complains also of excessive daytime sleepiness (especially including precipitous sleep attacks), cataplexy (see Chapter 80), and possibly hypnogogic hallucinations, narcolepsy should be suspected. Isolated sleep paralysis as the primary diagnosis is more likely if the patient does not complain of cataplexy and if his or her daytime status is more consistent with the kind of fatigue one expects following poor sleep. Recurrent sleep paralysis episodes on a given night and poor sleep hygiene resulting in frequently changing sleep–wake schedules (which can

---

★ At times muscles innervated by the cranial nerves are spared.

precipitate sleep paralysis in vulnerable individuals) can be the cause of the poor daytime status. Especially if the daytime fatigue/sleepiness is severe and chronic, however, more than the patient's report should be taken into consideration in establishing the diagnosis.

The patient who does not report sleep paralysis but who does report the auxiliary symptoms commonly associated with sleep paralysis should also be questioned about sleep paralysis. This will affect how the reported symptoms are understood. Conversely, the patient who presents with sleep paralysis should also be questioned about the presence of terrifying nighttime dreams that cause midcycle awakenings from sleep and/or the other known auxiliary symptoms. Because of fear of stigmatization, the patient may not spontaneously present with those additional symptoms. Once these latter symptoms are elicited, the patient can be reassured by explaining that they are part of the sleep paralysis disorder.

For the patient who does present with apparent sleep paralysis, it is useful for purposes of developing a treatment plan to assess what the patient's affective reaction is to sleep paralysis. The terror and dread that can be associated with sleep paralysis attacks can be severe and therefore emotionally debilitating.

Other differentials should also be considered before isolated sleep paralysis disorder is established as the diagnosis. Familial periodic (hypokalemic) paralysis should be ruled out. This occurs in genetically predisposed individuals as an autosomal dominant muscle disease (61). *Hyper*kalemic periodic paralysis should also be ruled out (62,63). The pathophysiology of the paralysis is understood to be depletion of tissue potassium in the muscular system owing to an exaggerated 24-h variation in potassium exchange. The attacks often occur during periods of rest so that the individual may wake up paralyzed as in isolated sleep paralysis. The connection of these attacks with depletion of serum potassium, their periodicity, and their provocation by high carbohydrate meals and alcohol assist in differentiation of familial hypokalemic paralysis from isolated sleep paralysis (3).

Sleep paralysis as an incomplete attack of nocturnal epilepsy should be ruled out. Conversely, but in a similar vein, isolated sleep paralysis should be ruled out for patients who present with twitching movements and apparent loss of consciousness during the sleep-onset period. These differentials generally require a clinical EEG carried out during the patient's normal sleeping hours for assessment.

Central nervous system lesions should also be ruled out either by objective criteria or on the basis of symptom, as appropriate. Ethelberg (64) described sleep paralysis in a patient with damage to the frontal pole secondary to a meningocerebral scar associated with a frontal epidermoid cyst. The patient, who was 45 years old when seen, had been kicked in the right frontal region at age 3. At age 25, he had a sensory seizure affecting his entire face. Between the ages of 39 and 45, he had right frontal hypnopompic headaches if he went to sleep in the supine position. Shortly after this, sleep paralysis—occurring only when the patient was in the supine position during the sleep-onset period—developed. During these episodes, his lips twitched (he was trying to call out), and he appeared to be asleep. The patient had no history of convulsive or psychomotor seizures. EEG showed a mild dysrhythmia with no localizing signs.

Given our experience with a single patient, sleep paralysis secondary to cocaine use also should be ruled out.

TREATMENT

Treatments proposed for isolated sleep paralysis fall largely into two camps: psychologic and physiologic.

There is one component of the sleep paralysis literature suggesting that sleep paralysis is psychogenic and the treatment of choice therefore psychologic. Van der Heide and Weinberg (29), studying sleep paralysis in air force men, saw sleep paralysis as a defense against passive–aggressive psychic conflict: "[It is] more than conceivable that the psychosexual organization of the patients formed the basis for their indecisiveness and for their sleep paralysis." They concluded that because the symptom occurred only just prior to sleep onset or upon awakening, psychosexual conflict likely is involved, that is, these are times when sexual urges are active and under less ego control. Schneck reports many cases of isolated sleep paralysis (31,32,65,66) for which he believed a passive–aggressive conflict was etiologic. Goode (38), Payn (7), and Liddon (15) made the same point. Sleep paralysis was seen as a compromise between fulfillment of and defense against sexual and hostile impulses. All these authors report that psychoanalytic treatment led to the resolution of the sleep paralysis.

Certainly psychologic support should be offered to patients experiencing profound anxiety, dread, and/or terror in response to the sleep paralysis. It should be explained to patients that in the majority of cases, relaxing while the sleep paralysis episode runs its course leads to a more rapid resolution than if the patient fights against it. However, this is not universally true. Further, even those patients who are aware that all of their previous attacks have been relatively brief in duration at times have difficulty suppressing this panic. The fear that the current sleep paralysis attack will persist indefinitely continues. Finally, if the sleep paralysis attack is associated with terrifying hypnogogic hallucinations, simple reassurance is at times insufficient.

Unfortunately, sleep paralysis is too little studied, and treatment approaches too little researched systematically, to permit further definitive recommendations regarding treatment.

Autohypnosis has been tried and may be useful. Nardi (67) reported two cases in which autohypnosis for desensitization to the accompanying anxiety was taught. According to Nardi, this also led to a decrease in the duration of the sleep paralysis episodes.

Pharmacologic interventions have been the most common. There is a single case study suggesting that insulin-induced hypoglycemia can lead to remission of sleep paralysis (4). This has not been followed up, however, and likely is not the treatment of choice. There is also a single case study of a 32-year-old woman who had frequent sleep paralysis accompanied by hypnagogic hallucinations who responded well to fluoxetine (68).

Tricyclic antidepressants are the most frequently used agents. Roth (69) reports that a patient with predormital sleep paralysis was successfully treated with imipramine, but that chlorimipramine and amitriptyline were more effective. Snyder and Ham (53) focused on serotonergic agents in the treatment of isolated sleep paralysis. Their work suggested that tricyclic antidepressants with the greatest capacity to block serotonin reuptake and L-tryptophan (which is a precursor of brain serotonin) were the most powerful suppressants of sleep paralysis. Amitriptyline (75–100 mg) in association with L-tryptophan (2–4 g) at h.s. were the most successful in eliminating sleep paralysis.

SCIENTIFIC ISSUES

Scientific issues raised by the existence of sleep paralysis (either in its isolated form or as a component of narcolepsy) are many. One set of questions focus on the implication of sleep paralysis for understanding REM sleep.

1. Does sleep paralysis in fact represent a component (or set of components) of the REM process dissociated from sleep?
2. If so, what are the factors that lead to this error in timing, with REM features occurring close to but outside the bounds of sleep?
3. More generally, what is the physiologic trigger for sleep paralysis, that is, what leads to the out-of-phase activation of the bulbar inhibitory region?
4. Possibly most important from a basic science perspective, what does this experiment in nature tell us physiologically and functionally about REM sleep?

Were the several sleep disorders assumed to be associated with REM sleep (including also cataplexy, Chapter 80, and REM sleep behavior disorder, Chapter 82) systematically to be compared and contrasted, these experiments of nature might provide tremendous depth to our understanding of the rather unique state of sleep called REM. These may also cast further light on the mechanisms of narcolepsy, which is understood by many to be a disorder of REM sleep.

Other questions more specific to sleep paralysis are whether predormital and postdormital sleep paralysis—in the isolated form and in the context of narcolepsy—represent distinct disorders (or subdisorders), and if so what can be learned by comparing and contrasting the potentially four distinct types of sleep paralysis? The presence of sleep paralysis in some portion of the population only a few times in a lifetime and in others as a primary disorder raises the question of whether the difference is qualitative or quantitative. The neural pathways that subserve the development of sleep paralysis and the associated chemistry are to date little explored.

With respect to narcolepsy, there are a number of further questions. Is the trigger for sleep paralysis in narcoleptics the same as for isolated sleep paralysis? Is sleep paralysis a necessary component of narcolepsy, arising from a presumed single error that gives rise to the remainder of the syndrome? Alternatively, is the sleep paralysis in narcoleptics an epiphenomenon secondary to the immediate disruptions of the sleep–wake cycle known to occur in narcolepsy? It is clear that the severe daytime sleepiness of narcoleptics is not a necessary association to sleep paralysis, as this is absent in patients with isolated sleep paralysis. In narcoleptics, to the degree that sleep paralysis is a component of a narcoleptic syndrome, what is it centrally that might code for the motor manifestations (sleep paralysis and cataplexy) and the sleep/sleepiness symptomatology?

How do we understand the frequent literature notations that stress, and especially poor sleep in association with stress, is a prime antecedent condition for the development of sleep paralysis? There are some additional data that suggest that, at least in nonnarcoleptics with sleep paralysis, something about a disturbance of the sleep–wake cycle can precipitate attacks. This association should be explored, but keeping in mind that not everyone with disturbed sleep–wake cycles develops this disorder.

Snyder (42) documented in case study format a single episode of sleep paralysis in association with jet lag. It is now fairly well-established that dissociations among different circadian rhythms can occur under specific conditions. Subjects have repeatedly been studied in time-free environments, wherein they self-determine lights-on and lights-off periods and sleep–wake periods. Under these circumstances, the period of the temperature cycle (τ, period from temperature minimum to temperature minimum) separates from the period of the sleep–wake curve, the temperature cycle generally describing a shorter τ than the sleep–wake curve (70). Called "internal desynchronization," this can lead to changes in the organization of sleep. Importantly, the probability of REM sleep appears to wax and wane with the temperature cycle. It is possible that these were factors in the development of Snyder's jet-lagged sleep paralysis patient. In other words, it is possible that for this individual jet lag led to a similar dissociation with specific implications for REM sleep. Sleep paralysis was the result, that is to say, an episode of some of the features of REM sleep dissociated from an actual sleep period.

Fukuda et al (11) also speculated that sleep paralysis arises most directly from a disturbed sleep–wake cycle that secondarily affects the relationship of the constituents of REM sleep to the sleep–wake cycle. They suggested that it is a physiologically reasonable consequence of a disturbed sleep–wake cycle rather than a pathologic phenomenon. With respect to its association to narcolepsy, the group found sleep paralysis in 57% of the 102 narcoleptics they studied. However, it was their impression that even in these cases sleep paralysis was an epiphenomenon of narcolepsy, arising secondary to the generalized sleep–wake disturbance specific to this disorder. They did not see it as a primary (and therefore necessary) reflection of the underlying pathophysiology of narcolepsy. This latter remains to be elucidated.

Instructively, the same group (44) carried out polysomnographic studies in two female college students with, and two without, *Kanashibara* after experimentally reversing their sleep–wake cycle. This appeared to precipitate a sleep-onset episode in one subject and one episode in another subject arising out of an awakening from REM sleep. A study by Takeuchi et al (71) was consistent with the possibility that REM disruption leading to sleep paralysis may be the mediating factor between stressful life circumstances and/or circadian rhythm disturbances. They were able to elicit a small number of sleep-onset episodes of sleep paralysis in normal subjects by forcing an awakening about 40 minutes into a period of NREM sleep that followed a REM episode. In 71.9% of these trials, a sleep-onset REM period (SOREMP) was produced upon the subjects' return to sleep. All but one of the induced episodes of sleep paralysis occurred during the SOREMP.

The clue provided by the recurrent mention in the literature of position-dependency for sleep paralysis has not been pursued. Single case studies and large scale epidemiologic studies alike recurrently note that sleeping in the supine position is a frequent antecedent condition. Nor has there, in this context, been particular use made of the oft-repeated fact that sleep paralysis episodes can be fully terminated by a light touch. Peterson's 1978 research (72) focusing on the medial and lateral reticulospinal pathways likely is pertinent in this regard. Reticulospinal neurons receive strong, direct input from the sensorimotor cortex. Control is of axial and proximal, not distal (i.e., finger) muscles. Input is from somatic afferent fibers. These are activated by hair bending. The majority are activated by touch, pressure, or tapping on the skin. This information may be useful in utilizing the clue that sleep paralysis can be broken by light touch. Further, a second source of input to reticulospinal neurons is from the semicircular canal, which finding may in the future permit us to make use of the common citing of the supine position as an antecedent condition for sleep paralysis.

The implication for an anatomic substrate of the finding of Weitzner (3) of amelioration of sleep paralysis through insulin-induced hypoglycemia also remains to be replicated and understood.

Reports of sleep paralysis and association hypnogogic hallucinations in association with a lesion of the frontal pole (64) may ultimately be useful in unraveling the neural pathways involved. We reiterate that even in this patient, sleep paralysis occurred almost exclusively when the patient became drowsy while in the supine position. For this patient, sleep paralysis occurred in the absence of hypnogogic hallucinations. Ethelberg postulated that the development of sleep paralysis secondary to this lesion might suggest possible output from the frontal area to descending inhibitory fibers. This case study certainly raises the possibility that a descending pathway originating outside of the classic cortical motor area, in the region of the frontal pole, might also mediate initiation of untimely paralysis proximal to but not within the sleep period.

With respect to neurochemical mediators, there is even less understanding of sleep paralysis. Many authors (73–75) have provided evidence that the monoamines are involved in inhibiting the development of REM sleep, and that acetylcholine is involved at least in the triggering if not the maintenance of REM sleep. It is difficult, however, to apply these findings to phenomena associated with REM sleep that occur outside the bounds of sleep and that do not invariably represent the full complement of events believed to be unique to this "sleep" state. The neurochemical models of REM sleep currently available do not easily lend themselves to understanding the dissociation of descending inhibition of alpha motor neurons and dream-like phenomena—as a unit—from the remainder of the sleep period. It is likely that with additional components added or with some modifications, however, that this might be accomplished. Sleep paralysis in association with hypnogogic hallucinations does not occur within subjectively experienced sleep, but they are clearly sleep related. Thus, further insight into these events might help in the articulation of sleep/wake mechanisms.

The majority of efforts to develop some understanding of the neurochemistry of sleep paralysis and hypnogogic hallucinations does use what is known about the neurochemistry of REM sleep as a starting point. Snyder and Ham (53) empirically observed the effects of numerous pharmacologic compounds on sleep paralysis. As described above, they found that serotonin reuptake blockers and exogenous L-tryptophan were most effective in ameliorating the disorder. Based on this, they speculated that sleep paralysis may be secondary to decreased levels of brain serotonin. However, the serotonin reuptake blockers used were primarily tricyclic antidepressants, which also to varying degrees block norepinephrine reuptake and are also acetylcholine antagonists to varying degrees.

Bell et al (41) viewed sleep paralysis as a hyperadrenergic symptom, with possibly hypersecretion of noradrenaline from the locus coeruleus. They also reported (46) a high probability association between daytime panic attacks and sleep paralysis, and postulated that the two disorders may share a common neurologic mechanism, again possibly involving the locus coeruleus. However, on the surface at least, this is contradictory to the prevailing view of REM sleep as an organized whole. Noradrenergic pathways arising from the locus coeruleus are understood as being antagonistic to the development of REM sleep, at least as an integrated whole.

In summary, sleep paralysis has not received a great deal of attention. For those studying narcolepsy, sleep paralysis has been only a minor player and therefore of relatively less interest than cataplexy. For those focused on the more severe sleep disorders, sleep paralysis because of its low rate of presentation to sleep disorders centers has not been central. Yet, by virtue of its characteristics, isolated sleep paralysis disorder may be a physiologic Rosetta stone. And when translated. . . .

REFERENCES

1. Aldrich MS. Cardinal manifestations of sleep disorders. In: Kryger MH, Roth T, Dement C, eds. Principles and practice of sleep medicine. 2nd ed. Philadelphia: WB Saunders, 1994:422.

2. Narcolepsy. In: International classification of sleep disorders: diagnostic and coding manual. Rochester, MI: American Sleep Disorders Association, 1990:38–43.

3. Sleep paralysis. In: International classification of sleep disorders: diagnostic and coding manual. Rochester, MI: American Sleep Disorders Association, 1990:166–169.

4. Weitzner HA. Sleep paralysis successfully treated with insulin hypoglycemia. Arch Neurol Psychiatry 1952;68:835–841.

5. Schneck JM. Sleep paralysis, a new evaluation. Dis Nerv Syst 1957;18:144–146.

6. Everett HC. Sleep paralysis in medical studies. J Nerv Ment Dis 1963;136:283–287.

7. Payn SB. A psychoanalytic approach to sleep paralysis. J Nerv Ment Dis 1965;140:427–433.

8. Roth B, Buvhova S, Berkova L. Familial sleep paralysis. Schweiz Arch Neurol Neurochir Psychiatr 1968;102:321–330.

9. Ness RC. The old hag phenomenon as sleep paralysis: a biocultural interpretation. Cult Med Psychiatry 1978;2:15–39.

10. Penn NE, Kripke DF, Scharff J. Sleep paralysis among medical students. J Psychol 1981;107:247–252.

11. Fukuda K, Myasita A, Inugama M, Ishihara K. High prevalence of isolated sleep paralysis: Kanashibari phenomenon in Japan. Sleep 1987;10:279–286.

12. Luck CL. Sleep disturbance (letter). J Am Med Assoc 1981;246:163–164.

13. Chodoff P. Sleep paralysis with report of two cases. J Nerv Ment Dis 1944;100:278–281.

14. Schneck JM. Henry Fuseli, nightmare and sleep paralysis. JAMA 1969;207:725–726.

15. Liddon SC. Sleep paralysis and hypnagogic hallucinations. Arch Gen Psychiatry 1967;17:88–96.

16. Macnish R. The philosophy of sleep. New York: Appleton, 1834.

17. Binns E. The anatomy of sleep; or, the art of procuring a sound and refreshing slumber at will. London: John Churchill, 1842.

18. Mitchell SW. On some of the disorders of sleep. Va Med Monthly 1876;2:769–781.

19. Pfister H. Uber storunge des erwachers. Berl Klin Wochenschr 1903;40:385–387.

20. Trömner E. Uber motorische schlafstorange. Ztschr Gesamte Neurol Psychiatr 1911;4:228.

21. Rosenthal C. Uber das verzogert psychomotorische erwachen, seine entstehung und seine nosologische bedenting. Arch Psychiatr 1927;81:159–171.

22. Lhermitte J, Dupont Y. Sur la cataplexie et plus specialement sur la cataplexie du reveil. Encephale 1928;23:424–434.

23. Wilson SAK. The narcolepsies. Brain 1928;51:63–109.

24. Levin M. The pathogenesis of narcolepsy, with a consideration of sleep paralysis and localized sleep. J Neurol Psychopathol 1933;14:1–13.

25. Daniels LE. Narcolepsy. Medicine 1934;13:1–22.

26. Krabbe E, Magnussen G. On narcolepsy. I. Familial narcolepsy. Acta Psychiatr Neurol 1942;17:149–173.

27. Lichtenstein B, Rosenblum AH. Sleep paralysis. J Nerv Ment Dis 1942;95:153–155.

28. Rushton JC. Sleep paralysis. Med Clin N Am 1944;28:945–959.

29. Van der Heide C, Weinberg J. Sleep paralysis and combat fatigue. Psychosom Med 1945;7:330–334.

30. Hudson JI, Manooch DS, Sabo AN, et al. Recurrent nightmares in posttraumatic stress disorder: association with sleep paralysis, hypnopompic hallucinations, and REM sleep. J Nerv Ment Dis 1991;179(9):572–573.

31. Schneck JM. Sleep paralysis: psychodynamics. Psychiatr Q 1948;22:462–469.

32. Schneck JM. Sleep paralysis. Am J Psychiatry 1952;108:921–923.

33. Yoss RE, Daly DD. Criteria for the diagnosis of the narcolepsy syndrome. Proc Mayo Clin 1957;32:320–328.

34. Roth B. Narkolepsie a hypersomnie s hlediska fysiologie spanku. Prague: Statni Zdravotnicke Nakladatelstvi, 1957:331.

35. Roth B. Narkolepsie und Hypersomnie vom Standpunkt der Physiologie des Schlafes. Berlin: VEB Ver. Volk Gesundheit, 1962:428.

36. Hishikawa DJ. Sleep paralysis. In: Guilleminault C, Dement WC, Passouant P, eds. Advances in sleep research. Vol. 3. New York: Spectrum, 1976:97–124.

37. Coleman RM, Roffwarg HP, Kennedy SJ, et al. Sleep–wake disorders based on a polysomnographic diagnosis: a national cooperative study. JAMA 1982;247:997–1003.

38. Goode GB. Sleep paralysis. Am Med Assoc Arch Neurol 1962;6:121–130.

39. Ohderi JU, Odejide DA, Ikucsan BA, Adeyemi JD. The pattern of isolated sleep paralysis among Nigerian medical students. J Natl Med Assoc 1989;81(7):805–808.

40. Spanos NP, McNulty SA, Dubreuil SC, Pires M. The frequency and correlates of sleep paralysis in a university sample. J Res Personality 1995;29(3):285–305.

41. Bell CC, Shakoor B, Thompson B, et al. Prevalence of isolated sleep paralysis in black subjects. J Natl Med Assoc 1984;76:501–508.

42. Snyder S. Isolated sleep paralysis after rapid time-zone change (jet lag) syndrome. Chronobiologica 1983;10:377–379.

43. De Jong JT. Sleep paralysis and anxiety related to sleep in various cultures. Tijdschr Psychiatr 1991;33(10):681–693.

44. Fukuda K, Inamatsu N, Kuroiwa M, Miyasita A. Personality of healthy young adults with sleep paralysis. Percept Mot Skills 1991;73:955–962.

45. Suarez A. Isolated sleep paralysis in patients with disorders due to anguish crisis. Actas Luso Esp Neurol Psiquiatr Cienc Afines 1991;19(1):58–61.

46. Bell CC, Dixie Bell DD, Thompson B. Panic attacks: relationship to isolated sleep paralysis (letter). Am J Psychiatry 1986;143:1484.

47. Ribstein M. Hypnagogic hallucinations. In: Guilleminault C, Dement WC, Passouant P, eds. Advances in sleep research. Vol. 3. New York: Spectrum, 1976:145–160.

48. Liddon SC. Sleep paralysis, psychosis and death. Am J Psychiatry 1970;126:1027–1031.

49. Schneck JM. Sleep paralysis and nocturnal seizure disorder (letter). JAMA 1982;247:303.

50. Brain WR. Sleep: Normal and pathological. Br Med J 1939;2:51.

50a. Contreras D, Steriade M. Cellular basis of EEG slow rhythms: a study of dynamic corticothalamic relationships. J Neurosci 1995;15:604–622.

51. Hishikawa Y, Kancho Z. Electroencephalographic study on narcolepsy. Electroencephalogr Clin Neurophysiol 1965;18:249–259.

52. Nan'no H, Hishikawa Y, Koida H, et al. A neurophysiological study of sleep paralysis in narcoleptic patients. Electroencephalogr Clin Neurophysiol 1970;28:382–390.

53. Snyder S, Ham G. Serotonergic agents in the treatment of isolated sleep paralysis. Am J Psychiatry 1982;39:1202–1203.

54. Hodes R, Dement W. Depression of electrically induced reflexes ("H-reflexes") in man during low voltage "sleep." Electroencephalogr Clin Neurophysiol 1964;17:617–629.

55. Kubota K, Iwamura T, Niimi Y. Monosynaptic reflex and natural sleep. J Neurophysiol 1965;28:125–138.

56. Shimizu A, Yamada Y, Yamamoto J, et al. Pathways of descending influence on H-reflex during sleep. Electroencephalogr Clin Neurophysiol 1966;20:337–347.

57. Holmes CJ, Jones BE. Importance of cholinergic, GABAergic, serotonergic and other neurons in the medial medullary reticular formation for sleep–wake states studied by cytotoxic lesions in the cat. Neuroscience 1994;62:1179–1200.

58. Magoun HW, Rhines R. An inhibitory mechanism in the bulbar reticular formation. J Neurophysiol 1946;9:165–171.

59. Broughton R. Circaesemidian sleep rhythms and its relationship to the circadian and ultradian sleep–wake. In Koella WP, Obal F, Shulz H, Visser P, eds. Sleep '86. New York: Gustav Fischer, 1988:41–43.

60. Hishikawa Y, Sumitsuji N, Matsumoto K, Kaneko Z. H-reflex and EMG of the mental and hyoid muscles during sleep with special reference to narcolepsy. Electroencephalogr Clin Neurophysiol 1965;18:487–492.

61. Sipos I, Jurkatt-Rott K, Horasztosi C, et al. Skeletal muscle D HP receptor mutations alter calcium currents in human hypokalaemic periodic paralysis myotubes. J Physiol 1995;483(2):299–306.

62. Baguero JA, Ayala RA, Wang J, et al. Hyperkalemic periodic paralysis with cordias dysrhythmia: a novel sodium channel mutation? Ann Neurol 1995;37(3):408–411.

63. Iaizzo PA, Quasthoff S, Lehmann-Horn F. Differential diagnosis of periodic paralysis aided by in vitro myography. Neuromuscul Disord 1995;5(2):115–124.

64. Ethelberg S. Sleep paralysis or post-dormital chalastic fits in cortical lesions of the frontal pole. Acta Psychiatr Neurol 1956;108(suppl):121–130.

65. Schneck JM. Personality components in patients with sleep paralysis. Psychiatr Q 1969;43:343–348.

66. Schneck JM. Sleep paralysis and spontaneous hypnotic paralysis. Percept Mot Skills 1970;31:16.

67. Nardi JJ. Treating sleep paralysis with hypnosis. Int J Clin Exp Hypn 1981;29:358–365.

68. Koran LM, Raghovan S. Fluoxetine for isolated sleep paralysis. Psychosomatics 1993;34(2):184–187.

69. Roth B. Narcolepsy and hypersomnia. In: Williams RL, Karacan I, eds. Sleep disorders: diagnosis and treatment. New York: John Wiley, 1978:29–60.

70. Moore-Ede MC, Czeisler CA, Richardson GS. Circadian timekeeping in health and disease. N Engl J Med 1983;309:469–476, 530–536.

71. Takeuchi T, Miyasita A, Sasaki Y, et al. Isolated sleep paralysis elicited by sleep interruption. Sleep 1992;15(3):217–225.

72. Peterson BW. Reticulo-motor pathways: their connections and possible roles in motor behavior. In: Asanuma H, Wilson VS, eds. Integration in the nervous systems: a symposium in honor of David PC Lloyd and Rafael Lorente de No. Tokyo: Igaku-Shoin, 1978:185–201.

73. Jouvet M. The role of monoamines and acetylcholine containing neurons in the regulation of the sleep–waking cycle. Ergeb Physiol 1972;64:166–307.

74. McCarley RW, Hobson JA. Neuronal excitability modulation over the sleep cycle: a structural and mathematical mode. Science 1975;189:58–60.

75. Sitaram N, Gillin JC. Acetylcholine: possible involvement in sleep and analgesia. In: Davis KL, Berger PA, eds. Brain acetylcholine and neuropsychiatric disease. New York: Plenum, 1979:311–343.

REM Sleep Behavior Disorder

J. Gila Lindsley

INTRODUCTION

True somnambulism—sleep walking—defines a gray area in the otherwise sharp distinction between sleep and wakefulness. The somnambulist carries out certain stereotypic behaviors, some of them quite complex, as if he or she were awake. Yet by polysomnographic criteria the somnambulist is cortically asleep. As described in Chapter 83, somnambulism is a dissociative state, arising out of the deepest stage of non-REM (NREM) sleep, variously called either stage 3–4 or delta sleep.

In some respects, the activities of persons with rapid eye movement (REM) sleep behavior disorder resemble those of the somnambulist. However, whereas the somnambulist is generally amnestic to his or her activities during the night and rarely has any cognition, mentation, or affect associated with the episodes, the person with REM sleep behavior disorder (RBD) is flooded with vivid images, cognitions, and often affects that are intimately related to the behavior he or she is carrying out while still asleep. The person seems literally to be acting out a dream and, in fact, may carry out highly complex behaviors.

HISTORY

Debuting in a surprise, unscheduled presentation at the 1985 meeting of the Association of Professional Sleep Societies, REM sleep behavior disorder (RBD) was first characterized by Schenck et al (1) for four male and one female patient. All had sought help because of repeated, violent self-inflicted and other injuries caused by the patients' behaviors while asleep. Before the advent of polysomnography, which is a procedure for recording during sleep physiologic events such as the electroencephalogram (EEG), electrooculogram (EOG), and the submental electromyogram (EMG), it would

have simply been assumed that these patients were somnambulists, that is, sleep walkers in the classical sense. With polysomnography available in 1985, however, an unexpected finding was made. It was demonstrated for all five patients that the behaviors arose out of REM sleep rather than representing an aggressive form of classic somnambulism. This phenomenon had never been documented before, and hence the unscheduled presentation of the surprising findings.

Follow-up neurologic evaluation of these patients indicated that for three (two men, one woman), there was a possibly relevant neurologic compromise; but neurologic assessments of the other two, designated idiopathic, were unremarkable (1). The authors' implicit working hypothesis was that RBD, as in the case of cataplexy, could be either idiopathic or secondary to an organic central nervous system (CNS) disorder. As will be developed below, however, subsequent findings years later among some patients for whom the disorder appeared to be idiopathic at the time of diagnosis raises the question whether even in apparently idiopathic cases there might not already be a developing CNS insult that could not be appreciated at the time of diagnosis.

This disorder found its place in the diagnostic category system of sleep disorders medicine five years after the initial report, in 1990, in the first International Classification of Sleep Disorders (2), three years after Schenck and his collaborators published an abstract describing five years of clinical experience with this disorder (3). Based upon the information available at the time of publication, the estimate was that approximately 60% of cases are idiopathic and that advanced age is an apparent predisposing factor. Schenck's group provided a comprehensive update six years later (4) that summarizes their first ten years of experience with REM sleep behavior disorder patients. Sensitization of sleep disorders clinicians to this disorder has in recent years led to the publication of numerous case reports, some of which extend the description of what appears to be a complex syndrome and some of which can be interpreted to challenge the early hypothesis that there may be an idiopathic form of RBD.

DESCRIPTION

In our own laboratory, we have seen three such cases.

Case 1

A 59-year-old woman, with the exception of some few probable episodes of "REM-walking" in childhood, had been an essentially normal sleeper until two years previously, about three years after she began receiving chemotherapy with thiotepa for bladder cancer. She and her husband relate her dream behavior to initiation of thiotepa. Her husband describes that she then became increasingly more active during sleep, more often injuring herself while acting out her dreams. Initially, injuries were largely bruises. The more active the dreams became, the more severe were her injuries. She described one such active dream in detail: "In my dream, I was riding a horse. In the dream, the horse faltered and was beginning to fall. To prevent myself from being crushed, I jumped from the horse. This resulted in my taking a nose dive from my bed against my bureau."

Case 2

A second patient presented with the complaint, "I am in danger of being evicted from my trailer court because of the raucous parties they say I hold at night." Reports by a relative indicated that the patient herself, while asleep, was the raucous party! The patient, during her sleep, had been extremely active. History revealed a prodrome of especially vivid, at times disruptive, dreams of 15 to 20 years (she was 64 years old when she first presented to us for help). In the laboratory, we had the opportunity to observe her motorically activated dreams. Our own nighttime technician's account of the experience captures, part of which is reproduced in Figure 82.1, its flavor.

Figure 82.2 depicts two consecutive pages from this second patient's record. The typical eye movements of REM sleep can be seen in the second and third channels. Intruding into this period, during which complete atonia of antigravity muscles and hypotonia of oropharyngeal muscles should be expected, are several phasic events: "laugh, sob. . . ." At one point, the woman was described as sitting up in bed, apparently dealing out cards cursing at "someone" who was cheating—all while continuing to be in REM sleep.

Case 3

A 65-year-old man was brought in by his wife because "he dreams of snakes, spiders, rats crawling up the bed. He swings and punches in his sleep, and sometimes hits me. Once, he

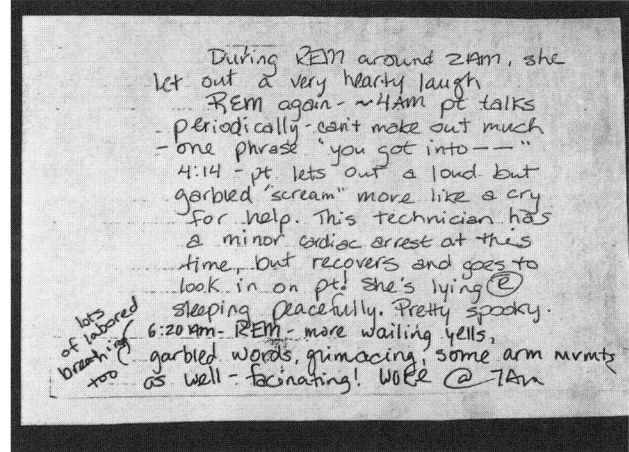

FIGURE 82.1   *Technician's account of sleeptime activities of patient with REM behavior disorder.*

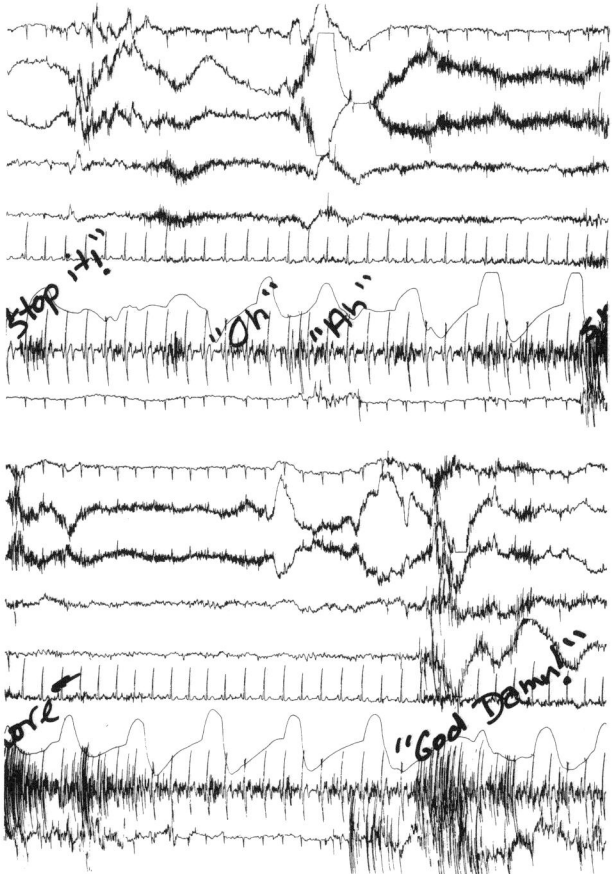

FIGURE 82.2   *Two epochs from record of a woman with REM behavior disorder. Note vocalizations and unusual muscle tonus, although this is REM sleep.*

had me by the neck and was choking me. He also talks sometimes when this happens, so I know that he seems to be acting out his dream." The patient was a recovering alcoholic with three years' sobriety when he presented for help; but his most motorically active dreams occurred when he was still actively drinking. The patient believes that the onset of his dream behaviors was at least 11 years earlier, when he already had been actively drinking for several decades.

We were not able to capture an elaborate sequence of this patient's dream behavior in the laboratory but were able to capture multiple episodes of significant compromise in the expected atonia of REM sleep. Figure 82.3, for instance, illustrates two consecutive pages from his record. The sustained elevation of submental EMG in association with a train of rapid eye movements and the lifting of his head while still in REM sleep show the compromised antigravity muscle atonia during this sleep state.

An unexpected feature of this third patient's history is suggestive either of compelling residues of dreams remaining once the patient has awakened, or, more likely, hallucinatory perceptual distortions:

*Upon awakening in the early A.M., I see in my bedroom vague forms of people and animals. These quickly disappear and become ordinary room furniture or plants or parts of the bedroom. Sometimes these animals or reptiles will seem to try to attack me and I will noisily defend myself.**

Such an episode was observed in the laboratory. When greeted by the technician in the morning, he "saw" a dog behind her. The "dog" eventually resolved into a common object. Curiously, the awakening was from delta, not REM, sleep. A lengthy episode of REM with sporadic lapses of atonia had preceded the delta period. The overt activity during sleep and the associated hallucinatory event both have responded very well to 0.5 mg of clonazepam at h.s.

Since the original finding by Schenck et al (1), reports in the literature of polysomnographically verified RBD have served to extend and to some degree further define the syndrome, its antecedents, and other of its aspects. Doghramji et al (6) reported three cases of REM behavior disorder. The polysomnographic studies also demonstrated an apparent release of atonia during REM sleep as reflected in gross, complex behaviors during this sleep stage. Tachibana et al (7) described the case of a Japanese man with RBD for whom sleep bruxism was a prominent symptom, leading them to suggest a common pathophysiology to RBD and certain types of sleep bruxism. There has not been a published follow-up on this observation in other patients or subjects. In another report (8), data from 14 RBD subjects

were interpreted to suggest abnormal autonomic activity and hyporeactivity during sleep and wakefulness for this disorder. As of this writing, reports are still too sparse to determine whether RBD can be idiopathic or if it is inevitably the result of CNS injury.

Salva and Guilleminault (9) described the sleep of two patients with olivopontocerebellar degeneration, both of whom demonstrated elevated chin EMG in their polysomnograms. In contrast to the early cases reported by Schenck et al (1,10), Doghramji et al (6), and those from our laboratory, in the Salva and Guilleminault patients the increased muscle tone was consistent throughout the recording period including REM sleep. This is in contrast to an escape from muscle atonia occurring only phasically during REM in association with eye movements. Nor did these patients complain of injuries occurring during sleep or of other factors associated with their sleep. Rather, their primary complaint was of daytime tiredness and sleepiness.

A variation on the theme of REM sleep behavior disorder was reported for a number of patients with multiple sclerosis in 1986 (11). Symptoms consistent with RBD were then reported for three patients with concurrent Shy-Drager syndrome, one with concurrent olivopontocerebellar atrophy, and two with no identifiable neurologic disease in 1988 (12). In 1989, magnetic resonance imaging (MRI) data for an additional six patients with polysomnographically diagnosed RBD were presented (13). For these patients, MRI of the brain identified probable lacunar infarcts in the periventricular region and/or the dorsal pontomesencephalic area, leading to the speculation that injury to the midrostral tegmental nuclei and/or to the tegmentoreticular tracts might be one cause of RBD. In 1990, Wright et al (14) offered a single case of a patient diagnosed with Shy-Drager syndrome who had concurrent RBD. The symptoms of progressive RBD had anticipated the development of Shy-Drager syndrome by many years.

In 1995, Tachibana et al (15) identified the polysomnographic signs of RBD in the absence of nocturnal behavioral complaints in five Japanese patients in an early stage of sporadic olivopontocerebellar atrophy. This led them to suggest that RBD might be an early sign of impending neurogenerative disease. The following year, Schenck's group (16) reported the results of a longitudinal study of 29 male patients initially diagnosed as having idiopathic RBD, 38% of whom were eventually diagnosed with a parkinsonian disorder. An additional 7% of the cohort eventually developed other neurologic disorders. Pareja et al (17) described the co-occurrence of what they describe as preclinical RBD and progressive supranuclear palsy in a woman who exhibited both somniloquy (sleep talking) and daytime speech inhibition. They suggested that somniloquy as well as yelling and limb jerking may be the chronologic prodrome to RBD. Following this, Schenck's group then found autopsy-confirmed evidence of Alzheimer's disease in one case of RBD (18), Plazzi et al (19) reported symptoms and

---

* This case may be similar to those reported by Gross et al (5), describing sleep disturbances and hallucinations in the acute alcoholic psychoses.

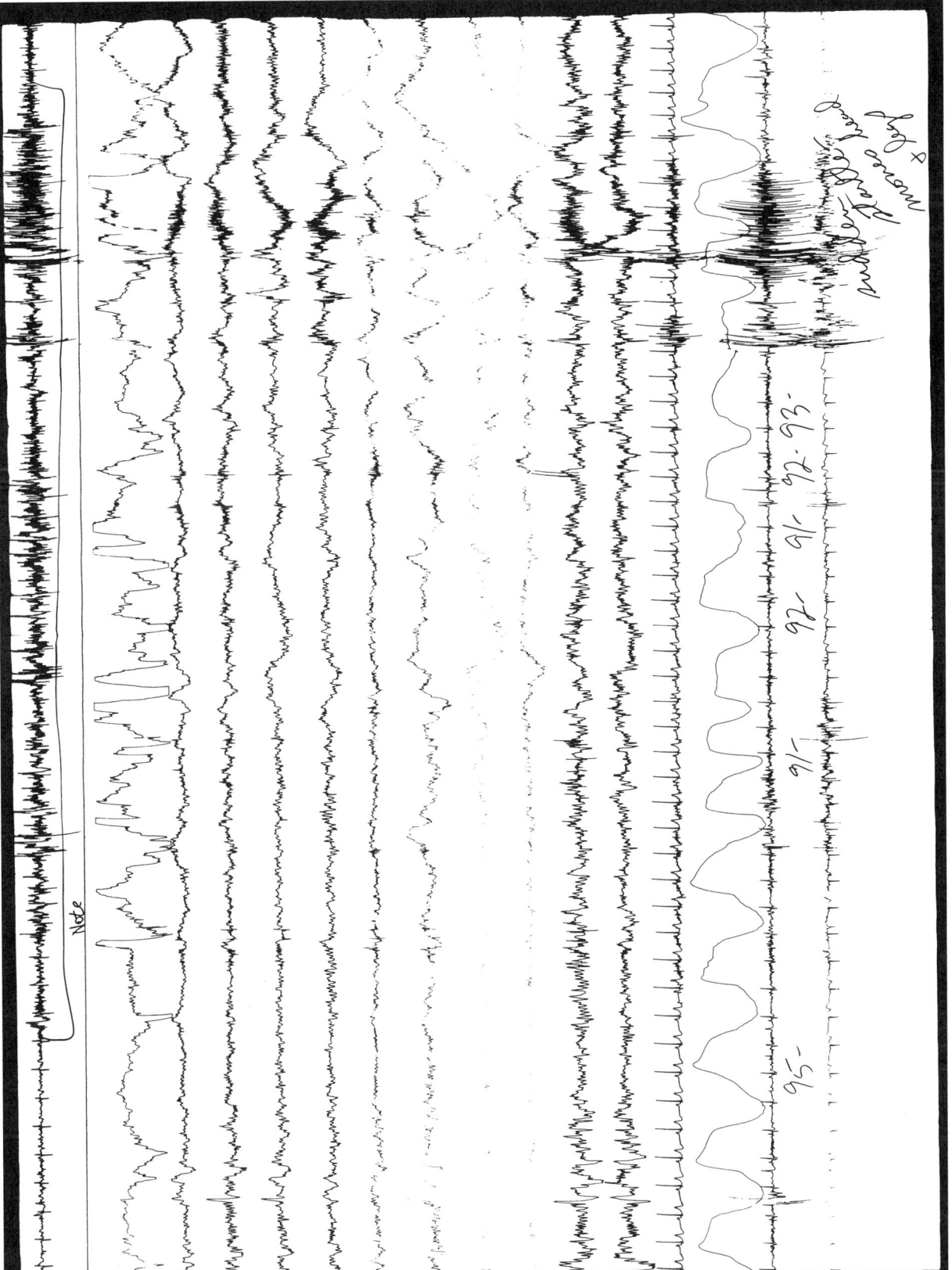

FIGURE 82.3 *REM episode beginning with appropriate atonia, proceeding into elevated submental EMG (first channel) in presence of rapid eye movements (third channel), and phasic episode terminated by head lifting.*

polysomnographic signs of RBD in 27 of 39 consecutive cases of multiple system atrophy patients, and Negro and Faber (20) reported the comorbidity of RBD and Lewy body disease in a single patient. Morfis et al (21) provided data to suggest that falling in association with nocturnal wandering may in some elderly patients be caused by RBD, with the implication that pharmacologic treatment of RBD (see below) may attenuate these incidents.

There have been some reports of polysomnographic signs and/or RBD clinical symptoms in patients without known gross lesion to the CNS but under circumstances than can suggest pathologic CNS involvement. Polysomnographic findings but in the absence of overt behavioral symptoms of RBD were found in 10 narcoleptic patients (22). Overt symptoms in combination with the polysomnographic signs of RBD were reported for one patient carrying a diagnosis of obsessive–compulsive disorder consequent upon the initiation of fluoxetine treatment, for whom the polysomnographic signs of RBD were still present at repeat polysomnography 19 months after fluoxetine discontinuation (23).

RBD has now been reported for a Chinese male (24) and for two children (25), without known indication of a concurrent neurologic disorder.

To our knowledge, other than some review papers (3,26), the foregoing are the entirety of the case reports available at this writing. It therefore is still premature to offer a conclusive characterization of this disorder, especially with respect to the possible cause–effect relationship between a variety of neurologic disorders and RBD, and especially with respect to the pathophysiology of the disorder. It is possible, and even likely, that the polysomnographic signs of RBD, with or without associated clinical symptoms, may be the final common outcome of a range of structural or functional disturbances of the CNS.

With that caveat, the following is a summary of the known characteristics.

1. The defining characteristic of the disorder is a failure of muscle atonia during REM sleep and consequent complex, often injurious, behaviors occurring while the patient is asleep. Dream material has generally seemed appropriate to the behaviors, suggesting the patients are acting out dreams.

2. Observable symptoms range from simple increase of muscle tone during REM sleep, and possibly nocturnal bruxism, to a range of behaviors: movement brought about by antigravity muscles, such as head lifting during REM sleep; talking, yelling, or jerking limbs during REM sleep; laughing and sobbing; punching, kicking, sitting, crawling, leaping out of bed; highly activated behaviors at times interactive with the bed partner, such as choking of the bed partner as described above.

3. There appears to be a concurrent dream disorder. Dreams become increasingly more vivid, unpleasant, action filled, and violent. The more violent behavioral activities

have a significantly higher probability of occurring in males. There is a suggestion that the increased activity and violence in patients' dreams may reflect feedback from incorporation of the actual movements into the dream, consistent with McCarly's activation–synthesis hypothesis (27). This remains to be determined.

4. The fully expressed disorder has been demonstrated in about one-third of the diagnosed patients to have been preceded by a definable prodrome of sleep talking, yelling, or limb jerking that began several decades before the frank onset of the sleep disorder. For instance, our patient whose REM behavior disorder may have been triggered by thiotepa treatment was described by her husband as having made movements with her hands as if she were unraveling yarn, and to "move" or twitch during a large amount of her sleeping time before the onset of the more violent movements.

5. Virtually all cases reported suffered varying degrees of injury during their sleep activities. Mahowald (28) estimated that 97% of the patient population sustained injuries during their sleep.

6. With respect to age of onset, increasing numbers of reports since the disorder was characterized would suggest that onset of REM sleep behavior disorder is in the later years, although the finding of RBD in children would suggest this is not inevitably so. Mean age of onset for the original sample is 55 years old, an average of 7 years earlier than their presentation for help. Schenck has documented a prodrome up to 27 years preceding frank development of the disorder, in the form of yelling and limb jerking (4).

7. The polysomnographic signs of RBD can be present in the absence of the overt behavioral syndrome. It will require more years of longitudinal study to determine whether the patients initially diagnosed with only the polysomnographic signs of RBD will eventually also develop the clinical symptoms.

8. At this writing, there is a tentative subclassification of REM sleep behavior disorder into an idiopathic form and one secondary to other medical disease. However, longitudinal study of patients originally classified as having the idiopathic form suggests that polysomnographic signs of RBD either in the presence or absence of the clinical behavior disorder may be a precursor to a diagnosable neurologic disease. The implication is that even before objective signs of the neurologic disease were appreciable the pathophysiology leading to its development may have secondarily created RBD. It must be kept in mind, however, that many of the neurologic diseases that eventually developed in these patients have an increasing probability of occurrence in an aging population, so that at this time there is not yet a way of assessing the possibility of a direct causal relationship between the pathophysiologies of RBD and of the variety of neurologic diseases under consideration.

9. Polysomnographic findings have been interesting. A large percentage of Schenck's patients have demonstrated periodic leg movements of sleep (see Chapters 56 and

66), occurring during NREM sleep throughout the night. This was true of two of our three patients; only the 65-year-old male patient was free of this. Periodic arm movements are variably represented as well. In addition, an even larger percentage of Schenck's patients showed limb movements/twitches that were aperiodic rather than periodic during NREM sleep. With respect to sleep architecture, 18% showed an increase over the age-normed range of total sleep time occupied by REM sleep and, perhaps a more robust finding, 78% showed an increase in percentage of total sleep time occupied by delta (slow-wave) sleep. This latter was true for our two female patients but not for the male patient. The former was true for none of our patients.

Another interesting aspect of the polysomnographic studies, as reported by Schenck's laboratory (25), was that although there seemed to be an increase in the density of eye movements during REM sleep, autonomic phasic event increase was not documented. Tachycardia, for instance, did not occur with the motor behavior. That is, sympathetic "paralysis" seemed to be sustained. The later data offered by Fereini-Strambi et al (8) would suggest in diagnosed RBD patients an unusual hyporesponsivity of the autonomic system not only during REM sleep but also during NREM sleep and during periods of waking as well. Perhaps the most interesting aspect of the polysomnograms of these patients was that release from atonia was episodic, not tonic. It had the highest probability of occurrence during trains of rapid eye movements. These abnormal episodes were sandwiched between segments of tonic REM with apparently normal atonia. (See, for instance, Fig 82.3.)

DIAGNOSIS

REM sleep behavior disorder should be suspected when a patient presents with recurrent episodes of extensive, complex motor activity clearly occurring during sleep, as described above, and especially when vivid dream material corresponding to the sleep-related activity is elicited from the patient at the time of the episode once he or she has awakened. It is not clear how best to select those patients with lesser behaviors during sleep (e.g., wringing of hands, twitches, and limb movements) who are at risk for developing violent, self-injurious behaviors during sleep. There is little information about the prodromal period other than what has been established historically by patients presenting with an already well-developed REM sleep behavior disorder. At this time we would recommend that if complex movements of any magnitude (simple but recurrent hand movements through the more violent complex motor activities) are observed in a patient, and especially if when awakened from these movements the patient relates dream material consistent with these movements, that the possibility of REM sleep behavior disorder should at least be considered. The suspicion index is increased if the patient is older and if there is a known neurologic disorder. The report

by Morfis et al (21) suggests that, in cases of nocturnal wandering associated with falls in elderly patients, the pharmacologically treatable disorder—RBD—should be considered in the differential.

Treatment planning relies upon a differential diagnosis between REM sleep behavior disorder and other sleep-related disorders that lead to similar symptomatology. The most probable differentials to consider are classic sleepwalking and sleep-related epileptic seizures. Polysomnography is essential for establishing the diagnosis. The expectation with sleepwalking is that the complex motor activity will arise from NREM sleep, generally delta sleep. Both this form of sleepwalking and delta sleep as well, however, are rare in the older individual. (For further consideration of the signs and symptoms of classic sleepwalking and differentials, see Chapter 83.) Polysomnography using an extended EEG montage is also useful in establishing the diagnosis of sleep-related epileptic seizures, on the basis of typical epileptiform activity occurring in association with the movements. Polysomnographic findings that are consistent with REM sleep behavior disorder are described in the first section of this chapter and will not be reiterated here. Other differentials to consider are night terrors (pavor nocturnus), periodic limb movements of sleep (see Chapter 84), paroxysmal nocturnal dystonia, and posttraumatic stress disorder (25).

The predilection of this disorder (as well as other sleep disorders such as sleep apnea and nocturnal myoclonus) for elderly patients suggests that it would be useful to screen all new older patients for sleep disturbance during the course of a routine history. A few simple questions regarding adequacy of sleep, adequacy of daytime alertness, and the presence/absence of unusual behaviors during sleep would indicate if the possibility of a primary sleep disorder should be pursued.

TREATMENT

A number of pharmacologic agents have been used for treating REM sleep behavior disorder patients. Schenck et al (25) have found clonazepam in the 0.5–1.5 mg dosage range at h.s. to have been the most consistently successful. The drug should be used cautiously if at all in patients with concurrent obstructive sleep apnea, however, because of possible respiratory depressant effects. Desipramine hydrochloride has met with some, albeit erratic, success, but is problematic in elderly patients. Various anticonvulsant, antidepressant, and sedative hypnotic drugs have not been useful in REM sleep behavior disorder (25). Doghramji et al (6) found that imipramine and trazedone produced transient improvement in their patients. However, consistent with Schenck's reported results, clonazepam in the 0.25–1.0 mg range at h.s. produced successful control in two of their three patients.

Bamford (29) reported the successful use of carbamazepine 100 mg orally three times a day for a 68-year-old

RBD patient. For this patient, carbamazepine did not produce aggravation of RBD, which its chemical relatives the tricyclic antidepressants, for theoretical reasons he cites, might have.

There have been reports of spontaneous improvement in some patients studied. In the case of our 65-year-old male patient, complete abstention from alcohol produced a lessening, but not complete control, of the disorder. Clonazepam treatment resolved the behavior disorder and associated hallucinatory perceptual distortions.

If medication is contraindicated, as it was for our patient who had been treated for bladder cancer with thiotepa, another possibility might be restraint. During one of the patient's two nights in our laboratory, a restraint was fashioned for her. It permitted her freedom of movement as long as she was recumbent but tightened and prevented further movement if she moved to sit or to leave her bed. This was associated with a lessening of the REM phasic tonicity during sleep. At follow-up a year and a half after her original study, she continued to use a restraint at home. She reported that this was associated not only with complete protection from self-injurious behavior but also with a change in her dream content. She reported that her dreams were less activated than they had been in the past. Also she reported that she awakened at night to find herself straining against the restraint considerably less frequently than she had in the past.

SCIENTIFIC ISSUES

The central clinical research issues are 1) is this a single disorder, or a symptom complex that can be the end result of diverse etiologies; 2) what is (are) this disorder's etiology; 3) how is the disorder best treated; and 4) in the event of several etiologies, what might be etiology-specific treatments. From a scientific perspective, perhaps the most interesting question in this regard is the etiology itself.

Longitudinal study of known RBD patients shows an increasingly larger cadre who, since diagnosis with idiopathic RBD, have been demonstrated to have a measurable insult to the nervous system or other significant medical disorders, but the remainder of these idiopathic patients studied appear not to have concurrent medical disorders. For those with insults to the nervous system specifically in the pontine area—an area known to be involved in the organization of REM sleep—the insult itself may be the etiology. However, for the remainder of that group, and for all of the patients with no apparent neurologic or other major medical disorder, one must assume that the etiology is more subtle. Altered chemistry (possibly the central cholinergic system) may be the primary causative agent. Other factors that can syndromically alter the values of pertinent indicator variables of REM sleep (e.g., tonicity, presence or absence of rapid eye movements, EEG) surely need to be sought.

Simply the existence of a sleep disorder for which a primary defining characteristic of REM sleep—muscle atonia—is compromised has profound basic research implications. Careful study of patients with this disorder, and comparison with experimentally produced REM without muscle atonia in research animals, likely will provide tremendous insight into the generators of this complex sleep state. Further, the disorder seems to have a predilection for older people, independent of presence or absence of known neurologic disease. Therefore, an understanding of the precise organizational mechanisms that go awry in this experiment of nature may increase insight regarding the aging brain.

The primary implication of a spontaneously occurring REM sleep without consistent atonia—and in fact *with* dramatic behavioral events—is that REM sleep is not a unitary event. The following discussion develops the thesis that the integrated state of REM sleep depends upon organization among multiple subordinate control systems.

Polysomnographic studies of REM sleep behavior disorder patients minimally support the notion that generation of tonic REM likely depends upon different mechanisms from phasic REM. The pertinent finding is that release (or, possibly, production) of the organized and often violent behavior occurs during phasic REM in association with trains of rapid eye movements. In these same patients, however, the integrity of tonic REM is spared. Even in animal research subjects, during a nonpathologic REM period subsets of physiologic events are specific either to tonic or to phasic REM sleep. During tonic REM, in addition to the decreased submental EMG, one finds increased hippocampal theta activity, increased brain temperature, olfactory bulb activity, and poikilothermia. During phasic REM, in addition to the defining characteristic of rapid eye movements, one finds interaural muscular activity, tongue movements, and pontogeniculooccipital (PGO) spikes. Whether or not these latter relate to auditory, motor, and visual events in the associated dreams, the point is that they indicate a normally occurring easing of atonia specific to phasic REM—paradoxically at a time when the inhibition of the H-reflex is at its greatest (see Chapter 81).

This distinction is supported by anatomic findings in animal studies (30–32) and with correlational research in a human narcoleptic sample (33). Other experimental data also point to differential control of tonic and phasic REM sleep. Ascending inhibitory output arising from the caudal spinal area, for instance, is implicated in the atonia of tonic REM, but appears to play no role in the atonia of phasic REM (31). Conversely, descending vestibular nuclei likely play an essential role in some of the phasic events of REM sleep, especially vegetative changes (phasic increase in pupillary diameter, phasic changes in heart rate) (29). Further, even within phasic REM, there may be more than one control system involved. These latter, vegetative, events of phasic REM are not affected in REM sleep behavior disorder.

Nor is it the case that tonic or phasic inhibition is unopposed during REM sleep. Despite the tonic descending inhibition of spinal motor neurons, descending pyramidal activity is as great as during relaxed wakefulness (30), this perhaps being manifest only during phasic REM. Tonic and phasic REM, therefore, are differentiable along multiple parameters. In the case of REM sleep behavior disorder, this distinction becomes particularly profound at least with respect to behavior and dream events (albeit not with respect to vegetative events). That is, minimally two subsystems proximally organizing these discrete aspects of REM sleep need be sought neurochemically to correspond to the already available anatomic data described.

Simple atonia during REM sleep versus inhibition of complex organized activity is another differentiating parameter. It has long been suspected, at least since the early work of Magoun and Rhines (34), that atonia during REM sleep was ultimately controlled by the bulbar inhibitory area. Later work by Holmes et al (35) would suggest that the ventromedial medullary reticular formation, which projects to spinal cord, is the bulbar locus most immediately involved with atonia of neck musculature and inhibition of gross motor activity during REM. Lesions at this level of the neuraxis produced both tonically increased neck muscle tonus throughout the REM period and overt movements (whole body and vigorous limb movements). Waking behavior, however, was not measurably affected.

Activation of the bulbar inhibitory region during REM is believed to depend upon output from the pontine segmental area (see more comprehensive discussion in Chapter 81). It is to the pontine tegmentum that overall executive function with respect to REM sleep is attributed. It is this area that is actually implicated in the overall choreography of REM sleep, including but not restricted to REM atonia. However, the pontine segmental area itself is differentiated with respect to muscle tonus and motor control during REM sleep. Different loci of the area are involved in different aspects of REM atonia; that is, REM sleep without muscle atonia is itself not a unitary phenomenon, at least in animal preparations. Depending upon the site of the lesion in the pontine segmental area, distinctly different behavioral repertoires are released during REM sleep. Hendricks et al (36) identified three different "syndromes" of release from atonia, each specific to the lesion site:

1. increased proximal limb and head movements without either head raising or coordinated behavior;
2. head raising, righting of forequarters, movement of head, neck, and forelimbs, staring and reaching, suggestive of an orienting response; and
3. violent phasic behavior superimposed upon periods of atonia.

The authors' conclusion is that simple release of atonia depends upon one set of lesions but that production of elaborate behavioral sequences depends upon additional damage. That is, pontine areas involved in orchestrating inhibition of alpha motor neurons are distinct from those involved in the release of highly organized behaviors. These highly orga-

nized behaviors are stereotypic, not interactive with the environment, and may well be organized at the level of the brainstem, possibly relying upon pontine input to the superior colliculus.

Earlier work by this same group (37) had shown that pontine segmental lesions in cats leading to REM without atonia also led to a significant increase in wake-time exploratory behavior of the animals. This is in distinction to the absence of measurable changes in daytime behavior reported by Holmes and co-workers in bulbar lesions producing REM muscular atonia (35).

With the foregoing in mind, we propose that there is a complex hierarchy, likely within the brainstem, regarding REM sleep control. The pontine segmental area as an integrated unit may well have ultimate executive control over REM sleep. However, there likely are one or several intermediaries between the pontine executive area and the local effector systems most immediately responsible for the events of REM sleep. This executive function seems to be only loosely coupled with each of the separable events of REM sleep, including but not restricted to motor control.

Closer inspection of REM sleep behavior disorder in association with sleep paralysis (see Chapter 81) and cataplexy (see Chapter 80) speaks even more elegantly to this point. Comparison among these spontaneously occurring movement disorders of sleep, so intimately associated with REM sleep (Table 82.1), demonstrate multiple double dissociations of various elements of REM sleep. Table 82.2 identifies the parameters along which these three disorders can be differentiated from each other and from REM sleep. These are time of occurrence, phasic EMG twitches, irregular respirations, locomotion and complex behavior, likely the atonia of oropharyngeal muscles, and state of consciousness. That is, when the full symptom pictures of these REM disorders are considered together, one sees a number of REM-related components that can be dissociated from each other, including but not restricted to motor components, and without a gross lesion.

With respect to relative neurochemistries, response of the disorders to pharmacologic agents with known effects on neurotransmitters may provide some information bearing upon the loci of the respective discrete control system defects. Mahowald and Schenck (28), for instance, speculated that clonazepam has been the most consistently effective in the treatment of REM sleep behavior disorder because of its effects on central dopaminergic and serotonergic pathways. Clonazepam may produce a presynaptic blockade of dopamine-mediated stereotypic behavior, thereby inhibiting it. The implied hypothesis is that the behavior released (or produced, presumably by brainstem structures) during REM sleep is dopaminergically mediated. Clonazepam also appears to increase serotonin synthesis. In that regard, Mahowald and Schenck cited the 1981 work of Hishikawa et al (38) indicating that both serotonin-depleting agents and lesions of serotonergic brain tissue lead to disinhibition of phasic REM processes and apparent hallucinatory behaviors. The

Table 82.1 Movement Disorders Associated with REM Sleep. Comparison of Symptom Constellation for Sleep Paralysis, Cataplexy, and REM Behavior Disorder (Characteristics Generally Shared by REM Sleep and the Three Movement Disorders of Sleep)

Individual Characteristics	REM Sleep	Sleep Paralysis	Cataplexy	REM Behavior Disorder
Rapid eye movements	Present at unpredictable times with varying density	Present during episodes	Unclear if present during episodes	Present during episodes, concurrent with REM sleep
Dreaming	Present	Hypnogogic/hypnopompic hallucinations may be dream equivalent; also, can be associated with frightening dreams	? Some	Unusually activated dreams (e.g., self-defense from an attacker)
Saw tooth waves (EEG)	Present, to varying degrees	Present, same distribution as REM sleep	Not reported	Present, frequency not reported
Complete atonia of antigravity muscles	Present with greatest suppression of H reflex during dense eye movements	Present, with caudorostral development during an episode	Present, with rostrocaudal development during an episode	Completely absent phasically but otherwise present during REM sleep

Table 82.2 Heterogeneity Among Disorders and REM with Respect to Characteristic

Individual Characteristics	REM Sleep	Sleep Paralysis	Cataplexy	REM Behavior Disorder
Time of occurrence	During sleep, usually at 90-min intervals	Just before sleep onset or upon awakenings	During wakeful time in the day	During phasic REM sleep
Phasic EMG twitches	Present, varying density and frequency	Not reported	Not reported	Throughout the sleep period
Irregular respirations	Especially with dense eye movements: apnea and tachypnea	Subjectively; experience of respiratory distress at times	Not reported	Not reported but "dreams" incorporate generalized arousal
Locomotion and complex behavior	Absent	Absent	Absent	Complex behavior, often vigorous locomotion, physically
Atonia of oropharyngeal muscles	Progressive with duration of REM sleep	May underly reports of respiratory distress	Not reported	Not reported
Sleeping, not subjectively aware	Sleeping, but afferent input may be incorporated into dreams	Subjectively awake; arousal greater than prior stage 1 sleep	Not reported. May progress to true sleep	Amnestic to behaviors
Duration of episode	Self-limiting. Length increase across sleep period	Seconds to minutes. Releases with light touch, name calling	Up to 15–20 min. Attack not responsive to stimulation	Self-limiting. Behaviors often awaken patient
Incidence	Always present in normal sleep	Narcoleptics: 8–57% of population. Idiopathic: seems transmitted through maternal line	Affects close to 100% of narcoleptics. Rare, idiopathic. Transmitted as unmixed autosomal dominant	Unknown. Some patients have rostral pontine/olivo/cerebellar lesions; others, neuropathy. Remainder idiopathic
Age of onset		Highly variable	Highly variable	Predilection for older patients. Mean age of onset 55 years old

implied hypothesis is that REM sleep behavior disorder may rely, in part, upon insult to the brain serotonin system. Pertinent in this regard, during REM sleep without atonia induced in animals by lesion, is that serotonergic dorsal raphe nuclei that normally are electrically silent become extremely active (39).

Table 82.3 presents a comparison of REM sleep with sleep paralysis, cataplexy, and REM sleep behavior disorder

as a function of cholinergic and serotonergic manipulations. Neurochemical manipulations such as these, especially with pure agonists and antagonists, would prove to be the more effective scalpel to dissect REM sleep control into its component parts were the large number of REM parameters that can vary independently all addressed simultaneously. Table 82.2 suggests features additional to the defining characteristics of the disorders that should be addressed. Clearly

Table 82.3 Relative Neurochemistries of REM Sleep and Movement Disorders Believed to be Associated with REM Sleep

Individual Characteristics	REM Sleep	Sleep Paralysis	Cataplexy	REM Behavior Disorder
Response to acetylcholine manipulation	Specific agonists decrease REM latency, more so with endogenous depression	No reported results of specific agonists or antagonists; tricyclic antidepressants reported variously to ameliorate, exacerbate, or have no effect	Orphenadrine (antagonist) ($n = 3$) had no effect. In canine models, some cholinoceptive receptors hypersensitive; muscarinic mimetic (arecoline) exacerbated it; muscarinic blockers reduced it	No specific agonists or antagonists studied
Response to serotonin manipulation	Agonist may modulate latency, spacing, and duration of REM	Small n case studies; some suspect tricyclic antidepressants with most serotonin. Reuptake block and L-tryptophan most effective as therapy. L-tryptophan most effective with AMI (? 2° to antiacetylcholine property)	Zimelidine (selective serotonin reuptake inhibitor) had potent anticataplectic effect ($n = 11$), but no effect on excessive daytime sleepiness	No specific agonist or antagonists studied. Suppression in some patients with desipramine. (Klonapin most effective.) $n = 4$

it would be important to use pharmacologic agents with a single locus of effect. Tricyclic antidepressants, unfortunately, affect several neurotransmitter systems.

SUMMARY

Perhaps the most critical scientific issue suggested by the natural occurrence of REM sleep behavior disorder, and fortified by a comparison of it with the other two sleep disorders under discussion, is that REM sleep is not a unitary event. Pontine structures possibly working in concert with each other may have ultimate executive control over the timing and constituents of REM sleep. However, this executive function seems to be only loosely coupled with apparently several systems that have proximal control over the multiple physiologic events of REM sleep.

The REM sleep-related movement disorders are instructive in this regard. Comparing and contrasting the multiple components of each disorder, one begins to identify what probably are the independently controlled components of REM sleep. That comparison, in turn, speaks to the need to seek the neurochemistries of REM sleep rather than *the* neurochemistry. The specific dissociable factors that fall out of such a comparison, combined with the anatomic research already done, provide added direction for that search.

REM sleep behavior disorder, perhaps even more than the other two sleep-related movement disorders, provides a unique opportunity. It is a naturally occurring abnormality of REM sleep. As such, furthering our understanding of this disorder may promote increased depth to our knowledge of REM sleep—the sleep state that more than any other has captured the imagination of both lay and scientific communities.

REFERENCES

1. Schenck CH, Bundlie SR, Mahowald MW. Human REM sleep chronic behavior disorders: a new category of parasomnia. Sleep Res 1985;14:208.
2. International classification of sleep disorders: diagnostic and coding manual. Rochester, MN: American Sleep Disorders Association, 1990:177–180.
3. Schenck CH, Bundlie SR, Patterson AL, et al. 5 years of clinical experience with 21 patients having chronic REM sleep behavior disorder (RBD). Sleep Res 1987;16:424.
4. Schenck CH, Mahowald MW. REM sleep parasomnias (review). Neurol Clin 1996;14(4):697–720.
5. Gross MM, Goodenough DG, Tobin M, et al. Sleep disturbances and hallucinations in the acute alcoholic psychoses. J Nerv Ment Dis 1966;142:493–514.
6. Doghramji K, Connell TA, Gaddy JR. Loss of REM sleep atonia: three case reports. Sleep Res 1987;16:327.
7. Tachibana N, Yamanka K, Kaji R, et al. Sleep bruxism as a manifestation of subclinical rapid eye movement sleep behavior disorder. Sleep 1994;17(6):555–558.
8. Ferini-Strambi L, Oldania A, Zucconi M, Smirne S. Cardiac autonomic activity during wakefulness and sleep in REM sleep behavior disorder. Sleep 1996;19(5):367–369.
9. Salva MA, Guilleminault C. Olivopontocerebellar degeneration, abnormal sleep, and REM sleep without atonia. Neurology 1986;36:576–577.
10. Schenck CH, Bundlie SR, Ettinger MG, Mahowald MW. Chronic behavioral disorders of human REM sleep: a new category of parasomnia. Sleep 1986;9:293–308.
11. Schenck CH, Slater GE, Sherman RE, et al. Multiple sclerosis and sleep: survey report and polygraphic detection of REM and NREM motor abnormalities. Sleep Res 1986;15:163.
12. Sforza E, Zucconi M, Petronneli R, et al. REM sleep behavioral disorders. Eur Neurol 1988;28(5):295–300.
13. Culebras A, Moore JT. Magnetic resonance findings in REM sleep behavior disorder. Neurology 1989;39(11):1519–1513.
14. Wright BA, Rosen JR, Buysse DJ, et al. Shy-Drager syndrome presenting as a REM behavioral disorder. J Ger Psychiatry & Neurol 1990;3(2):110–113.
15. Tachibana N, Kimura K, Kitajima K, et al. REM sleep without atonia at early stage of sporadic olivopontocerebellar atrophy. J Neurol Sci 1995;132(1):28–34.
16. Schenck CH, Bundlie SR, Mahowald MW. Delayed emergence of a parkinsonian disorder in 38% of 29 older men initially diagnosed with idiopathic rapid eye movement sleep behaviour disorder. Neurology 1996;46(2):388–393.

17. Pareja JA, Caminero AB, Masa JF, Dobato JL. A first case of progressive supranuclear palsy and pre-clinical REM sleep behavior disorder presenting as inhibition of speech during wakefulness and somniloquy with phasic muscle twitching during REM sleep. Neurologia 1996;11(8):304–306.

18. Schenck CH, Garcia-Rill E, Skinner RD, et al. A case of REM sleep behavior disorder with autopsy-confirmed Alzheimer's disease: postmortem brain stem histochemical analyses. Biol Psychiatry 1996;40(5):422–425.

19. Plazzi G, Corsini R, Provini F, et al. REM sleep behavior disorders in multiple system atrophy. Neurology 1997;48(4):1094–1097.

20. Negro PJ, Faber R. Lewy body disease in a patient with REM sleep disorder (letter). Neurology 1996;46(5):1493–1494.

21. Morfis L, Schwartz RS, Cistulli PA. REM sleep behaviour disorder: a treatable cause of falls in elderly people. Age Ageing 1997;26(1):43–44.

22. Schenck CH, Mahowald MW. Motor dyscontrol in narcolepsy: rapid-eye-movement (REM) sleep without atonia and REM sleep behavior disorder. Ann Neurol 1992;32(1):3–10.

23. Schenck CH, Mahowald MW, Kim SW, et al. Prominent eye movements during NREM sleep and REM sleep behavior disorders associated with fluoxetine treatment of depression and obsessive–compulsive disorder. Sleep 1992;15(3):226–235.

24. Chung KF, Wong MT. Rapid eye movement sleep behaviour disorder in a Chinese male. A N Z J Psychiatry 1994;28(1):144–146.

25. Schenck CH, Bundlie SR, Smith SA, et al. REM behavior disorder in a 10 year old girl and aperiodic REM and NREM sleep movements in an 8 year old brother. Sleep Res 1986;15:162.

26. Schenck CH, Bundlie SR, Patterson AL, et al. Rapid eye movement sleep behavior disorder: a treatable parasomnia affecting older adults. JAMA 1987;257:1786–1789.

27. McCarley RW. REM dreams, REM sleep, and their isomorphisms. In: Chase M, Weitzman ED, eds. Advances in sleep research. Vol. 8. Sleep disorders: basic and clinical research. New York: Spectrum, 1983:95–122.

28. Mahowald MW, Schenck CH. REM sleep behavior disorder. In: Kryger MH, Roth T, Dement WC, eds. Principles and practice of sleep medicine. New York: WB Saunders, 1987:389–401.

29. Bamford CR. Carbamazepine and REM sleep behavior disorder. Sleep 1993;16(1):33–34.

30. Aserinsky E. Sleep and altered states of consciousness: physiological activity associated with segments of the rapid eye movement period. Res Publ Assoc Res Nerv Ment Dis 1967;45:338–423.

31. Arduini A, Berlucchi G, Strata P. Pyramidal activity during sleep and wakefulness. Arch Ital Biol 1963;101:530–544.

32. Morrison AR, Bowker RM. A caudal spinal source of cervical and forelimb inhibition during sleep. Exp Neurol 1971;33:684–692.

33. Nan'no H, Hishikawa Y, Koida H, et al. A neurophysiological study of sleep paralysis in narcoleptic patients. Electroencephalogr Clin Neurophysiol 1970;28:382–390.

34. Magoun HW, Rhines R. An inhibitory mechanism in the bulbar reticular formation. J Neurophysiol 1946;9:165–171.

35. Holmes CJ, Jones BE. Importance of cholinergic, GABAergic, serotonergic and other neurons in the medial medullary reticular formation for sleep–wake states studied by cytotoxic lesions in the cat. Neuroscience 1994;62:1179–1200.

36. Hendricks JC, Morrison AR, Mann GL. Different behaviors during paradoxical sleep without atonia depend on pontine lesion site. Brain Res 1982;239:81–105.

37. Morrison AR, Mann GL, Hendricks JC. The relationship of excessive exploratory behavior in wakefulness to paradoxical sleep without atonia. Sleep 1981;4:247–257.

38. Hishikawa Y, Sugita Y, Lijima S, et al. Mechanisms producing "stage 1-REM" and similar dissociations of REM sleep and their relation to delirium. Adv Neurol Sci 1981;25:1129–1147.

39. Parmeggiani PL. Interaction between sleep and wakefulness. Waking Sleeping 1977;1:123–132.

Sleepwalking (Somnambulism)

PRAKASH S. MASAND   JEFFREY B. WEILBURG

INTRODUCTION

Until the early 1960s, sleepwalking (somnambulism) was thought to be a dissociative reaction related to dreaming. However, polysomnographic studies have demonstrated that sleepwalking occurs during sleep stages three and four, that is, during nonrapid eye movement (NREM) sleep rather than during dreaming or REM sleep. The somnambulist remains deeply asleep despite the motoric arousal. Thus, somnambulism has been called a disorder of arousal—for example, a pathologic arousal during sleep—and tends to be classified as a parasomnia in DSM IV along with nightmare disorder, sleep terror disorder, REM sleep behavior disorder, and sleep paralysis.

Sleepwalking is much more common in children than in adults. Ten percent to 15% of children between 5 and 12 years of age have had at least one episode. In the general adult population the prevalence of somnambulism is 1% to 6%, although a higher incidence is reported in patients with schizophrenia, hysteria, and anxiety neuroses.

Sleepwalking is also commonly associated with other parasomnias. Nearly one-third of somnambulists have nocturnal enuresis; one-tenth of childhood sleepwalkers and one-half of adult sleepwalkers have night terrors. Somnambulism affects both sexes equally and is four to six times more common in patients with Tourette's syndrome or migraine than in those without it.

CLINICAL FEATURES

Sleepwalking typically occurs during the first 3 hours of sleep when stages three and four of NREM are most prevalent. Adult sleepwalkers have episodes earlier in the night than do childhood sleepwalkers. The episodes last from 30

seconds to 30 minutes but can be longer in some instances. Rarely is there more than one episode per night.

In childhood, sleepwalking is usually a benign, self-limited condition. The first episode usually occurs before the age of 10 years and the last before age 15. Adult somnambulists have a later age of onset, almost three times as many episodes per year, frequent temporal association with stress or major life events, and more years of sleepwalking. Onset of sleepwalking in old age is uncommon and is usually a manifestation of organicity such as delirium, drug toxicity, and seizure disorder.

During a typical episode the subject will sit up in bed. Most children do not actually walk but may make repetitive movements. The sleepwalker may arise from the bed and walk about the room or even around the house, in rare instances leaving the house. During the episode the subject appears dazed, has a blank staring face, and movements are clumsy. He or she is relatively unresponsive to the communicative efforts of others. Children often walk to their parents' bedroom or to the toilet. Researchers disagree about the dexterity and degree of motor performance possible during a somnambulistic episode.

The lack of awareness makes sleepwalking potentially dangerous, particularly in adult sleepwalkers, who are twice as likely to injure themselves than children. Rarely, acts of violence toward others or sexual assaults have reportedly occurred during episodes, although this remains controversial.

On awakening from a sleepwalking episode, the somnambulist usually has no memory of the episode or only a vague awareness, although there may be a short period of confusion and disorientation.

In childhood sleepwalkers, daytime functioning is usually normal and psychologic testing does not demonstrate any consistent psychopathology. In contrast, 72% of adult sleep-walkers were given a psychiatric diagnosis compared with 33% of childhood sleepwalkers. The Minnesota Multiphasic Personality Inventory (MMPI) profiles of the adults showed active, outwardly directed behavioral patterns, suggestive of difficulties in handling aggression. Interestingly, the profiles did not support an interpretation of sleepwalking as "hysterical dissociation."

Adult sleepwalkers have shown more epochs containing hypersynchronous delta waves and more stage 3–4 sleep interruptions on polysomnography compared to normal controls. Occasional reports have described adult sleepwalking occurring exclusively in the premenstrual period or in association with sleep-related eating disorders.

ETIOLOGY

Genetic Causes

Monozygotic twins are concordant for sleepwalking six times more frequently than dizygotic twins. When a parent gives a history of sleepwalking, the child is six times more likely to be a sleepwalker than when neither parent sleepwalks. First-degree relatives of sleepwalkers are 10 times more likely to sleepwalk than the general population. Second- and third-degree relatives also have a greater risk of sleepwalking. Mothers of siblings who sleepwalk have a twofold risk for sleepwalking. A two-threshold multifactorial mode of inheritance has been suggested based on the above data.

Developmental Causes

The frequent onset of these disorders in childhood with termination by late adolescence strongly suggests the role of developmental factors such as delay in maturation. Also, the presence of sudden, rhythmic, high-voltage bursts of delta frequency during slow-wave sleep in sleepwalkers through age 16 indicates central nervous system (CNS) immaturity as a causative factor in childhood sleepwalkers.

Psychological Causes

Psychological factors are an important etiologic factor in adult sleepwalkers. In fact, most early work on the subject considered somnambulism as a form of dissociative hysteria. Many psychodynamic formulations were proposed including the acting out of latent homosexual conflicts, flight from oedipal temptation, defense against castration anxiety, breakthrough of infantile erotic attitudes, and aggressive and sexual motor activity aimed primarily at a fear-inspiring father. However, electroencephalographic (EEG) studies, MMPI profiles, and psychiatric interviews do not support the view that somnambulism is a dissociative reaction. There is considerable evidence, however, showing increased psychopathology and the role of stress and major life events in adult sleepwalkers.

Organic Causes

Fever and medications can precipitate sleepwalking episodes. Elevated temperature suppresses stages three and four of NREM sleep, sometimes followed by rebound, predisposing subjects to somnambulistic episodes. These are differentiated from delirium by their short duration, occurrence early in the night, and persistence after the febrile period.

DIFFERENTIAL DIAGNOSIS

Complex partial seizures (CPS) occurring during sleep should be included in the differential diagnosis, but it is very rare for CPS to present with somnambulism. Seizures can occur any time during the day or night and are brief in duration. Automatisms (e.g., chewing, swallowing, salivation) can be found with sleepwalking. A family history of sleepwalking or night terrors is usually absent in seizures. Sleep EEG can be a helpful tool.

Night terrors also occur during NREM sleep but are characterized by intense fear and panic, coupled with an initial scream.

Differentiation from hysterical dissociative phenomena such as amnesia, fugue states, and multiple personalities is important. Hysterical amnesia is an example of motivated nonrecall, that is to say, failure to retrieve an existing memory, whereas in sleepwalking little in the way of memory trace exists.

Various medications have been reported to precipitate somnambulistic episodes. These include thioridazine, lithium carbonate, diphenhydramine, chlorpromazine, thioxanthene, methylphenidate, chlorprothixene, methaqualone, zolpidem, and propranolol, or a combination of these agents.

Malingering can be differentiated when patients demonstrate various complicated goal-directed activities. Episodes usually last for more than 15 minutes and may occur at any time during the night. The activities require considerable planning, but the next day the patient claims amnesia for the episode. Larceny, sexual indiscretion, and antisocial activities are among the motives for such behavior.

Sleepwalking in the elderly is usually a sign of delirium or adverse effects of medication. REM sleep behavior disorder is a rare condition usually seen in elderly persons. It occurs during REM sleep with loss of REM atonia and is characterized by vigorous or violent behaviors usually accompanied by unpleasant dream content. There are usually multiple nightly events in contrast to somnambulism, which usually involves single nightly events.

TREATMENT

Most children outgrow sleepwalking, so parents may be simply reassured and instructed regarding safety. In adults, because sleepwalking episodes are potentially dangerous, a safe environment (e.g., sleeping on the first floor, bolts on the doors and windows, removal of dangerous objects) is sought. Attempts to interrupt the episode should be avoided as these may only frighten or confuse the somnambulist.

Case reports indicate that benzodiazepines, particularly diazepam and clonazepam, may be used to treat episodes of sleepwalking. Diazepam and clonazepam probably alter delta sleep physiology. Antidepressants including imipramine and paroxetine have also shown usefulness in treating sleepwalking.

In adults, a flexible psychotherapeutic approach is indicated in sleepwalkers with evidence of psychopathology. An important aspect of psychotherapy is to help the patient identify stressors and deal with frustrations in a healthy, nonaggressive manner. A number of techniques such as hypnosis, anticipatory awakening, and reciprocal inhibition have been described as alternative treatment modalities, but with inconsistent results.

GENERAL READING LIST

Berlin RM, Qayyum U. Sleepwalking: diagnosis and treatment through the life cycle. Psychosomatics 1986;27:755–760.

Broughton RJ. Sleep disorders: disorders of arousal? Science 1968;159:1070–1078.

Cooper AJ. Treatment of coexistent night terrors and somnambulism in adults with imipramine and diazepam. J Clin Psychiatry 1987;48:209–210.

Hupaya LVM. Seven cases of somnambulism induced by drugs. Am J Psychiatry 1979;136:985–986.

Jacobson A, Kales A, Lehmann D, et al. Somnambulism: all night electroencephalographic studies. Science 1965;148:975–977.

Kales A, Jacobson A, Paulson MJ, et al. Somnambulism: psychophysiological correlates I. All night EEG studies. Arch Gen Psychiatry 1966;14:595–604.

Kales A, Soldatos CR, Bixler EO. Hereditary factors in sleepwalking and night terrors. Br J Psychiatry 1980;137:111–118.

Kales A, Soldatos CR, Caldwell AB, et al. Somnambulism: clinical characteristics and personality patterns. Arch Gen Psychiatry 1980;37:1406–1410.

Kales JD, Soldatos CR, Vela-Bueno A. Treatment of sleep disorders III: enuresis, sleepwalking, night terrors and nightmares. Ration Drug Ther 1983;17:1–7.

Kavey NB, Whyte J, Resor SR, et al. Somnambulism in adults. Neurology 1990;40:749–752.

Mendelson WB. Sleepwalking associated with zolpidem. J Clin Psychopharm 1994;14:150.

Oswald I, Evans J. On serious violence during sleepwalking. Br J Psychiatry 1985;147:688–691.

Rauch PK, Stern TA. Life threatening injuries resulting from sleepwalking and night terrors. Psychosomatics 1986;27:62–64.

Schenck CH, Bundlie SR, Ettinger MG, et al. Chronic behavioral disorder of human REM sleep: a new category of parasomnia. Sleep 1986;9:293–308.

Schenck CH, Hurwitz TD, Bundlie SR, et al. Sleep related eating disorders: polysomnographic correlates of a heterogenous syndrome distinct from daytime eating disorders. Sleep 1991;14:419–431.

Schenck CH, Milner DM, Hurwitz TD, et al. A polysomnographic and clinical report on sleep related injury in 100 adult patients. Am J Psychiatry 1989;146:1166–1173.

Tachibana N, Sugita Y, Terashima Y, et al. Polysomnographic characteristics of healthy elderly subjects with somnambulism-like behaviors. Biol Psychiatry 1991;30:4–14.

Sleep Pathologies Associated with Nocturnal Movements

BRUCE L. EHRENBERG

HISTORY AND OVERVIEW

Willis described restless leg movements in relation to insomnia in 1685 (1), but Symonds was first to differentiate what he felt was a pathologic (abnormal) form of twitches during sleep from "common nocturnal jerks" (2). The latter probably represent what are now referred to as "sleep onset myoclonus," "hypnic jerks," or "sleep starts" and were considered "physiologic" (i.e., not pathologic) by Oswald (3). Symonds, when first describing his five clinical cases of "nocturnal myoclonus," was convinced that it represented a variant of epilepsy, although only one of his cases was said to have had "frank epilepsy" (poorly documented); indeed, he alluded to excessive amounts of the "common" jerks at night as a possible marker for families with "idiopathic epilepsy." However, his patients with the "pathologic" form all had insomnia, and in at least one case there was a clear periodicity of arousals at 1-minute intervals, these last two features being compatible with (but not diagnostic of) what should now be called "periodic limb movements of sleep" (PLMS) with associated insomnia. (The official term in the new International Classification of Sleep Disorders (4)—*periodic limb movements disorder*—does not include the word *sleep* and therefore lacks specificity.) Of note, Symonds' "epileptic" responded to trimethadione with much improved sleep, although one other patient did not respond to that drug; in any case, without polysomnographic and video documentation of the sleep and movement patterns, it is probable that there was a mixture of phenomena included among his patients. (The question remains whether there is an increased incidence of epilepsy among patients with leg twitches at night, but this has not been adequately studied to date. A full understanding of the complex relationship between disordered sleep and epilepsy is beyond the scope of this chapter, but has begun to receive more attention of late (5–7).)

In addition to the hypnic jerks mentioned above, other physiologic forms of nocturnal movements include the twitches of various body areas without synchrony, periodicity or symmetry, commonly found in normals during rapid eye movement (REM) sleep (8) and during stage 1 sleep (9). These physiologic forms must be carefully differentiated from the pathologic entities described below by the use of specific polygraphic recording techniques; they cannot be accurately diagnosed (or even guessed at) by the clinical history alone.

Lugaresi et al were the first to provide a polygraphically documented description of periodic movements in sleep of patients with daytime restless legs syndrome (RLS) (10) and of patients without RLS (11). In addition, his group has studied the behavior of other pathologic forms of myoclonus: spinal myoclonus and facial spasms that persist during sleep; cortically mediated epileptic myoclonus (including the rhythmic jerks of epilepsia partialis continua, the repeated partial motor seizures of Jacksonian epilepsy, and the extensive spasms of subacute sclerosing leukoencephalitis), which gradually decrease during the onset of sleep; and other abnormal movements, including those of extrapyramidal origin (e.g., choreoathetosis and hemiballismus) and those of subcortical and brainstem origin (e.g., palatal myoclonus and opsoclonus), which reliably disappear in sleep (12). Another extrapyramidal condition that diminishes during sleep is the tremor of Parkinson's syndrome. However, nocturnal limb twitches identical to those of PLMS may emerge in Parkinson's disease patients, and this was originally thought to be due to the treatment with L-dopa (13). More recently, it has been found that, at least in PLMS/RLS patients, L-dopa is a useful treatment for the leg movements (14), thus suggesting that the movements observed in parkinsonian patients are a nocturnal rebound phenomenon owing to the short half-life of the drug. In a similar vein, the dopaminergic blockers—phenothiazines and butyrophenones—are known to cause persistent akathisia (restless legs) and nocturnal movements that are strikingly similar to RLS and PLMS, respectively, and the latter may cause a marked sleep disruption (15). The fasciculations of amyotrophic lateral sclerosis and other diseases of the anterior horn cell (lower motor neuron) do not disappear in sleep; these phenomena are mediated at the spinal cord level.

There has emerged a syndrome of rather extreme REM-related movements often involving sustained and massive motion of limbs in an "acting out" fashion, as though the patient were physically involved in his dream; this may be seen in an "idiopathic" form (16) or with olivopontocerebellar degeneration (OPCD) (17) and may be related to a loss of the generalized inhibition of sustained motor activity normally found in the REM-sleep of humans after the newborn period. In another series of cases, REM behavior disorder has been linked to well-documented narcolepsy (18). More recent studies have shown that REM behavior disorder is not rare, and in long-term follow-up, the "idiopathic" or sporadic patient may turn out to develop a degenerative disorder.

Another, rather uncommon, group of disorders comprises the paroxysmal nocturnal dystonias (PND) (19,20). The attacks are characterized by repeated stereotyped episodes of dystonic, ballistic, or choreoathetoid movements during non-REM (NREM) sleep. The episodes may be short (15 to 60 seconds) and responsive to treatment with anticonvulsants, or prolonged (5 to 60 minutes) and unresponsive to anticonvulsant therapy (21). A relationship of the first type to true epileptic seizures is strongly suspected since seizures emanating from the supplementary (sensori-)motor area look similar and often have no associated abnormality

on the (ictal) electroencephalogram (EEG). In addition, there are two rare syndromes of paroxysmal daytime episodes that parallel the nocturnal variety: paroxysmal kinesigenic dystonia, which is similar to the short-duration PND attacks clinically and in response to anticonvulsants, and paroxysmal dystonic choreoathetosis, which mimics the long-duration PND attacks.

Other types of nocturnal motor activity that will be discussed in detail include sleep bruxism (see Chapter 85) and a recently described and as yet under-recognized entity of "fragmentary myoclonus in non-REM sleep," which may help fill some important gaps in the understanding of these phenomena.

DEFINITIONS AND METHODOLOGIES

PLMS

Periodic (limb) movements disorder (PMS is the former acronym, although PLMS emphasizes that the legs—and sometimes the arms—are involved and also avoids confusion with the premenstrual syndrome) is defined by Coleman et al (22) as "stereotyped, repetitive, nonepileptiform movements of the lower extremities occurring primarily in NREM sleep." The timing characteristics of the movements are defined differently by various authors but there is general agreement on a duration of 0.5 to 5.0 seconds (most patients average 2 seconds) and a repetition interval of 5 to 90 seconds (most patients fall between 20 and 40 seconds) (Fig 84.1). Some of the variation in definitions among early workers in the field can be seen in Table 84.1 (23).

More recently, specific standards for scoring leg movements in sleep have been published (30). Inter-rater

Table 84.1   Early Definitions of Nocturnal Myoclonus (PLMS)

Authors	Duration of Events	Number of Events per Series	Periodicity (Inter-event Interval)	Diagnosis of PLMS
Association of Sleep Disorders Centers, 1979 (24)	0.5–10.0 s	≥30 events	5–120 s of events	≥3 series
Guilleminault et al, 1975 (25)	0.5–15.0 s	≥3 events	>120 s	Not reported
Coleman et al, 1980 (22)	0.5–4.0 s	≥5 events	20–40 s	≥40 events/night
Coleman, 1982 (26)	0.5–5.0 s	≥4 events	4–90 s	≥5 events/h; criterion for diagnosis of "nocturnal myoclonus syndrome": ≥5 arousals/h sleep following myoclonus events
Wittig et al, 1983 (27)	Not reported	Not reported	Not reported	≥3 series of ≥30 events or "more but shorter series causing frequent awakenings or arousals"
Mosko et al, 1984 (28)	Not reported	Not reported	Not reported	Periodic leg movements for ≥45 min or 15% of sleep time
Scrima et al, 1985 (29)	Single spike to usually <5 s	No minimum number of events	No periodicity criterion	≥5 MAL (23) arousals per hour of sleep—must be just after MAL event

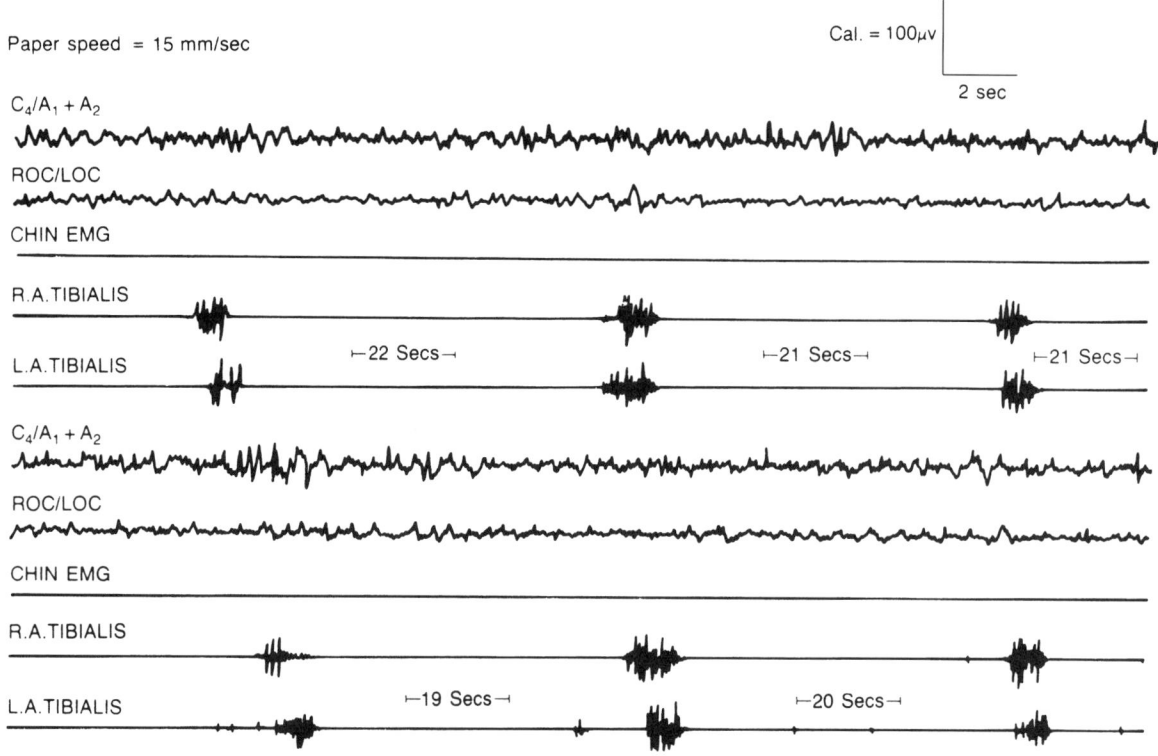

FIGURE 84.1 *Polysomnogram of PMS from the right and left legs during 2 minutes of stage 3 sleep in a 47-year-old man with chronic insomnia. The surface EMG is obtained from skin electrodes overlying the anterior tibialis muscles. ROC/LOC represents an eye movement channel from electrodes placed at the outer canthi of both eyes. From Coleman R, Pollak CP, Weitzman ED. Periodic movements in sleep (nocturnal myoclonus): relation to sleep disorders. Ann Neurol 1980;8:416–421.*

reliability has been studied, with good correlations found for the leg movements but lower correlations for the related arousals (31). Standards for scoring EEG arousals have also been published, but are complex and have been more difficult to fully implement (32).

The amplitude of the movements can be measured on the polysomnograph (PSG) tracing and a cut-off criterion of greater than 25% of a baseline full-effort contraction of the same muscle is now used. However, there are clearly some patients who have repeated arousals in association with very small electromyogram (EMG) bursts, and although some such cases may represent activity damped by the methods of recording or the location of the electrodes with respect to the muscle in question, there are occasional patients who have only minimal motor activity and yet have synchronized periodic arousals. This may help explain cases where the apparent movements are too few in number to cause the clinical EDS findings (usually such patients do have at least one series of large amplitude movements) and raises the question as to whether the motoric manifestations are sometimes merely an epiphenomenon of a fundamental central nervous system (CNS) sleep disturbance.

In the opposite extreme, there are patients with PLMS who have very violent kicks and may injure their bed partners or themselves. (In one personally attended case, the patient apparently kicked into the air so sharply that he hyperextended his leg, awakening with a swollen knee that required arthroscopic surgery.) There is evidence that some forms of chronic arthritis may be linked to PLMS (see below).

In addition to the legs, there may be involvement of other parts of the body (33), especially the arms. Some labs monitor multiple muscles on each of the four limbs, looking for any movement and applying criteria similar to that in Table 84.1; with such thorough monitoring, there may be a greater degree of detection of the periodic phenomena. Further, some labs require a minimum of 6 hours total sleep time, although this may be impractical with severe insomnia patients.

The usual joint movements that are seen involve dorsiflexion of the big toe or the ankle, or flexion of the knee or the hip, or combinations of these. (Indeed, it has been noted by one author that there may also be fanning of the smaller toes, thus simulating the Babinski and triple flexion responses (34); however, this is not a universal presentation.) Unlike most other movement disorders, which are abolished during even light stages of sleep, PLMS activity appears with the onset of sleep stages 1 or 2 (persistence for at least 4 serial repetitions and preferably into sleep stage 2 are important points in differentiating the "physiologic" form of Loeb et al (9)). There are no comprehensive studies showing the distribution of leg movements over the various sleep stages in large numbers of patients, but of the individual cases illustrated in the literature, some have had the largest amounts of leg movement activity in stages 3 and 4 and some have had the maximal activity in stage 2. Clinical experience shows that PLMS is usually most prevalent in stages 1 and 2, and is rare in REM sleep. However, the occurrence of PLMS in stages 3 and 4 is most helpful diagnostically since this virtually rules out "pseudo leg movements" due to sleep apnea (obstructive apneas almost never occur in deep NREM sleep).

The relationship of PLMS to RLS adds another perspective: in nine members of a family with RLS, the leg movements were recorded in wakefulness as well as sleep and showed a periodicity similar to that seen in PLMS, with the intermovement intervals gradually increasing as the patients became drowsy and then entered stage 2 sleep; the authors concluded that RLS and PLMS "represent two clinical manifestations of the same CNS dysfunction" (35).

When scoring PSG recordings for the number of periodic leg movements, it is necessary to eliminate those that are associated with the end of an apnea or hypopnea (32). This is particularly tricky when mild hypopneas are not detected owing to their minimal effects on the monitored respiratory parameters but an associated leg movement nevertheless occurs. (Added esophageal pressure monitoring is helpful here, in detecting the subtle hypopneas of patients with the upper airway resistance syndrome (36). There is less of a problem when the limb movements appear in, or are confined to, REM sleep—when PLMS activity is usually suppressed but compromised respirations are more likely to occur.

It is useful to note the number of times a leg movement is associated with a *full awakening*—usually defined as the appearance of an occipital alpha (8 to 12 Hz) rhythm for at least 60 seconds; an *incomplete awakening*—alpha for 15 to 60 seconds; or an *arousal*—variably defined as the appearance of occipital alpha activity for less than 15 seconds or sometimes any change in the sleep patterns indicative of an abrupt reduction in the depth of sleep. (The standard sleep-staging criteria (37) do not allow for the awake state to be counted as being present in any given 30-second epoch unless waking EEG activity is present for at least 15 seconds of that epoch. Thus, briefer arousals have to be counted separately lest one lose the information they convey about the degree of sleep disruption in the affected recording.)

Occasionally, there are large amounts of generalized 7 to 11 Hz activity during deep NREM sleep—the so-called alpha–delta pattern (38)—in patients with the fibrositis-fibromyalgia/chronic fatigue syndrome, in whom the EEG pattern is thought to represent unrefreshing, poor quality sleep; these patients may have alpha–delta with or without PLMS (39). Further, there may be confusion of some "normal" features of NREM sleep with certain subtle

arousal patterns: 1) prolonged spindles, 2) excessively repetitive K-complexes, and 3) bursts of increased delta (1 to 3 Hz) activity, although these are not universally accepted as signs of arousal (32). Such subtle arousals can be surmised when a physiologic event such as a leg movement is closely associated with a vertex V-wave or K-complex—EEG phenomena that are known to occur normally when externally applied stimuli disturb sleep. Lavie (40) has tried to further refine the concept of subtle EEG arousals by suggesting the term *microarousal* be applied whenever a "burst of . . . delta–alpha" or a "K-alpha complex" is seen; he has found each in association with episodes of disordered breathing during sleep.

There may be even more subtle levels of arousal that presently are not counted. Perhaps more widespread use of computerized spectral analysis equipment in sleep laboratories would allow better detection of such phenomena as 1) transient suppressions of delta activity in deep slow-wave sleep and 2) brief drops in the rate of spindle production in stage 2 sleep. Also, there may be a decrease in the quality of sleep when the PSG shows chronically low levels of delta or spindle activity during NREM sleep, although age-specific standards and better clinical correlates are needed for such a measure to become useful. Lack of attention to such EEG features of sleep recordings may account for some of the cases where PSG studies have failed to demonstrate the cause of daytime fatigue in patients clinically thought to have nonrestorative sleep, especially those whose MSLTs objectively demonstrate excessive daytime sleepiness.

The PLMS patient may present as having either a disorder of initiating or maintaining sleep (DIMS) or as having a disorder of excessive somnolence (DOES) according to the original terminology from the Association of Sleep Disorders Centers nosology (41). These two main categories may appear to be opposites and present an apparent paradox. Carskadon et al (42) found that PLMS is common in the elderly and even though their subjects did not complain of sleepiness, there was a substantial amount of daytime sleepiness on objective testing; Coleman et al (22) remarked that this "indicates that the concept of having a sleep–wake complaint is very subjective." Thus, the working diagnoses of insomnia (DIMS) and hypersomnolence (DOES) are usually based on the presenting complaint of the patient even though objective findings may not always corroborate the patient's experience. Indeed, the line between these two groups becomes quite blurred as one examines the situation closely: both groups have poor quality sleep of which they are aware, to various degrees, and the primary difference is the ability of the DIMS patients to maintain daytime alertness (excessively so?) while the DOES patients usually have poor sleep no matter when they attempt it (and more often than not, they feel compelled to). These two major headings have been eliminated in the new International Classification of Sleep Disorders, and the major entities, including PLMS, RLS, and the sleep apneas, are now called "intrinsic dyssomnias" (4).

Fragmentary (Pathologic) Myoclonus of NREM Sleep

A recent report by Broughton and Tolentino (43) has expanded the category of sleep movements to include those that are more truly "myoclonic" (less than 150 msec duration, over 50 μV amplitude) but that have heretofore been considered nonpathologic. (The original cases of Symonds ("sleep myoclonus") may have included some with this entity and thus we have come full cycle in the semantic tangle.) This disorder, called "fragmentary myoclonus of NREM sleep" (FMS) represents another form of movements during sleep that are associated with EDS, even in the absence of other sleep disorders. The definition requires that there be large amounts of myoclonic muscle activity, usually maximal in the legs (especially anterior tibialis) but also seen in upper limb muscles. The activity is quite random and does not appear to be restricted to stage 1 (like the "physiologic" variety of Loeb et al (9) or stage REM (44). The amount of activity is great—at least 100 events during any consecutive 20-minute period of stages 2, 3, or 4—compared to the finding in controls by Dagnino et al (45) of 10 events in 20 minutes of stage 1, or five events in 20 minutes of REM sleep. The study by Broughton et al (46) found four patients (out of 38) whose EDS could not be explained by any other sleep disorder including sleep apnea/hypopnea, typical periodic movements of sleep, or narcolepsy with or without cataplexy; one of the 34 other patients had insomnia rather than EDS and another had periodicity of the myoclonus, suggesting a linkage to PLMS.

One unexplained factor in these patients is that the sleep–wake complaints are out of proportion to the degree of apparent sleep disruption—in fact, the sleep architecture is often normal and essentially undisturbed, in contrast to the typical PLMS patient.

The distinction between spinal/extrapyramidal movement phenomena and PLMS/FMS is that the latter are the only cases of (presumed) origin above the level of the spinal cord that are persistent in sleep. Dagnino et al (45) showed that, at least for the physiologic variety (which may be an early or subclinical form of FMS), there is an absence of such activity in patients with a severed spinal cord or with severe cortical brain damage (as in a stroke) on the side controlling the limb in question. Etiologic mechanisms will be considered later in this chapter.

EPIDEMIOLOGY

PLMS is most prevalent in the elderly and shows a clear increase with age (Fig 84.2), although there have been many cases seen in young adults, and rarely even in infants as young as 18 months (personal observation). A survey of healthy seniors over age 60 has shown an incidence as high as 57% (but at least half of these had fewer than 5 movements per hour) (48). Other studies have shown incidences

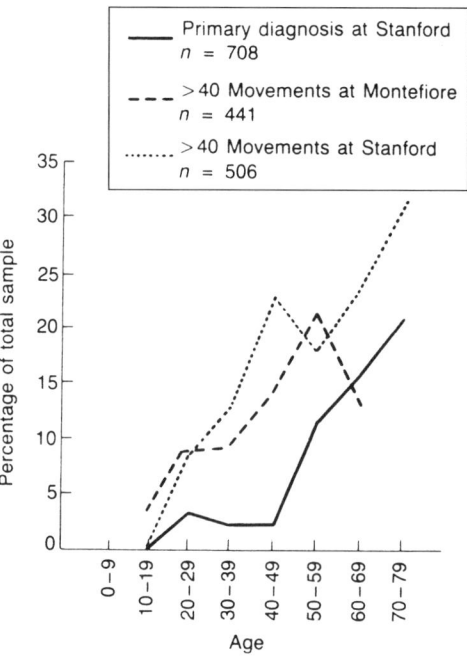

FIGURE 84.2 *Age-related prevalence by decades for diagnoses of PLMS in all newly referred patients (Stanford, 1978–79). Patients were included only when arousal with periodic leg movements was judged to be the cause of sleep–wake complaints (arousal index ≥5). Also shown are data on cases of 40 or more movements from this clinic and from another sleep disorders center (Montefiore Hospital). Regardless of whether PLMS is defined by a minimal number of movements or by the physician's judgment of the arousing effect of the movements, the prevalence of PMS increases with age. From Coleman RM, Miles LE, Guilleminault C, et al. Sleep–wake disorders in the elderly: a polysomnographic analysis. J Am Geriatr Soc 1981;29:289–296.*

of 37% to 53%, although these were of patients with sleep complaints (47,49). Among patients over age 60 with sleep problems, 18% in one study were eventually given the primary diagnosis of periodic movements or restless legs syndrome, and furthermore, longitudinal follow-up of such patients showed an increasing prevalence of nocturnal movements with aging (50) (Fig 84.2). Yet a study of mountain-dwelling nonagenarians in Vilcabamba, Ecuador, found a remarkable lack of either PLMS or sleep apnea (albeit, using only a four-channel ambulatory EEG recorder); these findings were used to explain the unusual longevity and general good health of the subjects (51). The authors attributed their findings to differences in familial or dietary and exercise factors.

PLMS is found in 3% to 26% of patients of all ages complaining of insomnia and about 1% to 12% of EDS patients, yet given the higher prevalence of PLMS among the elderly, even if only moderate and severe cases are counted, the rate of sleep complaints seems unexpectedly low. Some have speculated that the elderly are more likely to accept their lot owing to the prevailing geriatric stereotype of slowed function or lowered expectations of sleep quality (47,52).

There may also be less concern among retired persons about their ability to arise on as timely a basis as was previously necessary with their work-day schedule; but perhaps some who retire have already "slowed down" owing to the physiologic changes in their sleep quality. Those who haven't slowed down may chafe at the mandatory retirement age, which is based on the "average" individual and his or her ability as perceived by a society that has accepted the geriatric stereotype.

CLINICAL CORRELATES

Both insomnia and hypersomnolence (or EDS) are heard as complaints from patients with PLMS, thus raising the question as to how these symptomatic complaints are generated and how they differ. The tendency to daytime sleepiness is understandable, at least on a superficial level, since many of these patients have hundreds of leg movements at night, often leading to severely fragmented and disrupted sleep (although the patient is usually only vaguely aware of this); because this is a chronic condition, such patients may go for years without a good night's rest and their sleepiness may become profound. (This is more readily seen with sleep apnea patients since the apneas are likely to be associated with more severe arousals or disruptions of the sleep patterns.) On the other hand, patients with insomnia (PLMS–DIMS) are often found to have similarly disrupted nocturnal sleep, once sleep is achieved; they are often more aware of the awakenings, and although many such patients do not have severe sleep-onset latency problems, the ones that do (some of these are afflicted with daytime restless leg syndrome) are usually aware of the leg muscle activity as a factor in their insomnia.

Coleman et al (53) studied sleepiness in a group of seven mild-to-moderate PLMS patients ages 54 to 71; they found that over a 3-day period, sleepiness (as measured by the Stanford Sleepiness Scale (SSS) and by the Multiple Sleep Latency Test (MSLT) varied from pathologic to normal (and did so independently of the nocturnal sleep measures such as number of movements per hour or number of arousals per hour; they also found night-to-night variability in the number of arousals but the movements themselves were stable over all three nights. These findings demonstrate that the measures of daytime sleepiness (SSS and MSLT) may not always be accurate in PLMS patients, at least when the patients are not markedly somnolent (the one moderately severe case in the study did show a significant correlation between PLMS and sleepiness scores). Further, the number of arousals per hour of sleep did show a weak correlation with the subsequent day's degree of sleepiness as measured on the MSLT, and this correlation might have reached significance with a larger number of subjects (or, a greater percentage of the moderately to severely afflicted). Coleman and co-workers ended their discussion by calling for studies of new treatments for PLMS so that it can be determined if reducing the number of leg movements can indeed ame-

liorate the symptoms of sleepiness and fatigue. Since that article, a number of treatments have been developed that suppress the leg movements, improve the sleep quality, and reduce the EDS or insomnia (54,55) (see below, under Treatment).

A study by Rosenthal et al (56) showed that there are subtle but measurable differences in the sleep disruptions of DIMS and DOES patients: the sleepy patients had longer histories of subjective sleep trouble (average 22.4 years versus 14.3 years), shorter latencies to sleep onset, more total stages 3 and 4 sleep per night (average of 18.5 minutes compared to 10.9 minutes for DIMS), but more total arousals that were shorter in duration and more concentrated in clusters or series. Ohanna et al (57) found, conversely, that insomniacs had the greater number of leg movements per series; however, their cases were milder and their definition of "series" may have been different. Rosenthal's group also noted that insomnia patients had shorter intervals between individual movements, with a mean of less than 26 secs, while the hypersomnolent patients had more than 26 secs between movements; Ohanna and colleagues found a similar separation between the groups. However, Montplaisir et al (35) showed that the intermovement interval in familial RLS/PLMS with insomnia lengthens from 24 seconds in stage 1 sleep to 35 seconds upon entering stage 2 of sleep. Furthermore, Coleman et al (22) found that the greater the variability of the intermovement interval, the more disturbed the sleep. The reasons for these findings are not clear but Rosenthal et al (56) suggested two hypotheses: 1) the insomniacs are more sensitive to awakening stimuli during sleep (such as the leg movements may represent) while the hypersomnolent patients tend to sleep through the stimuli, or 2) the two groups represent two points on a continuum with the hypersomnolent patients having arrived at a more advanced stage and, after a period of chronically disturbed sleep, having developed EDS as well as shorter awakenings at night. One possible way to reconcile these ideas is as follows: the parts of the brain responsible for maintaining wakefulness are more active in the younger DIMS patients, thus keeping them more alert in the daytime but keeping them from sleeping as deeply or soundly at night (and often requiring sedatives). Thus, their "complaint" of insomnia may be the result of this greater perception of nocturnal sleeplessness, and their belief that a "good night's sleep" is considered an important sign of good health (as it is in most cultures) leads them to seek medical help. Alternatively, they may be experiencing persistent excessive activity from the CNS sleep center(s) that they perceive as fatigue that they must rely on their "waking system" to overcome (which, in younger patients, may be more resilient). The sleepy patients, on the other hand, may have a weaker waking system, worn out from age or from greater duration of illness, which is not able to overcome—without stimulant medications—the excessive sleep-induction activity from parts of the brain that have been chronically deprived of their normal functional cycles at night. The "weaker" waking system may be the result of genetics or age. (It is not as yet clear why the sleep-related parts of the brain function as they do or, indeed, why we sleep at all. Nonetheless, there is evidence in humans of "pressures" for both REM and NREM stages, when these are deprived, and the latter may be the stronger pressure of the two in PLMS (58).

Coleman and co-workers found a broad range of disorders among patients studied in a sleep center and found to have PLMS. In one early study (59) of 441 sleep clinic patients, they found fewer than 40 periodic movements (excluding those at the end of apneas) on all-night PSGs in 19% of insomniacs, 15% of sleep apnea patients, 10% of narcoleptics, 12% of patients with "other hypersomnias," and 9% of patients with other disorders including parasomnias and sleep–wake schedule disorders. This would appear to indicate either that PLMS is a nonspecific finding among patients with a variety of sleep complaints or, conversely, that the presence of PLMS may be a contributing factor in many different sleep disorders. In support of the latter is the finding of PLMS as the only factor disturbing sleep in a subgroup of those with daytime sleepiness as the presenting complaint. In addition, there are several studies that show an increased incidence of PLMS in narcolepsy (60,61), but other studies dispute the importance of the finding (62) or show no increase (22). One study (23) showed that up to 89% of narcoleptics have significant amounts of muscle activity in the legs during sleep (which the authors called "MAL," probably a combination of PLMS and the fragmentary myoclonus of Broughton and Tolentino (43)). Thus, much of the "phasic," brief, truly myoclonic activity that had been ignored prior to the findings of "FMS" by Broughton's group now may have to be considered as an additional factor when it occurs in large amounts (>300/h); and according to Broughton et al (46) this may not be a rare finding among sleep clinic patients. True PLMS are found with increasing frequency in elderly narcoleptics (22), but this may indicate merely that leg movements in such patients are more likely to develop with time owing to the effects of disrupted sleep–wake patterns on the internal circadian pacemaker, or perhaps in part because of medications being taken (63). It would be of interest, however, to further study the elderly narcoleptics to see if those who do not have PLMS represent a different subgroup. Another possibility is that the underlying tendency to develop PLMS is predetermined by heredity and that its determinants may be loosely linked to the HLA-DR2 locus that has been found prevalent in narcoleptics (64). Thus, sleep-related complaints may have to be viewed as the result of combinations of more than one type of underlying disorder.

Associated conditions found with RLS (and therefore presumably correlated with PLMS) include iron- and folate-deficiency anemias (65,66), neuropathies with diabetes (67) or amyloid (68), uremia (69), and normal pregnancy (70). In one study, PLMS was found surprisingly prevalent among childhood leukemics in remission; the patients had all received cranial irradiation and intrathecal methotrexate and

the authors suggested that the latter may alter central dopamine and serotonin function (71). Hypertension, which has been found frequently in association with sleep apnea syndrome (72,73), was present in 25% of the PLMS patients *without* sleep apnea in one study (22), but this finding has not as yet been verified. Cold temperature, especially of the feet, may sometimes be a predisposing factor according to Ekbom (74), and fevers were noted by some of his patients to abolish the movements. Although these same factors have not all been reported in association with PLMS, there is a report of improvement in nocturnal leg movements in a patient using thermal biofeedback (75), and one personally observed insomnia patient had her best sleep during treatment with interferon (an agent that induces fevers and hypersomnolence in humans and sleep in rabbits (76)).

Fibromyalgia/fibrositis syndrome (also called "rheumatic pain modulation disorder") has been found to be related to sleep disorders, most often PLMS and so-called alpha–delta sleep (39). The latter involves the appearance of large amounts of alpha activity during deep NREM sleep (stages 3 and 4, or delta sleep), and can be found in patients with other disorders including hypersomnolence, daytime sleepiness, eating disorders, and schizoid or affective disorders (38). Some fibrositis patients may respond to chlorpromazine or amitriptyline (39); but antipsychotics can cause or uncover PLMS and akathisia (77), which has several characteristics in common with RLS (78), while tricyclics may induce or worsen both daytime sleepiness and PLMS in susceptible individuals (79).

Sexual dysfunction and personality changes have been reported in patients with EDS due to sleep apnea syndrome (73), but there have been no similar reports with PLMS, though further studies are needed.

A study of three patients with atypical depression found sleep disruption by PLMS or alpha–delta activity and noted a response in all cases to valproate (80). In a preliminary report of an open-label uncontrolled study, a large group of patients diagnosed polysomnographically with PLMS had subjective improvement in sleep and daytime alertness from taking small bedtime doses of valproate (81). Other disorders in which PLMS may sometimes play a part include attention deficit disorder (pediatric (82) and adult (80) forms) and intractable migraine syndrome (80), as well as possibly epilepsy, toxemia of pregnancy, and senile dementia. Treatment of the sleep problem in each of the above has led to clinical improvement in the presenting condition and improved daytime alertness (personal observations), but such anecdotal cases need to be confirmed by large-scale controlled studies.

It might well be asked how a single—and largely hidden—disorder can be associated with so many clinical entities. However, most of these conditions are either the direct result of daytime somnolence or are indirectly caused by stress—possibly the stress of having to daily overcome excessive sleepiness accumulated after years of poor quality sleep. Indeed, additional clinical disorders related to stress, such as gastroduodenal ulcers, myocardial ischemia, hypertension, and stroke, all of which can be found among severe cases of sleep apnea, might be expected in the end stages of severe long-standing PLMS as well.

ETIOLOGY

As mentioned earlier in this chapter, the relationship of restless legs syndrome (RLS) to PLMS has been studied by Montplaisir et al (35), who found that there are close similarities in the phenomena, especially in familial cases. Although Weitzman thought PLMS was always present in the nocturnal sleep of patients with RLS, others have found occasional patients with RLS who do not have PLMS at night. Also, most PLMS patients do not complain of clearcut RLS. (However, if one asks PLMS patients detailed questions about daytime leg restlessness, the answers are occasionally positive, indicating that the clinical detection rate of RLS may be somewhat low.) Nevertheless there are several important aspects of these two entities indicating the possible sharing of at least some mechanistic factors between them. Most RLS patients do have severe PLMS and Montplaisir and co-workers found that the familial occurrence of RLS/PLMS follows a dominant pattern; in their study, the 62-year-old mother of the propositus showed severe RLS without PLMS (albeit her sleep was perhaps too severely disrupted to allow detection of PLMS) while the propositus' 3-year-old daughter (one of the youngest cases reported in the literature) had significant PLMS on one night's recording (with none on two other nights). The researchers also showed that, in the propositus, there was a periodicity to the daytime movements (if nonperiodic voluntary activities were ignored) that had an average intermovement interval of less than 20 seconds, while in stage 1 the mean interval increased to 24 seconds and during stage 2 to 35 seconds. (Coleman et al (22) noted the similarity of these periodicities to that of the "Mayer waves" found in day and night recordings of physiologic phenomena such as intracranial pressure.) Montplaisir et al (14) also noted an elevation of dopaminergic factors in the CNS of their propositus and suggest, in another study, that dopamine receptors may be reduced in sensitivity in these disorders.

Askenasy et al (83) have suggested that PLMS found in Parkinson's disease are the result of a basal ganglia dysfunction, although this is based in large part on the apparent improvement with appropriate anti-Parkinson medications. Wechsler et al (84) have recently shown that patients with PLMS have evidence of hyperexcitability in the patterns of their blink reflexes, somatosensory evoked responses, long latency motor responses, and H reflexes. They suggested that this is evidence of a disorder at the pontine level or above. This does not answer the question as to whether the PLMS is acting partly in a causal role via the effects of sleep deprivation or is merely another manifestation of a systemic hyperexcitability.

In discussing Smith's work (34) on the Babinski-like pattern of PLMS, Walters and Hening (85) suggested that since the Babinski sign usually occurs with damage to the pyramidal tracts as a release of central inhibitory activity, perhaps there is altered transmission in these tracts in PLMS.

There is a normal tendency for the "antigravity" muscles of the legs (gastrocnemii, quadriceps, glutei) to overpower the opposing muscles, and this may lead to contractures of these muscles in immobilized patients after a stroke or spinal cord damage or in any patients with chronic upper motor neuron dysfunction. Thus, there may be a "teleological need" for the opposing muscles to be exercised (particularly the anterior tibialis, since they oppose the gastrocnemii—the body's most powerful muscles). Heavy exercise in normals has been shown to improve stages 3 and 4 sleep (86) (possibly protective against sleep apnea as well as PLMS, both of which tend to be most pronounced in stages 1 and 2); exercise may also reduce the central drive for PLMS since it is known to reduce the daytime urge for movements in patients with RLS. Further, anecdotal cases in the author's experience demonstrate that some athletic patients note marked increases in nocturnal movements and disruption of their sleep with resultant EDS after sudden cessation of heavy daily exercise regimes owing to injury or severe illness. Thus, one testable hypothesis is that the steady deterioration in stages 3 and 4 and the great prevalence of PLMS in the elderly is in part related to reduced exercise levels, which generally decline with age in most cultures. This does not account for the occasional cases of severe PLMS found in some young adults and adolescents and even in the rare infant. Additional genetic or environmental factors may be needed to explain such "premature" cases. Coleman et al (22) noted that many patients with PLMS also have disturbances in their 24-hour sleep–wake (circadian) rhythms, and that the latter may be an underlying causative factor in PLMS. It is suggested in another study (80) that both types of sleep disturbance may be fundamentally related to an altered function of the circadian rhythm pacemaker in the suprachiasmatic nucleus (SCN), allowing for nocturnal encroachment of daytime-like CNS activity (leg movements or alpha activity in the EEG). Since the SCN has mostly gamma-aminobutyric acid (GABA) receptors (87), this may have bearing on the response to valproate, which is thought to enhance activity at these receptors (88). Another intriguing aspect of the circadian hypothesis is the close association of the daily temperature curve with the sleep–wake cycle; as previously mentioned, there are many PLMS patients who note "cold feet" (75), thus suggesting a disorder in the thermoregulatory center of the hypothalamus, perhaps in turn caused by an underlying SCN disturbance.

It has been argued that instead of being a *cause* of poor sleep, PLMS may be the *result*, or at least a parallel phenomenon, with no separate clinical import. This idea seems consistent with the findings of Bixler et al (89) of a 6%

incidence of PLMS (defined as 3 or more epochs of at least 30 consecutive leg-EMG bursts in a night) in a normal asymptomatic group averaging 40 years of age. However, their subjects had arousals with only 10% of the leg movements and this may explain why there were no sleep complaints; the patients with insomnia or EDS generally have arousals in association with 20% to 50% of the leg movements. Also, since the prevalence of PLMS rises with advancing age, perhaps Bixler's "asymptomatic" middle-aged cases will become tomorrow's overt cases.

TREATMENT

There have been a number of papers over the past 8 to 10 years that have begun to address the issue of treatment for PLMS (54,55,57,90). Drugs that affect the GABA-receptor have been the most effective, including the benzodiazepines, baclofen, and valproate. The most widely touted pharmacologic therapy employs the benzodiazepines, especially clonazepam, but these are also among the most popular sleep-inducing medications used in general practice and more recently have become popular among psychiatrists treating various disorders including depression (91). Indeed, since PLMS is found to be a cause of at least 15% of insomnia, it may well be that there are many undiagnosed PLMS patients who are nevertheless receiving an appropriate treatment and benefiting from it. PLMS patients who have hypersomnia or EDS, on the other hand, often have great difficulty with the sedative effects of the benzodiazepine class, and in fact some of these patients have had profoundly sedating responses to relatively minute doses of diazepam or other tranquilizers and sedative/hypnotic preparations (personal observation). The other major difficulty with the benzodiazepines is the tendency for patients to develop tolerance to the beneficial effects over time (91). This can be a devastating problem when attempts are subsequently made to withdraw the medication, since such a procedure will tend to severely exacerbate the underlying sleep disorder and cause other withdrawal effects such as tremors, headaches, nausea, and even seizures (all of these possibly brought out at least in part by the sleep disruption as well as the "denervation hypersensitivity" of the benzodiazepine receptor). This may account for some of the patients who are so severely addicted to these substances that they cannot tolerate being weaned. In fact, there may be a tendency for people with PLMS (and others with chronic severe sleep disturbances) to gravitate toward benzodiazepines when obtainable (or to alcohol as an alternative) and then to develop addictions to these substances after initially obtaining relief.

These problems, as well as the lack of a clear mechanism of action or studies showing adequate elimination of leg movements by these medications, have led to the search for more effective, less problematic therapies. Baclofen was found effective in one study, but interestingly, it did not decrease the number of leg movements; rather it seemed to improve the sleep by causing a greater dissociation between the leg movements and their tendency to produce sleep disruptions (92). One problem with this drug is its short duration of action, and the possibility exists that, like other agents that affect the GABA receptor, tolerance may develop. One class of agents that has been found to affect the GABA receptor but has not been specifically studied in patients with PLMS is the barbiturates (93), including phenobarbital, which are among the most widely prescribed sleep agents for decades. This class of drugs has undoubtedly been used in PLMS patients unknowingly (and perhaps successfully), but once again the problem of tolerance and abuse is well recognized with this group of medicines. Finally, valproate is a medication whose mechanism of action is not fully understood, although a number of studies have suggested that its anticonvulsant action involves some type of enhancement of GABA-receptor activity (88). The advantage of this medication is the lack of any known tendency for tolerance to develop, and since the drug has been available in Europe for 20 years, it seems likely that any abuse potential would have become clear by now. In preliminary studies with valproate, there appear to be a substantial number of PLMS patients—including some with RLS and some with narcolepsy–cataplexy—who experience improved daytime alertness (or reduced leg restlessness for RLS patients) for follow-up periods up to 2 years (unpublished data). It should be noted that PLMS patients with EDS may be extraordinarily sensitive to the sedative effects of valproate so that it is necessary to use nocturnal-only administration of relatively small doses of straight valproic acid (non-enteric-coated, shorter-acting form), aiming to achieve a morning-after serum level of less than 20 mg/L (80). Valproate has been used as a sleep-inducing agent in Europe (94–96) and indeed the patients who return with levels greater than 20 mg/L often complain of excessive daytime fatigue, headaches, and moodiness, probably related to a "hangover" effect of the drug (80). Another antiepileptic drug with a similar efficacy in open-label trials is gabapentin. This drug has some advantages in that its side effect profile is quite favorable, it doesn't interact with other medications, and it is not metabolized by the liver.

Other pharmacologic agents that have been used for sleep-consolidation include dopaminergic agonists such as L-dopa (14), bromocriptine (97), and gamma-hydroxybutyrate (98) (which has a presumed dopaminergic effect during withdrawal from each dose). The stimulants pemoline, methylphenidate, and d-amphetamine have long been used as daytime stimulants for those with EDS and are thought to act at dopaminergic receptors. Interestingly, some EDS patients who take these stimulants report that their nocturnal sleep quality seems improved, although a substantial number of those with or without known sleep disorders who use (or abuse) these drugs may *develop* insomnia, especially if the levels are significant during the night. The release of a long-acting or slow-release form of L-dopa/carbidopa for Parkinson's disease has turned out to be beneficial for many intractable PLMS patients. Studies by Coleman et al (22) initially showed that L-dopa might exacerbate PLMS but work by Montplaisir et al (14) demonstrated that during the first 2 hours of sleep there were beneficial effects, after which there was a rebound, causing an exacerbation of the PLMS. When gamma-hydroxybutyrate is used, the effect is the opposite, so that the drug is usually given in the evening, about 2 to 4 hours before bedtime, thus allowing the exacerbating effect on PLMS to wear off before bedtime and permitting the rebound (beneficial) effects to be concentrated in the first few hours of sleep (98). This may not be optimal for those PLMS patients whose worst sleep occurs in the latter half of the night, when the repeated bouts of leg movement activity may increase in intensity during the lighter stages of NREM sleep.

Interestingly, patients with true narcolepsy, who have been found to have from 10% to 75% incidence of PLMS (usually greater with age), may improve when treated with some of these same agents. The use of valproate, L-dopa (99), and gamma-hydroxybutyrate (98) has led to some amelioration of the sleep attacks, sometimes allowing reductions in stimulant dosages, suggesting that at least in some narcoleptics there may be a significant contribution of sleepiness from underlying PLMS.

Opiates form another class of agents that have been used successfully in PLMS as well as RLS, and codeine was effective in at least one study (100). Although these agents pose obvious difficulties with respect to tolerance and abuse potential, the authors claim that their patients tend not to deviate from the prescribed regimes. On the other hand, it is probably the least objectionable agent for use during pregnancy; stool softeners should be added to counteract the constipating effects of the opiate.

Adrenergic blocking agents have had some limited use in patients with sleep disorders. One patient with PLMS responded to an alpha-adrenergic blocker, phenoxybenzamine (101). Studies have shown a moderate—but not necessarily long-lasting—response to the beta-blocker propranolol in RLS (102), akathisia (103), and in narcolepsy (104). Clonidine, an alpha$_2$-adrenergic agonist, has been used for RLS (105).

Serotonergic agents such as L-tryptophan and 5-hydroxytryptophan have been used with some success in RLS (106) but have not been found useful in PLMS (107). Other therapies that have been found helpful in RLS that have not been demonstrated to work for PLMS include iron (66) and folate (108) (these worked even when a deficiency was not present), vitamin E (109), vasodilators (110), and aldehydes (111).

Another anticonvulsant that has been tried in PLMS is phenytoin (112). Carbamazepine has been used in RLS (113), but this agent is of limited use since it is a tricyclic

compound and may be expected to cause worsening of PLMS (79).

Patients with PLMS often complain of nocturnal leg cramps that may awaken them, but it has not been determined if the average patient that *presents* with recurrent nocturnal cramps has PLMS. Quinine has been used for many years for nocturnal cramps (114) and may be of use as an adjunctive therapy in PLMS patients.

Other drugs that have been found to cause or exacerbate RLS or PLMS include lithium (115), caffeine (116), terbutaline (117), and nifedipine (118) (other calcium channel blockers may also be suspect). As mentioned earlier, antipsychotic-neuroleptic drugs commonly cause akathisia (119), which is similar to RLS (77) and can be associated with a sleep disturbance (14) that may be the same as PLMS.

Clearly, the syndrome of PLMS, although probably ancient and recognized at least in some sense many years ago, has only very recently been adequately described, and the effective therapies are only just now being found and evaluated. Since this entity, at least when severe, has widespread effects on the sufferers, the impetus for more research—especially controlled drug trials—should continue to grow in the years to come.

REFERENCES

1. Willis T. The London practice of physick. London: Bassett and Crooke, 1685.
2. Symonds CP. Nocturnal myoclonus. J Neurol Neurosurg Psychiatry 1953;16:166–171.
3. Oswald I. Sudden bodily jerks on falling asleep. Brain 1959;82(1):92–103.
4. International classification of sleep disorders: diagnostic coding manual. Rochester, MN: American Sleep Disorders Association, 1990.
5. Sterman MB, Shouse MN, eds: Sleep and epilepsy. New York: Academic, 1982.
6. Hoeppner JB, Garron DC, Cartwright RD. Self-reported sleep disorder symptoms in epilepsy. Epilepsia 1984;25(4):434–437.
7. Kellaway P. Sleep and epilepsy. Epilepsia 1985;26(suppl 1):S15–S30.
8. Aserinsky E, Kleitman N. Regularly occurring periods of eye motility and concomitant phenomena during sleep. Science 1953;118:273–274.
9. Loeb C, Massazza G, Sacco G, Arnone A. Etude polygraphique des "myoclonies hypniques" chez l'homme. Rev Neurol (Paris) 1964;110(3):258–268.
10. Lugaresi E, Tassinari CA, Coccagna G, Ambrosetto C. Particularités cliniques et polygraphiques du syndrome d'impatience des membres inférieurs. Rev Neurol (Paris) 1965;113(5):545–555.
11. Lugaresi E, Coccagna G, Gambi D, et al. A propos quelques manifestations nocturnes myocloniques. (Nocturnal myoclonus de Symonds.) Rev Neurol (Paris) 1966;115:547–555.
12. Lugaresi E, Coccagna G, Mantovani M, et al. The evolution of different types of myoclonus during sleep. Eur Neurol 1970;4:321–331.
13. Klawans HL, Goetz C, Bergen D. Levodopa-induced myoclonus. Arch Neurol 1975;32:331–334.
14. Montplaisir J, Godbout R, Poirier G, Bédard MA. Restless legs syndrome and periodic movements in sleep: physiopathology and treatment with L-DOPA. Clin Neuropharmacol 1986;9(5):456–463.
15. Castaldo V. The effect of akathisia on sleep. A preliminary study. J Nerv Ment Dis 1968;146(6):498–501.
16. Schenck CH, Bundlie SR, Patterson AL, Mahowald MW. Rapid eye movement sleep behavior disorder. A treatable parasomnia affecting older adults. JAMA 1987;257(13):1786–1789.
17. Salva MAQ, Guilleminault C. Olivopontocerebellar degeneration, abnormal sleep and REM sleep without atonia. Neurology 1986;36:576–577.

18. Schenck CH, Mahowald MW. Motor dyscontrol in narcolepsy: rapid-eye-movement (REM) sleep without atonia and REM sleep behavior disorder. Ann Neurol 1992;32:3–10.

19. Lugaresi E, Cirignotta F. Hypnogenic paroxysmal dystonia: epileptic seizure or a new syndrome? Sleep 1981;4:129–138.

20. Lugaresi E, Cirignotta F, Montagna P. Nocturnal paroxysmal dystonia. J Neurol Neurosurg Psychiatry 1986;49:375–380.

21. Lugaresi E, Cirignotta F, Montagna P. Nocturnal paroxysmal dystonia. In: Kryger MG, Roth T, Dement WC, eds. Principles and practice of sleep medicine. Philadelphia: WB Saunders, 1989:410–421.

22. Coleman R, Pollak CP, Weitzman ED. Periodic movements in sleep (nocturnal myoclonus): relation to sleep disorders. Ann Neurol 1980;8:416–421.

23. Hartman PG, Scrima L. Muscle activity in the legs (MAL) associated with frequent arousals in narcoleptics, nocturnal myoclonus and obstructive sleep apnea (OSA) patients. Clin Electroencephalogr 1986;17(4):181–186.

24. Association of Sleep Disorders Centers. Diagnostic classification of sleep and arousal disorders. Sleep 1979;2:1–137.

25. Guilleminault C, Raynal D, Weitzman ED, Dement WC. Sleep-related periodic myoclonus in patients complaining of insomnia. Trans Am Neurol Assoc 1975;100:19–21.

26. Coleman RM. Periodic movement in sleep (nocturnal myoclonus) and restless legs syndrome. In: Guilleminault C, ed. Sleeping and waking disorders: indications and techniques. Menlo Park: Addison-Wesley, 1982:265–295.

27. Wittig R, Zorick F, Piccione P, et al. Narcolepsy and disturbed nocturnal sleep. Clin Electroencephalogr 1983;14:130–134.

28. Mosko SS, Shampain DS, Sassin JF. Nocturnal REM latency and sleep disturbance in narcolepsy. Sleep 1984;7:115–125.

29. Scrima L, Diaz O, Cabrera N, Hartman P. Arousals following any muscle activity in legs (MAL): in narcolepsy, apnea, and nocturnal myoclonus patients. Sleep Res 1985;14:213.

30. The Atlas Task Force: Recording and scoring leg movements. Sleep 1993;16:748–759.

31. Bliwise DL, Keenan S, Burnburg D, et al. Inter-rater reliability for scoring periodic leg movements in sleep. Sleep 1991;14:249–251.

32. The Atlas Task Force: EEG arousals: scoring rules and examples. Sleep 1992;15:173–184.

33. Lugaresi E, Coccagna G, Montavani M, Lebrun R. Some periodic phenomena during drowsiness and sleep in man. EEG Clin Neurophysiol 1972;32:701–705.

34. Smith RC. Relationship of periodic movements in sleep (nocturnal myoclonus) and the Babinski sign. Sleep 1985;8(3):239–243.

35. Montplaisir J, Godbout R, Boghen D, et al. Familial restless legs with periodic movements in sleep: electrophysiologic, biochemical, and pharmacologic study. Neurology 1985;35(1):130–134.

36. Guilleminault C, Stoohs R, Clerk A, et al. A cause of excessive daytime sleepiness: the upper airway resistance syndrome. Chest 1993;104:781–787.

37. Rechtschaffen A, Kales A, eds: A manual of standardized terminology, technique, and scoring system for sleep stages of human subjects. Washington: US Government Printing Office, 1968.

38. Hauri P, Hawkins DR. Alpha–delta sleep. EEG Clin Neurophysiol 1973;34:233–237.

39. Moldofsky H. Sleep and musculoskeletal pain. Am J Med 1986;81(suppl 3A):85–89.

40. Lavie P. Nasal breathing during sleep. In: Guilleminault C, Lugaresi E, eds. Sleep/wake disorders: natural history, epidemiology, and long-term evolution. New York: Raven, 1983:151–162.

41. Association of Sleep Disorders Centers. Diagnostic classification of sleep and arousal disorders. Sleep 1979;2:1–137.

42. Carskadon M, van den Hoed J, Dement W. Sleep and daytime sleepiness in the elderly. J Geriatr Psychiatry 1980;13(2):135–151.

43. Broughton R, Tolentino MA. Fragmentary pathological myoclonus in NREM sleep. EEG Clin Neurophysiol 1984;57:303–309.

44. Askenasy JJM, Yahr MD, Davidovitch S. Isolated phasic discharges in anterior tibial muscle: a stable feature of paradoxical sleep. J Clin Neurophysiol 1988;5(2):175–181.

45. Dagnino N, Loeb C, Massazza G, Sacco G. Hypnic physiological myoclonus in man: an EEG–EMG study in normals and neurological patients. Eur Neurol 1969;2:47–58.

46. Broughton R, Tolentino MA, Krelina M. Excessive fragmentary myoclonus in NREM sleep: a report of 38 cases. EEG Clin Neurophysiol 1985;61:123–133.

47. Coleman RM, Miles LE, Guilleminault C, et al. Sleep–wake disorders in the elderly: a polysomnographic analysis. J Am Geriatr Soc 1981;29:289–296.

48. Reynolds CF, Kupfer DJ, Taska LS, et al. Sleep of healthy seniors: a revisit. Sleep 1985;8(1):20–29.

49. Ancoli-Israel S, Kripke DF, Mason W, Kaplan OJ. Sleep apnea and nocturnal myoclonus in a senior population. Sleep 1981;4:349–358.

50. Coleman RM, Bliwise DL, Sajben N, et al. Epidemiology of periodic movements of sleep. In: Guilleminault C, Lugaresi E, eds. Sleep/wake disorders: natural history, epidemiology, and long-term evolution. New York: Raven, 1983:217–229.

51. Okudaira N, Fukuda H, Nishihara K, et al. Sleep apnea and nocturnal myoclonus in elderly persons in Vilcabamba, Ecuador. J Gerontol 1983;38(4):436–438.

52. Kripke DF, Ancoli-Israel S, Okudaira N. Sleep apnea and nocturnal myoclonus in the elderly. J Am Geriatr Soc 1982;29:289–296.

53. Coleman RM, Bliwise DL, Sajben N, et al. Daytime sleepiness in patients with periodic movements in sleep. Sleep 1982;5(suppl 2):S191–S202.

54. Moldofsky H, Tullis C, Quance G, Lue FA. Nitrazepam for periodic movements in sleep (sleep-related myoclonus). Can J Neurol Sci 1986;13(1):52–54.

55. Peled R, Lavie P. Double-blind evaluation of clonazepam on periodic leg movements in sleep. J Neurol Neurosurg Psychiatry 1987;50(12):1679–1681.

56. Rosenthal L, Roehrs T, Sicklesteel J, et al. Periodic movements during sleep, sleep fragmentation, and sleep-wake complaints. Sleep 1984;7(4):326–330.

57. Ohanna N, Peled R, Rubin A-HE, et al. Periodic leg movements in sleep: effect of clonazepam treatment. Neurology 1985;35(3):408–411.

58. Broughton R. Performance and evoked potential measures of various states of daytime sleepiness. Sleep 1982;5(suppl 2):135–146.

59. Coleman RM, Pollack CP, Weitzman ED. Periodic nocturnal myoclonus in a wide variety of sleep-wake disorders. Trans ANA 1978;103:230–233.

60. Baker TL, Guilleminault C, Nino-Murcia G, Dement WC. Comparative polysomnographic study of narcolepsy and idiopathic central nervous system hypersomnia. Sleep 1986;9(1):232–242.

61. Mosko SS, Shampain DS, Sassin JF. Nocturnal REM latency and sleep disturbance in narcolepsy. Sleep 1984;7:115–125.

62. Montplaisir J, Godbout R. Nocturnal sleep of narcoleptic patients: revisited. Sleep 1986;9(1):159–161.

63. Guilleminault C, Raynal D, Takahashi S, et al. Evaluation of short-term and long-term treatment of the narcolepsy syndrome with clomipramine hydrochloride. Acta Neurol Scand 1976;54:71–78.

64. Poirier G, Montplaisir J, Decary F, et al. HLA antigens in narcolepsy and idiopathic central nervous system hypersomnolence. Sleep 1986;9(1 part 2):153–158.

65. Norlander NB. Therapy in restless legs. Acta Med Scand 1953;145:453–457.

66. Ekbom KA. Restless legs syndrome after partial gastrectomy. Acta Neurol Scand 1966;2:79–89.

67. Gorman C, Dyck P, Pearson J. Symptoms of restless legs. Arch Intern Med 1965;115:155–160.

68. Heinze F, Frame B, Fine C. Restless legs and orthostatic hypotension in primary amyloidosis. Arch Neurol 1967;16:497–500.

69. Callaghan N. Restless legs syndrome in uremic neuropathy. Neurology 1966;16:359–361.

70. Ekbom KA. Restless legs. Acta Med Scand (suppl) 1945;158:1–123.

71. Kotagal S, Rathnow SR, Chu J-Y, et al. Nocturnal myoclonus—a sleep disturbance in children with leukemia. Dev Med Child Neurol 1985;27:124–127.

72. Kales A, Cadieux RJ, Shaw LC, et al. Sleep apnoea in a hypertensive population. Lancet 1984;2:1005–1008.

73. Guilleminault C, van den Hoed J, Mitler MM. Clinical overview of the sleep apnea syndromes. In: Guilleminault C, Dement WC, eds. Sleep apnea syndromes. New York: AR Liss, 1978.

74. Ekbom KA. Restless legs syndrome. Neurology 1960;10:868–873.

75. Ancoli-Israel S, Seifert AR, Lemon M. Thermal biofeedback and periodic movements in sleep: patients' subjective reports and a case study. Biofeedback Self Regul 1986;11(3):177–188.

76. Krueger JM, Dinarello CA, Shoham S, et al. Interferon alpha-2 enhances slow-wave sleep in rabbits. Int J Immunopharmacol 1987;9(1):23–30.

77. Munetz MR, Cornes CL. Distinguishing akathisia and tardive dyskinesia: a review of the literature. J Clin Psychopharmacol 1983;3:343–350.

78. Walters AS, Hening W. Clinical presentation and neuropharmacology of restless legs syndrome. Clin Neuropharmacol 1987;10:225–237.

79. Ware JC, Brown FW, Moorad PJ, et al. Nocturnal myoclonus and tricyclic antidepressants. Sleep Res 1984;13:72.

80. Pies R, Adler D, Ehrenberg BL. Sleep disorder associated with "atypical depression": response to valproate. J Clin Psychopharm (in press).

81. Ehrenberg BL. Valproate for periodic leg movements of sleep. Electroenceph Clin Neurophysiol 1991;79:65P.

82. Busby K, Firestone P, Pivik RT. Sleep patterns in hyperkinetic and normal children. Sleep 1981;4(4):366–383.

83. Askenasy JJ, Weitzman ED, Yahr MD. Are periodic movements in sleep a basal ganglia dysfunction? J Neural Transm 1987;70(3–4):337–347.

84. Wechsler LR, Stakes JW, Shahani BT, Busis NA. Periodic leg movements of sleep (nocturnal myoclonus): an electrophysiological study. Ann Neurol 1986;19(20):168–173.

85. Walters AS, Hening W. Clinical presentation and neuropharmacology of restless legs syndrome. Clin Neuropharmacol 1987;10(3):225–237.

86. Shapiro CM, Warren PM, Trinder J, et al. Fitness facilitates sleep. Eur J Appl Physiol 1984;53(1):1–4.

87. Borsook D, Richardson GS, Moore-Ede MC, Brennan MJ. GABA and circadian timekeeping: implications for manic–depression and sleep disorders. Med Hypotheses 1986;19(2):185–198.

88. Johnston D. Valproic acid: update on its mechanisms of action. Epilepsia 1984;25(suppl 1):S1–S4.

89. Bixler EO, Kales A, Vela-Bueno A, et al. Nocturnal myoclonus and nocturnal myoclonic activity in a normal population. Res Commun Chem Pathol Pharmacol 1982;36:129–140.

90. Boghen D. Successful treatment of restless legs with clonazepam. Ann Neurol 1980;8:341.

91. Cohen LS, Rosenbaum JF. Clonazepam: new uses and potential problems. J Clin Psychiatry 1987;48(suppl):50–56.

92. Guilleminault C, Flagg W. Effect of baclofen on sleep-related periodic leg movements. Ann Neurol 1984;15(3):234–239.

93. Olsen RW. GABA-drug interactions. Prog Drug Res 1987;31:223–241.

94. Boxer CM, Herzberg JL, Scott DF. Has sodium valproate hypnotic effects? Epilepsia 1976;17(4):367–370.

95. Schneider E, Ziegler B, Maxion H. Gamma-aminobutyric acid (GABA) and sleep. The influence of di-n-propylacetic acid on sleep in man. Eur Neurol 1977;15(3):146–152.

96. Puca FM, Genco S, et al. Il sonno di coreici cronici dopo terapia con valproato sodio. Boll Sco Ital Biol Sper 1984;60(5):989–992.

97. Walters AS, Hening WA, Kavey N, et al. A double-blind randomized crossover trial of bromocriptine and placebo in restless legs syndrome. Ann Neurol 1988;24:455–458.

98. Broughton R, Mamelak M. The treatment of narcolepsy–cataplexy with nocturnal gamma-hydroxybutyrate. Can J Neurol Sci 1979;6(1):1–6.

99. Bedard MA, Montplaisir J, Godbout R. Effect of L-DOPA on periodic movements in sleep in narcolepsy. Eur Neurol 1987;27(1):35–38.

100. Hening WA, Walters A, Kavey N, et al. Dyskinesias while awake and periodic movements in sleep in restless legs syndrome: treatment with opioids. Neurology 1986;36(10):1363–1366.

101. Ware JC, Pittard JT, Blumoff RL. Treatment of sleep related myoclonus with an alpha-receptor blocker. Sleep Res 1981;10:242.

102. Strang RR. The symptoms of restless legs. Med J Aust 1967;1:1211–1213.

103. Lipinski JF, Zubenko GS, Cohen BM, Barreira PJ. Propranolol in the treatment of neuroleptic-induced akathisia. Am J Psychiatry 1984;141:412–415.

104. Meier-Ewert K, Matsubayashi K, Benter L. Propranolol: long-term treatment in narcolepsy–cataplexy. Sleep 1985;8(2):95–104.

105. Handwerker JV, Palmer RF. Clonidine in the treatment of restless legs syndrome. N Engl J Med 1985;313:1228–1229.

106. Billiard M, Besset A, Passouant P, et al. Treatment of chronic insomnia: long-term follow-up. Sleep Res 1978;7:210.

107. Guilleminault C, Mondini S, Montplaisir J, et al. Periodic leg movement, L-DOPA, 5-hydroxytryptophan, and L-tryptophan. Sleep 1987;10(4):393–397.

108. Botez MI. Folate deficiency and neurological disorders in adults. Med Hypotheses 1976;2:135–140.

109. Ayres S, Mihan R. Leg cramps (systremma) and "restless legs" syndrome: response to vitamin E (tocopherol). Calif Med 1969;111:87–91.

110. Ekbom KA. Restless legs. A report of 70 new cases. Acta Med Scand (suppl) 1950;246:64–68.

111. Brenning R. Restless legs. Svenska Lakartidn 1957;54:2293.

112. Hogg PS. Three cases of "restless legs" or "Ekbom's syndrome" as seen in general practice. Practitioner 1972;209:82–83.

113. Telstad W, Sørensen Ø, Larsen S, et al. Treatment of the restless legs syndrome with carbamazepine: a double blind study. Br Med J 1984;288:444–446.

114. Quinine for "night cramps." Med Lett Drugs Ther 1986;28(726):110.

115. Heiman EM, Christie M. Lithium-aggravated nocturnal myoclonus and restless legs syndrome. Am J Psychiatry 1986;143(9):1191–1192.

116. Lutz EG. Restless legs, anxiety and caffeinism. J Clin Psychiatry 1978;39:693–698.

117. Zelman S. Terbutaline and muscular symptoms. JAMA 1978;239(10):930.

118. Keidar S, Binenboim C, Palant A. Muscle cramps during treatment with nifedipine. Br Med J (Clin Res) 1982;285(6350):1241–1242.

119. Barnes TRE, Braude WM. Akathisia variants and tardive dyskinesia. Arch Gen Psychiatry 1985;42:874–878.

Sleep Bruxism

Bruce L. Ehrenberg

INTRODUCTION

Although some people grind their teeth voluntarily in the daytime (often in association with anger), the term *sleep bruxism* properly refers to involuntary contractions of the masseter muscles causing grinding of teeth (often producing an easily detectable clicking sound) during nocturnal sleep. The patient is unaware of the problem and often it is first noted by a parent or sibling when it presents in childhood (as is often the case (1)), by a spouse or roommate in adulthood, or by the dentist who may note worn surfaces of the teeth. It is most easily detected during electroencephalography (EEG) if electrodes are placed over the temporalis muscles, which contract in conjunction with the masseters; this yields bursts of electromyographic (EMG) activity that are usually quite prominent ($>75\,\mu V$), last about 0.25 to 0.7 seconds each, and are repetitive two or more times in succession at a rate of about 1 Hz (once per second).

In a recent review of the subject, Hartmann described bruxism as occurring in clusters or episodes of rhythmic grinding of the teeth at 1 Hz and lasting for 5 seconds or longer (2). In a study of 16 patients with moderately severe damage to the surfaces of the teeth, Hartmann and colleagues found an average of 25 episodes of bruxism during polysomnograms (all-night EEG studies) (3).

The relationship of bruxism episodes to the stages of sleep has been debated recently. Earlier studies showed a preponderance during stage 2 and often with arousals that disturb the sleep (4–6). A more recent study has demonstrated that patients presenting with *destructive* bruxism (causing either detectable tooth damage or temporomandibular joint [TMJ] pain) tend to have most of their episodes of tooth-grinding during rapid eye movement (REM) stage, while occasional patients presenting with insomnia or hypersomnia can have equal amounts of

tooth-grinding during the night, but with the majority occurring during stage 2 (7). The authors went on to speculate that the reason for the destructiveness of teeth-grinding during REM stage is the loss of a protective influence from pterygoid muscles that normally oppose the masseters, but that are normally blocked disproportionately during this stage of sleep (along with most other voluntary skeletal muscles) (7).

EPIDEMIOLOGY

Some authors estimate a prevalence of bruxism at 5% to 20% of the population, but one author found signs and symptoms related to bruxism in 78% of a group of young adults (8). In another study, 30.7% of 1,052 dental patients had evidence of teeth-grinding (9). However, these figures represent the sum of both daytime and nocturnal teeth-grinding. Most dentists do not consider it necessary to treat the majority of teeth-grinders and only about 10% of bruxers are considered seriously enough afflicted for treatments such as mouthguards to be prescribed for nocturnal use (2).

Hartmann noted that bruxism "usually begins in late childhood or adolescence" and often disappears by age 40 (2). He also noted that both sexes are affected about equally and that a familial pattern is often seen, although the latter has not been studied in detail.

CLINICAL CORRELATES AND ETIOLOGIC FACTORS

A large proportion of the literature on bruxism emphasizes the relationship of daytime stresses to increased clinical occurrences of nocturnal bruxism, although most of the work on this aspect of bruxism is based on subjective reports by patients and their acquaintances. Indeed, many of the treatment approaches are aimed at psychotherapy, biofeedback, or muscle relaxation techniques in an attempt to reduce the stresses that have long been thought at fault by most workers in this field, although there are few carefully controlled studies of this rather common and often innocuous disorder.

Some recent work has begun to suggest that this entity has a physical as well as psychologic basis and that awareness of its presence in an individual may help uncover some important physiologic characteristics. Bruxism has been seen in association with sleep apnea, and in one study where sleep apnea patients were prospectively studied for teeth-grinding, there was a significant correlation between the amount of jaw clenching and the apnea–hypopnea index (number of respiratory events per hour); there was also a reduction in both phenomena when the patients were turned from supine to lateral decubitus position (10). Since position is known to affect sleep apnea, this suggests that bruxism may be caused by subtle apneas or appear in relation to the *arousals* triggered by the apneas, which are themselves "stressful" events.

Another common sleep disorder involves periodic leg movements (see Chapter 84), and this has been found in frequent association with teeth-grinding (7), although it is likely that these two phenomena occur in parallel rather than one causing the other. Indeed, one group (11) has suggested that the two entities are linked physiologically (when they occur independently of one another, they both may appear in bursts at the same rate of repetition, 20 to 40 seconds apart) and biochemically (they both have an increased incidence in Parkinson's disease patients receiving L-dopa therapy (12,13)). In addition, as with periodic leg movements, the tricyclic antidepressants may exacerbate bruxism (personal observations).

Hartmann et al (3) studied alcohol as an agent that can exacerbate bruxism and found, in a placebo-controlled sleep laboratory study, that four "drinks" before bedtime were followed by a significant amount of bruxism in sleep for over half of the subjects. He also noted that stimulants such as cocaine and amphetamines are reputed to exacerbate or cause bruxism.

There is a high incidence of bruxism (often during the daytime and in the awake state) in patients with severe mental retardation (14,15). This may be related to a generalized loss of inhibitory influences on such behaviors.

It has also been found in some individuals that jaw malformations or poor occlusive alignment of teeth can be a causative factor in bruxism (16). This has also been shown experimentally (17,18).

TREATMENT

Treatment should be restricted to those in whom a significant associated problem has developed (or has been found as a cause) since the disorder itself is only rarely severe enough to cause major dental problems. If dental problems such as malocclusion are found, these may be corrected if the problem is serious enough on its own merits; but if the treatment is to cause extensive alteration of one's jaw, it might be simpler to use a mouthguard if the grinding noise is the only major complaint.

A thorough sleep history looking for associated sleep disorders may be warranted. These are sometimes not recognized as problems by the patient yet may be a cause of significant morbidity later on, such as sleep apnea and its relation to hypertension (19,20). Otherwise, noninvasive treatment methods are preferable and may include biofeedback (21) or behavioral modification (22). A simple massage (23) and a review of progressive relaxation techniques may be just as effective and less expensive.

REFERENCES

1. Wigdorowicz-Makowerowa N, Grodzki C, Panek H, et al. Epidemiologic studies on prevalence and etiology of functional disturbances of the masticatory system. J Prosthet Dent 1979;41:76–82.
2. Hartmann E. Bruxism. In: Dryger MH, Roth T, Dement WC, eds. Principles and practice of sleep medicine. 1st ed. Philadelphia: WB Saunders, 1989:385–388.
3. Hartmann E, Mehta N, Forgione A, et al. Bruxism: effects of alcohol. Sleep Res 1987;16:351.
4. Tani K, Yoshii N, Yoshino I, Kobayashi E. Electroencephalographic study of parasomnia: sleeptalking, enuresis and bruxism. Physiol Behav 1966;1:241–243.
5. Satoh T, Harada Y. Tooth-grinding during sleep as an arousal reaction. Experientia 1971;27:785–786.
6. Satoh T, Harada Y. Electrophysiological study on toothgrinding during sleep. Electroencephalogr Clin Neurophysiol 1973;35:267–275.
7. Ware JC, Rugh JD. Destructive bruxism: sleep stage relationship. Sleep 1988;11(2):172–181.
8. Solberg WK, Woo MW, Houston JG. Prevalence of mandibular dysfunction in young adults. J Am Dent Assoc 1979;98:25–34.
9. Glaros AG. Incidence of diurnal and nocturnal bruxism. J Prosthet Dent 1981;45:545–549.
10. Phillips BA, Okeson J, Paesani D, Gilmore R. Effect of sleep position on sleep apnea and parafunctional activity. Chest 1986;90(3):424–429.
11. Montplaisir J, Godbout R, Boghen D, et al. Familial restless legs with periodic movements in sleep: electrophysiologic, biochemical, and pharmacologic study. Neurology 1985;35(1):130–134.
12. Coleman R, Pollak CP, Weitzman ED. Periodic movements in sleep (nocturnal myoclonus): relation to sleep disorders. Ann Neurol 1980;8:416–421.
13. Magee KR. Bruxism related to levodopa therapy. JAMA 1970;214:147.
14. Lundqvist B, Heijbel J. Bruxism in children with brain damage. Acta Odontol Scand 1974;32(5):313–319.
15. Richmond G, Rugh JD, Dolfi R, Wasilewsky JW. Survey of bruxism in an institutionalized mentally retarded population. Am J Ment Defic 1984;88(4):418–421.
16. Kirk GA. Bruxism in maxillary overdenture patients. J Prosthet Dent 1984;52(5):764.
17. Budtz-Jorgensen E. Occlusal dysfunction and stress. An experimental study in macaque monkeys. J Oral Rehabil 1981;8:1–9.
18. Rugh JD, Barghi N, Drage CJ. Experimental occlusal discrepancies and nocturnal bruxism. J Prosthet Dent 1984;51(4):548–553.
19. Kales A, Cadieux RJ, Shaw LC, et al. Sleep apnoea in a hypertensive population. Lancet 1984;2:1005–1008.
20. Guilleminault C, van den Hoed J, Mitler MM. Clinical overview of the sleep apnea syndromes. In: Guilleminault C, Dement WC, eds. Sleep apnea syndromes. New York, AR Liss, 1978.
21. Cassisi JE, McGlynn FD, Belles DR. EMG-activated feedback alarms for the treatment of nocturnal bruxism: current status and future directions. Biofeedback Self Regul 1987;12(1):13–30.
22. Cherasia M, Parks L. Suggestions for use of behavioral measures in treating bruxism. Psychol Rep 1986;58(3):719–722.
23. Rudrud E, Halaszyn J. Reduction of bruxism by contingent massage. Spec Care Dent 1981;1(3):122–124.

Childhood Disorders of Movement

Brainstem Myoclonus: Dancing Eyes, Dancing Feet

Marcel Kinsbourne

Most myoclonic states originate from cerebral cortex, with grossly abnormal electroencephalograms (EEG) featuring multifocal discharges. But an infrequently seen form of myoclonus has its own interest: the EEG is normal, the eyes jerk continually at random, and the pathogenesis, though not firmly established, appears to be an autoimmune reaction, usually in relation to remote malignancy.

Kinsbourne (1) reported the acute onset of intense, widespread, irregular, and continual myoclonus in six children aged 6 to 18 months. The shock-like muscular contractions reached a plateau of maximal intensity within 1 week and then continued at that level uncomplicated by any further disability until treatment was instituted. The children had had a nonspecific respiratory or gastrointestinal infection (or DPT vaccination in one case) within 48 hours of onset. The EEG was persistently normal disconfirming myoclonic epilepsy, and so was an airencephalogram and a cortical biopsy in one case.

The disorder was distinguishable from acute cerebellar ataxia (for which it might previously have been mistaken) by the unpredictable irregularity of the perturbations of muscular tone as well as by the oculomotor appearances. Rather than nystagmus, there were involuntary conjugate displacements of gaze unpredictable in their direction and amplitude, and as continual as the perturbation of somatic musculature. This ocular myoclonus was termed "dancing eyes." It corresponds to "opsoclonus," described in adults (2). In one case that resolved before the appropriate treatment was discovered, the condition continued for a matter of years and then "burned out," leaving the child motorically intact but moderately mentally retarded. The other children were given intermuscular adrenocorticotropic hormone (ACTH) and exhibited a dramatic relief of symptoms. The level of ACTH could be titrated down to a level at which the myoclonus would again begin to intrude and could then be

effectively maintained just above that level in most cases. The substitution of an oral corticosteroid was often successful. After 7 years it has been possible to stop the treatment without recurrence, but in several personally observed cases unsteadiness or clumsiness persisting into adolescence remained responsive to ACTH administration.

This syndrome has been since documented in well over 100 reported cases (3) and variously named opsoclonus–myoclonus, infantile polymyoclonia, syndrome of rapid, irregular movements of eyes and limbs in childhood, and Kinsbourne's syndrome. As in the original series the onset is typically acute, although at times ascending in severity for up to 7 days. The speediest spontaneous recovery has been after 3 months. Occasionally recovery is incomplete and followed by relapse. Subsequent to the resolution of the myoclonus, more than half the children are developmentally handicapped, often mentally retarded, usually dysarthric. Sometimes they have selective learning or attention disability.

Polymyography confirms the shock-like nonrhythmicity of the muscular contractions and concurrent EEG confirms the absence of any attending observable paroxysmal wave forms.

Autopsy studies of this condition are rare. Case 5 of Kinsbourne's series died at age 33 months. Only perivascular lymphocytic aggregations scattered in the brainstem were observed.

An autoimmune affliction of brainstem has been repeatedly suggested, initially by Kinsbourne, based on the dramatic ACTH response. Two of his patients had hypo-gamma-globulinemia, and another had complement fixation evidence of recent infection with lymphocytic choriomeningitis virus. Three patients of Dyken and Kolar (4) had cerebrospinal fluid lymphocytosis and immunoglobulin (Ig) abnormality. Bray et al (5) suggested that antibodies against neuroblastoma antigen may cross-react with a similar antigen in the cerebellar cells and thereby create damage. Most recently Noetzel et al (6) reported two such cases with serum antibodies directed against the 210 kDa neurofilament protein. Cawley et al (7) had previously described a child with IgG antibodies that stained peripheral nerve axons and a neurofibrillary component of Purkinje cells by immunofluorescence. Postmortem neuropathology has shown Purkinje neurons to be particularly affected (8). Neurofilaments are limited to neurons and a major element of their cytoskeletal structure. Neuroblastoma also contains immunoreactive filament proteins (9). This could explain the dramatic association between myoclonic encephalopathy and neuroblastoma first reported (10).

Since Solomon and Chutorian's (10) two cases, many examples of the association have been published. The localization of the neuroblastoma is disproportionately frequently thoracic and a substantial number of the patients have the benign variant, ganglioneuroblastoma. The prognosis of neuroblastoma in this syndrome was strikingly superior to that of neuroblastoma in general, even when adjusted for the young age of the child. Like the idiopathic variant, the myoclonus associated with neuroblastoma often responds to steroids and in most cases it also remits after tumor resection, although it has been repeatedly reported to recur subsequently. The long-term outlook relative to residual deficits seems little different from that of the idiopathic condition, regardless of tumor resection.

The syndrome of myoclonic encephalopathy of infancy is rather specific, particularly in the developmental stage during which it has its incidence of onset. It is questionable whether myoclonic syndromes occurring later in life are of similar etiology, let alone examples of the same condition. Brainstem myoclonic states in adults, including opsoclonus, do occur as a remote effect of various neoplasms. Hunter and Kooistra (11) report the neuropathologic findings in a 58-year-old woman with an opsoclonus–myoclonus syndrome. Structural lesions were limited to the cerebellum and inferior olives and there was severe selective depletion of Purkinje cells in the neo- and paleocerebellum. They pointed out that these changes are similar to those described in paraneoplastic cerebellar cortical degeneration (12), and the latter may coincide with opsoclonus–myoclonus (13). However, numerous documented cases of adult opsoclonus/myoclonus have occurred in the absence of neoplasia, including Hunter and Kooistra's own case. Etiologies include vascular accidents, encephalitis, degenerative diseases, and drug toxicity, among others. It would appear that the syndrome is related to cerebellar Purkinje cells and that the autoimmunity can be triggered by neuroblastoma antigen released from neuroblastoma, but also by various forms of direct brain damage. The postinfectious cases in adults seem to have a relatively benign course and are often transient (14).

REFERENCES

1. Kinsbourne M. Myoclonic encephalopathy of infants. J Neurol Neurosurg Psychiatry 1962;25:271–276.
2. Cogan DG. Opsoclonus, body tremulousness, and benign encephalitis. Arch Ophthalmol 1968;79:515–551.
3. Lott I, Kinsbourne M. Myoclonic encephalopathy of infants. In: Fahn S et al., eds. Advances in neurology. Vol. 43, Myoclonus. New York: Raven, 1986.
4. Dyken P, Kolar O. Dancing eyes, dancing feet: infantile polymyoclonia. Brain 1968;91:305–320.
5. Bray PF, Ziter FA, Lahey ME, et al. The coincidence of neuroblastoma and acute cerebellar encephalopathy. J Pediatr 1969;75:983–990.
6. Noetzel MJ, Cawley LP, James VL, et al. Anti-neurofilament protein antibodies in opsoclonus–myoclonus. J Neuroimmunol 1987;15:137–145.
7. Cawley LP, James VL, Minard BJ, et al. Antibodies to Purkinje cells and peripheral nerve in opsoclonia. Lancet, 1984:509–510.
8. Moe PG, Nellhaus, G. Infantile polymyoclonia–opsoclonus syndromes and neural crest tumors. Neurology 1970;20:756–764.
9. Trojanowski JQ, Lee VMY. Anti-neurofilament monoclonal antibodies: reagents for the evaluation of human neoplasms. Acta Neuropathol 1983;59:155–158.
10. Solomon GE, Chutorian AM. Opsoclonus and occult neuroblastoma. N Engl J Med 1968;279:475–477.
11. Hunter S, Kooistra C. Neuropathologic findings in idiopathic opsoclonus and myoclonus. J Clin Neuro-ophthalmol 1986;6:236–241.
12. Hensen RA, Urich H. Cancer and the nervous system: the neurologic manifestations of systemic malignant disease. Boston: Blackwell Scientific, 1982:346–367.
13. Ellenberger C, Campa JF, Netsky MG. Opsoclonus and parenchymatous degeneration of the cerebellum. Neurology 1968;18:1041–1046.
14. Digre KB. Opsoclonus in adults. Arch Neurol 1986;43:1165–1175.

Motor Dysfunction in Autism

Margaret L. Bauman

Early infantile autism is a behaviorally defined disorder that was initially described by Kanner in 1943 (1). By definition, clinical features of the syndrome are manifested by 36 months of age and include disordered language and cognitive skills; impaired social relatedness; abnormal responses to sensory stimuli; events, and objects; poor eye contact; an insistence on sameness; islands of rote memory; repetitive and stereotypic behavior; and a normal physical appearance (2). The prevalence rates are now estimated to be 10 to 13 per 10,000 and the disorder is more commonly seen in boys than girls by a ratio of 2.5 to 4.0 : 1 (3–5).

Although many autistic children have been described as developmentally disabled, most notably in language, relatively little attention has been paid to motor function, which for many years was considered to be intact. However, with increasingly careful clinical observation, descriptions of abnormal motor behavior have become more common and there is growing evidence that these abnormalities may be present very early in life. As infants and toddlers, many autistic children have been reported to stiffen or to push others away, seeming to prefer being alone (6). In addition, there is emerging evidence that unusual patterns of movement may be evident as early as 4 to 6 months of age. Teitelbaum and co-workers (Teitelbaum P, personal communication, 1997) systematically reviewed video tapes of 17 infants and toddlers later diagnosed as autistic and those of 12 normally developing children in order to assess the motor patterns involved in lying, righting, sitting, crawling, standing, and walking. Abnormalities were observed in many of the autistic children as early as 3 months of age and included an unusual shape of the mouth, poor eye–head coordination and, atypical righting responses.

Delays in the attainment of motor milestones have also been noted in approximately 50% of the cases studied (7). Many children, particularly the most severely impaired, have been reported to be delayed in learning to walk, using utensils, or dressing (6). Awkwardness, clumsiness, and impairment of neuromotor integration have been described (8). Some autistic children appear to have difficulty carrying out organized movements and seem unable to perform more than one motor task at a time (9,10). Hyperactivity, irritability, wakefulness, temper tantrums, and hand flapping, particularly with excitement or stress, have been consistently described. Neurologic "soft signs" have also been observed (11), the most common being choreiform movements of the extremities, poor balance and coordination, impaired finger–thumb opposition, and disordered articulation and word production. Mild intermittent dystonic postures of the hands and fingers have commonly been observed, and may be accompanied by choreoathetoid movements or superimposed upon repetitive and stereotypic behavior (12).

Abnormalities of muscle tone and reflexes have also been commonly reported but, when present, are usually symmetric in distribution. Muscle tone may be mildly decreased or, in some cases, increased. Deep tendon reflexes are generally decreased in most autistic children but have been reported to be increased in some. Unsustained clonus at the ankles may be seen with passive range of motion and plantar reflexes are generally flexor in uncomplicated cases (6,13,14).

In a study of 42 autistic children and young adults, Minderaa et al (15) reported an increased incidence of positive snout and visual rooting reflexes in comparison with age- and sex-matched controls. The visual rooting reflex appeared to be age-dependent, presenting primarily in younger autistic subjects and suggesting that the retention of this reflex might be a developmental phenomenon. The snout reflex, which usually disappears in normal infants after 6 months of age, was observed in 32 of the 42 autistic subjects studied. Whether these "primitive" reflexes were specific to retarded autistic individuals, in contrast to normally intelligent autistic and nonautistic retarded children, was not determined.

Some of the most notable of the motor behaviors associated with the diagnosis of autism are repetitive and stereotypic movements of the body, limbs, and fingers (16). These movements may include rhythmic rocking of the body from foot to foot while standing, rocking of the upper body while sitting, rhythmic flapping of the arms and hands, or repetitive flicking of the fingers in front of the eyes. Inanimate objects may be incorporated into this behavior such as string that is twirled, wheels of toys that are spun, or repetitive tapping of blocks, pencils, or eating utensils. These behaviors appear to serve no observable purpose, have been considered self-stimulatory in nature, and are usually difficult to eliminate. They appear most often among autistic children who are mentally retarded and are progressively less apparent with increased IQ. It has been noted, however, that even among normally intelligent autistic children stereotypies may be exacerbated during periods of stress on into adulthood. Repetitive behaviors have been similarly reported in normally developing children. In a study of 142 nonhandicapped youngsters, Troster (17) observed body rocking, head banging, hair twisting, nail biting, and facial movements. These stereotypies appeared to be associated with concentration, arousal, frustration, boredom, and distraction and seemed to stabilize the child's level of arousal in monotonous, frustrating, or overstimulating situations. Given these observations, it is possible that stereotypic behavior may be playing a similar role for autistic children.

Self-injurious behavior (SIB) is a singularly dramatic and dangerous motor activity seen in association with autism. These behaviors vary widely in severity and frequency of occurrence. In their mildest form, SIB may include light face slapping, hair pulling, face scratching, or hand biting. More serious injury may result from major head banging, hitting, or other forms of self-mutilation that may lead to fractures of the head, limbs, or ribs, retinal detachment, and deep cutaneous wounds that are often slow to heal because of recurrent trauma and that may become secondarily infected. As with the repetitive and stereotypic behaviors described above, SIB is very difficult to eliminate although consistent, well-monitored behavioral management programs may be helpful. In some cases, however, medical and physical restraints must be used in order to protect the patient from self-inflicted, potentially fatal injuries. Although the neurologic significance and etiology of SIB are not known, it has been suggested that, at least a subpopulation of self-abusive autistic individuals may have high concentrations of opioid peptides in their cerebral spinal fluid and may not perceive SIB as painful. Clinical studies using opioid antagonists to reduce the frequency of SIB initially showed promise but more recent investigations have led to inconsistent results (18).

Unusual gait patterns have been described in autistic individuals and have been linked to those frequently observed in association with extrapyramidal motor disorders. Studied by means of high-speed photography (12), autistic children have been noted to move their limbs more slowly through the gait cycle and to take shorter steps than their unaffected peers. They tended to walk with their head bowed, arms flexed at the elbows, and with symmetrically reduced or poorly coordinated movements of the upper extremities. Further, when walking, the autistic children tended to make contact with the ground first with their toes or in a flat-footed manner, rather than using the normal heel–toe pattern. In more extreme cases, "toe walking" was observed to be pronounced. "Striatal toes" seen unilaterally or bilaterally have also been noted, whereby the great toe may flex upward into a Babinski reflex position when the foot makes initial contact with the ground during walking. Postural adjustments for movement did not appear to be automatic, particularly during walking or when arising from a sitting to a standing position.

Postural control has been more specifically analyzed in 91 autistic children ages 6 to 20 years in comparison with normal subjects using a computerized posturographic procedure (19). In this study, autistic children appear to show a "paradoxical postural stress response" whereby they demonstrated better stability in more difficult positions with vision occluded and restricted somatosensory input. In addition, autistic subjects exhibited an unusual distribution of body weight over the toes and heels, showed excessively mobilized multiple control systems to sustain posture, were conspicuously unstable, and showed directionally inconsistent and sporadic lateral sway. The authors concluded that the presence of these postural patterns was most consistent with abnormalities arising from the mesocortex or the cerebellum.

Postural control in autistic children has been further studied in relationship to motion vision (20). It has been determined that humans make postural adjustments in response to optical flow and that infants react posturally to movements in their visual environment as soon as they are able to stand alone. Thus, visual proprioception plays a major role in the control of stance. Analysis of sway was evaluated in five autistic children, ages 4 to 7 years, in comparison with 12 age- and sex-matched controls using a force platform whereby changes in anterior-posterior and lateral positions were computed on-line. The autistic children were found to be significantly more posturally unstable than the nonautistic children and were substantially unreactive to visual motion. The authors hypothesized that inadequate modulation of motor and sensory output and deficits in sensory motor integration occurring early in development might contribute to these abnormalities of postural stability.

Further support for the presence of poor postural stability among autistic individuals was reported by Kaplan et al (21) in a study involving the relationship of vision to spatial orientation. In this study, the authors hypothesized that "ambient vision," which is important for the orientation of the body to the environment, movement, and depth, may be impaired in autistic persons. Thus, a defect in ambient vision could have an impact on the maintenance of body posture, locomotion, and the perception of self-motion. Some of the autistic subjects in this study, provided with "ambient lenses," showed clinical improvement in postural stability. However, the possible pathophysiology of this hypothesis remains as yet to be determined.

Delays in initiating, changing, or arresting a motor sequence and rapid fatigue during prolonged tasks have also been described. In a study of 36 autistic subjects analyzed in comparison with learning disabled and normal controls, the autistic children were found to have difficulty in goal-directed motor acts, even in very simple situations (22). Suggested causes for this skill deficit included an impairment of sequencing ability, failure to predict the consequences of the intended act, and impaired visual control of movement. It thus appeared that even very simple motor activities seem to depend upon a number of different processes related to "executive control" such as anticipatory planning, adjustment to external feedback, and coordination of multiple elements into a goal-directed sequence. While normal preschool children also showed deficits in handling goal-directed tasks, they demonstrated significant gains in "executive control" between 2 and 4 years of age, suggesting that the acquisition of improved motor control is a developmental phenomenon.

Expressionless faces with little spontaneous movement and poverty of bodily gesture have been frequently described in autistic individuals (23), and the failure to use gesture for communication purposes has been the subject of several clinical investigations (24,25). Initially, the absence of gestural usage was attributed to withdrawal or to a lack of intent to communicate. However, a deficit in body imitation skills that would preclude the learning of communicative gesture has been offered as an alternative hypothesis, which is supported by the observation that the learning and performance of complex coordinated motor tasks in high-functioning autistic children is difficult, thus suggesting a motor dyspraxia.

Recently, the use of sign language in relationship to motor functioning was investigated in a group of 14 low-functioning autistic children (26). It was determined that these children made formational errors primarily of hand-shape and movement and, to a lesser extent, in location. Eleven of the fourteen children were administered an apraxia test battery. Those showing the least evidence of apraxia demonstrated a relatively low rate of formational errors, while those showing the greatest difficulty with praxis produced relatively few signs and had the highest percentage of errors, particularly in movement. While there may be a variety of reasons why autistic children have trouble with communication, the authors suggested that deficits in motor functioning probably account for some of the difficulties these children experience when learning to sign.

In a study of 20 verbal and nonverbal autistic children, the verbal subjects were found to exhibit significantly better oroneuromotor function than those in the nonverbal group. Further, the verbal children demonstrated significantly greater abilities on the Pediatric Oral Motor Examination (POME) for eating behaviors, voluntary nonverbal oral abilities, and prespeech/speech tasks than the nonverbal children. Although both groups were delayed in oroneuromotor function, the nonverbal children showed the greatest degree of difficulty. Thus, both verbal and nonverbal autistic children were found to exhibit oroneuromotor deficits similar to those observed in other organically impaired, developmentally disabled children (27).

Nonmotor causes for limited gestural usage have also been postulated. In a recent study, Ohta (28) observed that autistic subjects consistently gave only partial responses to a gestural imitation test. Based on these results, the author suggested that the limited use of gesture in autism may not be motorically based but may result when the integration of a visual image is perceived as a series of parts rather than as a whole, resulting in partial or limited responses. Alternatively, Attwood et al (23) have suggested that autistic individuals do use some gesture to communicate, but only under specific circumstances. These authors noted that autistic children use nonverbal "instrumental gesture" in order to influence the behavior of others much as one would manipulate an object. For example, the autistic child might place his hand on a parent's hand in order to have that parent move or retrieve a desired object. In this study, in almost all cases, the "instrumental gestures" used spontaneously by autistic children seemed to serve the purpose of reducing or ending social contact. The autistic child never used "expressive gesture" that presupposed the communication of feelings, as in consoling someone who had been hurt. The authors concluded, therefore, that at least some of the limitation in gestural use by autistic children might be related to their impairment in understanding and communicating feeling states.

Several studies have shown an unusually high incidence of nonright-handers among autistic individuals (29–32). All studies to date seem to indicate that autistic children with mixed dominance generally function at a lower cognitive level than children with established hand dominance, while left-handers showed a trend toward superiority on cognitive assessment. It has been suggested that the poor performance of the children with mixed dominance implies bilateral central nervous system impairment. The relatively strong performance by the decidedly left-handed children remains unexplained.

Impairment of representational play with objects is a common characteristic of young autistic children and may, at least in part, be related to the automaticity of motor skills (33). Motor imitation tasks have been reported to be markedly delayed in a study of 6- to 10-year-old autistic subjects and were consistent with those observed in 2- to 3-year-old normal children (34). It has also been suggested that motor development in general may not proceed much beyond the 2- to 3-year level in many autistic individuals. Thus, although fine and gross motor skills in this disorder may be functional, many autistics often lack the coordination and dexterity that characterize normal motor maturation. In a study of 21 children with Asperger's syndrome and high functioning autism, Manjiviona and Prior (35) noted that almost half of their subjects were late in walking and most were described as awkward on fine motor tasks. These children demonstrated the most difficulty in controlling the force and direction of throwing a ball, suggestive of cerebellar dysfunction. Furthermore, half of the subjects had difficulty taking a slow, careful approach to tasks but instead tended to rush, seemingly unable to slow down. This pattern of motor control was most often observed during tasks requiring manual dexterity, such as cutting, and appeared to be similar to that associated with deficits in executive function (36).

As yet, it is difficult to fully explain the neurologic basis for the motor abnormalities and movement disorders observed in autism and their relationship to the morphologic features of the brain so far described in this disorder. None of the motoric impairments that have been reported would be considered essential to the diagnosis, and in some cases motor function has been said to be entirely normal. Although repetitive and stereotypic behaviors are perhaps the most common movement disorder associated with the autistic syndromes, these behaviors may also be seen in nonautistic and mentally retarded children and may be essentially absent in autistic individuals of normal intelligence. Dysfunction of the basal ganglia and regions of the medial frontal lobe cortex have been suggested as possible sites of abnormality based on postural and gait disturbances that have been noted (14). To date, however, no anatomic abnormalities have been found in these areas, or in the related nuclei of the thalamus, sensory association cortices, or vestibular system (37,38). The anterior cingulate gyrus has been found to be abnormal in some cases, but these findings have been inconsistent (39). Abnormalities of the brain in autism have been found in selected regions of the limbic system including the hippocampal complex, amygdala, mammillary body, and septal nuclei, and it is likely that the neuronal circuitry between these areas and the limbic and sensory association neocortical regions of the brain may affect not only cognitive and social function but motor development as well. Although abnormalities of the cerebellum and cerebellar circuits have been consistently observed microscopically and inconsistently described on imaging studies, the specific relationship of these findings to those in the limbic system and to the clinical features of autism remain unknown (40,41).

Animal studies have indicated that cerebellar and limbic abnormalities play an important role in the classic eye-blink conditioned response (motor learning) (42–44). The cerebellum has been determined to be essential for the learning of the conditioned eye-blink response (42,45) while the hippocampus appears to contribute to the reflex response by processing complex stimulus patterns (44). The classic eye-blink reflex has been similarly studied in a series of 11 autistic subjects, 7 to 22 years of age (46). Compared to controls, the autistic individuals learned the task at a more rapid rate.

At this time, motoric and movement abnormalities are being increasingly reported in autism and there appears to be a growing appreciation of the significant role that these impairments may be playing in the daily functioning of affected individuals. However, well-controlled, large population studies are lacking. With mounting evidence for an identifiable neuroanatomic substrate for the autistic syndromes including the presence of abnormalities of the cerebellum and cerebellar circuits, a closer look at motoric function in this disorder is warranted. We do not know, for example, whether motor development in autism follows a normal maturational sequence, nor do we know whether the changes in muscle tone, balance, coordination, dexterity, posture, and gait alter with increasing age. Although stereotypies, choreoathetosis, and dystonic posturing have been described, we do not know the spectrum or frequency of these movement disorders within the autistic syndromes nor their relationship, if any, to language, cognition, and social skills. Many questions remain and careful clinical longitudinal studies directed specifically toward the analysis of development as it relates to motor skills and movement patterns in autism are needed.

REFERENCES

1. Kanner L. Autistic disturbances of affective contact. Nerve Child 1943;2:217–250.
2. Diagnostic and Statistical Manual of Mental Disorders. 4th ed. Washington: American Psychiatric Association, 1994.
3. Bryson SE, Clark BS, Smith IM. First report of a Canadian epidemiological study of autistic syndromes. J Child Psychol Psychiatry 1988;29:433–445.
4. Tanoue Y, Oda S, Asano F, Kawashima K. Epidemiology of infantile autism in southern Ibaraki, Japan: differences in prevalence in birth cohorts. J Autism Dev Disord 1988;18:155–166.
5. Gilberg C, Steffenburg S, Schaumann H. Is autism more common now than ten years ago? Br J Psychiatry 1991;158:403–409.
6. DeMyer M, Hingtgen J, Jackson R. Infantile autism reviewed: a decade of research. Schizophr Bull 1981;7:388–451.
7. Wolf L, Goldberg B. Autistic children grow up: an eight to twenty-four year follow-up study. Can J Psychiatry 1986;31:550–556.
8. Sparrow SS, Rescorla LA, Provence S, et al. Follow-up of "atypical" children—a brief report. J Am Acad Child Adolesc Psychiatry 1986;25:181–185.
9. Wing L. The handicaps of autistic children—a comparative study. J Child Psychol Psychiatry 1969;10:1–40.
10. Wing L. Early childhood autism. Oxford: Pergamon, 1976.
11. Jones V, Prior M. Motor imitation abilities and neurological signs in autistic children. J Autism Dev Disord 1985;15:37–46.
12. Vilensky JA, Damasio AR, Maurer RG. Gait disturbances in patients with autistic behavior. Arch Neurol 1981;38:646–649.
13. Minshew NJ, Payton JB. New perspectives in autism, Part I: the clinical spectrum of autism. Curr Probl Pediatr 1988;18:563–610.
14. Maurer RG, Damasio AR. Childhood autism from the point of view of behavioral neurology. J Autism Dev Disord 1982;12:195–205.
15. Minderaa RB, Volkmar FR, Hansen CR, et al. Brief report: snout and visual rooting reflexes in infantile autism. J Autism Dev Disord 1985;15:409–416.

16. Schreibman L. Diagnostic features of autism. J Child Neurol 1988;3:SS7–64.
17. Troster H. Prevalence and functions of stereotyped behaviors in nonhandicapped children in residential care. J Abnorm Child Psychol 1994;22:79–97.
18. Herman BH, Hammock MK, Arthur-Smith A, et al. Naltrexone decreases self-injurious behavior. Ann Neurol 1987;22:550–552.
19. Kohen-Raz R, Volkmar FR, Cohen DJ. Postural control in children with autism. J Autism Dev Disord 1992;22:419–432.
20. Gepner B, Mestre D, Masson G, de Schonen S. Postural effects of motion vision in young autistic children. Cog Neurosci Neuropsychol 1995;6:1211–1214.
21. Kaplan M, Carmody DP, Gaydos A. Postural orientation modifications in autism in response to ambient lenses. Child Psychiatry Hum Dev 1996;27:81–91.
22. Hughes C. Brief report: planning problems in autism at the level of motor control. J Autism Dev Disord 1996;26:99–107.
23. Attwood A, Frith U, Hermelin B. The understanding and use of interpersonal gestures of autistic and Down's syndrome children. J Autism Dev Disord 1988;18:241–257.
24. Rutter M. The development of infantile autism. Psych Med 1974;4:147–163.
25. Bartak L, Rutter M, Cox A. A comparative study of infantile autism and specific developmental receptive language disorder. Br J Psychiatry 1975;126:127–145.
26. Seal BC, Bonvillian JD. Sign language and motor functioning in students with autistic disorder. J Autism Dev Disord 1997;27:437–466.
27. Amato J. Oroneuromotor, psycho-social, and symbolic functioning in verbal and nonverbal autistic children. Doctoral thesis. Columbia University, New York, 1991.
28. Ohta M. Cognitive disorders of infantile autism: a study employing the WISC, spatial relationship conceptualization, and gesture imitations. J Autism Dev Disord 1987;17:45–62.
29. Tsai LY. The relationship of handedness to the cognitive, language and visuo-spatial skills of autistic patients. Br J Psychiatry 1983;142:156–162.
30. Fein D, Waterhouse L, Lucci D, Synder D. Cognitive subtypes in developmentally disabled children: a pilot study. J Autism Dev Disord 1985;15:77–95.
31. Fein D, Waterhouse L, Lucci D, et al. Handedness and cognitive functions in pervasive developmental disorders. J Autism Dev Disord 1985;15:323–333.
32. Soper HV, Satz P, Orsini DL, et al. Handedness patterns in autism suggest subtypes. J Autism Dev Disord 1986;16:155–167.
33. Hammes JG, Langell T. Precursors of symbol formation and childhood autism. J Autism Dev Disord 1981;11:331–345.
34. Van Smeerdijk L. Childhood autism and the problem of imitation. Thesis. La Trobe University, Virginia, Australia.
35. Manjiviona J, Prior M. Comparison of Asperger's syndrome and high-functioning autism on a test of motor impairment. J Autism Dev Disord 1995;25:23–39.
36. Ozonoff S, Pennington BF, Rogers SJ. Executive function deficits in high functioning autistic individuals: relationship to theory of mind. J Child Psychol Psychiatry 1991;32:1081–1105.
37. Bauman ML, Kemper TL. Histoanatomic observations of the brain in early infantile autism. Neurology 1985;35:866–874.
38. Bauman ML, Kemper TL. Neuroanatomical observation of the brain in autism. In: Panksepp J, ed. Advances in biological psychiatry. Vol. I. 1995:1–26.
39. Bauman ML, Kemper TL. Limbic and cerebellar abnormalities—consistent findings in infantile autism. J Neuropath Exp Neurol 1988;17:369.
40. Courchesne E, Yeung-Courchesne R, Press GA, et al. Hypoplasia of cerebellar vermal lobules VI and VII in autism. N Engl J Med 1988;318:1349–1354.
41. Bauman ML, Kemper TL. Abnormal cerebellar circuitry in autism? Neurology 1989;39(suppl 1):186.
42. McCormick DA, Thompson RF. Cerebellum: essential involvement in the classical conditioned eyelid response. Science 1984;223:296–299.
43. Sears LL, Steinmetz JE. Acquisition of conditioned-related activity in the hippocampus is affected by lesions of the cerebellar interpositus nucleus. Behav Neurosci 1990;104:681–690.
44. Steinmetz JE, Lavond DG, Ivkovich D, et al. Disruption of classical eyelid conditioning after cerebellar lesions: damage to a memory trace system or a simple performance deficit? J Neurosci 1992;12:4403–4426.
45. Berthier NE, Moore JW. Activity of deep cerebellar nuclear cells during classical conditioning of nictitating membrane extension in rabbits. Exp Brain Res 1990;63:44–54.
46. Sears LL, Finn PR, Steinmetz JE. Abnormal classical eye-blink conditioning in autism. J Autism Dev Disord 1994;24:737–751.

Neuropathology of Autism

Margaret L. Bauman

More than 50 years have passed since Leo Kanner first described early infantile autism (1), a behavioral syndrome characterized by social isolation, disordered language, repetitive and stereotypic behavior, poor eye contact, an insistence on sameness, unusual islands of rote memory, and a normal physical appearance. For many years, autism was considered to be a psychodynamically determined disorder. Over the past 25 years, however, there has been mounting evidence for a neurologic basis for the syndrome and the strong belief that autism must have a definable neuroanatomic substrate.

Many regions of the brain have been hypothesized to be abnormal in autism. Early studies speculated that the thalamic nuclei (2), the basal ganglia (3), and the vestibular system (4) might be important in this disorder. With the advent of advanced medical technology, however, other areas of the brain have come under scrutiny. Positron emission tomography (PET) in autistic adults has shown reduced positive correlation patterns in frontal and parietal regions, as well as in the thalamus, caudate nucleus, lenticular nucleus, and insula, suggesting impairment of functional interaction between these regions (5). Using[31] P nuclear magnetic resonance spectroscopy, Minshew et al (6) have reported a decrease in phosphocreatine and adenosine triphosphate levels, a borderline decrease in phosphomonoesters, and increased phosphodiesters in the dorsal prefrontal cortex in high-functioning autistic adolescents and young adults. These findings suggest neuronal membrane alteration and altered energy metabolism in the frontal cortex. Further support for frontal lobe involvement has been provided by analysis of regional cerebral blood flow demonstrating frontal hypoperfusion in five autistic children, ages 3 to 4 years, which reverted to normal by the age of 6 to 7 years, a pattern that suggests delayed frontal maturation (7).

Other brain regions of interest have included structures of the posterior fossa and cerebellum where abnormalities of size have been reported with computerized tomographic (CT) and magnetic resonance imaging (MRI) techniques (8–11). However, these findings have been inconsistent (12). The medial temporal lobe has frequently been suggested as a potential site of abnormality in autism (13–16). Although early pneumoencephalographic findings seemed to support this notion (17), subsequent CT studies did not show definitive abnormalities (18–20). An MRI analysis of the cross-sectional size of the posterior hippocampus, measured in 33 autistic patients ages 5.9 to 42.2 years, failed to show any significant differences in size when compared with control subjects (21). More recently, an additional limbic system structure has been investigated in vivo. A PET study involving seven high-functioning autistic subjects found that the right anterior cingulate appeared to be significantly smaller and metabolically less active than that observed in normal subjects (22). The authors suggested that the abnormalities noted in this region of the cingulate might relate to the deficits in organization and executive function that have been observed in autism.

Despite interest in a possible underlying neuroanatomic substrate for this disorder, there have been relatively few morphologic investigations involving brain tissue obtained from autistic subjects. One of the first observations, reported in 1968, noted "slight thickening of the arterioles, slight connective tissue increase in the leptomeninges and some cell increase" in tissue obtained from a right frontal lobe biopsy (23). Some years later, Darby, in a review of 33 cases of childhood psychosis, suggested a possible relationship between limbic system lesions and the affective component of autism (24). However, no specific pathology was described. Subsequently, Williams et al (25) microscopically studied sections of hippocampus, parahippocampal gyrus, thalamus, hypothalamus, striatum, and midbrain tectum from four individuals with autistic behavior, looking primarily for cell loss and gliosis. No consistent abnormalities were noted. In the mid 1980s, Coleman et al (26) performed neuronal and glial cell counts in multiple cortical regions of an autistic brain and two age- and sex-matched controls and found no differences. These authors concluded that abnormalities during early stages of nervous system development and migration were unlikely in autism and that the probable pathologic process was more likely to occur later during the elaboration of neuronal processes and synapses. More recently, Guerin et al (27) reported their findings in the brain of a 16-year-old boy with severe mental retardation. Except for the presence of slight thickening of the meninges, mild ventricular dilatation, thinning of the corpus callosum, scattered perivascular lymphocyte infiltrates, and a few microglial nodules in the lower brainstem, no pathologic abnormalities were appreciated. The authors hypothesized that, given the lack of obvious findings on routine neuropathologic analysis, autism may be caused by excessive axonal elimination during brain development.

In the majority of studies performed to date, no obvious gross structural abnormalities of the brain have been observed at autopsy in association with autism (28). However, the presence of increased brain weight and brain volume have been reported in a significant number of cases in recent years. In an MRI study of posterior fossa structures, Piven et al (29) reported significantly increased mid-sagittal brain area in 15 high functioning autistic males. Similarly, Filipek et al (30) noted increased brain volume with MRI in 22 autistic individuals as compared with developmental language disordered subjects. These observations seem to be consistent with the report that the brains of three of four mentally handicapped autopsied autistic patients were found to be heavier than expected for age and sex (31). Further evidence of brain enlargement has been provided by an MRI study of 35 autistic subjects, ages 12 to 29 years, in which brain volume was found to be significantly enlarged in male but not female autistics as compared with controls (32). This volumetric increase appeared to predominantly involve the parietal, temporal, and occipital lobes. More recently, in this same series of autistic subjects, Piven et al (33) reported that the body and posterior subregions of the corpus callosum were significantly small relative to total brain size. The authors suggested that these findings may reflect abnormal connectivity of the cerebral cortex in autism or an increase in brain size that is unrelated to the size of the corpus callosum. In a series of 19 autopsied cases, Bauman and Kemper (34) reported that the brains of autistic subjects less than 12 years of age were heavier than expected for age and sex (35) by 100 to 200 g (p value 0.05), while those of subjects older than 18 years of age tended to weigh less than expected. However, in the older age group, the differences in weight and volume

as compared to normal subjects did not reach statistical significance. This observation, combined with patterns of microscopic abnormality that appear to differ with age, has led to the suggestion that the pathologic basis for autism may involve an ongoing process. At this time, the underlying mechanism responsible for these findings is not known nor is it clear how these observations may relate to the clinical features of autism. Macrocrania (head circumference greater than the ninety-seventh percentile) has been reported in approximately one-third of autistic children less than 16 years of age (36). Similar data is not available in adults. Further clinical and pathologic studies involving large numbers of subjects are needed to better understand the significance and nature of these findings.

Using the standardized technique of whole brain serial section (37), Bauman and Kemper have systematically studied the brains of nine well-documented autistic patients in comparison with identically processed age- and sex-matched controls (28). All brains studied showed no abnormalities of external brain structure or myelin. With the exception of the anterior cingulate gyrus, microscopic analysis of multiple cortical regions in all of the autistic cerebra demonstrated no abnormality of cortical lamination, neuronal size or number, or cellular migration, consistent with the findings of Coleman et al (26). In addition, a systematic survey of the basal ganglia, thalamus, hypothalamus, and basal forebrain failed to delineate any differences from the controls.

Microscopic abnormalities were noted in specific regions of forebrain and posterior fossa structures (28). Areas of the forebrain that were found to be involved were confined to the hippocampus, subiculum, entorhinal cortex, amygdala, anterior cingulate cortex, mammillary body, and septum, structures known to be related to each other by interconnecting circuits and that comprise a major portion of the limbic system of the brain. In comparison with controls, these areas of the autistic brains showed increased cell packing density (increased number of neurons per unit volume) and reduced nerve cell size bilaterally. Using the rapid Golgi technique, pyramidal neurons of areas CA1 and CA4 of the hippocampus were found to show reduced complexity and extent of dendritic arbors (38). In the amygdala, small cell size and increased cell packing density were most pronounced medially in the cortical, medial, and central nuclei, while the lateral nucleus appeared to be comparable to controls. The exception to this pattern was observed in the brain of a 12-year-old autistic boy with a history of significantly atypical behavior but normal intelligence (39). In this case, the findings of small cell size and increased cell packing density was less pronounced in the hippocampal complex when compared with that observed in more severely impaired subjects, but the entire amygdala was diffusely abnormal. This difference in severity and distribution of abnormality, when correlated with clinical features, may suggest that while all subjects showed limbic system findings, symptomatic manifestations among autistic individuals may vary according to the location and degree of underlying brain abnormality.

In the septum, reduced cell size and increased cell packing density were similarly noted in the medial septal nucleus (MSN) in all cases. However, the nucleus of the vertical limb of the diagonal band of Broca (NDB) showed unusually large, plentiful, but otherwise normal appearing neurons in all of the autistic subjects less than 12 years of age (28). In contrast, these same neurons were noted to be small and markedly reduced in number in all of the autistic patients older than 22 years of age.

Outside of the forebrain, abnormalities have also been noted in the cerebellum and cerebellar circuits in these same autistic brains. A variable reduction in the number of Purkinje cells and to a lesser extent granule cells was observed throughout the cerebellar hemispheres, predominantly in the posterolateral neocerebellar cortex and adjacent archicerebellar cortex, with sparing of the vermis (40–42). Similar to the findings noted in the NDB of the septum, the neuronal features of the globose, emboliform, and fastigial nuclei, located in the roof of the cerebellum, appear to differ with age. Small pale neurons that are reduced in number are seen in these nuclei of all of the autistic subjects older than 22 years. In all of the younger autistic brains, however, these same neurons as well as those of the dentate nucleus are enlarged in size and present in adequate numbers (28).

Areas of the principal inferior olive related to the abnormal cerebellar cortex failed to show evidence of the expected retrograde cell loss in the autistic brains. In subjects older than 22 years, the olivary neurons were present in adequate numbers but were abnormally small and pale. In all of the younger brains, these same cells were enlarged but were otherwise normal in appearance and number. In all of the autistic brains, the neurons of the inferior olivary nucleus tended to cluster at the periphery of the inferior convolutions, a pattern that has been reported in several disorders of prenatal origin associated with mental retardation (43,44).

Additional abnormalities have been described in the brainstem of autistic subjects and have included the presence of a widened fourth ventricle in one case (25) with corresponding thinning and elongation of the superior cerebellar peduncle. Imaging studies have yielded variable observations in regard to brainstem structure (29,45–47). Several autistic individuals with documented maternal thalidomide exposure between days 20 and 24 of gestation have been reported to have a variety of cranial nerve motor symptoms and ear malformations without evidence of other physical abnormalities (48). Based on these observations, Rodier et al (49) pathologically studied the brainstem of a 21-year-old autistic female. Although this patient had no history of intrauterine toxic exposure, abnormalities of the motor cranial nerves were found, including nearly complete absence of the facial nucleus and superior olive as well as shortening of the brainstem between the trapezoid body and

the inferior olive. These observations, along with experimental data from rats, suggest that injury occurring in the central nervous system (CNS) during or just after the closure of the neural tube could result in the selective loss of neurons derived from the basal plate of the rhombencephalon. If true, these findings might indicate that the etiologic factors (genetic and/or exogenous agents) for autism may occur very early in gestation at about the time of neural tube closure. The authors speculated that such an early injury might disturb the development of later-forming structures by altering the environment in which they develop or could directly disturb the anlage of those structures, resulting in abnormalities as development continues.

The major focus of the forebrain abnormalities so far observed in autism has been on the closely interrelated circuits of the hippocampus, subiculum, and entorhinal cortex and three areas directly related to them—the septum, mammillary body, and anterior cingulate gyrus. Both the hippocampal complex and the nuclei of the amygdala are related to the limbic neocortex, and both receive direct projections from the sensory association cortex. Further, the central and medial amygdalar nuclei provide a direct projection to the reticulate core of the basal forebrain and brainstem. Thus, the anatomic abnormalities in the forebrain of these autistic patients are in position to disrupt the circuitry, and consequently the function, of the hippocampal complex and amygdala as well as the limbic and sensory association neocortical areas and reticulate core of the brain to which they are related.

The behavioral significance of this circuitry has been demonstrated in experiments where lesions in these regions have produced decided effects on motivation, emotion, memory, and learning, many of which resemble behaviors seen in childhood autism. Purposeless hyperactivity, impaired social interaction, hyperexploratory behavior, and the inability to recognize or remember the significance of visually or manually examined objects have been observed following bilateral medial temporal lobe ablations in monkeys (50). Similar neurosurgical lesions in humans have resulted in these same behaviors (51). Further, hyperactivity, stereotypic motor behavior, and a disordered response to novel stimuli have followed bilateral removal of the hippocampus in animals (52,53). Bilateral surgical removal of the amygdala in monkeys has resulted in indiscriminate examination of objects, withdrawal from previously rewarding social interactions, loss of fear of normally aversive stimuli, and reduced ability to attach meaning to a specific situation based on past experience (54). Further support for the role of the amygdala and hippocampus in autism has been provided by Bachevalier and Merjanian (55) who, by bilaterally ablating these same structures in neonatal monkeys, created animals with striking autistic-like behavior.

Surgical lesions in monkeys, confined to the amygdala, have resulted in animals who exhibit a loss of fear to normally aversive stimuli, compulsive indiscriminate examination of objects, and withdrawal from formerly socially rewarding situations (54). These same animals have also shown a reduced ability to attach meaning to new environments based on past experience, resulting in poor adaptability to novel situations. Additional studies have indicated that bilateral ablations of the amygdala result in a severe impairment of cross-modal associative memory, suggesting that the amygdala may be important for the integration and generalization of information that is processed by multiple sensory systems in the brain, a frequently difficult task for autistic individuals (56).

In addition to behavior, the forebrain areas that have been noted to be abnormal in autism have been implicated in disturbances of memory and learning. Bilateral ablations of both the hippocampus and the amygdala have been connected with severe loss of recognition and associative visual memory in monkeys (57,58), which is more profound than that noted following the removal of either structure alone (57). Identical lesions have also resulted in marked impairment of tactile memory, suggesting that combined lesions of the amygdala and hippocampus result in a severe memory deficit that is at least bimodal and that is comparable to the global anterograde amnesia seen following medial temporal lobe surgery or pathology in humans (59). In 1991, however, Squire and Zola-Morgan reconsidered the hypothesized relationship of medial temporal lobe structures to memory (60). They noted that the severe memory loss, previously attributed to bilateral combined lesions of the hippocampus and amygdala, was the result of the inadvertent surgical damage to the cortical regions adjacent to the amygdala and not to the inclusion of the amygdala. Thus, the structures important to the medial temporal lobe memory system appear to include the hippocampal formation and related entorhinal, perirhinal, and parahippocampal cortices.

Two mechanisms for learning have been proposed. The first involves limbic structures that engage a feedback process with the cortex, linking different kinds of memories and experiences into "cognitive learning." The second system is believed to be independent of the limbic circuits and is related to stimulus–response repetition or "habit" learning. Mishkin and Appenzeller have suggested that the neural substrate for "habit" learning may include the striatum and neocortex of the cerebral hemispheres and have hypothesized that, in nonhuman primates, this substrate may be fully developed at birth. In contrast, the "cognitive system" may be more slow to mature (61). While the effect of an early disturbance to the limbic system structures is unknown, it is likely that curtailment of development and prenatally acquired lesions in these regions could disrupt or distort the acquisition and interpretation of information. Such a disturbance in information processing could potentially lead to the disordered cognition, language, and social interaction associated with autism. In contrast, the preservation of the habit memory system could account for the need for sameness, preoccupation with a narrow range of interests and

activities, and unusual memory for rote information observed in some autistic individuals. Studies have suggested that these two neural systems mature at different times in both human and nonhuman primates. The habit system appears to develop and become functional early in life, while the representational system develops later in childhood (62,63). Thus, it is possible that a developmentally abnormal neuronal circuitry involving the limbic system would have little impact on cognitive functioning during the first one to two years of life. With development, however, the effect of this disturbed circuitry may gradually become evident, leading to what appears to be a deterioration in social, language, and cognitive abilities, features frequently reported as part of the early history of childhood autism.

Areas of abnormality outside of the forebrain have been confined to the cerebellum and related inferior olive. The relationship of these lesions to those in the forebrain is unclear. In the neocerebellar cortex, bilateral symmetrical loss of Purkinje cells and granule cell neurons without evidence of significant gliosis has been observed in all brains studied to date. However, the degree to which the Purkinje cells are reduced in number is somewhat variable and appears to be unrelated to the severity of clinical symptoms, the presence or absence of seizures, or the use of medication. The absence of glial cell hyperplasia suggests that these lesions have been acquired early in development. In animal studies, Brodal (64) has noted a progressively decreasing glial response following cerebellar lesions at increasingly early ages. Moreover, the preservation of neurons in the principal inferior olive further supports the early origin of the cerebellar lesions. Retrograde loss of olivary neurons regularly occurs following cerebellar lesions in immature postnatal and adult animals (64) and in neonatal (65) and adult humans (66,67), presumably because of the close relationship of the olivary climbing fiber axons to the Purkinje cell dendrites (68). In the fetal monkey, it has been shown that prior to establishing their definitive relationship to the Purkinje cell dendrites, the olivary climbing fibers synapse in a transitory zone beneath the Purkinje cell layer of the cerebellar cortex called the "lamina dissecans" (69). Since in the human fetus this transient zone is no longer evident after 30 weeks' of gestation (70), it is likely that the cerebellar cortical lesions have their onset at or before this time. Further support for this interpretation has been provided by Goldman and Galkin (71). In an analogous situation, these investigators noted that, in the rhesus monkey, the expected retrograde cell loss of neurons in the medial dorsal nucleus of the thalamus failed to occur following prenatal lesions prior to, but not after, 106 days of gestation (71).

The relationship of the cerebellar lesions observed in the autistic brain to the clinical features of the disorder is unclear. In general, cerebellar dysfunction beginning early in life, including a congenital absence of the cerebellum, has been associated with few neurologic symptoms (65,72). Animal experiments have shown the existence of a direct pathway between the fastigial nucleus and the septal nuclei and the amygdala, and a reciprocal relationship with the hippocampal complex, suggesting that the cerebellum may play a role in the modulation of emotion and higher cortical function (73,74). Further, both animal and human studies have suggested a role for the cerebellum in the control of affective behavior (75) and functional psychiatric disorders (76). Experiments in rabbits have implicated the dentate and interpositus nuclei in learning and modulation of the classical conditioned reflex response (77) and similar findings have been reported in autistic children and adults (78). Thus, experimental studies suggest that the cerebellar lesions in adult animals may result in disturbances of emotion, behavior, and learning. The effect of similar lesions during development is as yet unknown.

It has been well established that the cerebellum is involved in the acquisition of some types of motor learning and in the regulation of motor coordination (79). It has also been suggested that the cerebellum may play a role in the control of motor and sensory timing (80). Accurate timing depends on the ability to predict when an event should occur and the establishment of synchrony between dynamic events. Research has suggested that the lateral cerebellar hemispheres and dentate nuclei play an important role in this function (81). Additional studies have indicated that the cerebellum may play a role in mental imagery, anticipatory planning (82), and in some aspects of language processing (83). The cerebellum has likewise been implicated in the control of attention, specifically the voluntary shift of selective attention between auditory and visual modalities, believed to be due to its relationship with the parietal association cortices through connections in the pons (84,85). More recently, studies in the cebus monkey have established that the dorsolateral prefrontal cortex, believed to be involved in "spatial working memory," is the target of output from the dentate nucleus of the cerebellum (86). This relationship to the prefrontal cortex suggests that the cerebellum is involved in the planning and timing of future behavior. In addition to these many functions, the cerebellum also appears to play a role in the regulation of the speed, consistency, and appropriateness of mental and cognitive processes, as well as the control and integration of motor and sensory information and activity (87).

The etiology of the abnormalities seen in the autistic brain is unknown. Four of the nine autistic subjects so far anatomically studied experienced seizures and received medication; the remaining patients did not. The neuroanatomic findings in all cases are similar, suggesting that neither seizure activity nor medication is a major factor. Further, the presence of preserved olivary neurons associated with significantly reduced numbers of cerebellar Purkinje cells, multiple areas of the forebrain showing increased cell packing density and reduced neuronal cell size, and an absence of gliosis are consistent with a curtailment of normal development. The preserved olivary neurons suggest that the process that caused these abnormalities occurred or began before birth.

Bauman and Kemper (88) have suggested that the presence of neuronal enlargement in the deep cerebellar and inferior olivary nuclei in all of the autistic subjects less than 12 years of age may indicate the presence of a retained fetal circuit between these two nuclear groups. It has been further postulated that this fetal circuit may be unable to sustain itself into adult life with resultant cell atrophy and loss in the older autistic brains. While this notion appears to support the concept of abnormal neuronal circuitry as the basis for the autistic syndrome, the validity of this hypothesis must be confirmed by future research.

More recently, Bailey et al (89) observed neuroanatomic abnormalities in the brains of six autistic subjects that were more widespread than previously reported. Four of the six brains were large for age and sex. Abnormalities were described in scattered cortical regions and in the brainstem, primarily in the inferior olive. Reduced numbers of Purkinje cells were observed in the cerebellar cortex, predominantly involving the hemispheres. Hippocampal findings were noted in only one case. The authors concluded that their findings did not support previous observations of localized neurodevelopmental abnormalities involving the limbic system and cerebellum in the autistic brain, and suggested that the involvement of the cerebral cortex may be important in this disorder.

Neuroanatomic abnormalities so far reported in autism have largely focused on the limbic system and cerebellar circuits—regions of the brain important to the processing of some types of complex information. These findings appear to be consistent with recent neuropsychologic studies reported in autistic subjects (90) in which the resulting data seem to support a multiple primary deficit model in which the deficit pattern within and across domains is reflective of the complexity of the information processing demands. Further, these studies support the concept that autism is a late information processing disorder with sparing of early information processing.

Given the absence of an animal model for research and the limited availability of autopsy material for neuroanatomic study, future expanded and more detailed neuroimaging techniques may offer improved opportunities for in vivo study of the brain. Much of the neuroimaging research to date has been devoted to measurements of area and volume in specific brain regions, most notably of the cerebellum. Although it was initially assumed that differences in the structural size of specific brain regions was a reflection of microscopic neuroanatomic abnormalities, it has become clear that imaging and histologic findings are not necessarily equivalent. In the cerebellum, for example, the histologic findings are the most marked in the posterior and lateral regions of the cerebellar hemispheres that have received little imaging attention. In contrast, the major MRI abnormality reported in the autistic brain has been hyoplasia of the vermis, a structure that has been found to be histologically normal. While there may be methodologic and technologic factors that have contributed to these inconsistent observations, it is also possible that at least some of the microscopic features in the autistic brain may be beyond detection by modern imaging techniques. In any case, there appears at this time to be a mismatch between the microscopic and imaging studies of the cerebellum and hippocampus in autism, and it is therefore prudent to interpret the results of imaging studies in this disorder with caution.

In summary, although abnormalities so far described in the autistic brain have shed little light on the pathogenesis of this disorder, the anatomic defects that have been described appear to have been acquired early in development and are located in areas of the brain that are critical to the development of normal behavioral, cognitive, and memory function. It is therefore possible that the neuronal circuitry of these affected regions, as well as that of the areas of the brain to which they are closely related, may be dysfunctional on a developmental basis, and that this disordered circuitry may be responsible, at least in part, for the clinical picture of autism.

REFERENCES

1. Kanner L. Autistic disturbances of affective contact. Nerve Child 1943;2:217–250.
2. Coleman M. Studies of the autistic syndromes. In: Katzman R, ed. Congenital and acquired cognitive disorders. New York: Raven, 1979:265–303.
3. Vilensky JA, Damasio AR, Maurer RG. Gait disturbances in patients with autistic behavior. Arch Neurol 1981;38:646–649.
4. Ornitz EM, Ritvo ER. Neurophysiologic mechanisms underlying perceptual inconsistency in autistic and schizophrenic children. Arch Gen Psychiatry 1986;19:22–27.
5. Horowitz B, Rumsey JM, Grady CL, Rapoport SI. The cerebral metabolic landscape in autism. Arch Neurol 1988;45:749–755.
6. Minshew NJ, Goldstein G, Dombrowski SM, et al. A preliminary 31P MRS study of autism: evidence for undersynthesis and increased degradation of brain membranes. Biol Psychiatry 1993;33:762–773.
7. Zilbovicius M, Garreau B, Samson Y, et al. Delayed maturation of the frontal cortex in childhood autism. Am J Psychiatry 1995;152:248–252.
8. Bauman ML, LeMay M, Bauman RA, Rosenberger PB. Computerized tomographic (CT) observations of the posterior fossa in early infantile autism. Neurology 1985;35(suppl 1):247.
9. Courchesne E, Yeung-Courchesne R, Press GA, et al. Hypoplasia of cerebellar vermal lobules VI and VII in autism. N Engl J Med 1988;318:1349–1354.
10. Courchesne E, Townsend J, Saitoh O. The brain in infantile autism. Neurology 1994;44:214–228.
11. Gaffney GR, Tsai LY, Kuperman S. Cerebellar structure in autism. Am J Dis Child 1987;141:1330–1332.
12. Filipek PA. Quantitative magnetic resonance imaging in autism: the cerebellar vermis. Current Opin Neurol 1995;8:134–138.
13. Boucher J, Warrington EK. Memory deficits in early infantile autism: some similarities to the amnestic syndrome. Br J Psychiatry 1975;67:73–87.
14. Delong GR. A neuropsychological interpretation of infantile autism. In: Rutter M, Schopler E, eds. Autism. New York: Plenum, 1978:207–218.
15. Damasio AR, Maurer RG. A neurological model for childhood autism. Arch Neurol 1978;35:777–786.
16. Maurer RG, Damasio AR. Childhood autism from the point of view of behavioral neurology. J Autism Dev Disord 1982;12:195–205.
17. Hauser SL, Delong GR, Rosman NP. Pneumographic findings in the infantile autism syndrome. Brain 1975;98:667–688.
18. Hier DB, LeMay M, Rosenberger PB. Autism and unfavorable left-right asymmetries of the brain. J Autism Dev Disord 1979;9:153–159.
19. Gillberg C, Svendsen P. Childhood psychosis and computed tomographic brain scan findings. J Autism Dev Disord 1983;13:19–32.
20. Creasey H, Rumsey JM, Schwartz, et al. Brain morphometry in autistic men as measured by volumetric computed tomography. Arch Neurol 1986;43:669–672.
21. Saitoh O, Courchesne E, Egaas MS, et al. Cross-sectional area of the posterior hippocampus in autistic patients with cerebellar and corpus callosum abnormalities. Neurology 1995;45:317–324.
22. Haznedar MM, Buchsbaum MS, Metzger M, et al. Anterior cingulate gyrus volume and glucose metabolism in autistic disorder. Am J Psychiatry 1997;154:1047–1050.
23. Aarkrog T. Organic factors in infantile psychosis and borderline psychosis. Retrospective study of 45 cases subjected to pneumoencephalography. Dan Med Bull 1968;15:283–288.
24. Darby JK. Neuropathologic aspects of psychosis in childhood. J Autism Child Schizoph 1976;6:339–352.
25. Williams RS, Hauser SL, Purpura DP, et al. Autism and mental retardation. Arch Neurol 1980;37:749–753.
26. Coleman PD, Romano J, Lapham L, Simon W. Cell counts in cerebral cortex of an autistic patient. J Autism Dev Disord 1985;15:245–255.
27. Guerin P, Lyon G, Barthelemy C, et al. Neuropathological study of a case of autistic syndrome with severe mental retardation. Dev Med Child Neurol 1996;38:203–211.
28. Bauman ML, Kemper TL. Neuroanatomical observations of the brain in autism. In: Panksepp J, ed. Advances in biological psychiatry. New York: JAI, 1995:1–26.
29. Piven J, Nehme E, Simon J, et al. Magnetic resonance imaging in autism: measurement of the cerebellum, pons and fourth ventricle. Biol Psychiatry 1992;31:491–504.
30. Filipek PA, Richelme C, Kennedy DN, et al. Morphometric analysis of the brain in developmental language disorders and autism. Ann Neurol 1992;32:475.
31. Bailey A, Luthert P, Bolton P, et al. Autism and megalencephaly. Lancet 1993;34:1225–1226.
32. Priven J, Arndt S, Bailey J, Andreasen N. Regional brain enlargement in autism: a magnetic resonance imaging study. J Am Acad Child Adolesc Psychiatry 1996;35:530–536.
33. Piven J, Bailey BS, Ranson BJ, Arndt S. An MRI Study of the corpus callosum in autism. Am J Psychiatry 1997;154:1051–1056.
34. Bauman ML, Kemper TL. Is autism a progressive process? Neurology 1997;48(suppl):285.
35. Dekaban A, Sadowsky D. Changes in brain weights during the span of human life: relation of brain weights to body heights and body weights. Ann Neurol 1978;4:345–356.
36. Woodhouse W, Bailey A, Rutter M, et al. Head circumference in autism and other pervasive developmental disorders. J Child Psychol Psychiatry 1996;37:665–671.
37. Yakovlev I. Whole brain serial histological sections. In: Tedeschi CG, ed. Neuropathology: methods and diagnosis. Boston: Little, Brown, 1970:371–378.
38. Raymond GV, Bauman ML, Kemper TL. Hippocampus in autism: a Golgi analysis. Acta Neuropath Scand 1996;91:117–119.
39. Bauman ML, Kemper TL. Limbic and cerebellar abnormalities are also present in an autistic child of normal intelligence. Neurology 1990;40(suppl 1):359.
40. Ritvo ER, Freeman BJ, Scheibel AB, et al. Lower Purkinje cell counts in the cerebella of four autistic subjects: initial findings of the UCLA-NSAC autopsy research report. Am J Psychiatry 1986;143:862–866.
41. Arin DM, Bauman ML, Kemper TL. The distribution of Purkinje cell loss in the cerebellum in autism. Neurology 1991;41(suppl 1):307.
42. Bauman ML, Kemper TL. Observations on the Purkinje cells in the cerebellar vermis in autism. J Neuropath Exp Neurol 1996;55:613.
43. Sumi SM. Brain malformation in the trisomy 18 syndrome. Brain 1980;93:821–830.
44. DeBassio WA, Kemper TL, Knoefel JE. Coffin-Siris syndrome: neuropathological findings. Arch Neurol 1985;42:350–353.
45. Gaffney GR, Kuperman S, Tsai LY, Minchin S. Morphological evidence for brain stem involvement in infantile autism. Biol Psychiatry 1988;24:578–586.
46. Hsu M, Yeung-Courchesne R, Courchesne E, Press GA. Absence of pontine abnormality in infantile autism. Arch Neurol 1991;48:1160–1163.
47. Hashimoto T, Tayama M, Murakawa K, et al. Development of the brainstem and cerebellum in autistic patients. J Autism Dev Disord 1995;25:1–18.
48. Stromland K, Nordin V, Miller M, et al. Autism in thalidomide embryopathy: a population study. Dev Med Child Neurol 1994;36:351–356.

49. Rodier PM, Ingram JL, Tisdale B, et al. Embryological origin for autism: developmental anomalies of the cranial nerve motor nuclei. J Comp Neurol 1996;370:247–261.
50. Kluver H, Bucy P. Preliminary analysis of functions of the temporal lobes in monkeys. Arch Neurol Psychiatry 1939;42:979–1000.
51. Terzian H, Delle-Ore G. Syndrome of Kluver and Bucy reproduced in man by bilateral removal of the temporal lobes. Neurology 1955;3:373–380.
52. Kimble DP. The effects of bilateral hippocampal lesions in rats. J Comp Physiol Psychol 1963;56:273–283.
53. Roberts WN, Dember WN, Brodwick M. Alteration and exploration in rats with hippocampal lesions. J Comp Psychiatry 1962;55:695–700.
54. Mishkin M, Aggleton JP. Multiple functional contributors of the amygdala in the monkey from the amygdaloid complex. In: Ben-Ari Y, ed. INSERM symposium, no. 20. Amsterdam: Elsevier North Holland Medical, 1981:409–419.
55. Bachevalier J, Merjanian PM. The contribution of medial temporal lobe structures in infantile autism: a neurobehavioral study in primates. In: Bauman ML, Kemper TL, eds. The neurobiology of autism. Baltimore: Johns Hopkins University, 1994:146–169.
56. Murray EA, Mishkin M. Amygdaloidectomy impairs crossmodal association in monkeys. Science 1985;228:604–606.
57. Mishkin M. Memory in monkeys is severely impaired by combined but not by separate removal of amygdala and hippocampus. Nature 1978;273:297–298.
58. Mahut H, Zola-Morgan S, Moss M. Hippocampal resections impair associative learning and recognition memory in the monkey. J Neurosci 1982;2:1214–1229.
59. Murray E, Mishkin M. Severe tactual memory deficits in monkeys after combined removal of the amygdala and hippocampus. Brain Res 1983;270:340–344.
60. Squire LR, Zola-Morgan S. The medial temporal lobe memory system. Science 1991;253:1380–1386.
61. Mishkin M, Appenzeller T. The anatomy of memory. Sci Am 1987;256:80–89.
62. Bachevalier J, Mishkin M. Effects of neonatal lesions of the amygdaloid complex or hippocampal formation on the development of visual recognition memory. Soc Neurosci Abstr 1991;17:338.
63. Overman W, Bachevalier J, Turner M, et al. Object recognition versus object discrimination: comparison between human infants and infant monkeys. Behav Neurosci 1992;106:15–29.
64. Brodal A. Modification of Gudden method for study of cerebral localization. Arch Neurol Psychiatry 1940;43:46–58.
65. Norman RM. Cerebellar atrophy associated with etat marbre of the basal ganglia. J Neurol Psychiatry 1940;3:311–318.
66. Holmes G, Stewart TG. On the connection of the inferior olives with the cerebellum in man. Brain 1908;31:125–137.
67. Greenfield JG. The spino-cerebellar degenerations. Springfield, IL: Charles C Thomas, 1954.
68. Eccles JC, Ito M, Szentagothai J. The cerebellum as a neuronal machine. New York: Springer, 1967.
69. Rakic P. Neuron-glia relationship during granule cell migration in developing cerebellar cortex. A golgi and electron microscopic study in macacus rhesus. J Comp Neurol 1971;141:283–312.
70. Rakic P, Sidman RL. Histogenesis of cortical layers in human cerebellum particularly the lamina dissecans. J Comp Neurol 1970;139:473–500.
71. Goldman PS, Galkin TW. Prenatal removal of frontal association cortex in the fetal rhesus monkey; anatomic and functional consequence in postnatal life. Brain Res 1978;152:451–485.
72. Blackwood W, Corsellis JAN. Greenfield's neuropathology. Chicago: Year Book Medical, 1976.
73. Heath RG, Harper JW. Ascending projections of the cerebellar fastigial nucleus to the hippocampus, amygdala and other temporal lobe sites; evoked potential, and histological studies in monkeys and cats. Exp Neurol 1974;45:268–287.
74. Heath RG, Dempsey CW, Fontana CJ, Myers WA. Cerebellar stimulation: effects on septal region, hippocampus and amygdala of cats and rats. Biol Psychiatry 1978;113:501–529.
75. Berman AJ, Berman D, Prescott JW. The effect of cerebellar lesions on emotional behavior in the rhesus monkey. In: Cooper IS, Riklan M, Snider RS, eds. The cerebellum epilepsy and behavior. New York: Plenum, 1974:277–284.
76. Heath RG, Franklin DE, Shraberg D. Gross pathology of cerebellum in patients diagnosed and treated as functional psychiatric disorders. J Nerv Ment Dis 1979;167:585–592.
77. McCormick DA, Thompson RF. Cerebellum: essential involvement in the classically conditioned eyelid response. Science 1984;223:296–299.
78. Sears L, Finn PR, Steinmetz JE. Abnormal classical eye-blink conditioning in autism. J Autism Dev Disord 1994;24:737–751.
79. Bloedel JR. Functional heterogeneity with structural homogeneity: how does the cerebellum operate? Behav Brain Sci 1992;15:666–678.
80. Keele SW, Ivry R. Does the cerebellum provide a common computation for diverse tasks? A timing hypothesis. Ann NY Acad Sci 1990;608:179–207.
81. Holmes G. The cerebellum in man. Brain 1939;62:1–30.
82. Leiner HC, Leiner AL, Dow RS. Cerebrocerebellar learning loops in apes and humans. Ital J Neurol Sci 1987;8:425–436.
83. Peterson SF, Fox PT, Posner MI, et al. Positron emission tomographic studies in processing of single words. J Cog Neurosci 1989;1:153–170.
84. Courchesne E, Akshoomoff NA, Townsend J. Recent advances in autism. In: Naruse H, Ornitz EM, eds. Neurobiology of infantile autism. Amsterdam: Excerpta Medica, 1992:111–128.
85. Akshoomoff NA, Courchesne E. A new role for the cerebellum in cognitive operations. Behav Neurosci 1992;106:731–738.
86. Middleton FA, Strick PL. Anatomical evidence for cerebellar and basal ganglia involvement in higher cognitive function. Science 1994;266:458–461.
87. Schmahmann JD. An emerging concept. The cerebellar contribution to higher function. Arch Neurol 1991;48:1178–1187.
88. Bauman ML, Kemper TL. Abnormal cerebellar circuitry in autism? Neurology 1989;39(suppl 1):186.
89. Bailey A, Luther T, Dean A, et al. A clinicopathological study of autism. Brain 1998;121:889–905.
90. Minshew NJ, Goldstein G, Siegel DJ. Neuropsychologic functioning in autism: profile of a complex information processing disorder. J Int Neuropsychol Soc 1997;3:303–316.

Rett Syndrome: A Clinical and Neurobiologic Overview

Leon S. Dure IV   Alan K. Percy

INTRODUCTION

In 1966, Andreas Rett (1) described a progressive disorder that occurred only in females and was characterized clinically by onset in infancy with autistic-like behavior, mental and growth retardation, gait ataxia/apraxia, loss of purposeful use of the hands with subsequent appearance of stereotyped hand movements ("hand washing"), seizures, scoliosis, intermittent hyperventilation/breath holding, and dementia (2–7). Since that time, this phenotype has been observed in more than 4,000 girls throughout the world, including some 2,000 or more in the United States and several hundred in Europe and Japan (8). Its suggested prevalence is 1 in 10,000 to 15,000 girls, about twice the age-specific prevalence of phenylketonuria (6,7,9). Involvement of males has been suggested, although rarely. Thus, Rett syndrome (RS) is a disorder combining mental retardation with associated abnormalities of movement, communication, and growth.

Despite convincing evidence that a genetic mechanism is involved, its gene locus is unknown. An X-linked disorder restricted to females has been postulated, but detailed examination of the X chromosome has failed to identify a candidate (8,10). Alternative genetic mechanisms have been proposed, but again no evidence is available. No relationship to fragile-X syndrome has been found (11). To date, no cytogenetic, biochemical, or molecular marker for the disorder is available, and its pathogenesis and etiology are unknown (6–8,12).

DIAGNOSIS

The diagnosis of typical or classic RS is based on well-established criteria most recently summarized by an international working group (13). These criteria (Table 89.1) are, and, however criteria (Table 89.1)

form the nucleus from which the recognition of variant forms of RS is now emerging.

The awareness of girls with variant expressions of RS features (15) has led to the systematic analysis of such children by Hagberg and Skjeldal (16). These authors have now elaborated a set of primary and secondary criteria (Table 89.2) for application in those girls or women who meet some, but not all, of the necessary criteria described in Table 89.1. In order to qualify as having variant RS, the child must demonstrate at least 3 of 6 main criteria and at least 5 of 11 supportive criteria (consideration is being given to extending this to 6 of 11). The emergence of this ever-expanding variant group underscores the importance of careful diagnosis and rigid classification of classic and variant forms of RS prior to entry into clinical studies or comparison trials.

Natural History

RS is now regarded as a developmental disorder based on its clinical profile and recent careful neuroanatomic analyses. While progressive neuromotor findings are typical, progressive dementia is not. Indeed, social and communication skills may actually improve after the initial period of regression. RS follows a clinical pattern that generally allows the identification of four more or less distinct clinical stages, as summarized in Table 89.3 (17,18). In spite of the generalized growth and mental retardation, many patients may survive into middle adulthood and beyond (2–5,7,8,17, 19).

Specific clinical issues to be considered in the natural history of RS include longevity, the stereotypies, irritability, sleep disturbances, seizures, breathing pattern irregularities, growth and feeding difficulties, ambulation, and scoliosis.

Table 89.1 Rett Syndrome Diagnostic Criteria

Necessary Criteria

1. Female gender is no longer included, as the possibility of undiagnosed male cases cannot be excluded (14).
2. Normal prenatal and perinatal period with psychomotor development that appears to be normal during the first (6–22) months of life.
3. Normal head circumference at birth, with subsequent deceleration of head growth between age 3 months and 4 years.
4. Early behavioral, social, and psychomotor regression with severely impaired expressive and receptive language and social interaction.
5. Loss of all but the most basic purposeful hand skills, with the appearance of stereotypic hand movements, e.g., handwringing, squeezing, clapping, mouthing, and "washing"/rubbing automatisms occurring between ages 1 and 4 years.
6. Appearance of gait apraxia and gait ataxia/apraxia at the same age.
7. Diagnosis tentative until 2 to 5 years of age.

Exclusion Criteria

1. Evidence of intrauterine or perinatally acquired brain damage.
2. Organomegaly or other signs of storage disease.
3. Congenital microcephaly or evidence of intrauterine growth retardation.
4. Retinopathy or optic atrophy.
5. Identifiable metabolic or other progressive neurologic disorder.
6. Acquired neurologic disorder due to infections or head trauma.

Source: Modified from Hagberg B. Rett syndrome: clinical peculiarities and biological mysteries. Acta Paediatr 1995;84:971–976 and Percy A. Rett syndrome: the evolving picture of a disorder of brain development. Dev Brain Dysfunct 1996;9:180–186.

Table 89.2 Diagnostic Criteria for Variant Rett Syndrome

Main Criteria

Loss of finger skills
Loss of babble/speech
Hand stereotypies
Loss of communication skills
Deceleration of rate of head growth
RS disease profile

Supportive Criteria

Breathing irregularities: hyperventilation and/or breath holding
Bloating/air swallowing
Teeth grinding (bruxism)
Gait dyspraxia
Scoliosis/kyphosis
Lower limb neurologic dysfunction
Feet disturbances: cold/bluish; *growth-impaired/dystrophic*
RS temporal pattern of EEG development from serial recordings
Unprovoked laughing/screaming spells
Pain indifference
RS eye pointing/eye communication

Source: Reproduced by permission from Hagberg BA, Skjeldal OH. Rett variants: a suggested model for inclusion criteria. Pediatr Neurol 1994;11:5–11.

Table 89.3 Clinical Stages in Classic Rett Syndrome

I. **Early-Onset Stagnation Stage (age 6–18 months)**
 Developmental arrest/stagnation
 Changed communication/interaction and eye contact
 Nonspecific personality changes
 Diminished play interest
 Hand waving: nonspecific/episodic
 Decelerated rate of head growth

II. **Rapid Regression Stage (age 1–4 years)**
 Psychomotor deterioration/regression
 Autistic manifestations
 Characteristic stereotypies
 Loss of hand skill/hand use
 Clumsy ambulation/apraxia/ataxia
 Irregular breathing: hyperventilation/breath holding
 Seizures

III. **Pseudostationary Stage (age 4–10 years)**
 Stabilization of communication problems
 Mental retardation, but emotional contact
 Slowly progressive gross motor dysfunction of variable degree
 Gait apraxia prominent
 Jerky truncal ataxia
 Seizures common

IV. **Late Motor Deterioration Stage (after age 5 years to adolescence or death)**
 Decreasing mobility: wheelchair bound
 Quadriparesis
 Increasing lower motor neuron signs
 Progressive scoliosis
 Progressive trophic foot disturbances
 "Improving" emotional contact
 Fewer seizures
 Growth retardation, but normal puberty
 Staring, unfathomable gaze

Source: Modified from Hagberg B, Witt-Engerstrom I. Rett syndrome: a suggested staging system for describing impairment profile with increasing age towards adolescence. Am J Med Genet Suppl 1986;1:47–59.

Longevity

Girls or women with Rett syndrome may have shortened life expectancy, and sudden, unexpected deaths have been described both in young children and in adults (6). Nevertheless, survival data from the Baylor Rett Center indicate only a modest number of excess deaths prior to age 20 to 25. Thereafter, the rate of death exceeds the normal population (70% surviving to age 35 versus >98% normally), but is far less than that in a multiply handicapped, institutionalized population (27%) (12,20).

The Stereotypies

The prominent clinical hallmark of Rett syndrome is the presence of hand stereotypies (6). Focus on these stereotypies should not ignore the presence of common but much less prominent stereotypic movements of the head and face as well as the feet. However, those involving the hands are the most dramatic and obvious. Each child develops her own specific movements, which may evolve over time both in character and in intensity. Typically, the movements involve hand washing or handwringing, but may also feature knitting-type activities. Other girls may have stereotypies with their hands held apart at the side or front of the chest, around the face or head, or with the arms extended. Various combinations of the movements may also be noted. Finger rubbing or flicking movements are common, and overlapping one finger on another may be seen. Some girls keep their hands in or near the mouth, and although they may not actually bite themselves, they will develop calluses or frank tissue breakdown from the frequent irritation and the fact that the hands are often wet.

The stereotypies are present during wakefulness, but not during sleep. They tend to be reduced markedly or absent during acute illnesses such as common respiratory infections and are often exaggerated or activated by new or stressful situations. They tend to be most florid during the latter portion of stage II and through stage III during childhood and adolescence, but do diminish in intensity and frequency with increasing age and particularly with entry into stage IV. During the initial phase of regression (stage II), hand stereotypies may be quite subtle and elusive.

Irritability

During the regression phase, extreme irritability with unconsolable crying for no apparent reason is the most difficult problem for parents (6). These periods may last for minutes or hours and, for many parents, may seem interminable. Overall, irritability may be prominent for many months or even more than one year, causing significant stress within the family. In later years, particularly during adolescence, similar inconsolable crying may be noted. During this period, attention should be directed toward the gastrointestinal and genitourinary tracts to obviate more chronic problems. Rupture in the gastrointestinal tract has been noted and may have resulted from chronic constipation and fecal impaction.

Sleep Disturbance

Abnormal sleep patterns are common in RS, with frequent interruptions of sleep and alterations in the normal sleep distribution pattern (6). In particular, rapid eye movement sleep tends to be reduced significantly, in some girls even being undetectable (21). Parents often note that girls with RS are awake in the night, simply lying quietly. At other times, they may hear inappropriate laughing or screaming.

Seizures

Initial reports suggested that seizures occur in a majority of girls with RS. More recent reports indicate that seizures are much less commonly encountered (12), perhaps as low as 25% to 30% of cases. Seizures may be generalized or complex partial. Many of the events considered to represent clinical seizures by parents and medical staff are in fact Rett behaviors. Long-term video-electroencephalogram (EEG) recordings have demonstrated clearly that these behaviors have no electrical correlate. Kerr (22) described so-called vacant spells in which behavioral arrest was not accompanied by any significant changes in the EEG. Conversely, electrographic seizures have been seen in association with subtle clinical events that were not recognized as such. Seizures tend to be present first in early childhood and be most frequent during school age, with a subsequent diminution through adolescence. Correspondingly, the EEG is typically normal during the first 2 years and follows a similar ontogeny (see below) (23–26). In a small percentage, seizures may occur early, beginning in infancy, and may have the character of infantile spasms or myoclonic epilepsy. These girls may, therefore, have obviously abnormal early development, making it difficult to define a specific pattern of regression prior to appearance of the more typical features of RS.

Breathing Irregularities

Abnormal breathing patterns during wakefulness, but not during sleep, are present in the majority of girls with RS (6). As in the hand stereotypies, these disturbances accelerate during stage II, are most active in stage III, decline in stage IV, and tend to increase with stress or strange surroundings and decrease with acute illness. They consist of hyperventilation, breath holding, or some combination of both. Breathing irregularities may be preceded or accompanied by forced expulsion of air (puffing) or saliva. Breath holding may last for many seconds and occasionally exceed one minute. PaO_2 levels may drop substantially during these periods. Substantial air swallowing may occur, with prominent bloating. The bloating disappears during sleep.

Growth and Feeding

Pervasive growth failure is another hallmark of RS (6). Acquired deceleration in the rate of head growth was first described by Rett himself. More recently, similar failure in weight and linear growth has been noted (27). Further, hand and foot growth also decelerates from expected normal patterns (28). Feeding is often a problem in terms of the efficiency of chewing and swallowing mechanisms and, consequently, results in inadequate caloric intake (29). Assistance with feeding by a parent or other care provider is essential. In some instances, gastrostomy feeding is necessary to provide adequate intake. As noted above, constipation can be extremely difficult and may require constant attention to preserve normal bowel function.

Ambulation

The large majority (80%) of girls with RS learn to walk, even if delayed in some instances (6). The minority that do not walk tend to be those with significant hypotonia. Ambulation may be lost or depressed during the regression phase and regained in some. About 60% (of the 80%), tend to retain ambulation through adolescence into adulthood.

Scoliosis

Scoliosis may be a major clinical challenge in girls with RS (6,30–34). In particular, the very hypotonic girls lacking ambulation commonly develop a progressive scoliosis of very high degree, leading to compromise of cardiorespiratory function. Scoliosis also occurs in ambulatory RS as well, and clinicians must be vigilant and enlist the aid of orthopedists, by at least age 5, to participate in the care. Bracing may be tried, but does not appear to be effective in preventing progression. Ultimately, surgery may be required. Although RS may suggest increased surgical morbidity, current experience indicates no special postoperative management problems beyond those typically noted with this major procedure.

Other Features

Indifference to pain is commonly noted by parents (6). No information exists indicating dysfunction of specific pain mechanisms. It appears rather that central appreciation of pain or the subsequent response to it is delayed and either does not occur or is not recognized by others. The feet and, to a lesser extent, the hands may be cold and bluish. This appears to be a function of excess sympathetic tone inasmuch as unilateral sympathectomy resulting from scoliosis surgery reverses the finding in the ipsilateral foot (6). Further, the foot also appears to increase its growth rate. Dystonic postures are common and may involve both the trunk and extremities (35). With time, these may become fixed deformities. On average, girls with RS enter puberty at the expected time. Gynecologic consultation may be indicated to manage this aspect. Pregnancy has occurred in RS.

Differential Diagnosis

In the absence of a specific biologic marker, the diagnosis of RS must be made after the careful consideration and exclusion of several other disorders. This is most critical during the rapid regression phase occurring in stage II between the age of 1 to 3 years. As described in Table 89.4, these disorders share features in common with RS, including rapid regression of development with loss of previously acquired skills, marked irritability and inconsolable crying or screaming, and, in some cases, acquired deceleration in the rate of head growth. Particular consideration should be given to infantile autism, the infantile form of neuronal ceroid lipofuscinosis (INCL), Angelman syndrome, and the rare chromosomal deletion syndrome (18,36). However, it is now clear that girls with RS do not fulfill diagnostic criteria for autism (37,38), and what was once the most common initial misdiagnosis for RS is now mentioned less often.

Table 89.4   Differential Diagnosis in Rett Syndrome

Disorder	Differential Diagnostic Modality
INCL	CT, EEG, EM of skin, conjunctiva, lymphocytes
Angelman syndrome	Genetic studies
Infantile autism	Clinical evaluation
Glutaric aciduria	Urine organic acids
Salla disease	Urine sialic acid
Encephalitis	CSF, EEG
Toxic encephalopathies	Exposure history
Epileptic encephalopathy (early RS variant)	Not available
Ataxic cerebral palsy	Clinical evaluation

EM = electron microscopy.

Source: Modified from Hagberg BA. Rett syndrome: clinical peculiarities, diagnostic approach, and possible cause. Pediatr Neurol 1989;5:75–83.

In the Nordic countries, INCL is, perhaps, the most pertinent and difficult differential diagnosis, occurring with an incidence of 1 in 13,000 in those of Finnish origin (36). INCL, now mapped to chromosome 1, has a 25% recurrence risk, making precise diagnosis critical for appropriate family counseling. Recurrence in RS is less than 1%. RS-like features were described recently in a child with a 3p− deletion (39). Thus, it is important to utilize appropriate diagnostic methodologies, including clinical findings, chemical and biochemical modalities, high-resolution chromosomal analysis, EEG, and tissue biopsy to differentiate these conditions from RS.

During late stages of RS, consideration should also be given to the neurocutaneous syndromes as well as the toxic and postinfectious encephalopathies and the static encephalopathies.

Laboratory Data

Routine laboratory studies to evaluate metabolic or chromosomal abnormalities, including blood, urine, and cerebrospinal fluid (CSF) studies, are unremarkable (3–8). The increased levels of ammonia described initially (1,2) were not confirmed by later studies. The electroencephalogram is always abnormal during the course of RS, although no specific EEG pattern has been identified (2–8,21,23,25,26,40). The EEG is often normal up to age 2 years, after which the typical initial abnormalities usually include slow (3–5/s), poorly organized waking background. Often, scattered or bilateral synchronous spikes or sharp waves may be found. Spike-wave complexes are rare in the beginning but spike-wave and slow spike-wave activity may dominate the record, particularly during sleep, for many years. With increasing age, the EEG abnormalities tend to decline, and ill-defined low-voltage records (26,39) and rare epileptiform abnormalities are more typical in adulthood (21). Polygraphic data show abnormal respiratory patterns during wakefulness, and abnormal sleep and EEG characteristics, with almost continuous spike-and-slow wave activity or epileptiform abnormalities during sleep (21,26).

RS patients have decreased percentages of rapid eye movement sleep and, during wakefulness, a pattern of increased respiratory rate and effort. The occurrence of disorganized breathing and compensatory hyperventilation during wakefulness with regular continuous breathing during sleep may suggest an impaired voluntary/behavioral respiratory control system (6,21).

Cranial computed tomography (CT) and magnetic resonance imaging (MRI) show normal findings in young RS patients, but mild to moderate generalized brain atrophy in advanced stages of illness (4–7). Clinical and neurophysiologic studies in early stages of RS give no indications of peripheral nerve involvement (2,4–6,41,42), while lower motor dysfunction with marked limb atrophy is well known to occur with increasing age (2,17,41). Signs of denervation have been reported in advanced stages of illness (2,4,41,42), while studies of somatosensory potentials suggest spinal denervation (motor neuron degeneration) (43). Myopathic signs have not been reported so far (41).

BASIC SCIENCE

Neurobiology of Rett Syndrome

Despite a plethora of clinical and laboratory investigations, answers to many of the key questions regarding the pathogenesis of RS are still unknown. Once thought to be a neurodegenerative disease with a primary metabolic abnormality (2), RS is now hypothesized to be the result of maturational arrest of the brain and is considered a developmental disorder primarily affecting the central nervous system. The following discussion will attempt to review the pertinent findings and to provide a synthesis of the current thinking about the processes operant in RS.

The cornerstone observations describing RS are by necessity pathologic. A number of autopsies have been performed on both early- and late-stage RS patients. Grossly, RS brains are normal, although small. Microscopically, there appears to be an abnormally increased packing density of neurons within RS brains, and the neurons themselves are reduced in size. These findings have bolstered the hypothesis that RS is a disorder of maturational arrest (44). If such an arrest plays a role in RS pathogenesis, microcephaly could be explained by the failure to undergo normal synaptic development and neuropil formation (45). In one of the first large series of RS brain autopsies (46), the findings included microcephaly with some evidence of cortical atrophy, hypopigmentation of the substantia nigra (Figs 89.1, 89.2) with concomitant decrease in tyrosine hydroxylase immunoreactivity (Fig 89.3), and ultrastructural evidence of abnormal neuronal morphology in the frontal cortex and caudate nucleus (Figs 89.4, 89.5). Later studies, albeit in only a few cases, have also determined nigral abnormalities (47), but it is unclear whether these changes are primary (neurodegeneration) or secondary (atrophy).

Ultrastructural analyses have been relatively more informative in RS, demonstrating abnormal dendritic branching in layer 3 and 5 pyramidal neurons in the frontal, motor, and subicular cortex, using a Golgi impregnation method (48). Belichenko (49,50), using vital dye injections, has also shown abnormal dendritic architecture in various regions of RS brain and, using a confocal imaging technique, has demonstrated regions of dendrites that are spineless, possibly suggesting a loss or absence of cortical synapses. In studies of dendritic and synaptic protein markers, an abnormality in the expression of microtubule-associated proteins (MAP) has been noted in the RS cortex (51). More extensive analysis of dendritic markers has shown an increase of MAP-2 in subcortical white matter, again with a decrease in the cortex, and a relative increase of the MAP-5 isoform in RS (51). All of these findings are supportive of an abnormality of synaptogenesis in RS, and perhaps of a maturational arrest. Despite these findings, however, it will be important in the future to delineate these changes further in RS cases and controls, particularly with respect to maturational aspects of cortical morphology.

In part due to the pathologic findings and in part to clinical observations, Nomura and colleagues proposed that a maturational defect in RS could be rooted in a disorder involving the biogenic amines dopamine (DA), norepinephrine (NE), and serotonin (5-HT) (52). Synthesized in a relatively small region within the brainstem or midbrain, each of these compounds functions as a neurotransmitter with widespread projections throughout the neuraxis. Subsequent investigations revealed a decrease in metabolites for NE, DA, and 5-HT in cerebrospinal fluid in RS (53,54). In postmortem brain, similar findings were described in RS in the substantia nigra, but not the cortex or putamen (55). However, other studies have failed to show any changes in CSF biogenic amine concentrations in RS (56,57), perhaps related to differences in the assay conditions or the choice of controls.

In postmortem studies of various neurotransmitter systems, indications of subtle disorders of cholinergic, dopaminergic, and glutamatergic receptors are reported. Choline acetyltransferase (ChAT) activity has been shown to be decreased in enzymatic assays (58,59). More recently, acetylcholine transport, as measured by vesamicol binding, has been shown to be decreased in RS tissue (60). Studies of dopamine markers have revealed a decrease in D_2 receptors, with relative preservation of D_1 receptors, in RS caudate (61). Finally, although previous analyses of glutamate receptor binding in homogenates were felt to demonstrate no changes when compared with controls (58), more recent studies using quantitative in vitro autoradiography indicate a selective decrease in α-amino-3-hydroxyl-5-methyl-4-

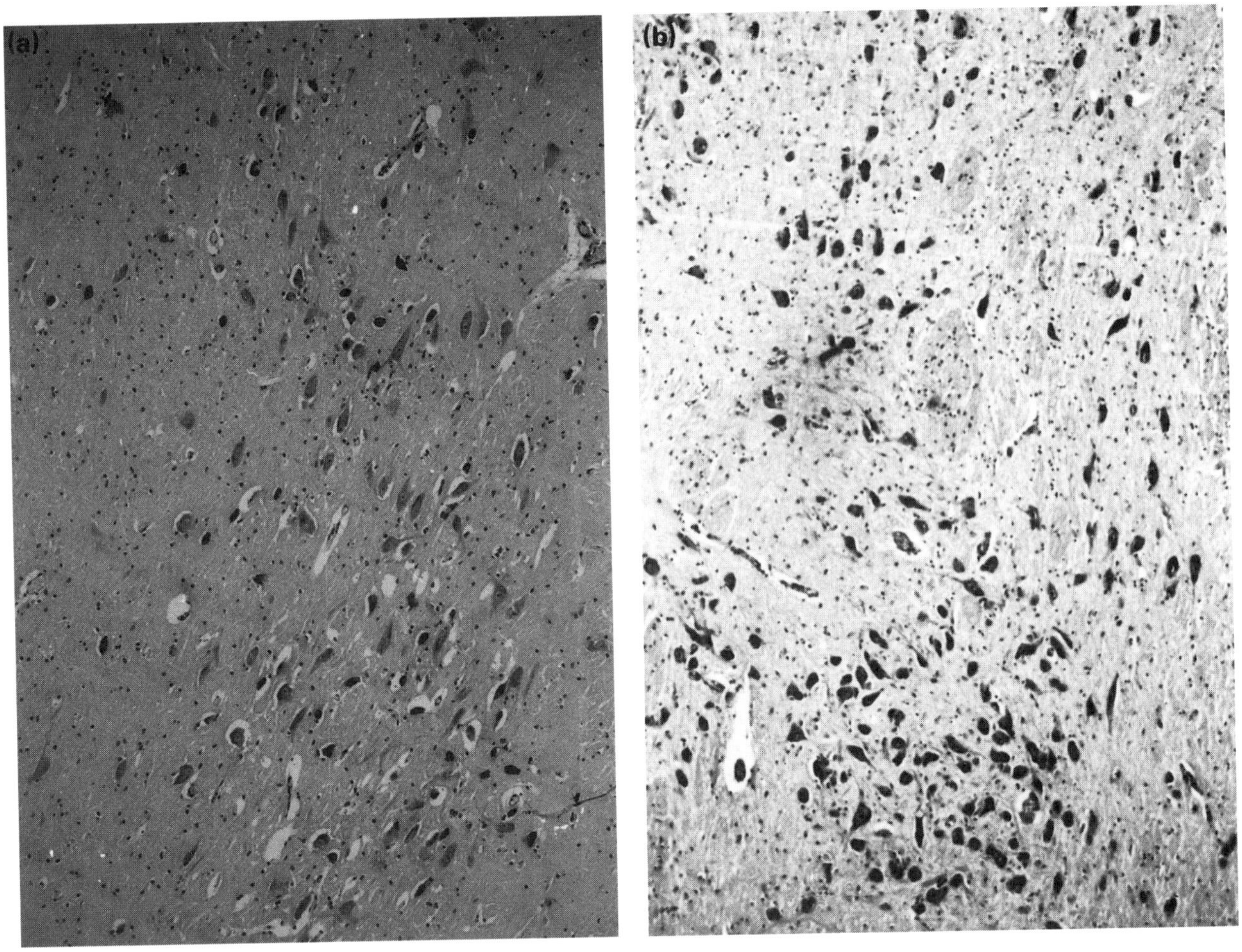

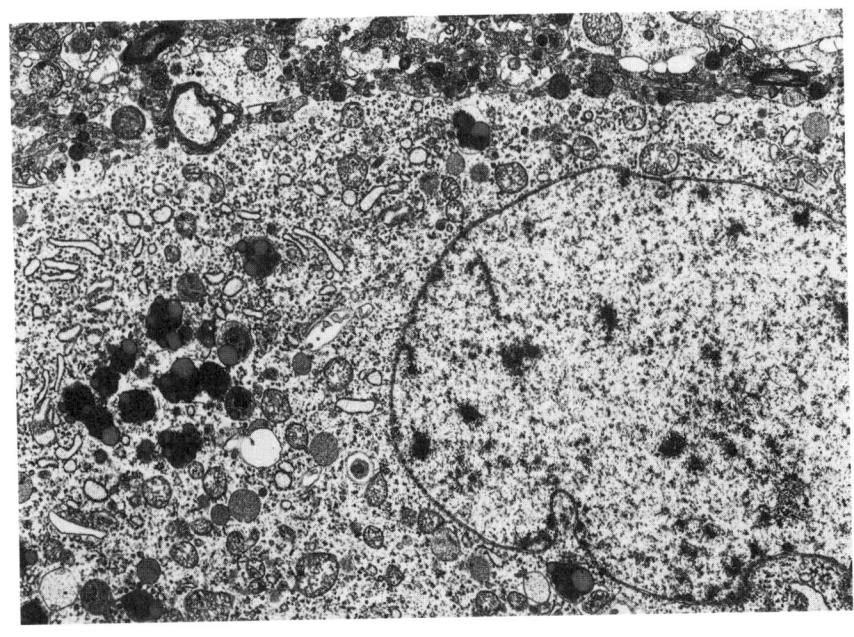

FIGURE 89.1 *(a) Substantia nigra in a 15-year-old girl with RS showing few pigmented neurons; (b) substantia nigra of 15-year-old control (Nissl, ×100).*

FIGURE 89.2 *Nigral cell of 11-year-old RS patient with regular cytoplasmic organelles but few neuromelanin granules showing normal triphasic substructure (×4500).*

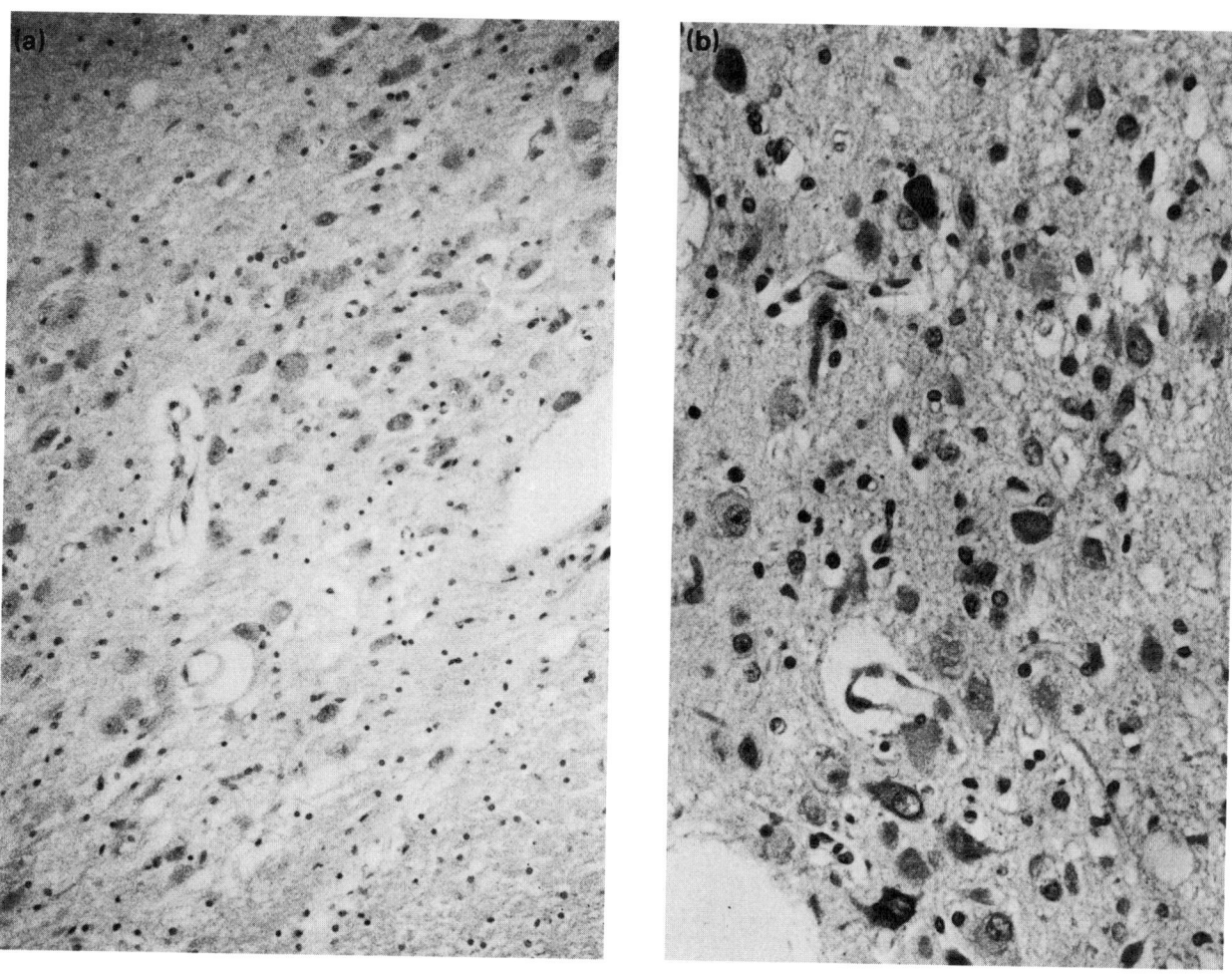

FIGURE 89.3 *Tyrosine hydroxylase immunoreactivity in subthalamic nucleus. (a) 17-year-old RS patient with negative reaction (PAP ×200). (b) 17-year-old control showing some strongly immunoreactive neurons (PAP method ×250).*

isoxazole-propionate (AMPA)-sensitive quisqualate receptors (62).

Despite the contradicting studies of urine and CSF biogenic amine metabolites, a wealth of clinical data suggest a role for biogenic amines in the pathophysiology of RS (4,63,64). Definitive studies of biogenic amine maturation, distribution, and function in RS remain to be performed.

Consonant with the findings of decreased brain weight and microcephaly, in vivo studies using quantitative MRI have demonstrated similar changes in brain. When compared with age- and gender-matched controls, cerebral volume is reduced in all brain areas in RS, typically secondary to changes in gray matter (65). Furthermore, these changes are most profound in the frontal cortex, caudate, and subicular cortex, as seen in pathologic studies. Interestingly, one study addressing cerebellar volume in RS found an age-related decrease in the cerebellum that was progressive, perhaps contributing to the evolving motor abnormalities seen in late-stage RS (66).

Other imaging modalities have been performed in RS patients to better delineate functional brain anatomy. Single photon emission computed tomography (SPECT), which has been used to analyze patterns of cerebral blood flow, demonstrates a diminution in frontal and temporoparietal regions, a pattern likened to that seen in the immature nervous system (67). Analysis of brain metabolites has been performed in RS using magnetic resonance spectroscopy. Although failing to demonstrate any changes in energy-related compounds (68), other studies have revealed a progressive decrease in *N*-acetyl-aspartate, which may indicate a secondary degenerative process causing a loss of gray matter (69). Clearly, further investigations will be necessary to more definitively characterize any metabolic changes in RS.

Proton emission tomography (PET) has come into use in RS to study receptor populations in vivo (70–72). Although used only in a few patients, the studies would seem to indicate a mild decrease in D_2 receptor populations,

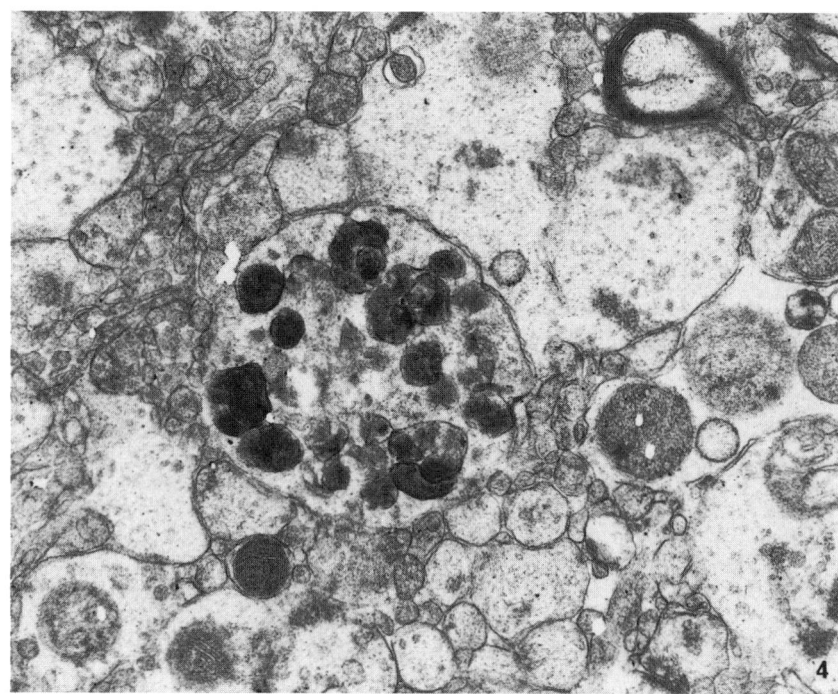

FIGURE 89.4   *Isolated abnormal neurite packed with granular bodies and mitochondria in the caudate nucleus of an 11-year-old RS patient (×18,000).*

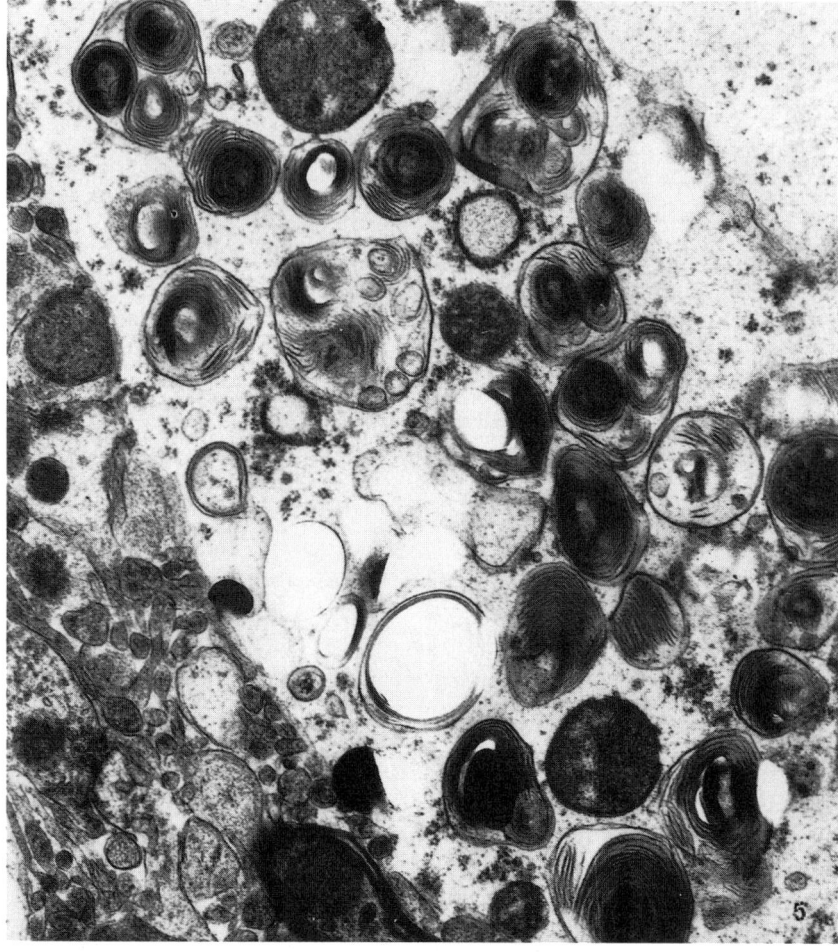

FIGURE 89.5   *Large mitochondria and dense or multilamellated bodies in degenerating axon of the caudate nucleus of an 11-year-old RS patient (×18,000).*

which is consistent with postmortem neurochemical data. Furthermore, if corrections for small brain size are incorporated, the loss of D_2 binding is even more striking and may point to a definitive pathologic marker in RS.

Finally, a number of other studies in RS have been performed, the significance of which is still under discussion. Following the clinical observation that RS patients demonstrate an apparent insensitivity of pain (73), beta-endorphins were measured in CSF. In numerous studies, the levels of beta-endorphins were decreased (74,75), but more extensive comparison with controls and other disease states demonstrated that this finding was not unique to RS (76). To examine the possibility of an excitotoxic process in RS, CSF glutamate has been measured in RS and been found to be elevated (77,78). However, no unifying hypothesis has emerged to take this into account, especially since no chronic neurodegenerative process appears to be operant in RS. Recently, low levels of nerve growth factor (NGF) have been reported in CSF (79). This finding is of some import, as it may represent corroboration for the hypothesis of a maturational arrest producing the pathologic changes seen in RS. To date, nevertheless, alterations in brain NGF have not been demonstrated, either at the cellular or molecular level.

In conclusion, RS is well studied but still poorly understood. Limitations to laboratory investigations of the neurobiology of this disease include some of its distinctive features: lack of a biologic marker identifying potential cases, a prolonged life span, and no clear genetic marker. Fortunately, the tools now available to neuroscientists will, in all likelihood, prove sufficient to provide an understanding of this disease, and continued investigations of RS will be successful in deriving an understanding of the pathogenesis of this disease.

MANAGEMENT

As the pathogenesis and etiology of RS are unknown, no definitive treatment specifically addressing the underlying defect(s) is presently available. Seizure management is necessary in many instances, but care must be directed to establishing and defining the seizure type and to being certain that the clinical behaviors are truly electrocortical seizures. Carbamazepine is usually effective, although alternative antiepileptic strategies may be required. Pharmacologic interventions for the movement disorder aspects of RS have been unrewarding (6). Vigilance must be employed regarding orthopedic problems. Surgery may be indicated in some.

The purpose of medical, occupational, physical, and music therapies in the treatment of these female patients showing severe mental, behavioral, and progressive physical handicaps and special communication problems is to maintain and redevelop functions and contacts with other family members and friends. This will require strong efforts by physicians, therapists, and parents (5,6,19,80). Attention to these habilitative aspects will minimize long-term problems.

CONCLUDING REMARKS

RS is an increasingly recognized neurodevelopmental disorder of females, commencing in infancy and characterized clinically by autistic-like behavior, stereotyped movements, acquired deceleration of rate of head growth, gait apraxia/ataxia, seizures, generalized growth and mental retardation, and later-onset dystonic rigidity. It is possibly related to a fundamental failure in neuronal maturation and interruption of normal synaptogenesis. Whereas the clinical diagnosis and staging of this condition are well established (5–8,13,14), laboratory studies are nonspecific. Despite extensive clinical, genetic, and laboratory studies, the gene locus, pathogenesis, and etiology of RS are unknown. The pathology of RS supports the concept of an arrest of normal development, the causative mechanisms of which remain poorly understood. The factors responsible for the severe aberrations of growth of both brain and body have not been identified. The molecular mechanisms underlying the movement disorders and related neuromediator dysfunctions in RS await further elucidation. Application of sophisticated techniques is needed for better elucidation of the genetic and molecular bases of this puzzling condition.

REFERENCES

1. Rett VA. Uber ein eigenartiges hirnatrophisches Syndrom bei Hyperammonamie im Kindesalter. Wein Med Wochenschr 1966;37:723–726.
2. Rett A. Cerebral atrophy associated with hyperammonemia. In: Vinken P, Bruyn G, eds. Handbook of clinical neurology. vol. 29. Amsterdam: Elsevier, 1977:305–329.
3. Hagberg B, Aicardi J, Dias K, Ramos O. A progressive syndrome of autism, dementia, ataxia, and loss of purposeful hand use in girls: Rett's syndrome: report of 35 cases. Ann Neurol 1983;14:471–479.
4. Nomura Y, Segawa M, Hasegawa M. Rett syndrome—clinical studies and pathophysiological consideration. Brain Dev 1984;6:475–486.
5. Opitz JM. The Rett syndrome. Am J Med Genet 1986;1:1–404.
6. Hagberg B. Rett syndrome—clinical and biological aspects. London: MacKeith, 1993:1–120.
7. Hagberg B. Rett syndrome: clinical peculiarities and biological mysteries. Acta Paediatr 1995;84:971–976.
8. Percy A. Rett syndrome: the evolving picture of a disorder of brain development. Dev Brain Dysfunct 1996;9:180–186.
9. Kozinetz CA, Skender ML, MacNaughton N, et al. Epidemiology of Rett syndrome: a population-based registry. Pediatrics 1993;91:445–450.
10. Ellison KA, Fill CP, Terwilliger J, et al. Examination of X chromosome markers in Rett syndrome: exclusion mapping with a novel variation on multilocus linkage analysis. Am J Hum Genet 1992;50:278–287.
11. Moore JW, Tuck-Muller CM, Murphy M, et al. Chromosome studies in 10 patients with the Rett syndrome. Am J Med Genet Suppl 1986;1:345–354.
12. Glaze DG. Commentary: the challenge of Rett syndrome. Neuropediatrics 1995;26:78–80.
13. Hagberg B, Goutieres F, Hanefeld F, et al. Rett syndrome: criteria for inclusion and exclusion. Brain Dev 1985;7:372–373.
14. Trevathan E, The Rett Syndrome Diagnostic Criteria Working Group. Diagnostic criteria for Rett syndrome. Am J Med Genet 1988;23:425–428.
15. Hagberg B. Clinical delineation of Rett syndrome variants. Neuropediatrics 1995;26:62.
16. Hagberg BA, Skjeldal OH. Rett variants: a suggested model for inclusion criteria. Pediatr Neurol 1994;11:5–11.
17. Hagberg B, Witt-Engerstrom I. Rett syndrome: a suggested staging system for describing impairment profile with increasing age towards adolescence. Am J Med Genet Suppl 1986;1:47–59.
18. Witt-Engerstrom I. Rett syndrome: the late infantile regression period—a retrospective analysis of 91 cases. Acta Paediatr 1992;81:167–172.
19. Witt-Engerstrom I. Rett syndrome in Sweden. Neurodevelopment, disability, pathophysiology. Acta Paediatr Scand 1990;(suppl):369.

20. Eyman RK, Grossman HJ, Chaney RH, Call TL. The life expectancy of profoundly handicapped people with mental retardation. N Engl J Med 1990;323:584–589.

21. Glaze DF Jr, Zoghbi H, Percy A. Rett's syndrome: characterization of respiratory patterns and sleep. Ann Neurol 1987;21:377–382.

22. Kerr A, Southall D, Amos P, et al. Correlation of electroencephalogram, respiration and movement in the Rett syndrome. Brain Dev 1990;12:61–68.

23. Glaze DF, Zoghbi H, Percy A. Rett's syndrome: correlation of electroencephalographic characteristics with clinical staging. Arch Neurol 1987;44:1053–1056.

24. Badr GG, Witt-Engerstrom I, Hagberg B. Brain stem and spinal cord impairment in Rett syndrome: somatosensory and auditory evoked responses investigations. Brain Dev 1987;9:517–522.

25. Hagne I, Witt-Engerstrom I, Hagberg B. EEG development in Rett syndrome. A study of 30 cases. Electroencephalogr Clin Neurophysiol 1989;72:1–6.

26. Ishizaki A, Inoue Y, Sasaki H, Fukuyama Y. Longitudinal observation of electroencephalograms in the Rett syndrome. Brain Dev 1989;11:407–412.

27. Schultz RJ, Glaze DG, Motil KJ, et al. The pattern of growth failure in Rett syndrome. Am J Dis Child 1993;147:633–637.

28. Schultz R, Glaze DG, Dunn K, et al. Hand and foot growth failure in Rett syndrome, Proceedings of World Congress on Rett Syndrome, Goteborg, Sweden, 1996.

29. Motil KJ, Schultz R, Brown B, et al. Altered energy balance may account for growth failure in Rett syndrome. J Child Neurol 1994;9:315–319.

30. Keret D, Bassett GS, Bunnell WP, Marks HG. Scoliosis in Rett syndrome. J Pediatr Orthop 1988;8:138–142.

31. Loder RT, Lee CL, Richards BS. Orthopedic aspects of Rett syndrome: a multicenter review. J Pediatr Orthop 1989;9:557–562.

32. Bassett GS, Tolo VT. The incidence and natural history of scoliosis in Rett syndrome. Dev Med Child Neurol 1990;32:963–966.

33. Guidera KJ, Borrelli J Jr, Raney E, et al. Orthopaedic manifestations of Rett syndrome. J Pediatr Orthop 1991;11:204–208.

34. Lidstrom J, Stokland E, Hagberg B. Scoliosis in Rett syndrome. Clinical and biological aspects. Spine 1994;19:1632–1635.

35. FitzGerald PM, Jankovic J, Percy AK. Rett syndrome and associated movement disorders. Mov Disord 1990;5:195–202.

36. Hagberg BA. Rett Syndrome: clinical peculiarities, diagnostic approach, and possible cause. Pediatr Neurol 1989;5:75–83.

37. Olsson B, Rett A. Autism and Rett syndrome: behavioural investigations and differential diagnosis. Dev Med Child Neurol 1987;29:429–441.

38. Percy AK, Zoghbi HY, Lewis KR, Jankovic J. Rett syndrome: qualitative and quantitative differentiation from autism. J Child Neurol 1988;3(suppl):S65–S67.

39. Wahlström J, et al. Congenital Rett syndrome phenotype—deletion short arm chromosome 3. Proceedings of World Congress on Rett Syndrome, Göteborg, Sweden, 1996. Eur Child Adolesc Psychiatr 1997;6:95.

40. Badr GG, Witt-Engerstrom I, Hagberg B. Neurophysiological findings in the Rett syndrome. I. EMG, conduction velocity, EEG and somatosensory-evoked potential studies. Brain Dev 1989;11:102–109.

41. Haas RH, Love S. Peripheral nerve findings in Rett syndrome. J Child Neurol 1988;3(suppl):S25–S30.

42. Oldfors A, Hagberg B, Nordgren H, et al. Rett syndrome: spinal cord neuropathology. Pediatr Neurol 1988;4:172–174.

43. Badr GG, Witt-Engerstrom I, Hagberg B. Neurophysiological findings in the Rett syndrome. II. Visual and auditory brainstem, middle and late evoked responses. Brain Dev 1989;11:110–114.

44. Bauman ML, Kemper TL, Arin DM. Microscopic observations of the brain in Rett syndrome. Neuropediatrics 1995;26:105–108.

45. Armstrong DD. The neuropathology of Rett syndrome—overview 1994. Neuropediatrics 1995;26:100–104.

46. Jellinger K, Armstrong D, Zoghbi HY, Percy AK. Neuropathology of Rett syndrome. Acta Neuropathol 1988;76:142–158.

47. Kitt C, Troncoso J, Price D, et al. Pathological changes in substantia nigra and basal forebrain neurons in Rett syndrome. Ann Neurol 1990;28:416–417.

48. Armstrong DD. The neuropathology of the Rett syndrome. Brain Dev 1992;14(suppl):S89–S98.

49. Belichenko PV, Oldfors A, Hagberg B, Dahlstrom A. Rett syndrome: 3-D confocal microscopy of cortical pyramidal dendrites and afferents. Neuroreport 1994;5:1509–1513.

50. Belichenko PV, Dahlstrom A. Studies on the 3-dimensional architecture of dendritic spines and varicosities in human cortex by confocal laser scanning microscopy and Lucifer yellow microinjections. J Neurosci Meth 1995;57:55–61.

51. Kaufmann WE, Naidu S, Budden S. Abnormal expression of microtubule-associated protein 2 (MAP-2) in neocortex in Rett syndrome. Neuropediatrics 1995;26:109–113.

52. Nomura Y, Segawa M, Higurashi M. Rett syndrome—an early catecholamine and indolamine deficient disorder? Brain Dev 1985;7:334–341.

53. Zoghbi HY, Percy AK, Glaze DG, et al. Reduction of biogenic amine levels in the Rett syndrome. N Engl J Med 1985;313:921–924.

54. Zoghbi HY, Milstien S, Butler IJ, et al. Cerebrospinal fluid biogenic amines and biopterin in Rett syndrome. Ann Neurol 1989;25:56–60.

55. Lekman A, Witt-Engerstrom I, Gottfries J, et al. Rett syndrome: biogenic amines and metabolites in postmortem brain. Pediatr Neurol 1989;5:357–362.

56. Lekman A, Witt-Engerstrom I, Holmberg B, et al. CSF and urine biogenic amine metabolites in Rett syndrome. Clin Genet 1990;37:173–178.

57. Perry TL, Dunn HG, Ho HH, Crichton JU. Cerebrospinal fluid values for monoamine metabolites, gamma-aminobutyric acid, and other amino compounds in Rett syndrome. J Pediatr 1988;112:234–238.

58. Wenk GL, Naidu S, Casanova MF, et al. Altered neurochemical markers in Rett's syndrome. Neurology 1991;41:1753–1756.

59. Wenk GL, O'Leary M, Nemeroff CB, et al. Neurochemical alterations in Rett syndrome. Dev Brain Res 1993;74:67–72.

60. Wenk G, Mobley S. Choline acetyltransferase activity and vesamicol binding in Rett syndrome and in rats with nucleus basalis lesions. Neuroscience 1996;73:79–84.

61. Wenk GL. Alterations in dopaminergic function in Rett syndrome. Neuropediatrics 1995;26:123–125.

62. Blue M, Hohmann C, Wallace S, et al. Excitatory and inhibitory neurotransmitter receptor expression is altered in Rett syndrome and in a mouse model for Rett syndrome. Soc Neurosci Abstracts 1996;22:1168.

63. Nomura Y, Honda K, Segawa M. Pathophysiology of Rett syndrome. Brain Dev 1987;9:506–513.

64. Nomura Y, Segawa M. Motor symptoms of the Rett syndrome: abnormal muscle tone, posture, locomotion and stereotyped movement. Brain Dev 1992;14(suppl):S21–S28.

65. Reiss AL, Faruque F, Naidu S, et al. Neuroanatomy of Rett syndrome: a volumetric imaging study. Ann Neurol 1993;34:227–234.

66. Murakami JW, Courchesne E, Haas RH, et al. Cerebellar and cerebral abnormalities in Rett syndrome: a quantitative MR analysis. AJR Am J Roentgenol 1992;159:177–183.

67. Nielsen JB, Lou HC, Andresen J. Biochemical and clinical effects of tyrosine and tryptophan in the Rett syndrome. Brain Dev 1990;12:143–147.

68. Nielsen JB, Toft PB, Reske-Nielsen E, et al. Cerebral magnetic resonance spectroscopy in Rett syndrome. Failure to detect mitochondrial disorder. Brain Dev 1993;15:107–112.

69. Hanefeld F, Christen HJ, Holzbach U, et al. Cerebral proton magnetic resonance spectroscopy in Rett syndrome. Neuropediatrics 1995;26:126–127.

70. Harris JC, Wong DF, Wagner HN Jr, et al. Positron emission tomographic study of D2 dopamine receptor binding and CSF biogenic amine metabolites in Rett syndrome. Am J Med Genet Suppl 1986;1:201–210.

71. Naidu S, Wong DF, Kitt C, et al. Positron emission tomography in the Rett syndrome: clinical, biochemical and pathological correlates. Brain Dev 1992;14(suppl):S75–S79.

72. Wagner HN Jr. Rett syndrome: positron emission tomography (PET) studies. Am J Med Genet Suppl 1986;1:211–224.

73. Brase DA, Myer EC, Dewey WL. Possible hyperendorphinergic pathophysiology of the Rett syndrome. Life Sci 1989;45:359–366.

74. Facchinetti F, Zappella M, Nalin A, et al. Plasma endorphins in Rett syndrome: preliminary data. Am J Med Genet Suppl 1986;1:331–338.

75. Myer EC, Tripathi HL, Brase DA, Dewey WL. Elevated CSF beta-endorphin immunoreactivity in Rett's syndrome: report of 158 cases and comparison with leukemic children. Neurology 1992;42:357–360.

76. Gillberg C, Terenius L, Hagberg B, et al. CSF beta-endorphins in childhood neuropsychiatric disorders. Brain Dev 1990;12:88–92.

77. Hamberger A, Gillberg C, Palm A, Hagberg B. Elevated CSF glutamate in Rett syndrome. Neuropediatrics 1992;23:212–213.

78. Lappalainen R, Riikonen R. High levels of cerebrospinal fluid glutamate in Rett syndrome. Pediatr Neurol 1996;15:213–216.

79. Lappalainen R, Lindholm D, Riikonen R. Low levels of nerve growth factor in cerebrospinal fluid of children with Rett syndrome. J Child Neurol 1996;11:296–300.

80. Moeschler JB, Charman CE, Berg SZ, Graham JM Jr. Rett syndrome: natural history and management. Pediatrics 1988;82:1–10.

Motor Disorders in Persons with Mental Retardation or Developmental Disabilities

Norberto Alvarez

DEFINITION, EPIDEMIOLOGY, AND ETIOLOGY

Mental retardation refers to those conditions in which there is a significant limitation in intellectual skills, whereas the term developmental disability is used when the individual cannot perform activities and roles as expected in a certain social environment. Frequently, mental retardation and developmental disabilities are present in the same person.

The American Academy on Mental Retardation defines four categories of risk factors that might be responsible for these conditions: biomedical, social, behavioral, and educational (1). To limit the scope of the definition in this chapter, we will limit the concept to conditions in which the brain injury is the consequence of prenatal, perinatal, or postnatal factors that occur in early life. In this context, the brain lesion will be considered static and not the consequence of progressive neurologic disorders. This is not to say that the clinical picture presented is static, since the motor signs change with the maturation of the brain; moreover, in many cases there is a delayed onset of movement disorders in persons with static brain lesions (2).

The spectrum of developmental disabilities varies from those cases with global cognitive deficits (e.g., severe mental retardation) to those individuals with disabilities limited to a particular area, such as seen in cases of learning disabilities. As a general term it includes other conditions that interfere with development, such as muscle disorders, epilepsy, or sensory impairments such as blindness and deafness.

The etiology of mental retardation is unknown in 24% to 40% of individuals with IQ below 50, and in as many as 45% to 62% of those individuals with IQ between 50 and 70 (3). In a small group of children, defined clinical disorders, mostly congenital or metabolic, can be identified (4,5).

Motor disorders of various kinds are commonly seen in persons with developmental disabilities, usually in association with other deficits (Table 90.1). Attempts to estimate the number of persons with developmental disabilities and motor disorders have several methodologic difficulties. The Education for All Handicapped Children Act has a broad definition, and 10% of the nation's children fit the criteria (6). However, this criteria includes children with disabilities such as epilepsy, learning disabilities, and emotional and other behavioral disorders that are not necessarily associated with motor disorders. For Kiernan and Bruininks (7), for example, 1% is a reasonable number for the prevalence of developmental disabilities for all ages in the general population; a similar figure (0.77%) was reported by Baird and Sadovnick (8). Data from the Metropolitan Atlanta Developmental Disabilities Study found that the prevalence of mental retardation among 10-year-old children was 1.2%. There were 0.84% of children with mild mental retardation (IQ 50 to 70), and 0.36% with severe mental retardation (IQ less than 50). The prevalence was higher in black children than in whites, and boys outnumbered girls (9).

The number of adults with developmental disabilities and movement disorders is not known. The United Cerebral Palsy Association estimates the number of adults in the United States with cerebral palsy, one of the most common associations of motor disorders and developmental disabilities, to be approximately 400,000.

In an outpatient neurology clinic set in an institution for adults with mental retardation, there were 21 persons (18%), out of 114 consecutive patients referred in a period of one year, with movement disorders (8 with tremors; 4, Parkinson's disease; 8, medication related; 1, dystonia), and 15 with gait disorders (10). This clinic evaluates acute new-onset problems and did not include persons with epilepsy or some

Table 90.1   Some Diseases Associated with Mental Retardation Where Movement Disorders Are a Prevalent Symptom

Ataxia
Congenital disorders
    Cerebellar malformations (agenesis, aplasia, dysplasia)
    Arnold-Chiari
Ataxia telangiectasia
Biotinidase deficiency
Metabolic
    Abetalipoproteinemia
    Argininosuccinic aciduria
    Hartnup disease
    Maple syrup urine disease (intermittent)
    Myoclonic epilepsy with ragged-red fibers
    Glutaric acidemia
    Isovaleric acidemia

Myoclonus
Aicardi's syndrome
Cerebral malformations
Myoclonic encephalopathy of infancy with or without neuroblastoma
Metabolic disorders
    Phenylketonuria
    Hyperglycinemia
    Maple syrup urine disease
    Menkes's syndrome
    Neuronal ceroid-lipofuscinosis
    Pyridoxine dependency
    Tay-Sachs disease
    Biotine deficiency
    Glutaric aciduria type I
    Myoclonic epilepsy with ragged-red fibers syndrome
Infectious disorders
    Encephalitis
    Postencephalitic syndromes
    Subacute sclerosis panencephalitis
Familial degenerative disorders
    Familial progressive myoclonic epilepsy
    Lafora body disease
    Alpers disease (progressive degeneration of the gray matter)
    Tuberous sclerosis

Dystonia
Cerebral palsy
Benign dystonia of infancy
Dyspeptic dystonia with hiatus hernia
Ataxia telangiectasia
Hallevorden-Spatz syndrome
Phenylketonuria
Medications
    Phenytoin
    Carbamazepine
    Tagamet
    Reglan

Chorea
Cerebral palsy
    Kernicterus
    Hypoxia-ischemia
Hyperkinetic syndrome
Infectious diphtheria
Infectious encephalitis (rubeola, mumps, varicella, St. Louis)
Canavan spongy degeneration
Cerebral lipidosis
Medications
    Phenytoin, carbamazepine, haloperidol, and other dopamine blockers

Monoplegia-Quadriplegia
Birth asphyxia
Hypoxic-ischemic encephalopathy
Neurodevelopmental malformations

movement disorders such as myoclonus or chronic choreoathetosis.

A recent study to evaluate the medical and functional status of adults with cerebral palsy found that 52 persons (51%) out of 101 had movement disorders (athetosis, chorea, or dystonia) (11). Also, 80 persons (79%) had dysarthria resulting from pseudobulbar cerebral palsy, and 26 previously ambulatory persons (26%) were no longer able to walk.

The prevalence of movement disorder in 1,227 persons with developmental disabilities living in an institution was as follows: dyskinesia, 48%; dystonia, 29%; akathisia, 13%; parkinsonism, 3%; and other paroxysmal movement disorders, 4% (12). Seventy-two percent had at least one movement disorder, but some persons had more than one. From the anatomic point of view, developmental disability

is a heterogenous condition. It is not uncommon to find grossly normal brains in persons with a mild degree of mental retardation; however, grossly abnormal brains are almost constantly associated with a severe degree of mental retardation.

The development of the brain is characterized by a succession of well-defined events—neural induction, proliferation, migration, and cytodifferentiation—most probably under genetic control. Many factors can have a disruptive influence leading to obvious brain malformations, such as agyrias, pachygyrias, different types of hydrocephalies, and microcephalies. On occasion, the pathologic changes are subtle, limited to the microscopic level. Milder forms of neuronal migration disorders (heterotopias, cortical dysplasias) are frequently seen in persons with mental retardation. Dendritic abnormalities have also been described in a variety of mental retardation disorders.

Cytoarchitectonic abnormalities result in disruption of brain circuitry and synaptic organization. Many abnormalities in neurons (in the distribution, number, or the morphology) have been described in association with mental retardation, in some cases related to particular syndromes (13). The subject is very complex, but as a matter of example, quantitation of dendritic branches in persons with Down syndrome showed that anomalies are age dependent. Fetuses and neonates have rather normal dendritic trees; abnormalities, such as reduced dendritic tree, aberrant dendritic spines, and decreased spine density, were more frequent in infants and older individuals. In Rett syndrome, there is a reduction in neuronal size, increased neuronal density, and a decreased dendritic tree. In unclassified forms of mental retardation, reduced dendritic trees, decreased spine density, and aberrant dendrites and spines are common features. However, one of the common features in mental retardation is the presence of both cortical and subcortical disturbances in the synaptic relationship and/or in the circuitry in the cerebral cortex (13).

In general, the treatment of persons with developmental disabilities with or without mental retardation has been in the hands of pediatricians and pediatric neurologists; but, with the present trend of placing persons with developmental disability in community settings and the expectation that services would be provided by community physicians, these patients will become more frequent in adult clinical practices. In 1970 there were almost 190,000 persons with a handicap or mental retardation living in institutions in the United States. By 1995, the number was reduced to approximately 63,000 (14).

The age of the population with mental retardation is also increasing. The average age of 47 persons that died in a residential institution for persons with mental retardation in the period 1992–1996 was 63.8 years (range 41–95 years). The average age in the institution was 53 (range 32–89 years) (N. Alvarez, personal observations).

CEREBRAL PALSY

This term is used to identify all those individuals in whom the main disability is in the motor area; it also implies that the injury to the brain is nonprogressive and has occurred before the brain was fully mature. The term cerebral palsy (CP) should not be used when a progressive neurologic disorder of the brain is suspected. Quite frequently other disabilities, such as mental retardation, epilepsy, and sensory deficits in hearing and vision, are present. The frequent association of motor dysfunction with other deficits—mental retardation in 60% of the cases, hearing and visual deficits in 10% to 15%, and epilepsy in 30% of the cases, to mention the most common ones—is an indication that CP is an expression of a continuum of central nervous system dysfunction.

The number of children (less than 18 years) with CP is estimated at around 100,000 (15), and there are approximately 5,000 new cases per year (16). There was hope that the improvement in obstetrical and neonatal care would decrease the incidence of CP; however, it does not seem to be the case, and there are some suggestions that the combination of CP and mental retardation might be more frequent than before (17,18). With good comprehensive services most of these children will reach adulthood. A recent study regarding the life expectancy of persons with cerebral palsy showed that 85% will reach 39 years of age. The survival rate was lower among people with profound mental retardation (19).

Cerebral palsy is the end result of many different conditions, and in almost 50% of the cases the cause of the brain damage is not found. Recent literature identified two major risk factors: low birth weight and asphyxia. In children born at term, CP is most often the consequence of prenatal conditions; in children born preterm, there is a combination of prenatal and perinatal factors. Twenty-eight percent of children with CP were born with a birth weight of less than 1,500 g (16). In almost half of the cases, the weight was less than 2,500 g, and babies born weighing 4,000 to 4,500 g had the lowest rate of CP (16). New technologies that facilitate the survival of infants with very low birth weight might have contributed to this shifting in prevalence.

Causes that interfere with uterine growth, such as infections (rubella, toxoplasmosis, cytomegalovirus); congenital malformations; maternal illnesses such as thyroid disorders; and chromosomal abnormalities might play an important role in the final outcome. Another factor potentially associated with CP is multiple birth, with CP being less frequent in singletons and increasing in frequency in twins and triplets.

Kernicterus, due to Rh incompatibility and subsequent hyperbilirubinemia, was the most common cause of athetoid cerebral palsy before the introduction of exchange transfusions. Presently, serious birth asphyxia is the more common cause of choreoathetotic movement disorders (20) and is often associated with spastic quadriplegia and mental retardation.

Birth asphyxia was considered as the leading cause responsible for CP; however, recent research suggests that only a small percentage of normal fetuses are severely injured during delivery (21). Even among newborns with low Apgar score and low pH, there is a high incidence of congenital malformations, suggesting that prenatal factors could have contributed to the perinatal problems.

Traditionally, the motor disorders observed in persons with CP are divided in two main groups: pyramidal, or spastic, and extrapyramidal, or dyskinetic, where movement disorders such as chorea, dystonia, athetosis, ballismus, and tremors are the main feature. There are two other types, the rigid form and the ataxic form, which are much less frequent. However, probably most, if not all, cases of CP have some degree of mixed symptoms and are asymmetric to some degree.

Approximately 70% to 80% of the cases are of the spastic type, which is further divided in several subgroups according to the topographic distribution of the spasticity. In the hemiplegic form only one side is involved, and usually the arm is more involved than the leg; in the diplegic type, even though the four extremities might be affected, the symptoms are predominant in the legs. When the four limbs are severely involved, the term used is quadriplegia; the term bilateral (double) hemiplegia is reserved for those cases in which the four extremities are involved but the upper extremities are more involved than the lower extremities. Other terms, such as triplegia and monoplegia, are also used. There is some value in establishing a difference since the topography and the type of cerebral palsy might suggest an etiology, associated deficits, and prognosis. For example, choreoathetosis in adults could be the consequence of kernicterus, and the cognitive deficit in this subgroup is not severe, but deafness is seen in 70% of the cases. However, a choreoathetotic form in a young child is more probably the expression of a more diffuse brain damage, and cognitive deficiencies are more severe. Children with unilateral hemiplegia have no or minimal cognitive deficits, but a high frequency of sensory deficits such as homonymous hemianopsia, deficits in stereognosis and position sense, and a high incidence of epilepsy. Children with quadriplegia have more severe cognitive deficiencies and epilepsy. Spastic diplegia is more often seen in premature children.

Spasticity as a clinical sign is characterized by increased resistance to passive movement and is elicited by rapidly moving a joint with subsequent sudden stretching of the tendons. Classically the resistance increases up to a point, followed by a sudden "give" (clasp knife phenomenon). The changes in muscle tone and posture are more constant during the day and are not much affected by the emotional state of the patient.

In the extrapyramidal hypertonicity type, the muscle tone is characterized by the "lead-pipe" phenomenon, a persistent uniform resistance observed as long as the passive joint is moved. Also, there is a great variability in the postures, which are markedly affected by the emotional state of the patient. Dystonias are characterized by persistent contractions of a muscle or a group of muscles that result in a fixed position. In the athetotic form, the involuntary activity is often produced as an overflow phenomenon from an attempted voluntary movement and is characterized by excessive muscular activity, mostly in muscles not involved with the task and directly antagonistic (22).

Deep tendon reflexes are exaggerated in both conditions and thus are not very useful to differentiate these two forms of muscle tone. Sustained ankle clonus is more often seen in the spastic form; however, it can also be seen in the extrapyramidal form. However, a prominent Babinski sign could be used to differentiate infants with CP from those with other delays.

In many instances it is difficult to define the type of cerebral palsy in early life, since the clinical picture changes as the child gets older. Furthermore, many infants with suspicious signs of cerebral palsy in early life might not show any symptoms at the age of 7. Children that will develop spastic CP are hypotonic at birth and might remain as such for the first 6 to 8 months of life. In many cases, the exact type of clinical picture cannot be defined until the child is 2 to 3 years old.

Newborns with bilirubin encephalopathy and kernicterus develop a high-pitched cry and opisthotonos in the first week of life, but by the sixth week the muscle tone might be normal. An analysis of videotapes obtained of infants between 5 and 8 months of age, with clear signs of athetoid cerebral palsy at age 3 years, showed some useful correlations (23). Most athetoid infants lay asymmetrically, and difficulties in taking a symmetric posture correlated with the severity of the motor disability later on in life. Other correlations were difficulty in extending the neck and supporting the weight with the arms, poor stability of the neck and trunk, difficulty in flexing the neck in traction response, and asymmetric opening of the mouth (23). Atypical choreoathetoid movements can be seen in the second year of life, and most such children have symptoms of chorea by the age of 3 years (24). Some infants exhibited the tension athetoid subtype characterized by a muscle tone that fluctuates between a rigid posture when the child is stimulated and a choreoathetoid movement when the child is relaxed. In teenagers or young adults the choreoathetoid syndrome changed, with predominance of dystonia as the main manifestation of movement disorder.

Besides the maturation of the brain, another important factor that interferes with movement is the number of medical complications, such as progressive scoliosis, nerve entrapments and secondary muscle atrophies, and contractures, that are frequently seen in these patients. Contracture is one of the most common complications, mostly of the spastic form. The contractures are probably the result of several factors, where degenerative changes in the joints and atrophy of the muscles involved might play an important role; however, intrinsic changes in the contractile properties of the muscles might also be important (25). Contractures are not limited to limb joints. The temporomandibular joints are also affected and might be responsible for a slow progressive deterioration of feeding skills (26). Long-lasting dystonic posturing can lead to several orthopedic complications, from fixed immobile joints to a severe degree of deformity in the joints and marked osteoarthritic disorders.

Radiculomyelopathy (27) and carpal tunnel syndrome (28) have been described in persons with long-standing choreoathetotic CP. The long-standing movement disorder with intense flexion, extension, and mostly rotation of the neck is probably the main factor in this condition. The dystonia accelerates the development of cervical spondylosis; this plus other local factors, such as spinal instability and, in some cases, congenital malformations of the spine, contributes to the cervical myelopathies and root compressions observed. The spondylitic changes in persons with dystonic CP are more often at the C3-C4 levels, joints more involved in the rotation of the head, than at the C4-C5 and C5-C6 level, joints more involved with flexion extension movement (27). Mechanical factors are also responsible for the carpal tunnel syndrome (28); in these cases a "double-crushed" syndrome can also be postulated. Less frequently, acquired cervical spine disease has also been described in persons with the spastic form of cerebral palsy with no choreoathetosis (29).

MANAGEMENT OF PATIENTS WITH CEREBRAL PALSY

The successful management of these patients requires a multidisciplinary approach. Different therapies can be utilized to increase the quality of life of persons with CP.

Several different medicines have been used with some benefit. Among the most frequently used medicines are benzodiazepines (mostly diazepam), dantrolene, oral and intrathecal baclofen, and recently botulinum toxin.

Orthopedic surgery is often needed to prevent or correct deformities or to facilitate motility.

Several forms of rehabilitative therapies based on theories such as neurodevelopmental treatments, sensory integration, patterning, and conductive education are used in the treatment of these children; however, there is no solid evidence supporting them.

Cerebellar stimulation showed improvement in spasticity and athetosis (30); however, the method is no longer used. Electrical stimulation showed increase in passive range of motion in children with hemiplegia; however, this technique still requires more evaluation (31).

DELAYED-ONSET MOVEMENT DISORDERS IN PERSONS WITH DEVELOPMENTAL DISABILITIES

There are several reports of patients with static brain lesions and minimal or no neurologic delay who present with movement disorders years after the time of the injury. Scott and Jankovic (32) reported their experience with 53 patients, 22 (42%) of whom experienced perinatal hypoxia/ischemia. The mean latency for the development of movement disorders was 27.6 ± 15.6 years. The mean latency was independent of the cause of the injury and decreased with age. It was 26.4 ± 16.3 years when the initial insult was at age 2 years or younger, 4.9 ± 7.8 years when the age of the initial insult was between 6 to 17 years, and 2.5 ± 4.9 years when the age of the insult was more than 25 years. The 22 patients with perinatal hypoxia/ischemia developed dystonia, which in 9 of them was generalized. Interestingly, generalized dystonia was not seen when the brain injury occurred after age 2 years. In addition, tremor

was observed in 12, parkinsonism in 4, and myoclonus in 3. Other neurologic signs such as spasticity and cognitive or motor delay were present before the movement disorder developed. Burke (33) described 4 patients with strong evidence of perinatal anoxia and a fifth with a question of anoxia who developed abnormal dystonic movement between 6½ to 14 years after the injury. Treatment options for these patients include botulinum toxin injections, trihexyphenidyl, tetrabenazine, benzodiazepines, oral and intrathecal baclofen, and thalamotomy.

Even though maturational processes in the brain are associated with the clinical changes observed in patients with cerebral palsy, this explanation does not apply for the delayed-onset movement disorder. The pathophysiology of this syndrome is poorly understood.

MILD NEUROMOTOR DISABILITIES

There is a group of children who present with fine and gross motor abilities that are significantly below what is expected on the basis of their age and cognitive functions. Usually the motor deficit presents early in development, interferes with academic achievement and quality of life, and has no neurologic diagnosis to explain the condition. There is a marked deficit in the performance of motor activities, as well as frequent mild dyskinesia. These children have been identified through the years by different terms, such as "clumsy child syndrome," "minimal cerebral palsy," "minimal brain damage," and "developmental disorders of motor functions" (34,35). The incidence between ages 5 and 7 years varies from 5% to 15% (34).

The etiology of these cases is not clear. Some studies showed some high family incidence of clumsiness in close relatives. Perinatal complications might also play a role; however, in most instances no clear organic basis is found.

The diagnosis is based on clinical symptoms. Several test batteries have been developed. They have mostly a neurodevelopmental approach, documenting the areas in which the child is delayed compared with normal standards. Once an expected skill is not present, usually at 1.5 or more standard deviation from the norm, it would be considered a "soft" neurologic sign. The reliability of these tests is variable; nevertheless, the documentation of these soft signs is a useful method to determine sensory and motor delays. Characteristically these children present with some deviation of the normal development in infancy; for example, they might never crawl, or show some delays in the acquisition of certain motor milestones like walking or riding a tricycle or a bike. The failures in fine motor coordination might be seen in tasks such as buttoning and unbuttoning shirts, tying shoes, or holding a pencil. Some of the motor deficiencies become more obvious as the child grows older. Sport activities are quite frequently of poor quality and difficult. Usually these children do not have focal neurologic signs; however, laterality might be changed. Some degree of hypotonia is seen in many but not all of these cases. Mental retardation is not a problem; however, difficulties in learning either due to the motor deficits or to other associated deficits are common, as well as psychological problems.

There are very few follow-up studies documenting the natural history of this disorder. The benign view that the child will mature and outgrow the symptoms is not sustained by recent publications (35–38). Follow-up studies done in teenagers who presented these symptoms at ages 6 to 7 years (35,36) found that the "clumsy" children had more motor disorders, behavior problems, and difficulties of social adaptation and were less competent in academic subjects than teenagers with no past history of clumsiness. Medical problems, including fractures, persistence of fine motor problems in maze-tracing tasks, and increased substance abuse, were also more frequent. With practice and training there is some control of the motor disorders and some degree of adaptation; however, since the basic deficiency persists, the difficulties might be seen again when these young adults need to learn new skills. In a group of recruits with clumsiness in childhood, there were difficulties under the stress of intense military training (39).

TARDIVE DYSKINESIA

The subject of tardive dyskinesia (TD) is described extensively in other chapters of this book. In this chapter tardive dyskinesia will be considered in relation to persons with developmental disabilities. Tardive dyskinesia is a well-recognized complication of the chronic use of psychotropic medications. Quite frequently persons with developmental disabilities also have psychiatric disorders, and the use of psychotropic medications is frequently indicated in this population. Neuroleptics are also used to treat behaviors such as aggression, stereotypies, and self-injury. In spite of a growing concern about the widespread use of neuroleptics in persons with mental retardation, recent reports failed to show a marked decrease in the use of these medications (40). However, a trend to use other medications instead of antipsychotics has also been observed (41).

A recent survey of 1,101 adults with mental retardation (42) living in group homes found that 297 (27%) of them received one or more psychotropic drugs for the treatment of behavioral or emotional disorders. Neuroleptic drugs, the most frequently associated with tardive dyskinesia, were prescribed in 21% of the cases. Other surveys found an incidence between 18% and 49% in the United States; interestingly, a prevalence of 19% was reported in England and 14% in New Zealand (42). The prevalence is much higher in persons living in institutions, where the mean is reported at 57.4%, with a range of 36.9% to 85.9% (40). Degree of handicap increases the incidence of movement disorder (43).

The evaluation of tardive dyskinesia in persons with mental retardation presents some methodologic problems. Some are related to the methods used to measure the move-

ment disorders. The AIMS, DISCUS, and Rockland scales have been used by different authors. Some, like Rao et al (44), have found clear differences in the prevalence using different scales in the same population. The AIMS showed a prevalence of 21%; the Rockland, 42%. The difference was also seen when the sex was evaluated: the AIMS showed no difference, but the difference was significant in the Rockland scale.

The level of cooperation of the individual is also an important factor. Evaluation of the DISCUS in 344 persons living in an institution showed very poor cooperation among persons with a profound degree of mental retardation (45). A complicating factor is the presence of parkinsonism, which can mask tardive dyskinesia, especially in the elderly. Rao found a significant association of TD and parkinsonism (44).

A major problem is the high frequency of abnormal movements observed in this population that are similar but probably not related to the use of neuroleptics. In a study involving 236 persons with mental retardation living in an institution (46), there was a significant amount of motor disorders in most of the patients. Of interest was the presence of orofacial movements in 71% of those treated with neuroleptics at the time of the study, 70% of those treated in the past, and in 52% of those never exposed to neuroleptics. Movements of the head, trunk, and limbs were found in 53% of those currently on medication, in 52% of those previously exposed, and in 32% of patients never exposed to neuroleptics. Perioral movements of the face were present in 34% of those receiving neuroleptics, 20% of those previously on neuroleptics, and in 27% of those never on neuroleptics. The quality of the movement disorder was similar in the different groups. Youssef and Waddington (47) found orofacial dyskinesia in patients with mental retardation never exposed to neuroleptics. Even though these movements were always more frequent in the treated group, these studies highlight the importance of having group controls in any study of TD in persons with brain damage.

Farren and Dinan (43) evaluated 61 women with mental retardation using the AIMS, and found that 39 (64%) had dyskinesia, predominantly orofacial, and 20 (33%) had lumbar or trunk dyskinesias. There was a significant increase in movement disorders when the degree of handicap increased, but it did not correlate with diagnosis, age, or exposure to neuroleptics. An evaluation of a large cohort of individuals over the age of 65 with no prior brain damage showed a low prevalence of akathisia (1.5%) and TD (0.22%), which were usually associated with organic mental disorders and not necessarily to antipsychotic medications (48). These findings suggest that cerebral damage by itself might be a factor in the presence of involuntary movement disorders.

In the psychiatric population, the prevalence of akathisia ranges from 12% to 75% (49). In persons with mental retardation, it is much lower, at 7% (50) to 13% (51). This is probably an underrepresentation due to the subjective component in akathisia rarely obtained in persons with mental retardation.

Neuroleptic malignant syndrome, a severe and potentially fatal complication of the use of psychotropic medications, has also been reported in persons with developmental disabilities. The mortality has deceased from 20% to 30% in early reports to almost zero due to more awareness, early diagnosis, and better acute treatment. However, a review (52) of 29 cases of neuroleptic malignant syndrome in persons with mental retardation found a fatality rate of 21% (6 cases), approximately twice that of persons without mental retardation. Neuroleptic polypharmacy was present in 55% of the patients.

STEREOTYPIES AND SELF-INJURIOUS BEHAVIOR

Persons with mental retardation frequently present with repetitive, patterned movements that are involuntary or seem to have no apparent function, have some rhythmicity, and might also have a ritualistic quality. Self-injurious behavior (SIB), on many occasions, consists of repetitive behaviors that might be considered as extreme cases of stereotypies, where the harmful consequences of the behavior, and not necessarily the topography, are the basis for the difference and the classification. Self-injurious behaviors and stereotypies are frequently observed together in persons with mental retardation (53).

Most of the information regarding stereotypies is based on observations performed in persons with mental retardation, psychiatric disorders, or brain damage; however, stereotyped behaviors are also seen in normal individuals. For example, body rocking, head banging, and thumb sucking are common behaviors in normal children, which in many cases persist during early childhood (54). Troster (55) studied the prevalence of stereotyped behaviors in 142 nonhandicapped children between the age of 10 months and 11 years living in residential care. The study showed that 82 (58%) of the children exhibited some stereotypies at least once a week, and 57 (40%) of them more than once a day. The frequency of the stereotypies decreased with age, but even in the age group of 9 to 11 years there were children that exhibited body rocking, thumb sucking, repetitive manipulation of objects, nail biting, hair twisting, and/or repetitive hand and finger movement. The behaviors were elicited under certain situations, suggesting an environmental component.

The prevalence of stereotyped behaviors in persons with a severe to profound degree of mental retardation living in institutions was reported to be between 32% and 60.9% (56,57). The prevalence in noninstitutionalized persons is much lower (53). A recent study reported 8% with self-injurious behavior and 6.5% with stereotyped behavior (58). However, in persons with mental retardation and autistic psychosis living in community settings, it can be as high as 22% (59).

Stereotypies in persons might have different manifestations, with a predominance of body rocking, waving and flapping of hands, staring, head banging, and touching, feeling, and smelling different objects, sometimes seen in a ritualistic fashion. They might be related to degree of mental retardation and nonambulatory status (60).

Stereotypies are also sensible to environmental factors. They might be elicited by frustrations, demands, new environments, and/or sensory stimulation. Predictable patterns of stereotypies have been reported in persons with profound and severe handicaps (61), in nonambulatory persons with profound mental retardation (56), or in those confined to cribs (62).

Self-injurious behavior might be considered as an extreme expression of these behaviors, and is quite frequently associated with stereotypies. Studies performed in institutionalized individuals have reported a prevalence between 10% and 15% (63) (it could be as high as 38% in public residential facilities), but much lower, between 1% and 2.5%, in the population with mental retardation living outside institutions (63). The degree of mental retardation, as well as institutionalization, correlates with the prevalence of self-injury. The role of age is not clear. The incidence is slightly higher in males than in females among persons with handicaps (64).

The presence of self-injurious behavior is one of the most frequent causes of failure in community placement. It also is very expensive to treat this condition; in the United States, it is calculated that the yearly cost is in the area of $100,000 per year per person.

The majority of individuals with self-injurious behavior exhibited more than one topography (58), and stereotypies are twice as frequent in persons with self-injurious behavior (58), suggesting some form of association. However, studies with naltrexone (65) that showed improvement in SIB with no improvement, and even an increase, in stereotypy suggest that the biochemical mechanism might be different. Bodfish et al (57) described a high co-occurrence of stereotypy, self-injurious behavior, and compulsions in institutionalized adults with a severe to profound degree of mental retardation. The occurrence of compulsions was associated with an increased prevalence of stereotypies in 30% and an increased prevalence of self-injury in 41%, and there were 30% of persons with both stereotypy and self-injury.

Some researchers believe that stereotypies and self-injurious behavior are the consequence of self-stimulatory behavior (66); others assume a developmental relationship from stereotypic to self-injurious behavior (67). Others have seen a communication function, a relationship with arousal in a poorly stimulated environment, or lack of proper stimulation in early life (61). Even though these two conditions are frequently observed in the same individual, presently the relationship between them is not clear (54).

The organic basis of these behaviors is not well known, but studies in animals and humans suggest that in some cases there might be a biological basis for these behaviors. Lewis et al (68) suggest that stereotypies are neurobiological, the consequence of brain damage in early age. The high incidence of paradoxical responses to sedative-hypnotic medications observed by Barron and Sandman (66) in persons with a profound degree of mental retardation and with both stereotypy and self-injurious behaviors was also considered an indication that there is a biological substrate, related, in their opinion, to the beta-endorphin system. A significantly lower blink rate index in persons with stereotypy than in controls might suggest a hypodopaminergic function (57). Dopamine D_2 and serotonin receptors, dysfunction of the basal ganglia, the mesolimbic system, and involvement of neuropeptides and endorphins have also been implicated in the pathogenesis of these stereotypies (69).

Excessive opioid brain activity was postulated as responsible for self-injurious behavior and stereotypies. Sandman et al (65) found that persons with mental retardation, stereotypies, and self-injurious behavior had higher morning levels of beta-endorphins than mentally retarded controls. Gilberg et al (70) found elevated beta-endorphins in cerebral spinal fluid. Beta-endorphins have many behavioral effects, including decreased perception of pain and euphoric effects. One theory suggests that insensitivity to pain is responsible for the behavior, and another suggests that an opiate high, induced by the release of beta-endorphins at the time of the SIB, is the basis of the abnormal behavior and considers the behavior as an addiction. None of these theories is proved. The beta-endorphin theory has been applied in practice with the use of the opiate antagonists naltrexone and naloxone. But the clinical results were inconclusive, with some reporting positive effects (65,71), while others reported negative effects (72) and also an exacerbation of the SIB. In general, studies done with naltrexone and good methodology found a favorable response in 50% of the cases (40). However, a double-blind placebo-controlled study (73) with naltrexone in adults with autism not only failed to show any improvement in self-injurious behavior but also showed an increase in stereotypies. This variability of the response might not necessarily mean that the blockers have no role but might suggest the possibility of subgroups of persons with SIB with some disregulation of the beta-endorphin system. These persons might be a small percentage of the total population, and for the time being there are no methods to distinguish responders from nonresponders. For example, improvement was observed in some studies involving persons with autism (74–76) but not in nonautistic persons with mental retardation (77).

Serotonin deficiency is also postulated as an explanation for SIB. However, fluoxetine, a serotonin reuptake inhibitor, has been reported as reducing SIB (78) as well as inducing SIB (79).

The use of medication for the treatment of these behaviors is still controversial but is very frequent. The combination of self-injurious behavior and stereotypy is second only to aggressive and destructive behavior as a category likely to result in drug treatment (63). There are some regional differences, however, and these medications seem to be more frequently used in the United States than in some European countries such as Germany (58).

Neuroleptics, commonly prescribed in persons with self-injurious behavior on the basis that the self-injurious behaviors are the consequence of hypersensitivity to the dopamine D_1 receptors, suppress self-injurious behavior but probably through a nonselective mechanism. Studies that measure other behaviors showed that they were also suppressed (40). Thioridazine in moderate doses might be helpful, but might be detrimental in high doses. The experience with chlorpromazine is mostly on the negative side, and the information regarding haloperidol is insufficient (63). The response might be related to the severity of the SIB. Subjects with high stereotypy rates responded better to thioridazine (80) and haloperidol (81) than those with low stereotypy rates. In general, the available data do not permit a definite conclusion. However, the neuroleptics do seem to be effective in specifically suppressing stereotyped behaviors (probably because the therapeutic dose for the treatment of stereotypies is lower than the dose that suppresses general behavior). Conversely, they do not seem to be a good choice for the treatment of self-injurious behaviors.

Different dopamine receptors might be related to behaviors that are different but might be present in the same individual; for example, D_1 receptors might be involved in SIB while D_2 receptors are involved in stereotypic behavior.

Other drugs used in the treatment of stereotypic behavior, including benzodiazepines, methylphenidate, amphetamines, reserpine, fenflurazine, naltrexone, and clonidine, showed some variable results, but in general on the negative side.

With all the contradictions regarding the use of medications and the side effects of the medications, the clinician is presented with a difficult task to balance potential benefits with side effects. In extreme cases where the aberrant behavior interferes with the quality of life, a more aggressive approach might be justified.

SPECIAL CASES

In most cases of persons with mental retardation and stereotypies, no particular diagnosis can be made. However, some well-defined clinical entities are commonly associated with these movement disorders and offer an opportunity to learn about the biological basis of them. The recognition of these patients suggests that there are some syndrome-specific behavioral phenotypes and might shed some light on the biological basis of these disorders. Rett's syndrome and autism are discussed in other chapters of this book. Studies done in males with fragile-X syndrome showed a specific behavioral profile that included stereotyped behaviors as one of the common features. In addition, hyperactivity and inappropriate speech were significantly higher than in controls. In this sample there was no correlation with IQ, and self-injurious behavior was not increased when compared with controls (82).

Smith-Magenis syndrome, the result of an interstitial deletion of the 17p11.2 chromosome, is characterized by a combination of clinical features that includes brachycephaly, midface hypoplasia, brachydactylia, ear malformations, and a mild to moderate degree of mental retardation. Most of these patients also present with severe aggressive and self-mutilatory behaviors, such as pulling out fingernails and toenails or inserting foreign bodies into bodily orifices. Head banging and hand biting are also common findings. A particular stereotyped behavior, probably pathognomonic of this syndrome, is the presence of a self-hugging in which the patients either hug themselves by crossing both arms tightly across their chests and simultaneously tensing the upper body, or they clasp their hands while interlocking the fingers and squeezing the arms against the chest (83).

Lesch-Nyhan syndrome, an X-linked recessive disorder of purine metabolism, is characterized by mental retardation, spasticity, extrapyramidal symptoms, and intense self-mutilation, lip biting being the most distressing. Self-injury occurs in the presence of intact pain sensation. These patients have elevated uric acid, but treatment that is effective in reducing the uric acid does not improve the behavior disorder. No neuropathologic basis was found to explain the symptoms in this disorder. Abnormal response of D_1 receptors in the striatum has been postulated as the biological basis for this behavior in Lesch-Nyhan syndrome (84). In some cases the self-mutilatory behavior improved with carbidopa-levodopa. Naltrexone, a pure opioid antagonist, might also decrease this behavior in Lesch-Nyhan syndrome. The serotonin precursor L-5-hydroxytryptophan failed to improve this condition (38).

The prevalence of obsessive-compulsive disorders in Prader-Willi syndrome may be 20 to 40 times higher than in persons with other causes of mental retardation (85) and could be similar to the prevalence reported in persons with profound to severe degrees of mental retardation and a variety of developmental disorders (86). Serotonin uptake inhibitors have been found effective in this condition (87).

The presence of these stereotypies in conjunction with other behavioral abnormalities is possibly related to organic problems, and they should not be considered mannerisms or physiologic events.

DRUG-INDUCED MOVEMENT DISORDERS

This issue is extensively covered in other chapters. Some relevant issues related to persons with brain damage will be reviewed here. One of the main issues is whether the presence of previous brain damage predisposes individuals to have more reaction to drugs. There are some descriptions of drug-induced movement disorders that seem to point in that direction.

Suzuki et al (88) described 20 patients, 7 of whom had mental retardation, who developed an insidious dystonic reaction that involved mostly the trunk, producing a bend to one side with rotation in the same direction. In addition, some patients turned in a direction opposite to the direction of walking. These symptoms were related to the use of different types of antipsychotic drugs. There was improvement with anticholinergic drugs. The presence of abnormal CT findings in 6 of the 7 patients with mental retardation and in 5 of the 13 patients with schizophrenia was an indication of the importance of a precondition for the development of this form of drug-induced tardive dystonia.

Patients with brain damage are at a higher risk of toxicity due to the chronic use of antiepileptic medications (89). Phenobarbital increases hyperactive behavior in children previously hyperactive (90,91). Behavior changes were described in association with several antiepileptic medications (92). Phenytoin induced (93) choreoathetotic movement disorder in persons with brain damage. Gabapentin was found to produce a similar disorder associated with facial dyskinesia in a 37-year-old male with severe mental retardation (94) and also in 3 out of 28 patients with severe neurologic deficit and chronic epilepsy treated with additional gabapentin (95).

Chronic use of valproic acid in monotherapy produced a reversible Parkinson's syndrome in several patients with epilepsy (96,97). Choreic movements were also described in persons with brain damage on chronic valproic acid therapy (98). Oculogyric crisis was reported in a patient with mental retardation while on carbamazepine and valproic acid (99).

REFERENCES

1. Coulter DL. Prevention as a form of support: implications for the new definition. Ment Retard 1996;34:108–116.
2. Scott LB, Jankovic J. Delayed-onset progressive movement disorders after static brain lesions. Neurology 1996;46:68–74.
3. McLaren J, Bryson SE. Review of recent epidemiological studies of mental retardation: prevalence, associated disorders, and etiology. Am J Ment Retard 1987;92:243–254.
4. Ozand PT, Gascon GG. Organic aciduria: a review, Part I. J Child Neurol 1991;6:196–219.
5. Gascon GG, Ozand PT, Brismar J. Movement disorders in childhood organic acidurias. Clinical, neuro-imaging and biochemical correlations. Brain Dev 1994;16(suppl):94–103.
6. U.S. Office of Special Education and Rehabilitation Services. Fifth annual report to Congress in the implementation of P.L. 94–142. Washington, DC: Government Printing Office, 1983.
7. Kiernan WE, Bruininks RH. Demographic characteristics. In: Kiernan WE, Stark JA, eds. Pathways to employment for adults with developmental disabilities. Baltimore, Paul H. Brookes, 1986.
8. Baird PA, Sadovnick AD. Mental retardation in over half-a-million consecutive livebirths: an epidemiological study. Am J Ment Defic 1985;89:323–330.
9. Murphy CC, Yeargin-Allsopp M, Decoufle P, Drews CD. The administrative prevalence of mental retardation in 10-year-old children in metropolitan Atlanta, 1985 through 1987. Am J Public Health 1995;85:319–323.
10. Alvarez N. Neurology. In: Rubin IL, Crocker AC, eds. Developmental disabilities: delivery of medical care for children and adults. Philadelphia: Lea and Febiger, 1989:130–159.
11. Murphy K, Molnar GE, Lankasky K. Medical and functional status of adults with cerebral palsy. Dev Med Child Neurol 1996;37:1075–1084.
12. Stone RK, May JE, Alvarez WF, Ellman G. Prevalence of dyskinesia and related movement disorders in a developmentally disabled population. J Ment Defic Res 1989;33:41–53.

13. Kauffman WE. Mental retardation and learning disorders. A neuropathological differentiation. In: Capute AJ, Accardo PJ, eds. Developmental disabilities in infancy and childhood. 2nd ed. vol 2, The spectrum of developmental disabilities. Baltimore: Paul H. Brooks, 1996:49–70.

14. Lakin CK, Prouty B, Smith G, Braddock D. Trends and milestones. Nixon goal surpassed—two-fold. Ment Retard, February 1996:67.

15. Kuban CK, Leviton A. Cerebral palsy. N Engl J Med 1994;330:188–195.

16. Cummings SK, Nelson KB, Grether JK, Velie EM. Cerebral palsy in four northern California counties, births 1983 through 1985. J Pediatr 1993;123:232–237.

17. Nicholson A, Alberman E. Cerebral palsy—an increasing contributor to severe mental retardation? Arch Dis Child 1992;67:1050–1055.

18. Stanley FJ. Cerebral palsy trends: implications for perinatal care. Acta Obstet Gynecol Scand 1994;73:5–9.

19. Crichton JU, Mackinnon M, White CP. The life-expectancy of persons with cerebral palsy. Dev Med Child Neurol 1995;37:567–576.

20. Rosembloom L. Dyskinetic cerebral palsy and birth asphyxia. Dev Med Child Neurol 1994;36:285–289.

21. Nelson KB. Epidemiology and etiology of cerebral palsy. In: Capute AJ, Accardo PJ, eds. Developmental disabilities in infancy and childhood. 2nd ed. vol 2, The spectrum of developmental disabilities. Baltimore: Paul H. Brooks, 1996:73–79.

22. Hallet M, Alvarez N. Attempted rapid elbow flexion movements in patients with athetosis. J Neurol Neurosurg Psychiatry 1983;46:745–750.

23. Yokochi K, Shimabukuro S, Kodama M, et al. Motor function of infants with athetoid cerebral palsy. Dev Med Child Neurol 1993;35:909–916.

24. Paine RS. The evolution of infantile postural reflexes in the presence of chronic brain syndromes. Dev Med Child Neurol 1964;5:345–360.

25. Hufschmidt A, Mauritz KH. Chronic transformation of muscle in spasticity: a peripheral contribution to increased tone. J Neurol Neurosurg Psychiatry 1985;48:676–685.

26. Pelegano JP, Nowysz S, Goepferd S. Temporomandibular joint contracture in spastic quadriplegia: effect on oral motor skills. Dev Med Child Neurol 1994;36:487–494.

27. Hirose G, Kadoya S. Cervical spondylitic radiculo-myopathy in patients with athetoid-dystonic cerebral palsy: clinical evaluation and surgical treatment. J Neurol Neurosurg Psychiatry 1984;47:775–780.

28. Alvarez N, Larkin C, Roxborough J. Carpal tunnel syndrome in athetoid-dystonic cerebral palsy. Arch Neurol 1982;39:311.

29. Reese ME, Msall ME, Owen S, et al. Acquired cervical spine impairment in young adults with cerebral palsy. Dev Med Child Neurol 1991;33:153–166.

30. Cooper IS, Rikland M, Amin I, et al. Chronic cerebellar stimulation in cerebral palsy. Neurology 1976;26:744–753.

31. Hazlewood ME, Brown JK, Rowe PJ, Salter PM. The use of therapeutic electrical stimulation in the treatment of hemiplegic cerebral palsy. Dev Med Child Neurol 1994;36:661–673.

32. Scott LB, Jankovic J. Delayed-onset progressive movement disorders after static brain lesions. Neurology 1996;46:68–74.

33. Burke RE, Fahn S, Gold AP. Delayed-onset dystonia in patients with "static" encephalopathy. J Neurol Neurosurg Psychiatry 1980;43:789–797.

34. Blondis TA. The spectrum of mild neuromotor disabilities. In: Capute AJ, Accardo PJ, eds. Developmental disabilities in infancy and childhood. 2nd ed. vol 2, The spectrum of developmental disabilities. Baltimore: Paul H. Brooks, 1996:199–208.

35. Loose A, Henderson SE, Elliman D, et al. Clumsiness in children—Do they grow out of it? A 10 year follow-up study. Dev Med Child Neurol 1991;33:55–68.

36. Hellgren L, Gillberg C, Gillberg IC, Enerskog I. Children with deficits in attention, motor control and perception (DAMP) almost grown up: general health at age 16 years. Dev Med Child Neurol 1993;35:881–892.

37. Gillberg IC, Gillberg C. Children with preschool minor neurodevelopmental disorders. IV. Behaviour and school achievement at age 13. Dev Med Child Neurol 1989;31:3–13.

38. Gillberg IC, Gillberg C, Groth J. Children with preschool minor neurodevelopmental disorders. V. Neurodevelopmental profiles at age 13. Dev Med Child Neurol 1989;31:14–24.

39. Shelley EM, Riester A. Syndrome of minimal brain damage in young adults. Dis Nerv Syst 1972;33:335–339.

40. Baumeister A, Todd ME, Sevin JA. Efficacy and specificity of pharmacological therapies for behavioral disorders in persons with mental retardation. Clin Neuropharmacol 1993;16:271–294.

41. Cable WJL, Martinazzi V, Steinberg RM. Changing patterns of psychotropic drug use in institutionalized mentally retarded individuals. Neurology 1996;46:2(suppl):A145–A146.

42. Aman MG, Sarphare G, Burrow WH. Psychotropic drugs in group homes: prevalence and relation to demographic/psychiatric variables. Am J Ment Retard 1995;5:500–509.

43. Farren CK, Dinan TG. Dyskinesia in mentally handicapped women: relationship to level of handicap, age, and neuroleptic exposure. Acta Psychiatr Scand 1994;90:210–213.

44. Murti Rao J, Cowie VA, Mathew B. Tardive dyskinesia in neuroleptic medicated mentally handicapped subjects. Acta Psychiatr Scand 1987;76:507–513.

45. Granger DA, Yurkunski JM, Miller NH, et al. Systematic dyskinesia examination of profoundly mentally retarded persons: cooperation and assessment. Am J Ment Defic 1987;92:155–160.

46. Rogers D, Cerci C, Bartlett C, Pocock P. The motor disorders of mental handicap. An overlap with the motor disorders of severe psychiatric illness. Br J Psychiatry 1991;158:97–102.

47. Youssef HA, Waddington JL. Involuntary orofacial movements in hospitalized patients with mental handicap or epilepsy: relationship to developmental intellectual deficit and presence or absence of long-term exposure to neuroleptics. J Neurol Neurosurg Psychiatry 1988;51:863–865.

48. Green BH, Dewey ME, Copeland JR, et al. Prospective data on the prevalence of abnormal involuntary movements among elderly people in the community. Acta Psychiatr Scand 1993;87:418–421.

49. Gross EJ, Hull HG, Lytton GJ, et al. Case study of neuroleptic-induced akathisia: important implications for people with mental retardation. Am J Ment Retard 1993;98:156–164.

50. Ganesh S, Murti Rao JM, Cowie VA. Akathisia in neuroleptic medicated mentally handicapped subjects. J Ment Defic Res 1989;33:323–329.

51. Stone RK, May JE, Alvarez WF, Ellman G. Prevalence of dyskinesia and related movement disorders in a developmentally disabled population. J Ment Defic Res 1989;33(pt 1):41–53.

52. Boyd RD. Neuroleptic malignant syndrome and mental retardation: review and analysis of 29 cases. Am J Ment Retard 1993;98:143–155.

53. Rojahn J. Self-injurious and stereotypic behavior of non-institutionalized mentally retarded people: prevalence and classification. Am J Ment Defic 1986;91:268–276.

54. Fee VE, Matson JL. Definition, classification and taxonomy. In: Luiselli JK, Matson JL, Singh NN, eds. Self-injurious behavior: analysis, assessment, and treatment. New York: Springer-Verlag, 1992:3–20.

55. Troster H. Prevalence and functions of stereotyped behaviors in nonhandicapped children in residential care. J Abnorm Child Psychol 1994;22:79–97.

56. Dura JR, Mulick JA, Rasnake KL. Prevalence of stereotypy among institutionalized nonambulatory profoundly mentally retarded people. Am J Ment Defic 1987;91:548–549.

57. Bodfish JW, Crawford TW, Powell SB, et al. Compulsions in adults with mental retardation: prevalence, phenomenology, and comorbidity with stereotypy and self-injury. Am J Ment Retard 1995;100:183–192.

58. Bojahn J, Borthwick-Duffy SA, Jacobson JW. The association between psychiatric diagnosis and severe behavior problems in mental retardation. Ann Clin Psychiatry 1993;5:163–170.

59. Lund J. Behavioral symptoms and autistic psychosis in the mentally retarded adult. Acta Psychiatr Scand 1986;73:420–484.

60. Kobe FH, Mulick JA, Rash TD, Martin J. Nonambulatory persons with profound mental retardation: physical, developmental, and behavioral characteristics. Res Dev Disabil 1994;15:413–423.

61. Guess D, Carr E. Emergency and maintenance of stereotypy and self-injury. Am J Ment Retard 1991;96:299–319.

62. Warren SA, Burns NR. Crib confinement as a factor in repetitive and stereotyped behavior in retardates. Ment Retard 1970;8:25–28.

63. Aman MG. Efficacy for psychotropic drugs for reducing self-injurious behavior in the developmental disabilities. Ann Clin Psychiatry 1993;5:171–188.

64. Johnson S. Epidemiology. In: Luiselli JK, Matson JL, Singh NN, eds. Self-injurious Behavior: analysis, assessment, and treatment. New York: Springer-Verlag, 1992:21–57.

65. Sandman CA, Barron JL, Chicz-DeMet A, DeMet EM. Plasma b-endorphine levels in patients with self-injurious behavior and stereotypy. Am J Ment Retard 1990;95:84–92.

66. Barron J, Sandman CA. Relationship of sedative-hypnotic response to self-injurious behavior and stereotypy in mentally retarded clients. Am J Ment Defic 1983;88:177–186.

67. Cataldo MF, Harris JC. The biological basis for self-injury in the mentally retarded. Anal Intervent Dev Disabil 1982:21–39.

68. Lewis M, Baumeister AA, Mailman RB. A neurobiological alternative to the perceptual reinforcement hypothesis of stereotyped behavior: a commentary on

"self stimulatory behavior and perceptual reinforcement." J Appl Behav Anal 1987;20:253–258.

69. Jankovic J. Stereotypies. In: Marsden DC, Fahn S, eds. Movement disorders 3. Oxford: Butterworth Heinemann, 1994:503–517.

70. Gillberg C, Teponius L, Lonnerholm G. Endorphin activity in childhood psychosis. Arch Gen Psychiatry 1985;42:780–783.

71. Sandman CA, Barron JL, Crinella FM, Donnelly J. The influence of naloxone on the brain and behavior of a self-injurious woman. Biol Psychiatry 1987;22:899–906.

72. Zingarelli G, Ellman G, Hom A, et al. Clinical effects of naltrexone on autistic behavior. Am J Ment Retard 1992;97:57–63.

73. Willemsen-Swinkels SHN, Buitelaar JK, Nijhof GJ, van Engeland H. Failure of naltrexone hydrochloride to reduce self-injurious and autistic behavior in mentally retarded adults. Double-blind placebo-controlled studies. Arch Gen Psychiatry 1995;52:766–773.

74. Campbell M, Adams P, Small AM, et al. Naltrexone in infantile autism. Psychopharmacol Bull 1988;24:135–139.

75. Taylor DV, Hetrick WP, Neri CL, et al. Effect of naltrexone upon self-injurious behavior, learning and activity: a case study. Pharmacol Biochem Behav 1991;40:79–82.

76. Walters AS, Barret RP, Feinstein C, et al. A case report of naltrexone treatment of self-injury and social withdrawal in autism. J Autism Dev Disord 1990;20:169–176.

77. Sandman CA, Datta PC, Barron J, et al. Naloxone attenuates self-abusive behavior in developmentally disabled clients. Appl Res Ment Retard 1983;4:5–11.

78. Markowitz PI. Effect of fluoxetine on self-injurious behavior in the developmentally disabled: a preliminary study. J Clin Psychopharmacol 1992;12:27–31.

79. King RA, Riddle MA, Chappell PB, et al. Emergence of self-destructive phenomena in children and adolescents during fluoxetine treatment. J Am Acad Child Adolesc Psychiatry 1991;30:179–186.

80. Aman MG, White AJ. Thioridazine dose effects with reference to stereotypic behavior in mentally retarded residents. J Autism Dev Disord 1988;18:355–366.

81. Aman MG, Teehan CJ, White AJ, et al. Haloperidol treatment with chronically medicated residents: dose effects on clinical behavior and reinforcement contingencies. Am J Ment Retard 1989;93:452–460.

82. Baumgardner TL, Reiss AL, Freund LS, Abrams MT. Specification of the neurobehavioral phenotype in males with fragile X syndrome. Pediatrics 1995;95:744–752.

83. Finucane BM, Konar D, Haas-Givler B, et al. The spasmodic upper body squeeze: a characteristic behavior in Smith-Magenis syndrome. Dev Med Child Neurol 1994;36:78–83.

84. Jankovic J, Cakey TC, Stout JT, Butler IJ. Lesch-Nyhan syndrome: a study of motor behavior and cerebrospinal fluid neurotransmitters. Ann Neurol 1988;23:466–469.

85. Dykens EM. DNA meets DSM: the growing importance of genetic syndromes in dual diagnosis. Ment Retard 1996;34:125–127.

86. Stein JJ, Keating J, Zar HJ, Hollander E. A survey of the phenomenology and pharmacotherapy of compulsive and impulsive-aggressive symptoms in Prader-Willi syndrome. J Neuropsychiatry Clin Neurosci 1994;6:23–29.

87. Dech B, Budow L. The use of fluoxetine in an adolescent with Prader-Willi syndrome. J Am Acad Child Adolesc Psychiatry 1991;30:298–302.

88. Suzuki T, Koizumi J, Moroji T, et al. Clinical characteristics of the Pisa syndrome. Acta Psychiatr Scand 1990;82:454–457.

89. Iivananinen M, Viukari M, Helle EP. Cerebellar atrophy in phenytoin-treated mentally retarded epileptics. Epilepsia 1977;18:375–386.

90. Ingram TTS. A characteristic form of overactive behaviour in brain damaged children. J Ment Sci 1986;102:550–558.

91. Ounsted C. The hyperkinetic syndrome in epileptic children. Lancet 1955;2:303–311.

92. Kalachnick JE, Hanzel TE, Harder SR, et al. Antiepileptic drug behavioral side effects in individuals with mental retardation and the use of behavioral measurement techniques. Ment Retard 1995;6:374–382.

93. Willmore LJ, Wheless JW. Adverse effects of antiepileptic drugs. In: Willie E, ed. The treatment of epilepsy: principles and practices. Philadelphia: Lea & Febiger, 1993:824–834.

94. Buetefisch CM, Gutierrez A, Gutmann L. Choreoathetotic movements: a possible side effect of gabapentin. Neurology 1996;3:851–852.

95. Chudnov RS, Lawson CD, Dewey RB. Choreoathetosis as a side effect of moderate-dose gabapentin therapy in severely neurologically impaired patients. Neurology 1996;46(suppl 2):A176.

96. Armon C, Shin C, Miller P, et al. Reversible parkinsonism and cognitive impairment with chronic valproate use. Neurology 1996;47:626–635.

97. Alvarez-Gomez MJ, Vaamorde J, Narbona J, et al. Parkinsonian syndrome in childhood after sodium valproate administration. Clin Neuropharmacol 1993;16:451–455.

98. Lancman ME, Asconape JJ, Penry JK. Choreiform movements associated with the use of valproate. Arch Neurol 1994;51:702–704.

99. Gorman M, Barkley GL. Oculogyric crisis induced by carbamazepine. Epilepsia 1995;36:1158–1160.

Special Topics

Chapter

Apraxia: A Disorder of Motor Programming

Robert T. Watson   Leslie J. Gonzalez Rothi   Kenneth M. Heilman

INTRODUCTION

Apraxia has been defined as a disorder of skilled movement not explained by inattention, lack of comprehension, weakness, sensory loss, basal ganglia tremor, altered tone, or cerebellar ataxia. In addition to defining apraxia exclusively by what it is not, we define apraxia inclusively by characteristic features of the abnormal behavior (1). This chapter will focus on what Liepmann termed ideomotor apraxia (IMA). Limb IMA is defined as the inability to correctly perform skilled movements due to incorrect placement and movement of the limb or digits in space and inappropriate sequencing and timing of individual muscle contractions. In this chapter we make the following points:

1. Abnormal movements of IMA are caused by a disturbance of motor programming.
2. Motor programming for transitive movements is almost always lateralized to the left hemisphere in right-handers.
3. Apraxia is a primary deficit resulting from pathologic lesions within a network of association regions and their connections to motor areas.

We primarily discuss ideomotor limb apraxia because this has been most thoroughly studied. However, other parts of the body, such as the lips, mouth, and tongue, may also be apraxic (e.g., buccofacial apraxia). In addition, there are other apraxic disorders of the limbs, including dissociation apraxia, conduction apraxia, ideational apraxia, conceptual apraxia, dressing apraxia, and constructional apraxia. Because dissociation and conduction apraxia are associated with production deficits, we will briefly discuss these disorders. Constructional and dressing apraxia are associated with

visual-spatial and perceptual disorders. Ideational and conceptual apraxia are more related to planning deficits than to production deficits. Therefore, these other forms of apraxia will not be discussed here.

Hugo Liepmann introduced the study of apraxia over 100 years ago (2–5). Liepmann's first case was a 48-year-old ambidextrous government official who was syphilitic, aphasic, and thought to be a "complete imbecile." By restraining this patient's apraxic right arm, Liepmann was able to prove that the seeming "imbecile" when using his left hand had instead a "relatively rich intelligence." At autopsy, lesions of the left frontal white matter, supramarginal gyrus, superior parietal lobule, and angular gyrus were present. There was also destruction of the corpus callosum, except for the splenium, and a more recent right parietal infarction. This case represented an example of relatively unilateral apraxia and was of value because Liepmann was able to demonstrate that neither asymbolia nor agnosia could explain how one hand could perform normally while the other was impaired. These observations encouraged Liepmann to study apraxia more thoroughly.

In 1905 Liepmann reported that of 42 patients with left hemiplegia, none were apraxic when using their right limbs. In contrast, 20 of 41 with right-sided weakness were apraxic when using their left limbs. Based on these observations, Liepmann concluded that in right-handed patients the left hemisphere had a special role in movement and should be considered the "action hemisphere" as well as speech hemisphere. The lesions inducing apraxia were located above the internal capsule, whereas capsular or subcapsular lesions produced weakness of contralateral limbs but not apraxia. He again noted that aphasia and apraxia were also dissociable, providing further evidence for his postulate that apraxia cannot be explained as an asymbolia.

IDEOMOTOR CALLOSAL APRAXIA

To support the hypothesis that the left hemisphere is dominant for programming skilled acts and directing the right hemisphere to carry out these acts with the left hand, Liepmann and Maas (2) described a patient with a corpus callosum lesion who was apraxic when using the left limbs. The patient, Ochs, was a 70-year-old right-handed carpenter who had a transcortical motor aphasia and severe right hemiplegia (the latter was caused by a left pontine infarction that prevented testing praxis in his right limbs). His left side had normal motility, as he could perform many overlearned automatic acts. However, he was unable to perform many goal-oriented movements with the left limbs. Autopsy revealed, in addition to the left pontine infarction, occlusion of the left anterior cerebral artery distal to its frontopolar branch with resultant infarction of the white matter below the supplementary motor area (SMA) extending back through the paracentral lobule to the precuneus. This infarction involved part of the cingulum and body of the corpus callosum and effectively destroyed the origin of the anterior three-quarters to four-fifths of callosal fibers from the left hemisphere. Without right-sided lesions, this case supported Liepmann's hypothesis of left hemisphere dominance for praxis in right-handers.

Subsequent clinical studies also supported the dominance of the left hemisphere for praxis in right-handers. When apraxia occurs in right-handers it almost always follows left hemisphere damage. When apraxia occurs in left-handers, it is usually caused by right hemisphere damage. The rare cases of apraxia in right-handers following right hemisphere damage and the less frequent occurrence of apraxia in left-handers following right hemisphere damage have led to the conclusion that the association between handedness and praxis is not absolute. However, crossed apraxia is less common than crossed aphasia (in right-handers there are more cases of aphasia than apraxia following right hemisphere lesions). Based on this discrepancy, it appears that in the general population of right-handers, the right hemisphere is more likely to be dominant for language than for praxis, and handedness is more closely associated with praxis than with language. However, because aphasia is more frequent than apraxia in right-handers following left hemisphere lesions, praxis may be more bilaterally represented than language.

Geschwind and Kaplan (6) reported a case of callosal disconnection that was somewhat different from the case reported by Liepmann. They reported a 41-year-old right-handed man with a left frontal glioma who underwent a left frontal lobe amputation and ligation of major branches of the anterior cerebral artery. After much of his postoperative aphasia and weakness had resolved, it was possible to demonstrate limb apraxia in his left hand. Although there was mild right weakness and a prominent right grasp reflex, the right limb was considered eupraxic. This patient's left-sided apraxia was present only when the patient performed in response to a verbal command. This patient was capable of imitating and using actual objects and tools flawlessly with his left hand. When callosotomy was introduced for the treatment of epilepsy, it was said to not cause any, or lasting, left-sided apraxia. If IMA did appear, it was considered to be caused by extracallosal damage. For example, the patients reported by Gazzaniga and his coworkers (7) who had callosal disconnection for the treatment of intractable epilepsy also had apraxia of their left hands to verbal command but not to imitation or with actual object use. This cast doubt on Liepmann's ideas of left hemisphere dominance for praxis because if the representations of skilled movement were stored in the left hemisphere of right-handers, then callosal disconnection should have induced an inability to perform skilled movements to command, imitation, and with actual objects.

However, we reported on a patient who did not have these additional factors (8). She was a 43-year-old right-handed woman who was healthy prior to suffering a spontaneous supracallosal hemorrhage of unknown etiology. This hemorrhage resulted in spasm of her anterior cerebral arteries. She had an infarction of the anterior three-quarters to four-fifths of the body of her corpus callosum that spared the genu and splenium (9). She was eupraxic with her right limbs but profoundly apraxic with her left. Initially she was unable to demonstrate the intended use of an object, as if her disconnected right hemisphere did not know what the object was for or even that it was to be used. We believe the term conceptual apraxia best describes her loss of knowledge of an object's use. She evolved into a severe and lasting ideomotor apraxic patient, meaning that the examiner could determine the goal of her acts but they were poorly performed, with performance being worse to verbal command, improving with imitation, and further improving with object use. She also had apraxic agraphia, without aphasic agraphia, isolated to the left hand. Unlike the patients of Liepmann and Maas (2) and Geschwind and Kaplan (6), who were unable to type or use anagram letters with their left hand, our patient could flawlessly type with her left hand, whereas attempted writing produced an illegible scrawl. As this patient had severe apraxia and apraxic agraphia isolated to the left hand without other abnormalities on neurologic examination, she provided strong support for Liepmann's hypothesis that the left hemisphere is dominant for praxis in right-handers and directs the right hemisphere for carrying out acts with the left hand. A similar case has been subsequently reported (10).

How can one then account for the two different apraxic syndromes associated with callosal disconnection: one where actual object use and imitation are impaired and the other where they are normal? Geschwind (11) posited that the variability in performance on imitating or using objects was determined by the degree of dominance for praxis. Just as there are variations in the degree of left hemisphere dominance for language, there may also be variations in the degree of praxis dominance. Geschwind and Kaplan's patient

(6) who could imitate and use actual objects normally was thought to have considerable motor skills in the right hemisphere that could be elicited by either somesthetic or visual input. Geschwind noted, however, that other patients may remain apraxic during imitation or object usage because their right hemisphere lacks the skill to normally carry out these movements without guidance from the left hemisphere.

We have termed the inability to correctly perform to verbal command with the preserved ability to imitate and use objects *dissociation apraxia* (1). We have reported patients with lesions confined to the posterior portions of the left hemisphere who had *verbal dissociation apraxia*. We have posited that these patients have an intrahemispheric deficit that prevents verbal stimuli from activating movement representations (12). DeRenzi and his coworkers (13) have described other patients who could pantomime to verbal command but were unable to pantomime to the visual or somesthetic presentation of stimuli. In these cases of *visual or somesthetic dissociation apraxia*, the verbal stimuli were able to access the movement representations, but the visual or somesthetic stimuli were not able to access these movement representations.

IDEOMOTOR APRAXIA ASSOCIATED WITH HEMISPHERIC LESIONS

Parietal Lobe

If the left hemisphere is dominant for mediating praxis in most right-handers, then where in the left hemisphere are these praxis mechanisms located? Liepmann originally considered the supramarginal gyrus of the parietal lobe to be the site containing the movement formulas, or space-time formula, for performing skilled movements. He later denied believing that there were praxis centers and proposed that white matter tracts below the supramarginal gyrus carried information about the nature of the desired movement from more posterior parieto-occipital regions. A posterior lesion would produce ideational apraxia, whereas a lesion in the region of the supramarginal gyrus would interrupt the underlying white matter and result in IMA. Geschwind also did not believe there was a praxis center containing memories of movements but instead felt that the auditory association cortex (Wernicke's area), visual association cortex, and somesthetic association cortex projected to the premotor cortex (PMC), which directed the primary motor cortex to execute the appropriate movements. A lesion disconnecting Wernicke's area from the motor area would result in a verbal-motor disconnection apraxia, a visual-motor disconnection would impair imitation, and a somesthetic-motor disconnection would impair the use of tools and objects. Lesions affecting all these connections would result in classic IMA.

It has been proposed that the inferior parietal lobe region contains the representations for the spatial and temporal features of some skilled movements (14). When asked to choose the target gesture from among three alternatives, patients with lesions including the supramarginal gyrus could not discriminate the correct act from foils demonstrated by the examiner. In contrast, those with apraxia from more anterior lesions were able to identify the correct performance. Patients with bilateral IMA from a dominant parietal lobe lesion therefore have IMA because of disruption of the memories of the spatial and temporal features of these movements rather than from disconnection. Rothi and coworkers (15) have posited that there may be two types of movement representations, one important for decoding afferent input (input praxicon) and one important for producing skilled movements (output praxicon). Ochipa et al (16) described a patient who was more impaired imitating gestures than performing gestures to commands and termed this disorder *conduction apraxia*. Such observations support the postulate that there are input and output movement representations and that these representations may be dissociated.

Premotor Cortex

It is not entirely clear how these temporal-spatial movement representations are transformed into motor programs. Liepmann thought the sensorimotor cortex programmed single simple movements and a lesion here caused what he termed melokinetic (limb-kinetic) apraxia. A lesion of primary sensorimotor cortex causes a loss of precise independent finger movement that is characteristic of pyramidal tract dysfunction. Geschwind believed that area 6 convexity premotor cortex programmed movements and directed area 4 to execute them, but he never reported a case of apraxia following a lesion confined to the left convexity premotor cortex. Apraxia from isolated convexity frontal lesions is rare. However, Barrett and coworkers (17) described a patient who had a unilateral convexity premotor cortex lesion and demonstrated a serious and disabling IMA. The patient appeared to have difficulty with the simultaneous programming of multiple joint movements. For example, when using a screwdriver one must rotate the arm at the elbow while simultaneously flexing the shoulder and extending the arm at the elbow. The patient also was impaired at making open-looped ballistic movements.

We have proposed that another important premotor area for programming certain distal skilled movements in right-handers is the left supplementary motor area (18). We reported two cases of bilateral IMA for transitive movements following left SMA infarctions. The first case was a 65-year-old right-handed man who had a transcortical motor aphasia, increased reflexes on the right with a right extensor plantar response, and a right grasp response. The remainder of his neurologic examination was normal. He had IMA for transitive movements of the limbs, with the left more involved than the right because of an associated callosal lesion. Only the distal components of transitive movements were abnormal. Intransitive movements, buccofacial movements, total body movements, and the proper sequencing of skilled limb acts were all normal. The examiners could always tell if the goal of his apraxic movements was correct, indicating that he did not have an ideational or conceptual apraxia. The patient recognized that his movements were incorrect and could always pick out the correct movement from foils performed by the examiners. The possibility that our patient may have had apraxia on the right because of damage to the left SMA and apraxia on the left because of the callosal lesions (sympathetic apraxia) seems unlikely, as our second patient (see Ref. 18 for details) had bilateral apraxia without a callosal lesion. We have seen two additional patients with bilateral IMA from left SMA lesions, and others have been reported (19).

DIAGNOSIS OF APRAXIA

Apraxia may be a sign of several disorders, including stroke, Alzheimer's disease, and other degenerative diseases such as cortical basal ganglia degeneration. Most patients with stroke or dementia rarely present with a chief complaint of apraxia and only rarely do their families notice that a loss of motor skills is interfering with daily routines. This unawareness of apraxia may occur for several reasons. Patients with apraxia may have anosognosia for their deficit (20). They also often have aphasia and a right hemiparesis so that abnormal performance with their left hand is attributed to clumsiness of the nondominant hand. Their families often anticipate the needs of the patient and do not allow them to use tools. For example, they cut their food for them, bathe them, and comb their hair. Finally, apraxia is typically worse when pantomiming to verbal commands and less apparent when using objects. Patients are not asked to pantomime by family members. Recognition of apraxia, therefore, requires specific praxis testing.

Because limb apraxia can be confused with, or obscured by, more elementary neurologic deficits, it is imperative to do a thorough neurologic examination. The patient must be sufficiently attentive and comprehend the verbal command to pantomime. Assessment of comprehension by asking the patient to perform complex limb movements may cause the examiner to mistake an apraxic error for a comprehension disorder. Comprehension may be tested in these patients by asking them questions that can be answered by yes or no answers or by pointing. Strength must be adequate to ensure that the movement disorder is not caused by weakness. However, even in the absence of severe weakness, an inability to perform precise independent finger movement (e.g., picking up a coin from a table using a pincher grasp) may suggest cortical spinal system dysfunction. Sensory function, particularly position sense, should also be intact. In addition, the poorly directed tactile exploration of objects in patients with astereognosis is not apraxia. Disorders of the basal ganglia and cerebellum as well as myoclonic or focal epilepsy

must be excluded. Any of these sensory or motor disorders confined to one side of the body does not prevent testing for apraxia on the other side.

For clinical purposes the discovery of apraxia is important because it provides lateralizing and localizing information. Our experience agrees with others that testing of transitive movements, those made in relation to tools and objects, is most informative, and abnormalities of these movements are indicative of left hemisphere dysfunction in the vast majority of right-handers.

Each patient should perform the five following praxis tests:

1. Pantomime to verbal command ("Show me how you would use a _____.")
2. Imitation of pantomime ("This is the way you use a _____. Now you do it.")
3. Use the object ("Here is the _____. Show me how to use it.")
4. Imitation of the examiner using the object
5. Discrimination of the correct pantomime done by the examiner

In this last test, the examiner demonstrates the correct pantomime among foils. One foil is usually a body part as object error (for example, using fingers as the blades of a scissor), another may be a poorly executed movement, and another may be an unrelated movement (for example, using a screwdriver instead of scissors).

For practical purposes, the finding of apraxia for transitive movements in a right-hander indicates a lesion in the left hemisphere. If a right-handed patient whose right limbs can be tested is found to have unilateral left-sided apraxia, then the diagnosis of a callosal lesion can be made. To localize a lesion within the left hemisphere, the dominant supramarginal gyrus region is suspected in an apraxic patient who cannot discriminate correct from incorrect gestures performed by the examiner. Patients with SMA or callosal lesions can comprehend and discriminate the correct act performed by the examiner. These patients also recognize their own apraxic errors.

Praxis errors can greatly vary in quality. We have classified these errors into two main types: content and production. Content errors involve the production of a pantomime whose content does not represent the target gesture (21). For example, the patient may pantomime hammering for the request to show the use of a toothbrush. Errors may be unrelated, as in hammer/toothbrush, or may be related, as in pantomiming hammering for sawing. Patients with ideational apraxia or conceptual apraxia, by definition, produce content errors. Sometimes patients with severe IMA produce limb movements so degraded as to make the content unrecognizable; however, they should rarely produce errors where the content of one gesture is substituted for another.

Production errors have been divided into two major subtypes: spatial and temporal. Patients with IMA make production errors. The spatial errors of production can be either body part as tool, postural (internal configuration), orientation, or movement. One of the most commonly noted errors is using a body part as a tool. For example, when a patient is asked to pantomime using a screwdriver, the index finger may be used as if it were the shaft of a screwdriver. Since individuals without brain damage are also noted to do this during praxis testing, it is imperative to instruct the patient to pretend to hold the imagined tool rather than using their hand or digit as the tool. People without apraxia correct this error with instruction, whereas patients with apraxia will not (22).

Patients with IMA also commonly make orientation or movement errors. Regarding the former, when asked to pantomime or use an object or tool, we normally orient the imagined or real tool or object with the imagined or real target of the tool's action. For example, in pantomiming the use of a bread knife, the patient may fail to keep the cutting movement in a stable (e.g., sagittal) plane. Each skilled act has a characteristic joint movement pattern. For example, when using a bread knife to cut a slice of bread, the arm is alternatively flexed and abducted at the shoulder while the forearm is extended at the elbow and then the shoulder is extended and abducted while the elbow is flexed. An aberration of this characteristic movement is considered a movement error. For example, the apraxic patient may fail to extend his elbow while his shoulder is flexing, thereby making stabbing rather than cutting movements. Patients with IMA also make temporal errors. These errors consist of a delay before initiating a movement and incorrect coupling of speed with specific joint movements (23). Some apraxic patients will also demonstrate abnormal sequencing of the individual muscle contractions that comprise a motor program.

Patients with conduction apraxia make more errors when imitating than they do when pantomiming to command, and patients with disassociation apraxia may fail to correctly respond to stimuli presented in one modality (e.g., speech) but perform almost flawlessly in other modalities (e.g., vision).

MANAGEMENT

The management of apraxic patients begins with determining etiology in order to prevent further progression, if possible. Little research effort has been directed at remediation of apraxia. The few studies that have been performed have shown that these disorders are amenable to direct intervention (24–29). However, the benefits gained from treatment appear to be specific to the items treated, and these gains do not appear to generalize to untreated items or to different settings. Therefore, the items selected for treatment should be of pragmatic significance.

BASIC SCIENCE

The importance of the left inferior parietal lobe in praxis has gained general support based entirely on clinical observations. Explanations of why or how this area stores the spatial and temporal features of skilled movements and participates in the execution of motor programs have not been provided. If homologies with nonhuman primate anatomy are correct, then the inferior parietal lobe is a convergence site of multimodal association cortices with projections to prefrontal and premotor cortex. These anatomic features are in keeping with this being a higher-order association region capable of serving complex functions like skilled movements. Mishkin et al (30) demonstrated in monkeys that there are two visual streams, a dorsal stream from the occipital lobe to the parietal lobe and a ventral stream from the occipital lobe to the ventral temporal lobe. Whereas the ventral stream, or "what" system, appears to be important for object recognition, the dorsal stream, or "where" system, appears to be important in topographic orientation. Watson and coworkers have noted that in monkeys these "what" and "where" systems appear to converge in banks of the monkey's superior temporal sulcus (31). These investigators also note that the convergence of the "what" and "where" systems may not be limited to the visual system but rather may also occur in other modalities (e.g., somesthetic). As previously stated, the type of praxis errors most often seen with left inferior parietal lesions are errors of transitive movements. Because transitive movements are those made in relation to tools, it follows that these are movements that must interact with a target of the tool's action (the object). Such actions are usually made in reference to extrapersonal space. For example, using a hammer means directing the hammer to a real or imagined nail that is located in the environment away from the body. In addition, to properly use a tool, one must have knowledge of the tool shape so that one can correctly position one's hand to properly hold the tool. Therefore, to know how to pantomime tool use, one would have to use and synthesize knowledge stored in both the "what" and "where" systems. The caudal banks of the monkey superior temporal sulcus are probably the precursor of the human inferior parietal lobe. The clinical observation that the parietal region is important in the mediation of transitive movements is supported by the observation that increased regional cerebral blood flow (rCBF) in this region occurs only when movements have an extrapersonal frame of reference (32).

The proposal that the SMA is part of a praxis system has more scientific support than exists for the inferior parietal lobe (18,33–35). The SMA is reciprocally connected with the primary somatosensory cortex and area 5 of the monkey. Reciprocal connections with monkeys' inferior parietal lobe (area 7) also exist. There are reciprocal connections bilaterally with the motor cortex (Brodmann's area 4 and 8), the convexity portion of premotor area 6, and to the opposite

SMA. The SMA has bilateral subcortical projections to the striatum, red nucleus, and medullary reticular formation and ipsilateral connections to the ventrolateral and centrum medianum nuclei of the thalamus and to the pontine nuclei. Projections to the cervical and lumbar spinal cord have also been shown. Electrophysiological studies further support the role of the SMA in motor behavior. Stimulation of the SMA induces complex movements that include distal features, rather than the localized movements associated with individual muscle contractions induced by area 4 stimulation. Single-unit recording in monkeys has shown some SMA units that fire before learned complex movements performed with either extremity. The *Bereitschafts* potential, or readiness potential, has its origins in the SMA (36). Finally, rCBF during performance of learned complex sequential movements is increased in the contralateral primary motor cortex and bilaterally in the SMA. Since this increased flow is restricted to the SMA when the subject thinks of the sequence without actual movement, it has been proposed that the SMA contains programs for some motor subroutines (35).

We believe that the left hemisphere is specialized for the motor programming needed to perform transitive movements, that is, those made in relation to objects and tools, and that the SMA has a special role in these movements (18). We have proposed that the postural support and proximal movements that accompany the distal features of a transitive movement are mediated by interactions of the SMA with subcortical structures. Since our patients had normal proximal movements and postural support, these must have bilateral control. The distal features of movements are probably primarily executed by the motor cortex (Brodmann's area 4).

With practice, a movement becomes automatic or routine and may be performed in an open-looped mode. Even though the SMA receives input from the somatosensory cortex, it does not respond to peripheral somatosensory feedback, suggesting that the SMA might be important in open-looped movements. Area 4 does respond to peripheral sensory feedback, but this responsiveness is reduced by SMA activity, and the SMA may force area 4 into an open-looped mode. We have studied a peripherally deafferented patient who was able, except for orientation errors, to correctly demonstrate the use of tools (37). This observation supports the hypothesis that, except for orientation, the learned programs for tool use can be executed in an open-looped mode without aid of peripheral sensory feedback. However, the orientation of a tool with the target of its action (e.g., a hammer with a nail) is dependent on sensory feedback and must be done in a closed-loop fashion. This feedback from the periphery is based on visual, auditory, and somesthetic cues that provide knowledge of where the target object and limb are positioned in space.

A striking feature of the SMA anatomy is its reciprocal connections with area 5, an area of higher-order proprioceptive function. This part of the superior parietal lobe

(SPL) also has increased rCBF during movements in extrapersonal space (32). Lesion studies in nonhuman primates have indicated that proprioceptive information without visual guidance may be important for performing movement via the SMA (38). Monkeys with bilateral SMA lesions were unable to relearn a sequence of three movements (pushing, pulling, and twisting a catch, needed to uncover a food well). These animals had no problem with initiation of movement or individual movements but could not sequence these acts. Animals with SMA lesions were also unable to reach out to a position based on proprioceptive cues. However, the animals could reach normally with visual guidance. The animals therefore did not have difficulty with motivation or triggering movements but instead with directing movements based on proprioceptive cues about their own activities (i.e., based on internal cues). This was in contrast to the convexity premotor cortex, which directs movements based on visual or auditory guidance (i.e., information provided by external cues). Except for orientation toward the target, transitive movements cannot be entirely mediated by visual or auditory cues. It is possible that apraxia in patients with SMA lesions is related to an inability to use proprioceptive information to guide the next movement based on information from the prior movement in a complex task such as tool use. Based on this postulate, it might seem that intransitive movements done in an open-looped mode would be equally susceptible to SMA damage. However, patients with left SMA lesions are unimpaired on intransitive movements. This suggests that the SMA is necessary for the programming of movements requiring the special features of tool use, whereas other movement programs are stored elsewhere or are redundantly represented.

It would be of interest to evaluate praxic errors where tools of different complexity are used and also to compare complex intransitive movements with more simple transitive movements. It would also be instructive to grade the severity of apraxia in relation to the degree of movement in an extrapersonal compared with an intrapersonal frame of reference (e.g., hammer compared with comb). These analyses would provide some insight into those features of transitive movements that are uniquely susceptible to left SMA damage. It is possible that the SMA is especially important for programming movements that combine extrapersonal (peripersonal) and intrapersonal frames of reference. Transitive movements are the most striking examples of this interaction.

Since the SMA does not respond to proprioceptive feedback, then how is proprioceptive information used for transitive movements? We have studied a patient with an SPL lesion who may help answer this question (39). Her movements were markedly worse without visual guidance, suggesting that she was dependent on visual feedback and that her movements were inadequately controlled by proprioceptive feedback. However, she had no abnormalities of proprioception. Specialized testing showed an impairment of visual-somesthetic transcoding. When performing an open-looped motor program, there is no dependence on peripheral feedback, but there is need for an internal system that compares efferent copy from the SMA with proprioceptive feedback and corrects mismatches. We proposed that the SPL is part of an internal feedback system to monitor whether a preprogrammed movement is being done correctly. A loss of this internal monitoring between the SMA and SPL could result in the spatial and temporal errors seen in our patients. The SPL has archicortical cytoarchitectonic features like the SMA and reciprocally connects with the SMA. The SPL also has reciprocal projections with the dorsal convexity premotor cortex (PMC) by which it might program movements dependent on closed-looped somatosensory guidance. In contrast, the inferior parietal lobe (IPL) has paleocortical cytoarchitectonic features similar to the ventral convexity PMC and has reciprocal connections with the ventral convexity PMC. The IPL receives visual input and is important for the location of objects in space. Thus, the IPL-ventral convexity PMC may be important for movements based on visual guidance. Our patient with the SPL lesion improved when she was able to observe her own gestures, suggesting that she could use visual guidance between her intact IPL and ventral PMC.

Although we originally posited that the SMA contains motor programs to direct transitive movements (18), there are several problems with this hypothesis. Since these movements are phylogenetically the most recent acquisition, it is paradoxical that they would be programmed by the archicortical, or the most ancient, motor area. In addition, when we postulated this function of SMA it was partly based on data from intracarotid ^{133}Xe rCBF measurements that indicated that the SMA was active only during complex movements but not during routine simple movements such as isolated finger flexion or isometric finger contraction (35). Positron emission tomography has subsequently shown that the SMA is active in association with all movements (40). These observations require reassessment of the SMA in praxis.

What does the left SMA do in this distributed modular praxis network? Since our patients were not particularly impaired in initiating movements, we do not believe that the left SMA is critical for activating or initiating the movement itself. Instead, when performing transitive movements, the patients made spatial and temporal errors typical of IMA. Although the SMAs have increased metabolism in association with all movements, this does not reveal their function. Furthermore, changes in metabolism or single-unit recordings do not indicate whether either SMA is necessary for performing specific movements or simply active because some type of movement, as yet undetermined, might occur. In other words, because the SMAs are active in association with simple finger movements does not mean that they are necessary for these movements. In fact, such movements are correctly done after an SMA lesion.

The type of movement probably determines whether an active cortical region is used to perform the movements. For transitive movements, the left IPL has the spatial and temporal memories for these movements and uses the SMA to transcode these features into a motor program. Other movements may use different motor regions for transcoding. For example, the posterior association cortex may direct movements based on external sensory guidance and use the convexity PMC to transcode this sensory information into a program for action. Some simple movements may be programmed directly by area 4 or subcortical structures. Perhaps the phylogenetically oldest structure, the SMA, has delegated certain types of movements to more recently developed motor areas. As the convexity PMC developed, it was primarily to program movements based on external guidance and to provide motor learning; area 4 developed for the execution of distal fractionated movements. The development of the motor cortex made tool use possible. The SMA is important for programming these movements for open-looped execution. The parietal lobe is important for representations of movements made in relation to an extrapersonal reference system. If a left parietal lesion occurs, then the memories for these movements are disrupted and the patient displays apraxia. However, if sensory associative regions are not also destroyed, the act is still performed and is recognizable, albeit with degraded spatial and temporal features. The patient does not recognize his or her incorrect movements. If an SMA lesion occurs, the executed act is similarly degraded, even though the patient recognizes that his or her performance is incorrect.

Since the convexity PMC depends on sensory guidance, it may be that improvement seen with imitation (vision) or object use (vision and somesthesis) in patients with IMA is related to accessing these programs in the left PMC in addition to programs being represented in the right hemisphere (11). However, after programs in the left PMC or right hemisphere are accessed, these areas are still incapable of executing the program in an open-looped fashion, and the movements remain apraxic. Perhaps object use is generally better than imitation because it provides both visual and somesthetic input to the PMC. To determine if this is true, the praxis errors during object use with the patient blindfolded would need to be compared with object use with vision or with imitation. The interactions of other cortical and subcortical structures that take place before and during a movement should be thought of as occurring in parallel to provide the correct tone, velocity, amplitude, force, and strength for the called-up program.

In right-handed people it is only lesions of the left parietal lobe, or SMA, that cause IMA for transitive movements. This suggests not only a specialized function of the SMA but also hemispheric dominance. The left SMA is important for internally generated motor programs rather than programs exclusively dependent on external sensory guidance. In addition, the SMA seems to have retained a special role in performing open-looped movements that use both intrapersonal and extrapersonal frames of reference. The use of tools (transitive movements) is the best example of such movements, and these movements are apraxic with left SMA lesions. These issues in relation to praxis will only be clarified by further clinical observations, basic science studies, and by comparing the effects of lesions within this network in the right hemisphere with those in the left hemisphere.

REFERENCES

1. Heilman KM, Gonzalez-Rothi LJ. Apraxia. In: Heilman KM, Valenstein E, eds. Clinical neuropsychology. 3rd ed. New York: Oxford University Press, 1993:141–163.
2. Liepmann H, Maas O. Fall von linksseitger Agraphie und Apraxie bein Rechtsseitiger Lahmung. J Psychol Neurol 1907;10:214–217.
3. Kimura D. Translations from Liepmann's essays on apraxia. Res Bull 1980:1–80.
4. Faglioni P, Basso A. Historical perspectives on neuroanatomical correlates of limb apraxia. In: Roy EA, ed. Neuropsychological studies of apraxia and related disorders. Amsterdam: Elsevier, 1985.
5. Brown JW. Apraxia—introduction and clinical description. In: Aphasia, apraxia and agnosia. Springfield: Charles C Thomas, 1974:151–160.
6. Geschwind N, Kaplan E. A human cerebral deconnection syndrome: a preliminary report. Neurology 1962;12:675–685.
7. Gazzaniga MS, Bogen JE, Sperry RW. Dyspraxia following division of the cerebral commissures. Arch Neurol 1967;16:606–612.
8. Watson RT, Heilman KM. Callosal apraxia. Brain 1983;106:391–403.
9. Watson RT, Heilman KM, Bowers D. Magnetic resonance imaging (MRI, NMR) scan in a case of callosal apraxia and pseudoneglect. Brain 1985;108:535–536.
10. Graff-Radford NR, Welsh K, Godersky J. Callosal apraxia. Neurology 1987;37:100–105.
11. Geschwind N. The apraxias: neural mechanism of disorders of learned movement. Am Sci 1975;63:180–195.
12. Heilman KM. Ideational apraxia—a re-definition. Brain 1973;96:861–864.
13. DeRenzi E, Faglioni P, Sorgato P. Modality-specific and supramodal mechanisms of apraxia. Brain 1982;105:301–312.
14. Heilman KM, Rothi LJ, Valenstein E. Two forms of ideomotor apraxia. Neurology 1982;32:342–346.
15. Rothi LJG, Ochipa C, Heilman KM. A cognitive neuropsychological model of limb praxia. Cogn Neuropsychol 1991;8:443–458.
16. Ochipa C, Rothi LJG, Heilman KM. Conduction apraxia. J Neurol Neurosurg Psychiatry 1994;57:1241–1244.
17. Barrett AM, Schwartz RL, Raymer AM, et al. Dyssynchronous apraxia. Neurology 1996;46:A383.
18. Watson RT, Fleet WS, Gonzalez-Rothi L, Heilman KM. Apraxia and the supplementary motor area. Arch Neurol 1986;43:787–792.
19. Mehler MF. Spectrum and lateralization of praxic deficits following supplementary motor area infarction. Neurology 1988;38:172.
20. Rothi LJG, Mack L, Heilman KM. Unawareness (anosognosia) of apraxic errors. Neurology 1990;40:202.
21. Rothi LJG, Mack L, Verfaille M, et al. Ideomotor apraxia: error pattern analysis. Aphasiology 1988;2:381–387.
22. Raymer AM, Maher LM, Founda A, et al. The significance of body part as tool errors in limb apraxia. J Int Neuropsychol Soc 1996;2:27.
23. Poizner H, Mack L, Verfaille M, et al. Three-dimensional computer graphic analysis of apraxia. Brain 1990;113:85–101.
24. Code C, Jaunt C. Treating severe speech and limb apraxia in a case of aphasia. Br J Disord Commun 1986;21:11–20.
25. Pilgrim E, Humphreys GW. Rehabilitation of a case of ideomotor apraxia. In: Riddoch MJ, Humphreys GW, eds. Cognitive neuropsychology and cognitive rehabilitation. Hove, UK: Erlbaum, 1994.
26. Cubelli R, Irentini P, Montagna CG. Reeducation of gestural communication in a case of chronic global aphasia and limb apraxia. Cogn Neuropsychol 1991;8:369–380.
27. Maher LM, Ochipa C. Management and treatment of limb apraxia. In: Rothi LJG, Heilman KM, eds. Apraxia: the neuropsychology of action. Hove, UK: Erlbaum, 1997.
28. Ochipa C, Maher LM, Rothi LJG. Treatment of ideomotor apraxia. J Int Neuropsychol Soc 1995;2:149.
29. Maher LM, Rothi LJG, Greenwald ML. Treatment gesture impairment: a single case. ASHA 1991;33:195.
30. Mishkin M, Ungerleider LG, Macko KA. Object vision and spatial lesion: two cortical pathways. Trends Neurosci 1983;6:414–417.
31. Watson RT, Valenstein E, Day A, Heilman KM. Posterior neocortical systems subserving awareness and neglect. Neglect associated with superior temporal sulcus lesions but not area 7 lesions. Arch Neurol 1994;51:1014–1021.
32. Roland PE, Skinhoj HOJE, Lassen NA, Larsen B. Different cortical areas in man in organization of voluntary movements in extrapersonal space. J Neurophysiol 1980;43:137–150.
33. Brinkman C, Porter R. Supplementary motor area of the monkey: activity of neurons during the performance of a learned motor task. J Neurophysiol 1979;42:681–709.
34. Goldberg G. Supplementary motor area structure and function: review of hypotheses. Behav Brain Sci 1985;8:567–616.
35. Roland PE, Larsen B, Lassen NA, Skinhoj HOJE. Supplementary motor area and other cortical areas in organization of voluntary movements in man. J Neurophysiol 1980;43:118–136.
36. Deecke L. Bereitschaftspotential as an indicator of movement preparation and supplementary motor area and motor cortex. In: Bock G, O'Connor M, Marsh J, eds. Motor areas of the cerebral cortex. CIBA Foundation Symposium, no. 132. Chichester: John Wiley, 1987:231–250.
37. Heilman KM, Mack L, Rothi LJG, Watson RT. Transitive movements in a deafferented man. Cortex 1987;23:525–530.
38. Passingham RE. Two cortical systems for directing movement. In: Bock G, O'Connor M, Marsh J, eds. Motor areas of the cerebral cortex. CIBA Foundation Symposium, no. 132. Chichester: John Wiley, 1987:151–164.
39. Heilman KM, Rothi LJG, Mack L, et al. Apraxia after a superior parietal lesion. Cortex 1986;22:141–150.
40. Rapcsak SZ, Rothi LJG, Heilman KM. Apraxia in a patient with atypical cerebral dominance. Brain Cogn 1987;6:450–463.

The Alien Hand

DAVID N. LEVINE

DEFINITION

The term *alien hand* has two related but distinct meanings in the neurologic literature. It means a patient's failure to recognize the actions of one of his hands as his own. It also refers to a patient's expression—verbal or nonverbal—that the actions of one of his hands are autonomous—not subject to his will—and that the hand is the agent of another being. Expressions of foreign control may occur without failure of recognition, but failure to recognize one's actions as one's own is usually accompanied by expressions of foreign control. Hence the failure to recognize the actions of one's limb as one's own can be considered an alien hand in the strong sense, whereas expression of foreign control is an alien hand in the weak sense.

HISTORY

The term alien hand was first used in the French literature, where it was defined in its strong sense. Brion and Jedynak (1) described "Le signe de la main étrangère" in four patients with tumor or vascular malformation involving the corpus callosum. Their first patient, a 41-year-old man,

> put on his shirt with difficulty, trying to find his sleeves behind his back, when by chance one hand grasped the other. He pulled, trying to disengage, and said "Let my hand go. You're preventing me from getting dressed."

Their second patient, a 56-year-old woman, was tested with her right hand holding her left behind her back: "What do you have in your right hand?" "A hand." "Whose is it?" "Not mine, anyway."

Brion and Jedynak defined the sign of the alien hand as the inability to recognize the left hand as one's own when the hands are clasped behind the back. The sign was present in the absence of any major defect of proprioception. The hand could be identified by touch as a hand but not as the patient's *own* hand. The sign was related in some way to hemiasomatognosia, but unlike the latter, the lack of recognition was selective for touch.

Brion and Jedynak emphasized the failure of recognition of the hand as one's own when the hand was encountered as a tactile object, as in their second patient. However, they also described the failure to recognize the left hand as one's own when it executed movements. Their first patient did not recognize his left hand as the one seizing his right hand. The failure in recognition was of the grasping hand that would not let go rather than of the object that was grasped, which was the other hand.

When "la main étrangère" was translated into the "alien hand" in the American neurologic literature, the meaning of the term changed from the strong sense of an objective failure to recognize authorship of movements to the weaker sense of an expression of a subjective feeling of foreign control. Bogen (2) described the alien hand in patients with transection of the corpus callosum as "a circumstance in which one of the patient's hands—the left hand in the right-handed patient—behaves in a way which the patient finds 'foreign,' 'alien' or at least uncooperative." He believed that this was possibly a minor form of intermanual conflict, a dissociative phenomenon in split-brain patients in which one hand acts at cross purposes to the other.

In fact, the feeling that movements of the left hand were of foreign origin was first reported by Goldstein (3), although he did not use the term alien hand. Goldstein's patient was a 57-year-old woman who suffered two strokes in a 2-year period. After the second stroke, her left leg could not move voluntarily. Her left arm was not paralyzed, but there was a strong grasp reflex, sensory loss to tactile and proprioceptive stimuli, and marked apraxia. The patient said that the arm

> did not belong to her but rather did what it wished. Once, the hand grabbed her throat and squeezed so tightly that she could tear it away only with much force. Likewise, it tore the bedsheets without her having willed it . . . She complained that the hand existed independent of her will. When it grabbed something, it would not let go. "I myself can do nothing with it. When I drink and it holds the cup, it will not loosen up, and [the liquid] spills. I hit it then and say, Keep still, my little hand" [laughs]. "There must be an evil spirit in the hand."

The patients described by Brion and Jedynak (1), Bogen (2), and Goldstein (3) all had lesions involving the corpus callosum, and the alien hand was on the left side. It was widely assumed that the alien hand was a manifestation of failure to transmit information from the dominant left hemisphere to the nondominant right hemisphere because of the callosal lesion. The right hemisphere, with uninjured motor areas, could still direct activities of the left arm, but not under the control of the left hemisphere, which controlled speech and much of the rest of the patient's behavior. The dominant left hemisphere was cut off from motor control of the left hand and from somatosensory information regarding its activities, accounting for the feeling that the movements of the left hand were foreign.

This view was called into question by Goldberg et al (4), who presented two patients with alien hand (in the weak sense) following left medial frontal cortex infarction. Their patients both had a strong right-sided grasp reflex and motor perseveration of the right hand. The affected hand would reach out to grasp objects, and the patients, although aware of the behavior, could not prevent its happening. Patient 2 reacted with dismay to such movements and indicated that she had not initiated the movements. She said that the arm "would not do what I want it to do." The important point of Goldberg and associates' paper is that in both cases the alien arm was the *right* arm, even though both patients were right-handed. This was inconsistent with the callosal disconnection theory, in which only the nondominant hand could be dissociated from the dominant hemisphere. Goldberg et al suggested that the alien hand sign was caused by damage to the contralateral medial frontal lobe, particularly the supplementary motor area. The latter was felt to program motor acts by matching the motor programs represented in the central gyri of lateral neocortex with inner drives and needs that are represented in limbic cortex. Previous cases attributed to callosal pathology might have been caused by damage to the nearby medial frontal cortex.

Subsequently, a case of ours (5) showed that an alien hand in the strong sense could be present without either callosal apraxia or a medial frontal grasp reflex. Our patient was a 79-year-old right-handed woman who awoke to find her left arm limp and feeling "like a dead fish." She had left homonymous hemianopia and severe left-sided somatosensory loss. Her left arm was grossly ataxic with no improvement in coordination by visual monitoring (opticosensory ataxia). There was no apraxia, in that movements of the left arm to command or in imitation were qualitatively correct, albeit very ataxic. Her symptoms were caused by a right temporo-occipital infarction, associated with occlusion of the posterior cerebral artery.

This patient treated her ataxic, insensate arm like an alien presence with hostile motivations. Occasionally the arm would spontaneously reach for her dressing gown or knock off her spectacles. At this time the patient would complain that the arm moved on its own and that "He wants to harm me." She often restrained the ataxic left arm with the normal right arm and later was observed to fondle and cajole the left arm, saying, "There, there, behave yourself now . . . Don't be naughty."

Recently, two cases similar to ours have been reported. Doody and Jankovic's (6) sixth patient was an 85-year-old woman with a large right temporo-occipital infarction and a lacunar infarction in the right internal capsule. The alien left hand showed "coarse movements" that were "goal directed, self destructive." The patient believed that the left hand was hostile and adjusted to it by treating it like her child. The patient of Ventura et al (7) was a 58-year-old woman with a right thalamic and internal capsule hemorrhage that caused left-sided somatosensory loss and hemianopia. The left hand was not recognized as her own when it was placed, behind her back, in her right hand. There were spontaneous levitating movements of the left hand, of which she reported that it was as if someone else were moving the arm.

DIAGNOSIS

The sign of the alien hand in the strong sense is present when a patient is unable to recognize that actions of his upper extremity are his own. This is best observed in the absence of vision. Brion and Jedynak (1) observed patients with their hands clasped behind the back. The patients could not discriminate whether their unaffected hand was being held by their own alien hand or by someone else's hand.

An alien hand in the weak sense is present when a patient says that the actions of one of his or her limbs are not subject to his or her will but are rather the products of a foreign intelligence. The patient may state this outright, or it may be revealed in his or her actions. The patient may struggle to restrain the uncooperative limb, punishing or admonishing it, or may otherwise personify it by talking to it or by referring to it in the third person.

When an alien hand in the strong sense is present, the belief in foreign control, even if not explicitly stated, is a genuine delusion. The first patient of Brion and Jedynak actually believed that someone else, not he himself, was holding onto his other hand. In contrast, the patient with an alien hand in the weak sense is not truly delusional. The expression of foreignness is more an "as if" expression than a statement implying belief. The arm behaves "as if" it were under foreign control. The expression is akin to that of a patient with derealization who, in stating that things are "unreal" is describing his or her state of mind more than he or she is expressing a belief that surrounding objects are illusory.

The sign of the alien hand resembles, but can generally be distinguished from, other conditions involving an abnormal attitude toward a limb. A patient with left hemiplegia may deny ownership of his or her left arm. This is commonly associated with denial of paralysis [anosognosia of Babinski (8)]. Encountering the inert and insensate limb, the patient, who believes himself fully mobile, may express the belief that the arm belongs to someone else or may believe it to be another object, such as a snake or a stick. Even when patients are aware of their paralysis, they may easily be deceived into mistaking their own hand for someone else's, or vice versa, if there is a major sensory loss in the affected limb. Some patients with chronic hemiplegia, without anosognosia or major sensory loss, personify the paralyzed limb, giving it a name, referring to it as "he" or "she," or addressing it as if it were a separate being, such as a pet or a child (9). Although the patient with an alien hand may share many of these behaviors of the patient with hemiplegia—failure to recognize by touch that the arm is his or her own, and personification of the arm—the arm is mobile and not paralyzed. The alien hand, as we have defined it, requires either lack of recognition or feeling of foreignness about movements of the affected limb.

Another symptom that must be distinguished from the alien hand is hemiasomatognosia. This refers to a patient's reporting that one side of the body or one limb is no longer there. This, again, may occur in patients with hemiplegia. At times the behavior is quite delusional, the patient believing that a limb has been surgically removed or asking the physician to help to find the missing limb. More often, however, the patient uses the expression of absence figuratively. Hemiasomatognosia may also occur in nonhemiplegic individuals. Most often this is in the context of a focal seizure, where the vivid sensation of absence of one side of the body may constitute part of the aura. The patient with an alien hand, like the hemiasomatognosic patient, lacks full appreciation of a body part. However, he or she does not feel that the limb is missing—that it no longer exists. Rather, he or she fails to appreciate what it is doing.

The alien hand has been reported to date in four clinical contexts:

1. Callosal lesions, particularly the body of the corpus callosum, caused by surgical transection, infarction, hemorrhage, or tumor. The nondominant hand is affected and may be alien in the strong as well as weak sense. Intermanual conflict is often prominent, and forced grasping is usually absent. Signs of interhemispheric disconnection are present,

most commonly apraxia, agraphia, and tactile anomia of the nondominant hand.

2. Infarction of the left medial frontal cortex, particularly the supplementary motor area. The contralateral, dominant right hand is affected and is alien in the weak sense. Forced grasping is prominent, as is motor perseveration of the affected hand, whereas signs of interhemispheric disconnection are absent.

3. Infarction or hemorrhage in the posterior right hemisphere, either temporo-occipital or posterior thalamic. The contralateral, nondominant left hand is affected and may be alien in the strong as well as weak sense. Its movements are ataxic, coarse, often levitating. Left somatosensory loss and left homonymous hemianopia are present. Forced grasping is absent, as are signs of interhemispheric disconnection.

4. Focal seizures, with the type of alien hand depending on the location of the underlying lesion. Leiguardia et al (10) reported four cases. Two involved lesions of the medial frontal cortex, one on the left and the other on the right. The contralateral arm groped and grasped purposefully and perseveratively, to the patient's dismay. The patients recognized the affected limbs as their own, although they moved involuntarily. The other two involved the parietal and the parietotemporal lobes, left and right respectively. The patients suddenly seemed unaware of the location and movements of the contralateral limbs, which seemed purposeless. The patient with the left-sided alien limb did not seem to recognize the limb as his own.

The lesions associated with the sign of the alien hand thus tend to involve the medial rather than the lateral portions of the cerebral hemisphere, perhaps because the latter commonly cause hemiplegia, precluding movement of the affected limb. The lesions—strokes and tumors—are readily imaged by computed tomography and magnetic resonance imaging scans.

PATHOGENESIS

There are several factors that contribute to a patient's expression that movements of a limb are autonomous and of alien origin. By definition the movements must be involuntary, that is, unintended by the patient. But clearly not all unintended movements are perceived as alien in origin. In the normal individual, movements of postural adjustment, fidgeting, and various habitual gestures occur frequently, without any intention or effort. These are not considered alien; in fact, most go completely unheeded by the individual. To be perceived as alien, the movements or their effects must be noticed, that is, the individual must be aware of their occurrence.

The criteria of awareness but lack of intention are still not sufficient to account for the sign of the alien hand. A mild tremor meets these criteria but is usually not reported as alien. It is generally the case that movements reported as alien are complex in the sense of appearing motivated, and interfere with the well-being or with the intended actions of the individual. Such acts include prehension of objects, including parts of the patient's clothing or body, or pushing aside and striking. Because such acts seem to be goal directed and because they are inconsistent with the patient's own goals, they are reported as alien.

Thus, the patient with medial frontal infarction, who has not only a tactile grasp reflex but also the more complex "instinctive grasp reflex" of Denny-Brown (11), cannot prevent the contralateral arm from reaching out for objects seen as he or she walks about. The inability to release the grasp can impede progress toward an intended destination. The result may be frustration, dismay, and forcible restraint of the offending arm by the one that is intact. The patient may express lack of control over the affected limb, using language that attributes to the limb a mind of its own.

Another consideration influencing the likelihood that a patient will attribute independent existence to one of his or her limbs may be the patient's underlying personality. Critchley (9) has pointed out that some patients tend to personify diseased organs—not just limbs, but also viscera (peptic ulcer, for example). Perhaps patients who tend to be gregarious, uninhibited, and playful (5) may be more inclined to personify an abnormal limb.

Under some circumstances, the alien hand may develop in the strong sense; that is, the patient may not merely express a feeling of lack of control but may also be genuinely unaware that movements of the alien limb are his or her own. These circumstances are not entirely clear, but to date the alien hand in a strong sense has been reported only in the nondominant extremity, associated either with lesions of the body of the corpus callosum or with posterior hemispheric lesions causing somatosensory loss and hemianopia. This suggests that for the alien hand to develop in the strong sense, the patient—or at least that aspect that speaks and dominates behavior—must be deprived of information about the activities of the affected limb. This is generally not the case with uncomplicated medial frontal infarction that spares both the corpus callosum and the sensory system. There the patient is aware that it is his or her limb that is grasping, even though the patient cannot prevent it. His or her expressions of foreignness are in principle no different from what might occur in other movement disorders of acute onset, such as myoclonus or chorea. Only the purposeful quality of the grasping predisposes to expressions of an alien intelligence.

After acute callosal section the left hemisphere, which is the source of speech and generally dominates the patient's behavior, is no longer in full control of movements of the left hand. These are mediated by the disconnected, non-dominant, right hemisphere. Moreover, the dominant hemisphere is also cut off from somatosensory input from the left hand. The patient is thus verbally unaware of what the left hand has done unless the action occurs in the right visual field. In circumstances such as those used by Brion and Jedynak (1)—hands out of sight, behind the back—the

patient may be verbally unable to determine whether actions of the left hand are his actions or those of another person.

A similar lack of information about activities of the affected limb was present in the cases (5) with marked somatosensory loss in the left hand and left hemianopia. In such cases, minor movements, of postural adjustment for example, may be grossly exaggerated so that the limb can strike the patient. Because the movements are unintended, and because the patients lack the sensory feedback to determine their origin once their exaggerated character brings them to notice, the patients genuinely do not know at first that they have been struck by their own arm.

Thus, the alien hand is probably not a single symptom/sign. It can at least be divided into strong and weak forms. The strong alien hand sign requires true lack of recognition that movements of a limb are one's own, that is, the inability to discriminate whether such a movement is one's own or that of another person. The weak alien hand sign involves verbal expression that the arm is autonomous or other behavior, such as personifying a limb, in which the patient treats the limb as though it had a life of its own.

MANAGEMENT

The alien hand sign, whether strong or weak, can be caused by a variety of diseases of the brain, including stroke, tumor, or trauma. The treatment of these various conditions is beyond the scope of this article.

From a symptomatic standpoint, the alien hand can be a source of dismay, anxiety, and frustration. These symptoms often respond to the physician's reassurance that such phenomena are not unexpected in the patient's illness and (in conditions such as stroke or callosal section) that improvement is likely.

Little that is more specific can be offered. Patients with an uncontrolled grasp reflex, who reach for things as they walk, can be treated by keeping the affected limb occupied during ambulation. For example, a cane can be held in the hand (4). The patient of Levine and Rinn (5), whose ataxic movements appeared to arise from exaggerated unintentional fidgeting or gesturing, appeared to respond to exercises in progressive muscle relaxation.

REFERENCES

1. Brion S, Jedynak CP. Troubles du transfert interhemispherique (callosal disconnection). A propos de trois observations de tumeurs du corps calleux. Le signe de la main étrangère. Rev Neurol 1972;126:257–266.
2. Bogen JE. The callosal syndrome. In: Heilman KM, Valenstein E, ed. Clinical neuropsychology. New York: Oxford University Press, 1979:308–359.
3. Goldstein K. Zur Lehre der motorischen Apraxie. J Psychol Neurol 1908;11:169–187, 270–283.
4. Goldberg G, Mayer NH, Toglia JV. Medial frontal cortex infarction and the alien hand sign. Arch Neurol 1981;36:683–686.
5. Levine DN, Rinn WE. Opticosensory ataxia and alien hand syndrome after posterior cerebral artery territory infarction. Neurology 1986;36:1094–1097.

6. Doody RS, Jankovic J. The alien hand and related signs. J Neurol Neurosurg Psychiatry 1992;55:806–810.

7. Ventura MG, Goldman S, Hildebrand J. Alien hand syndrome without a corpus callosum lesion. J Neurol Neurosurg Psychiatry 1995;58:735–737.

8. Babinski J. Contribution a l'etude des troubles mentaux dans l'hemiplegie cérébrale (anosognosie). Rev Neurol 1914;27:845–847.

9. Critchley M. Misoplegia, or hatred of hemiplegia. Mt Sinai J Med 1974;41:82–87.

10. Leiguardia R, Starkstein S, Nagues M, et al. Paroxysmal alien hand syndrome. J Neurol Neurosurg Psychiatry 1993;56:788–792.

11. Denny-Brown D. The nature of apraxia. J Nerv Ment Dis 1958;126:9–33.

Primitive Reflexes in Psychiatry and Neurology

Neil W. Kowall   Stephen A. Berman

GENERAL REMARKS AND DEFINITIONS

Primitive reflexes (PRs) are patterned motor responses to specific tactile stimuli that are normally present in infants, less frequently seen in normal adults, and found with greater frequency in the elderly and in those with assorted neuro-psychiatric disorders (1). Since they exist in hydranen-cephalic infants (2,3), their genesis is thought to rely on spinal and brainstem mechanisms. There is no unanimity of opinion regarding the definition of primitive reflexes. In general, a superficial tactile stimulus is applied to the face or hand and the reflex response is observed locally, with one exception (the palmomental reflex). Included within the category of reflexes elicited by tactile facial stimulation are perioral reflexes such as the suck, snout, and rooting reflexes. Reflexes involving ocular or periocular stimulation include the glabellar and corneomandibular reflexes. Reflexes elicited by hand (or foot) stimulation include the grasping and groping reflexes. The palmomental reflex is elicited by hand stimulation, the reflexive action being observed in the ipsilateral mentalis muscle. There has been a long debate concerning whether primitive reflexes found in adults without other evidence of neurologic impairment should be considered normal phenomena.

HISTORICAL REVIEW

John Hughlings Jackson originally posited a hierarchical concept of the nervous system, in which higher centers inhibit the reflexive function of more primitive or lower centers (4). Dysfunction at higher levels releases the sup-pressed activity of more primitive centers; so activities nor-mally seen in infants are lost as the nervous system matures, only to reappear in aging or illness.

The significance of primitive reflexes as indicators of disease has been controversial. The uncertain significance of perioral reflexes was noted as early as 1903 by Toulouse and Verpas (5), and the controversy regarding these reflexes persists today. The corneomandibular reflex was originally described by von Solder (6) in 1902 and subsequently redis-covered several times. He originally considered the reflex a reliable indicator of a pathologic process but subsequently found a less exaggerated form in half of normal subjects. Gordon and Bender (7) provide an extensive historical review of this reflex. The palmomental reflex was discovered by Marinesco and Radovici (8) in 1920 in a patient with amyotrophic lateral sclerosis and prominent corticobulbar signs. They also initially felt that this reflex was always associated with brain disease but later found the reflex in half of normal controls. Blake and Kunkle (9) provide a more extensive historical review of the palmomental reflex. The glabellar tap was first described by Overend (10) in 1896 and has been classically associated with Parkinson's disease. Pearce et al (11) review the literature concerning this reflex.

METHODS OF ELICITATION

Prior to elicitation of any primitive reflexes, some general points must be considered (1,12). The patient should not be anxious and the procedure should be explained. In all cases, except the corneomandibular and glabellar, the eyes should be closed.

Perioral reflexes include the suck, snout, and rooting reflexes (13). The suck reflex is elicited by stroking the lips with a tongue blade or flexed index finger. If the lips suck, the reflex is present. The snout reflex is elicited by firm pressure on the philtrum; pursing of the lips or pouting is a positive reflex. Alternatively, the philtrum may be tapped with a hammer. There may be puckering, protrusion, or elevation of the lower lip. The reflex does not fatigue. The corner of the mouth is stroked with a tongue blade to elicit the rooting reflex. Movement of the corner of the mouth to the object is a positive response.

Periocular reflexes are the glabellar tap and corneomandibular reflex. The glabellar tap is performed by tapping between the eyebrows with a finger and observing eyelid movement. There is no visual threat, and the patient is asked not to blink. Persistence beyond nine taps is considered abnormal. The corneomandibular reflex is produced by gentle backward pressure of the gloved index finger (12) or wick (1) on the cornea (12) with the eyelids held open. If positive, a brief deviation of the jaw away from the stimulated side due to action of the ipsilateral lateral pterygoid muscle is produced. This reflex rapidly fatigues.

Reflexes elicited by appendicular stimulation include the grasping and groping reflexes and palmomental reflex. The grasping and groping reflexes are tested by distracting the patient, who sits with hands on his or her lap, palms up, as the palms are stroked lightly. If the patient grasps the examiner's hands, he or she is asked not to. If the grasp response persists on repeat, it is considered positive. The palmomental reflex is performed by vigorous stroke of a thumbnail or key along the thenar eminence. The stimulus should be disagreeable but not painful (9). If the ipsilateral mentalis muscle contracts, the reflex is positive, even if it extinguishes. The reflex usually extinguishes after three or four trials and then returns in 30 seconds (12).

SIGNIFICANCE IN CLINICAL DIAGNOSIS

Normal Aging

There is a striking lack of consistency in the literature regarding the frequency of primitive reflexes in the normal population. Estimates range from 2% to 58% (9,12). Although, generally, each primitive reflex was originally considered abnormal by the author(s) who defined it, many practicing neurologists now interpret these signs either as variations of normal or as abnormalities so nonspecific they have virtually no impact on diagnosis or case management. Most typical are the positions of Franceschi (14) and Blake and Kunkle (9), who hold that primitive reflexes are only abnormal in the presence of other signs. Support for such a view can be found in the work of Reis (15), who found electrical evidence of a palmomental reflex in all patients examined if the stimulus was strong enough. Furthermore, he could elicit mentalis contraction following stimulation anywhere on the body surface. Because most abnormalities suggested by PRs increase in frequency with advancing age, the relationship between the primitive reflexes and aging itself has been a central part of the controversy. Jacobs and Gossman (12) found an age-related increase in the frequency of snout, corneomandibular, and palmomental reflexes. They

describe a characteristic pattern of appearance of these reflexes. The palmomental reflex appears earliest and most frequently and, like the snout reflex, may be found in isolation. The corneomandibular reflex was only found when one of these reflexes was also present. One or more of these three reflexes were found in about 50% of 105 normal subjects (aged 20–88). Koller and associates (16) found that the snout reflex and to a lesser extent the glabellar reflex are correlated with increasing age. The corneomandibular and glabellar reflex are much less frequent (<10%) and are more often associated with disease (16).

Franceschi (14), however, found no relationship between age and incidence of primitive reflexes, and Jensen et al (17) found that the palmomental reflex and glabellar tap did not increase in occurrence with increasing age. More recently, investigators have approached the issue by employing community-dwelling healthy controls as opposed to controls picked from hospitalized populations. A study by Nichols et al (18) and a very large study of 537 subjects by Waite et al (19) used rigorous batteries of medical and neurologic examinations to help ensure that the controls were healthy aged subjects. Neither study found an increase in primitive reflexes with aging. Despite methodologic differences between the studies, they both reached the conclusion that occurrence of primitive reflexes with aging was not the norm and that such changes probably represent actual disease. No study, however, has been able to demonstrate that such reflexes are diagnostic of any particular neurologic disease.

Localization of the presumed damage is speculative. For example, Gordon and Bender's study of the corneomandibular reflex agrees with the conclusions of Nichols et al and Waite et al in that they found only one weakly positive reflex among 300 normal controls (7). In attempting to localize the lesion in the abnormal patients, they concluded that this reflex could derive from both bilateral cerebral disease and suprapontine brainstem lesions. They also observed that 10% to 15% of patients have a corneomental response due to mentalis contraction. Ansink (20) examined the physiologic and pathologic basis of the corneomandibular, perioral, and palmomental reflexes. He concluded that the corneomandibular reflex often signifies damage to the ventral midbrain and that perioral and palmomental reflexes indicate increased reflex irritability due to diffuse cerebral insults.

The high incidence of corneomandibular reflex (34% of normal patients over 65) reported by Ansink probably relates to his use of intense and long-lasting corneal stimulation and mechanical measurement of jaw response. Likewise, the influence of intensity of stimulation and sensitivity of measurement probably explains the results of Reis (15), who used electrodiagnostic equipment to find a palmomental reflex in every subject. As these signs are standardly elicited, the largest, most recent, and best controlled studies indicate that a strong positive response for several primitive reflexes is not a normal adult finding, even in the aged. But, by themselves, such findings offer no etiologic and little anatomic specificity. We will next consider the primitive reflexes in the context of several nervous system diseases.

Dementia

Paulson and Gottlieb (1) found that primitive reflexes are of limited use as predictors of dementia and generally indicate diffuse bilateral and irreversible central nervous system disease. Tweedy et al (13) found that snout and grasp reflexes correlate with cognitive dysfunction, whereas glabellar, suck, root, and palmomental reflexes do not. They correlate better with computed tomographic (CT) evidence of ventricular dilatation than with cortical atrophy, suggesting that they indicate supranuclear motor dysfunction rather than dementia. Huff and Growdon (21) found that suck, snout, and grasp reflexes were associated with dementia, as determined by the Blessed Dementia Scale, independent of age. Jenkyn et al (22) found that the glabellar reflex and suck reflex were associated with diffuse cortical dysfunction as determined by neuropsychologic and mental function tests and neurologic examination. They suggested that these reflexes be used as part of a battery of 13 items to screen for diffuse cortical dysfunction. Koller et al (16) reported that snout and glabellar reflexes do not correlate with psychometric testing or atrophy on CT, although glabellar reflex was more common in demented patients. They concluded that they have little clinical value in evaluation of the elderly. Similarly, Moylan and Saldias (23) found no correlation between suck, snout, grasp, glabellar blink, and palmomental reflexes and atrophy on CT scan. Gordon and Bender (7) found that the corneo-mandibular reflex reflects corneomandibular hyperreflexia, most often as a result of severe bilateral cerebral or brainstem lesions associated with a decreased level of consciousness. Its localizing value is limited, but it is usually a result of suprapontine damage.

A large, more recent study by Molloy et al (24) examined 136 patients known to have Alzheimer's dementia (AD). They assessed both the cognitive status and the activities of daily living. Although the studies did not show a correlation between cognitive level and the existence of primitive reflexes, those with prominent primitive reflexes had more behavioral problems and more difficulties performing the activities of daily living. They also manifested more rigidity, gait abnormalities, and apraxia. It is possible that some of the older studies erred by considering only the presence or absence of primitive reflexes but not the preponderance of a combination of many PRs present simultaneously. Vreeling et al (25) compared three patient groups: normal aged, aged with vascular dementia, and aged with AD. Both of the dementia groups differed from the normal group in the preponderance of PRs. No individual reflex or group of reflexes could distinguish vascular dementia from AD, but there appeared to be a relationship between severity of dementia and the number of PRs present in a given

patient. Sinisi et al (26) studied 128 elderly individuals living in retirement homes. They examined for PRs and other neurologic and physical findings and used standardized scales such as the Hachinski dementia score and the Plutchik GRS score. They found that the simultaneous presence of the snout reflex, glabellar tap response, and palmomental reflex was highly correlated with the presence of dementia. With respect to following the cognitive decline of Alzheimer's patients, Franssen et al (27) found that both extrapyramidal and pyramidal signs, mainly expressed as bradykinesia, showed some correlation with cognitive impairment, but the PRs per se did not. Davous et al (28) found that rigidity and loss of optokinetic nystagmus correlated with the dementia severity in Alzheimer's disease. Thus, it appears that a large number of easily elicited PRs should raise a reasonable suspicion of a possible dementing illness, but they do not signify which type or the severity. Rigidity and bradykinesia, which are not PRs but which are easily elicited neurologic signs, may correlate somewhat with either the cognitive decline or, alternatively, with other aspects of functional impairment.

Parkinsonism

The glabellar reflex is usually present in Parkinson's patients (>80%) and often resolves with L-dopa therapy. Klawans and Paulson (29) consider the glabellar tap sign the best monitor of severity in Parkinson's disease (PD), and Klawans and Goodwin (30) found that L-dopa treament could abolish the sign. Pearce et al (11) examined the sensitivity and specificity of the glabellar tap reflex in parkinsonism and found a high degree of sensitivity but a lack of specificity. Many (13 in 56) patients with widespread cerebral pathology also had a positive reflex. They note that the palmomental reflex may be the first sign of Parkinson's disease. Gossman and Jacobs (31) found that the incidence of the palmomental and snout reflexes in parkinsonism patients was not different from age-matched controls, but that the corneomandibular reflex was 2.5 times more frequent in parkinsonism patients, suggesting that this reflex is pathologically exaggerated in parkinsonism. Maertens de Noordhout and Delwaide (32) found a palmomental reflex in 16% of controls and 71% of parkinsonian patients. They noted an increased incidence in patients with akinesia and a decreased incidence in patients with dyskinesia. Klawans and Paulson (29) also noted an increased incidence of the palmomental reflex in Parkinson's disease. Jensen et al (17) noted that the glabellar sign and the palmomental reflex are almost as frequent in intracranial disease that does not affect the basal ganglia as they are in basal ganglia disease, thus limiting their diagnostic value. Pearse and colleagues also consider primitive reflexes to be dependent nonspecifically on the degree of cerebral degeneration (11).

With respect to disease progression, the number and intensity of PRs appear to increase with time in patients with Parkinson's disease (33), and such changes probably correlate with worsening severity (34). The number of PRs present in the same patient appears to show correlation with cognitive decline, according to Vreeling et al (35), though the authors stress that the reflexes must be elicited and scored via a standardized protocol. In a study of the palmomental, snout, grasp, corneomandibular, and glabellar reflexes in patients with Parkinson's disease, the corneomandibular reflex was more frequently observed in demented Parkinson's disease patients than in the nondemented. The others, individually, did not appear to predict dementia in Parkinson's disease.

Psychiatric Disease

Keshavan and Yeragani (36) note that primitive reflexes may occur more frequently in patients with psychotic disorders than in normal subjects. They may correlate with the severity and chronicity of the psychosis, and longitudinal studies suggest that primitive reflexes may be reversible in schizophrenic and affective psychosis. Burra et al (37) report a case of atypical affective illness associated with snout, grasp, sucking, and glabellar tap reflexes that resolved on two separate occasions over a 2-year period after the psychosis was treated. The patient made a dramatic recovery, including loss of primitive reflexes, when electroconvulsive therapy was administered during the second admission. Lohr (38) reported two patients, aged 29 and 35, with criteria for schizophrenia according to the *Diagnostic and Statistical Manual of Mental Disorders, Third Edition*, who exhibited transient grasp reflexes. Huber and Paulson (34) found no association between grasp, palmomental, and corneomandibular reflexes and depression in patients with Parkinson's disease. Youssef and Waddington (39) reported an interesting association between PRs and tardive dyskinesias in patients with either schizophrenia or bipolar disorder. They speculate that an underlying developmental abnormality may underlie both PRs and tardive dyskinesias. An attempt to replicate these findings in a younger population of schizophrenic patients showed no association between PRs and tardive dyskinesia or cognitive dysfunction in the schizophrenic patients (40). However, it did demonstrate a high yield of PRs in the schizophrenic patients, and the authors suggest that the PRs in themselves could reflect either a neurodevelopmental abnormality or a neurodegeneration that may be related to the schizophrenia (40).

Trauma and Cerebrovascular Disease

Isakov et al (41) examined the palmomental, snout, and corneomandibular reflexes in patients after stroke or cranial trauma and found no difference from age-matched controls when each reflex was considered individually (43% versus 35%). All three reflexes were abnormal in 13% of brain-damaged subjects, compared with none of the 100 controls. Botvin et al (42) found that the presence of primitive reflexes was negatively related to favorable outcome after

stroke, but less so than mental status measures such as orientation and aphasia.

Mori and Yamadori (43) found that an ipsilateral unilateral grasp reflex was seen commonly (29%) in patients with right hemispheric damage but rarely (4%) in those with left hemispheric lesions. The lesion sites were either persylvian or subcortical.

HIV Disease

In recent years several studies of individuals positive for the human immunodeficiency virus (HIV) and matched HIV-negative controls have shown that HIV-positive persons, and especially those with frank acquired immunodeficiency syndrome (AIDS), have an increased incidence of primitive reflexes (44–47). Marder et al (47) studied 123 HIV-positive and 84 HIV-negative homosexual men for 4.5 years and found increased development of primitive reflexes as well as extrapyramidal signs in the HIV-positive group. Orefice et al (45) examined the snout, palmomental, and glabellar reflexes in 106 HIV-positive patients without neurologic symptoms and found a significant increase in the presence of one or more primitive reflexes in the HIV-1-positive individuals. In addition, two or more primitive reflexes were never seen in the HIV-1-negative group, but they were frequently observed in the HIV-1-positive group, particularly in the more advanced stages. The authors conclude that the primitive reflexes may be an important early sign of neurologic involvement. In a large study in Tanzania, a culture in which HIV-1 positivity is generally not associated with either homosexuality or injection of intravenous drugs, the presence of the suck reflex and the palmomental reflex was significantly increased in HIV-1-positive individuals compared with controls and was still higher in severely ill AIDS patients. The prevalence of the signs increased with the HIV stage and with the presence of AIDS-related neurologic disorders (44).

Two small studies, however, raise cautionary notes about the interpretation of the primitive reflex sings. Manji et al found that the presence of primitive reflexes did not, in isolation, serve as a marker for HIV encephalopathy in otherwise asymptomatic patients (48). And Madlener et al found that the presence of the palmomental reflex did not by itself predict the later development of encephalopathy in HIV patients (49). The study of Manji et al contained only 8 symptomatic AIDS patients, and the investigation of Madlener et al was able to follow up on only 47 of the original 143-patient group at 6 months and only 18 at 12 months. In addition, they did not study combinations of abnormal reflexes. Nonetheless, these latter two investigations remind us that correlation with the presence of an already known condition, or even with the stages of the condition, is not the same as the ability to make useful predictions about the course of the disease. We believe that more work must be done to evaluate the usefulness of the PRs in following the HIV-positive individual.

THEORETICAL IMPLICATIONS

Blake and Kunkle (9) theorized that the palmomental reflex is a fragmentary wince reaction. Reis (15) postulated that the palmomental reflex is a fragment of a general nociceptive response present normally. He elicited mentalis contraction following cutaneous stimulation anywhere on the body surface. As the stimulus intensity was increased, a wince was elicited. Jacobs and Gossman (12) also consider the palmomental, corneomandibular, and snout reflexes to be fragments of facial expression and emotion, such as wincing, startling, or crying, that are integrated in the brainstem. These fragmentary expressions are normally suppressed in the mature nervous system, only to be reexpressed by aging or by pathologic states that disinhibit the subsequently imposed inhibitory influences. The sensitivity of the glabellar response to treatment of Parkinson's disease has led to speculation that it is related to loss of inhibition mediated through dopaminergic pathways (50). However, an attempt by Huber and Paulson to correlate the response to dopamine levels in parkinsonian patients showed no relationship to blood levels of dopamine (50). In the future, it may be possible to test specific pathways using functional magnetic resonance imaging (MRI), positron emission tomography scan, or single photon emission computed tomography (SPECT) technology. Using electrophysiologic measurements of index finger abduction after cutaneous stimulation, Fuhr et al (51) showed weaker inhibition in PD patients. The inhibition could be partially normalized with dopaminergic treatment.

CONCLUSION

Our understanding of the significance of PRs has evolved somewhat from the late 1980s, at which time an editorial (52) stated that they were of uncertain value in the clinical examination of adult patients. The prior studies were done in the context of an earlier overestimation of the diagnostic value of PRs, and they showed, quite correctly, that individual abnormal reflexes could frequently be found in otherwise normal individuals. More recent work has differed in several ways. First, there has been more attention to standardization, not only of the tests for the PRs themselves but also in the choice of normal control groups. The best studies now use controls living in the community as opposed to patients with diseases other than the one under immediate consideration. Second, the investigators have asked more refined questions. Although the various studies are still rather individualistic in comparison with the large cooperative studies that have been done for stroke and heart disease, the following specific questions have been coherently addressed. Do the PRs occur as a part of normal aging? Can the PRs sensitively distinguish between a normal and an abnormal nervous system? Can the PRs distinguish between different abnormalities of the nervous system? If the abnormality is already known, can the PRs function as an index of disease

progress and/or adequacy of treatment? Finally, the recent studies have been much larger and, thus, there have been sufficient patients to examine the effect of multiple PRs present in the same patient as well as the ease in eliciting the reflexes.

We believe that some of the questions posed in the preceding paragraph now have reasonably firm answers. With respect to normal aging, one can state that it is quite unusual at any age for a normal individual to have several (i.e., three or more) easily elicited PRs of the type discussed in this review. As a corollary to this finding, it appears that the presence of several easily elicited PRs does serve as an indicator of the existence of some neurologic disease. Nevertheless, the clinician must be aware that no study has produced sensitivity and specificity data for the standard neurologic examination that would allow the calculation of a specific probability and confidence interval. The same, however, is true for most other signs (e.g., cogwheeling, Babinski sign, reflex asymmetry) elicited by the neurologic exam.

With respect to individual diseases, there is no good evidence that the PRs possess diagnostic specificity. Once the diagnosis is known, however, they may give useful insights. For example, the glabellar tap response may serve as a good indication of the progression of Parkinson's disease or the adequacy of treatment, particularly for the physician well experienced in following the disease. It is not clear, however, that exclusion of this sign from the diagnostic armamentarium would worsen the physician's diagnostic or therapeutic performance. Also, it has not been shown that a neophyte physician could substitute this sign for a more complete examination and thereby adequately monitor the Parkinson's patient without an extensive knowledge of the natural history of Parkinson's disease.

Another interesting possibility is that physicians might use the PRs to focus more attention on the nervous system of a patient with AIDS. Certainly, recent advances in AIDS treatment suggest that early treatment might now be beneficial, and one could theorize that treating central nervous system AIDS very early might forestall permanent damage. But the reader must also be aware that no study has demonstrated the usefulness of incorporating these signs into the treatment decision. Clearly, one must not interpret the absence of PRs as a reason to forego other, more definitive, examinations of the nervous system. Their presence, however, should certainly raise some concern.

In conclusion, we believe that the modern clinician should not dismiss the PRs as useless relics. In the specific contexts noted above, they appear capable of offering some useful clinical information. However, they still must be interpreted in the context of other findings from the history, the overall medical examination, and laboratory tests. In such a framework they may help to create a more complete picture of the clinical state of the patient and his or her response to the surrounding environment.

REFERENCES

1. Paulson G, Gottlieb G. Development reflexes: the reappearance of foetal and neonatal reflexes in aged patients. Brain 1968;91:37–52.
2. Hamby W. Hydranencephaly: clinical diagnosis, presentation of 7 cases. Pediatrics 1950;6:371–383.
3. Halsey J, Allen N, Chamberlin H. Chronic decerebrate state in infancy, neurologic observations in long surviving cases of hydranencephaly. Arch Neurol 1968;19:339–346.
4. Jackson JH. Evolution and dissolution of the nervous system. In: Taylor J, ed. Selected writings of John Hughlings Jackson. London: Hodder and Stoughton, 1932;2:3–118.
5. Toulouse ED, Verpas CL. La reflexe buccale. Compt Rend Soc Biol 1903;55:952–953.
6. Solder F von. Der corneomandibular reflex. Neurol Centralb 1902;21:111–113.
7. Gordon RM, Bender MB. The corneomandibular reflex. J Neurol Neurosurg Psychiatry 1971;34:236–242.
8. Marinesco G, Radovici A. Sur un reflexe cutane nouveau: Reflexe palmomentinnier. Rev Neurol 1920;27:237–240.
9. Blake JR Jr, Kunkle EC. The palmomental reflex. A physiological and clinical analysis. Arch Neurol Psychiatry 1951;65:337–345.
10. Overend W. Preliminary note on a new cranial reflex. Lancet 1896;i:619.
11. Pearce J, Aziz H, Gallagher JC. Primitive reflex activity in primary and symptomatic parkinsonism. J Neurol Neurosurg Psychiatry 1968;31:501–508.
12. Jacobs L, Gossman MD. Three primitive reflexes in normal adults. Neurology 1980;30:184–188.
13. Tweedy J, Reding M, Garcia C, et al. Significance of cortical disinhibition signs. Neurology 1982;32:169–173.
14. Franceschi M. Three primitive reflexes in normal adults. Neurology 1981;31:225. Letter.
15. Reis DJ. The palmomental reflex. A fragment of a general nociceptive skin reflex: a physiological study in normal man. Arch Neurol 1961;4:486–498.
16. Koller WC, Glatt S, Wilson RS, Fox JH. Primitive reflexes and cognitive function in the elderly. Ann Neurol 1982;12:302–304.
17. Jensen JPA, Gron U, Pakkenberg H. Comparison of three primitive reflexes in neurological patients and in normal individuals. J Neurol Neurosurg Psychiatry 1983;46:162–167.
18. Nichols ME, Meador KJ, Loring DW, et al. Age-related changes in the neurologic examination of healthy sexagenarians, octogenarians, and centenarians. J Geriatr Psychiatry Neurol 1994;7:1–7.
19. Waite LM, Broe GA, Creasey H, et al. Neurological signs, aging, and the neurodegenerative syndromes. Arch Neurol 1996;53:498–502.
20. Ansink BJJ. Physiologic and clinical investigations into 4 brain stem reflexes. Neurology 1962;12:320–328.
21. Huff FJ, Growdon JH. Neurological abnormalities associated with severity of dementia in Alzheimer's disease. Can J Neurol Sci 1986;13:403–405.
22. Jenkyn LR, Walsh DB, Culver CM, Reeves AG. Clinical signs in diffuse cerebral dysfunction. J Neurol Neurosurg Psychiatry 1977;40:956–966.
23. Moylan JJ, Saldias CA. Developmental reflexes and cortical atrophy. Ann Neurol 1979;5:499–500. Letter.
24. Molloy DW, Clarnette RM, McIlroy WE, et al. Clinical significance of primitive reflexes in Alzheimer's disease. J Am Geriatr Soc 1991;39:1160–1163.
25. Vreeling FW, Houx PJ, Jolles J, Verhey FR. Primitive reflexes in Alzheimer's disease and vascular dementia. J Geriatr Psychiatry Neurol 1995;8:111–117.
26. Sinisi L, De Michele G, Mansi D, et al. Relationship of neurological and psychological signs to physical and metabolic risk factors in elderly persons living in retirement facilities: a multidisciplinary approach. Funct Neurol 1989;4:277–282.
27. Franssen EH, Kluger A, Torossian CL, Reisberg B. The neurologic syndrome of severe Alzheimer's disease. Relationship to functional decline. Arch Neurol 1993;50:1029–1039.
28. Davous P, Lamour Y, Roudier M. Standardized neurologic study in senile dementia of Alzheimer's type [in French]. Encephale 1989;15:387–396.
29. Klawans HL Jr, Paulson GW. Primitive reflexes in parkinsonism. Confin Neurol 1971;33:25–32.
30. Klawans HL Jr, Goodwin JA. Reversal of the glabellar reflex in Parkinsonism by L-dopa. J Neurol Neurosurg Psychiatry 1969;32:423–427.
31. Gossman MD, Jacobs L. Three primitive reflexes in parkinsonism patients. Neurology 1980;30:189–192.
32. Maertens de Noordhout A, Delwaide PJ. The palmomental reflex in Parkinson's disease. Comparison with normal subjects and clinical relevance. Arch Neurol 1988;45:425–427.
33. de Groot MC, Trommel J, Gips CH. Developmental reflexes and parkinsonism in mentally disturbed aged: a 1-year follow-up study [in Dutch]. Gerontologie 1980;11:144–146.
34. Huber SJ, Paulson GW. Relationship between primitive reflexes and severity in Parkinson's disease. J Neurol Neurosurg Psychiatry 1986;49:1298–1300.
35. Vreeling FW, Verhey FR, Houx PJ, Jolles J. Primitive reflexes in Parkinson's disease. J Neurol Neurosurg Psychiatry 1993;56:1323–1326.
36. Keshavan MS, Yeragani VK. Primitive reflexes in psychiatry. Lancet 1987;i:1264. Letter.
37. Burra P, Powles WE, Riopelle RJ, Ferguson M. Atypical psychosis with reversible primitive reflexes. Can J Psychiatry 1980;25:74–77.
38. Lohr JB. Transient grasp reflexes in schizophrenia. Biol Psychiatry 1985;20:172–175.
39. Youssef HA, Waddington JL. Primitive (developmental) reflexes and diffuse cerebral dysfunction in schizophrenia and bipolar affective disorder: overrepresentation in patients with tardive dyskinesia. Biol Psychiatry 1988;23:791–796.
40. Barnes TR, Crichton P, Nelson HE, Halstead S. Primitive (developmental) reflexes, tardive dyskinesia and intellectual impairment in schizophrenia. Schizophr Res 1995;16:47–52.
41. Isakov E, Sazbon L, Costeff H, et al. The diagnostic value of three common primitive reflexes. Eur Neurol 1984;23:17–21.
42. Botvin JG, Keith RA, Johnston MV. Relationship between primitive reflexes in stroke patients and rehabilitation outcome. Stroke 1978;9:256–258.
43. Mori E, Yamadori A. Unilateral hemispheric injury and ipsilateral instinctive grasp reaction. Arch Neurol 1985;42:485–488.
44. Howlett WP, Nkya WM, Kvale G, Nilssen S. The snout and palmomental reflexes in HIV disease in Tanzania. Acta Neurol Scand 1995;91:470–476.
45. Orefice G, Carrieri PB, Troisi E, et al. Three primitive reflexes in HIV-1-infected individuals: a possible clinical marker of early central nervous system involvement. Acta Neurol (Napoli) 1993;15:409–415.
46. Thomas P, Pesce A, Vinti H, et al. Palmo-mental reflex and anti-HIV seropositivity [in French]. Ann Med Interne (Paris) 1989;140:740–741.
47. Marder K, Liu X, Stern Y, et al. Neurologic signs and symptoms in a cohort of homosexual men followed for 4.5 years. Neurology 1995;45:261–267.
48. Manji H, Connolly S, McAllister R, et al. Primitive reflexes and the bedside antisaccadic eye movement test in HIV asymptomatics—the Middlesex Hospital MRC Cohort Study. Int Conf AIDS 1992;8:104.
49. Madlener J, Enzensberger W, Herdt P, et al. Palmomental reflex in immunocompromised HIV patients. Int Conf AIDS 1993;9:429.
50. Huber SJ, Paulson GW. Influence of dopamine and disease severity on primitive reflexes in Parkinson's disease. Eur Neurol 1989;29:141–144.
51. Fuhr P, Zeffiro T, Hallett M. Cutaneous reflexes in Parkinson's disease. Muscle Nerve 1992;15:733–739.
52. Forgotten symptoms and primitive signs. Lancet 1987;i:841–842. Editorial.

Mirror Movements

ANDREW G. HERZOG   HERBERT F. DURWEN

INTRODUCTION

In 1874, Westphal (1) described in hemiplegic patients involuntary limb movements that were identical to simultaneous contralateral voluntary movements. In 1879, Erlenmeyer (2) applied to them the term "mirror movements." Since then, different reports have suggested that mirror movements have a number of characteristic features. They occur predominantly with finger movements (3–7). They are more prominent with increased effort of muscle contraction, repetition of movement, and in the setting of weakness (3–7). They can be voluntarily suppressed, at least to some extent. They are normally present during childhood (3–8), but can occasionally persist into adolescence and adulthood with (7,9,10) or without (4,11–17) associated neurologic or behavioral findings. Persistent mirror movements can be familial (18). Mirror movements appear under pathologic conditions in association with pyramidal deficits, especially in individuals with hemiplegia or evidence of congenital brain damage (19,20). They have also been described in association with Parkinson's disease (21), Klippel-Feil syndrome (16,22,23), Friedreich's ataxia (15), Arnold-Chiari malformation (16), and in phenylketonuria (24).

DEFINITION

Mirror movements represent a category of involuntary associated or synkinetic movements. They specifically refer to simultaneous, contralateral, involuntary, symmetric, identical movements that accompany voluntary movements. They do not include the widespread activation of contralateral limb muscles in association with great physical exertion or fatigue. Exaggeration of the hemiplegic posture with contralateral volitional activity is a common involuntary associated movement but is considered to be separate from mirror movements. Likewise, activation of ipsilateral synergistic muscles with voluntary movement in an intact or paretic limb represents another category of involuntary activity.

OCCURRENCE OF MIRROR MOVEMENTS

Mirror movements are most commonly encountered in the setting of congenital or acquired hemiplegia or hemiparesis. Although they are usually described in relation to cerebral lesions, they also occur with pyramidal lesions in the brainstem and spinal cord. Mirror movements generally occur when movements on the paretic side are associated with involuntary identical movements on the intact side. In some cases of hemiplegia, however, the affected side can move only with volitional movement of the intact side. Early reports suggested that associated movements occur in about 15% of hemiplegic cases (25). Recent surveys are lacking.

Mirror movements are also encountered in individuals with developmental or acquired lesions that disrupt interhemispheral connections, such as midline malformations and porencephaly, or in disorders of pyramidal tract decussation, such as the Klippel-Feil syndrome. In extrapyramidal disorders, particularly Parkinson's disease, it is generally movement of the intact side that is associated with involuntary movement of the contralateral affected side.

Contradictory data exist concerning the occurrence of mirror movements in the general population. Cernacek (26), for example, suggested that during spontaneous or conditioned muscle contraction, clinically inapparent contralateral electrical activity in symmetric muscles could be demonstrated in everyone by means of electromyographic recording. The electrical concomitants of mirror movements are called mirror activity. Some investigators (27), however, have not been able to find mirror activity in normal individuals at all, and others have documented it only under conditions of severe fatigue (28) or marked physical effort (28,29).

We addressed this issue in our own surface electromyographic investigation of mirror activity in 35 normal adult subjects. They were verbally requested to perform specific distal and proximal movements, sequentially using strong and weak efforts, as well as single tonic and repetitive phasic patterns of contraction on each side. All subjects demonstrated mirror activity on at least one trial on each side (Table 94.1). It was elicited significantly more often ($P < 0.001$) with distal than proximal movements (Table 94.2). Strong effort was associated with significantly more ($P < 0.001$) mirror activity than weak effort (Table 94.3). Repetition did not significantly increase the frequency of mirror activity (Table 94.4).

FACTORS THAT INFLUENCE THE OCCURRENCE OF MIRROR MOVEMENTS

All normal individuals may manifest mirror activity. Significant differences may nevertheless exist between normal individuals and ones with neurologic disorders. Such differences have already been proposed in a few reports (6,29,30). Not all movements are associated with mirror activity. Cernacek found mirror activity in 77.6% of all trials (30). Our investigation documented mirror activity in 44.4% of all trials. The large discrepancy between the two studies in the frequency of mirror activity, despite the use of sensitive electrical recording in each, underscores the likelihood that factors other than just movement may influence the occurrence of mirror activity.

Site

Mirror activity in normal subjects in our investigation (see Table 94.2) was significantly more frequent ($P < 0.001$) with movements of the first dorsal interosseus and abductor digiti minimi (54.3%) than the flexor digitorum communis and biceps brachii muscles (29.2%). This conclusion is consistent with Curschmann's (5) clinical observation in hemiplegic subjects that symmetric contralateral coactivation occurs primarily with abduction and adduction of the thumb and other fingers, whereas more proximal movements show the phenomenon less often. Hereditary mirror movements have also demonstrated this predilection for mirroring in distal muscles (4,7,12,14,15).

Table 94.1   Frequency of Mirror Activity with Verbally Elicited Movements in Normal Adults

Muscles	Total Number of Trials	Trials with Mirror Activity	
		Number	Percentage
First dorsal interosseus	514	214	41.6
Abductor digiti minimi	658	422	64.1
Flexor digitorum communis	433	99	22.9
Biceps brachii	330	124	37.6
Total	1,935	859	44.4

Table 94.2   Comparison of Verbally Elicited Mirror Activity Frequency Between Proximal and Distal Muscle Groups for Different Sides, Efforts, and Types of Movement

	Proximal Muscle Group[a]			Distal Muscle Group[b]			
	Total Number of Trials	Trials with Mirror Activity	Percentage	Total Number of Trials	Trials with Mirror Activity	Percentage	P Value
Sides							
All	763	223	29.2	1,172	636	54.3	<0.001
RD	191	46	24.1	299	123	41.1	<0.001
RND	185	55	29.7	294	152	51.7	<0.001
LD	188	59	31.4	281	188	66.9	<0.001
LND	199	63	31.7	298	173	58.1	<0.001
Effort							
Strong	424	186	43.9	627	441	70.3	<0.001
Weak	339	37	10.9	545	195	35.8	<0.001
Type of Movement							
Single tonic	397	114	28.7	580	317	54.7	<0.001
Repetitive	366	109	29.8	592	319	53.9	<0.001

RD, right dominant; RND, right nondominant; LD, left dominant; LND, left nondominant.
[a] Proximal muscle group consists of flexor digitorum communis and biceps brachii.
[b] Distal muscle group consists of first dorsal interosseus and abductor digiti minimi.

Table 94.3   Comparison of Verbally Elicited Mirror Activity Frequency Between Strong and Weak Effort Movements for Different Sides and Types of Movement

	Weak Effort			Strong Effort			
	Total Number of Trials	Trials with Mirror Activity	Percentage	Total Number of Trials	Trials with Mirror Activity	Percentage	P Value
Sides							
All	884	232	26.2	1,051	627	59.7	<0.001
RD	225	41	18.2	265	128	48.3	<0.001
RND	217	50	23.0	262	157	59.9	<0.001
LD	202	62	30.7	267	185	69.3	<0.001
LND	240	79	32.9	257	157	61.1	<0.001
Type of Movement							
Single tonic	485	137	28.2	492	294	59.8	<0.001
Repetitive	399	95	23.8	559	333	59.6	<0.001

RD, right dominant; RND, right nondominant; LD, left dominant; LND, left nondominant.

Table 94.4   Comparison of Verbally Elicited Mirror Activity Frequency Between Single Tonic and Repetitive Movements for Different Sites, Sides, and Effort

	Single Tonic Movement			Repetitive Movement			
	Total Number of Trials	Trials with Mirror Activity	Percentage	Total Number of Trials	Trials with Mirror Activity	Percentage	P Value
Sites							
Proximal	397	114	28.7	366	109	29.8	NS
Distal	580	317	54.7	592	319	53.9	NS
Sides							
All	977	431	44.1	958	428	44.7	NS
RD	247	79	32.0	243	90	37.0	NS
RND	244	108	44.3	235	99	42.1	NS
LD	237	125	52.7	232	122	52.6	NS
LND	249	119	47.8	248	117	47.2	NS
Effort							
Strong	492	294	59.8	559	333	59.6	NS
Weak	485	137	28.2	399	95	23.8	NS

RD, right dominant; RND, right nondominant; LD, left dominant; LND, left nondominant; NS, not significant.

The basis for the predilection of mirror movements to occur in distal muscles has not been established, and is not readily explained by existing models of mirror movements. Green (6) has advanced the hypothesis that mirror movements may result from a loss of lower motor neuron inhibition by the crossed pyramidal corticospinal tract and a concomitant release of the effects of older brainstem motor pathways, such as the rubrospinal tract. The argument is as follows. Mirror movements occur most commonly in distal muscles. Spinal motor neurons that innervate distal muscles are the sites of termination of crossed pyramidal corticospinal tract fibers. Mirror movements in childhood tend to disappear with maturation of the pyramidal system. Mirror movements appear most commonly in neurologic disorders that produce pyramidal deficits.

The rubrospinal tract has been implicated in mirror movements because in monkeys (31) it terminates in the vicinity of motor neurons that regulate distal muscle function. In humans, however, the role of the rubrospinal tract in mirror activity is in question because the magnocellular portion of the red nucleus, which constitutes the cells of origin of the rubrospinal tract, is small and the rubrospinal pathway has not been traced caudal to upper cervical segments of the spinal cord (32,33).

Mirror activity may be mediated by the incomplete decussation of the pyramidal tract. This was proposed independently by Ford (34) and Zulch and Muller (25). One objection to this notion, however, is that the ipsilateral pyramidal tract projects predominantly to motor neuron pools that innervate axial and proximal limb muscles (35) rather than the distal muscles that show the highest frequency of mirror activity.

Several groups of investigators have suggested that mirror movements may be the result of contralateral hemispheral activation via feedback or callosal mechanisms. Contralateral hemispheral activation has received some support from cerebral blood flow (36) and evoked potential (37) findings. Electrophysiologic measurements of mirror activity latency (6,29), however, make peripheral feedback an unlikely mechanism. Direct transcallosal activation of mirror movements by the motor cortex also seems unlikely since interhemispheral callosal connections exist predominantly between areas that represent axial and proximal limb muscles rather than distal muscles (38). Transcallosal activation of mirror movements via premotor or sensory association cortices, however, warrants further consideration and will be addressed later in this chapter.

Effort

Our data (see Table 94.3) show that movements carried out with strong effort (59.7%) were associated with significantly more ($P < 0.001$) mirror activity than those which were carried out with weak effort (26.2%). This finding is consistent with the data of previous clinical and electromyographic investigations (3,5–7,28–30,39). Curschmann (5) postulated that increased effort of movement is reflected by increased numbers of neural impulses that result in greater spread of motor activity to the contralateral side. He suggested that it was increased effort that accounted for the occurrence of more mirror activity with fatigue. Directly pertinent neuroanatomic and neurophysiologic data, however, are lacking.

Repetition of Movement

The data in our investigation (see Table 94.4) did not show a significant effect of repetition of movement on the occurrence of mirror activity, regardless of the task that was performed or the limb that was used. This is in contrast to the findings by Green (6), who demonstrated that successive hand movements were associated with progressively more marked mirror activity and progressively shorter onset latency. Green, however, recorded these findings in a hemiparetic population. Further studies are warranted, therefore, to determine if this discrepancy represents a difference between normal and hemiparetic individuals or differences in methodology and the control of factors, such as effort, which has already been shown to increase mirror activity.

Handedness, Dominance, and Side of Movement

A few reports have raised the possibility that cerebral dominance, handedness, or side of movement may influence the occurrence of mirror movements. The data, however, have been sparse and often contradictory, and the possible effects of these factors have not been firmly established (2,3, 5,11,26). Curschmann (5) observed in his clinical study that mirror movements in predominantly right-handed young adults occurred more frequently with left-sided conditioned movements. He found the opposite situation in a strongly left-handed man. Woods and Teuber (40) reported that in young children, mirroring was more common with conditioned movements of the right hand, but with increasing age, children established the reverse pattern. Cernacek (30) reported that mirror activity occurs significantly more often with movements of the dominant side. In ambidextrous individuals, the frequency of mirror activity was equal from both sides. He proposed the explanation that muscle contraction is stronger on the dominant side and, therefore, is associated with the activation of more neural units to threshold levels required for the occurrence of mirror activity. Hopf et al (29), however, did not find any significant difference in mirror activity frequency between movements of the dominant and nondominant sides.

We carried out an investigation (41) to evaluate the effects of handedness, dominance, and side of movement on the frequency of electromyographically recorded mirror activity that was associated with verbally elicited movements in 18 right- and 17 left-handed subjects. Handedness was defined according to the Edinburgh Inventory by Oldfield (42).

Left-handers showed a significantly higher frequency of mirror activity in intrinsic hand muscles regardless of whether the data for right- and left-sided movements were considered combined (59.2% versus 49.4%, $P < 0.01$) or separately (right, 51.7% versus 41.1%, $P < 0.01$; left, 66.9% versus 58.1%, $P < 0.05$) (Table 94.5). Left-sided movements were associated with a higher frequency of mirror activity for both right-handers (58.1% versus 41.1%; $P < 0.001$) and left-handers (66.9% versus 51.7%; $P < 0.001$) (Table 94.6). No significant difference in the frequency of mirror activity was found between movements carried out by the dominant (53.4%) and nondominant (54.9%) hands (Table 94.7).

No statistically significant effect of handedness, dominance, or side of movement was demonstrated on the frequency of mirror activity in proximal muscles (see Tables 94.5–94.7).

One possible explanation for the higher frequency of mirror activity with left-sided movements to verbal commands may be that mirror activity results from contralateral hemispheral activation, and language representation is strongly lateralized to the left hemisphere of the brain in the great majority of human adults (43,44). Fine finger movements of the type that were shown to be associated with

Table 94.5 Comparison of Verbally Elicited Mirror Activity Frequency Between Right- and Left-Handed Subjects for Different Sexes and Sides of Movement Analyzed Separately for Proximal and Distal Muscle Group Activation

	Right-Handed Subjects			Left-Handed Subjects			
	Total Number of Trials	Trials with Mirror Activity	Percentage	Total Number of Trials	Trials with Mirror Activity	Percentage	P Value
Proximal Muscles[a]							
Total	390	109	27.9	373	114	30.6	NS
Sex							
Male	175	61	34.9	174	69	39.7	NS
Female	215	48	22.3	199	45	22.6	NS
Side							
Right	191	46	24.1	185	55	29.7	NS
Left	199	63	31.7	188	59	31.4	NS
Distal Muscles[b]							
Total	597	296	49.4	575	340	59.2	<0.01
Sex							
Male	265	133	50.2	263	155	58.9	<0.05
Female	332	163	49.1	312	185	59.3	<0.05
Side							
Right	299	123	41.1	294	152	51.7	<0.01
Left	298	173	58.1	281	188	66.9	<0.05

NS, not significant.
[a] Proximal muscle group consists of flexor digitorum communis and biceps brachii.
[b] Distal muscle group consists of first dorsal interosseus and abductor digiti minimi.

Table 94.6 Comparison of Verbally Elicited Mirror Activity Frequency Between Right- and Left-Sided Movement for Different Sexes and Handedness Analyzed Separately for Proximal and Distal Muscle Group Activation

	Right-Sided Movement			Left-Sided Movement			
	Total Number of Trials	Trials with Mirror Activity	Percentage	Total Number of Trials	Trials with Mirror Activity	Percentage	P Value
Proximal Muscles[a]							
Total	376	101	26.9	387	122	31.5	NS
Sex							
Male	172	58	33.7	177	72	40.6	NS
Female	204	43	21.1	210	50	23.8	NS
Handedness							
Right	191	46	24.1	199	63	31.6	NS
Left	185	55	29.7	188	59	31.4	NS
Distal Muscles[b]							
Total	593	275	46.4	579	361	62.3	<0.001
Sex							
Male	268	121	45.1	260	163	62.7	<0.001
Female	325	154	47.4	319	198	62.1	<0.001
Handedness							
Right	299	123	41.1	298	173	58.1	<0.001
Left	294	152	51.7	281	188	66.9	<0.001

NS, not significant.
[a] Proximal muscle group consists of flexor digitorum communis and biceps brachii.
[b] Distal muscle group consists of first dorsal interosseus and abductor digiti minimi.

T a b l e   9 4 . 7   Comparison of Verbally Conditioned Mirror Activity Frequency Between Dominant and Nondominant Sides for Different Sexes and Sites of Movement

	Dominant Side			Nondominant Side			
	Total Number of Trials	Trials with Mirror Activity	Percentage	Total Number of Trials	Trials with Mirror Activity	Percentage	P Value
Proximal Muscles[a]							
Total	379	105	27.7	384	118	30.7	NS
Sex							
Male	170	59	34.7	179	71	39.6	NS
Female	209	46	22.0	205	47	22.9	NS
Distal Muscles[b]							
Total	582	311	53.4	592	325	54.9	NS
Sex							
Male	263	138	52.5	267	146	54.7	NS
Female	319	173	54.2	325	179	55.1	NS

NS, not significant.
[a] Proximal muscle group consists of flexor digitorum communis and biceps brachii.
[b] Distal muscle group consists of first dorsal interosseus and abductor digiti minimii.

different frequencies of mirror activity between the left and right side are regulated by the crossed corticospinal pyramidal system that originates in the motor cortex of the contralateral cerebral hemisphere, especially the precentral motor cortex. The data that suggest an important role for the crossed corticospinal pyramidal tract in mirror movements were cited previously. Wernicke's area in the left hemisphere is usually involved in the comprehension of spoken language. Anatomic and clinicopathologic data suggest that a verbal command to carry out finger movements using the right hand is probably transmitted from Wernicke's area to the premotor cortex in the same left hemisphere and then relayed to the ipsilateral precentral motor cortex, from whence pyramidal fibers send impulses to the spinal cord lower motor neurons that innervate muscles in the right hand (43). In order to carry out finger movements using the left hand, the command must be transmitted from Wernicke's area in the left hemisphere to the right precentral motor cortex (43). This probably involves transmission of information from Wernicke's area to the left premotor cortex and then, via the corpus callosum, to the premotor cortex and finally to the motor cortex of the right hemisphere (43,44). An alternative but less likely possibility involves transmission of information from Wernicke's area, across the callosum, to the corresponding cortex in the right hemisphere and from there to the ipsilateral premotor and precentral motor regions. The greater frequency of mirror activity associated with commands to move the left side, therefore, may be related to the bihemispheral activation required to convey verbal information to move the left side. In contrast, movements of the right hand may be mediated more unilaterally by the left hemisphere. The finding that mirror activity in left-handers, like right-handers, occurs sig-

nificantly more with movements of the left side may similarly be attributed to the predominant lateralization of language representation to the left hemisphere in 60% to 70% of left-handers (44).

The significantly greater frequency of mirror activity in left-handed individuals may also be related to the organization of the language representation in the brain. Left-handers have been shown by the Wada technique to have bihemispheral language representation in 15% to 30% of cases, in comparison with 4% among right-handers (44). This tendency for language to be presented in both hemispheres in left-handers may promote greater bihemispheral activation and more frequent mirror activity in the performance of finger movements to verbal commands. In the small minority of left-handers with strong right hemispheral representation of language, one would expect the findings to be the opposite from the right-handed population. A strong right hemispheral lateralization of language, therefore, may account for the findings in a left-handed man described by Curschmann (5), in whom mirror movements were more frequent with right-sided conditioned movements.

Side of movement and handedness were shown to have a significant effect on the frequency of mirror activity associated with verbally induced movements by distal but not proximal muscles. This finding may be related to differences in the regulation of distal and proximal movements by the motor system, language areas, or both. As stated earlier, fine finger movements of the type that were shown to be associated with different frequencies of mirror activity on the left and right sides are regulated predominantly by the pyramidal system that originates in the contralateral motor cortex. Movements by the proximal muscle group, in contrast, are regulated largely by extrapyramidal motor systems that receive input from widespread regions of the cerebral cortex. Previous reports (5) and our own data suggest that movements produced by these two systems differ in the frequency of mirror activity associated with them. Many apraxic patients who cannot carry out skilled finger and hand movements to command because of disconnections between Wernicke's area and the motor cortex can, nevertheless, carry out more proximal commands (43,45). This finding has led to the hypothesis that proximal movements may be carried out to command in apraxic patients by a nonpyramidal motor system descending from Wernicke's area (43,45).

Since the preservation of the ability to carry out proximal movements to command has also been demonstrated in some individuals with destruction of Wernicke's area or the entire left hemisphere, it has been proposed that the right hemisphere may have the capacity to comprehend proximal commands. In fact, the ability to carry out proximal commands may be a phylogenetically older capacity that developed in both hemispheres at some earlier stage of evolution before the full development of cerebral dominance (43). If each hemisphere has language and motor representation that can regulate proximal movements without bihemispheral activation, side of movement and handedness need not and do not exert a significant effect on the frequency of mirror activity observed with movements by proximal muscles.

CONCLUSIONS

Mirror movements are generally considered to represent a moderately uncommon phenomenon that reflects brain pathology attributable to midline developmental abnormalities or pyramidal lesions. Recent electromyographic data suggest that the phenomenon may be widespread and sensitive to a number of factors. The great variability of findings and apparent discrepancies in the literature may perhaps be reconciled by a consideration of these factors. Mirror activity may provide us with valuable information regarding the structural and functional organization of the normal brain, serve as an objective quantifiable marker for pathology, and offer a potential biofeedback modality for motor learning and rehabilitation.

ACKNOWLEDGMENTS

Supported in part by a grant from the Harvard Medical School Milton Fund and the DFG (Deutsche Forschungsgemeinschaft), 5300 Bonn, FRG.

REFERENCES

1. Westphal C. Uber einige bewegungserscheinungen an gelahmten gliedern. Arch Psychiatr Nervenheilk 1874;4:747–759.
2. Erlenmeyer FA. Die schrift—grundzuge—grundzuge ihrer physiologie und pathologie. Stuttgart: Bonz, 1879.
3. Abercrombie MLJ, Linton RL, Tyson RC. Associated movement in normal and physically handicapped children. Dev Med Child Neurol 1964;6:573–580.
4. Crawford C. Report of a family showing mirror movements. Austr Ann Med 1960;9:176–179.
5. Curschmann H. Beitrage zur physiologie und pathologie der kontralateralen mitbewegung. Dtsch Z Nervenheilk 1906;31:1–52.
6. Green JB. An electromyographic study of mirror movements. Neurology 1967;17:91–94.
7. Meyer BC. Report of a family exhibiting hereditary mirror movements and schizophrenia. J Neurol Ment Dis 1942;96:138–145.
8. Fog E, Fog F. Cerebral inhibition examined by associated movements. In: Byx M, McKeith R, eds. Minimal cerebral dysfunction. London: Sparties Society, Heinemann, 1963:52–57.
9. Freiman IS, Micheels L, Kahn RL. A hereditary syndrome characterized by mirror movements, left-handedness and organic mental defect. Trans Am Neurol Assoc 1949;74:224–226.
10. Woods BT, Eby MD. Excessive mirror movements and impulsive aggression: two facts of the same deficit? Biol Psychiatry 1982;17:23.
11. Drinkwater H. Obligatory bimanual synergia with allocheiria in a boy otherwise normal. Proceedings of the 17th International Congress of Medical Section XI, London, 1913:117.
12. Haerer AF, Currier RD. Mirror movements. Neurology 1966;16:757–760, 765.
13. Johnston PW. Hereditary mirror movements. Bull Los Angeles Neurol Soc 1948;13:119.
14. Rasmussen P, Waldenstroem E. Hereditary mirror movements: a case report. Neuropaediatria 1978;9:189–194.
15. Regli F, Filippa G, Wiesendanger M. Hereditary mirror movements. Arch Neurol 1967;16:620.
16. Schott GD, Wyke MA. Congenital mirror movements. J Neurol Neurosurg Psychiatry 1981;44:586–599.
17. Smith C. Mirror movements. Am J Dis Child 1947;73:175.
18. Haerer AF, Currier RD. Mirror movements. Neurology 1966;16:757–761.
19. Berlin I. Mirror movements. Report of two cases. Arch Neurol Psychiatry 1951;66:394.
20. Walshe FMR. On certain tonic or postural reflexes in hemiplegia with special reference to the so-called "associated movements" (Part I). Brain 1923;46:1–37.
21. Luttman E, MacLay WS, Stokes AB. Persistent mirror movements as a heredo-familial disorder. J Neurol Psychiatry 1939;10:349–356.
22. Baird PA, Robinson GC, Buckler W St J. Klippel-Feil syndrome: a study of mirror movements detected by electromyography. Am J Dis Child 1967;113:546.
23. Bauman GI. Absence of the cervical spine, Klippel-Feil syndrome. JAMA 1932;98:129.
24. Friedman R, Levinson A. Mirror movements in a case of phenylpyruvic oligophrenia. J Pediatr 1954;44:553–557.
25. Zulch KJ, Muller N. Associated movements in man. In: Vinken PJ, Bruyn GW, eds. Handbook of clinical neurology. vol. 1, Disturbances of nervous function. Amsterdam: North Holland, 1969:404–426.
26. Cernacek J. Paired activities of the hemispheres in the motor sphere. Csl Neurol 1959;22:221.
27. Chaco J, Blank A. Mirror movements in hemiparesis. Confin Neurol 1974;36:1–4.
28. Partridge MJ. Electromyographic demonstration of facilitation. Phys Therapy Rev 1954;34:1–7.
29. Hopf HC, Schlegel HJ, Lowitzsch K. Irradiation of voluntary activity to the contralateral side in movements of normal subjects and patients with central motor disturbance. Eur Neurol 1974;12:142–147.
30. Cernacek J. Contralateral motor irradiation—cerebral dominance. Arch Neurol 1961;4:61–68.
31. Lawrence DG, Kuypers HGJR. Pyramidal and nonpyramidal pathways in monkeys: anatomical and functional correlations. Science 1965;148:973.
32. Nathan PW, Smith MC. The rubrospinal and central tegmental tracts in man. Brain 1982;105:223–269.
33. Voss-Herlinger G. Taschenbuch der Anatomie III. 14th ed. Stuttgart: Fischer-Verlag, 1973:46.
34. Ford F. Disease of the nervous system. In: Infancy, childhood and adolescence. 3rd ed. Springfield: Charles C Thomas, 1952:309.
35. Ghez C. Introduction to the motor system. In: Kandel E, Schwartz J, eds. Principles of neural sciences. Amsterdam: Elsevier North-Holland, 1981:271.
36. Harati Y, Meyer JS, Wheeler AH. Neuroanatomical and neurophysiological explanations for mirror movements in Klippel-Feil syndrome derived from rCBF studies. In: International Congress series, no. 548. Amsterdam: Excerpta Medica, 1981:386.
37. Shibasaki H, Nagae K. Mirror movement: application of movement related cortical potentials. Ann Neurol 1984;15:299–302.

38. Brodal A. Neurological anatomy—in relation to clinical medicine. 2nd ed. New York: Oxford University Press, 1969:677.

39. Jelasic F, Ott B. Kontralaterale synkinesien. Klinische und elektromyographische untersuchungen bei ideopathischen und symptomatischen formen. Dtsch Z Nervenheilk 1969;195:187.

40. Woods BT, Teuber HL. Mirror movements after childhood hemiparesis. Neurology 1978;28:1152–1158.

41. Durwen HF, Herzog AG. The effect of handedness, dominance and laterality of movement on the frequency of mirror movements—an electromyographic investigation. Neurology 1985;35(suppl 1):180.

42. Oldfield RC. The assessment and analysis of handedness: the Edinburgh inventory. Neuropsychologia 1971;9:97.

43. Geschwind N. The apraxias: neural mechanisms of disorders of learned movement. Am Sci 1975;63:189–195.

44. Geschwind N. Disconnection syndromes in animal and man (Parts I and II). Brain 1965;88:237–294, 585–644.

45. Geschwind N. Preservation of axial movements to verbal command in cases of apraxia or comprehension deficit. Symposium on Corpus Callosum, Lyon, May, 1974:301–307.

The Periodic Paralyses: A Review

Robert H. Brown

INTRODUCTION

The periodic paralyses are inherited disorders characterized by episodic muscle weakness occurring with either abnormal levels of serum potassium or enhanced sensitivity to changes in serum potassium levels. These are conventionally subdivided into hypo- and hyperkalemic forms. A normokalemic category shares many features with the hyperkalemic form (1). As summarized by Engel (2), these potassium-sensitive periodic paralyses have many common attributes:

1. They are usually inherited as an autosomal dominant trait.
2. The paralytic episodes typically begin proximally and spread distally.
3. Episodes may be restricted to proximal foci or may be generalized and profoundly severe.
4. During paralytic episodes the affected muscles are inexcitable.
5. Either form of potassium-sensitive paralysis may be associated with myotonia as a chronic, interictal manifestation of the underlying disorder.
6. Exercise may trigger either generalized weakness or focal limb weakness; cold may also precipitate these attacks.
7. Rest following exertion exacerbates the weakness; on the other hand, exercise or warm-up may stop an episode.
8. In either form of the illness, permanent weakness may develop after repeated attacks.

Perhaps more than any other disorders in neurology, the periodic paralyses are particularly amenable to both biophysical modeling and analysis. These disorders have been the subject of several excellent reviews (2–6).

HYPOKALEMIC PERIODIC PARALYSIS

Clinical Manifestations

Although sporadic cases are reported, hypokalemic periodic paralysis is usually autosomal dominant with high penetrance (2,3). Attacks typically begin at about the time of puberty. Episodes are more frequent and severe early after onset of the disease and may diminish in intensity and number after the third decade. Males are usually more severely affected than females. As indicated in Table 95.1, precipitating factors include intense exercise, rest after exercise, ingestion of carbohydrates and sodium, exposure to cold, and excitement. The resulting weakness usually begins in the nighttime or early morning. Thus, a typical case is an athletic male in his early twenties who plays touch football late in the afternoon, consumes a pizza and beer or a sugary soft-drink, and goes to bed to awaken in the early morning unable to move. The limbs are most commonly involved, particularly proximally, but in rare cases there may be life-threatening diaphragmatic weakness or cardiac irritability; some authors describe a mortality risk of 10% or so (7). Rarely, myotonia (a sustained muscle contraction due to prolonged electrical irritability of the muscle membrane) may be present in affected individuals both during and between attacks. It is often confined to the eyelids (8). Closely related is paramyotonia congenita of von Eulenberg (below), in which there is more widely distributed, cold-induced myotonia, particularly of the eyelids and hands.

Laboratory Findings

During acute paralytic episodes there is a fall in serum potassium (though not always below the range of normal) in association with urinary retention of potassium, sodium, chloride, and phosphate ions (9). Thus, urinary concentra-

Table 95.1   Clinical Features of Periodic Paralyses

	Hypokalemic	Hyperkalemic
Onset	Puberty	Early childhood
Attack duration	Hours to days	Minutes to days
Interictal interval	Many hours to days	May be less than 1 h
Precipitating factors	Cold; rest after exercise; carbohydrates	Cold; rest after exercise; carbohydrate depletion; potassium
Ameliorating factors	Sustained mild exercise; potassium	Sustained mild exercise; carbohydrates
Provocative tests	Glucose and insulin; intra-arterial epinephrine	Potassium loading
Treatment		
Prophylactic	Low sodium diet; low carbohydrate diet; potassium; acetazolamide; dichlorphenamide; triamterene; spironolactone; diazoxide	Frequent carbohydrates; acetazolamide
Acute	Potassium p.p.; potassium i.v. (in mannitol)	Glucose, insulin; calcium gluconate β blockers

tions of these ions fall; urinary excretion of potassium may fall prior to an attack. There may also be reduced urine output. Concomitantly, there is an increase in total body water, with an apparent shift in water from the extra- to the intracellular compartment. The interictal concentrations of intramuscular sodium and potassium are, respectively, increased and either normal or decreased (9,10); these do not substantially increase during attacks perhaps because of the intracellular shifts in water. Physiologically, the paralyzed muscle is electrically inexcitable, with a subnormal transmembrane potential and normal contractility of the underlying myofibrillar apparatus. The physiologic defect producing these changes is not well defined, although studies (see below) have suggested a membrane defect, possibly of sodium conductance (g_{Na}).

Muscle Pathology

The development of histologic abnormalities in muscle in affected individuals tends to correlate with the duration and severity of the disorder; early in the disease the muscle may be entirely normal by light and electron microscopy. In advanced cases an irreversible vacuolar myopathy may develop, resembling the myopathy in individuals with severe potassium depletion (11). Engel has reported that several ultrastructural abnormalities may precede vacuolization, including duplication and dilation of the T tubules and dilation of the sarcoplasmic reticulum (12). Early vacuoles are derived from these constituents, may contain lamellae and amorphous material, and may be reduced nicotinamide adenine dinucleotide positive. Through contact with T tubules, evolving vacuoles may contain extracellular fluid whose rupture into the sarcoplasm may potentially be injurious to the muscle cell (for example, by elevating intracellular calcium levels). Some vacuoles are autophagic.

Differential Diagnosis

The major differential considerations in hypokalemic periodic paralysis are listed in Table 95.2. In cases with a clear family history the diagnosis is usually not in doubt. Very early or sporadic cases may pose a diagnostic challenge, particularly if the serum and urine potassium changes are not beyond the limits of normal. Fortunately, screening to exclude most of the entities in Table 95.2 is straightforward. Thyrotoxic periodic paralysis is usually sporadic and more common in Orientals; it is more male predominant than hypokalemic periodic paralysis (13). Serum and urine electrolyte shifts in thyrotoxic periodic paralysis are similar to those in hypokalemic periodic paralysis. Barium poisoning produces a toxic syndrome characterized by hemorrhagic gastroenteritis, cardiac irritability, seizures, and hypokalemic muscle paralysis. The hypokalemia correlates with an intracellular shift of potassium. This is believed to be a consequence of a block by barium of one or more potassium channels. In the face of sustained potassium influx via the sodium-potassium adenosine triphosphatase, a barium-induced reduction in potassium efflux will result in a net intracellular shift of potassium ions (14). Because the potassium (g_K) and chloride (g_{Cl}) conductances account for the normal, negative transmembrane potential in muscle, a reduction in g_K by barium might be expected to explain the observed depolarization (loss of normal transmembrane potential) of barium-toxic muscle.

Provocative Diagnostic Testing

In uncertain cases, provocation of hypokalemic weakness may be diagnostic. A hypokalemic challenge may be initiated by administration of oral or intravenous glucose, with insulin given either subcutaneously or intravenously. These

Table 95.2 Differential Diagnosis of the Periodic Paralyses

Hypokalemic	Hyperkalemic
Primary	**Primary**
Hypokalemic periodic paralysis	Hyperkalemic periodic paralysis
Paramyotonia congenita	Normokalemic periodic paralysis
	Paralysis periodica myotonia
Secondary	
Thyrotoxic periodic paralysis	**Secondary**
Barium-induced periodic paralysis	Potassium overload syndromes
Potassium-wasting syndromes	Muscle crush
Gastrointestinal	Renal insufficiency
Diarrhea	Adrenal insufficiency
Sprue	
Laxative abuse	
Endocrinologic	
Cushing's syndrome	
Conn's syndrome	
Bartter's syndrome	
Renal	
Metabolic alkalosis	
Thiazide therapy	
Licorice intoxication	
Hyperaldosteronism	
Metabolic acidosis	
Renal tubular acidosis	
Amphotericin B therapy	
Ammonium chloride ingestion	

measures may be augmented by salt loading or exercising the patient. Intra-arterial epinephrine, but not norepinephrine, characteristically induces a reduction in the amplitudes of evoked muscle action potentials and twitch tension in patients with hypokalemic periodic paralysis but not in controls or, in most cases, patients with thyrotoxic periodic paralysis (9).

Treatment

Acute attacks are treated with potassium, which in most instances may be given orally. If the oral route is problematic, potassium may be administered intravenously, preferably in mannitol because sodium- and glucose-containing solutions may worsen the hypokalemia. Low carbohydrate and low sodium diets may help prevent attacks. Potassium is also reported to be useful in prophylactic treatment, although this is controversial.

The carbonic anhydrase inhibitor acetazolamide is clearly prophylactic and may improve interictal strength. An analogous inhibitor, dichlorphenamide, may also be beneficial (15). The mechanism of action of these compounds is not clear. They may act through the carbonic anhydrase, whose inhibition produces a mild metabolic acidosis; this, in turn, increases egress of potassium from muscle. These compounds, like diazoxide, may also diminish insulin release after glucose loading and thereby decrease an insulin-induced

intracellular shift of potassium ions. These potential beneficial effects of the carbonic anhydrase inhibitors in hypokalemic periodic paralysis are partially countered by their kaliuretic effects; the latter may explain the use of these drugs in hyperkalemic periodic paralysis.

Drugs that promote renal retention of potassium, such as triamterene and the aldosterone antagonist spironolactone, are also preventive treatments. The mainstay of therapy for thyrotoxic periodic paralysis is the restoration of the euthyroid state; β-adrenergic blockers such as propranolol are prophylactic in this disease but not in primary hypokalemic periodic paralysis. In other forms of secondary hypokalemic paralysis, the goal of treatment is correction of the underlying disorder.

HYPERKALEMIC PERIODIC PARALYSIS

Clinical Manifestations

Like the hypokalemic form, hyperkalemic periodic paralysis (adynamia episodica heretidaria) is usually inherited as an autosomal dominant trait, although some sporadic forms are recognized (16,17). It typically begins before the age of 10 and is characterized by attacks that are briefer in duration and less severe than in the hypokalemic disorder; some attacks may last for more than a day. The weakness is often proximal. It is precipitated by cold, rest after exercise, fasting, and ingestion of potassium. Attacks are aborted by sustained, mild exercise and by eating frequent meals or snacks. By contrast with episodes of hypokalemic periodic paralysis, in hyperkalemic paralysis there may be paresthesias and myalgias. Cardiac irritability can arise during the hyperkalemia but is probably less life-threatening than in hypokalemic paralysis. Clinical and subclinical myotonia is frequent in some hyperkalemic patients and may be exacerbated both by cooling and potassium depletion. Hyperkalemic periodic paralysis may occur without myotonia, with myotonia, and with paramyotonia (cold-induced myotonia). The term paralysis periodica myotonia is sometimes used to describe patients with both hyperkalemic periodic paralysis and paramyotonia congenita (18).

Laboratory Findings

Serum potassium rises during paralytic episodes but may not exceed the normal upper limits; in this sense, the term "hyperkalemic" is imprecise. Urinary potassium losses increase. By contrast, serum sodium and chloride are either unchanged or fall (19). As Engel points out, these changes suggest increased efflux of potassium from and influx of sodium and chloride into muscle during the acute attacks (2).

Muscle Pathology

As in hypokalemic paralysis, there may be a vacuolar myopathy in hyperkalemic paralysis. It is said that the central vacuoles are larger in the former disorder, but this is not inviolate. The vacuolar changes may be irreversible and more pronounced in long-standing cases (2).

Differential Diagnosis

As listed in Table 95.2, the differential diagnosis includes the forms of hyperkalemic periodic paralysis with and without myotonia, normokalemic periodic paralysis, and secondary forms of hyperkalemic paralysis. The grouping of hyper- and normokalemic periodic paralysis is largely based on their similar sensitivity to potassium loading; it does not preclude the possibility that some forms of normokalemic paralysis may be fundamentally distinct.

Provocative Diagnostic Testing

Particularly in cases without a family history or major increments in potassium during weakness, it may be diagnostic to determine whether a potassium challenge provokes weakness. Potassium is given without glucose immediately after exercise during fasting.

It may also be diagnostic to challenge hyperkalemic periodic paralysis patients with exercise (e.g., 125 W on an ergometer for 30 minutes). Both normal and hyperkalemic patients developed mild hyperkalemia during the exercise, accompanied by some degree of acidosis. This hyperkalemia is not associated with paralysis. In normal individuals, rest following the exercise results in a normalization of the potassium level. In the hyperkalemic patients this also occurs but, within an hour or so, a second period of hyperkalemia follows, during which the patients become weak (18). It may be that acidosis prevents the paralysis during the initial hyperkalemia with exercise.

Treatment

Treatment of the acute episodes is directed at reduction of serum potassium levels. Glucose, insulin, and infusions of calcium gluconate are the primary modalities; acute reversal of paralysis has also been reported with the adrenergic compounds epinephrine and metaproterenol, salbutamol, and glucagon (20). Prophylaxis may be possible with frequent carbohydrate snacks or through the use of potassium-wasting diuretics such as thiazides or acetazolamide, which, as noted above, may have multiple effects on potassium homeostasis. Mineralocorticoids such as fludrocortisone may be beneficial.

PARAMYOTONIA (OF EULENBERG)

This disorder is characterized by cold-induced muscle stiffness or myotonia (21). It is usually inherited as an autosomal dominant disorder. By contrast with the myotonia in hypo- or hyperkalemic periodic paralysis, the myotonia in this disorder paradoxically worsens with sustained exercise. For this reason the disorder was designated paramyotonia.

PATHOGENESIS OF THE PERIODIC PARALYSES AND MYOTONIA

Ideally any description of the pathogenesis of these disorders will explain both the electrical behavior of the muscle cells during exposure to high and low potassium and observed alterations in overall potassium homeostasis. Moreover, an adequate model must explain the mechanism by which certain agents provoke and others ameliorate the illnesses. Numerous investigators have studied these phenomena in detail. In the last decade, the elegant electrophysiologic studies of Lehmann-Horn, Rudel, Ricker, and others have facilitated definition of the underlying membrane defects.

Hypokalemic Periodic Paralysis

Based on the Nernst equation for the potassium reversal potential, it was anticipated that the fall in extracellular potassium (K_e) during the paralytic episodes would be associated with muscle cell hyperpolarization. In fact, the opposite occurs. At the nadir of the hypokalemic spells the membrane is substantially depolarized, to a degree that suffices to explain the inexcitability of the muscle cell (22). Because the membrane resting potential, at which no net membrane current flows, is the sum of the potassium, chloride, sodium, and sodium-potassium pump (Na-K) currents, a low K_e might theoretically depolarize the membrane in several ways:

1. Reducing g_K and as a consequence outward current flow carried by potassium ions.
2. Reducing the hyperpolarizing Na-K pump current.
3. Increasing inward sodium currents.
4. Changing the balance of these such that, in the face of an abnormally elevated g_{Na}, a minor fall in potassium current flow would result in a significant net increment in inward current flow and depolarization.

The first possibility was supported by the model of barium-induced hypokalemic paralysis; barium reduces g_K presumably by interfering with potassium ion flow through a voltage-dependent potassium channel (14). With a fall in g_K the overall membrane conductance should be reduced. As a consequence, at any level of activity the Na-K pump should be more electrogenic and potentially of more than normal importance in maintaining the membrane potential. Thus, any condition that impaired Na-K pump function might precipitate depolarization (23). In particular, adrenergic agonists or insulin, which enhance Na-K pump activity, might reduce K_e to a level at which the pump shuts down; without the pump's electrogenic contribution to membrane potential, depolarization would result, as suggested by the second hypothesis above. Several considerations mitigate against this hypothesis. First, it is difficult to understand why pump inhibition induced by low K_e would not rapidly reverse as the membrane depolarizes; this depolarization should augment potassium efflux through voltage-sensitive potassium channels. The outflowing potassium ions should then potentially be available for reactivation of the pump. Second, it is not clear that the contribution of the Na-K pump to the membrane potential is enough to account for the observed depolarization with hypokalemia (24). Third, the degree of hypokalemia at which paralysis is observed is not adequate to cause inhibition of the pump (25). Fourth, and most important, by contrast with barium paralysis, in hypokalemic periodic paralysis the data strongly indicate that g_K is normal, whereas g_{Na} is increased (26).

The possibility that g_{Na} may be enhanced in hypokalemic periodic paralysis is strongly suggested by in vitro studies of biopsied affected muscle. Intracellular recording of affected muscle revealed a prompt depolarization to about −50 mV reproducibly induced by lowering K_e from 3.5 to 1.0 mmol (26). A similar depolarization was also seen when the fibers were cooled to 27°C or bathed in chloride-poor medium. The current-voltage (I-V) relationships of the membranes were normal under normal conditions. However, with either low K_e or low extracellular chloride (Cl_e) the relationship is shifted in the direction of increased inward current over all potentials studied, suggesting that the g_{Na} must be abnormally increased (Fig 95.1a–c). The available data do not allow one to determine whether g_{Na} is chronically elevated in a basal manner or it is somehow increased specifically by the reduction in K_e. The former seems more likely given that reductions of both K_e and Cl_e induce the depolarization and shift in I-V relationship. When normal skeletal muscle is bathed in potassium-free and chloride-free muscle, the fibers depolarize to about −50 mV, without an underlying abnormality of g_{Na} (27). This depolarization is not seen in normal muscle with reductions in either K_e or Cl_e alone. The resting g_K in these experiments may be gauged by the slopes of the I-V curves at the resting potential (about −80 mV). As Figure 95.1 shows, in hypokalemic periodic paralysis the slopes at about −80 mV are quite similar at potassium 3.5 and 1.0 mmol, suggesting that the g_K is similar at these K_e. Together, these results strongly suggest that the primary defect in these fibers in vitro is an abnormally high g_{Na}, possibly accentuated with hypokalemia.

This model potentially explains the effects of carbohydrates, insulin, and adrenergic stimulation on this illness. Thus, with carbohydrate consumption or the administration of glucose and insulin (known to provoke paralysis) (28), the resulting elevations in insulin levels should enhance Na-K pump activity, promoting a drop in K_e that would precipitate hypokalemic depolarization in affected muscle. In fact, studies of a hypokalemic periodic paralysis patient using euglycemic insulin clamp suggested abnormally high sensitivity of the Na-K pump to insulin (28). Insulin may also directly depress g_K. By the same token, stress or the administration of epinephrine, which also precipitates hypokalemic periodic paralysis, would enhance Na-K pump activity, with a similar result.

Other distinctive features of the hypokalemically paralyzed muscle in Figure 95.1a–c are noted. The authors postulated that the abnormally high g_{Na} might be a consequence of channels other than the voltage-sensitive sodium channel because tetrodotoxin (TTX) did not block the depolarization. Moreover, the antiarrhythmic drug tocainide, also thought to interact with the sodium channel, was not clinically beneficial in this disease. Finally, the authors found that the hypokalemic fibers are generally less excitable than normal fibers; with normal K_e, depolarizing currents produced fewer action potentials. Even with prehyperpolarization of fibers, the resulting action potentials had diminished overshoots, suggesting diminished excitability.

Hyperkalemic Periodic Paralysis with Myotonia

In vitro analysis of muscle from a patient with hyperkalemic periodic paralysis with myotonia revealed a normal resting potential (i.e., −80 mV) with normal K_e. With elevation of K_e to 6 mM there was enhanced excitability and, in some fibers, prolonged trains of spontaneous electrical activity (29). Strikingly, in some trains the abnormal electrical discharges arose alternately from two different potentials at about −65 mV and −45 or −50 mV. With further elevation of K_e to 7 mM, there was stable depolarization to about −45 mV in the majority of fibers. The addition of TTX totally reversed this depolarization, suggesting the depolarization was derived from an enhanced g_{Na}. This was also suggested by direct recording of increased intracellular sodium activity after depolarization with 7 mM K_e. In one patient, with normal K_e the muscle membrane I-V relationship was indistinguishable from controls. However, at K_e of 7 mM the hyperkalemic periodic paralysis muscle revealed a remarkable flattening of the I-V curve between −60 and −40 mV, possibly with a region of negative slope at about −40 mV (Fig 95.1d) (29). This suggests an augmented net inward current within this range of membrane potentials. One implication of the flattened I-V curve is that there may be metastable "resting potentials" between which the membrane may oscillate; this correlates well with the observed excitability arising from two different potentials under conditions of high K_e.

In muscle from another patient with hyperkalemic periodic paralysis with myotonia, the I-V relationship was abnormal even at normal K_e. The abnormality was again a greatly enhanced steady-state inward current above about −70 mV that was completely abolished by addition of TTX (Fig 95.1e) (30). In this patient's muscle, at 9 mM K_e the I-V curve was normal in the presence of TTX. Without TTX there was excessive inward current, again suggesting a defect in g_{Na}. Analysis of intracellular sodium activity suggested that in these muscles, depolarization activated a subsequently noninactivating, "slow" sodium current (30). It was

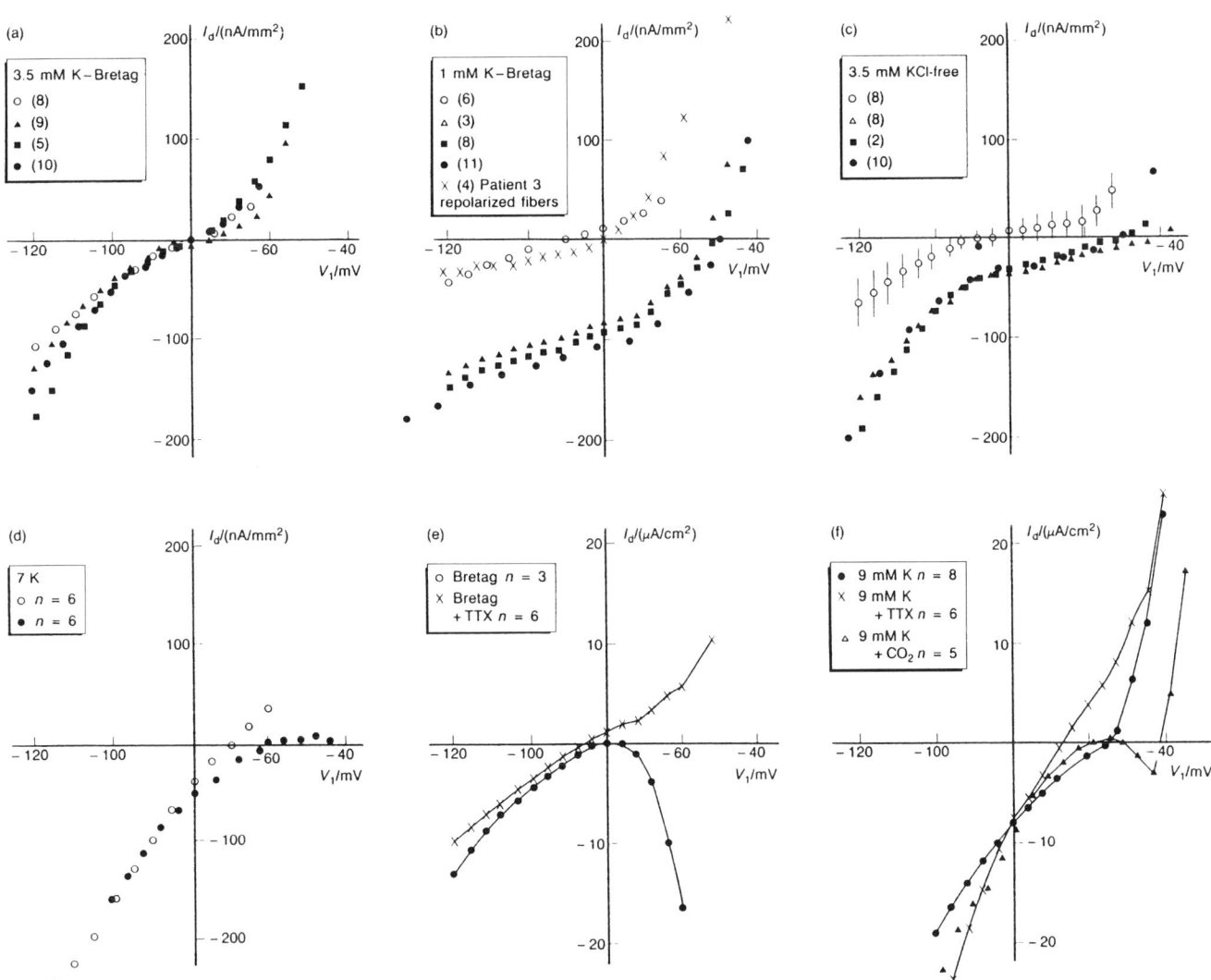

FIGURE 95.1   *Steady-state I-V relationships in periodic paralysis. (a–c) Hypokalemic periodic paralysis (26). (a) Normal K_e. (b) 1 mM potassium. (c) 3.5 mM K_e in chloride-free medium. Muscle from three periodic paralysis patients (●); normal muscle (○). The patients' muscles are normal at K_e = 3.5 mM potassium. When potassium is lowered, there is a downward shift in the I-V curve at all potentials, suggesting increased inward or decreased outward current contribution to the total membrane I-V profile. In (c), a similar I-V relationship is evident in chloride-free, 3.5 mM potassium medium. (d–f) Two cases of hyperkalemic periodic paralysis with myotonia (29,30). Muscle from periodic paralysis patient (●); control muscle (○). At 7 mM potassium the patient, but not the control, muscle demonstrates a region of flattening of the I-V curve from −40 to −60 mV; this region predisposes the membrane to electrical irritability, correlating with the patient's myotonia. In the second patient, (e) and (f) are normal and 9 mM potassium, respectively. Patient muscle without (●) and with TTX (∗). In (e), the patient's I-V profile demonstrates a pronounced inward current above −80 mV; this is abolished with TTX. As in (f) hyperkalemia induces depolarization, which is partially reversed by TTX. Increasing the P_{CO_2} further depolarizes the muscle and imposes a region of negative slope between −40 and −50 mV (△). These and related data suggest that depolarization of this patient's muscle activates an abnormally large inward current, probably a slow sodium current.*

not established whether these were abnormal or defective variants of the usual voltage-dependent "fast" sodium channel or a type of noninactivating slow sodium channel (31–33).

In studies of the second patient, low extracellular pH reversed the effect of K_e elevation on depolarization and paralysis (30,34). Cations such as calcium and hydrogen ions reduce surface negative charge on the membrane and thereby hyperpolarize the transmembrane potential. This shifts the measured voltage dependence of gates in the membrane in a positive-going direction. Depending on whether the predominant shift is on the activation or inactivation gates, titrating surface negative charge can either enhance or depress sodium current flow. In depolarized fibers, surface charge titration with lowered pH accentuates sodium current (30). This suggests that the clinical benefit of hydrogen and calcium ions (35) in periodic paralysis is mediated by enhanced g_{Na}. These points clearly have bearing on the clinical observation that patients may not have weakness during exercise or may delay paralysis by exercising;

exercise may produce low-grade acidosis. This may also explain the efficacy of acetazolamide in this disorder.

Hyperkalemic Periodic Paralysis Without Myotonia

Muscle from a patient with this disorder was generally not overly irritable and had a normal resting potential. At 10 mM K_e there was a depolarization beyond that expected from the Nernst equation, suggesting heightened conductance to a species such as sodium with a reversal potential well positive to that for potassium (29). In another case, the I-V relationship was not significantly different from normal even with 10 mM potassium (in a TTX-free medium). Although elevation of K_e to 10 mM did not dramatically alter these particular electrical properties of the muscle, it did render the fibers inexcitable. The basis was not fully defined, but these effects might be expected in a fiber with heightened g_{Na}.

As in the hypokalemic case (above), in hyperkalemic periodic paralysis the known exacerbating and beneficial effects, respectively, of fasting and carbohydrates might arise from interactions with the Na-K pump. In fasting, circulating levels of insulin are low and as a result there is little to drive the Na-K pump; hyperkalemia might be expected on this basis. With carbohydrate ingestion, insulin levels would rise and thereby augment Na-K pump activity. This, in turn, might enhance intracellular pumping of K_e, potentially precipitating hypokalemia and ameliorating the hyperkalemic paralysis.

Detailed electrophysiologic studies of muscle from patients with both hyperkalemic periodic paralysis and paramyotonia are rare. It is therefore difficult to speculate about mechanisms that might produce these disorders jointly. As recently suggested, a single gene defect may conceivably produce both syndromes, a possibility underscored by the fact that different members of the same family may manifest either hyperkalemic periodic paralysis or cold-induced paramyotonia (36). Rare families have been described in which members may have cold-induced paramyotonia, weakness inducible by oral potassium administration, and paradoxical hypokalemia during attacks of paralysis (37).

Paramyotonia Congenita

Muscle from these patients also demonstrates normal resting potentials. Here the central electrophysiologic finding is that fibers cooled to 27°C show a diffuse increment in inward current at all membrane potentials (38). When applied before fibers are cooled, TTX prevented depolarization; by contrast, TTX added after cooling did not cause repolarization. This diffuse increment in inward current is reminiscent of the abnormal sodium flux in hypokalemic periodic paralysis and contrasts the observation in hyperkalemic periodic paralysis with myotonia in which the increased sodium

current is restricted to membrane potentials above about −60 or −65 mV (Fig 95.2). In paramyotonia congenita, rewarming the chilled fiber did not by itself cause repolarization. Repolarization was seen if the reversal potential for chloride anions was briefly shifted in a negative direction by exposure to chloride-free media. On reperfusion with normal concentrations of chloride ions, repolarization was prompt. This observation could be interpreted to suggest a depolarizing shift of the chloride current reversal potential.

Other Forms of Myotonia

While available data in these studies implicate enhanced g_{Na} in the pathogenesis of myotonia, it should be recalled that there are other possible mechanisms (6,39). In myotonia congenita, as distinct from myotonic dystrophy, the primary defect appears to be a reduction in membrane g_{Cl}. With each muscle action potential, the egress of potassium from the cytoplasm into the extracellular fluid within the confined space of the T tubules increases K_e within those structures. After only a few action potentials, the tubular K_e accumulation may shift the reversal potential for potassium measurably in a positive direction. Inasmuch as the repolarizing muscle fiber has a high conductance, both the chloride and potassium and the increment in the potassium reversal potential do not affect the degree of repolarization; in effect, the chloride system provides a shunting conductance to ensure full repolarization. On the other hand, in the myotonic goat and patients with myotonia congenita, it appears that g_{Cl} is subnormal. Thus, the reversal potential for potassium determines the extent of repolarization; this will diminish after several action potentials. As the resting potential thereby shifts in a positive-going direction, the cell becomes more electrically irritable because the difference between the resting potential and the sodium threshold falls. This predisposes to additional action potential bursting and hence myotonia. Taken together, the periodic paralysis and myotonia congenita studies suggest that there may be several mechanisms whereby myotonia is produced. Moreover, they emphasize the interrelationship between the complex anatomy of the muscle cell and muscle membrane excitability.

APPROACHES TO MODELING OF PERIODIC PARALYSIS

Because the primary abnormalities underlying the periodic paralyses affect membrane excitability, a detailed understanding of the pathogenesis of these diseases should be enhanced by analysis of biophysical models of skeletal muscle membranes. Such quantitative models allow one independently to analyze the effect of each ion system or compartment on excitability and thereby assess whether a particular defect reproduces observed abnormalities of muscle cell excitation. A great limitation of such models is that they are inherently no more powerful than available

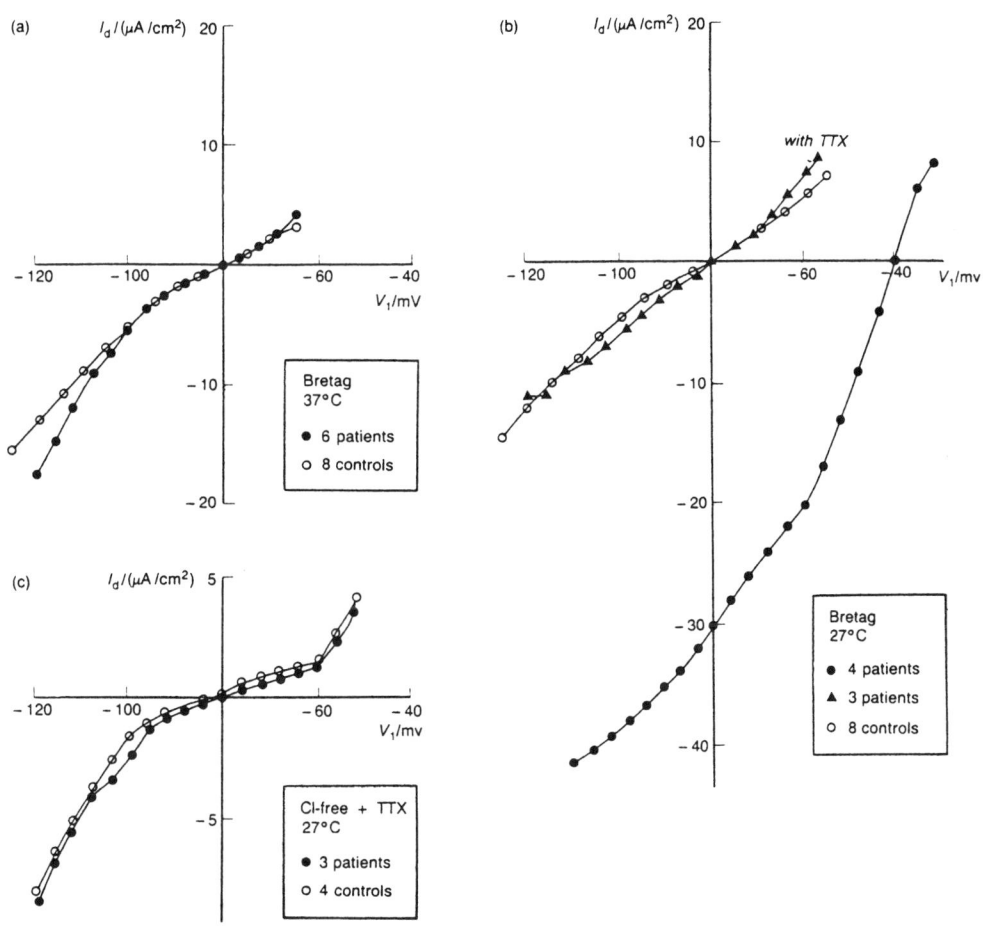

FIGURE 95.2 *Steady-state I-V relationships in paramyotonia congenita (38). At 37°C, patient (●) and control (○) muscle are indistinguishable (a). In four patients, cooling to 27°C induces a large inward current (b), which is entirely blocked by TTX (c).*

descriptions of pertinent membrane parameters. Ideally, a full membrane model will include all factors significantly modifying excitability: voltage-dependent ion channels (usually simulated using Hodgkin-Huxley equations), Na-K pump, the sodium-calcium (Na-Ca) pump, and intracellular compartments that can sequester or buffer concentrations of pertinent ions. This ideal has been most closely realized in the elegant modeling of heart muscle by DiFrancesco and Noble (40); detailed but somewhat less comprehensive models also exist for skeletal muscle (41,42). It is instructive to use even a simplistic simulation of the skeletal muscle ion-specific current-voltage relationships to model possible explanations for the periodic paralyses. Figure 95.3 illustrates a set of simulated steady-state *I-V* curves from a hypothetic muscle membrane. In each instance, the solid line is the total or net membrane current (I_{total}), representing the sum of sodium, potassium, and chloride currents. The *I-V* functions have been calculated to approximate the expected steady-state voltage dependence for each ion. Thus, in normal muscle, the chloride and potassium reversal potentials (E_{rev}) are at -100 mV; E_{rev} for sodium is $+20$ mV. The slope of the potassium current curve decreases slightly with increas-

ing membrane potential, reproducing a degree of anomalous rectification. Panels (a) and (c) are intended to represent normal total membrane *I-V* relationships, illustrating total and constituent ion currents. The only difference between (c) and (a) is the larger sodium current (i_{Na}) in (c).

In panels (b) and (d), hyperkalemic periodic paralysis is simulated respectively from models (a) and (c) by assuming that

1. hyperkalemia augments net inward i_{Na} by diminishing the voltage sensitivity of all the sodium channel inactivation gates,
2. E_K is shifted in a positive direction, and
3. the conductance of i_K increases K_e slightly.

The principal observation in (b) and (d) is that identical changes have quite different consequences, depending on the initial "normal" membrane model. In (b) there is membrane depolarization. In (d) there is both depolarization and flattening of the *I-V* curve, which has a region of negative slope between -30 and -60 mV. The latter renders the membrane unstable and might predispose to electrical irritability; the clinical consequence of the negative slope

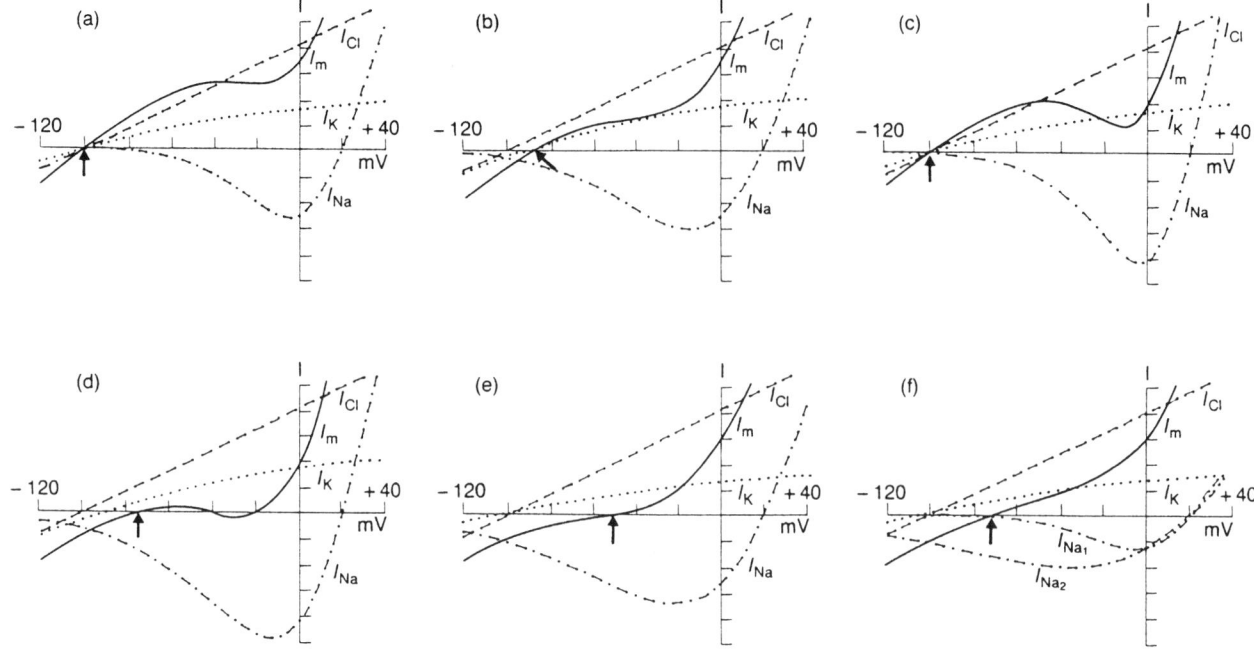

FIGURE 95.3   *Hypothetic I-V relationships in hypo- and hyperkalemic periodic paralysis. (a and c) Normal profile with differing sodium currents. (b) Simulates the effect of hyperkalemia on (a) with three assumptions: 1) the sodium current is augmented at negative potentials by diminishing the steepness of its voltage dependence, 2) the E_{rev} for potassium is shifted in a positive direction, and 3) the g_K is slightly increased. (d) Simulates the effect of hyperkalemia on (c) with the same three assumptions as in (b). As discussed in the text, the effects of these changes on the I-V profiles, and the possible clinical consequences, are determined both by the postulated disease-specific defect (altered I_{Na} voltage dependence) and the properties of the constituent ion systems. By analogy with (b) and (d), (e) models hypokalemic periodic paralysis by postulating that hypokalemia increases I_{Na} by reducing the voltage dependence of the sodium current. Hypokalemia is also assumed to shift the E_{rev} for the potassium current in the negative direction and slightly decrease g_K. (f) Simulates hypokalemic paralysis by assuming that in this autosomal dominantly inherited disease one-half of the sodium channels have a diminished voltage dependence and thus enhanced current flow at negative potentials. In both (e) and (f) the result is membrane depolarization. In each panel the arrowhead denotes the resting potential at which there is no net current flow.*

region might well be increased firing and myotonia. Thus, whether a given gene defect produces hyperkalemic paralysis with or without myotonia may be determined as much by the configuration of the other ion systems as by the defect itself.

In panel (e), hypokalemic periodic paralysis is simulated by assuming that

1. hypokalemia augments i_{Na} by diminishing the voltage sensitivity of all of the sodium channel activation gates,
2. E_{rev} for potassium is more negative, and
3. the overall g_K is decreased.

Panel (f) is an alternate simulation of hypokalemic periodic paralysis obtained by assuming that g_{Na} is increased in half of the sodium channels. This might occur in muscle heterozygous for a codominant mutation altering a critical, voltage-sensing region of the sodium channel. In this instance, the ratio of normal (I_{Na1}) to abnormal (I_{Na2}) sodium channels might well be 1:1.

By augmenting the g_{Na}, one may analogously simulate changes in the *I-V* curve in paramyotonia congenita. It should also be noted that this can be achieved by shifting

the chloride reversal potential in a depolarizing direction (data not shown). Indeed, the observation that paramyotonia congenita fibers in vitro can only be repolarized indirectly by altering the E_{rev} for chloride might be interpreted to implicate a primary g_{Cl} defect. While experimental data reviewed above implicate increased sodium influx in this disorder, it is not clear that this must result from a primary defect in g_{Na}. By depolarizing the membrane, a chloride shift could also increase i_{Na} flow. At all events, these considerations underscore the potential use of computer simulation in framing and testing hypotheses to explain excitability disturbances in muscle. A full skeletal muscle model, with descriptions of all variables governing excitation, including the confounding anatomy of the T-tubule system, would undoubtedly be a useful tool in the further analysis of disorders such as the periodic paralyses and myotonia.

MOLECULAR STUDIES IN PERIODIC PARALYSIS

As outlined above, an extensive literature implicates an abnormal sodium conductance in the pathogenesis of the periodic paralyses and paramyotonia congenita. In the last 2 years, this hypothesis has been tested directly using gene linkage and mutational analysis. In a large kindred with hyperkalemic periodic paralysis and myotonia, Fontaine et al (45) documented coinheritance of the disease with an allele associated with the adult isoform of the skeletal muscle sodium channel encoded on chromosome 17. This result has been confirmed in other large families by Ptacek et al (46) and Ebers et al (47). In Ebers' study (47), hyperkalemic periodic paralysis in families both with and without myotonia was linked to this channel. Similarly, in paramyotonia congenita, both Ptacek et al (48) and Ebers et al (47) have demonstrated linkage to this gene. The sodium channel was further implicated by patch clamp studies demonstrating distinctly abnormal behavior of single channels in affected but not control myotubes in vitro. When challenged with elevated extracellular potassium, a fraction of sodium channels in the affected myotubes became transiently noninactivating (49), a change which can be shown with Hodgkin-Huxley modeling to cause depolarization of the membrane and, through depolarization, inactivation of all of the sodium channels, including both normal channels and mutant channels not in a noninactivating mode (50). This inactivation of normally behaving channels constitutes a novel mechanism for dominant expression of a mutation and illustrates how an environmental factor (extracellular potassium concentration) can regulate expression of the mutation.

The linkage and patch clamp studies prompted a search for sodium channel mutations in the various affected families. At this time, four mutations have been identified, as shown in Figure 95.4, illustrating the proposed structure of the alpha chain of the sodium channel (51,52). This channel protein consists of approximately 2,000 amino acids that form four homologous domains, as indicated. Each domain consists of six membrane-spanning helices; these are thought to form a tetrameric structure with a central pore that is the channel itself. The fourth helix in each (hatch marked) is positively charged and appears to serve as a sensor of membrane field; these so-called S4 helices are critical in opening the channel (activation) after depolarization (53). Several lines of evidence indicate that the III–IV intracytoplasmic loop forms a loop or gate that pivots to inactivate the channel after it opens (53). Rojas et al (54) detected a methionine-to-valine transition near the cytoplasmic end of the sixth helix in the fourth domain, as shown, in the hyperkalemic paralysis family linked by Fontaine et al (45) to the muscle sodium channel (54). Ptacek et al (55) described a threonine-to-methionine substitution in the fifth helix in domain II in another hyperkalemic family. It is speculated that in each domain, the 5–6 extracellular loops may invaginate into the membrane to form the actual ion-passing pore. It is possible that this depends in some manner on an interaction of the inserted 5–6 loop with the inner extents of the fifth and sixth alpha helices, and that this interaction is in some manner modified by exposure to elevated extracellular potassium.

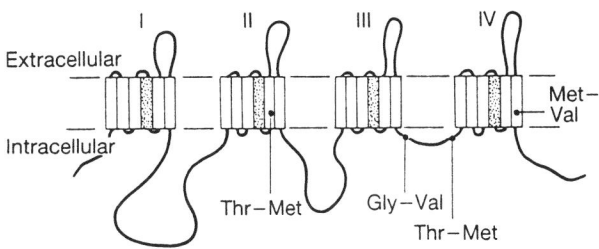

FIGURE 95.4 *Locations of skeletal muscle sodium channel mutations identified in hyperkalemic periodic paralysis and paramyotonia congenita. The alpha chain of the voltage-sensitive channel consists of approximately 2,000 amino acids that form four homologous membrane-spanning domains as shown. Each domain is composed of six helices; in each, the fourth helix is positively charged (hatched segment) and is believed to act as a voltage sensor that opens or activates the channel with membrane depolarization. Mutations identified in hyperkalemic periodic paralysis are situated toward the cytoplasmic ends of segment S5 in domain II and S6 in domain IV (methionine to threonine and methionine to valine, respectively); mutations causing paramyotonia congenita are located in the III–IV intracytoplasmic loop believed responsible for channel inactivation (glycine to valine and threonine to methionine).*

In four paramyotonia patients, two mutations have been identified in the III–IV intracytoplasmic loop, glycine to valine and threonine to methionine, as illustrated (56). The glycine-to-valine mutation is particularly intriguing because this disrupts a –gly–gly– pair that may serve as a hinge for pivoting; restriction of motion of this loop by the mutation may render its normal function more temperature dependent.

It is likely that there will be a family of mutations underlying these diseases involving both other sodium channel sites and other voltage-sensitive channels. Thus, McClatchey et al (57) have demonstrated that different hyperkalemic periodic paralysis families tend to have several different chromosome 17 haplotypes; the suggestion that these will have different mutations is underscored by the fact that, although seemingly linked to the sodium channel locus on chromosome 17, they do not have either of the two hyperkalemic paralysis mutations described to date. That there will be heterogeneity in these diseases is suggested further by the report of Fontaine et al (58) that hypokalemic periodic paralysis is not linked to the chromosome 17 sodium channel. Further, a voltage-dependent chloride channel has recently been found to underlie autosomal recessive myotonia in a mutant mouse (59); conceivably an analogous chloride channel will be implicated in other human myotonic diseases such as myotonia congenita.

CONCLUSIONS

There are several reasons to believe that the pathogenesis of the periodic paralyses will be clarified in the near future. First, technical advances in cellular electrical recording now allow detailed voltage clamp analysis of muscle fibers; this will undoubtedly improve our understanding of the primary electrophysiologic defects in periodic paralysis. Second, available molecular biologic methods permit isolation of genes encoding membrane constituents implicated in disturbances of excitability. As one example, the voltage-dependent sodium channel has now been cloned and sequenced (43,44). The hypothesis that some moiety of such molecules is defective in periodic paralysis can now be directly tested by a combination of methods, including immunofluorescence, immunoblotting, and RNA and DNA analysis. Finally, gene linkage analysis of periodic paralysis pedigrees offers another approach to defining the locus and nature of the defective gene. Though rare, families with periodic paralyses often are large, with several affected survivors, and thus are suited to traditional gene linkage analysis.

REFERENCES

1. Poskanzer DC, Kerr DNS. A third type of periodic paralysis with normokalemia and a favorable response to sodium chloride. Am J Med 1961;31:328–341.
2. Engel AG. Periodic paralysis. In: Engel AG, Banker BQ, eds. Myology. New York: McGraw-Hill, 1986:1843–1870.
3. Riggs JE. The periodic paralyses. In: Riggs JE, guest ed. Muscle disease. Philadelphia: WB Saunders, 1988:485–498.
4. Rudel R, Lehmann-Horn F. Membrane changes in cells from myotonia patients. Physiol Rev 1985;65:310–356.
5. Rudel R, Ricker K. The periodic paralyses. Trends Neurol Sci 1985;8:467–470.
6. Rudel R. The physiological basis of myotonia and the periodic paralyses. In: Engel AG, Banker BQ, eds. Myology. New York: McGraw-Hill, 1986:1297–1312.
7. Stubbs WA. Bidirectional tachycardia in familial hypokalemic periodic paralysis. Proc Roy Soc Med 1976;69:223–224.
8. Resnick JS, Engel WK. Myotonic lid lag in hypokalemic periodic paralysis. J Neurol Neurosurg Psychiatry 1967;30:47–51.
9. Engel AG, Lambert EH, Rosenem JM, Tauxe WN. Clinical and electromyographic studies in primary hypokalemic periodic paralysis. Am J Med 1965;38:626–640.
10. Shy GM, Wanke T, Rowley PT, Engel AG. Studies in familial periodic paralysis. Exp Neurol 1961;3:53–121.
11. Engel AG. Evolution and content of vacuoles in primary hypokalemic periodic paralysis. Mayo Clin Proc 1970;45:774–841.
12. Engel AG. Electron microscopic observations in primary and hyperthyroid periodic paralysis. Mayo Clin Proc 1966;41:797–808.
13. Engel AG. Thyroid function and periodic paralysis. Am J Med 1961;30:327–333.
14. Sperelakis N, Schneider MF, Harris EG. Decreased potassium conductance produced by barium toxicity in frog sartorius muscle. J Gen Physiol 1967;50:1565–1583.
15. Dalakas MC, Engel WK. Treatment of "permanent" muscle weakness in familial hypokalemic periodic paralysis. Muscle Nerve 1983;6:182–186.
16. Bradley WG. Adynamia episodica hereditaria. Brain 1969;92:345–378.
17. Gamstorp I. Adynamia episodica hereditaria. Acta Pediatr Scand 1965;45:1–126.
18. Ricker K, Rohkamm, Bohlen R. Adynamia episodica and paralysis periodica paramyotonica. Neurology 1986;36:682–686.
19. Streeten DH, Dalakos TG, Fellerman H. Studies on hyperkalemic periodic paralysis. Evidence of changes in plasma Na and Cl and induction of paralysis by adrenal glucocorticoids. J Clin Invest 1971;50:142–155.
20. Bendheim PE, Reale EO, Berg BO. Beta-adrenergic treatment of hyperkalemic periodic paralysis. Neurology 1985;35:746–749.
21. Becker PE. Genetic approaches to the nosology of muscle diseases. Myotonias and similar diseases. Birth Defects 1971;7:52–62.
22. Creutzfeld OD, Abbott PC, Fowler WM, Pearson CM. Muscle membrane potentials in episodica adynamia. Electroencephalogr Clin Neurophysiol 1963;15:508–515.
23. Layzer RB. Periodic paralysis and the sodium-potassium pump. Ann Neurol 1982;11:547–552.
24. Martin AR, Levinson SR. Contribution of the Na-K pump to membrane potential in familial periodic paralysis. Muscle Nerve 1985;8:359–362.
25. Daut J. Inhibition of the sodium pump in a guinea-pig ventricular muscle by dihydro-ouabain with effects on external potassium and sodium. J Physiol 1983;339:643–662.
26. Rudel R, Lehmann-Horn F, Ricker K, Kuther G. Hypokalemic periodic paralysis: in vitro investigation of muscle fiber membrane parameters. Muscle Nerve 1984;7:110–120.
27. Falk G, Landa JF. Effects of potassium on frog skeletal muscle in a chloride deficient medium. Am J Physiol 1960;198:1225–1231.
28. Minaker KL, Meneilly GS, Flier JS, Rose JW. Insulin-mediated hypokalemia and paralysis in familial hypokalemic periodic paralysis. Am J Med 1988;84:1001–1006.
29. Lehmann-Horn F, Rudel R, Ricker K, et al. Two cases of adynamia episodica hereditaria: in vitro investigation of muscle cell membrane contraction parameters. Muscle Nerve 1983;6:113–121.
30. Lehmann-Horn F, Kuther G, Ricker K, et al. Adynamia episodica hereditaria with myotonia: a non-inactivating sodium current and the effect of extracellular pH. Muscle Nerve 1987;10:363–374.
31. Chiu SY. Inactivation of sodium channels: second order kinetics in myelinated nerve. J Physiol 1977;273:573–596.
32. Almers W, Standfield PR, Stuhmen W. Slow changes in current through sodium channels in frog muscle membrane. J Physiol 1985;339:253–271.
33. Ruff RL, Simoncini L, Stuhmen W. Slow sodium channel inactivation in mammalian muscles: a possible role in regulating excitability. Muscle Nerve 1988;11:502–510.
34. Ricker K, Camacho LM, Grafe P, et al. Adynamia episodica hereditaria: what causes the weakness? Muscle Nerve 1989;12:883–891.
35. Engel AG, Lambert EH. Calcium activation of electrically inexcitable muscle fibers in primary hypokalemic periodic paralysis. Neurology 1969;19:851–858.
36. de Silva SM, Kuncl RW, Griffin JW, et al. Paramyotonia congenita or hyperkalemic periodic paralysis? Clinical features and electrophysiological features of each entity in one family. Muscle Nerve 1990;13:21–26.
37. Streib EW. Hypokalemic paralysis in two patients with paramyotonia congenita (PC) and known hyperkalemic/exercise-induced weakness. Muscle Nerve 1989;12:936–937.
38. Lehmann-Horn F, Rudel R, Ricker K. Membrane defects in paramyotonia congenita (Eulenburg). Muscle Nerve 1987;10:633–641.
39. Barchi RL. The myotonic syndromes. In: Riggs JE, ed. Neurologic clinics. vol. 6, Muscle disease. Toronto: WB Saunders, 1988:473–484.
40. DiFrancesco D, Noble D. A model of cardiac electrical activity incorporating ionic pumps and concentration changes. Philos Trans R Soc Scand 1985;307:353–398.
41. Adrian RH, Peachey LD. Reconstruction of the action potential of frog sartorius muscle. J Physiol 1973;235:103–131.
42. Adrian RH, Marshall MW. Action potential reconstruction in normal and myotonic muscle fibers. J Physiol 1976;258:125–143.
43. Catterall WA. Molecular properties of the voltage sensitive sodium channel. Ann Rev Biochem 1986;55:953–985.
44. Noda M, Shimiya S, Tanabe T, et al. The primary structure of the electrophorus electricus sodium channel detected with a cDNA sequence. Nature 1984;312:121–127.
45. Fontaine B, Khurana TS, Hoffman EP, et al. Hyperkalemic periodic paralysis and the adult muscle sodium channel gene. Science 1990;250:1000–1002.
46. Ptacek LJ, Tyler F, Trimmer JS, et al. Analysis in a large hyperkalemic periodic paralysis pedigree supports tight linkage to a sodium channel locus. Am J Hum Genet 1991;49:378–382.
47. Ebers GC, George AL, Barchi RL, et al. Paramyotonia congenita and hyperkalemic periodic paralysis are linked to the adult muscle sodium channel gene. Ann Neurol 1992;30:810–816.
48. Ptacek LJ, Timmer JS, Agnew WS, et al. Paramyotonia congenita and hyperkalemic periodic paralysis map to the same sodium channel gene locus. Am J Hum Genet 1991;49:851–854.
49. Cannon SC, Brown RH Jr, Corey DP. A sodium channel defect in hyperkalemic periodic paralysis: potassium induced failure of inactivation. Neuron 1991;6:619–626.
50. Cannon SC, Brown RH Jr, Corey DP. Hodgkin-Huxley modeling of myotonia in periodic paralysis (submitted).

51. Catterall WA. Molecular properties of the voltage sensitive sodium channel. Ann Rev Biochem 1986;55:953–985.
52. Noda M, Shimiya S, Tanabe T, et al. The primary structure of the electrophorus electricus sodium channel detected with a cDNA sequence. Nature 1984;312:121–127.
53. Stuhmer W, Conti F, Suzuki H, et al. Structural parts involved in activation and inactivation of the sodium channel. Nature 1989;339:597–603.
54. Rojas CV, Wang J, Schwartz LS, et al. A met-to-val mutation in the skeletal muscle NA+ channel alpha-subunit in hyperkalemic periodic paralysis. Nature 1991;354:387–389.
55. Ptacek LJ, George AL Jr, Griggs RC, et al. Identification of a mutation in the gene causing hyperkalemic periodic paralysis. Cell 1991;67:1021–1027.
56. McClatchey AI, Van den Bergh P, Pericak-Vance MA, et al. Temperature sensitive mutations in the III–IV cytoplasmic loop region of the skeletal muscle sodium channel gene in paramyotonia congenita. Cell 1992;68:769–774.
57. McClatchey AI, Tofatter J, McKenna-Yasek D, et al. Dinucleotide repeat polymorphisms at the SCN4A locus suggest allelic heterogeneity of hyperkalemic periodic paralysis and paramyotonia congenita. Am J Hum Genet 1992;50:896–901.
58. Fontaine B, Rouleua G, Haines J, et al. Hypokalemic periodic paralysis is not linked to skeletal muscle sodium channel gene on chromosome 17. Neuromuscul Disord (in press).
59. Steinmeyer K, Klocke R, Ortland C, et al. Inactivation of muscle chloride channel by transposon insertion in myotonic mice. Nature 1991;354:304–308.

Motor Control After Deafferentation

LEWIS SUDARSKY   DAVID M. DAWSON   JOSEPH BOSSOM

INTRODUCTION

Early animal studies describe a striking disturbance in motor behavior after the loss of somatic sensation in a limb. Studies by Mott and Sherrington (1) and Cooper and Denny-Brown (2) demonstrated loss of use and profound motor deficits after dorsal rhizotomy in primates. In his 1931 lectures, Sherrington summarized his experience with deafferentation in the monkey: "Willed movements are upset in the extreme . . . the desensitized limb is practically useless, for prehension quite so. The animal soon treats it as useless and as an encumbrance worse than useless" (3). Similar results were obtained by Twitchell in 1954 after bilateral C3-T3 dorsal rhizotomy. The limited movement that was seen in recovered animals was highly dependent on visual guidance (4).

A different outcome was observed by Munk in 1909. He deafferented one side and found considerable recovery of function, provided the good arm was bound. This forced the animal to use the operated side. The monkeys were able to use the arm to feed, though movements remained "ataxic, dysmetric, and clumsy" (5). In the studies of Taub and Berman, nearly all the dysfunction induced by unilateral deafferentation could be overcome by such encouragement and specific training (6). An extended period of immobilization of the normal arm was required to overcome the nonuse of the operated side. Taub showed that recovery of function was better after bilateral forelimb deafferentation. After bilateral procedures, animals were essentially forced to overcome the disincentives and limitations. Taub was quite emphatic about the level of skill the monkeys were able to reacquire. His subjects were described as capable of learning almost any task within the repertoire of a normal monkey, including prehensile grasp. "Even so demanding a task as picking up raisins from a shallow well between thumb and forefinger proved within their capabilities" (7). These claims have always been controversial, as there was no histologic verification of lesions. With even minimal sparing of sensory afferents, remarkable motor skills can be preserved.

Other studies of dorsal rhizotomy in primates from the 1970s established motor recovery well beyond that envisioned by Sherrington (3). In Bossom's studies good outcome was enhanced by improvements in surgical technique and perioperative care. Nonetheless, he stressed some limitations. Monkeys with deafferented upper limbs had an awkwardness (an "ataxia") in visually guided reaching behavior. Even in the most successful animals, normal elegance was never achieved. Animals with demonstrated proficiency in motor skills had a tendency not to use the limb in "free ranging" behavior (8,9). Polit and Bizzi studied the accuracy of highly trained forearm movements restricted to a single plane. Monkeys deafferented by dorsal rhizotomy were able to perform these movements with requisite precision, with and without visual guidance. Animals were also able to compensate for an unexpected displacement in position or load factor. However, some accuracy was lost in the deafferented animal when the spatial orientation of the apparatus was changed (10).

An extensive literature on lesions of the dorsal columns was critically reviewed by Wall in 1970 (11). Many negative studies have been done on sensation after dorsal column section, suggesting a redundancy of sensory afferent systems. The posterior columns are only one of the pathways contributing to somesthesia. Muscle spindle afferents in the spinocerebellar tracts, for example, are thought to be particularly important during movement. A disturbance in motor behavior after dorsal column section in monkeys was described by Gilman and Denny-Brown. They noted a lack of grasping, and a failure to use the affected arm after unilateral lesions. Upper limb movements were described as slow and inept during reaching behavior. Grooming movements were more precise (12). Wall speculated that the dorsal column pathway is essentially involved in active exploratory behavior, as opposed to passively acquired sensation. With ablation of sensory systems at a cortical level, the effects are more complex, as reviewed by Mountcastle. Prominent deficits are observed in the exploration of extrapersonal space (13).

In sum, the primate studies on deafferentation over the last century leave a sense of confusion about the nature of the deficit. With encouragement, considerable recovery of motor function appears possible in the deafferented limb, including the capability for some precision tasks. Yet the limb is regarded as somewhat useless by the animals, who occasionally neglect it in ordinary behavior. Some movements are done better than others. Disuse exceeds that which can be accounted for by the slight loss of dexterity and finesse.

HUMAN STUDIES

Early observations of motor disorder in humans without proprioception come from the nineteenth-century literature on tabetic neurosyphilis. "Locomotor ataxia" due to sensory loss was described by Romberg and others. The hallmark is a standing imbalance made worse by closure of the eyes. Gowers described oscillation of the bare feet and toes during stance, excess sway, and a slapping gait: "Often the feet are raised too high, thrown forward too far, brought down too suddenly, and the whole sole comes in contact with the ground at once." An imprecision was also described in the use of the hand. "It is impossible for the patient to button his coat, or to pick up a small object from the table; the fingers twist about in the attempt, and the grasp is not sustained; first one finger is felt to relax and then another" (14).

Foerster in 1911 and 1913 published his experience with a large series of cases in which the dorsal roots were resected over several segments (15,16). Variable motor function was observed; most of his patients had other neurologic deficits upon which deafferentation was superimposed. In none of his patients was motor function truly normal. Half a century later, Nathan and Sears studied the effects of dorsal rhizotomy on movement in the deafferented muscles in three patients. Observations were limited to the levator scapulae and diaphragm, and the more subtle problem of coordinated limb movement was not addressed. A brief period of nonfunction was reported, but ultimately recovery was observed in the respiratory muscles (17).

A most remarkable series of observations was reported by Rothwell et al in a man with severe sensory neuropathy (18). Experimental work indicates that a small proportion of afferent fibers traverse the ventral root, so the physiologic deficit in these patients may be somewhat more complete than that following dorsal rhizotomy. The patient, a 36-year-

old man, initially lost his proficiency at throwing darts. He progressed to the point that he was numb to the knees and unsteady in gait. Examination revealed that he had retained the ability to perform a large repertoire of fine movements. He could produce independent precise movements of the digits, and rapid alternating movements involving the hand and fingers. He was able to trace shapes in the air, with eyes open or closed, with a precision approaching normal subjects. But something was lost when translating these skills to the activities of daily living. The disparity was noted by Marsden et al:

> Despite the large range of laboratory tasks he could perform, his hands were relatively useless to him in daily life when undertaking fine tasks. He could only drink and feed himself with difficulty; writing and fastening buttons to dress himself were almost impossible (19).

This single case is perhaps the best studied in terms of motor skill. The investigators attempted to define the exact nature of the patient's incapacity. In the absence of visual guidance, a drift was evident in limb position over time. This was a cause of creeping error in tasks where maintenance of postural attitude was critical. The patient was also unable to adjust to changes in load during ongoing limb movement, a finding somewhat at odds with the studies of Polit and Bizzi in primates (10). This kind of load compensation may be important in the detailed workings of the human hand while writing, knitting, buttoning, and so on.

DESCRIPTION OF THE CLINICAL SYNDROME

The motor control disorder that follows deafferentation has four principal features.

1. There is a tendency toward disuse of the affected limb.
2. There is difficulty in the use of the hands. Patients exhibit clumsiness, misreaching, and pseudoathetosis.
3. There is a characteristic disorder of stance and gait.
4. Patients have difficulty with motor learning, and may not be fully able to use visual guidance systems to compensate.

In order to describe the core features of the syndrome in more detail, we include some reference to case material.

Patients with unilateral lesions prefer not to use the deafferented side. To some degree dysesthesias and pain may contribute to this preference, but some disuse is evident even in the absence of intrusive positive symptoms. Patients tend to describe the involved limbs as somewhat useless, even though they can master some manual skills with encouragement. Lesions of somatosensory pathways at a more rostral level also produce disuse, at least initially. With parietal lobe lesions, neglect is a prominent part of the syndrome (13).

A number of difficulties with precision are evident in the use of the hand. Patients have an awkwardness that interferes with fine manual skills. This is particularly evident in tasks where sensory and motor systems are interdependent, such as buttoning a shirt, writing, or manipulating tools. Lack of delicacy is also apparent in movements for which load compensation is a factor. Patients describe difficulty picking up a coffee cup without crushing it. Marsden and associates' patient described difficulty carrying a suitcase, and a constant need to check visually to be sure that he had not dropped it.

Writhing movements of the fingers are observed, enhanced by eye closure or aversion of gaze. These movements of the distal limb, called sensory pseudoathetosis, represent drift over time in feedback control of limb position. There is little to add to Gowers' description:

> If the patient attempts to hold out his hand in a fixed posture it is seen that [an] irregularity obtains; instead of a uniform balanced contraction the muscles contract and relax involuntarily, and slow unintended movements of the fingers result, sometimes closely resembling those of athetosis (14).

The same movements may occur in the foot, but not in the facial muscles.

A patient recently seen in our department illustrates many of these features.

Standing imbalance and gait disorder are common manifestations of sensory loss, though tabetic neurosyphilis has almost disappeared from contemporary practice. Drachman and Hart recognized this presentation in their classic paper on dizziness. They describe the patient, often diabetic, often elderly, whose imbalance is the product of multiple sensory deficits (21). A patient from our clinic with vestibular injury secondary to ototoxic drugs described severe standing imbalance. There was no vertigo, but walking required constant visual control and a railing, wall, or support surface to cling to. The dependence of postural support mechanisms on sensory information has been studied by Forssberg and Nashner (22) and Nashner et al (23). The system is highly dependent on information from muscle spindles and proprioceptive afferents.

Sudarsky and Ronthal identified sensory disorders as the cause of gait failure in 18% of cases, in a series of neurologic referrals for undiagnosed gait disorder in the elderly (24). Patients complain of vague dizziness or imbalance, though rarely active vertigo. The gait is wide based, with short steps and a tendency to be easily displaced, especially backward. An increased proportion of the gait cycle is spent in double limb stance, a biomechanical adaptation to failing balance (25). High stepping and slapping foot placement are sometimes observed, even in the absence of foot drop. The entire performance is much worse in the dark or with the eyes closed, and falls are common at night. Some such patients present with hip fracture.

The effect on motor learning is the most difficult to describe. Many fine motor tasks are thought to be largely preprogrammed, modified, and executed automatically by the nervous system when called. Such skilled actions—playing the piano is a good example—are too rapid to allow for sensory feedback during execution. There is great difficulty in the learning and initial acquisition of these so-called motor programs. This step requires trial and error and considerable effort, a difficulty to which anyone who has learned a new motor skill in adult life can attest. Obvious examples include serving a tennis ball, riding a bicycle, or eating with chopsticks.

Human patients with deafferentation or severe proprioceptive loss experience added difficulty learning new skills. Marsden et al related a story about a patient who purchased a new car sometime after the onset of his sensory disorder. Although previously able to operate a manual gearshift, he was unable to master the procedure in his new car. Operating the gearshift involves "learning the feel" of the car, something for which other sensory afferent information cannot substitute. Despite the motivation provided by expense, he ultimately gave up and made do with his old car (19).

Case Study

A 32-year-old woman, originally from Mexico City, developed an acute illness that would fall into the category of acute sensory ganglionopathy. Recovery was slow, but motor power returned adequately. She was left with a persistent, severe sensory loss of the type described by Asbury (20). Her sensory loss was nearly universal. She described herself as feeling as if she were in an astronaut's suit and covered with a thick layer of aluminum. Electrophysiologic studies done 3 years after the acute illness showed normal conduction velocity in motor fibers, and the amplitude of the muscle action potential was normal. In contrast, the amplitude of the evoked sensory action potential was depressed two orders of magnitude, and conduction velocity was slowed.

Her hand and finger use were inaccurate and slow. Sensory pseudoathetosis was present. Although she had no demonstrable position sense at proximal joints, her deficits seemed more evident in movements of the hands and fingers. She had trained herself to print and write using a pencil, using heavy pressure of her hand against the paper to prevent inaccurate movements. When her eyes were closed, she was completely unable to write and could not tell if she was making a mark on the paper. She could not button her clothes or tie her shoes. Interestingly, her reaching movements were relatively accurate and she was able to perform finger-to-nose testing with only modest impairment. When her eyes were closed and movement was repeated, it tended to resemble the prior movement quite closely. Her gait was slow and careful, wide based, with feet placed 12 to 18 inches apart. She wore heavy shoes with hard rubber heels, so that she could hear them strike the floor. She used visual correction and guidance to walk.

TREATMENT (MANAGEMENT) OF THE PATIENT

The described clinical syndrome may be observed with a variety of diseases, only some of which are treatable. In disorders of the peripheral nervous system, there is considerable capacity for regeneration and restoration of function. The general management and rehabilitation of the patient includes physiotherapy directed at learning new strategies for use of the limb. For the hand and arm, this generally involves the use of other afferent sensory systems to compensate. With good motivation and practice, a considerable repertoire of skilled movements can be reacquired.

For the trunk and legs, the emphasis is on gait training. Retraining balance has been attempted using sophisticated biofeedback techniques by Shephard et al (26). In most physical therapy departments, gait training heavily emphasizes assistive devices and sensible footwear to improve traction and widen the base of support.

SCIENTIFIC CONSIDERATIONS

A popular hypothesis suggests two modes for the organization and control of movement: automatic execution of preprogrammed movement, and movement under sensory feedback control. Wise and Evarts called these "open loop" and "closed loop" motor control (27). The terminology is borrowed from contemporary robotics, which has provided considerable inspiration for neurophysiologists.

Some precision tasks are done rapidly, in a preprogrammed fashion with little or no sensory feedback. According to this model, the neocortex supplies a goal for the movement, and a high-level specification is used to construct it from preprogrammed chunks. Typing and playing the piano are typical examples, in that the speed of finger movements does not allow for sensory guidance or a midcourse correction. Movements of this type are executed by pyramidal tract neurons essentially in an open-loop mode.

For other tasks, sensory feedback is essential. This dependence is particularly great for sensory-driven tasks such as exploratory behavior, eating with chopsticks, even buttoning or manipulating with the fingers. In this case, pyramidal tract neurons execute movement, but sensory feedback from the cerebellum and thalamus is used to refine ongoing movement. These open-loop systems are slower and have some propensity toward oscillation when disabled.

Studies of the anatomy by Wise and Strick support this dichotomy (28). The primary motor cortex (area 4) is the point of origin for the pyramidal tract neurons, the principal effector pathway. Nonprimary motor cortex includes two large cortical fields in the frontal lobe: the supplementary motor area (M2) and the premotor area. There is also speculation that the postcentral gyrus may have some role in movement. These areas enjoy distinct networks of subcortical connections. The basal ganglia (globus pallidus)

project largely to the supplementary motor area, via the ventrolateral thalamic nucleus. Presumably this is the pathway for automatic execution of preprogrammed movement (striatum → pallidum → ventrolateral thalamus → M2 → M1 motor cortex). The cerebellar connections are routed through a separate part of the thalamus to premotor and primary motor cortical fields. There are also direct connections from the postcentral gyrus (S1) to the precentral gyrus (M1). These pathways are better positioned to function in the sensory guidance of movement. Spinal afferents to the thalamus and cerebellum generate the peripheral feedback to close the loop.

There is also evidence that the cerebellum acts as a comparator in the execution and refinement of ongoing movement, that is, as a device that compares intention with performance. In studies of cerebellar afferents, Lundberg and Oscarsson demonstrated that the dorsal spinocerebellar tract reports on movement in progress. The ventral spinocerebellar tract, on the other hand, reflects the central command to motor neurons (29). In studies by Arshavsky et al, phasic activity normally seen in Clarke's column during locomotion was abolished by deafferentation, while the pattern of activity in the ventral pathway was unaffected by the loss of peripheral input (30). In normal functioning, the cerebellum can monitor these two pathways and help compensate for errors.

Studies for human cases are of special relevance to the scientific thought on this problem. Some highly skilled movements are retained after deafferentation, suggesting that they are done in open-loop mode. Other kinds of voluntary movement and motor learning are compromised by the degradation or absence of sensory feedback. Through studies such as these, we can begin to learn what anatomy is relevant to a particular task.

REFERENCES

1. Mott FW, Sherrington CS. Experiments upon the influence of sensory nerves upon movement and nutrition of the limbs. Proc R Soc Lond 1895;57:481–488.
2. Cooper, Denny-Brown D. Proc R Soc Lond 1927;102B:222.
3. Sherrington CS. Quantitative management of contraction in lowest level coordination. Brain 1931;54:1–28.
4. Twitchell TE. Sensory factors in purposive movement. J Neurophysiol 1954;17:239–254.
5. Munk H. Uber die Functionen von Hirn und Ruckenmark. Berlin: Hirschwald, 1909.
6. Taub E, Berman AJ. Avoidance conditioning in the absence of relevant proprioceptive and exteroceptive feedback. J Physiol Psychol 1963;56:1012–1016.
7. Taub E. Movement in nonhuman primates deprived of somatosensory feedback. Exerc Sport Sci Rev 1976;4:335–374.
8. Bossom J. Time of recovery of voluntary movement following dorsal rhizotomy. Brain Res 1972;45:247–250.
9. Bossom J. Movement without proprioception. Brain Res 1974;71:285–296.
10. Polit A, Bizzi E. Characteristics of motor programs underlying arm movements in monkeys. J Neurophysiol 1979;42:183–194.
11. Wall PD. The sensory and motor role of impulses travelling in the dorsal columns towards cerebral cortex. Brain 1970;93:505–524.
12. Gilman S, Denny-Brown D. Disorders of movement and behavior following dorsal column lesions. Brain 1966;89:397–418.
13. Mountcastle VB. Medical physiology. St Louis: CV Mosby, 1968:1415.

14. Gowers WR. Diseases of the nervous system. Philadelphia: Blakiston, 1888:290–291.

15. Foerster O. Uber die Beeinflussing spastischer Lahmingen durch die Resektion hinterer Ruckenmarkswurzeln. Dtsch Zeitschr Nervenheilkunde 1911;41:146–169.

16. Foerster O. On the indications and results of the excision of posterior spinal nerve roots. Surg Gynecol Obstet 1913;16:463–474.

17. Nathan PW, Sears TA. Effects of posterior root section on the activity of some muscles in man. J Neurol Neurosurg Psychiatry 1960;23:10–22.

18. Rothwell JC, Traub MM, Day BL, et al. Manual motor performance in a deafferented man. Brain 1982;105:515–542.

19. Marsden CD, Rothwell JC, Day BL. The use of peripheral feedback in the control of movement. In: Evarts E, Wise S, Bousfield D, eds. The motor system in neurobiology. Amsterdam: Elsevier, 1985:215–222.

20. Asbury AK. Sensory neuronopathy. Semin Neurol 1987;7:58–66.

21. Drachman D, Hart C. An approach to the dizzy patient. Neurology 1972;22:323–334.

22. Forssberg H, Nashner LM. Ontogenetic development of postural control in man. J Neurosci 1982;2:545–552.

23. Nashner LM, Black FO, Wall C. Adaptation to altered support and visual conditions during stance. J Neurosci 1982;2:536–544.

24. Sudarsky L, Ronthal M. Gait disorders among elderly patients. Arch Neurol 1983;40:740–743.

25. Sudarsky L, Simon S. Gait disorder in late-life hydrocephalus. Arch Neurol 1987;44:263–267.

26. Shephard NT, Telion SA, Smith-Wheelock M. Habitation and balance retraining therapy Neurol Clin 1990;8:459–476.

27. Wise S, Evarts E. The role of the cerebral cortex in movement. In: Evarts E, Wise S, Bousfield D, eds. The motor system in neurobiology. Amsterdam: Elsevier, 1986:307–314.

28. Wise S, Strick P. Anatomical and physiological organization of the non-primary motor cortex. In: Evarts E, Wise S, Bousfield D, eds. The motor system in neurobiology. Amsterdam: Elsevier, 1986:315–324.

29. Oscarsson O. Functional organization of spinocerebellar paths. In: Iggo A, ed. Handbook of sensory physiology. Vol. 2. New York: Springer-Verlag, 1973:339–380.

30. Arshavsky YI, Berkenglit MB, Fukson OI, et al. Origin of modulation in neurons of the ventral spinocerebellar tract during locomotion. Brain Res 1972;43:276–279.

Frontal Lobe Automatisms

GILBERT H. GLASER

INTRODUCTION

Involuntary disturbances of motion in epilepsy are almost infinite in variety. The characteristics of the movements and their extent and sequencing vary from the simple to the complex. When a patient develops a state of confusion or amnesia during or immediately following an epileptic seizure, but retains motor control and exhibits certain motor behaviors, these are said to be automatic and a state conveniently described as automatism (1). There may be varying degrees of interference with consciousness, but amnesia is usually complete. These movements then, associated with a seizure state and regarded as automatisms, are automatic, usually complex, and often bizarre, but frequently resemble voluntary activity. They may or may not be related to or stimulated by environmental influences. The international classification of seizures places automatisms in the category of complex partial seizures. These are most commonly regarded as of temporal lobe origin, especially from the deep temporal lobe, or hippocampal-amygdalar (limbic) origin. However, there has been increasing recognition, especially during the last two decades, that a number of such automatisms do arise from extratemporal, especially frontal lobe, structures, particularly those with limbic associations, but also more independently. As these have become more studied, certain observed phenomena tend to give them a more specific, characteristic entity. However, because of the physiologic developments of the spread of epileptiform activity during the seizure state throughout other brain structures, especially limbic, frequently definitive localization or even lateralization is difficult (2,3).

Historically, nonconvulsive seizures, such as automatisms, have been known since the writings of Hippocrates and Galen (4), but it was not until the early sixteenth century that epileptic automatisms were more clearly described.

Gowers (5) recognized automatisms, and the extensive work of Hughlings Jackson in the latter part of the nineteenth century (6) showed by careful pathologic studies in patients with specific seizures that most of these originated from the temporal lobe, not the frontal. Jackson also described, as had Bravais (7) previously, a simple localized motor clonic seizure form involving the extremities unilaterally. This, of course, is referred to as focal jacksonian epilepsy and is really a simple frontal lobe motor seizure of rolandic origin.

The extensive research of Penfield and Jasper during the late 1940s and early 1950s (1) involved meticulous study of patients with focal epilepsy in whom brain stimulation and electrocorticographic studies were carried out during operative intervention for the treatment of intractable focal seizures. In these studies, a number of patients were clearly found to have involvement of the frontal lobe and its component structures in motor automatisms. This early detailed characterization of frontal lobe automatisms described them as an automatic stereotyped behavior associated with amnesia. They were different from temporal lobe automatisms in that in those of frontal lobe origin there was a greater tendency to an invariable type of pseudovoluntary stereotyped activity. This type of activity, as presented by Penfield and Jasper, often involved tearing of clothing and choking movements at the throat, with resistance to attempts to stop these activities. The patient behaved in a confused manner, and occasionally during the seizure would wander about. Aversive movements and turning of the head and eyes, occasionally controversive, were frequent. Electrical stimulation of the frontal lobe cortex was shown by Penfield and Jasper (1) to produce many behavioral elements of the motor automatism associated with epileptiform discharges in the recorded electrocorticogram. A number of these patients were found to have the discharging focus in an intermediate region anterior to the motor cortex. Occasionally, the discharge would spread to the orbital region or rapidly to the opposite side. Certain cases had the frontal pole involved, when there was contusion or scar in that region.

An involvement of the supplementary motor cortex in frontal lobe automatisms in a certain number of patients also was first considered in detail by Penfield and Jasper (1). This region is anterior to the upper end of the precentral motor region, that is, the leg control area, and within the longitudinal fissure. Stimulations of this region produced aversive movements of the head and upper part of the body, usually turning to the side contralateral to the focus. Occasionally, however, the aversion was ipsilateral. When there was spread to the rolandic motor cortex region, there was more localized than generalized clonic motor activity, as in a generalized convulsion, and also a loss of consciousness. The supplementary motor cortex area within the longitudinal fissure has been studied by electrical stimulation, as well as analysis of epileptic discharging, with the production of the body movements, as described, along with vocalization. There have been extensive neurophysiologic investigations of this region, beginning with those of Horsley and Schafer (8), Leyton and Sherrington (9), and Foerster (10). A comprehensive survey of knowledge of basic and clinical research on the supplementary sensorimotor area is available. This survey includes information on supplementary sensorimotor area epilepsy with its characteristic automatisms, their differential diagnosis, and treatment (11).

CLINICAL CHARACTERISTICS AND DIAGNOSIS OF FRONTAL LOBE AUTOMATISMS

During the past 30 years and especially in the last decade, there has developed a body of knowledge that now tends to clarify the phenomena occurring in frontal lobe motor automatisms and enable their differentiation from those of temporal lobe origin. Extensive studies of frontal lobe anatomy, physiology, and seizures have been published recently (3,12,13). The early emphasis on the stereotyped nature of frontal lobe automatisms has been confirmed by a number of detailed investigations of significant numbers of patients (14–23). The motor automatisms associated with frontal lobe epilepsy only rarely show initial tonic or clonic activities that are simple in origin. The spread is rapid into the more complex stereotyped automatism. Most commonly, kicking, thrashing, and writhing movements occur, along with some rubbing and scratching movements of the arms and hands. Sexual automatisms, such as pelvic thrusting and genital manipulations, occasionally appear (19). There may be chewing movements and lip smacking. Complex posturing arm movements are frequent, especially in abduction positions. The leg movements often are aimless. Occasionally, they show bilateral coordinated activities. Bizarre facial expressions are frequent. There is often an

onset with a staring, frightened expression. Prominent autonomic changes are not found to be present, such as flushing pallor and piloerection. A complex partial seizure status epilepticus with prolonged frontal lobe automatisms continuing with prolonged confusion has been described in a number of cases (23). The vocalizations are frequently bizarre, with shouting and humming and squealing sounds, occasionally with obscenities. Frontal automatism seizures have had a duration of 15 to 30 seconds to a few minutes, but longer when there is secondary spread to other structures such as the temporal lobe.

The electroencephalogram has been found to vary from exhibiting slow wave focal discharges from a frontal region with just a lateralization to spike, polyspike, and spike and wave discharging focally, with occasional rapid generalization (1,3,12–14,17,19). Depth electrode encephalographic studies also have been carried out in these patients when under selected investigation for surgical treatment when the seizures became intractable to medication (12,13,21,22). Frequently, the scalp electroencephalogram does not show an adequate localization, but the depth recordings may show initial focal discharging from the orbital, median, frontal, and supplementary motor regions.

The pathology in the frontal lobe studied in structures removed surgically has shown small areas of encephalomalacia along with gliosis and sclerosis, dysplasia, and occasional tumor, particularly slow-growing gliomas, such as astrocytoma or oligodendroglioma.

Williamson et al (22) emphasized that although in both frontal and temporal lobe automatisms there may be a change in facial expression and complex illusional states at the onset of the seizure, the motor automatisms are more semipurposeful and have sexual features in the frontal lobe types. There is a more frequent occurrence of seizures in clusters, often many a day and often of brief duration. The stereotyped nature of the seizures is frequent and the vocalizations show a varying complexity. The postical period is relatively short with a rapid clearing. Rasmussen (18) studied the features of frontal lobe epilepsy in "pure culture" in 40 patients. He emphasized these automatisms as complex, stereotyped, and with vague and general body and postural movements. There was an absence of an aura in these patients, although some did have epigastric sensory symptoms.

The French group of Geier et al (15,16) reported extensive studies of patients prior to selection for neurosurgical treatment. The techniques of study have utilized combined depth electrodes, encephalography, and telemetry with video monitoring of the patients during the seizures. This type of investigation also has been used by others and summarized by Williamson et al (22). In these studies, again, the emphasis has been on the occurrence of stereotyped motor automatisms with frequent aversive or controversive deviations of the head and eyes before or after the more complex automatisms. Eupractic motor activity of one or both upper limbs has been described. The patients have shown either intelligible or unintelligible vocalizations and automatisms of mimicry, fear, laughter, and crying. The French investigators believe that the seizure activity developed in the frontal lobe eventually brings into play many numerous cortical and subcortical regions associated in the spread from the focus. The clinical characteristics of certain automatisms indicate that praxic, gnostic, and mnemic functions appear to be utilized during the automatisms, adjusting to what is happening in the immediate environment. Certain of the seizure phenomena are often seen to relate or apply to concrete objects in the surroundings. In one discussion, it is felt that this relation to objects is more than to other humans in the environment (15). A disassociation occurs in the environmental adaptation of the automatisms; that is, they are less adaptive to a reactivity to human influences than to the visualization or appearance of objects in the environment. This type of reactivity is also studied in relation to temporal lobe seizures and is worthy of more consideration in investigations of the phenomena of epilepsy in humans. The French group emphasize that these frontal lobe automatisms show difficulties in the succession and organization of series of movements, with a discontinuity of behavior in more prolonged seizures (16). Errors seem to multiply and the behavior becomes completely unadapted to the environment. These are especially seen when there is mesial or orbital-frontal discharge. However, the clinical aspects of the frontal lobe seizures are more particularly motor and less psychic, in differentiation from the temporal lobe complex partial seizure states. These workers conclude that through its seizures, the frontal lobe expresses one of its functions, especially that of triggering, adapting, and organizing movements.

It should be noted here that the clinical characteristics of the frontal lobe automatisms occasionally lead to the appearance of bizarre motor behavior that could be considered hysterical (23,24). This is especially so with frontal lobe seizures and automatisms in children, and when the episodes occur in association with sleep (24). The diagnostic evaluation to be carried out in these patients, of course, includes the initial establishment of the diagnosis of the presence of an epilepsy. This must be done by careful history, particularly the observation of the patient during the seizure or automatism, by individuals capable of reporting the phenomena in detail, as well as thorough medical and neurologic evaluations that could relate to the etiology. The recent development of more complex electroencephalographic technologies, particularly telemetering and ambulatory electroencephalographic cassette recording, is most helpful. Combined electroencephalography and video observation of patients enables the careful study of the motor and associated phenomena. Diagnostic imaging technology also has become extremely helpful in establishing focal origin; these include computed X-ray tomography, magnetic resonance imaging, and positron emission tomography, when available. When the patient's seizures become intractable to medical therapy, considerations of surgical intervention become paramount. It is then that more intensive electroencephalo-graphic monitoring is considered. The implantation of depth electrodes frequently enables delineation of a specific focus in patients where this may only be suggested by scalp electroencephalography or even when the latter shows generalized or equally bilateral discharges. Subdural electrodes laid over suspected areas are also currently utilized (12,13,25).

TREATMENT

Experience over time in the treatment of frontal lobe automatisms as part of the complex partial seizures stated in frontal lobe epilepsy has shown that these are difficult to treat pharmacologically. Total seizure control is possible, but is infrequent. Seizures can be limited by the careful use of drugs, paying particular attention to monitoring the drug levels in blood, and especially following the principles of using one drug at a time to the most optimally effective levels and, at the most, using two drugs. The drugs most used are carbamazepine, phenytoin, phenobarbital, primidone, and valproate. Each has its quota of problems in toxicity and side effects. Most effective has been carbamazepine, alone or in combination with one of the other drugs such as phenytoin or valproate. Also, phenobarbital or primidone in modest dosage occasionally is a useful adjuvant. In some cases, seizure limitation can be as effective as between 50% and 75%, but even this may be difficult to achieve.

When it is decided over a period of time, varying between 2 and 5 years, that the frontal lobe seizure state is intractable to medication, then directed neurosurgical treatment is considered, if a definitive focus can be found by the utilization of phased evaluations and diagnostic techniques as indicated above (12,13,25). The removal of such a focus has been reported to achieve focal seizure relief in 60% to 80% of the cases, in different series. It must be realized, however, that in many cases there may be bilateral or even more multiple foci, yet the removal of what may be considered the major focus can be effective. In some instances, corpus callosotomy may be helpful (12,13) in reducing the severity and frequency of the seizures.

REFERENCES

1. Penfield W, Jasper H. Epilepsy and the functional anatomy of the human brain. Boston: Little, Brown, and Co, 1954.
2. Schneider RC, Crosbey EC, Farhat SM. Extratemporal lesions triggering the temporal lobe syndrome. J Neurosurg 1964;22:246–263.
3. Manford M, Fish DR, Shorvon SD. An analysis of clinical seizure patterns and their localizing value in frontal and temporal lobe epilepsies. Brain 1996;119:17–40.
4. Temkin O. The falling sickness. Baltimore: Johns Hopkins Press, 1945.
5. Gowers WR. Epilepsy and other chronic convulsive disorders. London: J and A Churchill, 1881.
6. Jackson JH. Selected writings of John Hughlings Jackson. Vol. I, On epilepsy and epileptiform convulsions. Taylor J, ed. London: Hodder and Stoughton, 1931.
7. Bravais LF. Recershes sur les symptomes et le traitement de l'epilepsia hemipleagique. Unpublished thesis. Faculty of Medicine, Paris, 1827.
8. Horsley V, Schafer EA. A record of experiments upon the functions of the cerebral cortex. Philos Trans R Soc Lond 1886;179B:1–45.

9. Leyton ASF, Sherrington CS. Observations on the excitable cortex of the chimpanzee, orangutan, and gorilla. Q J Exp Physiol 1917;11:135–222.

10. Foerster O. The motor cortex of man in the light of Hughlings Jackson's doctrines. Brain 1936;59:135–159.

11. Luders H, ed. Supplementary sensorimotor area. Advances in neurology, vol. 70. New York: Raven Press, 1996.

12. Chauvel P, Delgado-Escueta AV, Halgren E, Bancaud J, eds. Frontal lobe seizures and epilepsies. Advances in neurology, vol. 57. New York: Raven Press, 1992.

13. Jasper HH, Riggio S, Goldman-Rakic PS, eds. Epilepsy and the functional anatomy of the frontal lobe. Advances in neurology, vol. 66, New York: Raven Press, 1995.

14. Ajmone-Marsan C, Goldhammer L. Clinical ictal patterns and electrographic data in cases of partial seizures of frontal-central-parietal origin. In: Brazier M, ed. Epilepsy: its phenomena in man. New York: Academic Press, 1973:235–258.

15. Geier S, Bancaud J, Talaraich J, et al. Automatisms during frontal lobe epileptic seizures. Brain 1976;99:447–458.

16. Geier S, Bancaud J, Bonis A, et al. The seizures of frontal lobe epilepsy: a study of clinical manifestations. Neurology 1977;27:951–958.

17. Ludwig B, Ajmone-Marsan C, Van Buren J. Cerebral seizures of probable orbito-frontal origin. Epilepsia 1975;16:141–158.

18. Rasmussen T. Characteristics of a pure culture of frontal lobe epilepsy. Epilepsia 1983;24:482–493.

19. Spencer SS, Spencer DD, Williamson PD, Mattson RH. Sexual automatisms in complex partial seizures. Neurology 1983;33:527–533.

20. Tharp R. Orbital frontal seizures. A unique electrographic and clinical syndrome. Epilepsia 1972;13:627–642.

21. Wieser HG. Electroclinical features of the psychomotor seizure. Stuttgart: Gustav Fischer–Butterworths, 1983.

22. Williamson PD, Spencer DD, Spencer SS, et al. Complex partial seizures of frontal lobe origin. Ann Neurol 1985;18:497–504.

23. Williamson PD, Wieser HG, Delgado-Escueta AV. Clinical characteristics of partial seizures. In: Engel J Jr, ed. Surgical treatment of the epilepsies. New York: Raven Press, 1987:101–120.

24. Stores G, Zaiwalla Z, Bergel N. Frontal lobe complex partial seizures in children: a form of epilepsy at particular risk of misdiagnosis. Dev Med Child Neurol 1991;33:998–1009.

25. Engel J Jr, ed. Surgical treatment of the epilepsies. New York: Raven Press, 1987.

Complex Motor Manifestations and Directed Aggression in Epilepsy

Robert C. Green   Orrin Devinsky

INTRODUCTION

The broad variety of experiential phenomenology in epilepsy offers tremendous opportunities to better understand the neurology of complex human behaviors. Spontaneous seizure discharges or focal electrical stimulation within the brain can produce simple involuntary motor movements as well as complex, semipurposeful sequences of motor action (automatisms). These same stimuli can evoke hallucinations or emotional experiences that provoke behavioral responses, such as running in response to ictal fear. One of the most controversial areas in behavioral neurology is the assessment of complex, seemingly purposeful motor behaviors in patients with epilepsy or suspected seizures. Recent developments in video-electroencephalographic (video-EEG) monitoring during seizures and in conjunction with electrical brain stimulation have permitted more precise electroclinical and anatomic correlations. However, despite its social, legal, and scientific importance, the evaluation of aggressive and violent behaviors remains particularly problematic. This chapter will review the literature of complex motor phenomenology in epilepsy with particular attention to the diagnosis and management of apparently purposeful motor behaviors such as directed violence.

EXCITATORY AND INHIBITORY FEATURES OF SIMPLE PARTIAL SEIZURES

Focal motor seizures were first described by Pritchard in 1822 (1) and are now understood to result from electrical discharges that stimulate neuronal groups in primary motor, premotor, or supplementary motor areas. Simple motor components of partial seizures include tonic, clonic, and myoclonic movements that are often described as jerking, twitching, quivering, drawing, or stiffening (2). Simple motor seizures usually involve the face, arm, or leg, but all smooth, cardiac, and skeletal musculature may be stimulated during partial seizures (3), and patients sometimes describe the feeling of an internal "movement" that cannot be seen. One of the largest series of simple motor seizures was described by Mauguiere and Courjon (4) in their study of 8939 epileptic patients over 3 years of age. In this population, 1153 (12.9%) had focal motor activity without march, 197 (2.2%) had focal motor activity with march, 581 (6.5%) had hemiconvulsions, and 465 (5.2%) had adversive seizures.

The role of inhibition in seizure-related behaviors was raised by Hughlings Jackson, who argued that elaborate mental states and complex actions occurred with overactivity of neural centers that are released from the control of other "higher centers" (5). Jackson opined that the complex behaviors during or after seizures were not a direct result of the discharging nerve cells, but a reflection of coordinated neural activity in areas not involved in the seizure spread. Jackson's contemporary, Bravais (6), first reported a transient hemiparesis following unilateral motor seizures, but Robert Todd's name was later given to the common clinical phenomenon of postictal paralysis (7). Early explanations of postictal paralysis cited exhaustion (7–9) or active inhibition (10,11), and more recent studies of this phenomenon have focused on a wide variety of membrane channel mechanisms (12). Todd's paralysis is not limited to motor weakness, but may also cause dysfunction in visual, somatosensory, language, and other cognitive functions and may contribute to motor hyperactivity, postictal agitation, and psychosis. Some complex behaviors, such as undressing, running, and wandering, may at times also be attributable to postictal inhibition. These symptoms may be distinguished by the characteristic time course of recovery after a known ictal event.

Partial seizures have historically also been recognized in the form of inhibitory seizures, that is, motor inhibition that is not a result of prior convulsive activity in the neurons subserving the affected muscle groups (11). Speech arrest is the most commonly recognized example of inhibited behaviors that can be produced by seizures or electrical stimulation of areas outside of the classic motor areas (13,14).

ICTAL AND POSTICTAL AUTOMATISMS IN COMPLEX PARTIAL SEIZURES

One of the first well-characterized cases of temporal lobe epilepsy is Jackson's report of Dr Z (15). The following description by that patient illustrates complex symptomology that was recognized to be a part of the epileptic seizure, even in the nineteenth century:

> I . . . have learnt . . . from friendly observers . . . my eyes have a vacant look as if they were not directed to anything near me, or indeed taking notice of anything in particular . . . I often say "yes" to any remark made to me . . . and . . . occasionally make a half-vocalised sound, whether addressed or not. This latter, I have been told, is somewhat like a modified and indistinct smacking of the tongue like a tasting movement, and is generally accompanied by a motion of the lower jaw. . . . Sometimes, specially if sitting I give one or two light stamps on the floor . . .

Complex partial seizures are associated with impairment of consciousness, and in most cases automatisms also occur. Impaired consciousness may be signaled by staring and arrest of ongoing behavior with diminished or absent responsiveness to verbal or gestural commands. Automatisms are semi-purposeful behaviors that require integrated motor functions (14,16). Automatisms may be divided into the following types:

1. Oroalimentary (lip smacking, chewing, swallowing, licking)
2. Facial (distorted facial expressions, frequently giving the appearance of fear)
3. Upper extremity (fumbling, clasping, grabbing movements of the hands; repetitive touching, scratching, or rubbing of objects or body parts)
4. Lower extremity-ambulatory (walking, running, bicycling movements of the legs, kicking)
5. Sexual (pelvic thrusting, masturbation)
6. Vocalization (sounds, words, or phrases) (17)

While automatisms are usually new actions, in some cases they are a continuation of ongoing behavior. For example, patients may continue to stir a pot of soup or shuffle a deck of cards.

In addition to this descriptive classification, automatisms have been categorized by localization of seizure onset and spread. Weiser divided complex partial seizures with temporal lobe onset into four electroclinical syndromes: temporobasal-limbic, temporal polar, opercular, and posterior temporal neocortical (18). According to this scheme, temporobasal-limbic seizures are often preceded by auras with initial preservation of consciousness. When the seizure discharge spreads to involve both temporolimbic regions, consciousness is usually impaired and automatisms with oroalimentary or complex gestural movements of the upper extremities occur. Postural changes as well as tonic and clonic movements may be observed during these seizures. Temporal polar seizures are similar to the basal-limbic seizures, but autonomic changes and oroalimentary automatisms tend to occur earlier. Opercular seizures are associated with focal clonic activity in the contralateral face or arm, auditory hallucinations, and aphasia. Complex auditory and vestibular hallucinations are the most characteristic features of posterior temporal neocortical seizures.

King and Marsan (19) reported the occurrence of motor phenomena in 159 (80%) of 199 patients with temporal lobe seizures by EEG criteria. From observations and patient histories, they documented adversive movements of the head or eyes as well as gestural, alimentary, verbal, ambulatory, and other complex automatisms. The most complex of these movements included changing clothes, lighting a cigarette, or rearranging objects in the room. These behaviors were more likely to be associated with anterior rather than posterior temporal foci, and usually were performed in a stereotyped fashion.

The diversity of clinical experiences in complex partial epilepsy and the relative insensitivity of interictal scalp EEG made more detailed characterizations of ictal phenomena difficult until the advent of recording techniques such as simultaneous closed-circuit television/video-EEG and the use of subdural and depth electrodes for stimulation and recording. These techniques were developed to assist in the localization and surgical resection of epileptic foci in patients with medically intractable epilepsy (20). The widespread use of video-EEG monitoring has provided vastly improved standards for distinguishing seizures from pseudoseizures and for understanding ictal and peri-ictal behaviors.

Early studies using simultaneous video-EEG monitoring clearly demonstrated complex motor events associated with seizure discharges. For example, Escueta et al (21) described 76 psychomotor seizures in 14 epileptic patients and separated attacks into those which began with total unresponsiveness (type I) and those which did not (type II). In both types, these authors described stereotyped automatisms (chewing, blinking, swallowing) progressing to "reactive" automatisms in which there was confusion and partial responsiveness to the environment along with coordinated, apparently purposeful activity (lighting a cigarette, drinking from a glass). Despite some responsiveness during the latter portions of the attacks, patients were generally amnestic for the entire period. Surface EEGs recorded during these attacks revealed focal epileptiform abnormalities during the unresponsive periods and sometimes during stereotyped automatisms, but bilateral temporal sharp and slow wave activity was usually seen during the clouded mental states associated with reactive automatisms. Subdural electrographic recordings following complex partial and secondary generalized tonic-clonic seizures usually demonstrate diffuse background attenuation, occasionally intermixed with sharp transients and spikes (22). In this study, postictal automatisms were common and included rubbing of the face, fumbling and picking movements of the hands, and oral movements. Resistive and aggressive behavior precipitated by environmental stimulation followed 4 of 16 generalized tonic-clonic seizures and 1 of 49 complex partial seizures in 10 patients.

The automatisms associated with frontal lobe seizures are among the most protean and bizarre reported (see Chapter 97). The frontal lobes are a quagmire for epileptologists who seek precise anatomic localization of seizures, because they cover such an extensive area and because seizures arising in the region tend to spread rapidly to temporal and contralateral areas. Despite these limitations, several electroclinical syndromes have been identified.

Seizures arising in the primary motor cortex produce focal clonic or tonic movements in the corresponding contralateral musculature. Epilepsia partialis continua (focal motor status) occurs with continuous seizure discharges from the motor cortex (18). In patients with temporal lobe epilepsy, simple motor phenomena usually occur late in the seizure, with electrical activity spreading to contralateral or frontoparietal structures (23).

Supplementary motor area seizures have been characterized by recording spontaneous events and by direct electrical stimulation (24). Discharges in this area produce speech arrest, forced vocalization (gutteral utterances, cries, phonemes, words), tonic posturing often followed by clonic movements of the contralateral or bilateral extremities, and deviation of the head and eyes to the opposite side (14,24,25). The "fencer's posture" (contraversive head and eye deviation with abduction, elbow flexion, and external rotation of the contralateral arm), in which the patient looks at their raised arm, is typical of supplementary motor area seizures. Consciousness is usually preserved unless secondary generalization occurs.

Seizures arising in other frontal regions produce less stereotyped manifestations. Electrocorticographic and depth electrode studies have documented ictal and interictal seizure foci in orbitofrontal, dorsolateral, frontal polar, and cingulate regions (26–31). Frontal lobe complex partial seizures from these sites may be characterized by prominent semipurposeful motor automatisms (e.g., sexual automatisms, hand clapping, rocking movements, finger snapping, bicycling movements of the legs, running), vocalization (e.g., shouting, screaming, cursing), and urinary

incontinence. Williamson et al (32) listed features that they considered characteristic of frontal lobe complex partial seizures:

1. frequent seizures, often appearing in clusters;
2. brief seizures, lasting approximately 30 seconds, but with episodes of complex partial status epilepticus;
3. paroxysmal onset and offset with little postictal confusion;
4. stereotyped episodes for each patient; and
5. bizarre automatisms often diagnosed as hysterical.

Following complex partial and generalized tonic-clonic seizures, patients are often confused and may perform complex behavioral sequences for which they are subsequently amnestic. Complex movements during the postictal period have not been the subject of extensive study, but many behaviors described during the ictal phase of temporal and frontal lobe complex partial seizures (e.g., sexual automatisms, shouting, repetitive touching movements) may occur after seizures as well. Poriomania, or prolonged ambulatory behavior in epileptic patients for which they are amnestic, may occur during an extended postictal period (33), and these episodes may be misdiagnosed as fugue states of psychiatric origin.

As described above, the electrical activity recorded in association with clinical seizures does not simply turn on and off, but is more likely to progress through stages that may appear different depending on whether recordings are from the surface, from the cortex, or from depth electrodes. Even in cases where depth electrodes are used, the features of the recording will depend on the proximity of the electrodes to the origin and spreading pathways of the seizure activity. Thus, the distinction between the ictus itself and the confusional states that characterize the postictal period may not always be clear under the best of circumstances. During some seizures, there may be cortical areas with active epileptiform discharges, although the complex behaviors may bear no relation to this activity. In contrast, EEG monitoring (scalp, subdural, depth) may fail to show any paroxysmal activity during a seizure.

Even prior to the use of sophisticated monitoring technology, it was clear that seizures could generate ictal emotions of fear, sadness, or even pleasure (34,35). This observation means that in addition to the possibility that complex or purposeful behaviors could arise out of postictal confusion, some complex behaviors could be direct responses to an ictal emotion. For example, a patient overwhelmed with ictal fear might strike out in the service of self-preservation that would be entirely appropriate to the emotions, if not the circumstances of the moment. Williams (35) specifically distinguished between movement occurring during postictal confusion and those he considered ictal, describing "elaborate coordinated movements which seem purposive" such as licking, laughing, sucking, grimacing, running, striking, and aggressive outburst among the forms of ictal experience. Numerous video-EEG studies of ictal events have confirmed the complexity of ictal events, but since even depth recordings cannot definitively determine when a seizure has ended, the symptomatic correlates of the postictal state have been much harder to distinguish.

PSEUDOSEIZURES

The variety of paroxysmal events associated with epilepsy has naturally led to the false presumption of seizure activity in patients who report unusual sensations or demonstrate motor movements suggestive of seizure activity. Historically, physicians since Hippocrates have struggled to classify seizure types and to sort out those which might be "nonepileptic" (36). The very term "pseudoseizures" implies that all such events can be cleanly divided into those caused by abnormal paroxysmal electrical discharges versus those that are of psychiatric etiology (psychogenic or hysterical seizures), whereas there are, in fact, a variety of nonepileptic, paroxysmal, illness-related behaviors that are frequently confused with epilepsy (Table 98.1). Also, in a small minority of patients, seizures are intentionally faked (factitious disorder or malingering).

Prior to simultaneous video-EEG recordings, the distinction between seizures and pseudoseizures rested on simplistic clinical determinants such as the patient's response to suggestion, pelvic thrusting, or the presence of incontinence (37–41). But as clinicians have come to appreciate the variability of authentic seizures, video-EEG monitoring has provided an invaluable new tool for these diagnostic dilemmas.

Reports of nonepileptic events verified by video-EEG demonstrate that pseudoseizures are common and frequently resemble epileptic seizures, with behavioral phenomena often mimicking simple and complex partial seizures as well as generalized tonic-clonic seizures. In approximately 10% to 20% of cases, patients with epileptic seizures also have coexisting pseudoseizures that can be more common and more refractory to therapy than their epileptic seizures (42–45). Activation procedures such as suggestion with saline injection may effectively elicit pseudoseizures (43,46–49). Conventional clinical assessment of pseudoseizures may be accurate in 67% to 80% of cases (43), suggesting that the discriminatory abilities of the bedside clinician are often quite good. Table 98.2 summarizes the characteristic clinical features of psychogenic seizures. Pseudoseizures are more likely to be characterized by the abrupt onset of symptoms, out-of-phase motor movements, prolonged duration, the absence of rigidity, and the presence of pelvic thrusting (47).

Video-EEG monitoring of seizures and pseudoseizures has demonstrated exceptions to each of these rules (50), and the common practice of reviewing only self-reported and observed events has been shown to miss important EEG information (51). Spike and seizure recognition programs may improve the value of this technique, but monitoring

Table 98.1   Nonepileptic Paroxysmal Disorders

I.   Cardiovascular
   A. Syncope
     1. Reflex (vasovagal, carotid sinus, glossopharyngeal)
     2. Respiratory (cough, Valsalva)
     3. Decreased cardiac output
       (a) Decreased left ventricular filling
         (i) Hypovolemia dehydration (orthostatic)
         (ii) Pulmonary embolism
       (b) Arrhythmias
       (c) Aortic stenosis
     4. Autonomic dysfunction (neurogenic, medication related)
   B. Breath-holding spells (cyanotic, noncyanotic)
   C. Mitral valve prolapse
II.   Cerebrovascular (transient ischemic attacks)
III.   Migraine
IV.   Movement disorders
   A. Tics, Tourette's syndrome
   B. Myoclonus
   C. Startle attacks (hyperexplexia)
   D. Chorea and paroxysmal choreoathetosis
   E. Stuttering attacks
   F. Spasmus mutans
V.   Sleep disorders
   A. Narcolepsy
   B. Night terrors (parvor nocturnus)
   C. Somnambulism
   D. Benign sleep jerks
   E. Periodic leg movements (nocturnal myoclonus)
VI.   Metabolic-toxic
   A. Endocrine
   B. Drug ingestion
VII.   Gastrointestinal disorders
VIII.   Psychiatric disorders
   A. Panic disorder
   B. Somatization disorder
   C. Dissociative disorder
   D. Intermittent explosive disorder (episodic dyscontrol)
   E. Psychogenic seizures (conversion disorder)
IX.   Malingering

remains the gold standard for the discrimination of seizures and pseudoseizures. It is important to note that in some cases, routine video-EEG monitoring, even with sphenoidal electrodes, may fail to reveal any paroxysmal changes in association with partial seizures, especially simple partial seizures (52,53).

DIRECTED AGGRESSION IN EPILEPSY

An enduring question in clinical epileptology has become the extent to which directed violence can occur during the ictus itself, and the circumstances in which violence committed by a patient with known or suspected epilepsy may be considered involuntary. Superstitious associations between

Table 98.2   Clinical Features of Psychogenic Seizures

Clinical Feature	Comment
Seizures induced by stress or specific settings (school, work, spouse)	Stress can precipitate epileptic seizures
Frequent seizures despite therapeutic levels of antiepileptic drugs	AED toxicity may exacerbate epileptic seizures or cause behavioral symptoms that appear psychogenic
Gradual onset of ictus (over minutes)	Epileptic seizures begin suddenly, but are often preceded by auras (usually <1 min) or premonitory symptoms of irritability or depression (hours)
Prolonged duration (>5 min)	Epileptic seizures usually last less than 5 min
Thrashing, struggling, crying, pelvic, side-to-side rolling, wild movements	Bizarre complex motor automatisms including thrusting can occur with frontal lobe CPS
Intermittent arrhythmic, out-of-phase jerking	During epileptic GTCS, jerking is rhythmic, in phase, and usually slows before stopping
Bilateral motor activity with preserved consciousness	Bilateral motor activity without unconsciousness may occur with epileptic seizures from the supplementary motor area
Clinical features fluctuate from seizure to seizure	Epileptic seizures are usually stereotypic
Absence of postictal confusion or lethargy after GTCS or CPS	There may be no postictal symptoms after frontal lobe, and less often, temporal lobe epileptic CPS
Postictal crying or shouting obscenities	Aggressive verbal and physical behavior may occur if patients are restrained after epileptic seizures

AED, antiepileptic drug; GTCS, general tonic-clonic seizures; CPS, complex partial seizures.

epilepsy and violence date back to antiquity, but the notion of aggressive behavior occurring either as an "epileptic equivalent" or during the postictal state was frequently described in clinical anecdotes during the late nineteenth and early twentieth centuries (5,54–56). For example, Maudsley (57) wrote, "If it (the deed) has been done with great violence, without indications of premeditation, without apparent motive and without secrecy, and if the accused person is discovered to be the victim of epilepsy, it is possible that it has been done in a paroxysm following an epileptic fit." This description emphasized the unplanned and excessive features of the presumptive fit, and carefully directed attention to the period following an epileptic seizure rather than to the ictus itself.

Scientific rationalization for the concept of discrete, involuntary directed violence in epileptic patients arose from numerous animal studies of aggressive and attack behaviors. Early in this century, experiments were published that demonstrated that brief, stimulus-bound fragments of attack behavior such as snarling and clawing could be elicited in decerebrate cats (58). In subsequent years, poorly directed "sham rage" was elicited in decorticate cats with minor stimulation and it was discovered that hypothalamic lesions or stimulations could modify the rage display (59–61). More recently, electrical and pharmacologic kindling of limbic areas has been found to modulate thresholds for spontaneous and hypothalamic stimulation-induced aggression in animals (62,63).

The limbic system is critical for understanding ictal and postictal behavioral changes, since this region is usually involved in the origin or spread of seizure activity and has a low threshold for epileptogenicity. Limbic areas represent a buffer zone between the hypothalamic and brainstem areas that execute drive-related behaviors (eating, drinking, sex,

aggression) and the cerebral cortex that regulates and cognitively reflects on behavior. Therefore, either hyperactivity or inhibition of specific limbic regions during seizures could strongly modulate behavior. For example, removal of the septum was shown to increase irritability and aggression in rats (64), and bilateral resection of the anterior temporal lobes produced placidity in monkeys (65,66) and humans (67,68). In humans, bilateral amygdalotomy can permanently reduce severe aggressive behavior in epileptics (69,70). Drawing on these observations from animal and human studies, early investigators of the human epileptic experience (14,34,35) believed that complex behaviors could be dissociated from provocation, intention, or even consciousness, and the stage was set for an emerging conceptualization of involuntary ictal violence.

The assessment of aggressive behaviors in epilepsy was complicated by the search for personality characteristics among epileptics. For example, Serafetinides (71) reported that of 100 patients requiring temporal lobectomy for medically refractory seizures, overt physical aggressiveness could be found in 36; he also reported that aggressiveness was more common in patients with left-sided seizure foci, early onset of seizure disorder, and cognitive impairment. A number of subsequent studies focused on the relationship of aggressiveness to epilepsy without attempting to distinguish ictal from nonictal features. In 100 children with temporal lobe epilepsy by EEG criteria, Ounsted (72) found outbursts of "catastrophic rage" in 36, noting that rage attacks were most highly correlated with early cerebral insult and early onset of seizures, rather than with the frequency or type of seizures. In a retrospective record review of 666 patients with temporal lobe epilepsy (16), only 47 (7%) were considered to be aggressive. In a similar review of 700 epileptic patients, Rodin (73) found only 34 (4.8%) who had committed aggressive acts, and noted that the presence or absence of psychomotor epilepsy was not a relevant variable. In a review of 212 patients referred to an EEG laboratory to be evaluated for aggressive behavioral outbursts, Riley and Niedermeyer (74) found minimally abnormal EEGs among only 6.6% of these patients, a rate comparable with that found among healthy adults. They concluded that most aggressive and rage behaviors could not be related to epilepsy. Devinsky and Bear (75) reported five patients with temporal lobe epilepsy in whom aggressive behavior occurred during the interictal period and was often associated with deepened emotionality and other behavioral changes. In each case the aggressive behavior occurred after the development of an epileptic focus clinically localized to the limbic system, and none of the patients had a history of developmental or sociologic factors associated with violent behavior. The issue of increased interictal aggression in a small subgroup of epileptic patients remains an area of great controversy.

Abnormal EEGs have been reported to be more frequent among habitually aggressive prisoners than among those who had committed a solitary aggressive crime (76), and to be more common among violent criminals (77) and murderers (78–80) than among the population at large. For example, Hill and Pond (78) described "unequivocable" epilepsy by clinical or EEG criteria in 18 of 105 murderers. Their review of these cases showed that epileptics were more likely than other criminals to murder children, and that none of the histories suggested that a seizure had taken place in conjunction with the crime. Indeed, most studies of criminals have concluded that there is a higher incidence of both epilepsy and of abnormal EEG among incarcerated prisoners, perhaps related to head trauma, but that prisoners with epilepsy are no more aggressive than those without epilepsy, as measured by review of the specific crimes (80,81), and that crimes committed during epileptic automatisms are extraordinarily rare (82–84).

The value of this early research was compromised by the fact that these studies were largely retrospective surveys of highly unrepresentative populations, using different historical and clinical measures to assess aggression, epilepsy, and EEG abnormalities. However, a consensus seems to emerge in which epilepsy and abnormal EEGs are overrepresented among criminal populations, but that violence is not more likely among epileptics than nonepileptics regardless of whether the subjects were in prison or had been evaluated at an epilepsy referral center.

Despite these limitations, a great deal of effort has been expended to prove or disprove the existence of "ictal violence" in which intentional and coordinated aggression directly results from an epileptic discharge. The attention to violence rather than to other complex seizure-related behaviors arises from the legal entanglements that have occurred when patients with epilepsy have pleaded diminished capacity due to seizures (85) and in the hopes that new insights might be gained about the neurobiologic

mechanisms of psychopathology in general and of violent behavior in particular (86). In a multicenter study of 5,400 patients from 16 centers who were screened for episodes of ictal violence, video-EEG studies of 19 violent patients were reviewed and described (87). This study emphasized the rarity of directed aggression during seizures, noting that although they clearly documented ictal violence, it was without exception "stereotyped, simple, unsustained." These authors proposed a rigorous set of criteria to be met before a crime could be determined to be the result of an epileptic seizure. A smaller report of monitoring studies in 15 patients with episodic aggression similarly concluded that none of the patients showed directed aggression during their seizures (88). Critics of these reports pointed out that any patients suffering from truly directed ictal violence were more likely to be triaged to the criminal justice system, where they would be far less rigorously studied, than the medical system (89). Yet, as noted above, it remains difficult to find convincing cases of ictal violence, even among criminal populations.

A number of case reports support the existence of directed ictal violence. Hindler (90) reported a murder that appeared to be ictal, although an EEG was never performed during an aggressive act. Marsh (91) reported one patient with "increased spike and wave discharges in the left nasopharyngeal region [sic] before and during the stereotyped aggressive motor behavior." Saint-Hilarie et al (92) reported two patients who had right temporal discharges on depth electrode studies in association with explicit and directed aggressive behaviors such as spitting and verbal and physical assaults. Smith (93) reported three patients with long-standing rage behaviors who demonstrated psychomotor seizures as recorded by depth electrodes in the right amygdala. Only one of these patients had surface findings, and in all three, rage episodes were preceded by a rising epigastric sensation. In this report, it was also claimed that a variety of environmental threats could provoke abnormal electrical discharges and coincident feelings of anger and rage. It should be noted that the differentiation of normal and abnormal patterns recorded from depth electrodes is not subject to the same well-accepted standards for interpretation as are scalp recordings.

In summary, the incidence of well-documented, directed ictal violence is vanishingly small, especially when one applies rigorous video-EEG monitoring criteria to substantiate such a case. It will remain difficult to dismiss the notion of ictal violence since complex partial seizures compromise consciousness to widely varying degrees and some interaction with the environment is clearly possible during and after seizures. Furthermore, the exact temporal course of the ictus is difficult to measure. In the confusional state that accompanies and follows many ictal events, patients do strike out, spit, curse, or throw items, and this violence may be "directed" against individuals participating in their restraint or care. To concede a connection between this clearly reactive type of violence and epilepsy is very different from the notion that temporolimbic seizures can drive otherwise peaceful patients to organized violent activity against unrelated individuals. The spectrum of reactive behaviors in any epileptic patient and the determinants of behavior in a state of impaired consciousness may also be affected by psychosocial variables such as drug use, coexisting psychiatric conditions, or previous socializing experiences with stress and aggression, as well as neurologic variables such as the presence of a coexisting developmental disability or structural lesion such as frontal damage due to head injury. The existing literature suggests that these factors are more relevant to violent behavior than the presence of seizures and that seizures may be more accurately regarded as one of many precipitants that lower the threshold of violent behavior under discrete circumstances. This interpretation would allow for the possibility that there are rare individuals in whom seizures are the most relevant factor in reducing their threshold for violence, but falls short of endorsing a model in which the seizure is somehow solely responsible for violent behavior.

REFERENCES

1. Pritchard J. A treatise on diseases of the nervous system. London, 1822.
2. Fincher E, Dowman C. Epileptiform seizures of Jacksonian character. Analysis of one hundred and thirty cases. JAMA 1931;97:1375–1381.
3. Devinsky O, Price B, Cohen S. Cardiac manifestations of complex partial seizures. Am J Med 1985;80:195–202.
4. Mauguiere F, Courjon J. Somatosensory epilepsy. Brain 1978;101:307–332.
5. Jackson JH. Temporary mental disorders after epileptic paroxysms. West Riding Asylum Med Rep 1875;5:105–122.
6. Bravais LF. Recherches sur les symptomes et le traitement de l'epilepsie hemiplegigue. Thesede Paris, 1827:118.
7. Todd R. Clinical lectures on paralysis, diseases of the brain, and other affections of the nervous system. Philadelphia: Lindsay and Blakiston, 1855.
8. Jackson J. On epilepsis and the after effects of epileptic discharges. West Riding Asylum Med Rep 1876;6:266–309.
9. Jackson J. On temporary paralysis after epileptiform and epileptic seizures: a contribution to the study of dissolution of the nervous system. In: Taylor J, ed. Selected writings of John Hughlings Jackson. New York: Basic Books, 1958:318–329.
10. Efron R. Post-epileptic paralysis: theoretical critique and report of a case. Brain 1961;84:381–394.
11. Gowers W. Epilepsy and other chronic convulsive disorders: their causes, symptoms and treatment. London: Churchill, 1881.
12. Dichter M, Ayala G. Cellular mechanisms of epilepsy: a status report. Science 1987;237:157–163.
13. Lesser R, Lueders H, Dinner D, et al. The location of speech and writing functions in the frontal language area: results of extraoperative stimulation. Brain 1984;107:275–291.
14. Penfield W, Jaspar H. Epilepsy and the functional anatomy of the human brain. Boston: Little, Brown and Co., 1954.
15. Jackson J. On a particular variety of epilepsy ("intellectual aura"), one case with symptoms of organic brain disease. Brain 1888;11:179–207.
16. Currie S, Heathfield K, Henson R, Scott D. Clinical course and prognosis of temporal lobe epilepsy: a survey of 666 patients. Brain 1971;94:173–190.
17. Sharbrough F. Complex partial seizures. In: Luders H, Lesser R, eds. Epilepsy: electroclinical syndromes. New York: Springer-Verlag, 1987.
18. Weiser H. Stereoelectroencephalographic correlates of focal motor seizures. In: Speckman E, Elger C, eds. Epilepsy and motor system. Baltimore: Urban and Schwarzenberg, 1983:287–309.
19. King D, Marsan C. Clinical features and ictal patterns in epileptic patients with EEG temporal lobe foci. Ann Neurol 1977;2:138–147.
20. Engel J. Approaches to localization of the epileptogenic lesion. In: Engel J, ed. Surgical treatment of the epilepsies. New York: Raven Press, 1987:75–100.
21. Escueta A, Kunze U, Waddell G, et al. Lapse of consciousness and automatisms in temporal lobe epilepsy: a videotape analysis. Neurology 1977;27:144–155.
22. Devinsky O, Kelly K, Sato S, et al. Postical behavior: a subdural electroencephalographic study. Epilepsia 1990;31:686.
23. Bossi L, Munari C, Stoffels C, et al. Somatomotor manifestations in temporal lobe seizures. Epilepsia 1984;25:70–76.
24. Penfield W, Welch K. The supplementary motor area of the cerebral cortex. A clinical and experimental study. Arch Neurol 1951;66:289–317.
25. Morris H, Dinner D, Luders H, et al. Supplementary motor seizures: clinical and electroencephalographic findings. Neurology 1988;38:1075–1082.
26. Ajmone-Marsan C, Ralston B. The epileptic seizure. Its functional morphology and diagnostic significance. Springfield: Charles C Thomas, 1957.
27. Mazars G. Cingulate gyrus epileptogenic foci as an origin for generalized seizures. In: Gastaut H, Jasper H, Bancaud J, Waltregny A, eds. The physiopathogenesis of the epilepsies. Springfield: Charles C Thomas, 1969:186–189.
28. Penfield W, Kristianson K. Epileptic seizure patterns. Springfield: Charles C Thomas, 1951.
29. Talairach J, Bancaud J, Geier S, et al. The cingulate gyrus and human behavior. Electroencephalogr Clin Neurophysiol 1973;34:45–52.
30. Tharp B. Orbital frontal seizures. An unique electroencephalographic and clinical syndrome. Epilepsia 1972;13:627–642.
31. Waterman K, Purves S, Kosaka B, Strauss E. An epileptic syndrome caused by mesial frontal lobe seizure foci. Neurology 1987;37:577–582.
32. Williamson P, Spencer D, Spencer S, et al. Complex partial seizures of frontal lobe origin. Ann Neurol 1985;18:497–504.
33. Mayeux R, Alexander M, Benson D, et al. Poriomania. Neurology 1979;29:1616–1619.
34. Daly D. Ictal affect. Am J Psychiatry 1958;115:97–108.
35. Williams D. The structure of emotions reflected in epileptic experience. Brain 1956;79:29–67.
36. Glaser G. Epilepsy, hysteria and possession: an historical essay. J Nerv Dis 1978;188:274–288.
37. Finlayson R, Lucas A. Pseudoepileptic seizures in children and adolescents. Mayo Clin Proc 1979;54:83–87.
38. Liske E, Forster F. Pseudoseizures: a problem in the diagnosis and management of epileptic patients. Neurology 1964;14:41–49.
39. Ramani V, Quesney L, Olson D, et al. Diagnosis of hysterical seizures in epileptic patients. Am J Psychiatry 1980;137:705–709.
40. Remick R, Wada J. Complex partial and pseudoseizures disorders. Am J Psychiatry 1979;136:320–323.
41. Riley T, Brannon W. Recognition of pseudoseizures. J Fam Pract 1980;10:213–220.
42. Desai B, Porter R, Penry J. The psychogenic seizure by video tape analysis: a study of 42 attacks in 6 patients. Neurology 1979;29:202–209.
43. King D, Gallagher B, Murvin A, et al. Pseudoseizures: diagnostic evaluation. Neurology 1982;32:18–23.
44. Lempert T, Schmidt D. Natural history and outcome of psychogenic seizures: a clinical study in 50 patients. J Neurol 1990;237:35–38.
45. Lesser R, Leuders H, Dinner D. Evidence for epilepsy is rare in patients with psychogenic seizures. Neurology 1983;33:502–504.
46. Cohen R, Suter C. Hysterical seizures: suggestion as a provocative EEG test. Ann Neurol 1982;11:391–395.
47. Gates J, Ramani V, Whalen S, Loewenson R. Ictal characteristics of pseudoseizures. Arch Neurol 1985;42:1183–1187.
48. Gulick T, Spinks I, King D. Pseudoseizures: ictal phenomena. Neurology 1982;32:24–30.
49. Luther J, McNamara J, Carwile S, et al. Psuedoepileptic seizures: methods and video analysis to aid diagnosis. Ann Neurol 1982;12:458–462.
50. Sussman N, Jackel R, Kaplan L, Harner R. Bicycling movements as a manifestation of complex partial seizures of temporal lobe origin. Epilepsia 1989;30:527–531.
51. Pierelli F, Chatrian G, Erdly W, Swanson P. Long-term EEG-video-audio monitoring: detection of partial epileptic seizures and psychogenic episodes by 24-hour EEG record review. Epilepsia 1989;30:513–523.
52. Devinsky O, Kelley K, Porter R, Theodore W. Clinical and electroencephalographic features of simple partial seizures. Neurology 1988;38:1347–1352.
53. Devinsky O, Sato S, Theodore W, Porter R. Fear episodes due to limbic seizures with normal ictal scalp EEG: a subdural electrographic study. J Clin Psychiatry 1989;50:28–30.
54. Echeverria M. On epilepsy: anatomo-pathological and clinical notes. New York: William Wood and Co., 1870.

55. Griesinger W. Mental pathology and therapeutics. London: New Sydenham Society, 1867.

56. Maudsley H. The pathology of mind. London: Macmillan, 1879.

57. Maudsley H. Responsibility in mental disease. London: Macmillan, 1906.

58. Woodworth R, Sherrington C. A pseudoaffective reflex and its spinal path. J Physiol 1904;31:234–243.

59. Bard P. A diencephalic mechanism for the expression of rage, with special reference to the sympathetic nervous system. Am J Physiol 1928;84:490–515.

60. Flynn J, Vanegas H, Foote W, Edwards S. Neural mechanisms involved in a cat's attack on a rat. In: Whalen R, Thompson R, Verzeano M, Weinberger N, eds. The neural control of behavior. New York: Academic Press, 1970:135–173.

61. Hess W, Akert K. Experimental data on role of hypothalamus in mechanism of emotional behavior. Arch Neurol Psychiatry 1955;73:127–219.

62. Post R, Weiss S, Clark M, et al. Seizures as an evolving process: implications for neuropsychiatric illness. In: Devinsky O, Theodore W, eds. Epilepsy and behavior. New York: Wley-Liss, 1991:361–388.

63. Siegel A. Aggression in epilepsy: animal models. In: Devinsky O, Theodore W, eds. Epilepsy and behavior. New York: Wiley-Liss, 1991:389–404.

64. Brady J, Nauta W. Subcortical mechanisms in emotional behaviors: affective changes following septal forebrain lesions in the albino rat. J Comp Physiol Psychol 1953;46:339–346.

65. Kluver H, Bucy P. Psychic blindness and other symptoms following bilateral temporal lobectomy in rhesus monkeys. Am J Physiol 1937;119:352–353.

66. Kluver H, Bucy P. An analysis of certain effects of bilateral temporal lobectomy in the rhesus monkey, with special reference to psychic blindness. J Psychol 1938;5:33–54.

67. Aichner F. Phenomenology of the Kluver-Bucy syndrome in man. Fortschr Neurol Psychiatr 1984;52:375–397.

68. Lilly R, Cummings J, Benson D, Frankel M. The human Kluver-Bucy syndrome. Neurology 1983;33:1141–1145.

69. Kiloh L, Gye R, Rushworth R, et al. Stereotactic amygdaloidotomy for aggressive behavior. J Neurol Neurosurg Psychiatry 1974;37:437–444.

70. Vaernet K, Madsen A. Stereotaxic amygdalotomy and basofrontal tractotomy in psychotics with aggressive behavior. J Neurol Neurosurg Psychiatry 1970;33:858–863.

71. Serafetinides E. Aggressiveness in temporal lobe epileptics and its relation to cerebral dysfunction and environmental factors. Epilepsia 1965;6:33–42.

72. Ounsted C. Aggression and epilepsy rage in children with temporal lobe epilepsy. J Psychosom Res 1969;13:237–242.

73. Rodin E. Psychomotor epilepsy and aggressive behavior. Arch Gen Psychiatry 1973;28:210–213.

74. Riley T, Niedermeyer E. Rage attacks and episodic violent behavior: electroencephalographic findings and general considerations. Clin Electroencephalogr 1978;9:131–139.

75. Devinsky O, Bear D. Varieties of aggressive behavior in temporal lobe epilepsy. Am J Psychiatry 1984;141:651–656.

76. Williams D. Neural factors related to habitual aggression. Consideration of differences between those habitual aggressives and others who have committed crimes of violence. Brain 1969;92:503–520.

77. Mark V, Ervin F. Violence and the brain. New York: Harper & Row, 1970.

78. Hill D, Pond D. Reflections on one hundred capital cases submitted to electroencephalography. J Ment Sci 1952;98:23–43.

79. Stafford-Clark D, Taylor F. Clinical and electro-encephalographic studies of prisoners charged with murder. J Neurol Neurosurg Psychiatry 1949;12:325–330.

80. Whitman S, Coleman T, Patmon C, et al. Epilepsy in prison: elevated prevalence and no relationship to violence. Neurology 1984;34:775–782.

81. Gunn J, Bonn J. Criminality and violence in epileptic prisoners. Br J Psychiatry 1971;118:337–343.

82. Gunn J. Criminal behaviour and mental disorder. Br J Psychiatry 1977;130:317–329.

83. Gunn J, Fenton G. Epilepsy, automatism, and crime. Lancet 1971:1173–1176.

84. Herzberg JL, Fenwick PBC. The aetiology of aggression in temporal-lobe epilepsy. Br J Psychiatry 1988;153:50–55.

85. Treiman D. Epilepsy and violence: medical and legal issues. Epilepsia 1986;27(suppl 2):S77–S104.

86. Stevens J, Hermann B. Temporal lobe epilepsy, psychopathology, and violence: the state of the evidence. Neurology 1981;31:1127–1132.

87. Delgado-Escueta A, Mattson R, King L, et al. Special report: the nature of aggression during epileptic seizures. N Engl J Med 1981;305:711–716.

88. Ramani V, Gumnit R. Intensive monitoring of epileptic patients with a history of episodic aggression. Arch Neurol 1981;38:570–571.

89. Pincus J. Violence and epilepsy. N Engl J Med 1981;305:696–698.

90. Hindler C. Epilepsy and violence. Br J Psychiatry 1989;155:246–249.

91. Marsh G. Neuropsychological syndrome in a patient with episodic howling and violent motor behaviour. J Neurol Neurosurg Psychiatry 1978;41:366–369.

92. Saint-Hilaire J, Gilbert M, Bouvier G, Barbeau A. Epilepsy and aggression: two cases with depth electrode studies. In: Robb R, ed. Epilepsy updated: causes and treatment. Chicago: Year Book Medical, 1980:145–176.

93. Smith J. Episodic rage. In: Girgis M, Kiloh LG, eds. Limbic epilepsy and the dyscontrol syndrome: proceedings of the first international symposium on limbic epilepsy and the dyscontrol syndrome. Amsterdam: Elsevier/North Holland Biomedical Press, 1980:255–265.

A New Role for the Cerebellum: The Modulation of Cognition and Affect

Jeremy D. Schmahmann

The possible role of the cerebellum in sensory, cognitive, and affective processing has long been overshadowed by interest in the cerebellar coordination of voluntary movement. Cerebellar motor disturbances are characterized by incoordination of the limbs (dysmetria), wide-based, unsteady, and lurching gait (ataxia), speech impairment (dysarthria), and a variety of disturbances of eye movements (such as nystagmus and overshoot and undershoot with attempted volitionally directed gaze). Midline lesions are characteristically associated with truncal ataxia, and lesions of the cerebellar hemispheres produce incoordination of the limbs. In degenerative diseases of the cerebellum, these motor phenomena are the major features of the clinical presentation. From the earliest days of clinical case reporting, however, instances of mental and intellectual dysfunction were described in the setting of cerebellar pathology (1,2). Investigators in the nineteenth and early part of the twentieth centuries lacked the necessary clinical and pathologic techniques to provide a clear understanding of their patients' lesions and psychiatric or cognitive disturbances. Consequently, their anecdotal clinical reports have been essentially ignored. Physiologists and anatomists in the first half of the twentieth century were not convinced that cerebellar function was confined to motor control. The cerebellum was shown to receive sensory projections from the periphery and from the cerebral hemispheres, as well as vagal, auditory, and visual input, and it was demonstrated that the cerebellum exerts some control in the sensory sphere and on autonomic functions. The results of these investigations indicated that the interpretation of cerebellar function suggested by the careful motor analyses of Babinski, Holmes, and others was too narrow. Snider (3), for example, believed that if the effects of experimental or clinical lesions of the cerebellum were analyzed by means of adequate physiologic and psychological tests, aspects of cerebellar function might be

unveiled beyond its role in motor control. He viewed the cerebellum as "the great modulator of neurologic function" and predicted for it a role not only in the field of neurology, but also in psychiatry.

There is now a sizable body of evidence, derived from anatomic, physiologic, theoretical, and functional neuroimaging studies, that links the cerebellum with nonmotor processing (4). Contemporary clinical investigations in patients have further supported this notion. Evidence is derived from the study of patients in whom there is a disorder of cognition and in whom a search has been made for the presence of previously unsuspected cerebellar pathology. In the complementary series of investigations, patients with cerebellar lesions have been studied by neuropsychological tests to determine the presence and nature of any impairment of cognition and emotion. An implicit assumption in most of these studies is that structure and function are tightly interwoven and that regions of the brain that are anatomically interconnected are functionally related.

This chapter provides a brief overview of some of the salient studies in the different disciplines within the neurosciences that have provided convincing evidence that the cerebellum is an integral component of the distributed neural circuitry subserving higher-order function, and therefore causally linked with definable clinical syndromes of altered behavior in adults and children.

PSYCHIATRIC DISORDERS AND STUDIES OF THE CEREBELLUM

The earliest reports of abnormal behaviors in association with cerebellar atrophy or agenesis described both emotional and intellectual dysfunction (Table 99.1). These anecdotal reports did not, for the most part, provide detailed clinical accounts of their patients' deficits, and the patho-

Table 99.1   Selected Clinical Reports from the Early Nineteenth Century
Until the Era of Anatomic Imaging

Investigator	Cerebellar Lesion	Behavioral Manifestation
Combettes, 1831	Agenesis	Delayed development, aberrant behavior
Andral, 1848	Agenesis, left hemisphere	"Imbecile, weakness of character"
Vulpian, 1866	Atrophy	Aberrant behavior
Otto, 1873	Agenesis	Low intelligence, aberrant/deviant behavior
Ferrier, 1876	Agenesis	Feeble minded
Doursout, 1891	Atrophy	"Idiocy, irritability, brutality"
Fusari, 1892	Near complete agenesis	Mental retardation ("grave imbecility")
Neff, 1894	Atrophy	Mental deficiency
Bond, 1895	Atrophy	"Foolishness"
Londe, 1895	Spastic ataxia/? Olivopontocerebellar atrophy	Mental difficulties
Claasen, 1898	Atrophy	Mental deficiency
Whyte, 1898	Friedreich's ataxia	Mental impairment
Anton, 1903 Anton and Zingerle, 1914	Agenesis	Delayed development, mental retardation
Batten, 1905	Agenesis	Mental retardation
Vogt and Astwazaturow, 1912	Hypoplasia of hemispheres	Mental retardation
Beyerman, 1917	Agenesis/"Congenital atrophy"	Mental retardation
Schob, 1921	Agenesis/"Congenital atrophy"	Mental retardation
Curschmann, 1922	Hereditary cerebellar ataxia	Mental impairment
Koster, 1926	Hypoplasia, cerebellar hemispheres	Mental retardation
Walter and Roese, 1926	Hereditary ataxia	Mental impairment
Santha, 1930	Agenesis/"Congenital atrophy"	Mental retardation
Scherer, 1933	Agenesis/"Congenital atrophy"	Mental retardation
Akelaitis, 1938	Cortical atrophy	Dementia (late stages)
Rubinstein and Freeman, 1940	Near complete agenesis	Mild mental retardation, poor recent memory, delusions
Knoepfel and Macken, 1947	Degeneration	Psychosis
Jervis, 1950	Agenesis/"Congenital atrophy"	Mental retardation
Schut, 1950	Olivopontocerebellar atrophy	Intellectual difficulty (late stages)
Mutrux et al, 1953	Agenesis/"Congenital atrophy"	Mental retardation
Gillespie, 1965	Degeneration with aniridia	Mental retardation ("oligophrenia")
Carpenter and Schumacher, 1966	Familial infantile cerebellar atrophy	Mental retardation
Aguilar et al, 1968	Ataxia-telangiectasia	Mental deficiency (late stages)
Joubert et al, 1969	Familial agenesis of the vermis	Mental retardation
Keddie, 1969	Cortical atrophy	Paranoid psychosis
Hoffman et al, 1971	Hereditary late onset cerebellar degeneration	Impaired intellect (late stages)
Landis et al, 1974	Olivopontocerebellar atrophy	Mild cognitive impairment

Source: Schmahmann JD. Rediscovery of an early concept. Int Rev Neurobiol 1997;41:3–27.

logic verification was rather scant in most cases. Both clinical neuropsychology and neuroimaging methods (in vivo and postmortem analysis) have advanced so much since these early reports that now they serve mostly to provide historical context to the discussion, but they cannot be seriously used as supporting evidence (1,2). In more recent times, Heath et al (5) observed increased neuronal discharges in the fastigial nucleus of an emotionally disturbed patient that correlated with the patient's experience of fear and anger. Heath (6) later produced amelioration of aggression in patients with severe emotional dyscontrol by chronically stimulating the cerebellar vermis through subdurally implanted electrodes. This technique was also employed by Riklan et al (7) for achieving seizure control but it relieved aggression, anxiety, and depression as well. Heath et al (8) performed computed tomography (CT) scans in schizophrenics and found abnormalities in the cerebellum in 40% of their 85 patients. The abnormal radiologic features were noted particularly in the cerebellar vermis and included atrophy in some cases and mass lesions in others. The cerebral hemispheres in these patients appeared radiographically normal. Vermal abnormalities in patients with schizophrenia were suggested by others as well (9–12). In 1981 Kutty and Prendes (13) described psychotic behavior in their adult patients who had cerebellar degeneration, and Hamilton et al (14) reported psychotic behavior and cognitive deficits in patients who were found at autopsy to have cerebellar degeneration, infarct, or tumor.

The search for a neurobiological substrate for autism was advanced by the finding of morphologic changes on autopsy in the amygdala as well as loss of neurons in the deep cerebellar nuclei, depletion of Purkinje cells throughout the cerebellar cortex and particularly in the posterior lobe, and abnormalities in the inferior olivary nucleus (15). Magnetic resonance imaging (MRI) studies have shown hypoplasia of vermal lobules VI and VII (the "neocerebellar vermis") (16) as well as of the cerebellar hemispheres (17). Children with attention deficit hyperactivity disorder have also been shown to have statistically smaller vermal lobules VI and VII on MRI (18), and a similar observation has been made in fragile X syndrome (19). These observations of morphologic changes in the cerebellum in diseases characterized by their psychopathology have been made in concert with the evolution of a new approach to the understanding of psychiatric disease, that is, in terms of the relationships between structure, chemistry, and function in the nervous system. The presence of cerebellar abnormalities in these disorders has been difficult to explain. Previous synthetic analyses (20–23) relied upon the early anatomic, physiologic, and behavioral literature as well as anecdotal case reports to account for a possible role of the cerebellum in the generation of these psychiatric disorders. The evolution of the many disciplines within the cognitive neurosciences, including neuropsychology, functional neuroimaging, and connectional anatomy, has aided the interpretation of these cerebellar findings in psychiatric diseases and has helped advance hypotheses regarding the nature of the cerebellar contribution to the psychopathology, as discussed below.

CEREBELLAR LESIONS AND DISORDERS OF COGNITION AND EMOTION

Neuropsychological Studies

In the past two decades neuropsychological tests have been performed in patients with degenerative cerebellar disorders. Patients with olivopontocerebellar atrophy (OPCA) were found by Landis et al (24) to have impairments in verbal and nonverbal intelligence, memory, and frontal system functions. Difficulties with concept formation, learning of paired associates, visual-spatial abilities, and general intellectual slowing were noted in the patients studied by Kish et al (25), Bracke-Tolkmitt et al (26), and Akshoomoff and Courchesne (27). Kish et al (28) further observed that the degree of cognitive impairment correlated with the severity of the ataxia. Botez-Marquard and Botez (29) reported a mild parietal-like syndrome with visual-spatial disturbances in their 15 OPCA patients, as well as longer visual and auditory reaction times. Cognitive deficits have been described in patients with Friedreich's ataxia (30,31), but this has not been a consistent observation.

Neuropsychological abnormalities in patients with cerebellar cortical atrophy have included impaired executive function demonstrated by increased planning times when performing the Tower of Hanoi test (32) and poor performance on tests of fluency and the initiation/perseveration subtest of the Mattis dementia rating scale (33). Additionally, a profound deficit was noted in the acquisition of implicit procedural and declarative knowledge in a fixed sequence visuomotor association task (34).

Wallesch and Horn (35) reported deficits in cognitive operations in three-dimensional space in patients who had tumors excised from the left cerebellar hemisphere. Visual-spatial disturbances were reported by Botez-Marquard et al (36) following infarction in the territory of the left superior cerebellar artery. Botez et al (37) had previously shown a number of cognitive deficits including visual-spatial impairments in a patient with chronic phenytoin intoxication. In single case reports of patients with right cerebellar infarction, linguistic processing was impaired as evidenced by agrammatism (38), decreased verbal fluency (39), and impaired error detection and practice-related learning of a verb-for-noun generation task (40).

Investigators have used patient populations to study specific hypotheses regarding cerebellar function in both motor and nonmotor domains. Cerebellar patients show deficits in their ability to learn motor skills such as rotor pursuit tasks (41) and prism adaptation (42), acquire classically conditioned eye blink reflexes (43–45), and judge the duration of short auditory stimuli or the velocity of moving visual stimuli (46). Cerebellar patients also have difficulty performing tasks that require shifts of attention between different modalities (47), and these results have been consistent with the suggestion that the cerebellum is important for anticipatory planning and prediction in a wide range of different behaviors.

Some observers have reached different conclusions regarding the performance of their patients with cerebellar dysfunction on tests of cognition. In a study of 15 hereditary and 24 sporadic cases of OPCA, Berent et al (48) found that patients had a full-scale IQ on the WAIS-R test of 93.46 ± 13.19 compared with the control subjects, who scored 113.72 ± 12.68. The conclusion of the authors of this study was that the 20-point difference between controls and patients could be ascribed to the fact that the controls were a highly educated group and that motor dysfunction and depression accounted for the impaired performance of the patient group. This raises questions concerning the choice of controls in that study, an important consideration in determining if the patients are impaired. In a study of patients with cerebellar stroke, Gomez-Baldarrain et al (49) were unable to document cognitive deficits except for mild impairments of naming. The patients and controls in this group had a mean educational level of eight years, and the controls were regarded as being normal if their mini-mental state fell at or above a level of 23 (out of a possible score of 30), regardless of age. These authors subsequently reported (50) that patients with unilateral cerebellar infarction demonstrated impairments of procedural learning on a serial reaction time task independent of the motor incapacity resulting from the cerebellar stroke.

Some cognitive functions appear to be spared in cerebellar lesions. Patients with cerebellar degeneration were studied by Dimitrov et al (51), and tests of selective attention, spatial attention, spatial rotation, and memory for temporal order were preserved. As discussed below, there are likely to be differences in clinical presentation of patients who have slowly progressive cerebellar degeneration as opposed to those who have acute loss of cerebellar tissue resulting from stroke. These case reports and studies stress the point, however, that ongoing clinical investigation is required to determine specifically what functions are impaired in patients with cerebellar injury, and what is the time course of these deficits.

Clinical Investigations

A persistent concern shared by investigators and clinicians is that there are very few descriptions of clinically relevant cases that address the possibility of a cerebellar contribution to nonmotor behaviors. It has been argued that detection of subtle behavioral deficits only by neuropsychological tests in patients with cerebellar lesions may be insufficient grounds to warrant a revision of the understanding of the role of the cerebellum in nervous system function. New evidence regarding the consequences of cerebellar lesions on behavior addresses this issue directly.

Posterior Fossa Syndrome in Children

For some years surgeons have been struck by the development of mutism in approximately 15% of children 1 to 4 days following resection of tumors of the cerebellar vermis (52–54). In the study of Pollack et al (53), the mutism was associated with an almost stereotyped response, with the children lying curled up in bed and whining inconsolably without speaking intelligible words. They seemed unable to initiate voluntary eye opening. They were unwilling or unable to eat, had difficulty initiating the chewing or swallowing process, and displayed an impairment of oral motor coordination. Speech returned to normal by 4 months following the surgery, but during the recovery phase the children spoke in a dysarthric and whispered or high-pitched voice. Neuropsychological studies showed difficulties in initiating and completing age appropriate motor responses and impairments in recent memory, attention span, and problem-solving abilities. This posterior fossa syndrome occurs almost exclusively with resection of midline cerebellar mass lesions via an inferior vermian incision, but not with resection of large hemispheric lesions. Pollack (55) has suggested that the syndrome may result from edema, inflammation, or focal hypoperfusion around the resection cavity and may reversibly compromise the functioning of the deep cerebellar nuclei and/or their afferent and efferent connections.

Cerebellar Cognitive Affective Syndrome in Adults

We studied 20 patients with lesions confined to the cerebellum prospectively over a 7-year period to determine if there are clinically relevant behavioral changes in adults with acquired cerebellar lesions (56). Thirteen patients had stroke, three had postinfectious cerebellitis, three had cerebellar cortical atrophy, and one was studied following excision of a midline tumor. All patients received neurologic examinations and bedside mental state tests, and most underwent neuropsychological testing. A pattern of clinically relevant behavioral changes was found that could be diagnosed at the bedside and quantified by neuropsychological tests. These deficits conformed to an identifiable syndrome, that we termed the *cerebellar cognitive affective syndrome*. It is characterized by the following:

1. Disturbances of executive function, including deficient planning, set-shifting, abstract reasoning, working memory, and decreased verbal fluency.
2. Impaired spatial cognition, including visual-spatial disorganization and impaired visual-spatial memory.
3. Personality change characterized by flattening or blunting of affect, and disinhibited or inappropriate behavior.
4. Linguistic difficulties, including dysprosodia, agrammatism, and mild anomia.

The net effect of these disturbances in cognitive functioning is a general lowering of overall intellectual function.

These impairments are present on routine bedside mental state tests and on standardized neuropsychological tests of cognitive function (Figs 99.1 to 99.3). They are not so subtle as to be detected only on high-level cognitive tests. Rather, they are clinically relevant and noted by family members and medical staff. The observed impairments cannot be explained by difficulties with motor control. In many cases motor incoordination was very mild as determined by clinical observation. Moreover, tests that are highly demanding of motor function were not administered to patients with moderate or severe dysmetria. Motor incapacity does not account for abnormalities of verbal IQ score (where responses are verbal and are untimed); impairment of Picture Arrangement and Picture Completion (where the motor requirement is minimal); and poor performance on the Boston Naming Test. On tests with a significant motor component (Rey Copy, Trail Making, Porteus Mazes) patients do not have difficulty drawing the lines. Rather their errors result from poor planning, and in the Mazes task they would often go into blocked paths and require several attempts to find the correct solution. This difficulty suggests that these patients have trouble with planning and integration of cognitive responses.

The neurobehavioral presentation in our patients was more pronounced and generalized in those with bilateral or large unilateral infarctions in the territory of the posterior inferior cerebellar arteries, and in those with subacute onset of pancerebellar disorders such as occurs with postinfectious cerebellitis. It was less evident in patients with more insidious disease (slowly progressive cerebellar degenerations), in the recovery phase (3 to 4 months) after acute stroke, and in those with restricted cerebellar pathology (small-branch occlusions affecting the anterior lobe of the cerebellum or the rostral part of the posterior lobe supplied by the superior cerebellar artery). Lesions of the posterior lobe are particularly important in the generation of the disturbed cognitive behaviors. The vermis is consistently involved in patients with pronounced affective presentations. The anterior lobe seems to be less prominently involved in the generation of these cognitive and behavioral deficits. One patient with an autonomic syndrome had a lesion involving the medial posterior lobe, including the fastigial nucleus.

Cerebellar Cognitive Affective Syndrome in Children
Early case studies of agenesis and hypoplasia of the cerebellum reported an association with mental retardation or emotional disability (1,2). More recent reports include the description of mania in a child with cerebellar degeneration (57), and Joubert et al (58) described mental retardation in children with dysplasia of the cerebellar vermis. We have been impressed particularly by the language delay as well as

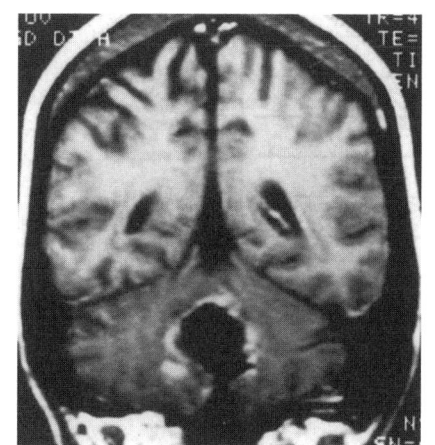
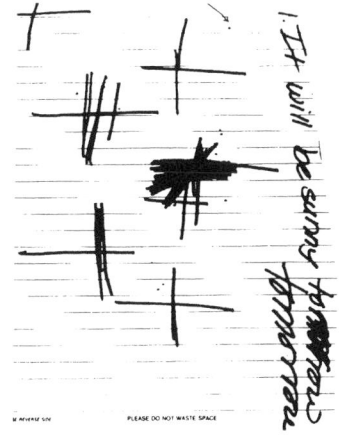
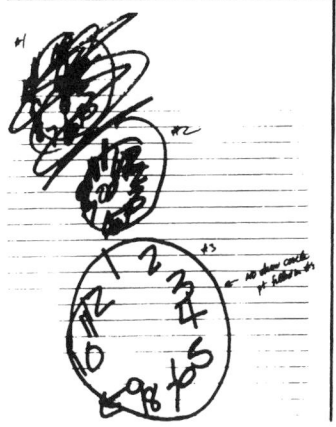
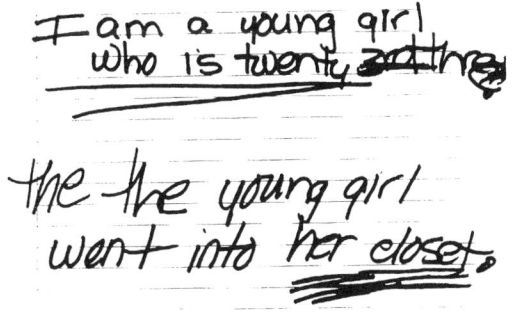

FIGURE 99.1 *T1-weighted coronal MRI of the brain of a patient following excision of a midline cerebellar ganglioglioma, and her responses when asked to draw a clock, bisect a line, and write a sentence. (Reproduced by permission from Schmahmann JD, Sherman JC. The cerebellar cognitive affective syndrome. Brain 1998;121:561–579.)*

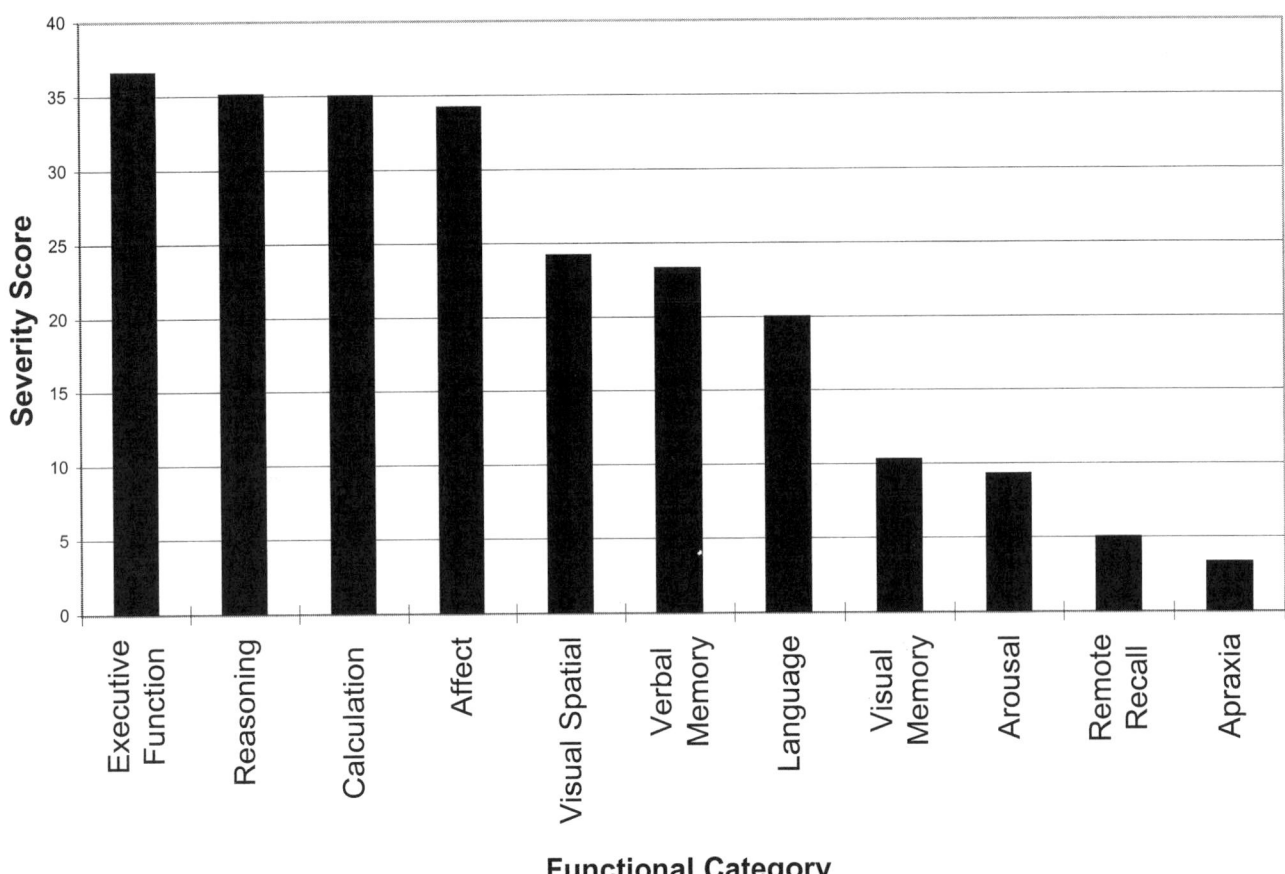

FIGURE 99.2   *Bar graph depicting the deficits found on bedside mental state testing in patients with cerebellar lesions. The degree of impairment on the individual tasks within each functional category was graded on a 3-point scale, from mild to severe. The severity score indicates the relative degree of impairment within the functional categories. (Reproduced by permission from Schmahmann JD, Sherman JC. The cerebellar cognitive affective syndrome. Brain 1998;121:561–579.)*

oculomotor apraxia in patients with Joubert syndrome and cerebellar agenesis (unpublished data). Apart from the observations of children with the posterior fossa syndrome characterized predominantly by postoperative mutism, little is known regarding the behavioral effects of acquired cerebellar lesions in the pediatric population. Most studies of the neurobehavioral consequences in children treated for posterior fossa tumors have essentially documented the combined effects of tumor, radiation, and chemotherapy. In the reports of children with astrocytomas (59,60), almost one-half of the patients who did not receive radiation showed serious behavioral, academic, or intellectual deficits, such as memory, language, or visual-spatial problems.

The finding of a cerebellar cognitive affective syndrome in adults led Levisohn et al (61) to investigate the behavioral consequences of tumor resections in children. In this study, a retrospective analysis was performed of the clinical evaluations and neuropsychological test results in 19 children (ages 3 to 14, mean age 8 years, 2 months) who had undergone resection of cerebellar tumors. Eleven had medulloblastomas involving the vermis; seven had astrocy-

tomas in the cerebellar hemisphere; and one child had an ependymoma near the midline. The children showed characteristic behavioral deficits, including difficulties with language initiation, such as reluctance to engage in conversation and long response latencies. Language impairments were seen in children with damage to the right hemisphere and included impaired verbal fluency and word-finding difficulties. Digit Span scores were poor in many patients, with deficits notable particularly in sequencing and planning as well as perseveration and difficulty maintaining set. Impairment of initiation was a common feature and resulted in poor confrontation naming and story retrieval. Visual-spatial deficits were prominent, and verbal memory deficits were accompanied by a failure to organize and encode verbal or visual-spatial material. Impaired regulation of affect was seen in children with extensive damage to the vermis. Five patients exhibited the posterior fossa syndrome. Dissociation between fine-motor and cognitive deficits was seen such that four patients without cognitive deficits had fine-motor deficits, and one without fine-motor deficits had visual-spatial deficits and mild word-

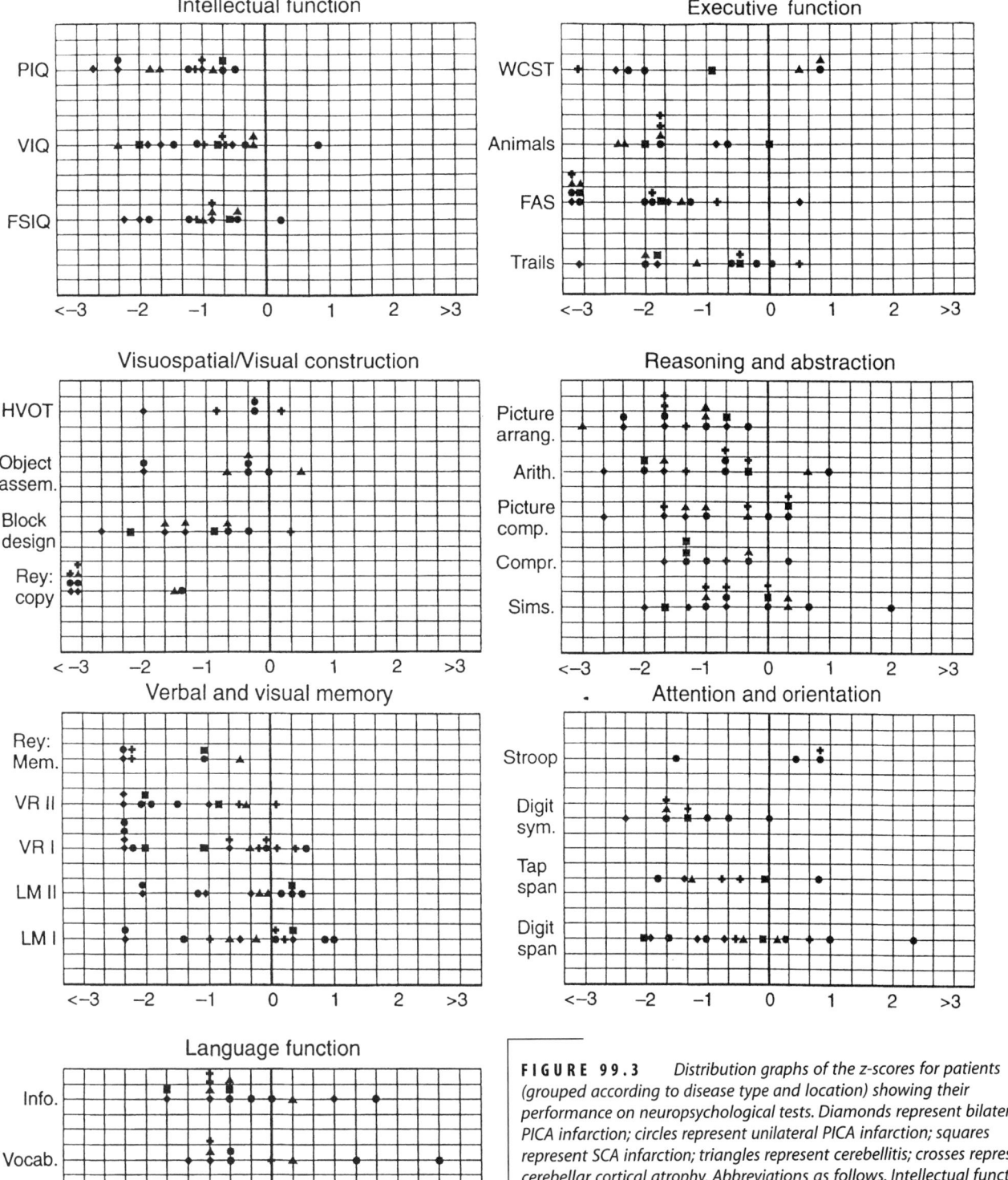

FIGURE 99.3 *Distribution graphs of the z-scores for patients (grouped according to disease type and location) showing their performance on neuropsychological tests. Diamonds represent bilateral PICA infarction; circles represent unilateral PICA infarction; squares represent SCA infarction; triangles represent cerebellitis; crosses represent cerebellar cortical atrophy. Abbreviations as follows. Intellectual function: Picture, Verbal and Full Scale Intelligence Quotient. Executive function: Wisconsin Card Sorting Test, Animal naming, F-A-S-verbal fluency test, Trails A and B. Visuospatial/Visual Construction: Hooper Visual Orientation Test, Object assembly. Reasoning and Abstractions: Picture arrangement, Arithmetic, Picture completion, Comprehension, Similarities. Verbal and Visual Memory: Rey Complex figure memory, Visual Reproduction I and II, Logical Memory I and II. Attention and Orientation: Digit symbol. Language function: Information, Vocabulary, Peabody Picture Vocabulary Test—Revised, Boston Naming Test. (Reproduced by permission from Schmahmann JD, Sherman JC. The cerebellar cognitive affective syndrome. Brain 1998;121:561–579.)*

finding problems. These deficits in visual-spatial skills, expressive language, initiating and sequencing of responses, verbal memory, and modulation of affect were similar to the observations in the adult population and suggest that the cerebellar cognitive affective syndrome is valid also in the pediatric population.

Anatomic Correlates

The cognitive and affective abnormalities in adults and children with cerebellar lesions are in many instances similar to those usually encountered in patients who have disorders of the cerebral hemispheres, and particularly of the association and paralimbic regions, or disorders of the subcortical area with which they are interconnected. Thus, disturbances of executive function are usually encountered in patients with lesions of the prefrontal cortex; visual-spatial deficits are seen following damage to the parietal lobe; decreased verbal fluency and linguistic processing difficulties are seen in the

setting of either frontal or temporal lobe pathology; impaired visual-spatial sequencing accompanies lesions of the right temporal lobe; and changes in affect and motivation commonly reflect disturbances in limbic-related regions in the cingulate and parahippocampal gyri (62–64). The presence of these cognitive deficits in patients with cerebellar lesions can be better understood when viewed in light of the anatomic connections linking the cerebral association areas and paralimbic regions with the cerebellum.

The cerebrocerebellar anatomic circuitry (Fig 99.4) consists of feedforward limb (the corticopontine and pontocerebellar pathways) and a feedback limb (the cerebellothalamic and thalamocortical systems). Anatomic investigations in the monkey have revealed pontine projections from sensorimotor cortices (65,66). More recently, strong and highly organized projections to the pons have been shown to arise from association areas in the dorsolateral and dorsomedial prefrontal cortex (67,68), posterior parietal regions (65,66,69,70), superior temporal polymodal (71),

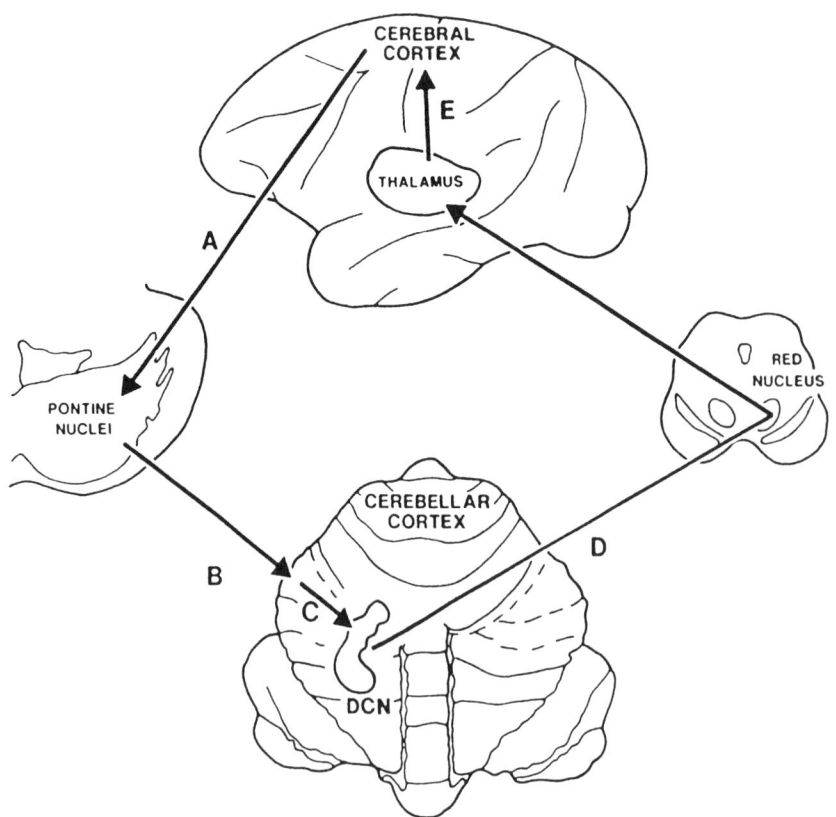

FIGURE 99.4   *Diagram of the anatomic circuits linking association areas and paralimbic cortices of the cerebral hemispheres with the cerebellum. The feedforward limb of the cerebrocerebellar circuit consists of the corticopontine projection (A) that carries this higher-order information (as well as sensorimotor inputs) from the cerebral cortex to the nuclei in the ventral pons, and the axons of the pontine neurons that convey this information via the pontocerebellar pathway (B) to the cerebellar cortex. The feedback limb of the cerebrocerebellar system originates in the cerebellar corticonuclear projection (C), and continues in a rostral direction as the deep cerebellar nuclei (DCN) send their axons to the thalamus [the cerebello-thalamic projection (D)] via the red nucleus, to which en passant terminals are distributed. The thalamic projection back to the association cortices (E) completes the feedback circuit. (Reproduced by permission from Schmahmann JD. The cerebellum in autism: clinical and anatomic perspectives. In: Bauman ML, Kemper TL, eds. The neurobiology of autism. Baltimore: Johns Hopkins University Press, 1994:195–226.)*

posterior parahippocampal (72) and dorsal prestriate regions (72,73), as well as from the cingulate gyrus (74). These anatomic findings (Fig 99.5) are in agreement with earlier physiological observations, such as those of Allen and Tsukuhara (75) and Sasaki et al (76), indicating the presence of parietal and prefrontal lobe connections with the cerebellar cortex. Furthermore, the medial mamillary bodies (implicated in memory) and deep layers of the superior colliculus (important for attention) have projections to the pons (77) and reciprocal connections with the cerebellum (78). Anatomic studies also reveal direct and reciprocal connections between the hypothalamus and cerebellum (78), and early physiological studies concluded that the cerebellum contributes to the limbic circuitry including septal nuclei and hippocampus (3,79–81). The details of the pontocerebellar projections have yet to be elucidated but the known anatomy of this system (82) is in agreement with the conceptual notion that the associative cortices are linked with the more recently evolved lateral cerebellar hemispheres (83–85). The cerebellar feedback loop through thalamus to the cerebral cortex appears to be directed not only to sensorimotor cortices, but also to the same associative areas from which the feedforward limb originates (Fig 99.6) (86–89). The demonstration of this associative cerebrocerebellar circuitry has led to the suggestion that the cerebellum is incorporated into the neural systems that subserve such higher-order behavior as working memory, executive function, visual-spatial abilities, linguistic processing, memory, attention, and emotional modulation (1,90). The neuropsychological and affective disorders in patients with cerebellar lesions are likely to be a consequence of disruption of these anatomic connections.

The projections from the associative and paralimbic regions of the cerebral cortex are funneled through the cerebrocerebellar circuit within multiple parallel but partially overlapping loops in the corticopontine pathway. These channels of information converge with topographic ordering within the basilar pontine nuclei, and this precise organization is probably present also in the pontine projections to the cerebellar cortex, although this still remains to be demonstrated for the associative inputs. These streams of information are acted upon by the cerebellar corticonuclear microcomplexes (91) and then transmitted via the deep cerebellar nuclei back to both specific and nonspecific thalamic nuclei, before returning to the cerebral cortex (88,90). The cerebrocerebellar system in this view then consists of discretely organized parallel anatomic subsystems that serve as the substrates for differentially organized functional subsystems (or loops) (36) within the framework of distributed neural circuits (68). The cerebellar contribution to these different subsystems may facilitate the production of harmonious motor, cognitive, and affective/autonomic behaviors. The hypothesis derived from this anatomic model is that disruption of the neural circuitry linking the cerebellum with the associative and paralimbic cerebral regions prevents the cerebellar modulation of functions subserved by the

affected subsystems, thus producing the observed behavioral deficits.

Functional Imaging

There continues to be an air of excitement about the ability to perform in vivo studies of the neuroanatomic basis of human behavior with functional neuroimaging. This modality has had a major impact on the understanding of, and interest in, the cerebellum. The demonstration of cerebellar activation during the performance of cognitive tasks established that narrow notions of the cerebellum as a motor control device were no longer tenable. Theoretical, anatomic, and clinical observations predicted cerebellar activation by some cognitive tasks on positron emission tomography (PET) and fMRI (functional MRI) studies. The extent to which the results of the imaging experiments would challenge the old hypotheses, however, could not have been imagined. They have dramatically altered the conventional understanding of cerebellar function.

Cerebellar activation has been observed during tests of language function including verb-for-noun substitution (Fig 99.7) (92) and synonym generation (93). Other cognitive tasks that have been studied specifically for the degree to which they produce cerebellar activation include working memory (Fig 99.8) (94,95), verbal memory (96,97), classical conditioning (98), mental imagery (99–101), shifting attention (Fig 99.9) (102), cognitive planning (103), sensory discrimination (104), and emotional modulation (105–109). The cerebellum is also activated during the early phases of acquisition of a motor skill (110–112), a finding supported by the recent demonstration that procedural learning is impaired in patients with focal cerebellar lesions (39). Some generalizations concerning the anatomic distribution within the cerebellum of these different functions can be derived such that crus I (of the ansiform lobule) on the right and vermal lobe VIIA-f (the folium) are activated during linguistic tasks, and shifting attention seems to activate crus I anterior on the left (according to the atlas of Schmahmann et al, reference 112a). Nevertheless, the precise organization of these cognitive and affective functions remains to be elucidated.

We recently performed a meta-analysis of the functional imaging studies that produce cerebellar activation by cognitive tasks (113). Fraught with methodologic considerations as this approach may be, it nevertheless provided a first glimpse of what appears to be a topographically organized map within the human cerebellum. Motor and nonmotor sites are represented in different regions. The anterior lobe is predominantly motor related, but most of the cognitive processing occurs within lobule VI and crus I of the ansiform lobules as well as in vermal lobules VI and VII. The flocculonodular lobe and caudal vermis are mostly concerned with eye movements. This analysis also revealed that cognitive tasks are frequently associated with more than one site of cerebellar activation and that there is an interdigita-

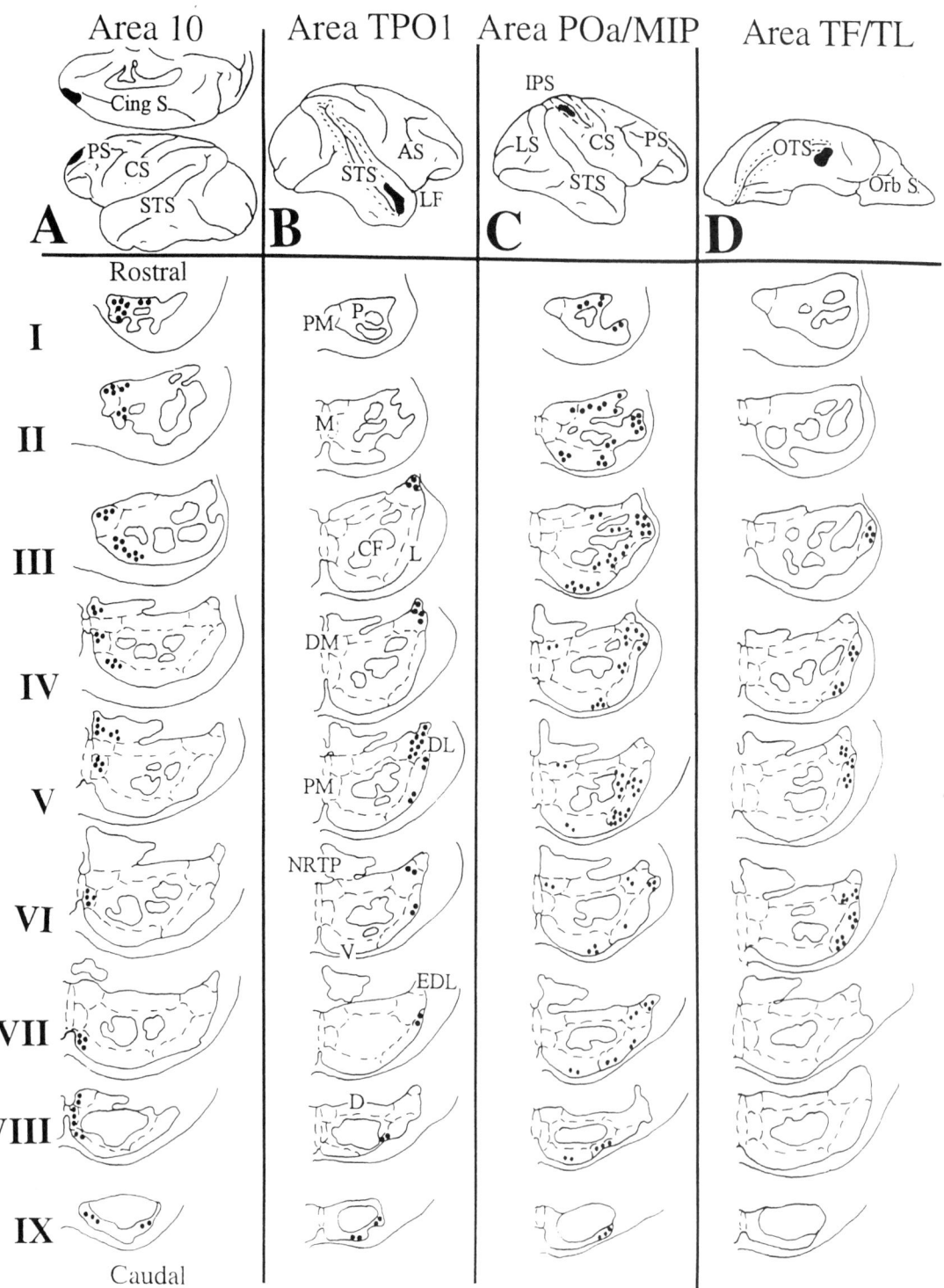

FIGURE 99.5   *Diagram of the projections to the basis pontis from selected regions within the cerebral association areas. Each cerebral area is connected with a unique and distributed subset of pontine neurons. The projections appear to be arranged in an interdigitating, but not overlapping manner. Radiolabeled amino acids (shaded black area in the cerebral hemispheres) were placed in the medial and lateral parts of the rostral prefrontal cortex in (A); in the cortex buried within the rostral upper bank of the superior temporal sulcus in (B); in cortex buried within the lower bank of the intraparietal sulcus in (C); and in the parahippocampal gyrus in (D). The label was transported in an anterograde fashion and terminated (black dots) in the ipsilateral half of the basis pontis from rostral level I to caudal level IX. (Reproduced by permission from Schmahmann JD. From movement to thought: anatomic substrates of the cerebellar contribution to cognitive processing. Human Brain Mapping 1996;4:174–198.)*

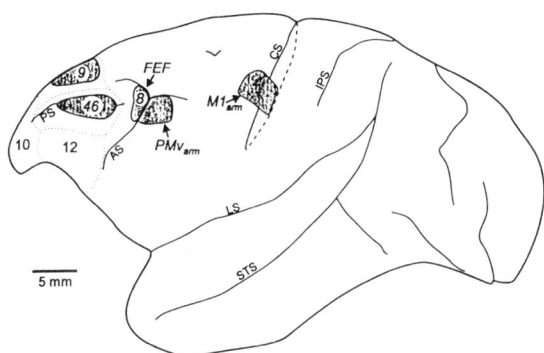

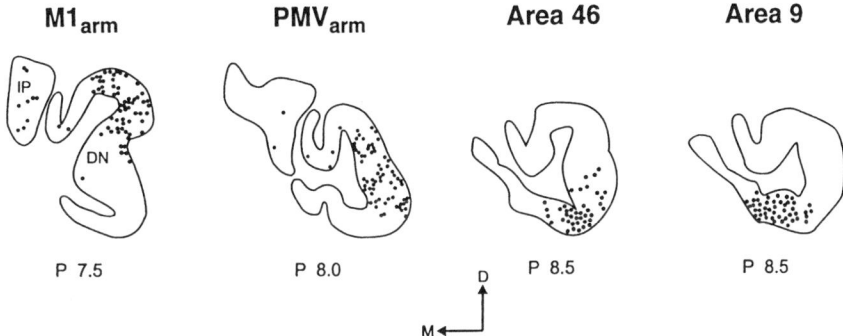

M1_{arm}   **PMV_{arm}**   **Area 46**   **Area 9**

P 7.5   P 8.0   P 8.5   P 8.5

FIGURE 99.6   *Lateral view of a cebus monkey brain (top) to show the location of injections of McIntyre-B strain of HSV1 in the primary motor cortex, ventral premotor cortex, and areas 9 and 46. The resulting retrogradely labeled neurons in the cerebellar dentate nucleus (bottom) are indicated by solid dots. (Adapted from Middleton FA, Strick PL. Cerebellar output channels. Int Rev Neurobiol 1997;41:61–82.)*

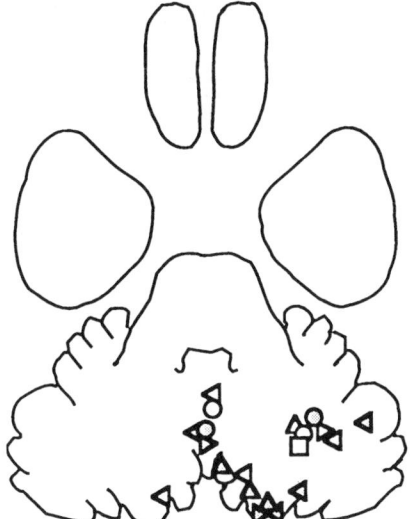

Petersen et al. (1989)
◁   generate verbs for visual words
Petersen et al. (1989)
▷   generate verbs for auditory words
Raichle et al. (1994)
△   generate verbs for visual nouns
Martin et al. (1995)
□   generate verbs for pictures
Grabowski et al. (1996)
○   generate verbs for visual nouns

Klein et al. (1995)
◁   generate synonyms
Klein et al. (1995)
▷   generate rhymes
Klein et al. (1995)
△   generate translations
Buckner et al. (1995)
○   generate stem completions

FIGURE 99.7   *Activation sites in the cerebellum across verb generation tasks. The locations of significant cerebellar activations found across five different verb generation studies are shown by black-outlined symbols, and the foci of activation found in several other verb generation tasks are indicated by gray-filled symbols. In most cases, the generation tasks were compared to a word-reading or object-naming task. All foci are plotted onto a transverse cerebellar section 26-mm below a transverse plane through the anterior and posterior commissures. (Reproduced by permission from Fiez JA, Raichle ME. Linguistic processing. Int Rev Neurobiol 1997;41:233–254.*

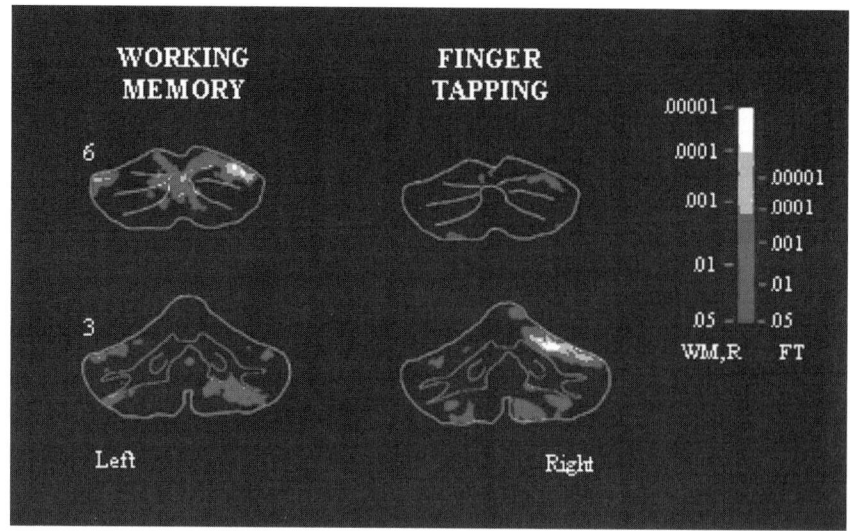

FIGURE 99.8 *Functional MRI scans (averaged across subjects) in selected oblique coronal sections of the cerebellum showing that different areas are activated by working-memory and by finger-tapping tasks. Lighter shades represent areas that exhibited increased activation in high relative to low load conditions (in working memory) or during finger tapping relative to rest. The gray scale on the right represents the significance levels (one-tailed p values) of averaged Z scores and is scaled differently for finger tapping than for working memory. (Adapted from Desmond JE, Gabrieli JD, Wagner AD, et al. Lobular patterns of cerebellar activation in verbal working-memory and finger-tapping tasks as revealed by functional MRI. J Neurosci 1997;17:9675–9685.)*

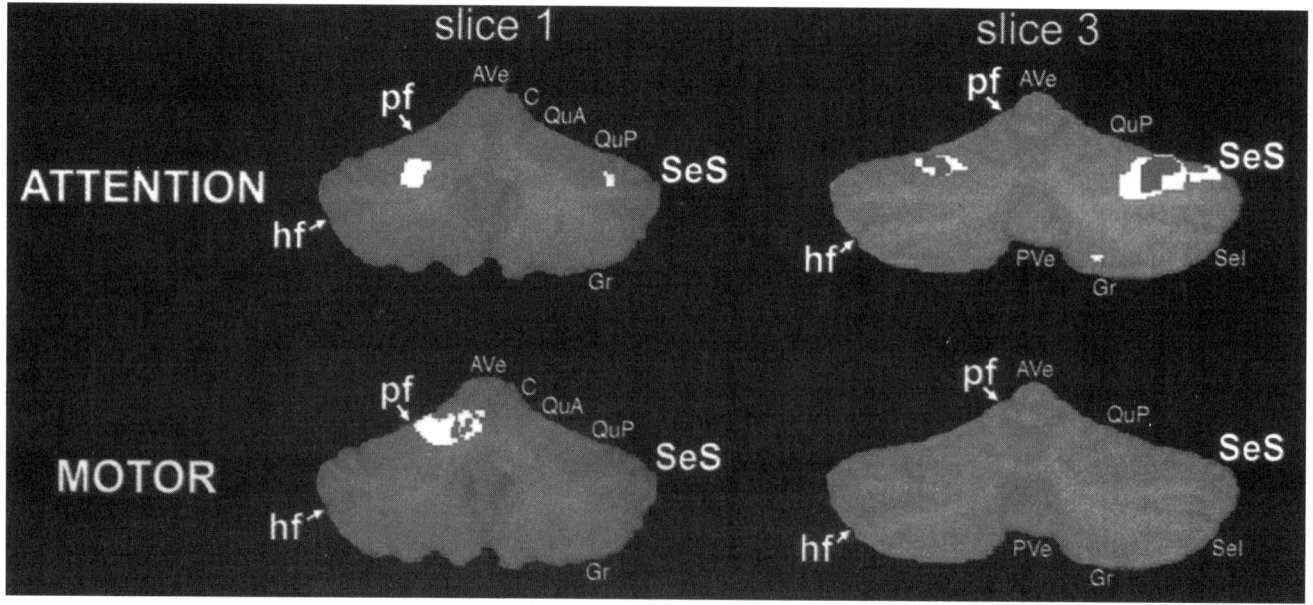

FIGURE 99.9 *Functional activation studies of the cerebellum show that tasks of attention-shifting and of motor performance activate different areas. Positron emission tomographic maps of the most common sites of activation across subjects were overlaid on averaged coronal anatomical images of anterior (slice 1) and posterior (slice 3) sections of the cerebellum. During the task that required shifts of attention, activation was seen in the left superior posterior part of the cerebellum (HVI and crus I of the ansiform lobule, termed* posterior quadrangular lobe *and* superior semilunar lobe *in this figure). During the motor performance, the anterior cerebellar lobe was activated. (Reproduced by permission from Courchesne E, Allen G. Prediction and preparation, fundamental functions of the cerebellum. Learning and Memory 1997;4:1–35.)*

tion and some overlap of activation sites, suggesting focal convergence zones within broad functional domains.

Other Supportive Evidence

There is a rich history of physiologic and behavioral investigations in animals suggesting that the cerebellum participates in sensory, autonomic, and behavioral functions. This body of work has been revisited in Dow and Moruzzi (114), Watson (20), and Schmahmann (1,2). The role of the archicerebellum and fastigial nucleus in autonomic responses and complex emotional behaviors (6,115–120), the critical incorporation of the anterior interpositus nucleus in classical conditioned learning (44,121–123), and the disruption of visual-spatial skills in cerebellar lesioned models (124,125) have been early and consistent indicators of nonmotor cerebellar functions. More recently, neurons in the cerebellar dentate nucleus of monkeys have been shown to be activated by a working memory task (89), and rats with hemicerebellectomy have been shown to have impairments in procedural memory (39).

WHAT IS THE CEREBELLAR ROLE IN HIGHER-ORDER FUNCTION?

It now appears that the cerebellum is involved in the organization of higher-order function. But what is the fundamental role of the cerebellum in these complex behaviors, be they motor, sensory, cognitive, affective, or autonomic? "Dysmetria of thought" is the concept that we proposed as the fundamental mechanism underlying disorders of intellect and emotion resulting from cerebellar dysfunction (1,90). When cognitive performance, affect, and autonomic function are considered in the light of the understanding of cerebellar motor deficits, then intact cerebellar function facilitates actions harmonious with the goal, appropriate to context, and judged accurately and reliably according to the strategies mapped out prior to and during the behavior. In this view, the cerebellum detects, prevents, and corrects mismatches between intended outcome and perceived outcome of the organism's interaction with the environment. In the same way as the cerebellum regulates the rate, force, rhythm, and accuracy of movements, so may it regulate the speed, capacity, consistency, and appropriateness of mental or cognitive processes. In this model, the cerebellar contribution to cognition is one of modulation rather than generation, correlating with the suggestions of Snider (3) that the cerebellum is the great modulator of neurologic function, of Heath (6) that the cerebellum is an emotional pacemaker for the brain, and of Ito (126) that the cerebellum serves to prevent, detect, and correct errors of thought in the same way as it does for errors of movement. In agreement with Leiner et al (83,84) that the cerebellum serves as a multipurpose computer designed to smooth out performance of mental operations, we have suggested that the cerebellum serves as an oscillation dampener, maintaining function steadily around a homeostatic baseline. When the cerebellar component of the distributed neural circuit is lost or disrupted, the oscillation dampener is removed. Mental processes are imperfectly conceived, erratically monitored, and poorly performed. There is an unpredictability to social and societal interaction, a mismatch between reality and perceived reality, and erratic attempts to correct the errors of thought or behavior. This concept of dysmetria of thought facilitates a new approach to the psychoses, because it focuses on aberrations of the cerebellum (1,90). Other investigators have adopted this anatomically based model in considering the cognitive and affective deficits that characterize schizophrenia (127).

A number of other hypotheses about the role of the cerebellum in cognitive and emotional behaviors have been proposed, some of which are briefly summarized here. Readers are referred to Schmahmann (4) for full discussion of these hypotheses by their principal proponents. Ivry (46) and others have maintained that the problems of coordination and mental functions that patients with cerebellar lesions experience can be understood as a problem in controlling and regulating the temporal patterns of movement and behavior. Thus the timing capabilities of the cerebellum are not limited to the motor domain but are utilized in perceptual tasks that require the precise representation of temporal information. In the view of Courchesne and Allen (128) the cerebellar role in motor and nonmotor behaviors is that the cerebellum is a master computational system that is able to anticipate and adjust responsiveness in a variety of brain systems in order to achieve goals determined by cerebral and other subcortical systems. These investigators have supported their view that the cerebellum is important for the coordination of the direction of selective attention by demonstrating impairments in this function in patients with cerebellar strokes and also in autistic individuals. The notions of Bower (129) that the cerebellum is involved in monitoring and adjusting the acquisition of most of the sensory data on which the rest of the nervous system depends has prompted functional imaging studies that have provided support for this view. This concept holds that rather than being responsible for any particular behaviorally related function, the cerebellum instead facilitates the efficiency with which other brain structures perform their own function.

In an analogous but slightly different view, Paulin (130) has stated that cerebellar function can be explained by assuming that it is involved in constructing neural representations of moving systems. Thus, the cerebellum could be a neural analog of a dynamic state estimator. The state estimator hypothesis according to Paulin would explain the participation of the cerebellum in controlling, perceiving, and imagining systems that move. Thach (131) has proposed that there is a context response linkage performed by the cerebellum in both motor and nonmotor areas of behavior. In this view, through practice, an experiential context automatically evokes a certain mental action plan. This plan could be in the realm of thought but would not necessarily lead to execution. Thus the specific cerebellar contribution to higher function would be one of context linkage and the shaping of responses to trial and error learning. Ito (132) has conceptualized the cerebellar involvement in thought based on the analogy between movement and thought from the viewpoint of control systems. In this view, the cerebellar corticonuclear microcomplex is connected to neuronal circuits involved in thought and may represent a dynamic or an inverse dynamic model of a mental representation. The cerebellum is designated as a regulatory organ subserving different executive functions and it is defined by its error-driven adaptive control mechanism and the model-building capability that is based on it. Thus Ito extended the error detection mechanism identified for the vestibulo-ocular reflex to the cerebellar regulation of thought and other aspects of higher function. The anatomically based models have been used in our own conceptualization of the role of cerebellum and higher function, as reported in Schmahmann (1,90) and as described above. Leiner et al (83,84) have also adopted an anatomically based approach and regarded the cerebrocerebellar system like the circuitry in a versatile computer. Thus the cerebellum is able to perform a large repertoire of computations on a wide range of information to which it has access. Each module in the lateral cerebellum is able to communicate with the cerebral cortex by sending out signals over its segregated bundle of nerve fibers, which is a powerful way of communicating information. The bundling of fibers enables a high level of discourse to take place between the cerebellum and cerebral cortex using internal languages that are capable of conveying complex information about what to do and when to do it.

The cerebellum is also involved in such diverse behaviors as skill learning, classical conditioning, spatial event processing, and autonomic and vasomotor regulation in addition to the clinical manifestations already documented. The anatomically based model in which anatomic loops subserve functional subsystems within the larger framework of the associative, paralimbic, and autonomic cerebrocerebellar communication is compatible with different functional hypotheses. It remains to be determined whether the concept of dysmetria of thought as an overarching functional hypothesis derived from the error detection model can also subsume these other functional hypotheses.

In the clinical studies performed to date, there is a suggestion of dissociation between motor, cognitive, and affective consequences of discrete cerebellar lesions, perhaps indicating that there is topographic organization of behavioral functions within the human cerebellum. Disturbances of affect, for example, have been more pronounced following lesions of the posterior vermis. Executive and visual-spatial abnormalities as well as linguistic difficulties have been more prominent following lesions of the posterior lobe. Motor deficits have been more pronounced in ante-rior lobe lesions, whereas the cognitive consequences of anterior lobe lesions have been limited. More precise structure–function correlations await the analysis of a larger group of patients with focal cerebellar lesions in order to develop more significant clinical–anatomic correlations than has been possible from the sample sizes studied to date. Such clinical investigations would test the hypothesis that different regions of the cerebellum subserve distinct cognitive functions (1,90). The results of functional imaging experiments provide support for the notion that different cognitive functions have different anatomic loci within the cerebellum. Linguistic processing, for example, appears to be concentrated in the vermal lobules VI through VII and the hemispheric extensions of these areas, that is, HVI and crus I of the ansiform lobe (40). This hypothesis has also been supported by functional imaging studies showing separate cerebellar regions of activation for motor and nonmotor functions (see, for example, Allen and Courchesne (102); Desmond et al (95)).

CONCLUSIONS

The descriptions of clinically relevant cognitive and affective changes resulting from cerebellar lesions indicate that the discussion concerning the role of the cerebellum in higher-order function has direct relevance for patient care. They also provide an opportunity to study these questions in the patient population. The demonstration of a characteristic behavioral syndrome resulting from acquired lesions of the cerebellum, the cerebellar cognitive affective syndrome, provides documentation of clinically relevant cognitive deficits in patients with pathology restricted to the cerebellum. Furthermore, the presence of cerebellar activation by cognitive tasks brings the cerebellum into the realm of behavioral neuroscience, and quite possibly also into the domain of psychiatric illness. The fact that there is a distributed topography of cognition in the cerebellum indicates that this is not an epiphenomenon. Rather, the cerebellum appears to be an essential node in the distributed neural circuitry subserving cognitive operations. The multiple discrete channels of information leading into the cerebellum from the cerebral cortex and directed back to the cerebral hemispheres by the cerebellar nuclei provide the anatomic substrate to support the findings documented in clinical and functional imaging studies. The new clinical and experimental data challenge the long-held assumption that the cerebellum is an exclusively motor control device. This realization has relevance for the understanding of how the structures of the brain support mental operations. It is important also at a practical clinical level because it allows patients and their families to comprehend behavioral effects of cerebellar lesions, and it facilitates the diagnosis and management of cognitive and affective consequences of focal cerebellar lesions.

ACKNOWLEDGMENTS

The author is grateful to Ms. Amy Hurwitz and Ms. Marygrace Neal for their assistance in preparing this work. Supported in part by the A. J. Berman Neurosurgical Research Fund.

REFERENCES

1. Schmahmann JD. An emerging concept: the cerebellar contribution to higher function. Arch Neurol 1991;48:1178–1187 and 1992;49:1230.
2. Schmahmann JD. Rediscovery of an early concept. Int Rev Neurobiol 1997;41:3–27.
3. Snider RS. Recent contributions to the anatomy and physiology of the cerebellum. Arch Neurol Psych 1950;64:196–219.
4. Schmahmann JD. The cerebellum and cognition. Int Rev Neurobiol 1997; 41.
5. Heath RG, Cox AW, Lustick LS. Brain activity during emotional states. Am J Psychiat 1974;131:858–862.
6. Heath RG. Modulation of emotion with a brain pacemaker. J Nerv Ment Dis 1977;165:300–317.
7. Riklan M, Marisak I, Cooper IS. Psychological studies of chronic cerebellar stimulation in man. In: Cooper IS, Riklan M, Snider RS, eds. The cerebellum, epilepsy and behavior. New York: Plenum Press, 1974.
8. Heath RG, Franklin DE, Shraberg D. Gross pathology of the cerebellum in patients diagnosed and treated as functional psychiatric disorders. J Nerv Ment Dis 1979;167:585–592.
9. Weinberger DR, et al. Cerebellar pathology in schizophrenia: a controlled postmortem study. Am J Psychiat 1980;137:359–361.
10. Moriguchi I. A study of schizophrenic brains by computerized tomography scans. Folia Psychiat Neurol Jpn 1981;35:55–72.
11. Lippmann S, et al. Cerebellar vermis dimensions on computerized tomographic scans of schizophrenic and bipolar patients. Am J Psychiat 1981;139:667–668.
12. Joseph AB, Anderson WH, O'Leary DH. Brainstem and vermis atrophy in catatonia. Am J Psychiat 1985;142:352–354.
13. Kutty IN, Prendes JL. Single case study. Psychosis and cerebellar degeneration. J Nerv Ment Dis 1981;169:390–391.
14. Hamilton NG, et al. Psychiatric symptoms and cerebellar pathology. Am J Psychiat 1983;140:1322–1326.
15. Bauman ML, Kemper TL. Neuroanatomic observations of the brain in autism. In: Bauman ML, Kemper TL, eds., The neurobiology of autism. Baltimore: Johns Hopkins University Press, 1994:119–145.
16. Courchesne E, et al. Hypoplasia of cerebellar vermal lobules VI and VII in autism. N Engl J Med 1988;318:1349–1354.
17. Murakami JW, et al. Reduced cerebellar hemisphere size and its relationship to vermal hypoplasia in autism. Arch Neurol 1989;46:689–694.
18. Berquin PC, et al. Cerebellum in attention-deficit hyperactivity disorder. Neurology 1998;50:1087–1093.
19. Mostofsky SH, et al. Decreased cerebellar posterior vermis size in fragile X syndrome: correlation with neurocognitive performance. Neurology 1998;50:121–130.
20. Watson PJ. Nonmotor functions of the cerebellum. Psychol Bull 1978;85:944–967.
21. Frick RB. The ego and the vestibulocerebellar system. Psychoanal Q 1982;51:93–122.
22. Snider RS. Cerebellar pathology in schizophrenia—cause or consequence? Neurosci Behav Rev 1982;6:47–53.
23. Taylor MA. The role of the cerebellum in the pathogenesis of schizophrenia. Neuropsychiat Neuropsychol Behav Neurol 1991;4:251–280.
24. Landis DMD, et al. Olivopontocerebellar degeneration. Arch Neurol 1974;31:295–307.
25. Kish SJ, et al. Cognitive deficits in olivopontocerebellar atrophy: implications for the cholinergic hypothesis of Alzheimer's dementia. Ann Neurol 1988;24:200–206.
26. Bracke-Tolkmitt R, et al. The cerebellum contributes to mental skills. Behav Neurosci 1989;103:442–446.
27. Akshoomoff NA, Courchesne E. A new role for the cerebellum in cognitive operations. Behav Neurosci 1992;106:731–738.
28. Kish SJ, et al. Neuropsychological test performance in patients with dominantly inherited spinocerebellar ataxia: relationship to ataxia severity. Neurology 1994;44:1738–1746.
29. Botez-Maquard T, Botez MI. Cognitive behavior in heterodegenerative ataxias. Eur Neurol 1993;33:351–357.
30. Fehrenbach RA, Wallesch C-W, Claus D. Neuropsychological findings in Friedreich's ataxia. Arch Neurol 1984;41:306–308.
31. Botez-Maquard T, Botez MI. Olivopontocerebellar atrophy and Friedreich's ataxia: neuropsychological consequences of bilateral versus unilateral cerebellar lesions. Int Rev Neurobiol 1997;41:388–411.
32. Grafman J, et al. Cognitive planning deficit in patients with cerebellar atrophy. Neurology 1992;42:1493–1496.
33. Appollonio IM, et al. Memory in patients with cerebellar degeneration. Neurology 1993;43:1536–1544.
34. Pascual-Leone A, et al. Procedural learning in Parkinson's disease and cerebellar degeneration. Ann Neurol 1993;34:594–602.
35. Wallesch C-W, Horn A. Long-term effects of cerebellar pathology on cognitive functions. Brain Cogn 1990;14:19–25.
36. Botez-Maquard T, Leveille J, Botez MI. Neuropsychological functioning in unilateral cerebellar damage. Can J Neurol Sci 1994;21:353–357.
37. Botez MI, et al. Reversible chronic cerebellar ataxia after phenytoin intoxication: possible role of cerebellum in cognitive thought. Neurology 1985;35:1152–1157.
38. Silveri MC, Leggio MG, Molinari M. The cerebellum contributes to linguistic production: a case of agrammatic speech following a right cerebellar lesion. Neurology 1994;44:2047–2050.
39. Molinari M, Leggio MG, Silveri M. Verbal fluency and agrammatism. Int Rev Neurobiol 1997;41:325–339.
40. Fiez JA, et al. Impaired non-motor learning and error detection associated with cerebellar damage. Brain 1992;115:155–178.
41. Sanes JN, Dimitrov B, Hallett M. Motor learning in patients with cerebellar dysfunction. Brain 1990;113:103–120.
42. Thach WT, Goodkin HP, Keating JG. The cerebellum and the adaptive coordination of movement. Annu Rev Neurosci 1992;15:403–442.
43. Woodruff-Pak DS. Classical conditioning. Int Rev Neurobiol 1997;41:342–365.
44. Solomon PR, Stowe GT, Pendlebury WW. Disrupted eyelid conditioning in a patient with damage to cerebellar afferents. Behav Neurosci 1989;103:898–902.
45. Daum I, et al. Classical conditioning after cerebellar lesions in humans. Behav Neurosci 1993;107:748–756.
46. Ivry R. Cerebellar timing systems. Int Rev Neurobiol 1997;41:556–571.
47. Courchesne E, et al. Impairment in shifting attention in autistic and cerebellar patients. Behav Neurosci 1994;108:848–865.
48. Berent S, et al. Neuropsychological changes in olivopontocerebellar atrophy. Arch Neurol 1990;47:997–1001.
49. Gomez-Baldarrain M, et al. Diaschisis and neuropsychological performance after cerebellar stroke. Eur Neurol 1997;37:82–89.
50. Gomez-Baldarrain M, et al. Effect of cerebellar lesions on procedural learning in the serial reaction time task. Exp Brain Res 1988;120:25–30.
51. Dimitrov M, et al. Preserved cognitive processes in cerebellar degeneration. Behav Brain Res 1996;79:131–135.
52. Van Dongen HR, Catsman-Berrevoets CE, van Mourik M. The syndrome of "cerebellar" mutism and subsequent dysarthria. Neurology 1994;44:2040–2046.
53. Pollack IF, Polinko P, Albright AL, et al. Mutism and pseudobulbar symptoms after resection of posterior fossa tumors in children: incidence and pathophysiology. Neurosurgery 1995;37:885–893.
54. Kingma A, et al. Transient mutism and speech disorders after posterior fossa surgery in children with brain tumors. Acta Neurochir 1994;131:74–79.
55. Pollack IF. Posterior fossa syndrome. Int Rev Neurobiol 1997;41:412–432.
56. Schmahmann JD, Sherman JC. The cerebellar cognitive affective syndrome. Brain 1998;121:561–579.
57. Cutting JC. Chronic mania in childhood. Case report of a possible association with a radiological picture of cerebellar disease. Psych Med 1976;6:635–642.
58. Joubert M, et al. Familial agenesis of the cerebellar vermis. A syndrome of episodic hyperpnea, abnormal eye movements, ataxia, and retardation. Neurology 1969;19:813–825.
59. LeBaron S, et al. Assessment of quality of survival in children with medulloblastoma and cerebellar astrocytoma. Cancer 1988;62:1215–1222.
60. Packer RJ, et al. A prospective study of cognitive function in children receiving whole-brain radiotherapy and chemotherapy: 2-year results. J Neurosurg 1989;70:707–713.

61. Levisohn L, Cronin-Golomb A, Schmahmann JD. Neuropsychological sequelae of cerebellar tumors in children. Soc Neurosci Abstr 1997;23:496.

62. Critchley M. The parietal lobes. New York: Hafner Press, 1953.

63. Fuster JM. The prefrontal cortex: anatomy, physiology and neurophysiology of the frontal lobe. New York: Raven Press, 1980.

64. Mesulam MM. Principles of behavioral neurology. Philadelphia: FA Davis, 1985:1–405.

65. Brodal P. The corticopontine projection in the rhesus monkey. Origin and principles of organization. Brain 1978;101:251–283.

66. Glickstein M, May JG, Mercier BE. Corticopontine projection in the macaque: the distribution of labelled cortical cells after large injections of horseradish peroxidase in the pontine nuclei. J Comp Neurol 1985;235:343–359.

67. Schmahmann JD, Pandya DN. Prefrontal cortex projections to the basilar pons: Implications for the cerebellar contribution to higher function. Neurosci Lett 1995;199:175–178.

68. Schmahmann JD, Pandya DN. The cerebrocerebellar system. Int Rev Neurobiol 1997;41:31–60.

69. May JG, Anderson RA. Different patterns of corticopontine projections from separate cortical fields within the inferior parietal lobule and dorsal prelunate gyrus of the macaque. Exp Brain Res 1996;63:265–278.

70. Schmahmann JD, Pandya DN. Anatomical investigation of projections to the basis pontis from posterior parietal association cortices in rhesus monkey. J Comp Neurol 1989;289:53–73.

71. Schmahmann JD, Pandya DN. Projections to the basis pontis from the superior temporal sulcus and superior temporal region in the rhesus monkey. J Comp Neurol 1991;308:224–248.

72. Schmahmann JD, Pandya DN. Prelunate, occipitotemporal, and parahippocampal projections to the basis pontis in rhesus monkey. J Comp Neurol 1993;337:94–112.

73. Fries W. Pontine projection from striate and prestriate visual cortex in the macaque monkey: an anterograde study. Vis Neurosci 1990;4:205–216.

74. Vilensky JA, Van Hoesen GW. Corticopontine projections from the cingulate cortex in the rhesus monkey. Brain Res 1981;205:391–395.

75. Allen GI, Tsukahara N. Cerebrocerebellar communication systems. Physiol Rev 1974;54:957–1008.

76. Sasaki K, Oka H, Matsuda Y, et al. Electrophysiological studies of the projections from the parietal association area to the cerebellar cortex. Exp Brain Res 1975;23:91–102.

77. Aas J-E, Brodal P. Demonstration of topographically organized projections from the hypothalamus to the pontine nuclei: an experimental study in the cat. J Comp Neurol 1988;268:313–328.

78. Haines DE, Dietrichs E. An HRP study of hypothalamo-cerebellar and cerebello-hypothalamic connections in squirrel monkey (*Saimiri sciureus*). J Comp Neurol 1984;229:559–575.

79. Anand BK, Malhotra CL, Singh B, Dua S. Cerebellar projections to the limbic system. J Neurophysiol 1959;22:451–458.

80. Harper JW, Heath RG. Anatomic connections of the fastigial nucleus to the rostral forebrain in the cat. Exp Neurol 1973;39:285–292.

81. Snider RS, Maiti A. Cerebellar contribution to the Papez circuit. J Neurosci Res 1976;2:133–146.

82. Brodal P. The pontocerebellar projection in the rhesus monkey: an experimental study with retrograde axonal transport of horseradish peroxidase. Neuroscience 1979;4:193–208.

83. Leiner HC, Leiner AL, Dow RS. Does the cerebellum contribute to mental skills? Behav Neurosci 1986;100:443–454.

84. Leiner HC, Leiner AL. How fibers subserve computing capabilities: similarities between brains and machines. Int Rev Neurobiol 1997;41:535–553.

85. Dow RS. Contribution of electrophysiological studies to cerebellar physiology. J Clin Neurophysiol 1988;5:307–323.

86. Schmahmann JD, Pandya DN. Anatomical investigation of projections from thalamus to the posterior parietal association cortices in rhesus monkey. J Comp Neurol 1990;295:299–326.

87. Schmahmann JD, Pandya DN. Anatomic organization of the basilar pontine projections from prefrontal cortices in rhesus monkey. J Neurosci 1997;17:438–458.

88. Middleton FA, Strick PL. Anatomical evidence for cerebellar and basal ganglia involvement in higher cognitive function. Science 1994;266:458–461.

89. Middleton FA, Strick PL. Cerebellar output channels. Int Rev Neurobiol 1997;41:61–82.

90. Schmahmann JD. From movement to thought: anatomic substrates of the cerebellar contribution to cognitive processing. Human Brain Mapping 1996;4:174–198.

91. Ito M. The cerebellum and neural control. New York: Raven Press, 1984.

92. Petersen SE, Fox PT, Posner MI, et al. Positron emission tomographic studies of the cortical anatomy of single-word processing. Nature 1988;331:585–589.

93. Klein D, Milner B, Zatorre RJ, et al. The neural substrates underlying word generation: a bilingual functional-imaging study. Proc Natl Acad Sci USA 1995;92:2899–2903.

94. Klingberg T, Roland PE, Kawashima R. The neural correlates of the central executive function during working memory—a PET study. Human Brain Mapping 1995(suppl. 1):414.

95. Desmond JE, Gabrieli JD, Wagner AD, et al. Lobular patterns of cerebellar activation in verbal working-memory and finger-tapping tasks as revealed by functional MRI. J Neurosci 1997;17:9675–9685.

96. Grasby PM, Frith CD, Friston KJ, et al. Functional mapping of brain areas implicated in auditory-verbal memory function. Brain 1993;116:1–20.

97. Andreasen NC, O'Leary DS, Arndt S, et al. Short-term and long-term verbal memory: a positron emission tomography study. Proc Natl Acad Sci USA 1995;92:5111–5115.

98. Logan CG, Grafton ST. Functional anatomy of human eyeblink conditioning determined with regional cerebral glucose metabolism and positron emission tomography. Proc Natl Acad Sci USA 1995;92:7500–7504.

99. Ryding E, Decety J, Sjoholm H, et al. Motor imagery activates the cerebellum regionally—a SPECT rCBF study with tc-99m HMPAO. Cogn Brain Res 1993;1:94–99.

100. Mellet E, Crivello F, Tzourio N, et al. Construction of mental images based on verbal description: functional neuroanatomy with PET. Human Brain Mapping Supplement 1995;(suppl 1):273.

101. Parsons LM, Fox PT, Downs JH, et al. Use of implicit motor imagery for visual shape discrimination as revealed by PET. Nature 1995;375:54.

102. Allen G, Courchesne E. Attentional activation of the cerebellum independent of motor involvement. Science 1997;275:1940–1943.

103. Kim SG, Ugurbil K, Strick PL. Activation of a cerebellar output nucleus during cognitive processing. Science 1994;265:949–951.

104. Gao J-H, Parsons LM, Bower JM, et al. Cerebellum implicated in sensory acquisition and discrimination rather than motor control. Science 1996;272:545–547.

105. Reiman M, Raichle ME, Robins E. Neuroanatomical correlates of a lactate-induced anxiety attack. Arch Gen Psychiatry 1989;46:493–500.

106. Bench CJ, Friston KJ, Brown RG, et al. The anatomy of melancholia. Focal abnormalities of cerebral blood flow in major depression. Psych Med 1992;22:607–615.

107. Dolan RJ, Bench CJ, Scott RG, et al. Regional cerebral blood flow abnormalities in depressed patients with cognitive impairment. J Neurol Neurosurg Psychiat 1992;55:768–773.

108. George MS, Ketter TA, Parekh PI, et al. Brain activity during transient sadness and happiness in healthy women. Am J Psychiatry 1995;152:341–351.

109. Mayberg HS, Liotti M, Jerabek PA, et al. Induced sadness: a PET model of depression. Human Brain Mapping Supplement 1995;(suppl 1):396.

110. Seitz RJ, Roland PE. Learning of sequential finger movements in man: a combined kinematic and positive emission tomography (PET) study. Eur J Neurosci 1992;4:154–165.

111. Jenkins IH, Brooks DJ, Nixon PD, et al. Motor sequence learning: a study with positron emission tomography. J Neurosci 1994;14:3775–3790.

112. Doyon J. Skill learning. Int Rev Neurobiol 1997;41:273–296.

112a. Schmahmann JD, Doyon J, Holmes C, et al. An MRI atlas of the human cerebellum in Talairach space. Neuro Image 13:S122.

113. Schmahmann JD, Loeber RT, Marjani J, Hurwitz AS. Topographic organization of cognitive functions in the human cerebellum. A meta-analysis of functional imaging studies. NeuroImage 1998:S721.

114. Dow RS, Moruzzi G. The physiology and pathology of the cerebellum. Minneapolis, MN: University of Minnesota Press, 1958.

115. Zanchetti A, Zoccolini A. Autonomic hypothalamic outbursts elicited by cerebellar stimulation. J Neurophysiol 1954;17:475–483.

116. Peters M, Monjan AA. Behavior after cerebellar lesions in cats and monkeys. Physiol Behav 1971;6:205–206.

117. Berntson G, Potolicchi S Jr, Miller N. Evidence for higher functions of the cerebellum: eating and grooming elicited by cerebellar stimulation in cats. Proc Natl Acad Sci USA 1973;70:2497–2499.

118. Cooper IS, Amin L, Gilman S, Waltz JM. The effect of chronic stimulation of cerebellar cortex on epilepsy in man. In: Cooper IS, Riklan M, Snider RS, eds. The Cerebellum, epilepsy and behavior. New York: Plenum Press, 1978:119–172.

119. Reis DJ, Doba N, Nathan MA. Predatory attack, grooming and consummatory behaviors evoked by electrical stimulation of cat cerebellar nuclei. Science 1973;182:845–847.

120. Berman AJ, Berman D, Prescott JW. The effects of cerebellar lesions on emotional behavior in the rhesus monkey. In: Cooper IS, Riklan M, Snider RS, eds. The Cerebellum, epilepsy and behavior. New York: Plenum Press, 1978:277–284.

121. Thompson RF. The neural basis of basic associative learning of discrete behavioral responses. Trends Neurosci 1988;11:152–155.

122. Woodruff-Pak D, Thompson RF, Logan CG. Neurobiological substrates of classical conditioning across the life span. NY Acad Sci 1990;608:150–178.

123. Topka H, Valls-Sole J, Massaquoi SG, Hallett M. Deficit in classical conditioning in patients with cerebellar degeneration. Brain 1993;116:961–969.

124. Lalonde R, Manseau M, Botez MI. Spontaneous alternation and habituation in Purkinje cell degeneration in mutant mice. Brain Res 1987;411:187–189.

125. Molinari M, Petrosini L, Dell'Anna ME, Gianetti S. Hemicerebellectomy induces spatial memory deficits in rats. Soc Neurosci Abstr 1991;17:919.

126. Ito M. Movement and thought: identical control mechanisms by the cerebellum. Trends Neurosci 1993;16:448–450.

127. Andreasen NC, Paradiso S, O'Leary D. "Cognitive dysmetria" as an integrative theory of schizophrenia: a dysfunction in cortical-subcortical-cerebellar circuitry? Schizophrenia Bull 1998;24:203–218.

128. Courchesne E, Allen G. Prediction and preparation, fundamental functions of the cerebellum. Learning and Memory 1997;4:1–35.

129. Bower JM. Control of sensory data acquisition. Int Rev Neurobiol 1997;41:489–513.

130. Paulin MG. Neural representations of moving systems. Int Rev Neurobiol 1997;41:515–533.

131. Thach WT. On the specific role of the cerebellum in motor learning and cognition: Clues from PET activation and lesion studies in man. Behav Brain Sci 1996;19:411–431.

132. Ito M. Cerebellar microcomplexes. Int Rev Neurobiol 1997;41:475–487.

Factitious Movement Disorders: Thoughts on a Difficult Problem

ROBERT R. YOUNG   ANTHONY B. JOSEPH

Much of the terminology used to describe movement disorders is, for several reasons, unsatisfactory. Because of the ancient, but still persistent, mind–brain dichotomy, many have tried to segregate movement disorders into those two categories. Most movements and some movement disorders *are* generated by mental processes, but others are not.

With advances in neuroscience and neuropsychiatry, it is becoming increasingly difficult to differentiate between what were in an earlier, simpler time called abnormal movements due to an organic brain disorder and those due to psychiatric or psychogenic disorders. Torticollis, now generally acknowledged to be a focal, cervical dystonia, was once thought to be caused by an urge to turn the head to avoid seeing something particularly traumatic. Torsion dystonia and the movements of complex partial seizures were also misdiagnosed as psychogenic. Stuttering was once treated by psychoanalysis. Even today, oculogyric crises caused by risperidone have been mistaken for a behavioral disorder.

Ultimately, of course, the psychiatric brain and the neurologic brain will prove to be the same, utilizing the same molecular, cellular, and systemic neurobiologic mechanisms. The differentiation between organic and psychiatric disorders will be less hotly debated, but factitious (defined as artificial, not natural) movement disorders will still exist and present some of the most difficult diagnostic and therapeutic problems. The patient described by Batshaw et al (1) (see also our Preface to the first edition, p. xvii) with Munchausen's syndrome, who was thought to have torsion dystonia, is a particularly good example of how well-meaning physicians can make inappropriate management decisions.

Shell shock, a common cause of tremor and paralysis in World War I, is clearly a psychogenic disorder, as are the abnormal movements seen in patients and actresses demonstrated by Charcot as hysterics. Fahn et al (2) define psy-chogenic movement disorders as abnormal movements that do not result from a known organic cause but are caused by psychological conditions. While that may be true, it is not a particularly helpful definition. Unusual or unpleasant psychological conditions are to be found everywhere, but how can we know if they cause the abnormal movements we are asked to manage? What is the known organic cause for essential tremor, spasmodic dysphonia, torsion dystonia, and so on? They are universally thought to be organic movement disorders but are still without demonstrated laboratory, neuroimaging, neuropathologic, or neurochemical abnormalities. Stress makes most movement disorders temporarily worse and in sleep, the ultimate form of relaxation, almost all of them disappear. Where does psychology end and neurology begin?

Rather than debate definitions and argue for various philosophical positions, we should begin by asking how can one best manage a given movement disorder. How can one recognize a factitious movement disorder? Unfortunately we do not have objective definitions of which movements can and which cannot be seen with disorders of various regions of the nervous system. We rely upon recognizing as organic those syndromes which we have seen many times before (e.g., essential tremor). We then are forced to make a judgment about whether the movements before us are inappropriate or inconsistent with those we have seen before.

Did the movements have a sudden onset with an obvious external cause or a reason for them to result in secondary gain of some type? Do the movements fluctuate inordinately during the exam and do they disappear when the patient is distracted? Are they absent when the patient thinks no one is looking? Have there been periods of spontaneous remission when the abnormal movements have completely disappeared for days? Can they be relieved by suggestion, psychotherapy, the use of placebos or placebo-like maneuvers? None of these criteria are truly objective and completely satisfactory in the modern scientific milieu in which physicians in most specialties practice. Nevertheless, if psychotherapy satisfactorily treats the movement disorder, the question of etiology no longer matters.

Is there a history of psychiatric illness, not necessarily of a conversion disorder or hysterical personality disorder, which were rare in the patients described by Deuschl et al (3), but of multiple functional somatic diseases, other psychosomatic diseases, or dissociative symptoms such as astasia–abasia, amnesia, or hypesthesia?

Attempts have been made to develop positive criteria for factitious movements based on the clinical examination or physiologic laboratory testing rather than relying on negative criteria such as outlined above. In considering tremor, perhaps the simplest movement disorder, Deuschl et al (3) used quantitative accelerometry (with and without weights added to the limb) and polyelectromyography to arrive at two criteria they felt were unique for factitious tremors. The first, their coactivation sign, is sudden increased muscle tone, felt clinically or recorded electromyographically, that precedes by approximately 300 milliseconds the development of tremor and persists as long as the tremor does; when the increased tone disappears, the tremor also disappears. The second is an increase in tremor amplitude when the limb (usually the hand) is loaded with 500 or 1,000 grams. Under these conditions, the amplitude usually decreases in essential tremor or the tremor of Parkinson's disease. Others have used accelerometry or electromyography (EMG) to document changes in amplitude or frequency of abnormal movements during the course of an examination, when the patient is distracted or is asked to make repetitive or complex movements with the noninvolved limb (4,5).

Ideally, if the movements are factitious, a positive, objective psychiatric diagnosis should be made, such as of conversion disorder, somatization disorder, factitious disorder, malingering, etc. This proves to be difficult at the present time but may become more useful in the future.

The scientific status of the movement disorder field is unsatisfactory and disappointing; we cannot describe what we see in objective quantifiable terms so that our colleagues and students can identify these movements with assurance from first principles. We still need senior experienced clinicians to recognize and differentiate between real movement disorders and factitious movements. This reliance on senior clinicians may be emotionally rewarding for the professor but, in reality, it is a testimony to the failure of our specialty to be as objective as most of the rest of medicine.

Finally, management of factitious movement disorders is not simple or easy. Many of these patients respond poorly per primum, and others relapse frequently. Physical therapy or pharmacotherapy may have striking short term effects, but unless they are combined with intensive psychotherapy, long-term relief of symptoms is unlikely.

When in doubt, as all of us often are in the clinic, it is better to say, "I'm not sure what this is. Let's try this and see what happens." The tendency to be avoided is the urge to pontificate ex cathedra.

REFERENCES

1. Batshaw ML, Wachtel RC, Deckel AW, et al. Munchausen's syndrome simulating torsion dystonia. N Engl J Med 1985;312:1437–1439.
2. Fahn S, Greene PE, Ford B, Bressman SB. Handbook of movement disorders. Philadelphia: Current Medicine, 1998.
3. Deuschl G, Koester B, Luecking CH, Scheidt C. Diagnostic and pathophysiological aspects of psychogenic tremors. Mov Disord 1998;13:294–302.
4. Williams DT, Ford B, Fahn S. Phenomenology and psychopathology related to psychogenic movement disorders. Adv Neurol 1996;65:231–257.
5. Elble RJ, Koller WC. Tremor. Baltimore: Johns Hopkins University, 1990.

Note: Page numbers in *italics* refer to illustrations; page numbers followed by t refer to tables.